Melvin A. Shiffman (Editor)

Mastopexy and Breast Reduction

Melvin A. Shiffman (Editor)

Mastopexy and Breast Reduction

Principles and Practice

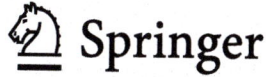

Melvin A. Shiffman, MD, JD
Department of Surgery
Tustin Hospital and Medical Center
17501 Chatham Drive
Tustin, CA 92780–2302
USA

ISBN 978-3-662-51857-1   ISBN 978-3-540-89873-3 (eBook)
DOI 10.1007/978-3-540-89873-3
Springer Dordrecht Heidelberg London New York

© 2009 Springer-Verlag Berlin Heidelberg
Softcover re-print of the Hardcover 1st edition 2009
This work is subject to copyright. All rights are reserved, whether the whole or part of the material is concerned, specifically the rights of translation, reprinting, reuse of illustrations, recitation, broadcasting, reproduction on microfilm or in any other way, and storage in data banks. Duplication of this publication or parts thereof is permitted only under the provisions of the German Copyright Law of September 9, 1965, in its current version, and permission for use must always be obtained from Springer. Violations are liable to prosecution under the German Copyright Law.

The use of general descriptive names, registered names, trademarks, etc. in this publication does not imply, even in the absence of a specific statement, that such names are exempt from the relevant protective laws and regulations and therefore free for general use.

Product liability: The publishers cannot guarantee the accuracy of any information about dosage and application contained in this book. In every individual case the user must check such information by consulting the relevant literature.

Cover design: eStudioCalamar, Figueres/Berlin

Printed on acid-free paper

Springer is part of Springer Science+Business Media (www.springer.com)

Foreword

The Breast: The center of emotional attraction, the source of nourishment, and means of seduction are some of the many possible definitions of this precious feminine attribute. Since ancient times, the female breast has had an important role for women and society in general. It is up to art to glorify it and it is the artist's job to find an ideal shape for it. Works of art survive as testimony to the evolution and transformation of the breast. Since prehistoric times, the cult of the Great Mother has settled in this place. The breast thus becomes the focus of the renewal of life and its cycles. It is the symbol of fertility and abundance and symbolizes life's renewal. The breast then is the center of the magical, wonderful forces that rule the world. The numerous statuettes typically with ample bosoms and emphasizing sexual organs testify to the powerful role that women played in the Egyptian, Minoan, Syrian, and Mesopotamian cultures. When the masculine element prevailed over the feminine, the breast became the creative principle of the universe. The Great Mother became the wife or the daughter. The breast was no longer a magical place. The statuettes were certainly feminine but they were not known for their beauty. Images of a marked yet less powerful sensuality were created instead.

From the Great Mother to Isis to Juno and finally to the cult of the Christian Virgin Mary, the breast is the quality of the feminine. In art, the breast becomes a true obsession. Greek art with its soft breasted Venuses started this trend. Each historic period and each artist has given its/his own interpretation of the attribute: ephebic for Memling and Piero di Cosimo, asexual for Botticelli, solemn and porcelain-like for Cranach, appetizing and well-shaped Giorgione and Titian's Venuses of the sixteenth century that finally indulge in pleasure. They established the trend of the alluring sensual girls who give themselves. The breast is opulent in the seventeenth century, unconventional for Fragonard, uninhibited for Goya, and offered in Manet.

The shape changes, the meaning changes. The shape is not only the manifestation of the age but also of moral qualities. The matter changes, perception changes. What remains unchanged today is the centrality of this precious attribute. It is now deprived of its old symbolic meanings, yet it is still an element of great charm, power, and seduction. In our time, there is indifference towards its history and origins. There seems to be no interest in recreating the sacred relationship between breast and magical powers: only the seductive and sexual qualities remain. We are surrounded by images of curvy women building their success around their generous breasts. What used to be creation is now aggressiveness.

The objective of plastic surgery is to reconstruct a peaceful relationship between the feminine and its external shape and to reestablish body harmony. Although even today plastic surgery is not regarded as having any artistic value, it would be advisable to start thinking about its objectives. Unlike sculpture or painting, surgery does not deal with amorphous matter but with live matter. Wood or marble grain is replaced by tissues, capillaries, muscles, and flesh. Live matter is in constant transformation. As the artist fixes his unstable desire forever in a permanent shape, in the same way the contemporary surgeon moulds the flesh to satisfy women's wishes. The breast is once again the center of the feminine. Surgery, like a work of art, must follow the principles of harmony. Their instruments are the same: proportion, harmony, symmetry, and shape. The artist-surgeon has to understand the body in which a shape will be created. He creates his own sculpture: the breast as a work of art on a living body. Woman as a live sculpture representing art in progress is live art.

Giorgio Fischer

Preface

Beautifying the breast with mastopexy, and/or breast reduction are some of the goals of the aesthetic surgeon to bring a better quality of life to the female (and sometimes the male) patient. Women desire to be more attractive by having breasts that meet their own expectations. What makes the aspects of the breast attractive can be driven by the female body as portrayed in magazines, posters, advertisements, movies, and videos as well as the male's attitude toward buxom women and women dressing in clothes that exaggerate the breast fullness. The surgeon performing mastopexy and/or breast reduction must understand the patients' driving force to change the shape or contours of their breasts. At the same time the patients' desires and expectations should be evaluated.

Surgical procedures in mastopexy and breast reduction are constantly changing with hopes of improving the results. The patients are looking for less scars, if possible, and safety in performance of the surgery. Breast reduction is the only aesthetic procedure of the breast (if one can call this an aesthetic procedure rather than correction of a medical problem) where patients are mainly satisfied with the reduction in volume that relieves their pain and discomfort and allows them to find clothes that fit properly without having to seek specially made sizes. These patients usually do not care about the scars. However, as aesthetic surgeons we try to reduce the scars in all patients if possible.

This book is an attempt to bring to the student, novice, and experienced breast surgeon as many of the various techniques as possible that are available in mastopexy and breast reduction including old, new, and modifications of the surgical procedures. There is a discussion of the procedures with indications, technical aspects, and possible complications. The anatomy of the breast, history of mastopexy and breast reduction, principles of mastopexy and breast reduction, preoperative care, postoperative care, avoidance and treatment of complications, and medical legal aspects are discussed.

The contributors have been carefully selected from international experts to bring to the reader a variety of ideas, new and old. It is hoped that the reader will begin to appreciate the magnitude of information that is available that will help in deciding the type of surgery that can be used in correcting the problems of ptosis, macromastia, gigantomastia, and breast asymmetries.

USA, 2009   Melvin A. Shiffman

Contents

Part I   Breast Anatomy

1   **Mammary Anatomy** 3
    Michael R. Davis

Part II   Preoperative

2   **Preoperative Consultation** 11
    Melvin A. Shiffman

3   **The Sitting, Oblique, Supine (SOS) Marking Technique for Mastopexy
    and Breast Reduction** 13
    Fahmy S. Fahmy

4   **Prediction of Weight in Breast Reduction Surgery** 19
    Nicole Z. Sommer, Elvin G. Zook

5   **Carpal Tunnel Syndrome in Women Undergoing Breast Reduction** 23
    Luis R. Pernia, Genelle Pernia

6   **Extent of Symptoms Preoperatively and Success of Breast Reduction
    for Symptomatic Macromastia: Personal Experiences** 29
    Judith B. Zacher

7   **Mammograms in Cosmetic Breast Surgery** 37
    Melvin A. Shiffman

Part III   Mastopexy

8   **History of Mastopexy** 43
    Jorge I. de la Torre, James N. Long, Luis O. Vásconez

9   **Principles of Mastopexy** 49
    Melvin A. Shiffman

10 **Treatment of Pseudoptosis** 51
    Frank Schneider-Affeld

11 **Crescent Mastopexy** 55
    Robert A. Shumway

12 **Benelli Concentric Mastopexy** 65
    Frank Schneider-Affeld

13 Short Scar Mastopexy with Flap Transposition:
    The Concept of the Biological Implant in Cosmetic Breast Surgery 73
    Moshe S. Fayman

14 Double Flap Technique: An Alternative Mastopexy Approach 97
    Andreas Foustanos

15 The Triple-Flap Interposition Mammaplasty 103
    Alberto Magno Lott Caldeira, Georg Bernhard Roth

16 "Flip-Flap" Mastopexy and Breast Reduction 115
    Robert S. Flowers, Adil Ceydeli

17 L-Wing Superior Pedicle Vertical Scar Mammaplasty 121
    Norbert Pallua, Erhan Demir

18 Fascial Suspension Mastopexy 129
    Ram Silfen, Morris Ritz, Graeme Southwick

19 Internal Mastopexy 145
    J. Dan Metcalf

20 Combined Mastopexy/Augmentation 149
    Alan A. Parsa, Natalie N. Parsa, Fereydoun D. Parsa

21 Breast Augmentation and Mastopexy: How to Select and Perform the
    Techniques Minimizing Complications 163
    Lázaro Cárdenas-Camarena

22 Vaser®-Assisted Breast Reduction and Mastopexy 179
    Maurice P. Sherman

23 Periareolar Mammaplasty for the Treatment of Gynecomastia with Breast Ptosis 189
    *Marco Túlio Rodrigues da Cunha, José Fernando Borges Bento,
    Antonio Roberto Bozola*

24 Mastopexy Complications 195
    Melvin A. Shiffman

Part IV Combined Mastopexy and Breast Reduction

25 Boustos' Technique of Periareolar Mastopexy and Breast Reduction 201
    Jacques Faivre

26 Dermal Purse String Reduction Mastopexy 207
    Franco Marconi, Filippo Brighetti

27 Breast Reduction/Mastopexy with Short Inverted T Scar 215
    Toma T. Mugea

28 Regnault B Mastopexy: A Versatile Approach to Breast Lifting and Reduction 231
    Howard A. Tobin

29 Mastopexy/Reduction and Augmentation without Vertical Scar 237
    Sid J. Mirrafati

30	**Breast Reduction and Mastopexy with Vaser in Male Breast Hypertrophy** *Alberto Di Giuseppe*	241

Part V Breast Reduction

31	**History of Breast Reduction** *Melvin A. Shiffman*	251
32	**Principles of Breast Reduction Surgery** *Melvin A. Shiffman*	257
33	**The Use of Epinephrine in Breast Surgery** *Michael S.G. Bell*	259
34	**Choosing a Technique in Breast Reduction** *Donald A. Hudson*	263
35	**Breast Reduction Techniques and Outcomes** *Courtney Crombie, Irfan Ibrahim Galaria, Colette Stern, W. Bradford Rockwell*	267
36	**Breast Reduction Algorithm Using TTM Chart** *Toma T. Mugea*	275
37	**Template-Goniometer for Marking the Wise Keyhole Pattern of Reduction Mammaplasty** *Dirk Lazarus*	291
38	**Individualized Wise Keyhole Pattern: An Aid in Reduction Mammaplasty of the Asymmetric Breasts** *Aycan Kayikçioğlu, Yücel Erk*	293
39	**Double Dermal Keyhole Pattern** *Elie Frederic Harouche*	297
40	**Deepithelialization in Breast Reduction: A Simple Technique** *Pierre F. Fournier*	301
41	**A Specially Designed Ruler and a Triangular Suture to Simplify Reduction Mammaplasty** *Gottfried Wechselberger, Petra Pülzl*	305
42	**Endoscopic Mastopexy and Breast Reduction** *Marco Aurelio Faria-Correa*	309
43	**Reduction Mammoplasty: The Use of Contact Tip ND:YAG Laser** *Jung I. Park*	317
44	**Axillary Reduction Mammaplasty** *Yhelda Felicio*	325
45	**Periareolar Mammaplasty with Transposition of Flaps** *Pedro Djacir Escobar Martins, Pedro Alexandre da Motta Martins, David Ponciano de Sena, Marcelo Marafon Maino*	333

46	**Inverted Keel Resection Breast Reduction** 341
	Ivo Pitanguy, Henrique N. Radwanski

47	**Superior Vertical Dermal Pedicle for the Nipple–Areola** 351
	Antonio Carlos Abramo

48	**Liposuction and Superior Pedicle** 361
	Felix Giebler, Eva Giebler

49	**Superior Medial Pedicle Breast Reduction and Auto Augmentation** 365
	Mike Huntly, Ronald Finger

50	**Reduction Mammoplasty with the Supero-Lateral Dermoglandular Pedicle Technique** ... 371
	Lázaro Cárdenas-Camarena

51	**Superior–Medial Pedicle Technique for Large Breast Reduction** 387
	Jorge I. de la Torre, James N. Long, Luis O. Vásconez

52	**The Central Mound Technique for Reduction Mammaplasty** 395
	Bret R. Baack

53	**Central Mound Technique for Breast Reduction** 401
	Richard C. Hagerty, Andre Uflacker

54	**The Robbins Inferior Pedicle Reduction Mammaplasty** 407
	Richard J. Restifo

55	**Modification of the Inferior Pedicle Technique** 415
	Sanjay Azad

56	**Short Scar Periareolar Inferior Pedicle Reduction Mammaplasty** 421
	Richard J. Restifo

57	**Reduction Mammaplasty using Inferior Pedicle Technique Combined with Dermal Suspension** 429
	Hülya Aydin, Burçak Tümerdem Uluğ

58	**Mckissock Bipedicle Breast Reduction** 435
	Melvin A. Shiffman

59	**Strömbeck Technique** 441
	Pierre F. Fournier

60	**Medial and Inferior Bipedicle Breast Reduction for Gigantomastia and Mammary Hypertrophy** 451
	Nicolae Antohi, Cristina Isac, Vitalie Stan, Tiberiu Bratu

61	**Modified Biesenberger Dual Pedicle Technique of Breast Reduction** 465
	Lloyd N. Carlsen

62	**Mammaplasty with a Circular Folded Pedicle Technique** 471
	Waldir Teixeira Renó

63	**The Modified Robertson Reduction Mammaplasty** 483
	Elvin G. Zook, Nicole Z. Sommer

64	**"Owl" Incision Technique Reduction Mammaplasty** *Oscar M. Ramirez, Sung Yoon*	489
65	**Regnault B Technique** *Robert F. Garza, Patricio Andrades, Jorge I. de la Torre, Luis O. Vasconez*	497
66	**Vertical (Lejour) Breast Reduction** *James F. Thornton, Paul D. McCluskey*	503
67	**Liposuction and Vertical Breast Reduction** *Felix Giebler*	511
68	**The Circumvertical Reduction Mammaplasty** *A. Aldo Mottura*	515
69	**Eliminating the Vertical Scar in Breast Reduction** *Simon G. Talbot, Julian J. Pribaz*	521
70	**The Bipolar Technique: Short Inframammary Scar Mammaplasty** *Vicente De Carolis*	533
71	**Breast Shaping by an Isolated Tissue Flap** *Matthias Voigt, Christoph Andree*	545
72	**Free Nipple Areolar Graft Reduction Mammaplasty** *Anthony Erian, Amal Dass*	555
73	**Liposuction Breast Reduction** *Martin Jeffrey Moskovitz*	563
74	**Breast Reduction with Ultrasound-Assisted Liposuction** *G. Patrick Maxwell, Allen Gabriel*	569
75	**Vaser-Assisted Breast Reduction** *Alberto Di Giuseppe*	575

Part VI Complications of Breast Reduction and Mastopexy

76	**Complications of Breast Reduction** *Melvin A. Shiffman*	593
77	**Late Sequelae of Breast Reduction** *Nicholas G. Economides*	601
78	**Breast Feeding After Breast Reduction** *Arnis Freiberg*	609
79	**Alteration of Nipple and Areola Sensitivity by Reduction Mammaplasty** *Schlenz Ingrid, Rigel Sandra, Schemper Michael, and Kuzbari Rafic*	613
80	**Prevention of the Inverted Teardrop Areola Following Mammaplasty** *Geoffrey G. Hallock, John A. Altobelli*	621

81 **Prevention of Teardrop Areola and Increasing Areola Projection in Inferior Pedicle Reduction Mammoplasty** 625
Meltem Ayhan, Metin Görgü, Bulent Erdoğan, Zeynep Sevým

82 **Correction of the High-Riding Nipple After Breast Reduction** 629
Greg Chernoff

83 **Zigzag Glanduloplasty to Reduce Flatness of Lower Pole of Breast Following Breast Reduction** 631
Felix Giebler

84 **Recurrent Deformities After Breast Reduction and Mastopexy** 635
Saul Hoffman

85 **Recurrent Mammary Hyperplasia** 639
James F. Thornton, Paul D. McCluskey

86 **Repeat Reduction Mammaplasty** 645
Donald A. Hudson

87 **Breast Reduction and Cancer in the Gland Remnant** 647
Beniamino Palmieri, Giorgia Benuzzi, Alberto Costa

88 **Breast Cancer and Reduction Mammoplasty** 657
David A. Jansen, Mary Catherine Ghere, Mark Lee, Madeline O. Jansen

89 **Skin Circulation in the Nipple After Bipedicle Dermal Flap Reduction** 671
Leif Perbeck

90 **Complications in Augmentation Mastopexy** 675
Mervin Low

Part VII Miscellaneous

91 **Medical Legal Aspects** 681
Melvin A. Shiffman

92 **Editor's Commentary** 687
Melvin A. Shiffman

Subject Index 689

List of Contributors

Antonio Carlos Abramo, MD, Ph.D.
Head Professor of the Post-Graduate Course of ACA
Institute of Assistance in Plastic Surgery of São Paulo
sponsored by Brazilian Society of Plastic Surgery
and Brazilian Medical Association at the General Hospital São Luiz - Unit Morumbi
Rua Afonso de Freitas, 41
641 04006-052, Sao Paulo SP
Brazil
E-mail: acabramo@abramo.com.br

John A. Altobelli, MD
The Lehigh Valley Hospitals
1230 S. Cedar Crest Blvd., Suite 202
Allentown, PA 18103
USA
E-mail: jaaltobelli@aol.com

Patricio Andrades, MD
Research and Clinical Fellow
Plastic and Reconstructive Surgery
Division of Plastic Surgery
The University of Alabama at Birmingham
510 20th Street South
1164 Faculty Office Tower
Birmingham, AL 35294-3411
USA
E-mail: patomed@tutopia.com

Christoph Andree, MD
Klinik für Plastische und Ästhetische Chirurgie
und Interdiziplinäres Brustzentrum
Bismarckallee 17
79098 Freiburg im Breisgau
Germany

Nicolae Antohi, MD
Associate Professor of Plastic Surgery
Head of the Department of Plastic Surgery
Hospital for Plastic Surgery and Burns
Esthera Medical Centre
University for Medicine and Pharmacy "Carol Davila"
Washington Str., 48A, Sector 1
Bucharest, Romania
E-mail: nantohi@hotmail.com

Hülya Aydin, MD
Professor, Department of Plastic, Reconstructive and Aesthetic Surgery
Faculty of Medicine
Istanbul University
Valikonagý cad. Kucukpamuk apt., 135/9
Nisantasý, Istanbul
Turkey
E-mail: drhulyaaydin@yahoo.com

Meltem Ayhan, MD
Talatpasa bulvari 7/2 Alayunt apt.
Alsancak, Izmir
Turkey
E-mail: meltem_2002@yahoo.com

Zeynep Aytug, MD
Ziya Gokalp blv. No: 10/14
Alsancak Izmir
Turkey
E-mail: zaytug@yahoo.com

Sanjay Azad, MD
7 Sibton Lane, Oadby,
Leister LE2 5UA
UK
E-mail: sanjay_azad@hotmail.com

Bret Baack, MD
Chair, Division of Plastic and Reconstructive Surgery
UNM Health Sciences Centre, 2211 Lomas Blvd.
NE Albuquerque, NM 87131
USA
E-mail: bbaack@salud.unm.edu

Michael S.G. Bell, MD
1919 Riverside Drive, Ottawa, ON
Canada K1H 1A2
E-mail: msgbell@cyberus.ca

José Fernando Borges Bento, MD
Avenida Santos Dumont
2312 Uberaba, MG- 38.050-400
Brazil
E-mail: jfb@uberabafactoring.com.br

Georgia Benuzzi, BSc
Department of General Surgery
University of Modena Medical School
Policlinico Di Modena, via Del Pozzo 71
41100, Modena
Italy

Antonio R. Bozola, MD, PhD
Avenida Jose Munia, 7075 São Jose do Rio Preto
SP- 15.085-350
Brazil
E-mail: bozola@bozola.com.br

Tiberiu Bratu, MD, PhD
Professor of Plastic Surgery
University of Medicine and Pharmacy "Victor Babes"
County Hospital Timisoara
Casa Austria, Str. I. Bulbuca 10
Romania

Filippo Brighetti, MD
Via Croara 7/F,
40068 San Lazzaro di Savena (BO)
Italy
E-mail: umcplast@yahoo.it

Alberto Mango Lott Caldeira, MD
Rua Visconde de Pirajá
414 Grupo 1012, 22410-002 Ipanema
Rio de Janeiro, RJ
Brazil
E-mail: albertocaldeira@uol.com.br

Lázaro Cárdenas-Camarena, MD
Professor, Unit of Plastic Surgery
Guadalajara University
Guadalajara, Mexico
Av. Chapalita 1300 Col. Chapalita
CP 45050 Guadalajara
Jalisco
México
E-mail: plassurg@mail.udg.mx

Lloyd N. Carlsen, MD
Assistant Clinical Professor
Department of Surgery
The Cosmetic Surgery Hospital
McMaster University
4650 Highway #7
Woodbridge, ON
Canada L4L 1S7
E-mail: josie@cosmeticsurgeryhospital.com

Adil Ceydeli, MD
Bay Medical Centre
Division of Plastic Surgery
801 E. 6th St, Suite 302
Panama City, FL 32401
USA
E-mail: adilc@excite.com

Greg Chernoff, MD
9002 N. Meridian St.
Suite 205
Indianapolis, IN 46260
USA
E-mail: greg@drchernoff.com

Alberto Costa, MD
Breast Service
Ospedale Fondazione Maugeri
Largo Maugeri, Pavia
Italy

Courtney Crombie, MD
Professor of Surgery
Division of Plastic Surgery
University of Utah
30 North 1900 East 3B205
Salt Lake City, UT 84132
USA
E-mail: *courtney.crombie@hsc.utah.edu*

Marco T.R. Da Cunha, MD, PhD
Rua Alfen Paixão
180 Ap. 202
Uberaba - MG - CEP 38.060-230
Brazil
E-mail: *cunhamarco@hotmail.com*

Pedro Alexandre Da Motta Martins, MD
Chief of Plastic Surgery Service
Department of Plastic Surgery
São Lucas Hospital
Pontifícia Universidade Católica do Rio Grande do Sul
Porte Alegre, RS
Brazil
and
Centro Clínico da PUC
Av. Ipiranga, 6690 - Conj 514
CEP 90610-000, Porto Alegre, RS
Brazil
E-mail: *pemar@pucrs.br*

Amal Dass, MD, MBChB, BAO(Ire), MRCS(Edin)
Fellow in Cosmetic Surgery
Blk 10B, Braddell View, #02-06, S, 579721
Singapore
amaldass_2000@yahoo.com

Michael Davis, MD
Division of Plastic Surgery
Birmingham School of Medicine, University of Alabama
510 20th Street South, 1164 Faculty Office Tower
Birmingham, AL 35294-3411
USA
E-mail: *drcutmd@aol.com*

Yhelda de Alencar Felicio, MD
Clínica Yhelda Felicion
Cirugia Plástica e Reconstrutora
Rua Professor Dias da Rocha N:1200
Aldeota CEP 60170-310
Fortaleza, Ceará, Brazil
E-mail: *yheldafelicio@secrel.com.br*

Vincente De Carolis, MD
Alonso de Cordova 2600 Dp. 21
Vitacura, Santiago
Chile
E-mail: vdecarolis45@gmail.com,
vdecarol@entelchile.net

Jorge I. De La Torre, MD
Associate Professor and Program Director
UAB, Division of Plastic Surgery
The University of Alabama at Birmingham
510 20th Street South
1164 Faculty Office Tower
Birmingham, AL 35294-3411
USA
E-mail: jdlt@uab.edu

David P. De Sena, MD
Resident, Department of Plastic Surgery
São Lucas Hospital
Pontifícia Universidade Católica do
Rio Grande do Sul
Av. Ipiranga, 6690 - Conj 514
CEP 90610-000, Porto Alegre, RS
Brazil
E-mail: dublesena@hotmail.com

Erhan Demir, MD
Department of Plastic Surgery
and Hand Surgery
Burn Centre, University Hospital
RWTH Aachen
Pauwelssstr 30
52074 Aachen
Germany
E-mail: erhan_demir@t-online.de

Alberto Di Giuseppe, MD
Via Simeoni, 6
60122 Ancona
Italy
E-mail: adgplasticsurg@atlavia.it

Nicholas G. Economides, MD
Instructor, Department of Surgery
Division of Plastic Surgery (1981–1996)
Chief of Plastic Surgery
Baptist Memorial Hospital
Memphis TN (1983–1992)
and
Chair, Division of Plastic Surgery
Holzer Clinic (current)
Holzer Clinic
90 Jackson Pike
Gallipolis, OH 45631
USA
E-mail: Neconomides@holzerclinic.com

Bulent Erdogan, MD
Associate Professor
Ankara Numune Research and Education Hospital
Department of Plastic Surgery
Ankara Numune Egitim Arastirma Hastanesi, Ankara
Turkey
E-mail: drbulenterdogan@yahoo.com

Anthony Erian, MD
Private Practice: Orwell Grange
43 Cambridge Road
Wimpole, Cambridge
UK
E-mail: erian@erian.demon.co.uk

Yücel Erk, MD
Professor and Chief
Department of Plastic and Reconstructive Surgery
Hacettepe University Medical Faculty
38 Sokak 4-4, 06500 Bahçelievler
Sihhiye, Ankara
Turkey
E-mail: yerk@hacettepe.edu.tr

Fahmy S. Fahmy, MD
Department of Plastic Surgery
Countess of Chester Hospital
Liverpool Road, Chester
Cheshire CH2 1UL
UK
E-mail: plasticsurgfahmy@aol.com

Jacques Faivre, MD
23 rue Vital
75116 Paris
France
E-mail: isa.faivre@wanadoo.fr

Marco A. Faria-Correa, MD
Department of Plastic and
Reconstructive Surgery
Catholic University Hospital
Centro Clinico do HSLPUC
Av. Ipianga 6690 conj 520, Cep:90.610.000
Porto Alegre, Rio Grande do Sul
Brazil
E-mail: drmarco@singnet.com.sg,
drmarco@fariacorrea.com.br

Moshe S. Fayman, MD
Department of Surgery
Division on Plastic Surgery
Suite 17, Rosebank Clinic, 14 Stutrdee Ave
Rosebank, Johannesburg
P.O. Box 1708, Parklands 2121
South Africa
E-mail: info@doctorfayman.co.za

Ronald Finger, MD
5356 Reynolds Street, Suite 505
Savannah, GA 31405-6017
USA
E-mail: plasticmike@msn.com

Giorgio Fischer, MD
Via della Camiluccia 643
00135 Rome
Italy
E-mail: giorgiofischer@flashnet.it

Robert S. Flowers, MD
677 Ala Moana, Suite 1011
Honolulu, HI
USA
E-mail: info@flowersclinic.com

Pierre F. Fournier, MD
Private Practice of Aesthetic Plastic Surgery
55 boulevard de Strasbourg
75 010 Paris
France
E-mail: pierre.fournier27@wanadoo.fr

Andreas Foustanos, MD, CCBC
Assistant Professor
Dimokrition University, Greece
Assistant Professor
Carol Davila University, Bucharest
Romania
and
Chief of the Department of Plastic Surgery
IASSO Hospital, Athens
Greece

Arnis Freiberg, MD
Professor Emeritus
Department of Surgery
University of Toronto
Hand Program 2 East, University Health Network
Western Division, Toronto Western Hospital
399 Bathurst Street
Toronto, ON
Canada M5T 258
E-mail: arnis.freiberg@uhn.on.ca

Allen Gabriel, MD
Director of Clinical Research
Loma Linda University Medical Centre
Department of Plastic Surgery
Loma Linda University
11175 Campus Street Suite 21126
Loma Linda, CA 92350
USA
E-mail: gabrielallen@yahoo.com

Irfan I. Galaria, MD, MBA
Chief Resident
Division of Plastic Surgery
University of Utah,
30 North 1900 East 3B205
Salt Lake City, UT 84132
USA
E-mail: irfan.galaria@hsc.utah.edu

Robert F. Garza, MD
Chief Resident
Plastic and Reconstructive Surgery
Division of Plastic Surgery
The University of Alabama at Birmingham
510 20th Street South, 1164 Faculty Office Tower
Birmingham, AL 35294-3411
USA
E-mail: robertfgarza@yahoo.com

Mary C. Ghere, BS
2808 Calhoun St.
New Orleans, LA 70118
USA
E-mail: melliot@tulane.edu

Eva Giebler, MD
Vincemus-Klinik,
Brückenstraße 1a
25840 Friedrichstadt/Eider
Germany
E-mail: info@vincemus-klink.de

Felix-Rüdiger G. Giebler, MD
Vincemus-Klinik,
Brückenstraße 1a
25840 Friedrichstadt/Eider
Germany
E-mail: info@vincemus-klink.de

Metin Gorgu, MD
Chief, Izmir Atatürk Research and Education Hospital
Department of Plastic Surgery
Izmir Ataturk Egitim Arastirma Hastanesi
Basin Sitesi, Izmir
Turkey
E-mail: metingorgu@estetik.tv

Richard C. Hagerty, MD
261 Calhoun St., Suite 200
Charleston, SC 29401
USA
E-mail: dukehagerty@aol.com

Geoffrey G. Hallock, MD
1230 S. Cedar Crest Blvd.
Allentown, PA 18103
USA
E-mail: pbhallock@cs.com

Elie Frederic Harouche, MD
Columbia University College of Physicians and Surgeons
903 Park Avenue
New York, NY 10021
USA
E-mail: harouche@aol.com

Saul Hoffman, MD
51 Hidden Ledge Road
Englewood, NJ 07631
USA
E-mail: shoffman2001@aol.com

Donald A. Hudson, MD
Head, Department of Plastic
Reconstructive and Maxillofacial Surgery
Groote Schuur Hospital
OMB H51
Observatory 7925
Cape Town
South Africa
E-mail: donald.hudson@ uct.ac.za

Mike Huntly, MD
5356 Reynolds Street, Suite 505
Savannah, GA 31405-6017
USA
E-mail: plasticmike@msn.com

Cristina Isaac, MD, PhD
Assistant Professor of Plastic Surgery
University Hospital for Plastic Surgery and Burns
University of Medicine and Pharmacy "Carol Davila"
Calea Grivitei 218, Sector 1
Bucharest
Romania
E-mail: inaisaac@yahoo.com

David A. Jansen, MD
3900 Veterans Memorial Blvd
Metairie, LA 70002
USA
E-mail: djansenmd@hotmail.com

Madeline O. Jansen
227 Hector Avenue
Metairie, LA 70005
USA
E-mail: djansenmd@hotmail.com

Aycan Kayikçioğlu, MD
Associate Professor
Department of Plastic and Reconstructive Surgery
Hacettepe University Medical Faculty
38 Sokak 4-4, 06500 Bahçelievler
Sihhiye, Ankara
Turkey
E-mail: akayikci@hacettepe.edu.tr

Rafic Kuzbari, MD, PhD
Department for Plastic and Reconstructive Surgery
Wilhelminenspital
Montleartstrasse 37
1160 Vienna
Austria
E-mail: rnk@aon.at

Dirk Lazarus, MD
86 New Church Street, Tamboerskloof
Cape Town 8001
South Africa
E-mail: lazarus@plasticsurgery.co.za

Mark Lee, MD
Tulane University School of Medicine
Division of Plastic Surgery
1430 Tulane 22
New Orleans, LA 70112
USA
E-mail: noteto_mark@yahoo.com

James N. Long, MD
Associate Professor
Division of Plastic Surgery
University of Alabama at Birmingham 510 20th Street
South FOT-1164
Birmingham, AL 35294
USA
E-mail: james.long@ccc.uab.edu

Mervin Low, MD
2549 Eastbluff Drive, #295
Newport Beach, CA 92660
USA
E-mail: drmlow@gmail.com

Marcelo Maino, MD
Chief Resident
Department of Plastic Surgery
São Lucas Hospital
Pontifícia Universidade Católica do Rio Grande do Sul
E-mail: mmaino@terra.con.br

Franco Marconi, MD
Via delle Lame, 61
40122 Bologna
Italy
E-mail: francomarconi.francomarc@tin.it

Pedro D.E. Martins, MD
Chief of Plastic Surgery Service
Pontificia Universidade Catolica do Rio Grande do Sul
Porte Alegre, RS
Brazil and Centro Clínico da PUC, Av. Ipiranga
6690 - Conj 514, CEP 90610-000, Porto Alegre, RS
Brazil
E-mail: pemar@pucrs.br

G. Patrick Maxwell, MD, FACS
Clinical Professor of Surgery
Loma Linda University Medical Centre
Department of Plastic Surgery
Loma Linda University
11175 Campus Street Suite 21126
Loma Linda, CA 92350
USA

Paul D. McCluskey, MD
Chief Resident
UT Southwestern Department
of Plastic Surgery
2707 Cole Ave #442
Dallas, TX 75204
USA
E-mail: pmccluskey2@yahoo.com

Dan Metcalf, MD
12400 St. Andrews Dr.
Oklahoma City, OK 73120
USA
E-mail: jdan1@mac.com

Sid J. Mirrafati, MD
3140 Redhill Avenue
Costa Mesa, CA 92626
USA
E-mail: drmirrafati@youngerlook.com

Martin J. Moskovitz, MD
Image Plastic Surgery LLC
140 Route 17 North, Suite 105
Paramus, NJ 07652
USA
E-mail: drm@imageps.com

Aldo Mottura, MD
Centro de Cirugia Estetica
Friuli 2110
5016 Cordoba
Argentina
E-mail: amott@esteticamottura.com

Toma T. Mugea, MD, PhD
Professor, Plastic and
Aesthetic Surgery
Oradea Medical
University, Oradea
Romania
and
Medestet Clinic
9/7 Cipariu Square,
Cluj-Napoca
Romania
E-mail: drmugea@medestet.ro

Norbert Pallua, MD, PhD
Professor and Chairman
Department of Plastic
Reconstructive and Hand Surgery
Burn Centre
University Hospital of the RWTH
Aachen University
Pauwelsstr., 30
52057 Aachen
Germany
E-mail: npallua@ukaachen.de

Beniamino Palmieri, MD
Professor, Department of Surgery
University of Modena and Reggio Emilia
Via del Pozzo, 71
41100 Modena
Italy
E-mail: palmieri@unimo.it

Jung I. Park, MD
9305 Calumet Avenue, Suite A2
Munster, IN 46321-2888
USA
E-mail: jungilparkmd@hotmail.com

Alan A. Parsa, MD
Seton Hall University School of Graduate
Medical Education at St. Francis Medical Centre
Trenton,
905 Nottinghill Lane
Hamilton, NJ 90869
USA
E-mail: a_parsa@hotmail.com

Don Parsa, MD
Professor of Surgery, Chief
Plastic Surgery Division
John A. Burns School of Medicine
University of Hawaii
1329 Lusitana Street, Suite 807
Honolulu, HI 96813
USA
E-mail: fdparsa@yahoo.com

Leif Perbeck, MD, PhD
Assistant Professor
Department of Surgery, Karolinska Institutet
Karolinska University Hospital, Solna
171 76 Stockholm
Sweden
and
Huddinge University Hospital
141 86 Huddinge
Sweden
E-mail: leif.perbeck@karolinska.se

Genelle Pernia, MD
PGY2, Montgomery Family Medicine Residency Program
Montgomery, AL 4371, Narrow Lane Rd., Ste 100
Montgomery, AL 36116
USA
E-mail: docnelle@aol.com

Luis R. Pernia, MD
Professor of Surgery
University of Alabama at Birmingham
Tuscaloosa Campus
100 Towncenter Blvd.
Tuscaloosa, AL 35406-1833
USA
E-mail: peribeca@dbtech.net, cavuofthesky@aol.com

Ivo Pitanguy, MD
Ivo Pitanguy Clinic, Rua Dona Mariana 65
Rio de Janeiro 22280-020
Brazil
E-mail: pitanguy@pitanguy.com.br

Julian Pribaz, MD
Professor of Surgery
Harvard Medical School
Brigham and Women's Hospital
75 Francis St.,
Boston, MA 02115
USA
E-mail: jpribaz@partners.org

Petra Pülzl, MD
Department of Plastic and Reconstructive Surgery
Innsbruck Medical University
Anichstrasse 35
6020 Innsbruck
Austria
E-mail: Petra.puelzl@i-med.ac.at

Henrique N. Radwanski, MD
Ivo Pitanguy Clinic
Rua Dona Mariana 65
Rio de Janeiro 22280-020
Brazil
E-mail: dr.henrique@pilos.com.br

Oscar M. Ramirez, MD
Esthetique Internationale
2219 York Road, Suite 100
Timonium, MD 21093
USA
E-mail: drramirez@ramirezmd.com

Waldir Teixeira Renó, MD
Cirurgia Plástica D'América
Rua Paissandú, 368, Centro Guaratinguetá
Sao Paulo
Brazil
E-mail: renosurg@uol.com.br

Richard J. Restifo, MD
59 Elm Street, Suite 560
New Haven, CT 06510
USA
E-mail: restifo@rrestifo.msn.com, rrestifo@msn.com

Sandra Rigel, MD
FA für Plastische,
Ästhetische und
Rekonstruktive Chirurgie
Laurenzerberg 2
1010 Wien
Austria
E-mail: sandra.rigel@womanandhealth.com, www.womanandhealth.com

Morris Ritz, MD (MB, BCh, FCS, FRACS)
Melbourne Institute of Plastic Surgery
253 Wattletree Road
Malvern 3144
Victoria
Australia
E-mail: morrisr@melbplastsurg.com

W. Bradford Rockwell, MD
Associate Professor of Surgery
Chief, Division of Plastic Surgery
University of Utah Health
Sciences Centre
University of Utah, 30 North 1900
East 3B205
Salt Lake City, UT 84132
USA
E-mail: brad.rockwell@hsc.utah.edu

Georg Bernhard Roth, MD
Rua Visconde de Pirajá
414 Grupo 1012, CEP 22410-002 Ipanema
Rio de Janeiro, RJ
Brazil
E-mail: gbroth@web.de

Michael Schemper, MD, PhD
Institute for Clinical Biometry
Special Department for Medical
Statistics
Medical University of Vienna
Spitalgasse 23
1090 Vienna
Austria
E-mail: michael.schemper@meduniwien.ac.at

Ingrid Schlenz, MD
Consultant, Department for Plastic
and Reconstructive Surgery
Wilhelminenspital
Montleartstrasse 37
1160 Vienna
Austria
E-mail: ingrid.schlenz@wienkav.at

Frank Schneider-Affeld, MD
Großflecken 68
24534 Neumünster
Germany
E-mail: info@con-tur.de

Maurice P. Sherman, MD
12845 Pointe Del Mar Way
Suite 100
Del Mar, CA 92014
USA
E-mail: info@drsherman.com

Melvin A. Shiffman, MD, JD
17501 Chatham Drive
Tustin, CA 92780-2302
USA
E-mail: shiffmanmdjd@yahoo.com

Robert Shumway, MD
9834 Genessee Avenue
Suite 225
La Jolla, CA 92037
USA
E-mail: shumwayinst@sbcglobal.net

Ram Silfen, MD
3 Ammon Vetamar
Tel Aviv 69930
Israel
E-mail: rsilfen@gmail.com

Nicole Z. Sommer, MD
Assistant Professor
Division of Plastic Surgery
Southern Illinois University School of Medicine
P.O. Box 19653
Springfield, IL 62794-965
USA
E-mail: nsommer@siumed.edu

Graeme Southwick, MD
Melbourne Institute of Plastic Surgery
253 Wattletree Road
Malvern 3144
Victoria
Australia
E-mail: graemes@melbplastsurg.com

Vitalie Stan, MD, PhD
Plastic Surgeon
University Hospital for Plastic Surgery and Burns
Calea Grivitei 218, Sector 1
Bucharest, Romania
E-mail: vitalie_stan@yahoo.com

Colette Stern, MD
Chief Resident/Plastic Surgery
Division of Plastic Surgery
University of Utah
30 North 1900 East 3B205
Salt Lake City, UT 84132
USA
E-mail: colette.stern@hsc.utah.edu

Simon G. Talbot, MD
Resident
Plastic Surgery, Harvard Combined Program
University of Auckland
USA
E-mail: sgtalbot@partners.org

James F. Thornton, MD
Associate Professor
Department of Plastic and Reconstructive Surgery
University of Texas Southwestern Medical Centre
1801 Inwood Rd, Suite WA 4.220
Dallas, TX 75390-9132
USA
E-mail: james.thornton@utsouthwestern.edu

Howard A. Tobin, MD
Facial Plastic and Cosmetic Surgery Centre
6300 Regional Plaza, Suite 475
Abilene, TX 79606, USA
E-mail: drtobin@newlook.com

Andre Uflacker, MD
College of Medicine
Medical University of South Carolina
Charleston, SC
USA
and
548 Overseer's Retreat,
Mt. Pleasant, SC 29464
USA
E-mail: uflacke@musc.edu

Burçak Tümerdem Uluğ
Department of Plastic and Reconstructive Surgery
Istanbul University, Bağdat cad., Hatboyu sok
Feneryolu, Özgen apt, 151/12, C blok, 34724
Kadıköy, Istanbul
Turkey
E-mail: burcaktumerdem@yahoo.com, burcaktumerdem@hotmail.com

Luis O. Vasconez, MD
Professor and Chief
Division of Plastic Surgery
University of Alabama at Birmingham
1813 Sixth Avenue, South MEB-524
Birmingham, AL 35294,
USA
E-mail: luis.vasconez@ccc.uab.edu

Matthias Voigt, MD
Praxis für Plastische Chirugie Freiburg
Bismarckallee 17
79098 Freiburg
Germany
E-mail: voigt.zoppelt@t-online.de

Gottfried Wechselberger, MD
Universitäts für Plastische und Wiederherstellungschirurgie
Medizinische Universität Innsbruck
Anichstrasse 35
6020 Innsbruck
Austria
E-mail: gottfried.wechselberger@i-med.ac.at

Sung W. Yoon, MD
5530 Wisconsin Avenue, Suite 1152
Chevy Chase, MD 20815
USA
E-mail: drsungyoon@yahoo.com

Judith B. Zacher, MD
43585 Monterey Avenue
Palm Desert, CA 92260-9342
USA
E-mail: jbzmd@aol.com, office@zachermd.com

Elvin G. Zook, MD
Professor and Chair
Plastic Surgery Institute, Southern Illinois University School of Medicine
747 North Rutledge Street, P.O. Box 19653
Springfield, IL 62794-9653
USA
E-mail: ezook@siumed.edu

Part I
Breast Anatomy

Mammary Anatomy

Michael R. Davis

1.1 Introduction

A thorough understanding of breast development and anatomy is a requirement for modern plastic surgeons. Advanced techniques of reduction mammaplasty, mastopexy, augmentation, and reconstruction demand comprehensive knowledge of the now detailed descriptions of breast architecture. As a complicated physiologic and esthetic structure, the form and function of the breast weighs heavily on a woman's psyche. Significant improvements or complications can impact greatly on self image for better or worse. Optimizing results and avoidance of complications take root in the knowledge of breast anatomy. Only then can a plastic surgeon engage his full creativity in sculpting the breast form.

1.2 Development

As a cutaneous appendage, the breast takes its origin from the ectoderm. The breast bud begins differentiation during weeks 8–10 along the milk ridge. The normal human breast develops over the fourth intercostal space of the anterolateral chest wall (Fig. 1.1). Supernumerary nipples and breasts can occur anywhere along the milk ridge from the axilla to the groin. Statistically they are most common near the left inframammary crease.

Following a brief period of activity shortly after birth in response to maternal hormones, breast development becomes dormant until the onset of puberty. Pubertal onset is becoming ever earlier in modern society, but currently occurs at approximately 9 years of age. Typically, by the age of 14, parenchymal growth has extended to its mature borders. These include the sternum medially, the anterior border of the latissimus dorsi laterally, the clavicle superiorly, and the inframammary crease inferiorly. These represent approximate anatomic landmarks that are not rigidly defined borders. Breast tissue can extend across the midline and beyond the inframammary crease. An extension of breast tissue normally penetrates the axillary fascia into the axillary fat pad and is termed the "Tail of Spence." Mature breast morphology projects off the chest wall in a conical fashion with its apex deep to the nipple–areola complex.

Development of overall breast shape is multifactorial. Breast form is dependent on fat content and location, muscular and skeletal chest wall contour, and skin quality. These structures display complex attachments and interactions to result in the final form. Breast shape and size is unique to each individual and is determined largely by heredity.

1.3 Parenchyma

Embedded within the fibrofatty stroma lies the glandular portion of the breast. Glandular structure consists of millions of lobules clustered to comprise approximately 20–25 lobes. Interlobular ducts come together to form approximately 20 main lactiferous ducts. Lactiferous sinuses collect milk, and specialized ducts within the nipple transmit milk to the surface (Fig. 1.2). Glandular size remains relatively constant from individual to individual. The bulk of the breast consists of fat. Subcutaneous fat as well as interlobular fat content determines texture, contour, and density.

The breast parenchyma is encompassed and supported by an intricate fascial system. The superficial fascial system is variable and sometimes indistinct from the overlying dermis anteriorly. Fat content of the subcutaneous tissue between the dermis and superficial fascia determines the clarity of these structures. Continuous with the superficial fascia is a deep component which separates the parenchyma from the pectoral fascia as well as fascia overlying adjacent muscles. Interposed between the superficial and deep components of the superficial fascial system are fascial extensions termed Cooper's ligaments. Anchored to the muscular fascia, these ligaments act to suspend the parenchyma. Attenuation of these tissues is largely responsible for ptosis.

M.A. Shiffman (ed.), *Mastopexy and Breast Reduction: Principles and Practice*,
© Springer-Verlag Berlin Heidelberg 2009

4   1 Mammary Anatomy

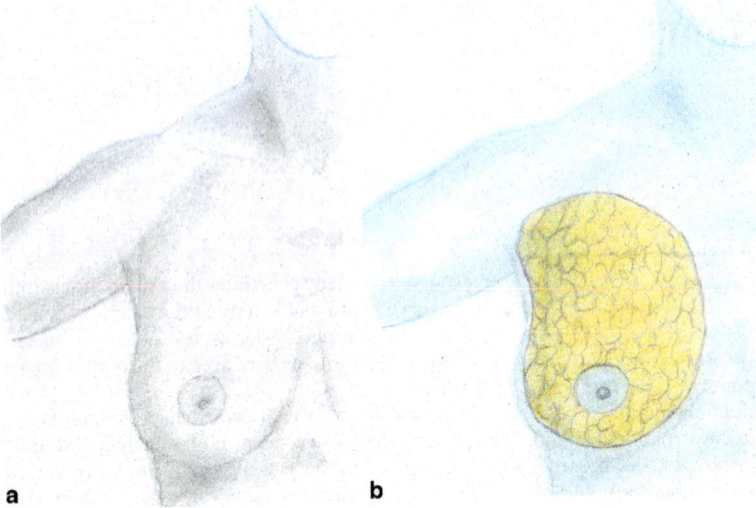

Fig. 1.1 a, b The breast overlies the anterolateral chest wall containing primarily glandular tissue and fibrofatty stroma

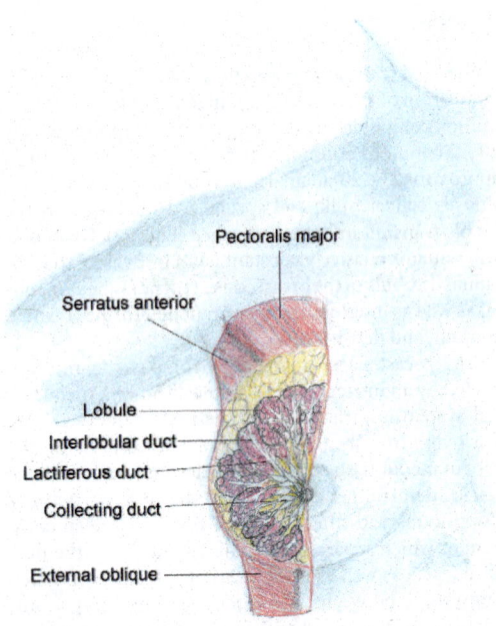

Fig. 1.2 Glandular breast tissue is lobular in structure with 20–25 lobes each drained by a lactiferous duct. Milk then enters collecting ducts followed by lactiferous sinuses prior to exiting the nipple

1.4
Musculature

At its foundation, the breast sits on prominent musculature that also impacts form and physiology. The five primary muscle groups that lie deep to the breast are pectoralis major and minor, serratus anterior, upper external oblique, and upper rectus abdominis. Perforating these structures are the breast's primary arterial, venous, nerve, and lymphatic supply.

1.5
Skeletal Support

Breast symmetry and form are also dependent on normal skeletal support. The breast overlies the anterolateral thorax principally over ribs 2–6. Conditions that manifest chest wall abnormalities such as pectus excavatum and carinatum, Marfan's syndrome, and Poland's syndrome can present a challenge in optimizing breast esthetics. It is also important to take note of changes in chest wall contour induced by plastic surgical intervention such as breast augmentation.

1.6
Arterial Supply

Breast tissue possesses a rich blood supply from multiple arterial sources (Fig. 1.3). These sources collateralize within the breast to make a redundant system with

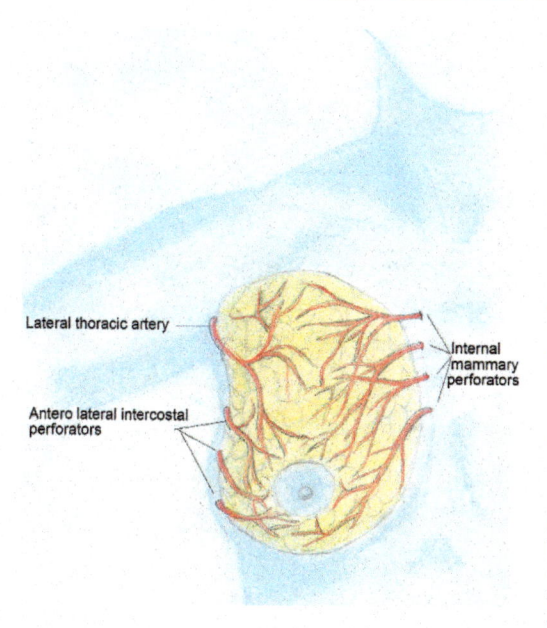

Fig. 1.3 Blood supply: the arterial supply to the breast is supplied predominantly by perforators from the internal mammary artery followed by the lateral thoracic and anterolateral intercostal arteries

significant clinical implications. Division of parenchyma is safe, provided one of the several primary axes is preserved.

Entering the superomedial portion of the breast over intercostal spaces 2–6 are perforators from the internal mammary artery. These vessels supply the medial pectoralis muscle prior to entering the breast tissue and overlying skin. The dominant perforators emanate from the second and third intercostal spaces. These should be spared during reduction mammoplasty using the superomedial pedicle. Of note, they are occasionally of adequate caliber for use as recipient vessels for free flap breast reconstruction.

Supplying the breast superolaterally is the lateral thoracic artery, also termed the external mammary artery. This vessel originates from the axillary artery and enters the breast from the inferior axilla. It distributes its main branches in the upper outer quadrant of the breast.

Intercostal vessels represent an additional important blood supply to the breast. The lateral breast receives anterior intercostal arteries from the third through sixth interspaces. These perforate the serratus anterior just lateral to the pectoral border. Lateral intercostal vessels enter the breast at the anterior margin of the latissimus dorsi to supply the lateral breast and overlying skin.

Medial intercostal perforators are responsible for directly supplying the inferomedial and central parenchyma inferior to the nipple. These perforators course upward through the breast tissue to supply the gland and are one source for nipple–areola complex perfusion.

1.7
Venous Drainage

Two systems of veins drain the breast. The subdermal venous plexus above the superficial fascia is quite variable and represents the superficial system. These veins arise from the periareolar venous plexus. Within the parenchyma, the superficial system anastomoses with the deep system. Deep venous drainage of the breast corresponds with the arterial supply. Venous perforators following internal mammary perforators drain via the internal mammary vein to the innominate vein. Lateral thoracic veins or external mammary veins drain into the axillary vein. Intercostal veins drain via the azygos vein into the superior vena cava.

1.8
Innervation

Mammary innervation is dense and has considerable redundancy (Fig. 1.4). In addition to the abundant general cutaneous sensitivity, the central portion of the breast including the nipple–areola complex serves as an erogenous zone and therefore is supplied by fibers contributing to a sensual character. Just as with the perfusion of the breast, innervation of the skin comes from all directions.

Superiorly the cervical plexus contributes fibers that course beneath the platysma to innervate the upper portion of the breast. These fibers course in the subcutaneous tissue and can be elevated and preserved with skin flaps of proper thickness.

Intercostal segmental nerves contribute the remainder of breast sensation and should be viewed as the primary sensory nerves. Through the interdigitations of the serratus anterior emanate the third through sixth anterolateral intercostal nerves. They enter the lateral breast at the lateral pectoral margin. Entering the medial breast along with the internal mammary perforators are contributions from the second through sixth anteromedial intercostal nerves. As with the anterolateral intercostal nerves, they contribute sensation to the nipple–areola complex.

Fig. 1.4 Innervation: branches of the cervical plexus supply the superior breast. The anteromedial and anterolateral intercostal nerves supply the mass of the breast inferiorly from their respective directions

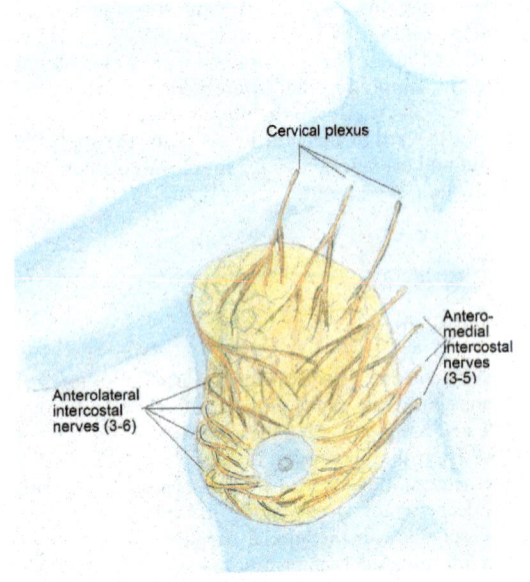

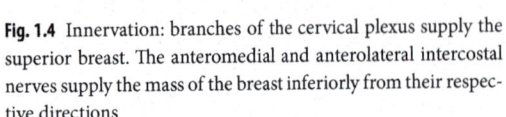

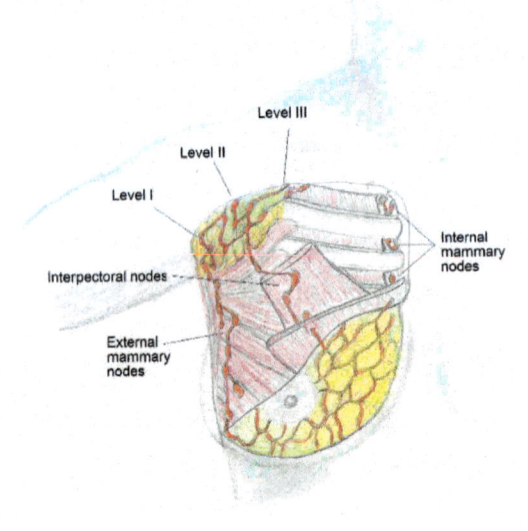

Fig. 1.5 Lymphatic drainage: lymphatic flow from the parenchyma coalesces first in the subareolar plexus, then is directed predominantly to the axilla. Medial lymphatics are directed to the internal mammary nodes or to the contralateral breast. Inferior lymphatics may enter the subperitoneal plexus

1.9
Lymphatics

Lymphatic drainage of the breast has been extensively studied for its oncologic implications (Fig. 1.5). Breast surgeons of all disciplines should have an intimate knowledge of lymphatic anatomy within the breast.

The predominance of lymph from the mammary gland passes along interlobular lymphatic vessels to the subareolar plexus. Lymph is then directed primarily toward the axillary lymph nodes (75%) coursing along the venous drainage. Lateral lymphatics course around the edge of the pectoralis major to enter the pectoral nodal group. Additional lymphatics route through the pectoral muscles leading to the apical nodal group. From the axilla, lymph drains into the subclavian and supraclavicular nodes.

The medial portion of the breast contributes lymphatic vessels, which drain via the parasternal or internal mammary nodes. They follow internal mammary perforators. There are occasional lymphatic contributions to the contralateral breast. Inferior lymphatics may enter the rectus sheath and drain into subperitoneal plexus.

1.10
Nipple–Areola Complex

As mentioned previously, the nipple–areola complex deserves special attention for its unique esthetic, sensual, and lactational function. It is an area of dense perfusion and innervation. Every attempt should be made to preserve these meaningful functions. Secondary to its physiologic redundancy, the nipple–areola complex can be reliably preserved with attention to anatomic principles.

Importantly, the blood supply to the nipple–areola complex is both parenchymal and subdermal. The varied dermoglandular pedicles used in reduction mammaplasty and mastopexy thus preserve potential lactation and perpetuate redundant perfusion. The subdermal plexus encompassing the nipple–areola complex serves to directly perfuse the skin of the nipple and areola.

The nipple itself represents the apex of the mammary gland. Specialized contractile lactiferous ducts within the nipple facilitate lactation. Montgomery's glands, which reside in the areola, lubricate the nipple–areola complex functioning primarily during lactation. Clinically they appear as small nodules distributed throughout the areola and should be preserved.

The nipple serves as a port of entry for bacteria into the mammary gland. Bacteria can be cultured from throughout the glandular portion of the breast. Thus, division of the gland as in most breast surgery can elaborate bacteria (typically *Staphylococcus epidermidis*). Bacterial prophylaxis should be strongly considered in any breast surgery, especially with implant placement.

Part II
Preoperative

Preoperative Consultation

Melvin A. Shiffman

2.1 Introduction

The physician patient relationship is established in the first consultation with the patient. The patient has to find out about the procedure to be followed and any of its problems as well as decide if the surgeon is competent and friendly. The medical record should be thorough and complete.

2.2 History

The present complaint and what is desired to relieve the problem should be elicited. This includes possible symptoms, especially related to possible breast reduction, such as back, shoulder, and/or neck pain as well as feelings of heaviness of the breasts and irritation in the breast folds. There may be neurologic symptoms such as numbness or pain in the hands as carpal tunnel syndrome can occur in patients with large breasts [1].

The past medical and surgical history is important to obtain so that possible problems can be avoided. This should include medical disorders such as heart or lung problems, diabetes mellitus, bleeding disorders or easy bruising, chronic neurologic disorders, allergies, and prior difficulties with anesthesia. Particular attention should be paid to prior breast surgeries and it would be wise to obtain the operative reports to see what was done and what techniques were used. If the prior records are not available, the surgeon should record what efforts were made to obtain the records. Previous breast irradiation should warn the surgeon about possible reduction in blood supply to the area treated.

Family history should be obtained with respect to any cancer, especially breast and ovarian cancer. If there is a strong history of breast and/or ovarian cancer, referral to a medical oncologist or genetic counselor would be wise to find out what the risks are for this patient to get cancer of the breast.

2.3 Physical Examination

If the patient is to have general anesthesia or intravenous sedation, the heart and lungs should be examined. The breast examination should be done in detail with the patient sitting and lying down. The breasts should be observed for nipple retraction and/or breast indentations, which may be indicative of an underlying cancer. Careful palpation for masses or tenderness is to be performed.

Measurements should be taken from the sternal notch and/or mid clavicle to nipples and nipples to midline. To determine the extent of ptosis, measurement should be made from the inframammary fold to the lowest part of the breast. If the breasts are very large, there should be measurement from the inframammary fold to the top of the new areola position. This will help to determine if nipple areolar transplant is necessary.

2.4 Explanation of Possible Risks

The patient should be given enough information in order to make a knowledgeable decision as to whether or not to have the procedure. The procedure recommended should be explained to the patient as well as any viable alternatives. The possible risks and complications of the recommended procedure and the alternatives should be described. It is not necessary for the surgeon to do the whole explanation himself/herself, although if he/she does, there will be better rapport with the patient. The surgeon should be able to answer any questions that remain after the discussion.

Sometimes, the patient may come from a distance and cannot come for a consultation until the day of surgery. The author prefers to see the patient the night before surgery if this is the case, as the patient will almost always come in (if flying) the day before surgery. Enough time, before surgery, should be taken to explain to the patient the surgery, alternatives, and possible risks and complications. Otherwise it leaves little time for the patient to contemplate whether or not the surgery is appropriate for him/her.

The patient may request preoperative and postoperative photos of prior patients. Usually the surgeon shows only the best results. There may be a need to show some of the bad results such as asymmetry or poor scars (hypertrophic or keloid).

Give written preoperative and postoperative instructions as well as oral explanations of both. Smoking should be discontinued at least 2 weeks before and 2 weeks after surgery. Estrogens should be discontinued 3 weeks before and 2 weeks after surgery, as estrogens increase the risk of thromboembolism. Aspirin and nonsteroidal anti-inflammatory drugs (NSAIDs) should be stopped 2 weeks before and 2 weeks after surgery. There are many herbals that should not be taken before and after surgery [2].

Make sure the patient understands the need for careful follow-up after surgery in order to detect complications in a timely fashion.

2.5
Medical Records

Record everything in detail, including discussions, phone calls, and missed appointments. Instruct your employees to record on the medical chart all discussions, presence of tobacco smell, and complaints. Return all calls in a timely fashion and record the date and time. The medical record is your best defense in case of litigation.

References

1. Pernia LR, Ronel DB, Leeper JD, Miller HL: Carpal tunnel syndrome in women undergoing reduction mammaplasty. Plast Reconstr Surg 2000;105(4):1314–1319
2. Shiffman MA: Dangers of herbs when performing surgery. Int J Cosm Surg Aesthet Derm 2000;2(2):95

The Sitting, Oblique, Supine (SOS) Marking Technique for Mastopexy and Breast Reduction

Fahmy S. Fahmy

3.1 Introduction

Macromastia can cause considerable emotional and physical stress. The problem of macromastia has been the subject of the efforts of many plastic surgeons since late nineteenth century. In United States alone nearly 40,000 women undergo breast reduction each year [1].

Breast reduction presents both artistic and technical challenges. The surgery aims to reduce the vertical and horizontal planes, shape the parenchyma, reposition the nipple–areola complex, and resect redundant skin. The surgery on paired organs has the added challenge of symmetry. The added effect of recumbence alters the shape and position of the breast. The classic breast shape, as we know it, exists in the erect posture. Much of the outcome of our work as plastic surgeons is determined by preoperative planning and designing. The availability of numerous marking techniques of breast reduction and mastopexy and the abundance of further modifications over the last decennia are clear indications that none of these techniques have proved to be ideal.

The majority aim to achieve some degree of precision in determining the angle between the two vertical limbs. This ultimately affects the amount of tissue resected and the postoperative shape. Few, if any, of such techniques have gained total popularity or acceptance by the plastic surgeons. The freehand marking technique is probably the most widely used technique. Devices as templates [2, 3] shaped wires, goniometers, and geometrical techniques have also been recommended [4–9]. Some of these devices have stood the test of time; others have been modified or abandoned.

The free hand technique, being the most widely used, requires experience and practice in order to achieve the desired results. Multiple devices have been created to facilitate markings, including templates, keyhole patterns, goniometers, etc. The standard pattern with a fixed angle of 110° between the two segments was further modified by McKissock [10] to allow for adjustment of the angle to the widely variable breast shapes. The wire keyhole pattern marking is influenced by the surgeon's experience [11].

The standard patterns and devices are rigid methods that may achieve symmetrical markings, not necessarily symmetrical outcomes. They do not account easily to preexisting breast asymmetry. Devices may also be not readily available in all hospitals. This factor could be a disadvantage to the surgeon who practices in more than one hospital.

The inherent difficulties of these techniques, the lack of flexibility, and the need to memorize different measures and mathematical calculations on some occasions made me alter my approach in the preoperative marking. Over the last 15 years, I have developed the sitting, oblique, supine (SOS) marking technique. This method is dependent on the natural breast fall and is aimed to guide the required angle between the two vertical limbs, each breast on its individual merits. It would be applicable in most breast reduction and mastopexy surgery; however, it is used largely in the inferior pedicle technique.

3.2 The SOS (Sitting, Oblique, Supine) Marking Technique

The patient is marked preoperatively in three positions.
1. *Sitting*: This position is adopted to mark the midline, midclavicular point (usually 7.5 cm from the sternal notch) and the breast meridian (Fig. 3.1). The breast meridian is marked as a straight line joining the midclavicular point to the current nipple–areolar complex (NAC) extending down to the inframammary fold. The superior limit of the vertical limbs is then marked with reference to the inframammary fold. This marks the possible future position of the NAC. The distance from the midclavicular point to the superior limit of the vertical limbs is then measured and the same measure is used to mark the contra-lateral NAC.

M.A. Shiffman (ed.), *Mastopexy and Breast Reduction: Principles and Practice*,
© Springer-Verlag Berlin Heidelberg 2009

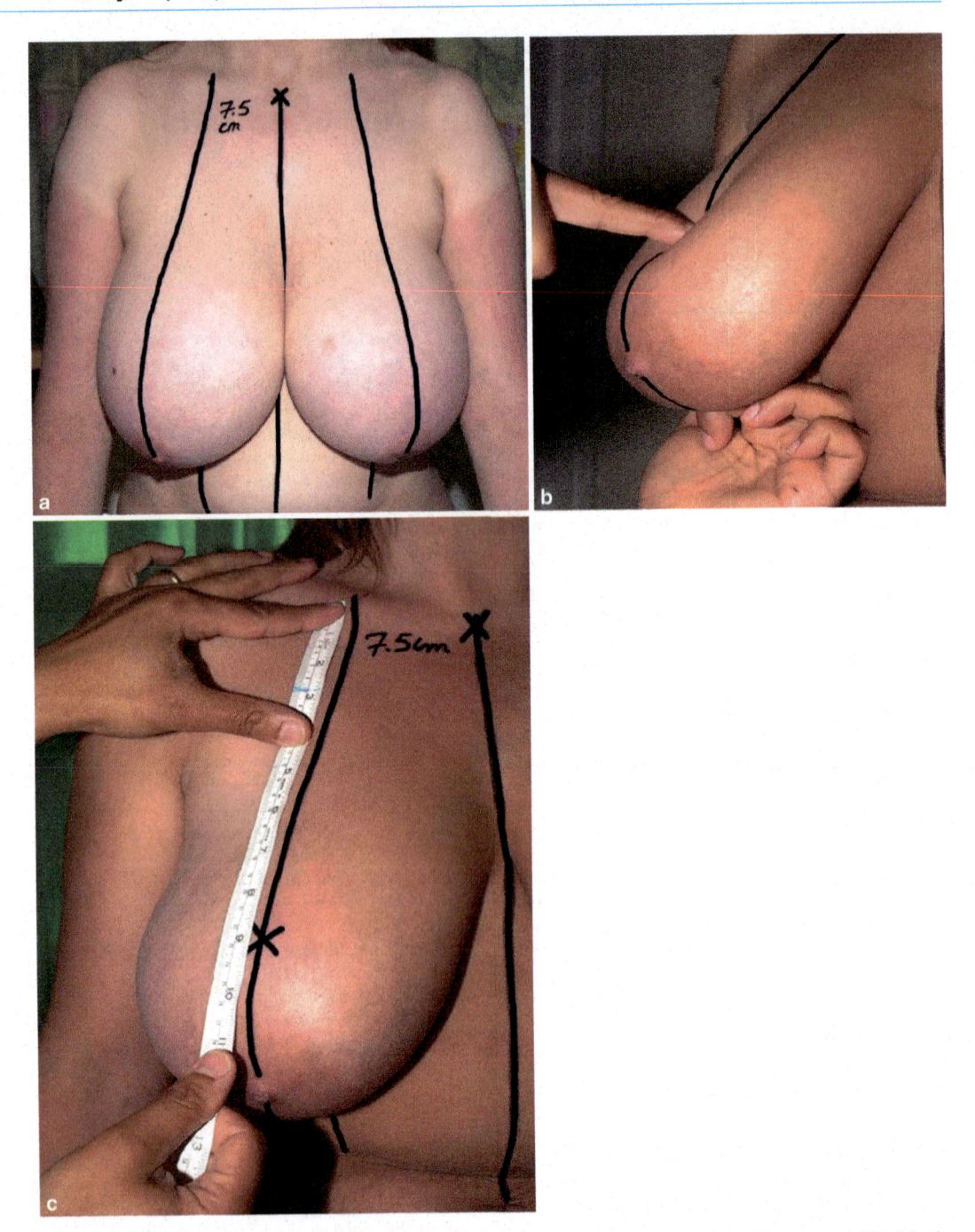

Fig. 3.1 Patient in sitting position. (**a**) The breast meridian marked from the midclavicular point, usually 7.5 cm lateral to the sternal notch. (**b**) The superior limit of the vertical limb marked with reference to the inframammary fold. (**c**) The contralateral NAC is marked at the same distance from the midclavicular point

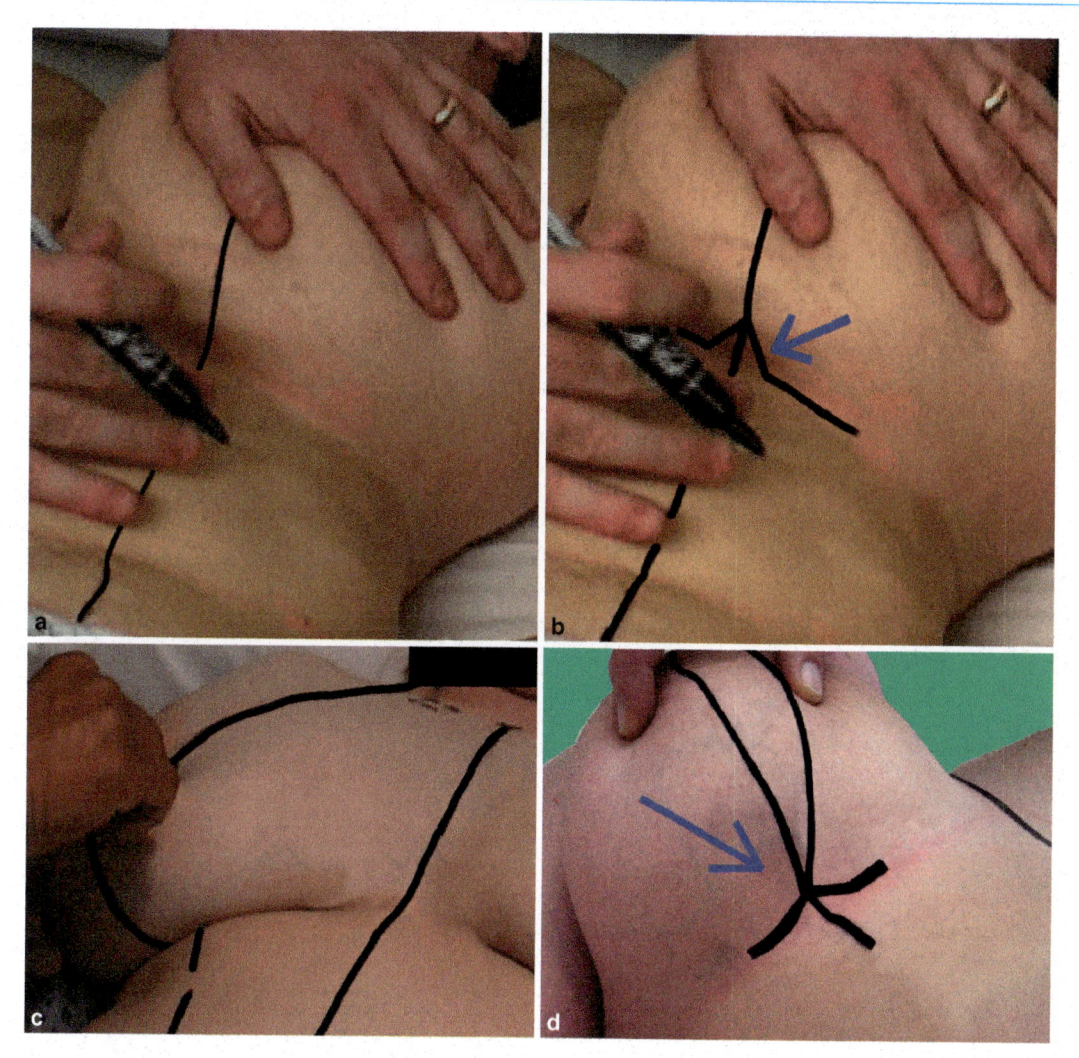

Fig. 3.2 Patient in the supine position. (**a**) Gentle pressure on the breast mound clearly defines the inframammary fold. (**b**) Marking of the inframammary fold, arrow pointing to the dart. (**c**) Marking of the medial limb. (**d**) Marking of the medial limb completed

2. *Supine*: The supine position is used to mark the inframammary fold incision and the medial limb of the vertical markings (Fig. 3.2). While the patient is lying flat, the inframammary fold is marked with a very gentle pressure on the breast mound. Every effort should be made intra-operatively to minimize the length of the future inframammary scar. A "dart" coinciding with the breast meridian is marked along the inframammary incision line. This aids in reducing tension on the wound at the time of skin closure. While remaining in the supine position, the breast will naturally fall laterally. A straight line is drawn joining the superior limit of the vertical limbs to the dart. This will indicate the medial limb of the vertical limbs.

3. *Oblique (Left and Right)*: The oblique position is mainly to mark the lateral limb of the vertical markings (Fig. 3.3). The patient is marked in the left and right oblique position. In the left oblique position, the right breast will naturally adopt a medial position. A straight line is marked joining the superior limit of the vertical limb to the dart. This marks the lateral limb of the right breast. While in the right oblique position, the left breast will adopt a medial position. A straight line is marked joining the superior limit of the vertical

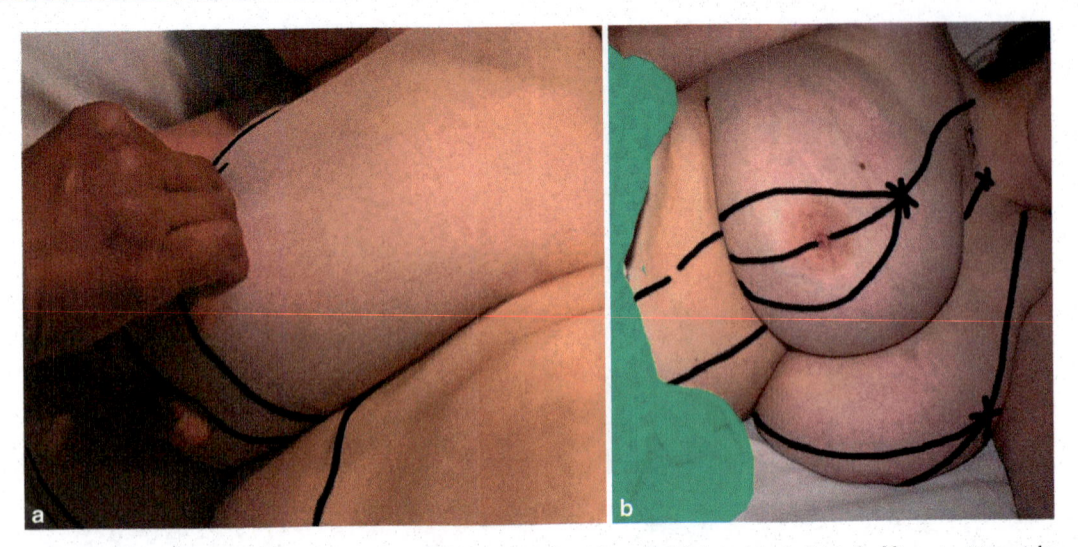

Fig. 3.3 Patient in the oblique position. (**a**) Right oblique position, marking the left lateral limb. (**b**) Left oblique position, right lateral limb marked

    limbs to the dart. This marks the lateral limb of the left breast.
4. Finally, the patient is returned to the sitting position. The medial and lateral vertical limbs are measured at a length of 7 cm from the superior limit of the vertical limbs.

The above are all the required preoperative markings (Fig. 3.4). I now tend to join the vertical limbs to the medial and lateral ends of the inframammary marking intra-operatively. This is carried out in "a cut as you go" fashion aiming at avoiding dog-ears and also reducing the length of the inframammary scar. The new NAC is usually marked towards the end of the procedure, after the resection is completed.

    The lower margin of the NAC is approximately 4–5 cm cephalad from the inframammary fold dart.

    The SOS marking is a versatile technique dependent on the natural breast fall. The breast is viewed as a dynamic organ requiring the individual analysis of each breast (Fig. 3.5). The natural fall of the breast spontaneously generates the desired angle between the vertical limbs, accounting for any existing asymmetries (Fig. 3.6).

    Marking the patient in the supine position has the added advantage of clearly identifying the inframammary fold. Marking in the sitting position only, as referred to in other techniques, may present difficulty in marking the inframammary fold in large ptotic breasts.

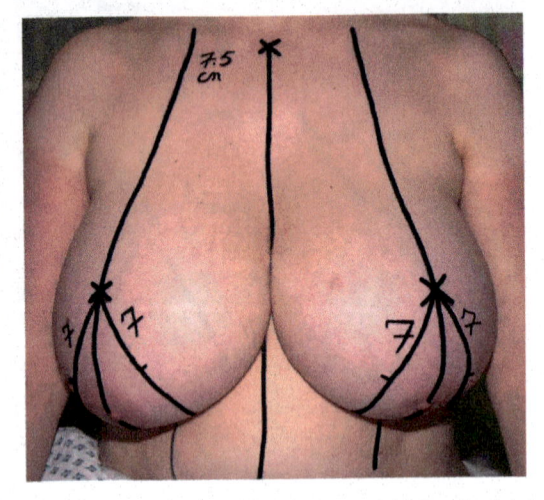

Fig. 3.4 Patient in sitting position marking the length of the vertical limbs

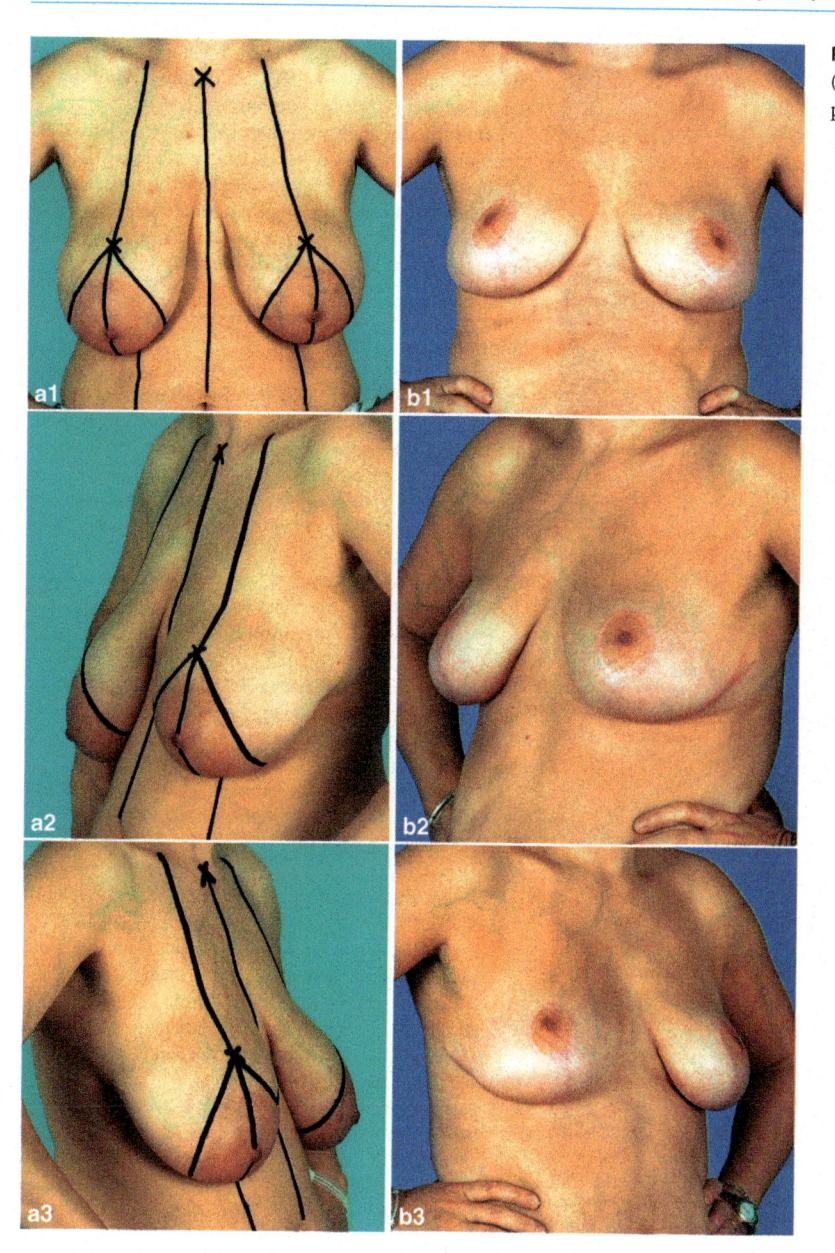

3.2 The SOS (Sitting, Oblique, Supine) Marking Technique   17

Fig. 3.5 (*a1-3*) Preoperative. (*b1-3*) Six months postoperative

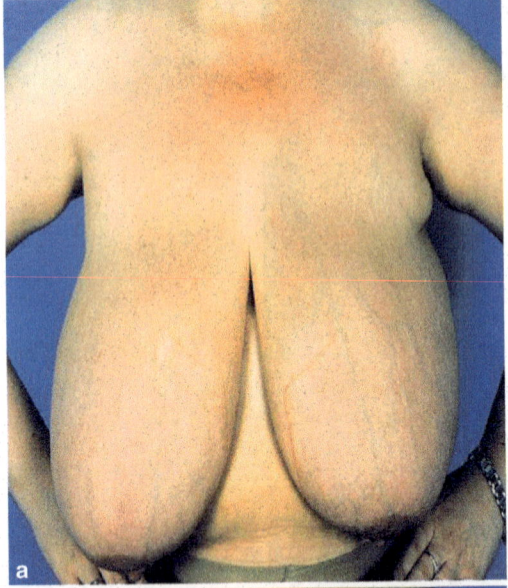

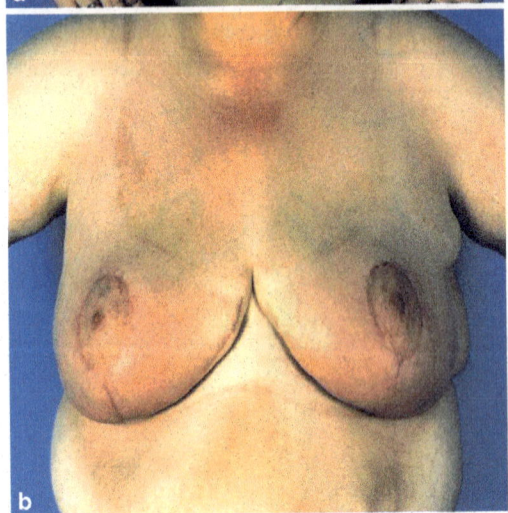

Fig. 3.6 (**a**) Preoperative showing asymmetry. (**b**) Six months postoperative right breast reduction

There are no specific devices required in this technique. There is no need to memorize any particular reference points apart from the three standard landmarks: the inframammary fold, the sternal notch, and the mid clavicular point. There is minimal handling of the breast, hence minimizing human errors.

Undoubtedly, there is a learning curve for any new technique. The SOS in my view is relatively easy to learn for the beginners and easy to adopt by the experienced. It is readily available, not requiring major alterations in our current practice and accounts for the great diversities in the shape and size of the breasts.

References

1. Goldwyn RM, Courtiss EH: Reduction mammaplasty by the inferior pedicle (pyramidal) technique. In: Goldwyn RM (ed), Reduction Mammaplasty. Boston, Little, Brown & Co. 1990, pp 255–266
2. Wise RJ: A preliminary report on a method of planning the mammaplasty. Plast Reconstr Surg 1956;17(5): 367–375
3. Palumbo SK, Shifren J, Rhee C: Modifications of the Lejour vertical mammaplasty: analysis of results in 100 consecutive patients. Ann Plast Surg 1998;40(4): 354–359
4. Courtiss EH, Goldwyn RM: Reduction mammaplasty by the inferior pedicle technique. An alternative to free nipple and areolar grafting for severe macromastia or extreme ptosis. Plast Reconstr Surg 1977;59(4):500–507
5. Kavka S: A simple device for marking the areola in vertical mammaplasty. Plast Reconstr Surg 1999;103(7):2087
6. Mendez-Fernandez MA: An easy-to-make, easy-to-use device for preoperative marking for reduction mammoplasty and mastopexy. Ann Plast Surg 1991;26(6): 602–603
7. Lazarus D: A new template-goniometer for marking the wise keyhole pattern of reduction mammaplasty. Plast Reconstr Surg 1998;101(1):171–173
8. Beer GM, Morgenthaler W, Spicher I, Meyer VE: Modifications in vertical scar reduction. Br J Plast Surg 2001;54(4):341–347
9. Paloma V, Samper A, Sanz J: A simple device for marking the areola in Lejour's mammaplasty. Plast Reconstr Surg 1998;103(7):2134–2135
10. McKissock PK: Reduction mammaplasty by the vertical bipedicle flap technique. Clin Plast Surg 1976;3(2): 309–320
11. Gasperoni C, Salgarello M: Preoperative breast marking in reductio0n mammaplasty. Ann Plast Surg 1987;19(4): 306–311

Prediction of Weight in Breast Reduction Surgery

Nicole Z. Sommer, Elvin G. Zook

Many studies showing the benefits of reduction mammaplasty have been reported; however, insurance companies have become more cost conscious and have made increasing efforts to deny this procedure. Spector and Karp [1] state that insurance companies often do not cover breast reductions that remove less than 1,000 g total (500 g of tissue from each side). However, their study shows that women who have less than 1,000 g of total weight removal, or even less than 750 g of totally removed, demonstrate "substantial relief of macromastia associated symptoms" and significant improvement in quality of life.

Seitchik and Schnur [2, 3] have recommended that the insurance companies base the minimum gram resection requirement on the patients weight and height rather than on an arbitrary number applied to all patients. Seitchik [2] found there was a correlation between body weight and a specimen weight of 0.68. He concluded that three levels of minimal volume resection should replace the one volume minimum. He proposed the weight resection correlations as follows: (1) Body weight less than 60 kg, 400 g resection. (2) Body weight 61–79 kg, 700 g resection. (3) Body weight >80 kg, 1,000 g resection. Schnur [3] gives percentiles of weight removal based on body surface area. The patient's body surface area, obtained by a graph of height and weight, determines the volume of breast tissue that must be removed to be above certain percentiles for all women having reductions. Below the fifth percentile is considered cosmetic, and above the 22nd percentile is considered medically necessary.

Once the plastic surgeon decides that the patient will benefit from reduction, he must determine how much breast tissue will be removed for insurance approval. The patient with a large body frame and large breast volume would certainly be above the 500 g requirement by many insurance companies and will not be a problem. The problem lies in the patient who is of smaller frame or height with the same proportion of breast tissue to body size as the larger patient. The conundrum that the plastic surgeon faces is how to accurately predict the weight of breast tissue to be removed. If the insurance companies will give preapproval, or disapproval, the patient knows whether the procedure will be covered and allow for financial planning. The surgeon should make every effort to be as accurate as possible with this prediction and not over-inflate the weight prediction to obtain coverage. If overestimation of weight to be removed occurs and the final weight by pathology of the specimen is less, the insurance company may refuse to pay the procedure charges because of the discrepancy.

A very good representation of this situation is presented by Becker [4] who gives many of the methods by which insurance companies try to avoid payment of claims. The absurdity of the insurance company guidelines is pointed out by Goldwyn [5]. If companies are going to make their determination by a predicted amount of weight to be removed, it would be helpful if the plastic surgeon had a simple reliable way of predicting the weight to be removed.

One of the more accurate methods for breast volume measurement is water displacement. The individual, while kneeling over a table, lowers her breast into a fluid container of known volume and the displacement is measured [6]. Others have placed containers over the breast and filled empty area with fluid [7–10]; discs [11], cones [12], thermoplastic casts [13, 14] have been described, but have limitations of maximum volume. Various anthropomorphic breast measurements [15–19] have all been proposed to determine breast volume but do not determine breast weight.

Three-dimensional imaging of the breast including mammography, [20] biostereometric measurements [21–29], and magnetic resonance imaging (MRI) have been reported as accurate measurements of breast volume, but require special equipments not always available to the surgeon. Bulstrode et al. [30] compared volume measurements determined by mammograms, thermoplastic molding, MRI, Archimedes principle, and anatomical measurements. They determined that the same methods should be used to compare volumes before and after for each patient, as it was unreliable to compare volume measurements using different techniques in the same patient. They concluded that mammogram measurements were reasonably accurate and that thermoplastic molding "showed promise." Kovacs [31] showed that MRI had the highest precision in volume calculation. Caruso et al. [32] compared the cost of the Gossman–Rowdner device with casting and MRI,

M.A. Shiffman (ed.), *Mastopexy and Breast Reduction: Principles and Practice,*
© Springer-Verlag Berlin Heidelberg 2009

and found that the Gossman–Rowdner device was much more cost-effective. However, this is a volume displacement method and has inaccuracies due to the differences in the weight of a fatty breast compared to a glandular breast. Comparing fatty vs. glandular breasts shows that they may have the same volume, but very different weights. All of these imaging techniques predict volume but do not help the surgeon to accurately predict weight of the breast tissue.

Sommer et al. [33] performed a retrospective review of 266 breast reduction patients, recording height, weight, and simple breast measurements, predicted weight to be resected and postoperative resected tissue weight. They measured the distances from the mid sternal notch to the nipple and the mid sternal notch to the inframmary fold in an attempt to predict weight of removal. With breast reductions greater then 600 grams per side and sternal notch to nipple distance >28.5 cm, the equation predicted the resected weight to be >500 g 80% of the time. However, between the critical 400 and 600 g range, which is most important for insurance approval, the prediction rate was only 50%. The prediction of weights, less than 400 g, was also found to be inaccurate.

They compared the predictability of the measurement with the senior author's estimate of the weight to be removed. The senior author used his past experience, manual examination, and evaluation of the breast as fatty vs. glandular to estimate preoperatively the amount of breast tissue to be resected. Estimation by the senior author in breast reductions >500 g was accurate 94% of the time.

4.1
Conclusions

There is no truly accurate method to predict weight to be removed in breast reduction. Volume measurements are reasonably accurate but do not measure weight. The experience of the surgeon in predicting weight to be removed appears to be the simplest and most accurate method for predicting weight removal. It is important that young surgeons predict preoperatively, record the weights, and then compare them with the weights removed to improve their ability to predict the weight to be removed.

References

1. Spector J, Karp N: Reduction mammaplasty: a significant improvement at any size. Plast Reconstr Surg 2007;120(4): 845–850
2. Seitchik MW: Reduction mammaplasty: criteria for insurance coverage. Plast Reconstr Surg 1995;95(6):1029–1032
3. Schnur P, Schnur E, Petty PM, Hanson TJ, Weaver AL: Reduction mammaplasty: an outcome study. Plast Reconstr Surg 1997;100(4):875–883
4. Becker H: Breast reduction insurance denials. Plast Reconstr Surg 2004;114(6):1687
5. Goldwyn RM: Breast reduction absurdum. Plast Reconstr Surg 1998;102(1):246
6. Schultz R, Dolezal R, Nolan J: Further application of Archimedes' principle in the correction of asymmetrical breasts. Ann Plast Surg 1986;16(2):98–101
7. Tezel E, Numanoglu A: Practical do-it-yourself device for accurate volume measurement of breast. Plast Reconstr Surg 2000;105(3):1019–1023
8. Bouman F: Volumetric measurement of the human breast and breast tissue before and during mammaplasty. Br J Plast Surg 1970;23(3):263–264
9. Wilkie T, Ship A: Volumetric breast measurement during surgery. Aesth Plast Surg 1977;1:301–305
10. Tegtmeier R: A quick, accurate mammometer. Ann Plast Surg 1978;1(6):625–626
11. Palin WE Jr, Fraunhofer J, Smith DJ Jr: Measurement of breast volume: comparison of techniques. Plast Reconstr Surg 1986;77(2):253–254
12. Grossman A, Roudner L: A simple means for accurate breast volume determination. Plast Reconstr Surg 1980;66(6):851–852
13. Campaigne BN, Katch VL, Freedson P, Sady S, Katch FI: Measurement of breast volume in females: description of a reliable method. Ann Human Biol 1979;6(4):363–367
14. Edsander-Nord A, Wickman M, Jurell G: Measurement of breast volume with thermoplastic casts. Scand J Plast Reconstr Surg Hand Surg 1996;30(2):129–132
15. Kanhai R, Hage J: Bra cup size depends on band size. Plast Reconstr Surg 1999;104(1):300
16. Westreich M: Anthropomorphic breast measurement: protocol and results in 50 women with aesthetically perfect breasts and clinical application. Plast Reconstr Surg 1997;100(2):468–479
17. Sigurdson L, Kirkland S: Breast volume determination in breast hypertrophy: an accurate method using two anthropomorphic measurements. Plast Reconstr Surg 2006;118(2):313–320
18. Regnault P, Daniel RK: Breast reduction. In: Regnault P, Daniel K (eds), Aesthetic Plastic Surgery. Principles and Techniques. Boston, Little Brown 1984, pp 499–538
19. Turner A, Dujon D: Predicting cup size after reduction mammaplasty. Br J Plast Surg 2005;58(3):290–298
20. Kalbhen C, McGill J, Fendley P, Corrigan K, Angelats J: Mammographic determination of breast volume: comparing different methods. AJR Am J Roentgenol 1999;173(6): 1643–1649
21. Sheffer D, Price T, Loughry C, Bolyard B, Morek W, Varga R: Validity and reliability of biostereometric measurement of the human female breast. Ann Biomed Eng 1986;14(1):1–14

22. Loughry CW, Sheffer DB, Price TE Jr, Lackney MJ, Bartfai RG, Morek WM: Breast volume measurements of 248 women using biostereometric analysis. Plast Reconstr Surg 1987;80(4):553–558
23. Loughry CW, Sheffer DB, Price TE, Einsporn RL, Bartfai RG, Morek WM, Meli NM: Breast volume measurement of 598 women using biostereometric analysis. Ann Plast Surg 1989;22(5):380–385
24. Galdino G, Nahabedian M, Chiaramonte M, Geng J, Klatsky S, Manson P: Clinical applications of three-dimensional photography in breast surgery. Plast Reconstr Surg 2002;110(1):58–70
25. Nahabedian M, Galdino G: Symmetrical breast reconstruction: is there a role for three-dimensional digital photography? Plast Reconstr Surg 2003;112(6):1582–1590
26. Losken A, Seify H, Denson D, Pardes AA Jr, Carlson G: Validating three-dimensional imaging of the breast. Ann Plast Surg 2005;54(5):471–476
27. Nahabedian M: Discussion: validating three-dimensional imaging of the breast. Ann Plast Surg 2005;54(5):477–476
28. Kovacs L, Eder M, Papadopulos N, Biemer E: Validating 3-dimensional imaging of the breast. Ann Plast Surg 2005;55(6):695–696
29. Kovacs L, Eder M, Hollweck R, Zimmermann A, Settles M, Schneider A, Udosic K, Schwenzer-Zimmerer K, Papadopulos NA, Biemer E: New aspects of breast volume measurement using 3-dimensional surface imaging. Ann Plast Surg 2006;57(6):602–610
30. Bulstrode N, Bellamy E, Shrotria S: Breast volume assessment: comparing five different techniques. The Breast 2001;10(2):117–123
31. Kovacs L, Eder M, Hollweck R, Zimmermann A, Settles M, Schneider A, Endlich M, Schwenzer-Zimmerer K, Papadopulos NA, Biemer E: Comparison between breast volume measurement using 3D surface imaging and classical techniques. The Breast 2007;16(2):137–145
32. Caruso MK, Guillot T, Nguyen T, Greenway F: The cost effectiveness of three different measures of breast volume. Aesthetic Plast Surg 2006;30(1):16–20
33. Sommer NZ, Zook EG, Verhulst SJ: The prediction of breast reduction weight. Plast Reconstr Surg 2002;109(2):506–511

CHAPTER 5

Carpal Tunnel Syndrome in Women Undergoing Breast Reduction

Luis R. Pernia, Genelle Pernia

5.1
Introduction

Women with mammary hypertrophy who present for reduction mammaplasty have several well-described musculoskeletal complaints, but a high prevalence of carpal tunnel syndrome had not been reported in the past. One hundred fifty-one patients, who underwent reduction mammaplasty from 1994 to 1996 were identified from a plastic surgery practice. To this group was added a convenience sample of 64 women volunteers with relatively smaller breasts (brassiere cup size B or smaller). The entire group was questioned about specific symptoms and examined using standard provocative tests. Carpal tunnel syndrome was defined as the coexistence of symptoms and at least two physical examination findings. Its association with breast size, age, race, and body mass index was examined. Stepwise logistic regression was used to determine which physical characteristics were predictive of the condition. Carpal tunnel syndrome was found in 30 patients (19.9%) (95% confidence interval, 13.8–27.1) and in none of the women in the convenience sample. Breast size and, to a lesser degree, body mass index were found to be highly significant predictors of carpal tunnel syndrome. After controlling for breast size, race was also significant. Breast size displayed an independent risk ratio of 6.67 when comparing the upper quartile of size to the lower quartiles. There was a markedly higher prevalence of carpal tunnel syndrome in women who presented for reduction mammaplasty than in those with smaller breasts. Breast size was a significant predictor of carpal tunnel syndrome.

5.2
History

Women with mammary hypertrophy have several well-described musculoskeletal complaints, including back pain, shoulder grooving from bra straps, headache, and neck pain [1–7]. Little had been reported on upper extremity neurologic symptoms caused by excessive breast size. Two articles reported ulnar nerve paresthesias in approximately 15% of their patients and one group reported symptoms of hand numbness or pain in 22.6% of their patients [8–10]. It has been our experience that upper-extremity neurologic symptoms in women with mammary hypertrophy occur much more frequently than reported. The distribution of symptoms is mostly along the median nerve, as in carpal tunnel syndrome.

5.3
Methods

All women who were presented to a solo plastic surgery practice in Tuscaloosa County, Alabama, for reduction mammaplasty from January 1994 to June 1996 were evaluated for inclusion in the study. The racial composition of the patient group was compared with the demographic composition of Tuscaloosa County as reported in the 1997 data from the US Bureau of the Census. Of the 169 women who presented for reduction mammaplasty, two were excluded for having undergone previous shoulder surgery involving the brachial plexus. Three women were excluded for having significant osteoarthritis in the cervical spine or wrists, which precluded their undergoing provocative testing for carpal tunnel syndrome. In addition, 13 women were excluded because of either incomplete testing or incomplete historical data.

Physical characteristics were determined, including age, race, body mass index, and breast size. Body mass index was calculated as the weight in kilograms divided by the square of the height in meters. Breast size was measured in centimeters from sternal notch to each nipple, with the patient sitting and unclothed; the average of both breasts was used in our analyses. The mean and range for age, breast size, and body mass index were calculated.

M.A. Shiffman (ed.), *Mastopexy and Breast Reduction: Principles and Practice*,
© Springer-Verlag Berlin Heidelberg 2009

The 151 patients enrolled in the study were interviewed for symptoms of carpal tunnel syndrome and were administered Tinel's, Phalen's, and Reverse-Phalen's tests during their physical examination. The interview and examination occurred before they underwent reduction mammaplasty. Positive symptoms were defined as pain, weakness, numbness, tingling, or burning along the radial palm or the first three fingers. In the Tinel test, the examiner tapped over the carpal tunnel at the wrist. In the Phalen test, the subject held her wrists maximally flexed for 60 s and in the Reverse-Phalen test, the wrists were held maximally extended for 60 s. A positive result was recorded if there was any tingling or paresthesia in the radial palm or in the first three fingers. We designated those women who had both symptoms and at least two positive physical examination findings as having carpal tunnel syndrome. The prevalence was determined for each physical characteristic: breast size, body mass index, age, and race. Confidence intervals were determined using a standard statistical formula [11].

A convenience sample of women volunteers with brassiere cup size B or smaller was drawn from the staffs of several hospitals in the Tuscaloosa area. The volunteers were not randomly selected. The same physical characteristics were determined as for the patient group. The volunteers were interviewed for symptoms of carpal tunnel syndrome and were tested in the same manner as the patients. The same interviewers were used as for the patient group. None of the volunteers had a history of either shoulder surgery or osteoarthritis. Carpal tunnel syndrome was defined in the same way as for the patients.

5.4 Complications

Because the volunteers were not randomly selected and because the patient and volunteer groups differed significantly, direct comparisons could not be made. Instead, a combined group of both the relatively large-breasted patients and relatively small-breasted volunteers was used to test the association of carpal tunnel syndrome with the various physical characteristics. Body mass index was categorized into normal (less than 25.0 kg m^{-2}), overweight (25.0–29.9 kg m^{-2}), and obese (greater than 30.0 kg m^{-2}) according to the 1998 National Heart, Lung, and Blood Institute criteria [12]. Breast size was divided into the quartiles observed in the study (less than 23.0 cm, 23.1–30.0 cm, 30.1–35.0 cm, and greater than 35.0 cm). Age was treated as a continuous variable. Logistic regression analysis was used in a stepwise fashion to determine predictors of carpal tunnel syndrome. The statistical package used was Statistical Package for the Social Sciences (release 4.1 for IBM VM/CMS).

5.5 Results

The characteristics of the patient and volunteer groups are listed in Table 5.1. The patient ages ranged from 13 to 64 years, with a mean of 32.8 years. Almost all patients were either Caucasian (89 patients, 58.9%) or African-American (61 patients, 40.4%). One patient was Hispanic. There was a higher proportion of Caucasians in the volunteer sample. Tuscaloosa County is mostly urban (71%) and contains a population of approximately 160,760, with 71% Caucasian, 28% African-American, and 1% other [13]. This racial composition is similar to that of our patient group, although African-Americans are somewhat over-represented.

Body mass index in the patients ranged from 20.8 to 54.2 kg m^{-2}, with a mean of 33.5 kg m^{-2}. The average of breast sizes in individual patients ranged from 24.8 to 47.5 cm, with a mean of 34.1 cm. These characteristics are similar to those of patients in other series of women undergoing reduction mammaplasty [9, 10, 14, 15].

The distribution of carpal tunnel symptoms and physical examination findings among patients and volunteers is listed in Table 5.2. Of the 151 women who presented for reduction mammaplasty, neurologic symptoms of carpal tunnel syndrome were reported by 129 (85.4%). Three had symptoms that were not in the distribution of the median nerve. Three women in the volunteer group (4.7%) reported neurologic symptoms of carpal tunnel syndrome. Eight of the volunteers had

Table 5.1 Characteristic of patients and volunteers

	Patients ($n = 151$)	Volunteers ($n = 64$)
Race		
Caucasian	89 (58.9%)	56 (87.5%)
African-American	61 (40.4%)	8 (12.5%)
Other	1	0
Age (years)		
Mean ± SD	32.8 ± 11.2	39.1 ± 12.3
Range	13–64	15–60
Breast size (cm)		
Mean ± SD	34.1 ± 5.0	20.4 ± 2.4
Range	24.8–47.5	14.0–24.5
Body mass index (kg m^{-2})		
Mean ± SD	33.5 ± 7.0	24.4 ± 3.9
Range	20.8–54.2	17.7–33.7

Table 5.2 Distribution of patients and volunteers with combination of carpal tunnel symptoms and physical examination findings

	Patients (n = 151)	Volunteers (n = 64)
Carpal tunnel symptoms	129 (85.4%)	3 (4.7%)
At least two physical findings	32 (21.2%)	2 (3.1%)
At least two physical findings and symptoms for carpal tunnel syndrome	30 (19.9%)	0 (0.0%)
Symptoms and no physical examination findings	25 (16.6%)	2 (3.1%)
At least two physical examination findings and no symptoms	2 (1.3%)	9 (14.1%)

symptoms that were not in the distribution of the median nerve. Two patients and nine volunteers who had two or more physical examination findings of carpal tunnel syndrome did not have related symptoms. There were 30 patients (19.9%, 95% confidence intervals, 13.8–27.1%) who met our criteria for carpal tunnel syndrome: two or more positive physical examination findings, in addition to neurologic symptoms, along the distribution of the median nerve. None of the volunteers met the criteria.

Table 5.3 lists the prevalence of carpal tunnel syndrome according to age, race, body mass index, and breast size in the combined group of patients and volunteers. Body mass index and breast size were characteristics significantly associated with carpal tunnel syndrome ($p = 0.015$ and $p < 0.001$, respectively). The mean age of those without carpal tunnel syndrome was 34.4 years, compared with 36.5 years for those with carpal tunnel syndrome ($p = 0.37$).

The difference in prevalence between the races was not significant ($p = 0.56$). In a multivariate analysis adjusting for age, race, body mass index, and breast size

Table 5.3 Prevalence of carpal tunnel syndrome according to various patient characteristics

	Total	Carpal tunnel syndrome[a]	Percent	95% confidence intervals (%) Lower	Upper
Patients	151	30	19.9	13.8	27.1
Controls	64	0	0	0	0
Race					
Caucasian	145	21	14.5	9.2	21.3
African-American	69	8	11.6	5.1	21.6
Breast size (cm)					
14.0–23.0	55	0	0.0	0.0	6.5
23.1–30.0	48	7	14.6	6.1	27.8
30.1–35.0	57	5	8.8	2.9	19.3
35.1–47.5	55	18	32.7	20.7	46.7
Body mass index (kg m^{-2})					
<25.0	53	2	3.8	0.5	13.0
25.0–29.9	53	6	11.3	4.3	23.0
>30.0	69	22	20.2	13.1	28.9

[a]Positive symptoms and at least two physical findings

of the combined patient and volunteer groups, only breast size and race were significant predictors of carpal tunnel syndrome ($p = 0.003$ and $p = 0.04$, respectively). The adjusted risk ratio for the highest quartile of breast size compared with the lower two quartiles was 8.43 (the lower two quartiles of breast size were combined because there were no cases of carpal tunnel syndrome in the lowest quartile). The adjusted risk ratio for the highest quartile of breast size compared with the third quartile was 6.33. Caucasians compared with African-Americans had an adjusted risk ratio of 2.92. Breast size displayed an independent risk ratio of 6.67 when comparing the upper quartile of size to the combined two lower quartiles.

A forward stepwise logistic analysis was performed to investigate the best predictors for carpal tunnel syndrome. Only breast size ($p < 0.0001$) and race ($p = 0.03$) were significant. The adjusted risk ratios for the highest quartile of breast size compared with the combined lower two quartiles was 10.11. The adjusted risk ratio compared with the third quartile was 6.12. For Caucasians compared with African-Americans, the adjusted risk ratio was 3.02.

5.6 Discussion

Many manifestations of excessively large breasts are well recognized and may include painful chronic mastitis, lower cervical pain, backache, hypertrophic arthritis of the lower cervical vertebrae, postural changes such as kyphosis and compensatory lordosis, grooving and irritation of the shoulders from brassiere straps, submammary intertrigo, thoracic outlet syndrome, and lack of self-esteem [1–7, 16]. Several recent articles describing outcome results of reduction mammaplasty have mainly compared techniques, discussed postoperative complications, and determined patient satisfaction. Most symptoms are relieved rapidly, and most patients have a high degree of satisfaction with the surgical results [10, 13–15, 17–25]. In our series, we found a high incidence of upper-extremity neurologic symptoms, mostly in the distribution of the median nerve.

Consensus criteria for the classification of carpal tunnel syndrome in epidemiologic studies were recently elaborated. It was determined that the combination of electrodiagnostic findings and symptom characteristics provides the most accurate diagnosis, and in the absence of electrodiagnostic studies, a combination of symptom characteristics and physical examination findings provides the greatest diagnostic information. This combination of symptoms and physical examination findings was reported to have a sensitivity of 0.12, a specificity of 0.97, and a positive predictive value of 0.31, assuming a prevalence of carpal tunnel syndrome of 10% [26]. In the absence of electrodiagnostic data, we defined carpal tunnel syndrome as recommended by the consensus criteria, and we required the presence of two positive physical examination findings. Although our results suggest that having mammary hypertrophy increases the risk of carpal tunnel syndrome, this result may be due to other factors that are associated with both carpal tunnel syndrome and mammary hypertrophy. Medical disorders related to carpal tunnel syndrome have been reviewed recently. In addition to older age, the diseases most commonly associated with carpal tunnel syndrome include hypothyroidism, diabetes mellitus, wrist osteoarthritis, and obesity [27]. Other than obesity, these risk factors were not addressed in our study. We found that breast size was a much better predictor of carpal tunnel syndrome than was body mass index, even after adjusting for body mass index, age, and race. It is likely that carpal tunnel syndrome is the result of a complex interaction between systemic susceptibilities and internal and external mechanical forces.

The 1988 National Health Interview Survey of 44,233 persons determined the prevalence of carpal tunnel syndrome in the general population of women in the United States. The telephonic survey was conducted by the National Center for Health Statistics and classified the prevalence of carpal tunnel syndrome into two categories: "self-reported" carpal tunnel syndrome and "medically called" carpal tunnel syndrome. Respondents had medically called carpal tunnel syndrome if they had worked within the previous 12 months and had seen a health care provider, that is, physician, chiropractor, physical therapist, or other, for prolonged hand discomfort, pain, burning, stiffness, numbness, or tingling in the hand, wrist, or fingers for 20 or more days or at least 6 consecutive days in the past year and had been told it was carpal tunnel syndrome. By this definition, the national female prevalence was only 0.67% (95% confidence interval, 0.51–0.82). The study authors believe this finding was reasonably accurate because the questions used to elicit a positive response were limited to people who had prolonged hand discomfort and because the respondents volunteered the term "carpal tunnel syndrome" without a leading question [28].

Prevalence and confidence intervals from our study were far higher than the prevalence reported in the 1988 National Health Interview Survey. Despite the statistical difficulties inherent in comparing such different groups, it is unlikely that they would account for the large difference in the prevalence of carpal tunnel syndrome. Although race by itself was not a significant predictor of carpal tunnel syndrome, after adjusting for breast size, there was a noted difference between Caucasians and African-Americans. This may be related to differences in types of occupation and will be the subject of further investigation by examining carpal tunnel rates in different breast size categories.

5.7
Conclusions

It is unclear why breast hypertrophy should lead to the development of neurologic signs and symptoms. Kaye [8], although describing symptoms in an ulnar nerve distribution, attributed the findings in his patients to a type of thoracic outlet syndrome where the lower trunk of the brachial plexus was compressed against the first rib. Others have described the effects of mammary hypertrophy on the skeletal system and have speculated that tingling, numbness, and weakness in the arms may result from brachial plexus compression between the coracoid process of the scapula and the rib cage as forward depression of the shoulders tilts the coracoid downward. The pectoralis minor muscle could be mostly responsible for moving the coracoid forward and narrowing the space through which the brachial plexus travels. The pressure from brassiere straps for the elevation of heavy breasts can contribute to the compression of the brachial plexus as well [29, 30].

Our findings of a high prevalence of carpal tunnel syndrome in women who present for reduction mammaplasty could be important in helping to establish criteria for third-party reimbursement for the procedure. There is little in medical literature to help insurers develop objective criteria for reimbursement; there is no precise definition or diagnostic criteria for macromastia or pathologic breast hypertrophy. Because of the large number of body types and the variety of physical changes that occur with aging, it is difficult to determine the size at which breast enlargement becomes pathologic in any individual or group of large-breasted women. Many precertification requirements, such as back pain or the interpretation of a preoperative photograph, are subjective. Insurance companies are usually reluctant to reimburse patients unless certain criteria are met, such as specific amounts of breast-tissue resection or reduction in bra cup size. Such criteria have been challenged by noting that the procedure is usually performed to relieve painful symptoms and physical signs of breast hypertrophy rather than for primarily cosmetic or emotional reasons. Relief of symptoms is independent of body weight, body surface area, body mass index, and amount of breast tissue removed [17, 22, 31–33].

In our evaluation of women with mammary hypertrophy who presented for reduction mammaplasty, the prevalence of carpal tunnel syndrome was 19.9% when the condition was defined as the coexistence of symptoms and two physical examination signs. This represents a greatly increased risk of having carpal tunnel syndrome as compared with women in the general population. Breast size was a significant predictor of carpal tunnel syndrome, much better than was body mass index, and remained significant after adjusting for other physical characteristics [34]. This increased incidence correlating breast hypertrophy and carpal tunnel syndrome has also been corroborated by others, with electrophysiological studies finding a prevalence of 22% [35].

References

1. Stark RB: Plastic Surgery. New York, Harper and Row 1962
2. Rees TD: Plastic surgery of the breast. In: Converse JM (ed.), Reconstructive Plastic Surgery. Philadelphia, Saunders 1964
3. Conway H: Mammaplasty: analysis of 110 consecutive cases with end-results. Plast Reconstr Surg 1952;10(3):303–315
4. Clarkson P: Appearance, cosmetic surgery and mental health. Lond Clin Med J 1965;20:37–49
5. Kohn F, Dalrymple J: Plastic reconstruction of the enlarged breast: report of a new technique. Br J Plast Surg 1967;20(2):184–198
6. Barsky AJ, Kahn S, Simon BE: Principles and Practice of Plastic Surgery, 2nd Ed. New York, McGraw-Hill 1964
7. Maliniac JW: Breast Deformities and Their Repair. Baltimore, Waverly Press 1950
8. Kaye BL: Neurologic changes with excessively large breasts. South Med J 1972;65(2):177–180
9. Brown DM, Young VL: Reduction mammoplasty for macromastia. Aesthetic Plast Surg 1993;17(3):211–223
10. Schnur PL, Schnur DP, Petty PM, Hanson TJ, Weaver AL: Reduction mammaplasty: an outcome study. Plast Reconstr Surg 1997;100(4):875–883
11. Ostle B, Malone LC: Statistics in Research, 4th Ed. Ames, Iowa, Iowa State University Press 1988
12. Clinical Guidelines on the Identification, Evaluation, and Treatment of Overweight and Obesity in Adults. National Institutes of Health, National Heart, Lung, and Blood Institute June, 1998
13. Estimates of the population of counties by race and Hispanic origin: July 1, 1997. Population Estimates Program, Population Division, U.S. Bureau of the Census. Washington, D.C. 20233
14. Dabbah A, Lehman JA Jr, Parker MG, Tantri D, Wagner DS: Reduction mammaplasty: an outcome analysis. Ann Plast Surg 1995;35(4):337–341
15. Gonzalez F, Walton RL, Shafer B, Matory WE Jr, Borah GL: Reduction mammaplasty improves symptoms of macromastia. Plast Reconstr Surg 1993;91(7):1270–1276
16. Dubuisson AS: Dept. of Neurosurgery, CHU Liege, Belgium. The Thoracic Outlet Syndrome http://www.medschool.lsuhsc.edu/neurosurgery/nervecenter/TOS.html#anchor1091716 [NerveCenter 4(2), 1999]
17. Pers M, Nielsen IM, Gerner N: Results following reduction mammaplasty as evaluated by the patients. Ann Plast Surg 1986;17(6):449–455
18. Kinell I, Beausang-Linder M, Ohlsen L: The effect on the preoperative symptoms and the late results of Skoog's reduction mammaplasty. Scand J Plast Reconstr Surg Hand Surg 1990;24(1):61–65

19. Raispis T, Zehring RD, Downey DL: Longterm functional results after reduction mammaplasty. Ann Plast Surg 1995;34(2):113–116
20. McMahan JD, Wolfe JA, Cromer BA, Ruberg RL: Lasting success in teenage reduction mammaplasty. Ann Plast Surg 1995;35(3):227–231
21. Muller FE: Late results of Strombeck's mammaplasty: a follow-up study of 100 patients. Plast Reconstr Surg 1974;54(6):664–666
22. Bolger WE, Seyfer AE, Jackson, SM: Reduction mammaplasty using the inferior glandular "pyramid" pedicle: experiences with 300 patients. Plast Reconstr Surg 1987;80(1):75–84
23. Serletti JM, Reading G, Caldwell E, Wray RC: Long-term patient satisfaction following reduction mammaplasty. Ann Plast Surg 1992;28(4):363–365
24. Davis GM, Ringler SL, Short K, Sherrick D, Bengtson BP: Reduction mammaplasty: longterm efficacy, morbidity, and patient satisfaction. Plast Reconstr Surg 1995;96(5):1106–1110
25. Shakespeare V, Cole RP: Measuring patient-based outcomes in a plastic surgery service: breast reduction surgical patients. Br J Plast Surg 1997;50(4):242–248
26. Rempel D, Evanoff B, Amadio PC, de Krom M, Franklin G, Franzblau A, Gray R, Gerr F, Hagberg M, Hales T, Katz JN, Pransky G: Consensus criteria for the classification of carpal tunnel syndrome in epidemiologic studies. Am J Public Health 1998;88(10):1447–1451
27. Atcheson SG, Ward JR, Lowe W: Concurrent medical disease in work-related carpal tunnel syndrome. Arch Intern Med 1998;158(14):1506–1512
28. Tanaka S, Wild DK, Seligman PJ, Behrens V, Cameron L, Putz-Anderson V: The US prevalence of self-reported carpal tunnel syndrome: 1988 National Health Interview Survey data. Am J Public Health 1994;84(11):1846–1848
29. Letterman G, Schurter M: The effects of mammary hypertrophy on the skeletal system. Ann Plast Surg 1980;5(6):425–431
30. Kendall H, Kendall F, Boynton D: Posture and Pain. Baltimore, Williams & Wilkins, 1952, pp 156–159
31. Seitchik MW: Reduction mammaplasty: criteria for insurance coverage. Plast Reconstr Surg 1995;95(6):1029–1032
32. Schnur PL, Hoehn JG, Ilstrup DM, Cahoy MJ, Chu CP: Reduction mammaplasty: cosmetic or reconstructive procedure? Ann Plast Surg 1991;27(3):232–237
33. Position Paper: Reduction Mammaplasty: Recommended Criteria for Third-Party Payer Coverage. Socioeconomic Committee, American Society of Plastic and Reconstructive Surgeons, June, 1994
34. Pernia LR, Ronel DN, Leeper JD, Miller HL: Carpal tunnel surgery in women undergoing reduction mammaplasty. Plast Recontr Surg 2000;105(4):1314–1319
35. Iwuagwu O, Bajalan A, Platt A, Stanley P, Reese R, Drew P: Macromastia and carpal tunnel syndrome: is there an association? Aesthetic Plast Surg 2006;30(5):535–537

Extent of Symptoms Preoperatively and Success of Breast Reduction for Symptomatic Macromastia: Personal Experiences

Judith B. Zacher

6.1 History

There has been more than enough published data written over the last 15 years to put to rest the question of whether or not reduction mammoplasty alleviates the symptoms of excessively large breasts. In 1989, the medical director of Nationwide Insurance Company challenged me by refusing to authorize re-imbursement for breast reductions on the grounds that there was nothing in the literature proving its effectiveness, a stance that, in today's milieu of "evidence-based medicine," was, though counter-intuitive, correct. The following quotes are from the Group Claims and Cost Containment office of Nationwide Insurance and from Dr. Paul Metzger, then the medical director of Nationwide Insurance, in response to a preauthorization request for reduction mammoplasty, respectively. "It is the opinion of our Medical Director that all breast reduction is cosmetic in nature unless there has been evidence of breast disease, documented endocrine dysfunction, breast asymmetry, or hypertrophy related to puberty. The medical staff has reviewed all of the information received for the claim, again and can find no evidence of any of the above listed conditions as pre-operative diagnosis. Also, while this information does indicate complaints of back and shoulder pain, we have no medical literature on file to document that breast size and weight contribute to this type of pain. Therefore, no benefits can be allowed for this reduction mammoplasty procedure." "In the particular issue with reduction mammoplasty, the literature supplied to us and a review of the world literature as obtained from MEDLARS has failed, in our opinion, to document that reduction mammoplasty is other then cosmetic surgery.... The issue of back, neck, and shoulder pain remains controversial. Our experience suggests that most patients undergoing reduction mammoplasty for these symptoms develop the same or similar symptoms several years after the plastic procedure. I have personally reviewed the literature that we obtained from MEDLARS and can find no statistical studies as a 3 or 5 year follow-up. In fact, the longest follow-up that I find is six months."

This attitude stimulated my colleagues, Drs. Ronald Berggren and Ann Miller, and I to answer the implied challenge Nationwide Insurance gave us, with one of the early studies proving how wrong they were. A review of over 20 articles published since the late 1980s demonstrates the fact that mostly all patients get significant relief of symptoms of macromastia after their surgery, that the results are long lasting, that there is no reliable predictor of who will benefit the most, and that most women report a much higher quality of life postoperatively. All techniques of breast reduction, whether the more common Wise pattern [1], short scar [2], or liposuction technique [3], are equally successful in relieving the symptoms if an appropriate amount of weight is removed.

Many authors such as Collins et al. [4] and Miller et al. [5] have pointed out that body weight, height, bra size, grams of resection, and distance from clavicle to nipple–areolar complex, all parameters that insurance companies demand for prior authorization, have no significant relationship to the relief of symptoms. Bra size is not a reliable indicator of breast size as many women wear smaller cup sizes than they fit to avoid the cantilevered-out-front look (think projection) and thus will have breast overflow in their cleavage or axillary areas (Fig. 6.1). These women are, as Oprah Winfrey would say, "in cup (size) denial." Many women just refuse to wear a bra with a triple D or larger cup as a matter of principle, and others claim that the bras that do fit are too expensive or are unattractive. Most "pretty" bras are not made in sizes larger that 36C. There is enough variation in actual size and shape from one brand of bra to another to eliminate bra "size" as a reliable indicator of breast volume. Women after healing from any esthetic or reconstructive breast surgery should be seen by a professional bra fitter to help get the best support and postoperative appearance.

M.A. Shiffman (ed.), *Mastopexy and Breast Reduction: Principles and Practice,*
© Springer-Verlag Berlin Heidelberg 2009

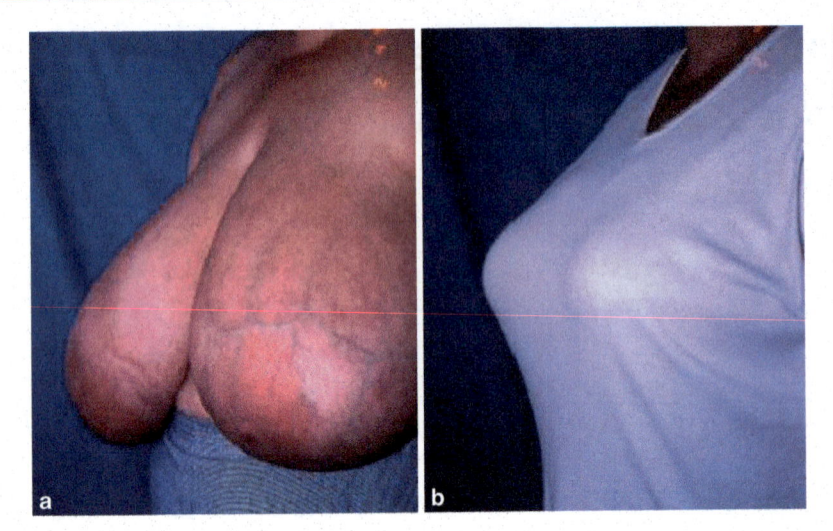

Fig. 6.1 (a) Patient without bra. (b) "Cantilevering" (projection) with bra

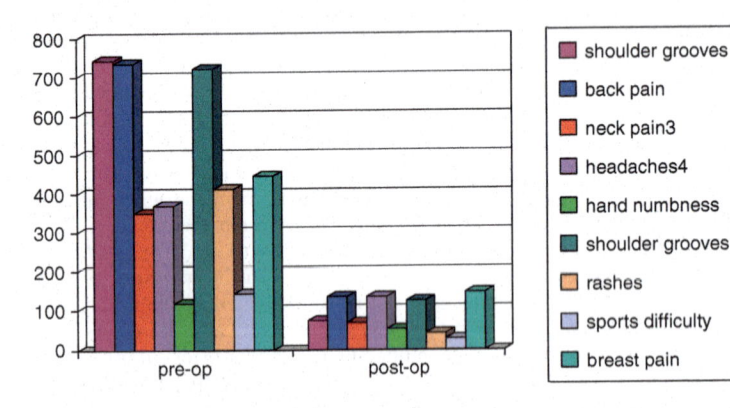

Fig. 6.2 Symptom cluster before and after breast reduction in 10 studies with 1,078 patients (not all studies asked the same questions)

All studies show dramatic disappearance of preoperative pain complaints, that is, shoulder pain, neck and upper back pain, lower back pain, breast pain, hand numbness, and frequent headaches (Fig. 6.2). But these are all subjective complaints, and the point at which large breasts cause or contribute to this constellation of symptoms is unique to each woman [6]. Unfortunately, no study has been done questioning a random group of large-breasted women (not those seeking reduction) regarding their symptoms. One study, Netscher et al. [7], attempted to do this by questioning 88 college student volunteers about breast related symptoms and comparing them with women requesting breast reduction and women seeking breast augmentation. The women seeking reductions scored vastly higher on the complaints of neck and back, and shoulder pain, and skin rashes than the "normal" group or the augmentation group. The university student group had only a small percentage of large-breasted women. Sigurdson et al. [8] organized focus groups of large-breasted women to discuss their symptoms and concluded that younger women were bothered more by psychological symptoms and older women were more bothered by physical complaints. However, the women enrolled in this study were those who were on the waiting list for breast reduction surgery.

If large breasts always caused these difficulties, plastic surgeons' waiting rooms would be overwhelmed. The reasons for this are multiple and varied: for instance, some women do like their big breasts and the attention they garner, while others are afraid of any elective surgery and yet others are afraid of the scars. Many women have told me that their families were against the surgery because it goes against what God has given them, others lack the financial ability or insurance coverage to have the surgery and of course, some women do not even know such surgery is an available option. For example, in early 2007, a morbidly obese young woman consulted me regarding the possibility of an abdominoplasty. When I suggested that she was an excellent candidate for gastric by-pass surgery instead, she appeared to have no idea what I was talking about.

Bruhlmann's study [6] suggested a direct relationship between the weight of tissue resected and the relief of symptoms, and Gray [9] reported "complete resolution of symptoms in all patients" after liposuction breast reduction. But others like Miller et al. [5] and Collins et al. [4]) feel that the best objective signs that the patient will benefit from reduction mammoplasty are shoulder grooves (Fig. 6.3) and inframammary rashes (Fig. 6.4). Infra-mammary and cleavage rashes are also extremely bothersome to these women, who find they must resort to various powders, antifungal creams, Kleenex, and even to tucking wash clothes under their bras. Hot, humid weather and hot flashes contribute to this misery.

Glatt [10] observed that the frequency of bra strap–shoulder grooves is not related to the patient's weight. In an attempt to determine the frequency of bra strap grooves, I reviewed the preoperative photos of 100 consecutive women coming to my office in the last 6 years seeking breast reduction surgery and judged that only 32 had significant grooves, and my associate Suzanne Quardt, M.D., rated them higher at 53. There was definitely no relationship between the size of their breasts or their body weight, and the development of grooves. Grooves occur in some patients but not in others, with similar size breasts (Fig. 6.5). This may be more of a sociological phenomena, with some women determined to lift their large breasts up to make their appearance smaller and to fit better into clothes, while other women just give up. Paradoxically, a few women had deeper grooves on the side of their smaller breast (Fig. 6.6).

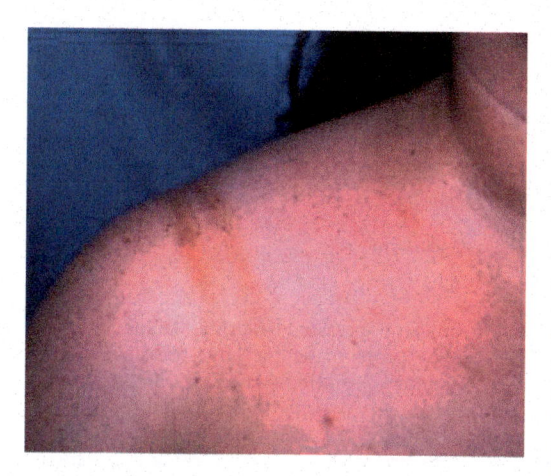

Fig. 6.3 Shoulder grooves

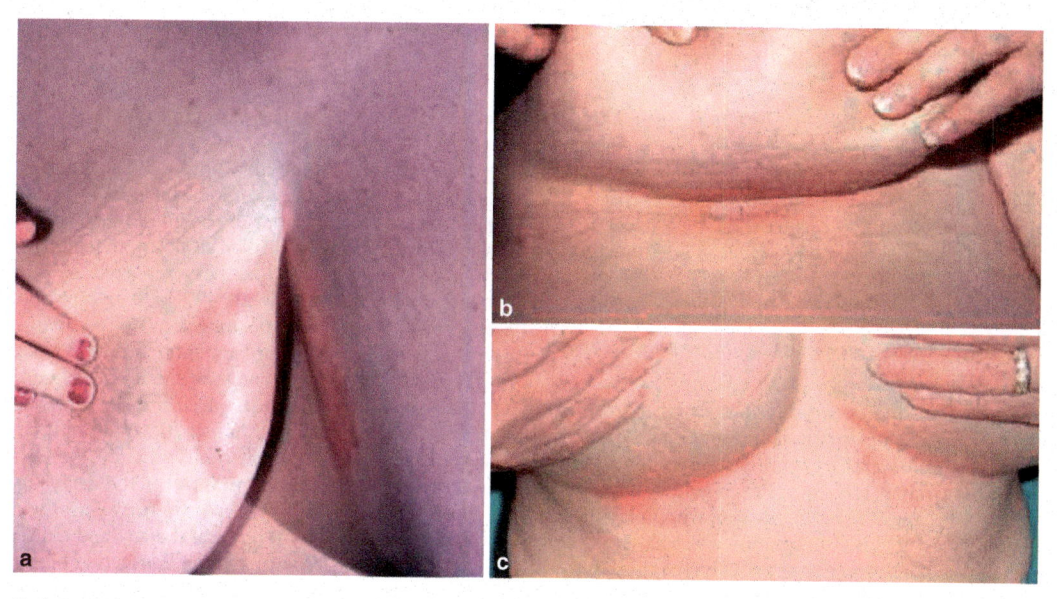

Fig. 6.4 a-c Cleavage rash

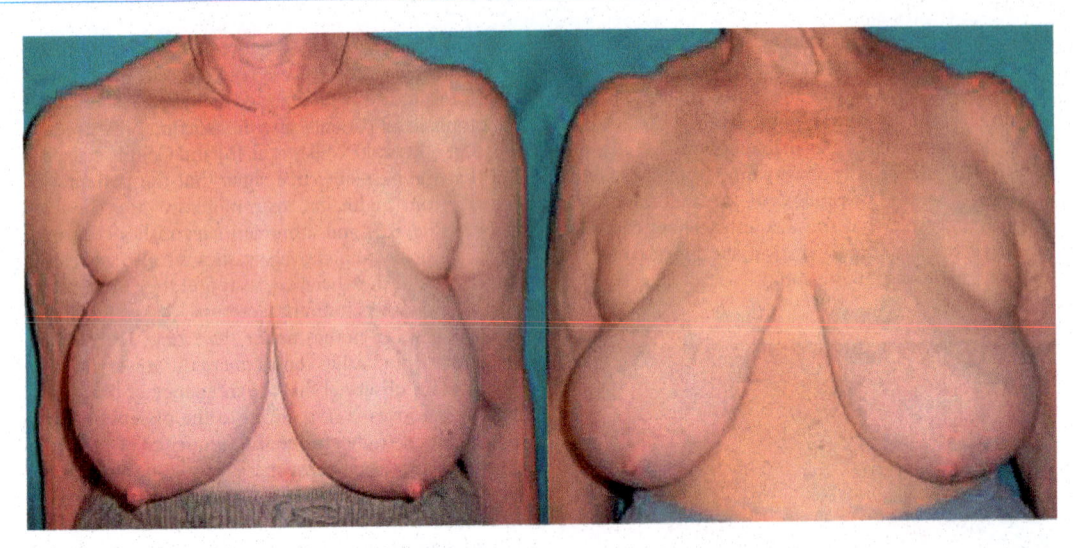

Fig. 6.5 Both patients have similar size breasts but patient on the right has shoulder grooves

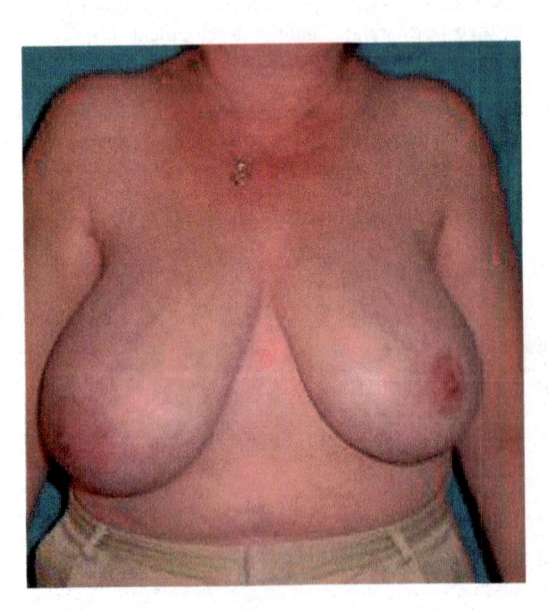

Fig. 6.6 Deep shoulder groove on side (*left*) with smaller breast

Mostly, all studies indicate that a high percentage of women seeking breast reductions have difficulty with physical exercise: running, aerobics, dancing, horse back riding, tennis, and even golf. Large breasts can get in the way of hand crossing while playing the piano (imagine Liszt's Paganini Etudes). They can even make some yoga positions challenging, that is, the salavasana or locust pose. The famous choreographer, George Ballanchine, is rumored to have refused to hire any large-breasted ballerinas. Domestic activities can be problematic for large-breasted women, such as laundry or putting away dishes. Sigurdson et al. [8] reported on two women who burned their breasts leaning over the stove. Even sedentary occupations can add to breast discomfort, working at a desk or keyboard, the weight of large breasts pulling on the shoulders is aggravated. Many patients have reported having to wear two bras to get support for any sports. Insurance companies have demanded that women get closer to their ideal body weight before authorizing reduction surgery. Some women will even admit that they have allowed themselves to gain weight in an attempt to minimize the relative appearance of their large breasts. Obviously, this is problematic, in that it is reasonable to assume that both exercise and diet are necessary for weight reduction, and most fat burning exercises are simply out of the question for these women. In the study by Miller et al. [5], there was a 63% increase in physical activity reported by the patients postoperatively; while 49% were overweight preoperatively, 40% were postoperatively. The operation clearly leads to an improvement in these women's overall health. Overweight women should be encouraged that weight loss efforts after surgery will not significantly adversely affect the esthetic results of their new breasts (Fig. 6.7).

Attempts have been made to quantify the degree of preoperative pain felt by patients by surveying their usage of pain medications, physical therapy, and chiropractic treatments. In their paper on liposuction breast reduction, Marcos et al. [11] detailed the efficacy (or nonefficacy) of nonsurgical methods to relieve the

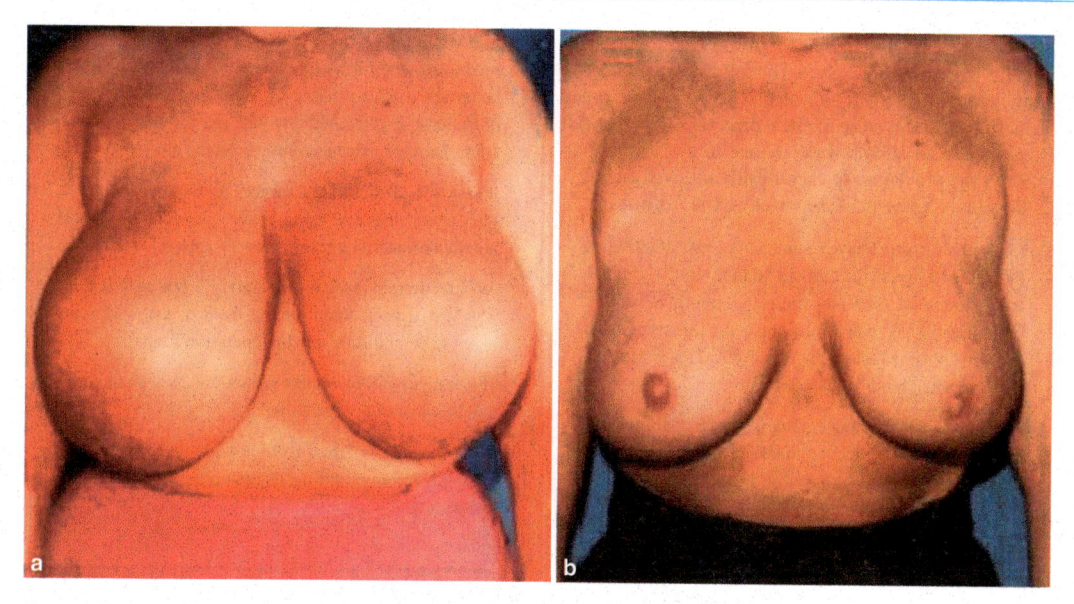

Fig. 6.7 (a) Patient prior to breast reduction. (b) Following breast reduction and weight loss

symptoms of large breasts. These therapies included physical therapy, strengthening, torso stretching, relaxation exercises, heat applications, back braces, custom bras, chiropractic treatments, weight loss, and NSAIDS. Weight loss provided permanent relief in 30% of those women, in their study, who were able to loose weight. Chiropractic, hydrotherapy, custom bras, and strengthening helped 5% each. The remaining therapies were equally temporary or provided no relief. I personally have received many demands from insurance companies wanting to know exactly what conservative therapies the women have tried before they will authorize surgery, and so this is valuable information. The techniques and benefits of chiropractic treatments are unknown to this author, but many patients are referred to plastic surgeons by their chiropractor (or orthopedic or spine surgeon) for reduction surgery after unsuccessful attempts to otherwise relieve their upper back and neck pain.

Although not every study reviewed asked patients about hand pain or numbness, there was a 17–40% incidence in those reported, with significant improvement postoperatively (Fig. 6.2). This phenomenon has not been explained. Iwuagwu et al. [12] studied women with macromastia, indicating a higher than normal incidence of carpal tunnel syndrome in these women but, despite clinical improvement, with no significant change in their postoperative nerve conduction studies. In a different paper, Iwuagwu [13] showed that "pulmonary function improves following breast reduction and the improvement correlated with specimen weight resected." This helps explain why patients, preoperatively, have said that they cannot sleep lying down flat, feeling suffocated, and why so many patients report a higher level of physical activity postoperatively.

The longevity of the symptom improvement after breast reduction is borne out in 12 of the studies reviewed that included long-term follow-up ranging from 2 to 10 years. Of the 18 studies that included the time of follow up for symptom relief evaluation, the earliest was 6 months post-op before the patients were included and questioned. The average follow-up time of the 2,185 patients reported collectively was 3.4 years. McMahan's [14] report on the long-term success of breast reductions in teenagers bears this out with an average follow-up time of 5.9 years and some as long as 20 years.

6.2
Psychosocial Aspects

The psychosocial aspects of this surgery cannot be emphasized enough. Despite a culture that values large breasts (329,000 augments done in the United States in 2006 according to Plastic Surgery News), many women with naturally oversized breasts hate it when people "talk to their breasts instead of their eyes" or are insulted when men think they are "easy" just because they are large-breasted. The joy these women experience being able to buy attractive bras off the rack, clothes that fit, blouses that tuck in, and have buttons that do not pop open cannot be ignored. Perhaps it will be useful to let the patients speak for themselves. The following are excerpts from letters written by women, who have had breast reduction surgery, to the medical director of Nationwide Insurance in an attempt to convince him of the importance of the procedure to their health and well-being.

Personal Experiences Reported to the Author

(Since the surgery) I have resumed my physical activities, I am able to run, swim, bike, and dance regularly, which are good for me both physically and emotionally. I am very grateful that my insurance company recognized abnormally large breasts for the physical handicap that they are, albeit not a "traditional" one.

I certainly was not too enthusiastic about going thru surgery but in order to alleviate further medical problems, pains, discomfort etc. it was the only choice to make…. I quickly recovered, feel great and am a new person.

My breasts were very tender and so sore and painful for many years. Sometimes I could hardly put my dishes in the cupboard because of the pain….My only regret is that I did not have it 10 years earlier.

Believe me, I do not take surgery lightly. In fact, this is the only surgery I've had. Since then I have been comfortable physically for the first time in years. Please try to imagine going through life with two huge, heavy drooping bags attached to your chest. It effected every waking moment of my life and now I feel comfortable.

Many people didn't understand why at 17 I was subjecting myself to this kind of operation. But the feelings I had were strong enough to convince me that it was the right thing to do. In addition to the physical aspects of my large breasts I got nasty and demeaning comments on my "appearance". After the operation I stood up straight physically as well as mentally.

I, like many other women have worked for many years in an office. The constant sitting and immobility in addition to the extra weight of my large bust have caused me to suffer chronic back and shoulder pain for more than 20 years. Since surgery I have not had one back-ache and my shoulder pain is gone.

Drug addiction, alcoholism and pregnancy are all by choice and are usually covered by insurance. Over-size breasts are NOT by choice, I guarantee you. If you would like to know how this feels, go to the grocery and buy 2 four pound grapefruit, then try and buy a bra to fit. Wear this for approximately 24 hours and then maybe you will understand the pain.

The size of my breasts made it impossible to lay on my back because I had trouble breathing in this position. I was embarrassed because of my size and that people made fun of me. My back and neck trouble were noticeably better the day I got home from the hospital, and now I don't have any trouble. My self esteem has improved 100%. I am not ashamed of my breasts, I am proud now.

It took several years after surgery to have the courage to start exercising and getting over the fear that those horrible breasts would somehow re-appear.

As I recovered from the operation I felt as if a great weight had been lifted off the front of me… My only regret is that I didn't have the operation sooner.

This last year, following my reduction has been the most painless year of my adult life.

(Before surgery) I had trouble with my balance with climbing and even riding a motorcycle. I just thought I was a klutz.

References

1. Cruz-Korchin N, Korchin L: Vertical versus Wise pattern breast reduction: patient satisfaction, revision rates, and complications. Plast Reconstr Surg 2003;112(6):1573–1578
2. Spector JA, Kleinerman R, Culliford AT, Karp NS: The vertical reduction mammaplasty: a retrospective analysis of patient outcomes. Plast Reconstr Surg 2006;117(2): 374–381
3. Moskovitz MJ, Muskin E, Baxt SA: Outcome study in liposuction breast reduction. Plast Reconstr Surg 2005;116(5): 1558–1559
4. Collins ED, Kerrigan CL, Kin M, Lowery JC, Striplin DT, Cunningham B, Wilkins EG: The effectiveness of surgical and nonsurgical interventions in relieving the symptoms of macromastia. Plast Reconstr Surg 2002;109(5):1556–1566
5. Miller AP, Zacher JB, Berggren RB, Falcone RE, Monk J: Breast reduction for symptomatic macromastia: can objective predictors for operative success be identified? Plast Reconstr Surg 1995;95(1):77–83
6. Bruhlmann Y, Tschopp H: Breast reduction improves symptoms of macromastia and has a long-lasting effect. Ann Plast Surg 1998;414(3):240–245
7. Netscher DT, Meade RA, Goodman CM, Brehm BJ, Friedman JD, Thornby J: Physical and psychosocial symptoms among 88 volunteer subjects compared with patients seeking plastic surgery procedures to the breast. Plast Reconstr Surg 2000;105(7):2366–2373
8. Sigurdson L, Mykhalovskiy E, Kirkland SA, Pallen A: Symptoms and related severity experienced by women with breast hypertrophy. Plast Reconstr Surg 2007;119(2):481–486
9. Gray LN: Update on experience with liposuction breast reduction. Plast Reconstr Surg 2001;108(4):1006–1010
10. Glatt BS, Sarwer DB, O'Hara DE, Hamori C, Bucky LP, LaRossa D: A retrospective study of changes in physical

symptoms and body image after reduction mammaplasty. Plast Reconstr Surg 1999;104(2):590–591
11. Moskovitz M, Muskin E, Baxt S: Outcome study in liposuction breast reduction. Plast Reconstr Surg 2004;114(1):55–60
12. Iwuagwu O, Bajalan A, Platt A, Stanley P, Reese R, Drew P: Macromastia and carpal tunnel syndrome: is there an association. Aesthetic Plast Surg 2006;30(5):535–547
13. Iwuagwu OC, Platt AJ, Stanley PW, Hart NB, Drew PJ: Does reduction mammaplasty improve lung function test in women with macromastia? Results of a randomized controlled trial. Plast Reconstr Surg 2006;118(1):1–6
14. McMahan JD, Wolfe JA, Cromer BA, Ruberg RL: Lasting success in teenage reduction mammaplasty. Ann Plast Surg 1995;35(3):227–231

Mammograms in Cosmetic Breast Surgery

Melvin A. Shiffman

7.1 Introduction

The use of preoperative and postoperative mammograms in cosmetic surgery has never been standardized. There appears to be some consensus that at least preoperative mammograms should be obtained according to the recommendations of the American Cancer Society for screening mammography. Women at average risk should begin monthly self-breast examination at age 20, clinical breast examination every 3 years from age 20 to 39, and annual mammogram and clinical breast examination starting at age 40 [1]. There is no specific surveillance strategy for women at higher risk for breast cancer, but these patients may benefit by earlier initiation of screening, screening at shorter intervals, and screening with additional methods such as ultrasound or magnetic resonance imaging [1].

7.2 Preoperative Mammogram

The purpose of a preoperative mammogram is to detect any significant disorder of the breast(s) prior to cosmetic surgery so that the problem can be resolved before surgery or during surgery. Also, the mammogram is a baseline for detecting abnormalities after the cosmetic surgery.

The incidence of new breast cancer cases is increasing at a yearly rate and was estimated to be 203,500 in 2002 [2] and 211,300 in 2003 in the United States [3].

It is essential to detect cancer early so that cosmetic procedures of the breast do not cut across, distort, diminish the opportunity for cure, or limit the usefulness of lumpectomy in the treatment of the cancer. Breast cancer is now being detected earlier in the development of the tumor, at a smaller size, and with a better prognosis for cure through the use of mammograms.

The detection of a fibroadenoma is significant since carcinoma may occur within the fibroadenoma [4–10]. The average age for fibroadenoma is 23 while the average age for carcinoma in the fibroadenoma is 43 [4].

A new tumor after age 35 should be biopsied (most commonly with stereotactic needle biopsy). Under age 35, a fibroadenoma would need to be biopsied or excised if it continues to grow.

The 18 to 39-year-old patient group is the most common age group for which the question of performing preoperative mammograms is most often debated. This age group has not had a high incidence of breast cancer, but there is presently a higher incidence than previously reported because of earlier diagnosis. The average breast cancer tumor size in the author's practice was 3.0 cm from 1964 through 1984 and from 1985 to 2006 it was 2.0 cm, showing that earlier diagnosis was being made through mammographic screening methods and better patient awareness of the need for regular examinations. Breast cancer has been reported in patients under the age of 30 [11]. The youngest patient with cancer seen by the author was 16 years of age. An argument by the radiologist has been that the youthful breasts have marked dysplasia on mammograms that prevents the detection of some abnormalities. By increasing the radiation slightly to eliminate some of the dysplastic changes, a mammogram can be performed that will then focus on architectural distortion and calcifications.

Patients with a significant family history of breast cancer should begin to have annual mammograms 10 years before the youngest age of the individuals in the family with the cancer. If a patient with a significant family history desires breast augmentation, then the patient must be forewarned of the problems of the implant, which may reduce the chances of early detection of cancer, and consideration given to placing the implants beneath the pectoralis major muscle.

7.3 Postoperative Mammograms Following Cosmetic Breast Surgery

Following cosmetic breast surgery, routine mammograms (6–12 months postoperatively) help to formulate a baseline for the future detection of breast cancer. Surgery involving the breasts can result in architectural distortion from scars and calcifications.

7.4
Cosmetic Surgeries

7.4.1
Breast Augmentation

The insertion of implants through areola or periareolar incisions usually involves dissection through the breast tissues that may result in architectural scars within the breast tissue. Axillary, inframammary, and umbilical approaches do not usually breach the breast tissue itself. Calcifications have been reported in the fibrous capsule (around the implant) but do not resemble the calcifications seen with breast cancer [12–17]. For implants in place for more than 12 years, 52.5% of those ruptured showed calcification but only 10.0% of intact implants showed calcification [13].

Fat transfer into the breast parenchyma is no longer performed [18]. The fat for augmentation is now injected beneath, into, and above the pectoralis muscle, although the patient should be forewarned of the possibility of inadvertent injection into the breast itself. The calcifications around a fat cyst are easily diagnosed as benign [19]. Stippled calcifications of fat necrosis following fat injection appear circular and smooth and can usually be distinguished by an experienced mammographer from calcifications found with cancer. If there is any question, the calcified area can be sampled through stereotactic needle biopsy under local anesthesia.

Kinoshita [20] found that in some magnetic resonance (MR) findings of fat necrosis, it was difficult to distinguish benign from malignant lesions. Kurtz et al. [21] studied MR findings in patients with fat necrosis and found that all of the 15 fat necrosis (FN) displayed fat-isointense signal on T1-weighted and on proton-weighted, fat-suppressed sequences. They were delineated by a more or less wide rim of low signal intensity with a sharp border to the center. After intravenous injection of gadopenetate dimeglumine, they showed no increase in signal intensity in the center and no increase, or a minor increase, of the rim. Ultrasound could not distinguish FN from recurrent tumor in six cases, although seven looked like atypical cysts. MR-mammography was felt to be a promising method for diagnosis of FN.

Bilgen et al. [22] studied 126 fat necrosis lesions in 94 patients. They found on the mammograms radiolucent oil cysts (34 or 26.9%), round opacity (16 or 12.6%), asymmetrical opacity or heterogenicity of the subcutaneous tissues (20 or 15.8%), dystrophic calcifications (5 or 3.9%), and suspicious spiculated mass (5 or 3.9%). Follow-up mammograms showed curvilinear calcifications in five, decreased density in six, rounded opacities disappearing with another two, more coarse dystrophic calcifications in 11, asymmetrical opacities becoming vague in six and an oil cyst and coarse calcifications developing in one, and spiculated mass developing a small radiolucent oil cyst in the center in one. On the sonograms, the lesions were solid in 18 (9.5%), anechoic with posterior acoustic enhancement in 21 (16.6%), anechoic with posterior acoustic shadowing in 20 (15.8%), cystic with internal echoes in 14 (11.1%), cystic with mural nodule in 5 (3.9%), had increased echogenicity of the subcutaneous tissues in 34 (26.9%), and were normal in 14 (11.1%). Follow-up ultrasound showed 18 of the 29 had increased subcutaneous tissue echogenicity turned back to normal, while in the remaining 11 small cysts had formed. In the 19 solid appearing masses, 15 showed decreases in size while four remained stable (biopsy disclosed fat necrosis). The four complex masses showed increase in size and appeared more cystic. It was concluded that knowledge of the mammographic and ultrasound appearance of fat necrosis and evolution of these patterns may enable imaging follow-up and reduce the number of biopsies.

7.4.2
Breast Reduction

In breast reduction, there is cutting into and removal of areas of breast tissue that may result in significant scarring, architectural distortion, and calcifications, usually from fat necrosis [23]. Miller et al. [24] noted that after reduction mammoplasty, all patients are left with a linear scar between the nipple and inframammary fold that accounts for the frequent finding of skin thickening along the lower breast. Fat necrosis presents as an irregular calcified mass. Brown et al. [25] noted that asymmetric densities were present in approximately half the patients. Parenchymal calcifications were apparent in 50% of patients after 2 years. Four out of 42 patients had biopsies for suspicious densities, which were benign on pathology.

Abboud et al. [26] have reported that breast reduction using liposuction has been associated with calcifications from fat necrosis. Sixty patients with breast reduction, 34 with and 26 without liposuction were studied. There was a 6–30 month follow-up and calcifications were noted in 11%. Deep intraparenchymal calcifications were more frequent after liposuction and most (5 of 7) were macrocalcifications. None could be confused with malignant calcifications because they were more scattered, more regular, and less numerous. If there is any question as to the cause of the calcifications, stereotactic needle biopsy should be performed. Alterations in breast tissue resulting from the use of UAL were a thickened dermal undersurface, markedly thickened vertical collagenous fibers with intact lymphatic vessels and intact blood vessels [27].

The use of ultrasound-assisted liposuction for breast reduction has not been found to be injurious to the breast tissue but still may be associated with calcifications [28, 29].

7.4.3
Mastopexy

Breast lift (mastopexy) does not usually disturb the breast parenchyma unless there is some breast tissue reduction. The lift is mainly a skin reduction with release of the breast from the underlying muscle to reorient the breast into a higher position.

7.5
Discussion

Preoperative mammograms are a screening technique to detect abnormalities before performing cosmetic surgery. There is some argument that cosmetic surgery is an elective procedure being performed on a healthy patient and there should be a more detailed workup with mammography to protect the patient even in the young age group before breast surgery. This would mean that every patient, no matter what age, should have a preoperative mammogram prior to cosmetic breast surgery [30]. Peras [31] reported that in 1,149 cases of cosmetic surgery, early diagnosis of breast cancer was possible in 34 cases by the use of mammography. He strongly recommended that a policy of mandatory preoperative mammography be implemented so that all patients can be protected from a potentially lethal disease by early detection.

It is the surgeon's choice whether to order a preoperative mammogram prior to cosmetic breast surgery on a patient under the age of 40. Once requested to have a preoperative mammogram, patients who refuse may safely be operated upon, but the refusal should be noted in the medical record. This will help to protect the physician if there is future litigation. It is also the physician's choice whether to do cosmetic breast surgery on a patient over the age of 40 who refuses a preoperative mammogram. The patient should be fully informed of the possible consequences of missing a significant abnormality.

Postoperative mammograms will protect the patient by obtaining a baseline for future reference. However, there are many patients who do not come back to the surgeon for follow up mammography because they feel fine and do not wish to be bothered with the procedure or the cost. The surgeon probably should document in the medical record that the postoperative mammogram had been suggested.

The patient who has a significant family history of breast cancer should be counseled on the possibility of future breast cancer and the possible need for genetic testing prior to any cosmetic procedure on the breast. If genetic testing is positive for BRCA1 or BRCA2, there is a 50–90% lifetime risk of developing breast cancer [32–35]. If the genetic abnormality is present, there is a variety of early detection and prevention programs available [36]. Patients at any age with a significant family history should have a mammogram before any cosmetic breast surgery is contemplated. The problems of early diagnosis of breast cancer that may be present if augmentation mammoplasty or any other cosmetic procedure of the breast is performed should be thoroughly explained prior to making any decisions about surgery.

References

1. Smith RA, Saslow D, Sawyer KA, Burke W, Costanza ME, Evans WP III, Foster RS Jr, Eyre HJ, Sener S, et al.: American Cancer Society guidelines for breast cancer screening: Update 2003. CA Cancer J Clin 2003;53(3):141–169
2. Jemal A, Thomas A, Murray T, Than M: Cancer statistics. CA Cancer J Clin 2002;52(1):23–47
3. Jemal A, Murray T, Samuels A, Ghafoor A, Ward E, Thun MJ: Cancer statistics. CA Cancer J Clin 2003;53(1):5–26
4. Durso EA: Carcinoma arising in fibroadenoma: a case report. Radiology 1972;102:565
5. Buzonowsaki-Konakry K, Harrison EG, Payne WS: Lobular carcinoma arising in fibroadenoma of the breast. Cancer 1975;35:450–456
6. Azzopardi JG: Problems in breast pathology. Philadelphia, W.B. Saunders 1979
7. Pick PW, Iossifides IA: Occurrence of breast carcinoma within a fibroadenoma. A review. Arch Pathol Lab Med 1984;108(7):590–594
8. Schnitt SJ, Connolly JL: Pathology of benign breast disorders. In: Harris JR (ed) Diseases of the Breast, 2nd edn. Philadelphia, Williams & Wilkins 2000, pp 75–93
9. Botta P-G, Cosimi MF: Breast lobular carcinoma in a fibroadenoma of the breast. Eur J Surg Pathol 1985;11:283–285
10. Diaz NM, Palmer JO, McDivitt RW: Carcinoma arising within fibroadenomas of the breast. A clinicopathologic study of 105 patients. Am J Clin Path 1991;95:614–622
11. Tabbane F, el May A, Hachiche M, Bahi J, Jaziri M, Cammoun M, Mourali N: Breast cancer in women under 30 years of age. Breast Cancer Res Treat 1985;6(2):137–144
12. Peters W, Smith D, Lugowski S, Pritzker K, Holmyard D: Calcification properties of saline-filled implants. Plast Reconstr Surg 2001;107(2):356–363
13. Peters W, Pritzker K, Smith D, Fornasier V, Holmyard D, Lugowski S, Kamel M, Visram F: Capsular calcification associated with silicone breast implants: incidence, determinants, and characterization. Ann Plast Surg 1998;41(4):348–360

14. Peter W, Smith D: Calcification of breast implant capsules: incidence, diagnosis, and contributing factors. Ann Plast Surg 1995;34(1):8–11
15. Schmidt GH: Calcification bonded to saline-filled implants. Plast Reconstr Surg 1993;92(7):1423–1425
16. Young VL, Bartell T, Destouet JM, Monsees B, Logan SE: Calcification of breast implant capsule. South Med J 1989;82(9):1171–1173
17. Nicoletis C, Wlodarczyk B: A rare complication of breast prosthesis: calcification of the periprosthetic retractile capsule. Ann Chir Plast Esthet 1983;28(4):388–389
18. Fulton JE: Breast contouring with "gelled" autologous fat: a 10-year update. Int J Cosm Surg Aesthet Derm 2003;5(2):155–163
19. Rocek V, Rehulka M, Vojacek K, Kral V: Fat necrosis of the breasts with ring calcification. Acta Univ Palacki Olomuc Fac Med 1982;102:143–147
20. Kinoshita T, Yashiro N, Yoshigi J, Ihara N, Narita M: Fat necrosis of breast: a potential pitfall in breast MRI. Clin Imagine 2002;26(4):250–253
21. Kurtz B, Achten C, Audretsch W, Rezai M, Zocholl G: MR mammography of fatty tissue necrosis. Rofo Fortschr Geb Rontgenstr Neuen Bildgeb Verhfahr 1996;165(4):359–363
22. Bilgen IG, Ustum EE, Memis A: Fat necrosis of the breast: clinical, mammographic, and sonographic features. Eur J Radiol 2001;39(2):92–99
23. Baber CE, Libshitz HI: Bilateral fat necrosis of the breast following reduction mammoplasties. Am J Roent 1977;128:508–509
24. Miller CL, Feig SA, Fox JW: Mammographic changes in reduction mammoplasty. Am J Roent 1987;149:35–38
25. Brown FE, Sargent SK, Cohen SR, Morain WD: Mammographic changes following reduction mammaplasty. Plast Reconstr Surg 1987;80(5):691–698
26. Abboud M, Vadoud-Seyedi J, De May A, Cukierfajn M, Lejour M: Incidence of calcifications in the breast after surgical reduction and liposuction. Plast Reconstr Surg 1995;96(3):620–626
27. Di Giuseppe A: Ultrasound-assisted liposuction for breast reduction. In: Shiffman MA, Di Giuseppe A (eds) Textbook of Liposuction: Principles and Practice. New York, Marcel Dekker 2004
28. Lejour M, Abboud M: Vertical mammoplasty without inframammary scar and with liposuction. Perspect Plast Surg 1990;4:67
29. Lejour M: Reduction of large breasts by a combination of liposuction and vertical mammoplasty. In: Cohen M (ed) Master of Surgery: Plastic and Reconstructive Surgery. Boston, Little Brown 1994
30. Jackson R: Personal communication. April 24, 2003
31. Perras C: Fifteen years of mammography in cosmetic surgery of the breast. Aesthetic Plast Surg 1990;14(2):81–84
32. Taucher S, Gnant M, Jekesz R: Preventive mastectomy in patients at breast cancer risk due to genetic alterations in the BRCA1 and BRCA2 gene. Langenbecks Arch Surg 2003;388(1):3–8
33. Winer EP, Morrow M, Osborne CK, Harris JR: Malignant tumors of the breast. In: DeVita VT, Hellman S, Rosenberg SA (eds) Cancer: Principles & Practice of Oncology. Philadelphia, Lippincott Williams & Wilkins 2001, pp 1651–1717
34. Ford D, Easton D, Bishop, Narod SA, Goldgar DE: Risks of cancer in BRCA1 mutation carriers. Breast Cancer Linkage Consortium. Lancet 1994;343(8899):692–695
35. Struewing JP, Hartge P, Wacholder S, Baker SM, Berlin M, McAdams M, Timmerman MM, Brody LC, Tucker MA: The risk of cancer associated with specific mutations of BRCA1 and BRCA2: among Ashkenazi Jews. N Engl J Med 1997;336(20):1401–1408
36. Grann VR, Panegeas KS, Whang W, Antman KH, Neugut AI: Decision analysis of prophylactic mastectomy and oophorectomy in BRCA1-positive or BRCA2-positive patients. J Clin Oncol 1998;16(3):979–985

Part III
Mastopexy

History of Mastopexy

Jorge I. de la Torre, James N. Long, Luis O. Vásconez

8.1
Introduction

The goal of mastopexy surgery is to elevate breast tissue, orient the nipple areolar complex properly, and improve symmetry of the breasts in order to maximize the aesthetics of the breasts. Various procedures and modifications have been suggested to improve the appearance of sagging or ptotic breasts. Breast ptosis is seen as Cooper's ligaments and the dermis become lax and gravity causes descent of breast tissue and the nipple areolar complex. A variety of factors can contribute to these phenomena. Patients with heavy breasts are more prone to ptosis because of excessive breast weight. Postpartum changes leave the suspensory ligaments and skin stretched following lactational engorgement and subsequent parenchymal atrophy. Postmenopausal patients demonstrate atrophy of breast tissue, dermal thinning, and loss of skin elasticity. Patients who have undergone massive weight-loss often lose breast volume and are left with redundant, loose breast tissue and skin resulting in breast ptosis. The removal of breast implants can similarly leave the breast envelope empty and lax.

8.2
Surgical Anatomy: A Historical Perspective

The dimensions of the breast vary depending on the patient's body habitus and age. In 1955, Penn [1] described measurements to locate the nipple–areolar complex (NAC) using a distance of 21 cm from the sternal notch to each nipple and between the two nipples, forming an equilateral triangle. The nipple location should be tailored to each individual however and a sternal notch-to-nipple distance of 21–23 cm with an inferior limb distance of 5–7 cm have been described as the ideal limits particularly when considering surgical correction of ptosis.

The arterial blood supply has a medial component supplied by the internal mammary artery and the lateral thoracic artery supplies the lateral aspect. In addition, there are several perforating arteries from the third through seventh intercostal arteries, which can be preserved from the chest wall to help insure viability of the NAC. Venous drainage is via the superficial system just under the dermis and from the deep system that accompanies the arterial supply. Lymph drainage is primarily via the retromammary lymph plexus located on the pectoral fascia. Early procedures which did not appreciate this anatomic relationship involved wide undermining of the skin and led to a very high rate of tissue necrosis [2].

Sensory innervation of the breast is provided by the intercostals and brachial plexus. Nipple sensation is provided by the third through fifth anterior cutaneous nerves and the fourth and fifth lateral intercostal nerves. Of these, the fourth anterior intercostal nerve is regarded by most authors as most contributory. The incidence of permanent injury to nipple sensation has dropped with technical refinements [3] to a fairly infrequent occurence if not rare outcome in patients undergoing mastopexy procedures [4].

In 1976, Regnault [5] presented a classification system for breast ptosis, which has seen various modifications over time.

The most commonly used systems are the following:
- Grade 1: Mild ptosis – Nipple just below inframammary fold but still above lower pole of breast
- Grade 2: Moderate ptosis – Nipple further below inframammary fold but still with some lower pole tissue below nipple
- Grade 3: Severe ptosis – Nipple well below inframammary fold and no lower pole tissue below nipple; "Snoopy nose" appearance
- Pseudoptosis – Inferior pole ptosis with nipple at or above inframammary fold; usually observed in postpartum breast atrophy

8.3
Early Techniques

Plastic surgery of the breast has been documented as early as 1669 when descriptions of postmastectomy reconstruction were reported. Some 200 years later, Velpeau, in 1854 [6], published his analysis of mastoptosis. Descriptions of the modern mastopexy procedure were first seen as early as the nineteenth century. Many

M.A. Shiffman (ed.), *Mastopexy and Breast Reduction: Principles and Practice*,
© Springer-Verlag Berlin Heidelberg 2009

of these early approaches offered a significant basis for the techniques that are currently used. Although the techniques mirrored those of reduction mammoplasty, the emphasis was on correcting ptosis of the breast. Most of these procedures involved elevation of the breast mound using suspension techniques. Pousson's technique (1897) [7] and Verchere's [8] mammoplasty (1898) both relied on direct excision of skin superior to the nipple areolar complex. With closure, the nipple and breast gland were elevated providing a simple solution to breast ptosis. Dehner utilized a semilunar resection of the superior breast tissue and split the pectoralis muscle so the breast tissue could be anchored to the periosteum of the ribs. In 1882, the inframammary incision was first described to facilitate tumor excision. It was implemented to facilitate mastopexy and reduction mammoplasty and was eventually utilized by Passot in 1925 [9].

Various pedicles to support the nipple areolar complex were described by the 1930s. Further evolution in mastopexy resulted in the refinement of both technique and analysis. One of the earliest techniques involved a two-stage approach, which Joseph described in 1925 [10]. The first stage transposed the nipples to their final location using broad and reliable pedicles. Shape and symmetry were ignored until the second procedure, performed several weeks later. The second procedure involved removing excess lower pole, shaping and lifting the breast, as well as maximizing symmetry between the two sides.

Kraske [11] described his innovative single-stage technique in 1923. In retrospect, it first utilized many of the principles of the modern mastopexy and reduction operations. This technique removed lower pole breast tissue and avoided extensive undermining of the skin from the breast parenchyma. The breast tissue and overlying skin were tightened with the excess tissue laterally excised, leaving a traditional inverted T scar. Unfortunately, because the results were considered suboptimal, it fell out of favor. In contrast, despite an extremely high rate of postoperative complications, one of the most popular techniques in the first half of the twentieth century was the Biesenberger procedure [12]. This approach employed wide undermining of the skin and excision of the lateral portion of the breast, with rotation of the medially based nipple pedicle to a more superior position. The skin was then tightened around the gland to provide shape.

8.4
Evolution of the Modern Approach

An anatomic-based approach was ultimately adopted and Strombeck described a bilateral horizontal pedicle in 1960 [13]. Primarily implemented for reduction of breast volume, a significant resection was performed cephalad to the horizontal pedicle. The pedicle was then imbricated along a vertical line from the nipple areolar complex extending inferiorly. This glandular tightening is similar to the vertical type reductions utilized currently and in addition helped establish the principle of maintaining the attachments between breast parenchyma and skin. Skin resection and closure was performed to remove excesses rather than to tighten or lift the breast, again a key feature of current mastopexy techniques.

The McKissock [14] vertical bipedicle technique similarly offered a robust de epithelialized pedicle to supply the nipple. Resection was performed medially and laterally as well as beneath the cephalic portion of the thick vertical pedicle. The pedicle was folded on itself to allow mobilization of the NAC, and the thick dermal–parenchymal flaps were then closed. The vertical bipedicle technique eventually evolved into the inferior pedicle technique described by various authors [15, 16]. This approach may currently be the most widely used technique, particularly for reduction mammaplasty. It has been applied to mastopexy procedures; however, a criticism of the approach is that the pedicle tends to drop, leading to recurrent ptosis and a boxy appearance of the breast. Alternatively, the superior pedicle first described by Weiner in 1973 [17] eliminated the inferior portion of the vertical bipedicle reduction. The limitation of this approach is the distance which the nipple can be safely transposed. As the long superior pedicle is folded to elevate the nipple, the vascular supply is compressed and the risk of nipple slough is increased.

Just as the vertical bipedicle led to vertically oriented single pedicle techniques, the Strombeck operation was the precursor of the lateral and medial pedicle procedures. Originally described by Skoog [18], the lateral procedure required resection of the medial and inferior quadrants of the breast.

The medial pedicle was also adapted from Strombeck's horizontal bipedicle technique. At the present, it is one of the most popular techniques employed for reduction mammaplasty. It lends itself quite well for mastopexy procedures. This approach can be combined with the vertical closure with ease.

While the importance of shaping the gland was recognized, significant emphasis was still placed on the "skin brassiere". These techniques used tightening of the skin envelope to shape and lift the breast parenchyma [19, 20]. Unfortunately, these approaches did not provide durable results. To avoid the dermal stretching that can occur with dermal mastopexies, both permanent and absorbable mesh have been used to reinforce the breast parenchyma with an internal brassiere [21, 22]. The Benelli round block or periareolar purse string mammoplasty uses a permanent suture rather than mesh to lift the breast tissue [23]. In patients with limited breast ptosis, it effectively limits scarring and provides elevation [24]. Subsequent descriptions have demonstrated reliable and safe results using mesh to reshape the breast mound [25]. Most recently, the use of acellular dermal matrix has been employed to avoid the use of prosthetic material, providing a more natural texture to the breast while achieving excellent early results. This approach also provides an effective method of covering prosthetic breast implants and has been used in reconstructive efforts as well [26, 27].

8.5 Current Concepts

Autologous mastopexy procedures require rearrangement of the breast tissue with minimal volume reduction. Some of the techniques for reduction mammaplasty are more readily adaptable to this purpose than others. As indicated, the vertical reductions reliably perfused the nipple with limited transposition of the NAC. Mobilization of the remaining tissue can be effected from deep to the superior pedicle. Additional procedures to recreate breast fullness using autologous tissue have been described using the dual pedicle dermoparenchymal mastopexy and the deepithelialized transverse rectus abdominis muscle, using the "Flip-Flap" mastopexy [28, 29]. Lateral and inferior pedicles have been used to autoaugment the breast as well. Placement of the autologous tissue flap deep to a strip of pectoralis muscle is reported to improve shape and maximize longevity of the lift. The use of the vertical bipedicle flap has also reemerged, reported to minimize scarring while preserving a more robust blood supply to the nipple. Khan [30] described a vertical scar bipedicle technique combined for minimal scarring and robust blood supply to the nipple–areolar complex as a further option for Mastopexies.

The vertical mastopexy eliminates the inframammary scar and was introduced by Lassus [31] using the superior pedicle. Subsequent modification was done by Lejour [32] to include the use of liposuction. The purpose was to reduce the length of the scar that extends beyond the inframammary fold onto the chest wall. The most recent modifications of the vertical mastopexy are based on the Hall-Findlay technique [33]. Her proposal of a superior medial pedicle has led to the growing popularity of the vertical mastopexy. The superior medial pedicle can be combined with autoaugmentation using either an inferior pedicle or a lateral pedicle. This tissue normally discarded in the reduction mammaplasty is suspended deep to the nipple and securely suspended to avoid recurrent ptosis.

The vertical-only incision has been advocated as minimizing scars, but has also seen modification to address its deficiencies. The Y-Scar vertical mammaplasty is an alternative to reduce further scar length [34]. Loustau et al. [35] used the Owl-technique combined with the inferior pedicle in mastopexies. More recently, the addition of a short inframammary scar has reduced the revision rate of the vertical mastopexy procedures. The inframammary resection is of particular value in those patients who have significant skin excess.

A variety of methods have been utilized to augment atrophic or hypoplastic breast tissue. These include percutaneous injection of foreign material (such as paraffin or silicone) and implantation of free dermal fat grafts. The advent of breast prostheses allowed the use of an implant to augment breast volume in combination with lifting procedures [36]. Although augmentation mammoplasty does not truly lift the breast, mild cases of ptosis, particularly those with involutional breast changes, can be corrected with breast augmentation alone. Moderate ptosis can be corrected using a circumareolar donut mastopexy including the round block techniques with the use of an implant [37]. The combination of volume increase and limited tightening allows correction of more significant ptosis than either approach alone. Improper implementation of this approach can lead to undesirable results, including widened periareolar scars. Moderate grade 2 ptosis can be addressed using circum-vertical mastopexy procedures, including the Regnault B technique and Lejour/Lassus techniques. Severe grade 2 ptosis and grade 3 ptosis usually require inverted T incisions regardless of the pedicle used even with an implant placed. Pseudoptosis can be addressed by augmentation and/or skin excision at the lower pole and nipple transposition can often be avoided.

Patients who have previously undergone augmentation mammoplasty can develop breast ptosis related to the implants that cause thinning of the skin, atrophy of the breast tissue, and stretching of the suspensory ligaments. These changes can drive the patients to the point where they request reoperation. Recent literature has criticized the concept of concurrent breast augmentation and mastopexy. Spear [38] cited an increased risk of infection, implant exposure, change in nipple sensibility and poor positioning of either the nipple or the implant. Primary augmentation plus mastopexy was found to have a significantly higher complication rate than primary augmentation alone. Handel [39] states that secondary mastopexy in the previously augmented breast does carry increased risks, due to the adverse effects of implants on mammary structures, but that with proper planning and attention to detail, most patients will achieve good outcomes.

The massive weight loss patient presents unique challenges, due to their severely redundant and inelastic skin envelopes, significant nipple ptosis, and prominent lateral skin rolls [40]. Losken and Holtz [41] describe a technique using the principles of Lejour and Hall-Findley and the application of the superomedial pedicle technique. This approach faciliates glandular plication in the lower pole, providing autoaugmentation of the upper pole. Graf et al. [40] describe the use of a loop of the pectoralis muscle to elevate and secure the breast tissue in a higher position. In the case of bariatric patients, an extended thoracic wall flap is tunneled under the muscle loop, which reduces the lateral roll and autoaugments the deflated bariatric breast. Various authors have described the use of an intercostal artery perforator flap in massive weight loss patients [42, 43]. The spiral flap employs a long pedicle based on intercostal perforators to integrate the upper body lift with mastopexy augmentation for upper torso enhancement after massive weight loss [44].

8.6 Conclusions

Currently there are many excellent options to achieve reliable and aesthetic outcomes for ptosis correction of the breast. Augmentation mammoplasty lack of volume and minimal ptosis. The round block technique is useful for limited ptosis and can be combined with placement of a prosthesis for augmentation. Perhaps the most versatile approach is the current incarnation of the vertical mastopexy. It affords use of medial or superior pedicle, can include autoaugmentation and even with short scar inframammary resection limits scarring while obtaining excellent results.

The future of mastopexy surgery lies in the ability to obtain lasting results using minimally invasive techniques. Endoscopic procedures that suspend the breast tissue and minimize apparent scarring have been developed but have limited indications. Alternatively, development of scar reduction, either through closure techniques or with postoperative treatments (i.e., laser treatments), offers patients the opportunity to undergo an ideal procedure for body contouring while minimizing visible scarring.

References

1. Penn J: Breast reduction. Br J Plast Surg 1955;7:357–371
2. Adair FE, Munzer JT: Fat necrosis of the female breast. Am J Surg 1947;74:117
3. Rees TD: Plastic surgery of the breast. In: Converse J (ed) Reconstructive Plastic Surgery. Philadelphia, W.B. Saunders 1977
4. Gonzales F, Brown FE, Gold ME, Walton RL, Shafer B: Preoperative and postoperative nipple areolar sensibility in patients undergoing reduction mammaplasty. Plast Reconstr Surg 1993;92(5):809–814
5. Regnault P: Breast ptosis. Definition and treatment. Clin Plast Surg 1976;3(2):193–203
6. Velpeau AALM: Traite des maladies du sein et de la region mammaire. Paris, Victor Masson 1854
7. Pousson M: De la mastopexie. Bull Mem Soc Chir Paris 1897;23:507
8. Vechere F: Mastopexie laterale contre la mastoptose hypertrophique. Med Mod 1989;9:340
9. Passot R: La correction esthetique du prolapsus mamarie par la procede de la transposition du mamelon. Presse Med 1925;33:317
10. Joseph J: Zur operation de hypertorphischen Hangeburst. Dstch Med Wochenschr 1925;51:1103
11. Kraske H: Die operation de atrpischen and hypertorphischen hangeburst. Munchen Med Wochenschr 1923;70:672
12. Biesenberger H: Blutversorgung and zirkulare umschnedung des warzenhofes. Zentralb Chir 1928;55:2385
13. Strombeck JO: Mammaplasty: report of a new technique based on the two-pedicle procedure. Br J Plast Surg 1960;13:79–90
14. McKissock PK: Reduction mammaplasty with a vertical dermal flap. Plast Reconstr Surg 1972;49(3):245–252
15. Ribero L: A new technique for reduction mammaplasty. Plast Reconstr Surg 1975;55(3):330–334
16. Robbins TH: A reduction mammaplasty with areolar-nipple based on an inferior dermal pedicle. Plast Reconstr Surg 1977;59(1):64–67
17. Weiner DL, Aiache AE, Silver L, Tittiranonda T: A single dermal pedicle for nipple transposition in subcutaneous mastectomy, reduction mammaplasty, or mastopexy. Plast Reconstr Surg 1973;51(2):115–120
18. Skoog T: A technique of breast reduction. Transposition of the nipple on a cutaneous vascular pedicle. Acta Chir Scand 1963;126:453–465
19. Aufricht G: Mammaplasty for pendulous breasts. Empiric and geometric planning. Plast Reconstr Surg 1949;4(1):13–29
20. Goulian D Jr: Dermal mastopexy. Plast Reconstr Surg 1971;47(2):105–110
21. Johnson GW: Central core reduction mammoplasties and Marlex suspension of breast tissue. Aesthetic Plast Surg 1981;5(1):77–84
22. Auclair E, Mitz V: Repair of mammary ptosis by insertion of an internal absorbable support and periareolar scar. Ann Chir Plast Esthet 1993;38(1):107–113
23. Benelli L: Technique de plastie mammaire: le "round bloc." Rev Fr Chir Esthet 1988;50:7
24. Benelli L: A new periareolar mammaplasty: the "round block" technique. Aesthetic Plast Surg 1990;14(2):93–100
25. Góes JC, Landecker A, Lyra EC, Henríquez LJ, Góes RS, Godoy PM: The application of mesh support in periareolar breast surgery: clinical and mammographic evaluation. Aesthetic Plast Surg 2004;28(5):268–274
26. Breuing KH, Colwell AS: Inferolateral AlloDerm hammock for implant coverage in breast reconstruction. Ann Plast Surg 2007;59(3):250–255

27. Gamboa-Bobadilla GM: Implant breast reconstruction using acelluar dermal matrix. Ann Plast Surg 2006;56(1): 22–25
28. Weiss PR, Ship AG: Restoration of breast contour with autologous tissue after removal of implants. Ann Plast Surg 1995;34(3):236–241
29. Flowers RS, Smith EM Jr: "Flip-flap" mastopexy. Aesthetic Plast Surg 1998;22(6):425–429
30. Khan UD: Vertical scar with the bipedicle technique: a modified procedure for breast reduction and mastopexy. Aesthetic Plast Surg 2007;31(4):337–342
31. Lassus C: A technique for breast reduction. Int Surg 1970;53(1):69–72
32. Lejour M: Vertical mammaplasty and liposuction of the breast. Plast Reconstr Surg 1994;94(1):100–114
33. Hall-Findlay EJ: A simplified vertical mammaplasty: shortening the learning curve. Plast Reconstr Surg 1999;104(3):748–759
34. Hidalgo DA: Y-scar vertical mammaplasty. Plast Reconstr Surg 2007;120(7):1749–1754
35. Loustau HD, Mayer HF, Saarrabayrouse ML: The owl technique combined with the inferior pedicle in mastopexy. Aesthetic Plast Surg 2008;32(1):11–15
36. Gonzalez-Ulloa M: Correction of hypotrophy of the breast by means of exogenous material. Plast Reconstr Transplant Bull 1960;25:15–26
37. De Benito J, Sanza IF: Periareolar techniques for mammary reduction and elevation. Aesthetic Plast Surg 1993;17(4):311–316
38. Spear SL, Boehmler JH IV, Clemens MW: Augmentation/mastopexy: a 3 year review of a single surgeon's practice. Plast Reconstr Surg 2006;118(7 Suppl):136S–147S
39. Handel N: Secondary mastopexy in the augmented patient: a recipe for disaster. Plast Reconstr Surg 2006;118 (7 Suppl):152S–163S
40. Graf RM, Mansur AE, Tenius FP, Ono MC, Romano GG, Cruz GA: Mastopexy after massive weight loss: extended chest wall-based flap associated with a loop of pectoralis muscle. Aesthetic Plast Surg 2008;32(2):371–374
41. Losken A, Holtz DJ: Versatility of the superomedial pedicle in managing the massive weight loss breast: the rotation-advancement technique. Plast Reconstr Surg 2007;120(4):1060–1068
42. Van Landuyt K, Hamdi M, Blondeel P, Monstrey S: Autologous breast augmentation by pedicled perforator flaps. Ann Plast Surg. 2004;53(4):322–327
43. Kwei S, Borud LJ, Lee BT: Mastopexy with autologous augmentation after massive weight loss: the intercostal artery perforator (ICAP) flap. Ann Plast Surg 2006;57(4):361–365
44. Hurwitz DJ, Agha-Mohammadi S: Postbariatric surgery breast reshaping. The spiral flap. Ann Plast Surg 2006;56(5): 481–486

CHAPTER 9

Principles of Mastopexy

Melvin A. Shiffman

9.1 Introduction

The techniques of mastopexy have evolved over many years. There are certain principles involved in the performance of mastopexy that may help to prevent some complications and reduce litigation.

9.2 Principles

1. Obtain all records of prior breast surgery and review the surgical reports prior to performing mastopexy.
   a. Be aware of the incisions used for a prior breast augmentation.
2. Obtain a preoperative mammogram on all patients (at least those over age 35–40).
   a. This may diagnose a cancer or other tumor that may need treatment before or at the same time as the mastopexy.
3. Obtain preoperative photographs on all patients.
   a. This will substantiate preoperative asymmetry or other deformities.
4. Learn all types of mastopexy and their indications.
   a. There is no universal mastopexy that will solve the problems in every patient.
5. Record preoperative measurements.
   a. Sternal notch and/or mid clavicle to nipples.
   b. Nipples to midline.
   c. Extent of ptosis: the degree of ptosis and/or measurement from nipple to inframammary fold and inframammary fold to lowest point of breast.
6. Always mark the breast for skin incisions and excisions before surgery.
   a. Mark with the patient sitting or standing.
   b. Doing mastopexy and breast augmentation without marking increases the risk of asymmetry (Fig. 9.1).

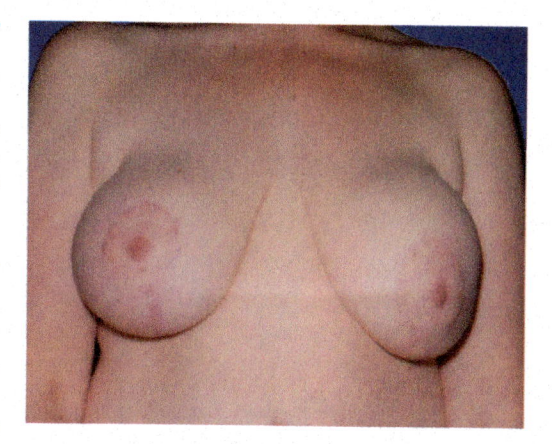

Fig. 9.1 Asymmetry with left breast lower than right after mastopexy and breast augmentation. There were no preoperative skin markings performed

7. Plan the type of mastopexy to fit the degree of ptosis.
   a. Severe ptosis cannot usually be treated adequately with a crescent mastopexy or Benelli "Round Block" mastopexy except with repeat procedures.
8. Plan to see the patient on the first postoperative day to evaluate for possible hematoma or nipple areolar cyanosis.
9. Smoking should be stopped at least 2 weeks before and 2 weeks after surgery to prevent postoperative necrosis.

9.3 Conclusions

Surgeons should be aware of the principles that will help reduce possible complications and avoid possible litigation.

M.A. Shiffman (ed.), *Mastopexy and Breast Reduction: Principles and Practice,*
© Springer-Verlag Berlin Heidelberg 2009

Treatment of Pseudoptosis

Frank Schneider-Affeld

10.1 Introduction

The breast changes as a result of aging, weight, fluctuations in weight, pregnancies, and breastfeeding. Sagging of the glandular body, breast envelope, and the nipple–areola complex (NAC) normally occurs synchronously and is described by Renault's Grade I to III ptosis classification. This classification describes the changes seen in the majority of breasts. The length of the thorax and the height of the SMF are, for the most part, not taken into account. Thus only absolute measurable parameters such as the distance of the nipples from the sternal notch provide signs of changes that are regarded by the observer as harmonious ("pleasing to the eye") or disharmonious.

Changes to the three criteria, glandular body, envelope, and height of the NAC, may occur asynchronously, although this is not frequent. This typically results in pseudoptosis and glandular ptosis or sagging of the breast following surgery (bottoming out).

In the case of pseudoptosis, only the volume of the breast changes, that is, the glandular body becomes smaller. The envelope and position of the NAC remain unchanged. Consequently, the upper half of the breast becomes concave in shape, the projection of the breast is reduced, and the lower half of the breast loses elasticity and thus sags without there being an increase in the nipple to submammary fold (N–SMF) distance. It looks like ptosis, but in fact is not.

With glandular ptosis, on the other hand, the volume, that is, glandular body, and the position of the NAC are both stable, while the envelope in the bottom section increases in length and bulges downward. N–SMF distance has increased.

The same changes occur with so-called bottoming out, in particular, following surgery using the inverted T technique and other mastopexy techniques, although this is less frequent.

10.2 History

Early literature did not report on pseudoptosis or glandular ptosis. These conditions were defined for the first time in 1976 by Renault [1]. In the case of pseudoptosis, he recommended a "simple small augmentation" as the treatment of choice. In the same context he warned against augmentation as treatment for other forms of ptosis. He referred to glandular ptosis as partial ptosis and recommended the modified B technique, a vertical mastopexy without repositioning of the NAC that is combined, where appropriate, with glandular body reduction, as the technique of choice.

In 1990, Benelli recommended augmentation for the correction of mammary hypotrophy and ptosis and was obviously referring here to pseudoptosis.

Brink endeavored to describe pseudoptosis in greater detail but did not make any proposals for treatment.

10.3 Technique and Complications

Pseudoptosis is defined as a reduction in the size of the glandular body. This results in an envelope that is too large relative to the glandular body and thus hangs loosely around the latter. Projection and upper filling decrease (Figs. 10.1–10.4).

The logical means of correction is augmentation, which serves to give back the envelope any lost volume. If there are reservations as to the use of silicone prostheses, the envelope can alternately be reduced in order to adapt it to the reduced volume. Crescent mastopexy (CM) is an ideal way of achieving this and this technique serves, in particular, to tighten the lower half of the breast and the scarring that is left behind is barely visible. The upper half of the breast benefits less from this type of intervention because, for the most part, the glandular body has involuted. "Upper pole fullness" cannot be achieved with CM.

In the case of glandular ptosis or "bottoming out," as it is called when referring to a side effect of mastopexy, the lower half of the breast is overstretched and manifests itself in a longer nipple-to-fold distance. The position of the NAC remains unchanged and there is also no change in the volume of the glandular body, although it has undergone sagging. As a consequence, the pressure on the lower half of the breast has increased (Fig. 10.5).

M.A. Shiffman (ed.), *Mastopexy and Breast Reduction: Principles and Practice*,
© Springer-Verlag Berlin Heidelberg 2009

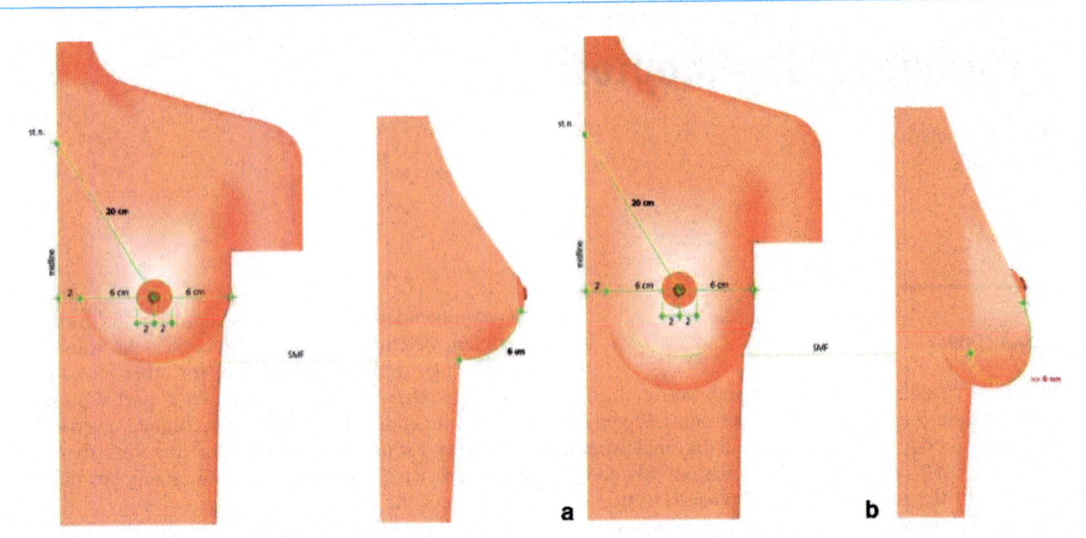

Fig. 10.1 The "attractive" breast. Distance measured from sternal notch to nipple (St.n.–N), 20 cm; nipple (N), 3 cm above SMF; NAC–SMF, 6 cm; *Projection*, +; *Upper filling*, +

Fig. 10.3 Glandular ptosis. St.n.–N, 20 cm; N, 3 cm above SMF; NAC–SMF, > 6; Projection, +; Upper filling, +

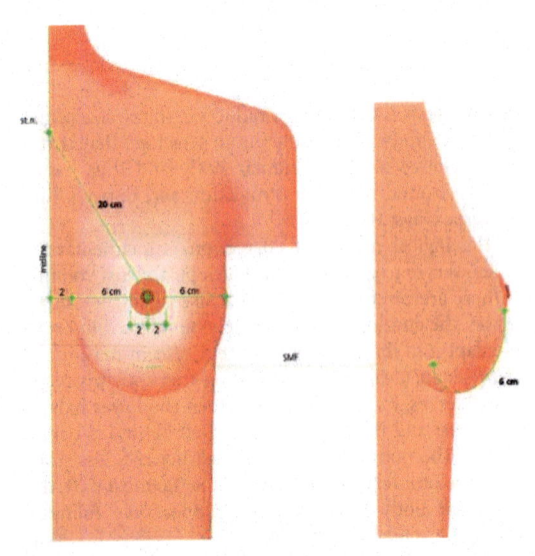

Fig. 10.2 Pseudoptosis. St.n.–N, 20 cm; N, 3 cm above SMF; NAC–SMF, 6 cm; Projection, Upper filling

To correct this condition, the envelope must be tightened and the glandular body fixed further up by means of glandular rearrangement. This is normally achieved using a standard vertical mastopexy technique, and so visible scars are left on the lower part of the breast.

Without glandular fixing, a recurrence can be expected within a short period of time.

Bottoming out is the same as glandular ptosis by definition. Various authors define pseudoptosis or glandular ptosis as separate conditions.

10.4
Discussion

In the majority of cases, the breast will begin to sag as a woman ages due to a reduction in content, loss of elasticity, or overstretching of the envelope, and sagging of the NAC. These changes occur at the same time and have been defined by Renault as Grade I to III ptosis. The definitions are still completely valid today. Special cases involving asynchronous changes are referred to as pseudoptosis and glandular ptosis or "bottoming out."

Increasing hypoplasia of the glandular body is thus the sole cause of pseudoptosis (Figs. 10.1 and 10.2). During consultations it is important to draw attention to the fact that pseudoptosis is not actually ptosis in the normal sense but "merely" refers to a loss of volume. In the mirror, the upper half of the breast has a concave appearance and the lower half of the breast appears to sag due to a lack of volume. As a consequence, corrective measures will restore the lost volume by a "small augmentation" as described by Renault in 1976.

Alternately, or in cases where there are acceptance problems with silicone prostheses, CM is an ideal choice. This technique allows the envelope to be tightened

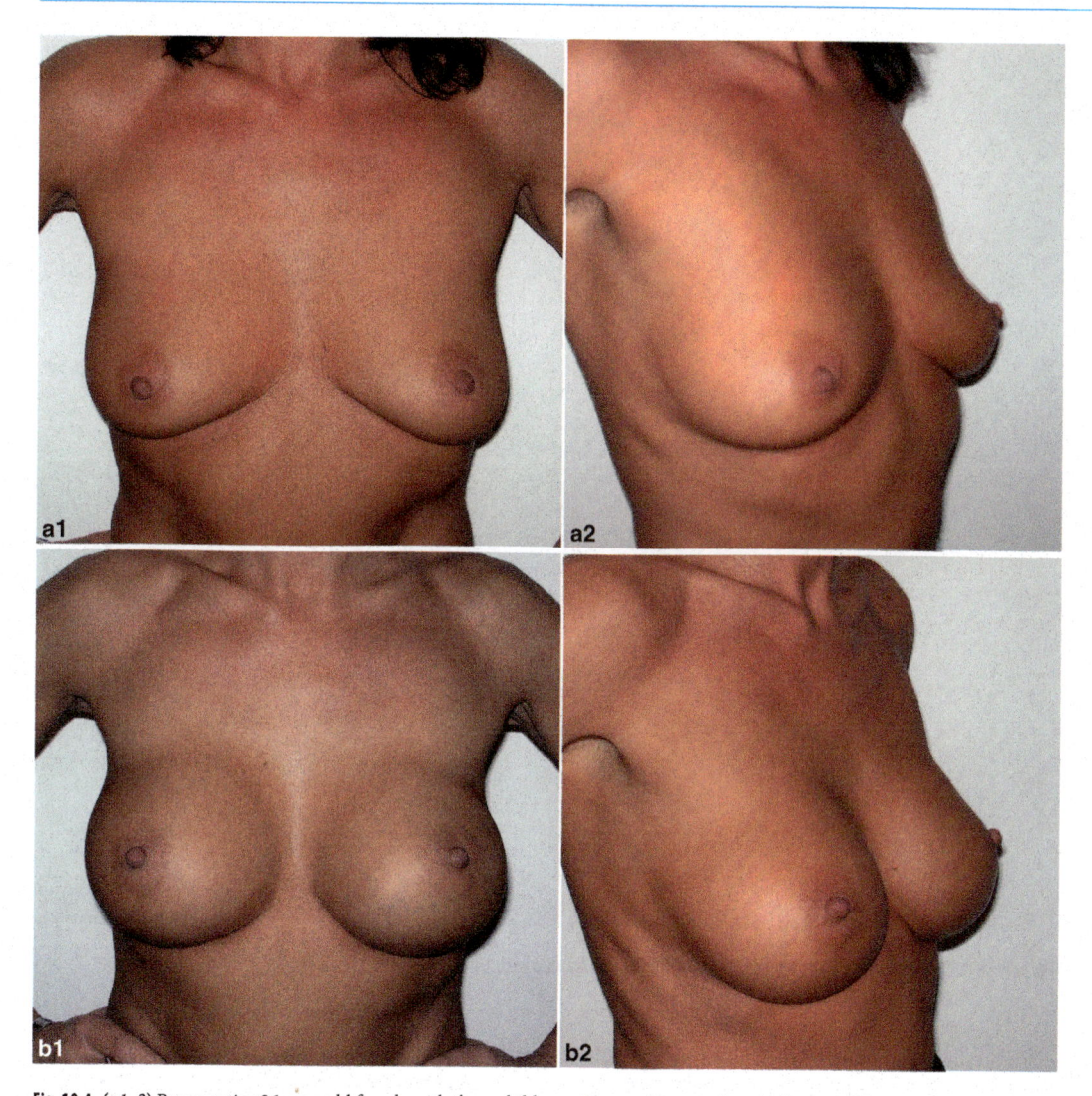

Fig. 10.4 (*a1, 2*) Preoperative 36-year-old female with three children with pseudoptosis (*b1, 2*) Three months postoperatively

slightly, but without having a major effect on the upper half of the breast in terms of upper pole fullness.

As the transitions to Grade I ptosis are fluid, eccentric CM] also enables the NAC to be lifted. It is this measure in particular that often significantly improves the appearance of the breast, because the correct position of the NAC plays a key role in ensuring a "pleasing" final result.

In the case of glandular ptosis (Fig. 10.3), the problem lies in the lower half of the breast, while the upper half and the NAC are both stable. Any corrective measure must thus tighten the overstretched skin and reduce the downward pressure caused by gravity.

The inverted T technique or scar-sparing modifications thereof are able to tighten the envelope in the lower section. Although on its own this measure would help in the short term, in the long term it would not provide stability. Fixing of the glandular body on the pectoral fascia is thus a mandatory part of this corrective technique. Visible scars in the lower part of the breast cannot be avoided.

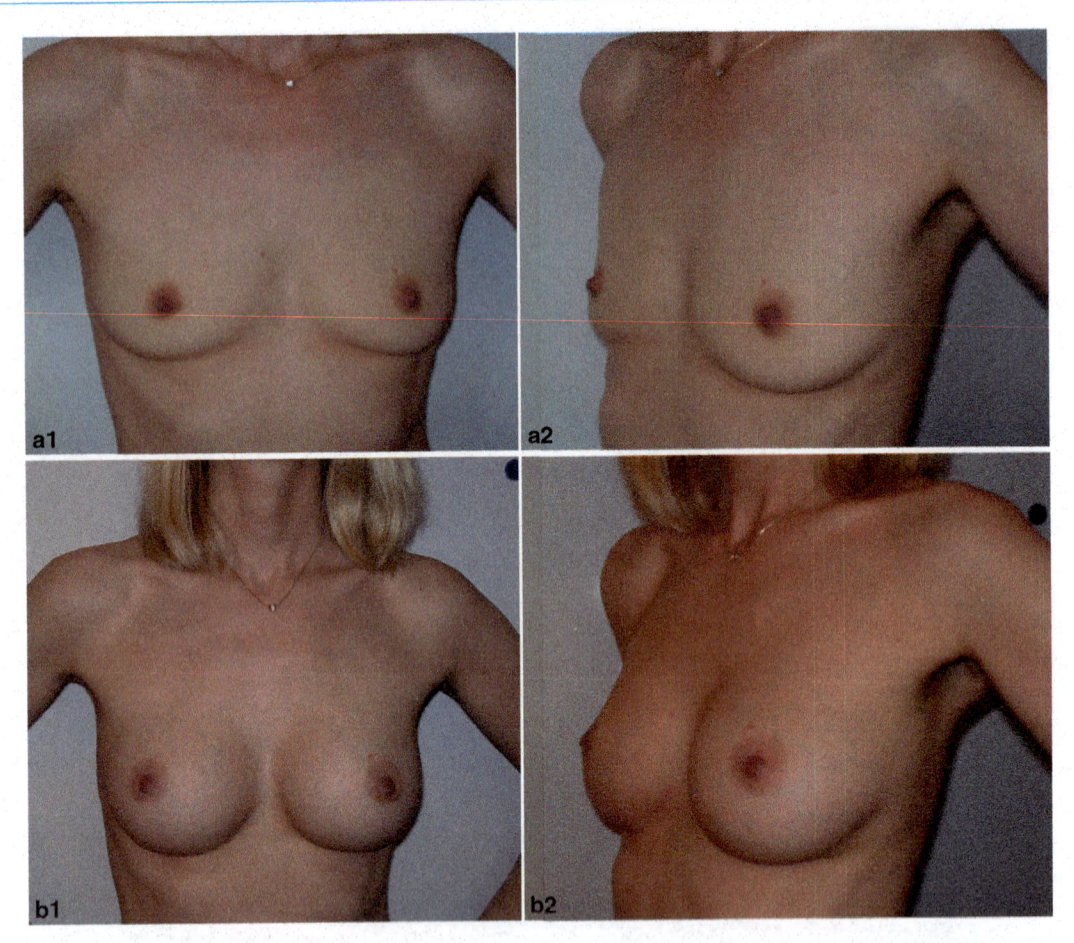

Fig. 10.5 (*a1, 2*) Bottoming out preoperatively of 38-year-old female with two children (*b1, 2*) Eighteen months postoperatively

Bottoming out after mastopexy surgery or reductions is identical to glandular ptosis. It occurs most frequently after the inverted T technique.

In pre-Grade I ptosis breasts, correction of the height and size of the NAC can be easily performed. With pseudoptosis, in particular, a high level of success and satisfaction can be achieved with minimal surgery.

Note:
1. The abbreviation CM for crescent, concentric, and eccentric mastopexy has been retained because it is in common use.
2. All measurements relate to the "ideal proportions" of an "attractive" breast.
3. Changes are marked in red.

Crescent Mastopexy

Robert A. Shumway

Breast surgery is one of the most difficult operations in cosmetic surgery because it should produce a beautiful, symmetrical, and durable result with minimal scarring.

—Madeleine Lejour [1]

11.1 Introduction

Aesthetic breast surgery has become an increasingly important part of the practice of cosmetic surgery since the middle of the twentieth century. A truly beautiful breast without obvious surgical scars is paramount in the minds of all surgeons performing cosmetic breast surgery. However, in the past, "traditional" mastopexy has often left unacceptable scars on the breast. Therefore, cosmetic surgeons must endeavor to correct breast ptosis without creating extensive and undesirable scarring on the breast. In accordance with these lofty goals, the areolar crescent and extended crescent mastopexy procedures have been formulated.

These versatile crescent breast lifts may be performed with or without concurrent breast augmentation and will provide consistent and reliable aesthetic results in nearly all age categories. To accomplish these goals, the crescent is used to optimize the position and appearance of the nipple–areola complex (NAC) by improving its symmetry, reducing NAC ptosis, and correcting nipple malposition by utilizing a shallow, intradermal, semicircular, or extended periareolar skin excision and closure. Crescent nipple lift with breast mastopexy is applicable for many different breast sizes and shapes. It eliminates the full circumareolar, vertical, and horizontal components used in other types of mastopexy procedures. The crescent lift can be used to reshape a breast or reposition the NAC to a more suitable position on the mammary mound, especially following breast augmentation. After augmentation, the breast will not only be larger, but will exhibit substantially different dimensions and proportions relative to the NAC. Thus, nipple lifting can create a completely different breast appearance [2]. The improved breast geometry and new shape will help create a more satisfactory aesthetic result for the patient who possesses newly augmented breasts.

Crescent mastopexy is reproducible, easy to learn, and can be performed on multiple future occasions throughout a patient's lifetime without creating additional scarring. All conscientious surgeons can master the crescent lift in conjunction with routine breast augmentation while using any of the four standard surgical approaches (transumbilical, periareolar, transaxillary, or inframammary). The technique is very effective for patients who exhibit glandular ptosis or grade I ptosis. The extended crescent mastopexy with appropriate breast augmentation will be required for grade II ptosis. Multiple crescent NAC lifts may be required for grade III ptosis with augmentation. Certainly, other types of mastopexy surgeries must be offered to any patients who exhibit grade III breast ptosis, along with a frank discussion of all future mastopexy scars. These "other mastopexies" will, of course, incur much more scarring [3]. The author has been very successful in aesthetically improving grade III breast ptosis by using appropriately sized implants (suitable for the patient's measured thorax) while applying the aggressive "extended" crescent mastopexy approach. The overall result is a well-placed NAC with a camouflaged, superficial, semiareolar surgical incision that can heal best at the NAC–breast skin junction. This chapter will now summarize a technique for achieving a balanced, beautiful breast without the obvious breast scars inherent in the traditional inverted "T" and vertical mastopexies [4].

11.2 History

Aubert published the first mammaplasty procedure in 1923 [5]. He was the first surgeon recorded to have performed an operation that reduced the size of the breast while relocating the NAC. To achieve his results, he undermined breast skin widely. Soon other doctors followed his example. Later, the popular Biesenberger [6] procedure borrowed many of Aubert's surgical principles, which were applied by numerous surgeons from the 1930s to the 1980s. However, there were many complications with these surgeries, such as skin and fat necrosis, NAC necrosis, glandular necrosis, hematomas, seromas, infections, and scarring. The root of these complications was related to the extensive undermining of skin from the gland, coupled with glandular disarticulation from the muscle. By the 1960s, Pitanguy [7] and others had

M.A. Shiffman (ed.), *Mastopexy and Breast Reduction: Principles and Practice,*
© Springer-Verlag Berlin Heidelberg 2009

developed a safer operation with better results by using "enbloc" gland resection, less skin undermining, and transposition of the NAC on dermoglandular flaps. By 1970, Lassus [8] determined that skin and glandular tissue should not be elevated. He felt that surgeons must preserve the integrity of Cooper's ligaments in order to produce a safer and longer lasting result.

Now, our modern day crescent lifts allow surgical transposition of the NAC without any tissue undermining whatsoever. Dermoglandular flaps are only used as needed when extensive manipulation of the NAC is warranted with very extended crescent lifts [9]. In short, the crescent concept of "less is more" applies today.

11.3 Anatomy and Technique

To appreciate the crescent mastopexy technique, we must first understand the relevant breast anatomy. The NAC epidermis is highly pigmented, with moderate wrinkling which allows for excellent incisional camouflage. The nipple's dermis, which has an extremely high collagen concentration (excellent for surgical support), contains apocrine sweat glands and numerous sebaceous glands with relatively few hair follicles. Around 15–25 milk ducts enter the nipple base and dilate to create the milk sinuses (well below any crescent surgical incisions). These sinuses terminate into cone-shaped ampullas. The circular areola surrounding the nipple varies greatly in diameter between 20 and 60 mm (Fig. 11.1). The areolar skin also contains sebaceous glands, sweat glands, Montgomery glands, and lanugo hair. Deep in the NAC (again, well below our surgical incisions) are smooth muscle fibers arranged in radial and circular connective tissue bundles, which are oriented longitudinally along lactiferous ducts. These fibers travel up into the nipple and cause nipple erection, areolar contraction, and evacuation of the milk sinuses [10]. By way of anatomical reasoning, crescent mastopexies will not interfere with future lactation or breast feeding.

The great majority of breast parenchyma, which is in no way violated by crescent mastopexy, extends from the level of the second or third rib down to the inframammary fold at the sixth or seventh rib [11]. The breast also extends laterally from the sternum to the anterior axillary line. The tail of Spence includes a variable amount of breast parenchyma (10–30% by volume) and is situated up in the axilla. The deep posterior surface of the gland lies on top of the superficial portion of the deep thoracic fascia (DFT), which is an extension of Scarpa's fascia inferiorly. It overlies the pectoralis major, rectus abdominus, external abdominal oblique, and serratus anterior muscles. The deep portion of the DFT lies beneath these muscles.

The breast tissue itself is enveloped by the superficial fascia of the anterior thoracic wall, which is an extension of Camper's fascia. This superficial fascia is continuous inferiorly with the superficial abdominal fascia of Camper and is continuous superiorly with the superficial cervical fascia. The superficial layer of this anterior superficial thoracic fascia (STF) is connected to the dermis and can be used to effectively suspend the NAC superiorly: this is why the crescent mastopexy technique is surgically possible and why it can provide a long lasting result. This suspension technique is used to mold and contour the shape of the breast [12]. The superficial fascial connection to the dermis is where the strength of crescent lifting and closure is derived. The deep layer of the STF lies directly above the pectoralis major muscle fascia and, most importantly, the superficial layer of the STF with the overlying dermis link to the deep layer of the STF by way of the ligaments of Cooper [13]. Cooper's ligaments are fibrous and elastic prolongations that divide the mammary gland itself into multiple septa and give it suspensory support. The breast parenchyma is made up of 15–25 lobes of glandular tissue separated throughout by Cooper's ligaments and surrounded by fat. Each lobe empties into a separate milk duct that terminates in the nipple as mentioned earlier.

Arterial blood supply to the breast consists of three main systems: the lateral thoracic artery, the internal mammary artery, and the intercostal arteries [14]. The chief arterial blood supply to the NAC comes from the branches off the lateral thoracic and internal mammary arteries. They both travel in the subcutaneous breast tissue and communicate, in an arcade-like fashion, with one another around and beneath the periareolar region. Small vessels reach the nipple base and give off a fine areolar network to the areolar skin. Thereafter, they ascend into the nipple in a circular fashion and arborize in the superior two-thirds of the nipple. None of the above arterial structures are compromised with crescent mastopexy.

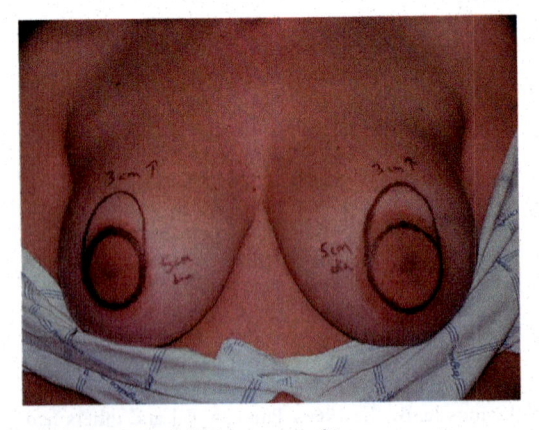

Fig. 11.1 NAC variability/crescent markings

The venous drainage of the breast has both a superficial and deep system [15]. This superficial venous system lies just deep to the superficial layer of the STF of the breast. Transverse veins make up 90% of areolar venous return. They run medially in the subcutaneous tissues and then join perforating vessels that empty into the internal mammary vein. The longitudinal veins make up the other 10% of venous return and ascend up to the suprasternal notch and empty into the superficial veins of the lower neck. The deep venous system of the breast involves perforating branches of the internal mammary vein, tributaries from the axillary vein, and perforating branches of the posterior intercostal veins. None of these veins are compromised by the crescent mastopexy procedure.

The sensory innervation of the breast varies somewhat among women [16]. The NAC is always innervated by the anterior and lateral cutaneous branches of the third, fourth, and/or fifth intercostal nerves. However, the distribution, size, and number of these nerves vary. For example, the fourth lateral intercostal cutaneous nerve branch, which is the most consistent nerve to innervate the NAC, supplies the nipple in about 93% of breasts [17]. In 79% of mammary glands, it is the only lateral nerve to the nipple. Fortunately, the crescent lift will not damage any of the nerves that supply the breast.

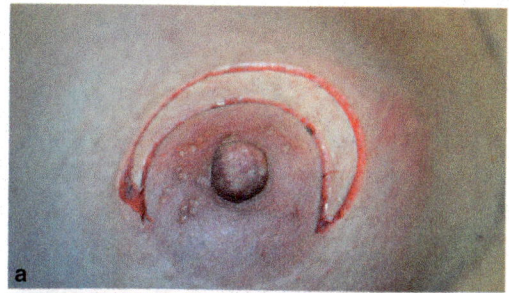

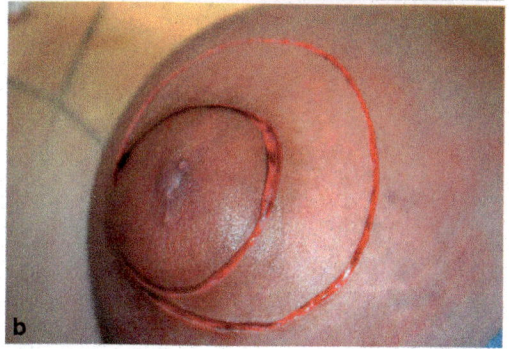

Fig. 11.2 (**a**) Extended crescent. (**b**) Generous extended crescent

11.4 Technique

The crescent skin excision can be generous (5–8 cm in width) or very restricted (Fig. 11.2). Additionally, one breast may need more skin excised than the other breast (Fig. 11.3). The author generally performs the initial lift on the more ptotic side first and then matches the second side with the first excision. The more extensive the breast ptosis, the more aggressive will be the crescent lift in width and length. The "extended crescent" can become very aggressive, almost circumareolar in shape. This will achieve the greatest amount of superficial breast tissue removal and lift. Traditionally, the standard crescent incision is semicircular in nature and can be rotated as needed if medialization of the NAC lift is also desired (Fig. 11.3). The depth of the incision and subsequent skin excision do not traverse the complete depth of the dermis. This "half-depth" excision leaves the reticular dermis intact so that our superficial skin excision simply disarticulates the papillary dermis from the reticular dermis. Therefore, deepithelialization actually means removal of the epidermis and portions of the papillary dermis while leaving the reticular dermis bed intact over the underlying fat and breast tissue. As the reticular dermis is closely attached to the underlying superficial layer of the anterior STF and Cooper's ligaments link this structure to the deep layer of the above fascia, one can understand why the crescent mastopexy has such strength and capacity to lift. The reticular dermis is attached to the deeper Cooper's ligaments and the closure itself causes lift without undermining breast skin (Fig. 11.4) [18].

Crescent mastopexy lifts may be used in concert with breast augmentation by any approach. The author often uses the TUBA method to avoid dissection through breast parenchyma. Alternatively, a superior–medial periareolar incisional approach to breast augmentation can be used, which is well camouflaged within the crescent lift incision (Fig. 11.5). After deepithelialization at the papillo-reticular dermal junction, a beautiful white fibrous layer of reticular dermis should be present. The surgical orientation of our crescent can be used to perform a number of actions, for example, (1) NAC lifting, (2) NAC shifting medially or laterally, (3) NAC reduction, (4) repositioning the NAC inferiorly, or (5) a combination of the above procedures.

The arc length of the crescent arch (and therefore its closure) is dependent on the diameter and the circumference of the NAC. The extended crescent mastopexy can be accomplished using a "near" circumareolar incision by sparing the inferior aspect of the NAC. The author

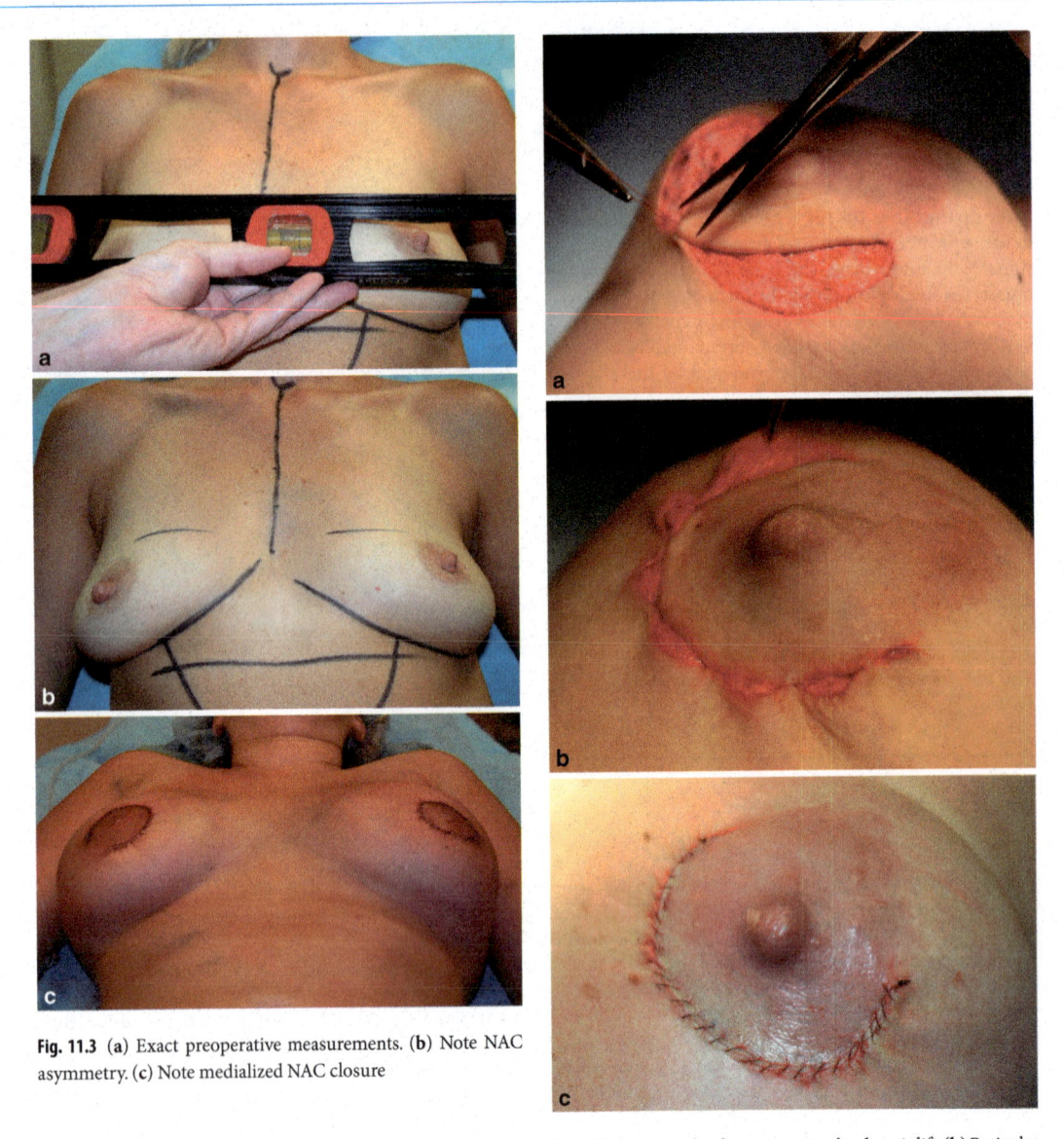

Fig. 11.3 (a) Exact preoperative measurements. (b) Note NAC asymmetry. (c) Note medialized NAC closure

Fig. 11.4 (a) Reticular dermis to reticular dermis lift. (b) Reticular dermis closure. (c) Final closure

has purposely avoided the Bennelli purse-string suture closures and has thus eliminated any Bennelli suture breast flattening with its associated NAC de projection. He has also been able to avoid skin puckering problems. The crescent extension allows for excellent closure with a more aggressive lift, similar to a Benelli lift, but without the purse-string suture [19].

The crescent closure is vital to the lift process and its overall results. Six to eight centimeter lifts are possible with the extended crescent mastopexy on larger breasts. Usually, one breast is different from the other in size, shape, and NAC orientation because "breasts are sisters not twins [20]." The author has tried many types of possible crescent closures. For example, A 3-0 or 4-0 Monocryl interrupted dermal closure with tiny horizontal mattress suture "bites" works nicely (Fig. 11.6). Vicryl sutures may extrude through the skin before they dissolve and the author avoids this braided suture material. The closure is done in an interrupted fashion by the "half to half to half" technique until a sufficient lift and wound

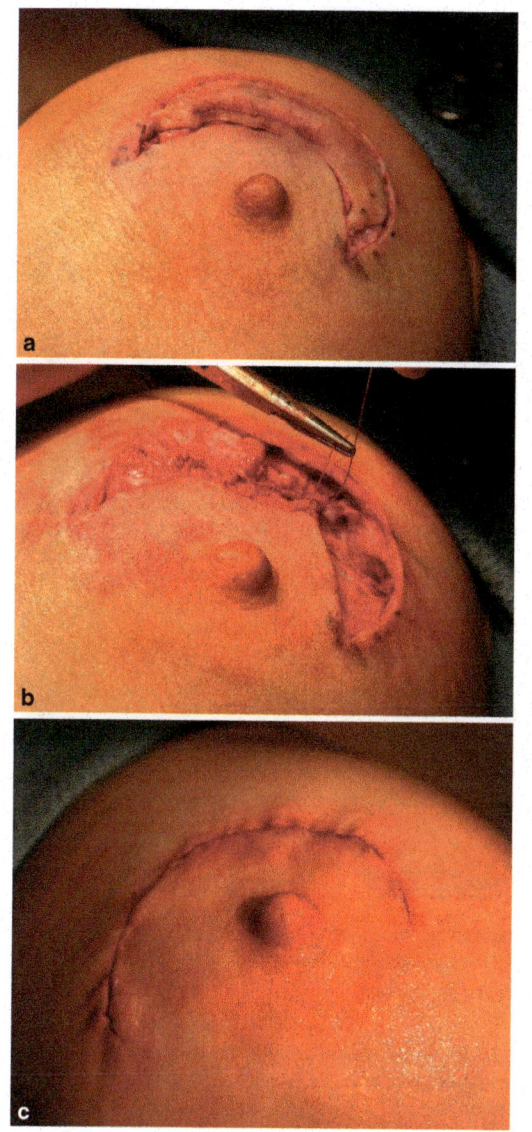

Fig. 11.5 (a) Periareolar approach camouflaged within crescent. (b) Periareolar closure within crescent. (c) Dermal closure over periareolar/crescent lift approach

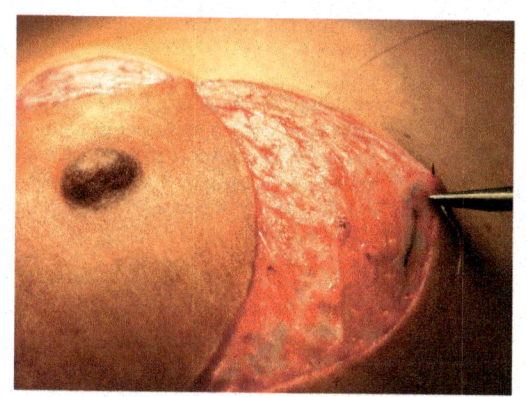

Fig. 11.6 Small horizontal mattress "bites" with Monocryl

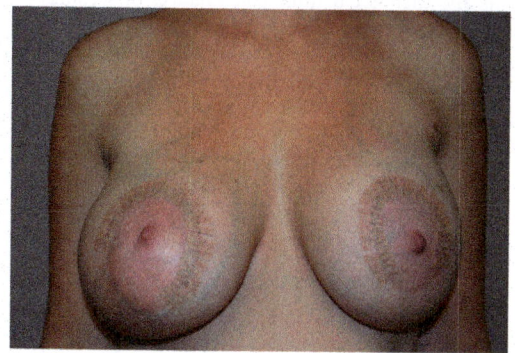

Fig. 11.7 Micropore Steri-Strips

approximation is achieved. Thereafter, a subcuticular 4-0 nylon suture will usually finish the closure. Sometimes, 6-0 or 5-0 interrupted nylon can also be used superficially. Another approach, especially on firm breasted nulliparous women, is to use a running locked 5-0 nylon or 5-0 plain gut suture over the initial 3-0 or 4-0 Monocryl sutures. Antitension closure methods with help from the surgical assistant, by the pinch technique, are very important. This will improve the suture line closure. Another option, after performing a secondary subcuticular closure, is the intraoperative use of the sterile, flesh colored steri-strips, along with benzoin or mastasol, as a third layer of closure (Fig. 11.7). Care should be taken not to allow any nonsterile adhesive solution to touch the incision site. Generally, 7–14 days of wound healing is allowed before using sterile Steri-Strips on the crescent wound. By this time, the incision is healing well without increasing the chance of chemical irritation or topical infection. Also, the fresh closure can be better monitored by visual inspection without Steri-Strips or the need to constantly replace them. Frequent Steri-Strip replacement can make tiny tears in a recent wound closure. Later, after the wound has matured and Steri-strips are no longer needed, topical antiscarring agents such as Cicaplast® or Mederma® may be used.

The crescent lift scar can be excised later if healing is suboptimal secondary to hypertrophic scarring. It is wise to wait about 6 months before re-excision and closure of any hypertrophic scars, as this will give the best chance for improved healing. Monofilament suture material for closure should be used. Occasionally, intradermal triamcinalone injections may be needed at alternate-week intervals. The crescent mastopexy procedure can be performed over and over again throughout the lifetime of the patient, if needed, by using the same process.

11.5 Complications

Complications from "traditional" mastopexy operations are numerous, while the crescent lift mastopexy has far less problems or complications. There are no concerns of failed glandular flaps or fat necrosis with crescent lifts and there are definitely no chances of seromas or hematomas from a nipple lift procedure. However, periareolar scarring can be significant (Fig. 11.8) and NAC hyperpigmentation or hypopigmentation can also occur (Fig. 11.9). Dehiscence, local wound infection, and NAC necrosis are certainly possible but extremely rare. Asymmetry is possible and can take the form of improper NAC placement on the breast mound. The correct vertical height, diameter, and shape of the NAC are challenging symmetries to create, but, most certainly, can be achieved (Fig. 11.10). The loss of nipple sensation should not be a problem with crescent mastopexy, as the lateral cutaneous intercostal nerves are not disrupted. Lactation and breast-feeding should be unaffected as no glandular disruption occurs with crescent lifts. Any under-corrected lift can be improved by a future secondary surgery using the previous incision lines under local anesthesia or conscious sedation. It is

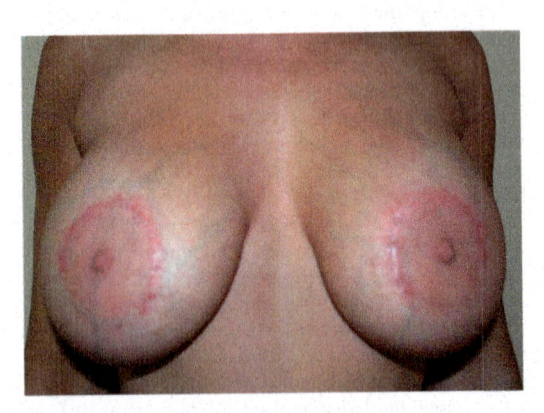

Fig. 11.8 Significant periareolar scarring (Vicryl suture)

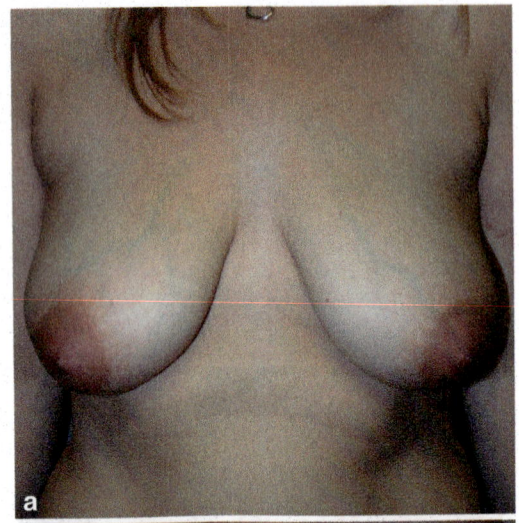

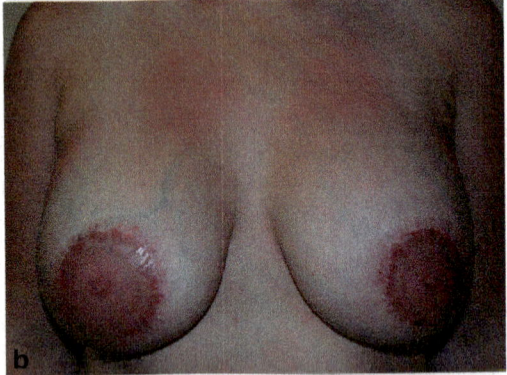

Fig. 11.9 (a) Preoperative transumbilical breast augmentation and extended crescent mastopexy. (b) Moderate postoperative hyperpigmentation

best to wait 6 months before attempting a secondary crescent procedure.

11.6 Discussion

The crescent mastopexy and the modified extended crescent mastopexy techniques are very effective for patients who exhibit glandular ptosis and grade I NAC ptosis (Fig. 11.11). Grade II ptosis can be treated with breast augmentation while using the extended NAC crescent lift (Fig. 11.12). However, grade III ptosis may respond best to vertical or inverted "T" mammaplasties

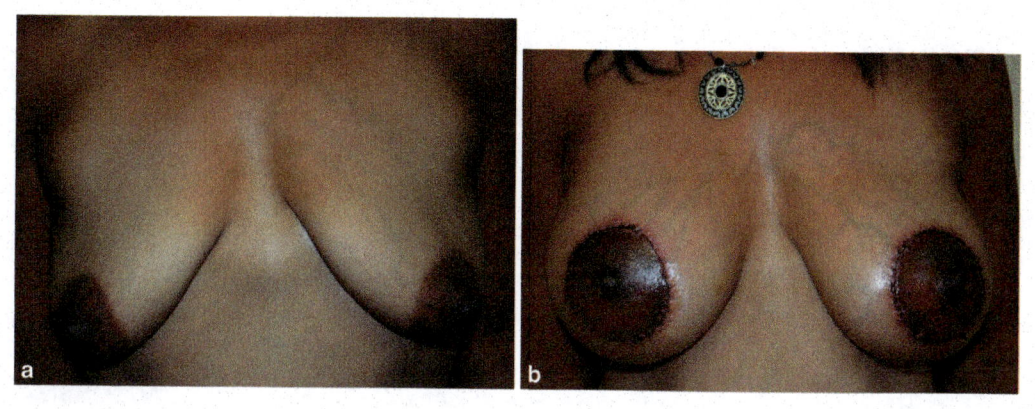

Fig. 11.10 (a) Preoperative transumbilical breast augmentation and extended crescent lift. (b) Postoperative efforts to achieve symmetry

and the surgeon must be the judge and jury (Fig. 11.13). In any case, it is important to match the type of lifting needed to accomplish specific goals. The surgeon should do the least amount of surgery possible and yet try to achieve the maximum amount of improvements. In other words, "less can be more." Moreover, simply placing large subglandular implants into a ptotic breast will not treat the underlying problem. A large prepectoral implant may fill a deflated breast envelope, but there is no actual lifting of the NAC or mammary gland itself. Over time, the breast will become more ptotic with the weight of prepectoral implants because many of the supporting fibers of Cooper will have been disrupted. Large subglandular implantations may lead to further ptosis in the future.

It is always much wiser to use appropriately sized implants for each patient. One must determine the correct base width/height of the breast and use the full spectrum of low, medium, or high profile saline or silicone implants, in your implant decision-making, to achieve the desired cup size. Thereafter, the surgeon should further determine how much lifting is needed. The crescent and extended crescent mastopexy with appropriate implantation will produce excellent, long lasting results for patients who exhibit up to grade II nipple ptosis. The use of multiple crescent lifts, or the possible application of more aggressive mastopexy procedures, should be discussed with patients who possess grade III ptosis. In any event, all patients must know the exact location and extent of any expected breast scars.

11.7 Conclusions

The crescent mastopexy and extended crescent mastopexy are powerful surgical tools that can be successfully combined with suitably chosen breast augmentation cases. There are minimal complications compared to other mastopexy procedures [21]. The exceptional versatility of these types of lifts can be used to correct nipple asymmetry, improve NAC positioning, and perform areolar reductions. Problems with breast feeding, skin puckering, loss of sensation, scarring, hematoma, seroma, necrosis, and wound healing delays or infections are

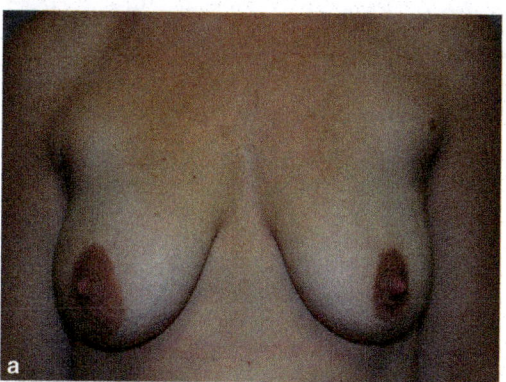

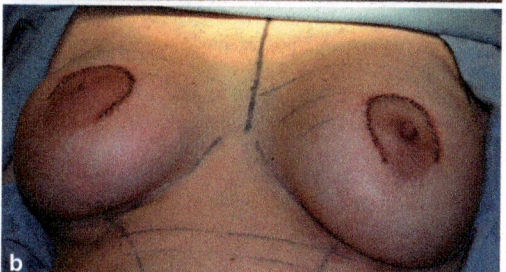

Fig. 11.11 (a) Grade I ptosis. (b) Grade I ptosis after transumbilical breast augmentation/crescent lift

62   11 Crescent Mastopexy

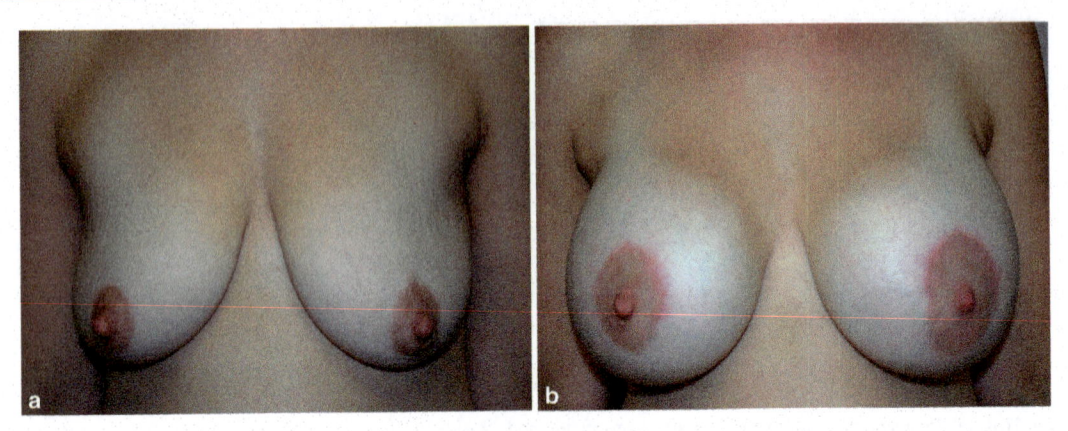

Fig. 11.12 (**a**) Grade II ptosis. (**b**) Grade II ptosis after transumbilical breast augmentation/aggressive crescent mastopexy

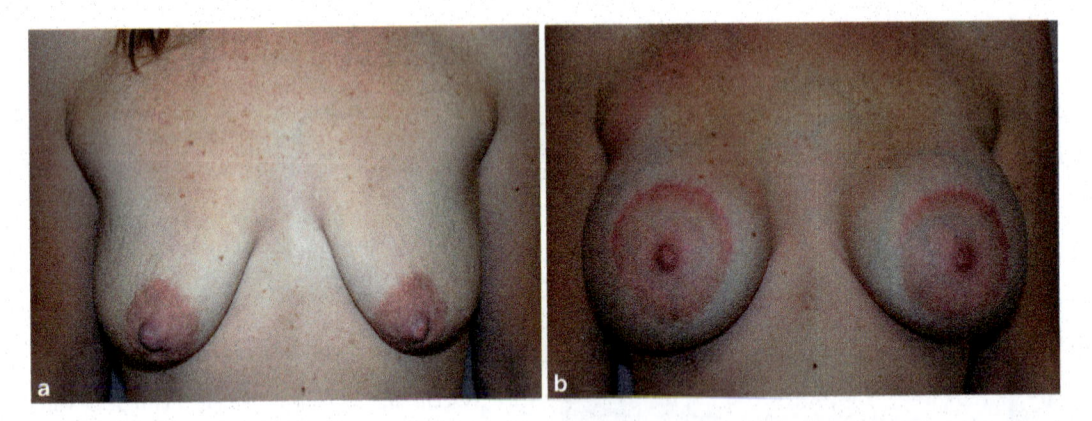

Fig. 11.13 (**a**) Grade III ptosis. (**b**) Grade III ptosis after transumbilical breast augmentation and extended crescent mastopexy

almost nonexistent. The crescent lift can be mastered by all well-trained cosmetic surgeons and may be repeated a number of times without additional scarring. The scar from a crescent mastopexy is "as good as it gets." In conclusion, the use of the crescent and extended crescent mastopexy should be in the repertoire of every cosmetic breast surgeon. If appropriately used, the crescent lift "elevates" us a little closer to the ideals endorsed by Lejour and many other prominent cosmetic breast surgeons the world over: beautiful, symmetrical breasts without scars.

References

1. Lejour M: Vertical mammaplasty: update and appraisal of late results. Plast Reconstr Surg 1999;104(3):771–781
2. Lejour M: Vertical mammaplasty and liposuction of the breast. Plast Reconstr Surg 1994;94(1):100–114
3. Skoog T: A technique of breast reduction: transposition of the nipple on a cutaneous vascular pedicle. Acta Chir Scand 1963;26:453–465
4. Strombeck JO: Mammaplasty: report of a new technique based on the two pedicle procedure. Br J Plast Surg 1960;13:79–90
5. Aubert V: Hypertrophie mammaire de la puberte. Resection pertielle restauratrice. Arch Franco Belges Chir 1923;3:284–289
6. Beisenberger H: Deformitaten und Kosmetische Operationen der Weiblichen Brust. Mandrich, Vienna 1931
7. Pitanguy I: Breast hypertrophy. Transactions of the International Society of Plastic Surgeons, 2nd Congress. Livingstone, Edinburgh, UK 1960, p 509

References

8. Lassus C: A technique for breast reduction. Int Surg 1970;53(1):69
9. Skoog T: Plastic Surgery: New Methods and Refinements. Stockholm, Almquist and Wiksell 1974
10. Hamilton WJ: Textbook of Human Anatomy, 2nd edn. London, McMillan 1966
11. Serafin D: Anatomy of the breast. In: Georgiade NG (ed) Reconstructive Breast Surgery. St. Louis, Mosby 1976, pp 18
12. Wuringer E, Mader N, Posch E, Holle J: Nerve and vessel supplying ligamentous suspension of the mammary gland. Plast Reconstr Surg 1998;101(6):1486–1493
13. Cooper AP: On the anatomy of the breast. London, Longman, Orme, Green, Brown and Longmans 1840
14. Maliniac JW: Arterial blood supply of the breast. Arch Surg 1943;47:329
15. Chang WH, Petry JJ: The breast an atlas of reconstruction. London, William & Wilkins 1984, pp 1–9
16. Craig RD, Sykes PA: Nipple sensitivity following reduction mammaplasty. Br J Plast Surg 1970;23(2):165–172
17. Farina MA, Newby BG, Alani HM: Innervation of the nipple areola complex. Plast Reconstr Surg 1980;66(4):497–501
18. Lockwood T: Reduction mammaplasty and mastopexy with superficial fascial system suspension. Plast Reconstr Surg 1999;103(5):1411–1420
19. Benelli L: A new periareolar mammaplasty: the "round block" technique. Aesthetic Plast Surg 1990;14(2):93–100
20. Mangubat AE: Personal communication. American Board of Cosmetic Surgery Review Course, Dallas, TX 4th March 2000
21. Cruz-Korchin N, Korchin L: Vertical versus wise pattern breast reduction: patient satisfaction, revision rates and complications. Plast Reconstr Surg 2003;112(6):1573–1578

Benelli Concentric Mastopexy

Frank Schneider-Affeld

12.1 Introduction

Breast ptosis cannot be prevented. Depending on tissue quality, pregnancies, weight, fluctuations in weight and other strains, an organ that ideally points forward will, as it becomes less firm, bow to gravity and sag downward. Lifestyle and the media have both played a role in propagating an ideal that is seen in women aged about 20, provided the aforementioned factors are not experienced. The aim of corrective surgery is to recreate the ideal (Fig. 12.1) and lift the nipple areolar complex (NAC), as well as achieve long-term stability. Ideally, such an intervention should not be visible to others, that is, there should be no conspicuous scarring.

Renault's classification of ptosis (1976) [1] is still valid today. Some authors have made modifications or have pointed to dependencies relative to weight [2].

While in the US, the inverted T technique has remained the preferred surgical standard, in South America and Europe, scar-sparing, vertical, and circumareolar techniques have been developed. The appeal of the latter techniques lies in the single scar that, ideally, is discretely positioned on the margin of the areola, at the border between the darker and lighter skin. This would be fine if there were not certain limitations, which are listed and discussed in this chapter. Given the right indication and technique, circumareolar mastopexy (CM) is an extremely satisfactory operation for both the patient and the physician (Fig. 12.2a, b).

12.2 History

Dieffenbach [3] reported in 1848 on esthetic breast surgery involving a "small" incision in the submammary fold (SMF). It was not until 80 years later that the first attempts were made to improve the appearance of the breast by removing skin above the NAC to lift the NAC [4–6]. A number of further incisions served to lift the breast envelope.

In 1969, Hinderer [7] reported for the first time on a circumareolar surgical technique. He restricted himself to patients with minor ptosis. Other authors followed suit [8–11]. These new techniques were principally developed in South America and Europe and were used, in part, on patients with more severe ptosis [12–14]. In the US, however, for understandable and often legal reasons, the inverted T remained the standard operation.

Despite the attraction of abstaining from a vertical scar, these new techniques were often difficult to reproduce or led to a flattening of the projection and problems in the area around the circumareolar scar with scar hypertrophies, scar spreading, and flattening of the NAC.

After "palpating" the limits, today the circu-mareolar technique is, as a rule, restricted to grade I or maximum grade II ptosis, with limited skin resection and limited NAC lifting, glandular rearrangement for internal stabilization of the breast, and the mandatory purse-string suture with nonabsorbable material.

If consideration is given to these principles and patients are chosen critically in terms of skin quality and breast size, then CM today has a rightful place in the correction of minor to moderate ptosis (I°–II°), and is frequently combined with breast reduction or augmentation, although the latter combination is viewed critically [15].

12.3 Technique

CM attempts to combine a correction of the position of the NAC with barely visible scarring on the outer margin of the areolas, that is, on the border between the pigmented and unpigmented skin with, as far as possible, stabilization of the inner breast, that is, the usually glandular tissue of the breast.

Renault [1] developed a ptosis classification that is still valid today and is based on the level of the NAC and the lower breast contour, both in relation to the SMF (Table 12.2).

While the NAC can be lifted via the removal of a crescent-shaped section of skin from 9 to 3 O' clock, with a concentric incision pattern, in addition to possible reduction of the NAC, the breast envelope can also be tightened. In the case of eccentric incisions, the "crescent" effect can additionally be utilized (Fig. 12.2a). All corrections are performed by means of de-epithelialization.

M.A. Shiffman (ed.), *Mastopexy and Breast Reduction: Principles and Practice,*
© Springer-Verlag Berlin Heidelberg 2009

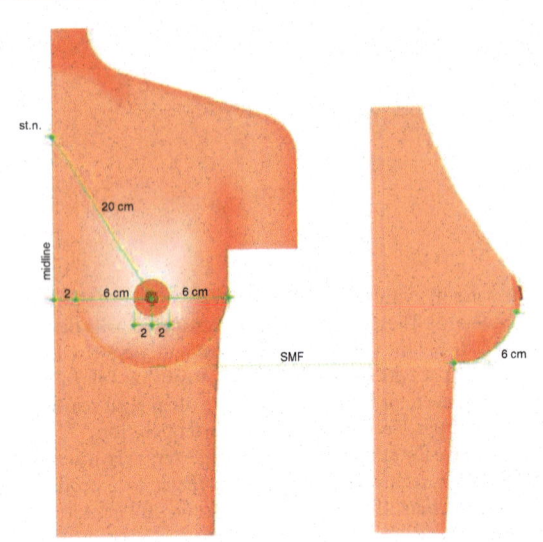

Fig. 12.1 The "Pretty" breast

Table 12.1 Renault's classification of Ptosis

I° (minor)	Nipple level with SMF
II° (moderate)	Nipple below SMF but above lower breast contour
III° (severe)	Nipple below SMF but level with lower breast contour
Glandular Ptosis	Nipple above SMF, glandular body below SMF
Pseudoptosis	Nipple above SMF, glandular body below SMF, hypoplasia

The tightening of the breast envelope can, at least with limited skin resection, only be achieved very discretely.

12.4 A Critical Comment on the "Ideal" Breast Shape

Renault's classification is still used today as the diagnostic basis for therapeutic measures for correcting ptotic breasts. His classification does not take weight or skin quality into account. The definition of glandular ptosis is not realistic in this regard. A large, that is, heavy breast must, with just a few exceptions, lie in the bottom portion, with the silhouette below the SMF. The medial, lateral, and lower radii of the "ideal" breast should all be approximately 6 cm. If the breast sags but retains these proportions, the appearance remains harmonious. The definition "glandular ptosis" is justified only when the lower radius extends to >6–7 cm. The perception of an ideal breast where the glandular body is normally above the SMF warps reality and creates the false impression among physicians and patients of a pathological condition that in reality is none and therefore does not require correction.

Scar widening or scar hypertrophy (Figs. 12.4, 12.5), deformation (Fig. 12.6) and flattening (Fig. 12.7) of the NAC, and wrinkling (Fig. 12.8) are typical consequences of skin resection. To minimize this risk, the diameter of the skin resection should be at most twice as large as that of the new NAC [16, 17].

The human skin is elastic and will "give" in the long run, even if the skin is closed using a good technique. As the scar is subjected to tension even with moderate skin resection, additional stabilization measures are required.

Both Peled [8] in 1985, followed by Benelli [13] in 1990 (round block), reported on the so-called pursestring suture. (Fig. 12.9) Here, the large outer ring is drawn together via a 38–42 sizer using nonabsorbable suture and tightened into a recessed knot.

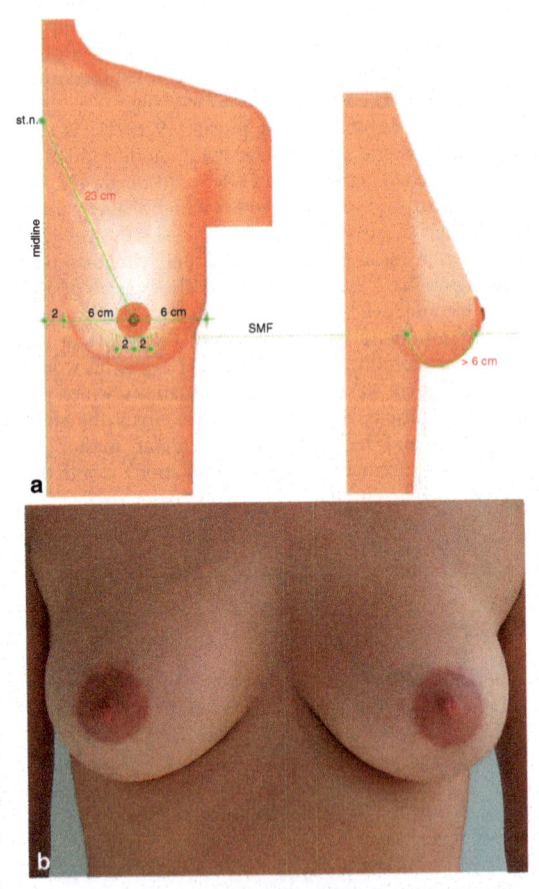

Fig. 12.2 (**a**) Minor Ptosis (I°). (**b**) Minor Ptosis (I°) 2 years after eccentric mastopexy with good result (Photo from H. Meyer, Hamburg)

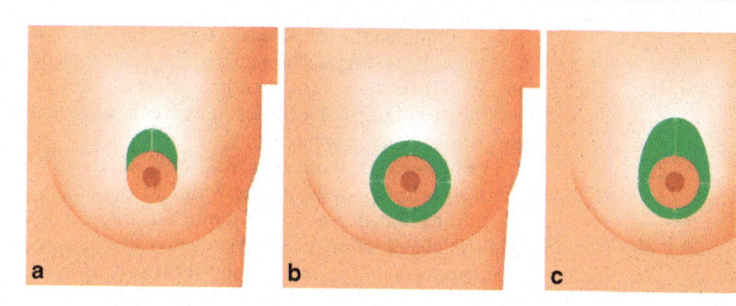

12.4 A Critical Comment on the "Ideal" Breast Shape

Fig. 12.3 Excision patterns: (**a**) Crescent. (**b**) Concentric. (**c**) Eccentric

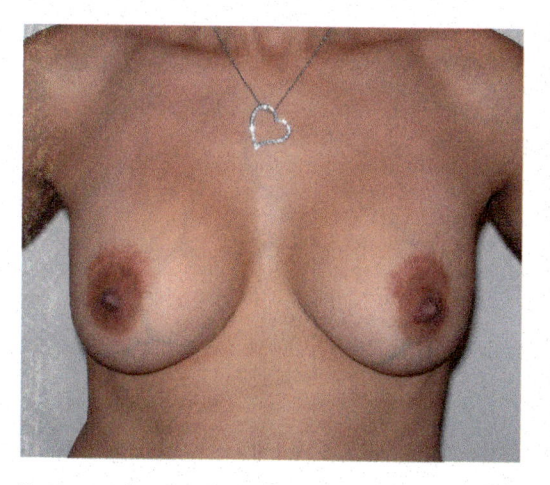

Fig. 12.4 Scar hypertrophy 6 months after crescent mastopexy

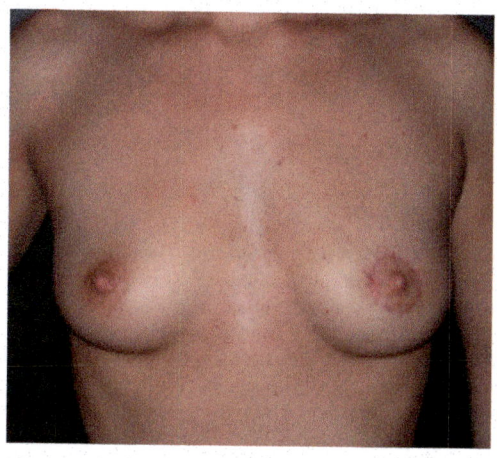

Fig. 12.6 Wrinkling of left side after eccentric mastopexy

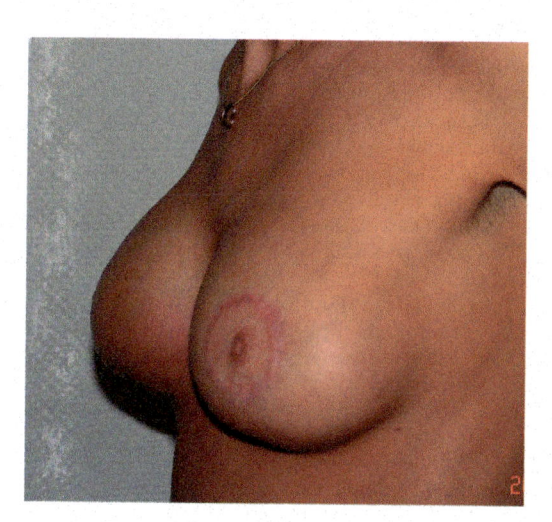

Fig. 12.5 Scar hypertrophy and flattening of the breast after eccentric mastopexy and breast augmentation

Today this is regarded as mandatory. Some authors, however, go beyond these generally accepted levels of skin tightening [7, 13].

Further stability is achieved via glandular rearrangement (or reshaping). With this technique, after appropriate mobilization, the mammary gland is normally fixed to the pectoral fascia using nonabsorbable sutures [7, 12, 17–21]. Periosteal fixation has also been described (Benelli [13]). Glandular rearrangement is generally recommended.

The additional insertion of nets to act as an internal bra has been published by Goes [12] and Bustos [14]. On the whole, however, this has been received with caution. The goal of all these measures is long-term stability, an improved projection, and upper pole fullness.

As a rule, it can be said that the size, that is, the weight, of breasts is inversely proportional to long-term performance. This applies to both the body's own tissue and foreign tissue (implants).

Inconspicuous scars, as seen with CM, at the expense of a good projection and long-term stability, are a poor solution. In the case of mild ptosis and small-to-

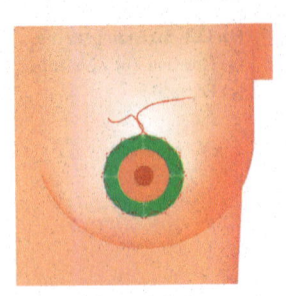

Fig. 12.7 Pursestring

medium-sized breasts, however, there are a large number of options available. CM is by far the best solution.

12.5
Complications

If CM is indicated to correct ptosis, it must be carefully considered to what extent shape and long-term performance could be negatively affected. The different views of patients and physicians must be discussed prior to making any decision. Although the satisfaction of the patient must be given priority, the latter is unable to assess long-term performance and the frequency of side effects. When given the choice, patients invariably prefer the circumareolar scar to the vertical scar, in the belief that the scar will not be visible on them.

It is the physician's task during preoperative briefing to get the patient to consider not easily recognized changes in the decision making process. To do this, however, he must be aware of facts that sometimes go beyond his own scope of experience.

First and foremost, wide and, in part, hypertrophic scars are stated to have an incidence of more than 50%. Revision surgery is required slightly less frequently to correct such scarring, and with vertical techniques the incidence of such revision surgery is considerably lower (CM: 50%, vertical techniques: 18–25%) [22]. Further complications include flattening of the projection and flattening of the NAC. Glandular "bottoming out" is, in contrast, less frequent compared with the vertical techniques [22]. Based on a review of nine earlier publications, it can be concluded that despite consistent use of purse-string suture, scar widening and deformation of the shape of the NAC are the main long-term criticisms (Table 12.2) [7, 13, 17, 19-24]. Hinderer thus always included a scar revision after 3–6 months in the primary operation. Nevertheless, he too conceded that in principle, a better shape and projection can be achieved with the vertical techniques.

Depending on the invasiveness, especially in the case of the glandular surgical component, the circulation and nerve supply (sense) of the NAC may be compromised.

As with all operations, the less invasive the intervention, the fewer the complications.

The following statements meet with general agreement: additional augmentation with CM extends the indications but increases the number of side effects. Additional reduction with CM reduces the number of side effects and stabilizes long-term performance [15].

12.6
Discussion

The idea of improving the projection in the long-term and lifting the NAC with barely visible scarring is fascinating and, if properly indicated, highly satisfactory for both the patient and the surgeon. However, the stumbling blocks are the details.

Three questions are raised:
1. How far may the NAC have sagged down from the "ideal position," that is, how many centimeters can the NAC be raised?
2. To what extent can the shape of the envelope be changed without causing injury to it as a result of vertical scarring? What effect does this have on the projection?
3. How stable are such efforts in the long term?

Eccentric incisions around the NAC (Fig. 12.3c) are performed most frequently. This allows the NAC to be raised between 1 cm and a maximum of 3 cm (if necessary in several steps) and also reduced in size to conform to the "ideal proportions" of 38–42 mm.

The NAC can only be lifted if the position of the nipple is either level with the SMF or projects over it. That means 3 cm or less. Almost all authors agree that if the NAC is positioned below the SMF in the projection, vertical tightening becomes necessary [16, 17, 19, 20, 22–25]. Circulation and innervation of the NAC are in no way compromised by de-epithelialization on its own.

In 1985, Peled [8] described the purse-string suture with nonabsorbable suture (12.9 formerly 12.7!) material for closing skin defects for the first time. In the case of mastopexy, this suture joins the outer, that is, larger, circumference with the smaller circumference, that is, the new margin of the NAC.

To additionally increase the strength of the scar, an indication of its limited durability, some authors recommend doubling or even tripling this pursestring suture

Table 12.2 Complications of concentric mastopexy

	Rohrich 06	Spear 01	Benelli 98	Brink 93	Baran 01	Hinderer 01	Elliott 02	Card.-C. 06	Gruber 06
N°	487	?	98	93	?	203	Since 6 years	196	9
NAC-widening		×	×			×			
NAC-flattening		×	×		×	×		14 Patients	0
Scar-widening	62%	×	0.20%		×			24 Patients	2 Patients
Scar-hypertrophy	50%	×			×			2 Patients	1 Patient
Wrinkling				Occasionally		×	1 Patient		
Rupture of suture				2 Patients			1 Patient		
Reduced long time stability								24 Patients	
Misshaped breast					×				
Revision	50%					Always			

[7, 27]. Today, this suture, with or without reinforcement, is regarded as mandatory for CM.

Although tightening of the envelope by removing preferably large concentric or eccentric skin portions sounds attractive, it does have its limitations. While Benelli and Hinderer [7, 13] perform surgery on all grades of ptosis, the majority of authors point to the limitations that Spear defined for the first time in 1990 in his guidelines [16]. According to these, the diameter of the skin resection should be at most twice as large as that of the new NAC. Loose skin (tuberous breast) and a large NAC allow this limiting value to be exceeded [17]. The inevitable wrinkling is thus kept to a minimum and, because it is not particularly pronounced, disappears after several months without the need for additional corrective surgery. In addition, a narrow dissection zone around the excision serves to smooth the unavoidable wrinkles. In risk cases, however, this may also jeopardize the blood circulation of the NAC.

The NAC itself is comprised of soft, elastic skin. The measures outlined above reduce the tendency for scar widening and flattening of the NAC due to continual tension to <50% [22]. This must at least be regarded as a partial success of this procedure. The existence of a "fibrous scar" as postulated by Benelli, which offers additional strength and durability, could not be confirmed. Attempts by Carreras to replace the purse-string suture (nonabsorbable) with slow-absorbing sutures and to hope for the above-mentioned stability from internal scar formation or to remove the purse-string suture after an extended period of time have not resulted in the desired stability [23].

CM should be combined with glandular rearrangement. This is regarded as mandatory or, at the very least, advisable by many surgeons [7, 12, 17–20, 27, 28].

This internal rearrangement reduces the pressure from the lower portions of the breast and increases the pressure in the central and upper portion where, as a rule, it is normally found in women aged 20, prior to pregnancy.

Excision of the glandular body can further reduce tissue pressure, that is, relieve skin strain, while so the elasticity of the skin causes the envelope to shrink, making it appear smaller [24]. All skin is elastic. There are nevertheless major genetic differences and, above all, cases of prior lesion, for example, following pregnancies and fluctuations in weight (striae). A typical indicator for good or poor skin retraction is the involution of the abdominal wall following pregnancies.

The insertion of meshes to stabilize the glandular body is probably a measure with good long-term results [12, 14]. This approach, however, is rightly criticized as it reduces the effectiveness of mammography controls and causes image artifacts [26, 29]. One in nine women will develop breast cancer at some point in their lives, so prevention must be given priority over esthetic aspects.

In the case of glandular ptosis, the effectiveness of CM is limited. With glandular body bottoming out, that is, a NAC–SMF distance of >7 cm, vertical surgical techniques are required [7, 17, 18, 22, 25], unless the patient is willing to sacrifice this type of tightening and accept bottoming out in the lower portion of the breast to avoid scarring. Provided that the NAC is at the "ideal level" and the projection is esthetically pleasing, this shape is regarded as harmonious [19]. The correct level of the NAC is far more important than the tautness of the lower portion of the breast in terms of esthetics. This is already normally the case with large breasts, that is, the glandular component of the ptosis becomes greater with increasing cup size, that is to say, with heavier breasts.

Upper pole fullness is a special aspect; in America this is requested and even demanded, whereas in Northern Europe, a somewhat straighter upper silhouette is seen as attractive and natural. For the "dirndl" (a Southern German traditional dress worn in Munich that will enhance the upper breast curve), upper pole fullness can be simulated using standard push-up bras. The glandular component of CM can be easily adjusted slightly to meet these requirements.

The limits of CM are determined by the individual's skin quality, that is, a genetic component, and the prior strains to which the skin has been subjected, following pregnancies and fluctuations in weight. The presence of striae is often a sign of such strains.

As a rule, large and heavy breasts are less stable in the long term. On the one hand, there is a desire for a good, forward-pointing projection and, on the other hand, the reality of a load which is pulled down by gravity. It is therefore recommended that good-quality bras be worn for sporting as well as day-to-day activities as the breast does not contain muscular tissue that can be strengthened.

The idea of replacing lost tissue by means of augmentative surgery is particularly appealing. The projection is improved and the position of the NAC is changed by rotating upward and forward. Tightening of the breast is only possible to a very limited extent with this technique, as the cause of the ptosis is the increased softness of the tissue, which is a result of age or pregnancy. This softness cannot be remedied by increasing the volume. Rather, a double contour is formed where the soft tissue hangs above the correctly positioned implant. Tightening of the envelope with CM is only possible in a very restricted number of cases, and in many cases, a vertical component cannot be avoided.

The population of women who have undergone augmentation or lifting has aged. The number of requests for re-lifts or removal of the prosthesis has increased.

Revision surgery following augmentation and/or mastopexy is not without risks due to reduced blood circulation. The lower tissue pedicle is, as a result of the pressure, normally thinner than the upper pedicle, which means that the upper pedicle is essentially responsible for supplying the NAC. Whether with or without reaugmentation, the extent to which the NAC can be moved as part of CM is restricted to 1–2 cm.

Undercutting should remain near the surface and not go too deep in order not to jeopardize the supply in the remaining structures [30, 31]. Where there is doubt, a two-step approach is the safest solution [32].

The main goal of our work is patient satisfaction. The patient group is particularly challenging; the patients may have problems with ageing and not always realistic expectations. Surgeons often make a more positive assessment of the surgical results than the patients themselves [15, 20]. First and foremost, it is the scarring that negatively affects the assessment [33] however, the size of the breast and the amount of lift achieved also have a relatively negative effect on the way the outcome is viewed [22, 32]. Indeed, half of all patients would like minor or major revision surgery, although there is certainly a large chasm between this wish and its implementation [15].

A number of aspects must be reconciled with CM, including symmetry, scarring, shape and size of the NAC, position of the NAC and, if relevant, implant factors. One must at least discuss whether omission of the implant factor would reduce the complication rate and, as such, increase patient satisfaction [15]. Augmentation would then have to be performed in a second operation. The time required and costs involved argue against two-step surgery.

Since the issue of scarring is so important in patient assessments, it is hardly surprising that many CM patients prefer this technique despite the poorer projection achieved. In retrospect, however, if scar formation is inconspicuous, the question of shape comes to the fore again. "The scar doesn't bother me, it is the shape that's important": (patient's comment following vertical mastopexy).

It is clear that a CM gold standard does not exist. Correct decisions require intensive, time-consuming, and honest dialog between the patient and physician. The road to achieving the final goal must be calculable for both parties.

12.7
Conclusions

The appeal of CM lies in the single scar because, ideally, it is discretely positioned on the margin of the areola, at the border between the darker and lighter skin. However, three aspects need to be considered:
1. Limitation of the amount of skin resection and thus also NAC lifting
2. As far as possible, glandular rearrangement
3. A mandatory purse-string suture of nonabsorbable material

The main complications are widening of the NAC, flattening of the NAC, scar widening, scar hypertrophy, and flattening of the projection. The frequency of revision surgery to correct these problems is as high as 50%. Nevertheless, patient satisfaction is greater than with vertical techniques. CM is often combined with breast reduction or augmentation. The latter procedure is not without controversy.

If consideration is given to the above-mentioned principles and patients are chosen critically in terms of skin quality and breast size, then CM is an extremely satisfactory surgical procedure for both the patient and the physician.

References

1. Renault P: Breast ptosis. Definition and treatment. Clin Plast Surg 1976;3(2):193–203
2. Pinsky MA: Radial plication in concentric mastopexy. Aesthetic Plast Surg 2005;29(5):391–399
3. Dieffenbach JF: Die Operative Chirurgie, Leipzig, Brockhaus Verlag 1848
4. Eitner E: Kosmetische operationen – ein kurzer leitfaden für den praktiker, Wien. J Berlin, Springer 1932
5. Holländer E: Die opperation der mammahypertrophie und der hängebrust. Dtsch Med Wochenschr 1924; 41:1400
6. Joseph J: Zur operation der hypertrophischen hängebrust. Dtsch Med Wochenschr 1925;51:1103–1105
7. Hinderer UT: Circumareolar dermo-glandular plication: a new concept for correction of breast ptosis. Aesthetic Plast Surg 2001;25(6):404–420
8. Peled IJ, Zagher U, Wexler MR: Purse-string suture for reduction and closure of skin defects. Ann Plast Surg 1985;14(5):465–469
9. Erol ÖO, Spira M: A mastopexy technique for mild to moderate ptosis. Plast Reconstr Surg 1980;65(5):603–609
10. Gruber RP, Jones HW Jr: The "Donut" mastopexy: indications and complications. Plast Reconstr Surg 1980;65(1):34–38
11. Felicio Y: Mammoplastia de reducción con solo una incisión periareolar. Cir Plast Ibero-Latinoamer 1986;13:3
12. Sampaio Góes JC: Periareolar mammoplasty: double-skin technique with application of mesh support. Clin Plast Surg 2002;29(3):349–364
13. Benelli L: A new periareolar mammoplasty: the "round block" technique. Aesthetic Plast Surg 1990;14(2):93–100
14. Bustos RA: Periareolar mammaplasty with silicone supporting lamina. Plast Recontr Surg 1992;89(4):646–657
15. Spear SL, Pelletiere CV, Menon N: One-stage augmentation combined with mastopexy: aesthetic results and patient satisfaction. Aesthetic Plast Surg 2004; 28(5):259–267
16. Spear SL, Kassan M, Little JW: Guidelines in concentric mastopexy. Plast Reconstr Surg 1990;85(6):961–966
17. Spear SL, Giese SY, Ducic I: Concentric mastopexy revisited. Plast Reconstr Surg 2001;107(5):1294–1299

18. Rohrich RJ, Thornton JF, Jakubiets RG, Jakubiets MG, Grünert JG: The limited scar mastopexy: current concepts and approaches to correct breast ptosis. Plast Reconstr Surg 2002;114(6):1622–1630
19. Brink RR: Management of true ptosis of the breast. Plast Reconstr Surg 1993;91(4):657–662
20. Elliott LF: Circumareolar mastopexy with augmentation. Clin Plast Surg 2002;29(3):337–347
21. Quiao Q, Sun J, Liu C, Liu Z, Zhao R: Reduction mammoplasty and correction of ptosis: dermal bra technique. Plast Reconstr Surg 2003;111(3):1122–1130
22. Rohrich RJ, Gosman AA, Brown SA, Reisch J: Mastopexy preferences: a survey of board-certified plastic surgeons. Plast Reconstr Surg 2006;118(7):1631–1638
23. Baran CN, Peker F, Ortak T, Sensöz Ö, Baran NK: Unsatisfactory results of periareolar mastopexy with or without augmentation and reduction mammoplasty: enlarged areola with flattened nipple. Aesthetic Plast Surg 2001;25(4):286–289
24. Gruber R, Denkler K, Hvistendahl Y: Extended crescent mastopexy with augmentation. Aesthetic Plast Surg 2006; 30(3):269–274
25. Biggs TM: Concentric mastopexy revisited. Discussion. Plast Reconstr Surg 2001;107(5):1300
26. McKissock PK: Periareolar mammaplasty with silicone supporting lamina. Discussion. Plast Reconstr Surg 1992;89(4):658–659
27. Becker H: The dermal overlap subareolar mastopexy: a preliminary report. Aesth Surg J 2001;21(5):423–427
28. Ritz M, Silfen R, Southwick G: Fascial suspension mastopexy. Plast Reconstr Surg 2006;117(1):86–94
29. Spira M: Crescent mastopexy and augmentation. Discussion. Plast Reconstr Surg 1985;75(4):542–543
30. Rohrich RJ, Beran SJ, Restifo RJ, Copit SE: Aesthetic management of the breast following explantation: evaluation and mastopexy options. Plast Reconstr Surg 1998;101(3):827–837
31. Handel N: Secondary mastopexy in the augmented patient: a recipe for disaster. Plast Reconstr Surg 2006; 118(7 Suppl):152–163
32. Spear SL: Secondary mastopexy in the augmented patient: a recipe for disaster. Discussion. Plast Reconstr Surg 2006;118(7 Suppl):166–167
33. Fayman MS, Potgieter E, Becker PJ: Outcome study: periareolar mammaplasty patients' perspective. Plast Reconstr Surg 2003;111(2):676–684

Short Scar Mastopexy with Flap Transposition: The Concept of the Biological Implant in Cosmetic Breast Surgery

Moshe S. Fayman

13.1
Introduction

The goal of mastopexy is defined as reconstructing an aesthetically pleasing breast by remodeling the breast mound, by repositioning the nipple–areola complex (NAC) in an appropriate position, and by reducing a large areola to a proportionate size. The use of breast tissue as a biological implant is a novel idea that entrusts the surgeon with a powerful tool to sculpt the contour of the breast. The concept can be applied in various manners to obtain specific aesthetic goals.

13.2
History

Regnault defined breast ptosis as a descent of the breast gland, skin, and nipple from the chest wall. She proposed a classification system based on the relationship between the NAC and the submammary fold [1]. Brink distinguished true ptosis from glandular ptosis, pseudoptosis, and parenchymal maldistribution [2].

A multitude of techniques and algorithmic approaches proposed in the literature to correct breast ptosis attest the disagreement on the ideal solution [3–9]. Concerns related to scaring [10], asymmetry, "bottoming out," and more continue to haunt patients and surgeons alike [11].

The milestone technique for mastopexy and reduction mammaplasty was based on the key-hole incision as popularized by Wise [12].

Attempts at reducing scaring led to the introduction of periareolar incision by Andrews et al. [13], and other authors further developed this technique [14, 15]. The periareolar mastopexy was criticized for three reasons: flattening of the breast, widening of the periareolar scar, and early recurrence of the ptosis. Technical solutions offered in an attempt to address those issues included the Benelli periareolar suture [16, 17] and the internal mesh proposed by Goes [18, 19]. Qiao et al. and Gulyas proposed an internal "dermal bra" as an alternative to the mesh [20, 21]. Problems related to purse string suture rupture, exposure, and removal were reported in up to 10% of the cases [20, 22, 23].

Lassus, Peixoto, Lejour, and Chiari popularized the vertical mastopexy [24–30]. This approach was designed to improve breast projection by approximating the medial and lateral pillars of the breast through the vertical incision. A caudal "dog ear" resulted occasionally, which prompted Maharchac et al. to introduce a short inframammary incision [31].

The issue of projection of the breast was addressed by Fayman et al. [32] who proposed the use of dermoglandular breast flaps as biological implant. Rearrangement of breast tissue was proposed by Hall-Findlay and Hammond and others [21, 33–35].

13.3
Surgical Technique

The concept of using a flap transposition as a biological implant in mastopexy represents a philosophy rather then a rigid technique. The technique can be adapted in various manners in pursuit of specific aesthetic goals. It can be utilized in conjunction with a variety of nipple–areola supporting pedicles. The author employed this approach with superior, inferior, supero-medial, and supero-lateral pedicles. This technique was employed in mastopexy as well as in breast reduction procedures. It was used in cases of vertical mastopexy (moderate to mild ptosis), vertical mastopexy with a short horizontal scar (moderate to severe ptosis), and with a key hole pattern mastopexy (severe to extreme ptosis).

The following technical description will offer guidelines rather then a rigid "cook-book" recipe.

M.A. Shiffman (ed.), *Mastopexy and Breast Reduction: Principles and Practice,*
© Springer-Verlag Berlin Heidelberg 2009

13.3.1
Vertical Mastopexy

The patient is marked for a vertical mastopexy. The NAC is marked for reduction to the desired size (diameter of 35–45 mm) and the arch of the planned incision that represents the circumference of the proposed areolar is marked accordingly (Fig. 13.1a–e). The NAC is elevated on a breast tissue pedicle to a distance of 21–24 cm from the sternal notch on the breast meridian according to the patient's build. The inferior margin of the skin excision is placed some 2 cm cephalad to the inframammary fold on the breast meridian. The width of the skin excision varies according to the size of the breast and also must take into consideration whether reduction is planned.

A decision is also made as to whether to mobilize the nipple–areola complex as a superior, supero-medial, supero-lateral, or inferior pedicled flap (Figs. 13.1 and 13.2). Superior pedicle is adequate when NAC elevation is minimal (less then 2 cm). Supero-medial and supero-lateral pedicles are easier to transpose when a more substantial elevation is required. These pedicles allow transposition and thus prevent nipple retraction, which can occur when the superior pedicle is folded upon itself.

Inferior pedicle is selected when the NAC is placed close to the lower border of the breast.

The variations of the concept can be utilized as follows:
1. *Superior pedicle techniques*: Mastopexy with the nipple–areolar elevated on a superior, supero medial, or supero lateral pedicle. The lower pole of the breast is used for volume enhancement as an inferiorly pedicled flap behind the NAC. When the transposition flap is sufficiently long, it does produce sustainable upper pole fullness (Figs. 13.1f–h and 13.3–13.7)
2. *Inferior pedicle techniques*: The inferior pedicle bears the inherent risk of "bottoming out." In the authors view, inferior pedicle is the pedicle of choice when the NAC is pre-operatively placed close to the caudal

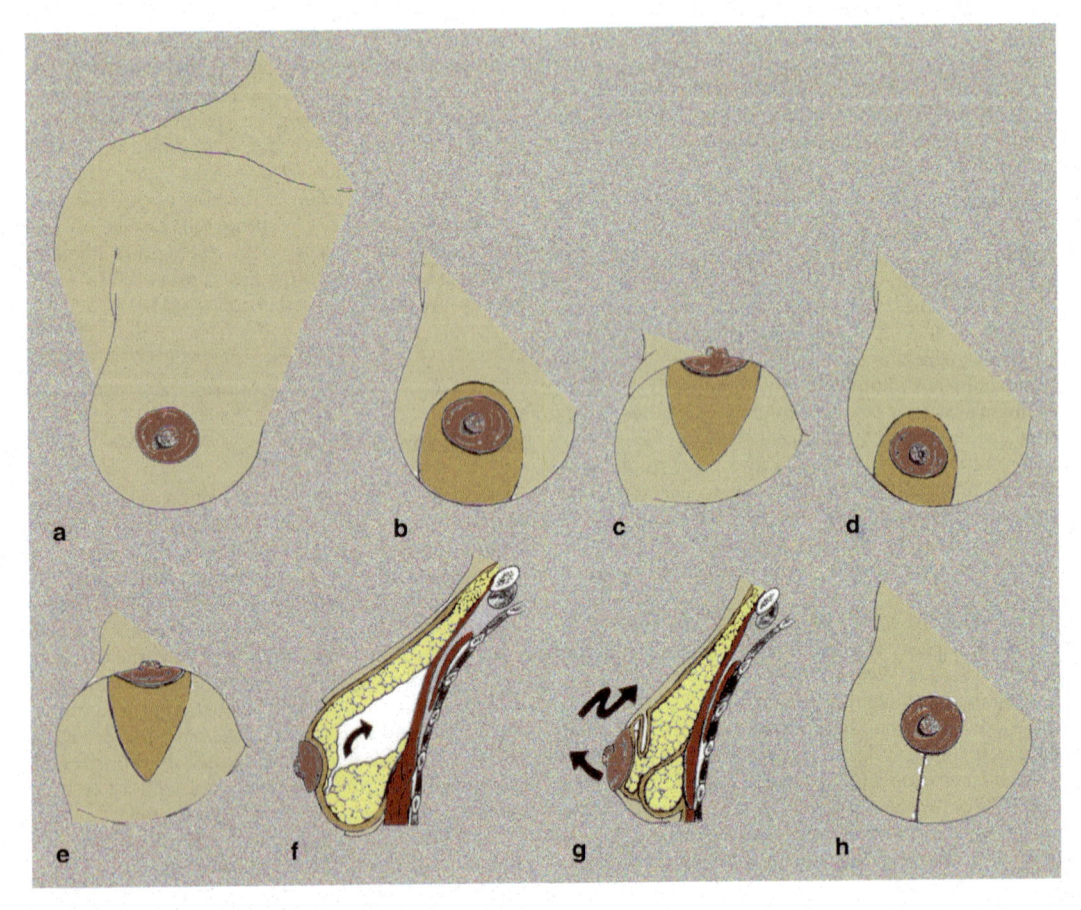

Fig. 13.1 (a–h) Superior pedicle

13.3 Surgical Technique   75

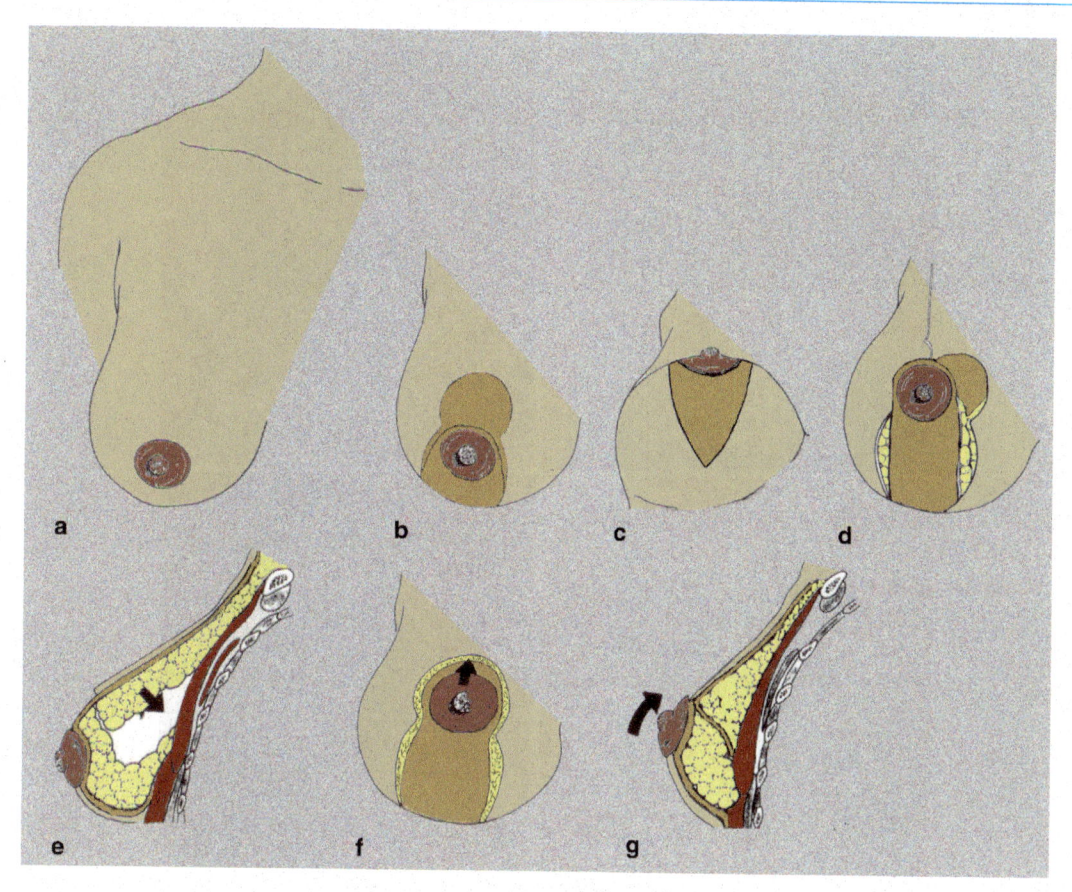

Fig. 13.2 (a–g) Inferior pedicle

border of the breast (Fig. 13.2). On this occasion, the inferior pedicle is substantially shorter than its superior counterpart, and carries a minimal risk of "bottoming out." When dealing with a short inferior pedicle, the blood supply of the flap appears superior to a long superior flap, adding to its attractiveness (Figs. 13.8 and 13.9).

3. *Extended superior pedicle techniques*: Mastopexy or breast reduction with the NAC mobilized as a superior, supero medial, or supero lateral pedicled flap. Continuation of the flap into the infra areola area is folded upon itself behind the NAC to increase projection (Figs. 13.10 and 13.11). This variation is useful in secondary cases that were primarily operated through a submammary incision. The old scar often severs the pedicle of the inferiorly pedicled dermo glandular flap, thus compromising its vascular supply. The extension of the superior flap is considered safer then an inferiorly pedicled dermoglandular flap with a scar across its pedicle.

The procedure is performed with the patient under a combination of local and IV sedation or general anesthesia. Deepithelialization is followed by incision and mobilization of the flaps. Dissection continues to the pre pectoral fascia to allow folding of the dermo glandular transposition flap (The "biological implant") behind the NAC. If the inferior flap technique is used, then the flap is anchored anterior to the breast parenchyma, which has been deepithelialized cephalad to the NAC. The superior flap is anchored to the pectoralis fascia. The medial and lateral breast pillars are approximated, and the skin is closed. Drains are seldom used. Adhesive dressing is utilized for 2–3 days and then just dry gauze is applied and held in position by means of a supportive brazier. Scar care includes massaging and application of silicone sheathing until scars mature.

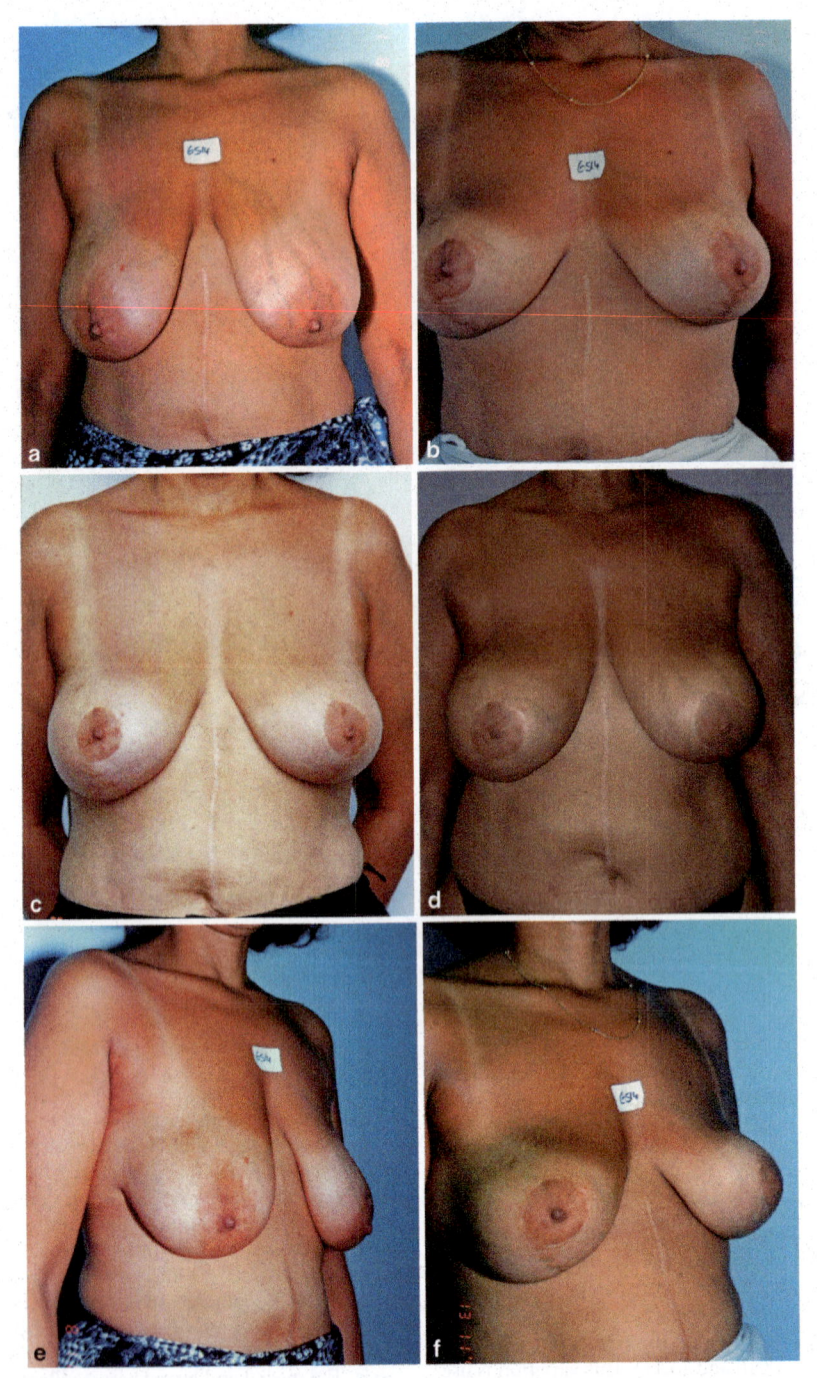

Fig. 13.3 A 42-year-old patient, mother of two underwent mastopexy through a vertical incision. NAC was mobilized as a supero lateral flap. The central portion of the breast was used as a biological implant behind the NAC. Sequential photographs of the patient were taken 1, 8, and 13 years after surgery. During this period, the patient underwent weight gain of 15 kg. The photos reveal that the breast flap maintained its position throughout this time and weight changes. This case illustrates the durability and longevity of the breast flap as a biological implant. (**a**) Pre op front view; (**b**) 1 year post op; (**c**) 8 years post op; (**d**) 13 years post op; (**e**) pre op oblique view; (**f**) 1 year post op;

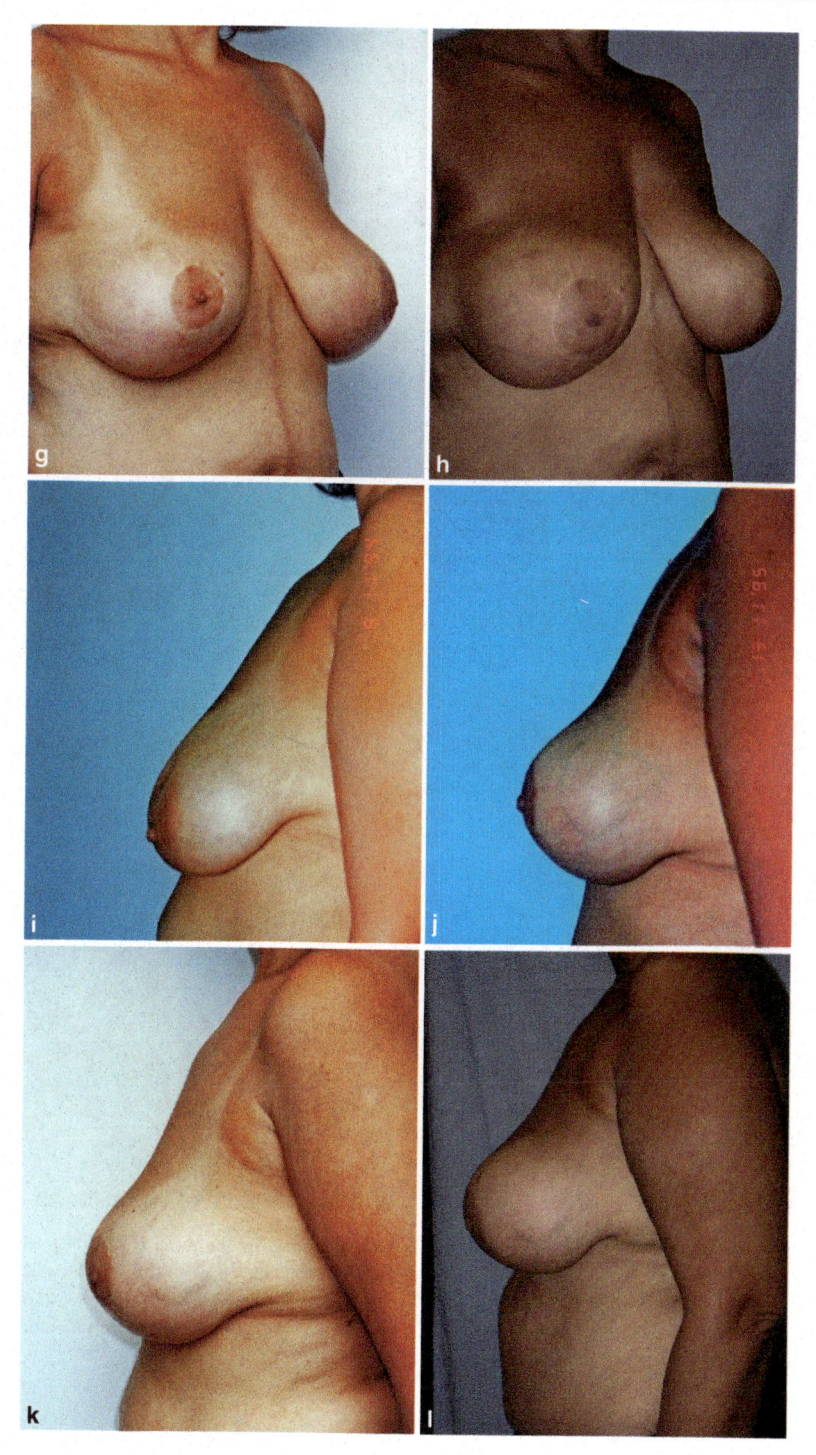

Fig. 13.3 *(continued)* (**g**) 8 years post op; (**h**) 13 years post op; (**i**) pre op lateral view; (**j**) 1 year post op; (**k**) 8 years post op; (**l**) 13 years post op

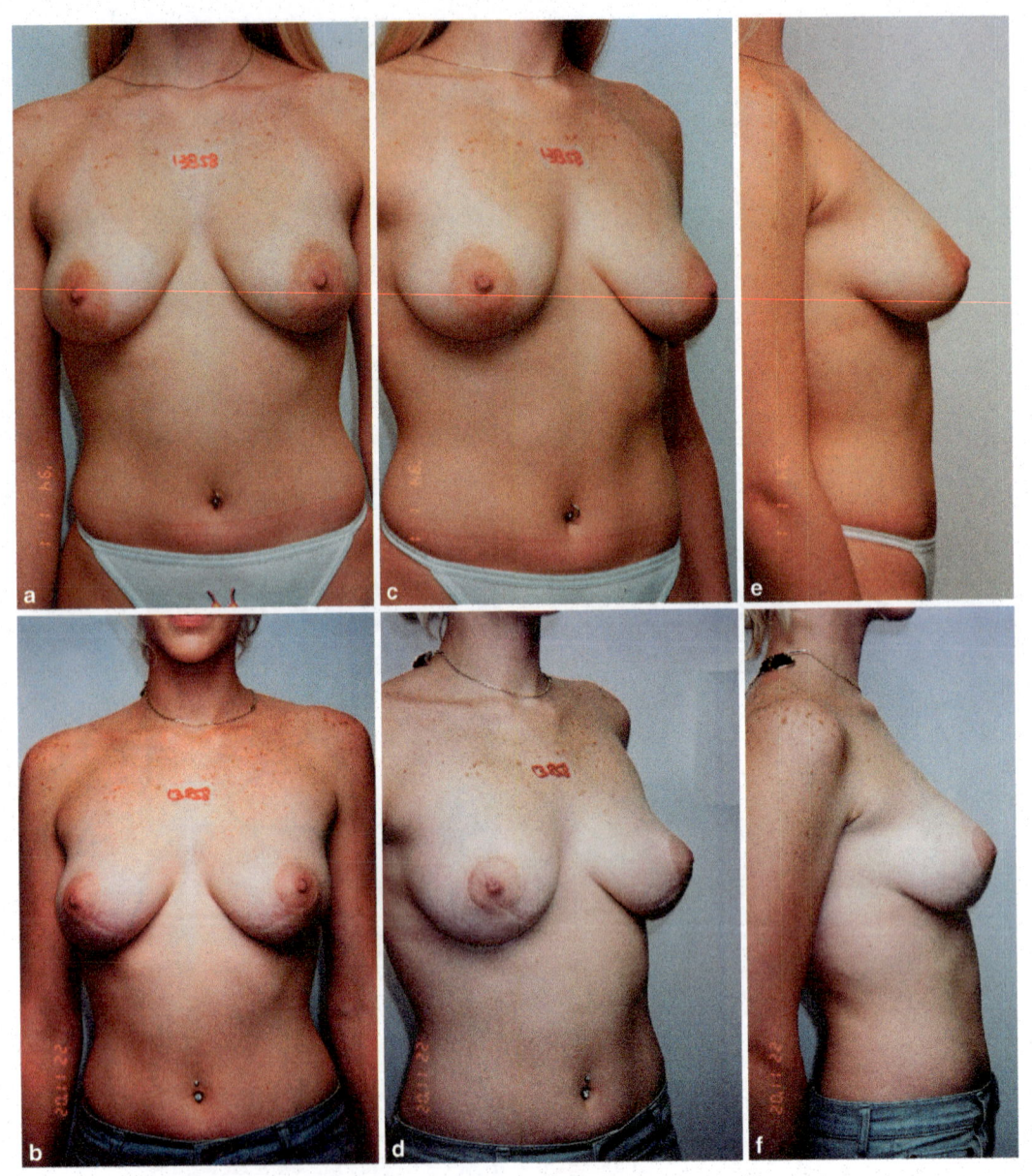

Fig. 13.4 This patient underwent a vertical incision masto-pexy. NAC diameter was reduced to 45 mm. The inferiorly pedicled dermoglandular flap was used as a biological implant behind the NAC flap. Twenty-two months after surgery she depicts a pleasing aesthetic improvement. Note some improvement of her upper pole fullness limited by the reach of the relatively short inferior flap. (**a**) Front view pre op; (**b**) front view 22 months post op; (**c**) oblique view pre op; (**d**) oblique view 22 months post op; (**e**) lateral view pre op; (**f**) lateral view 22 months post op

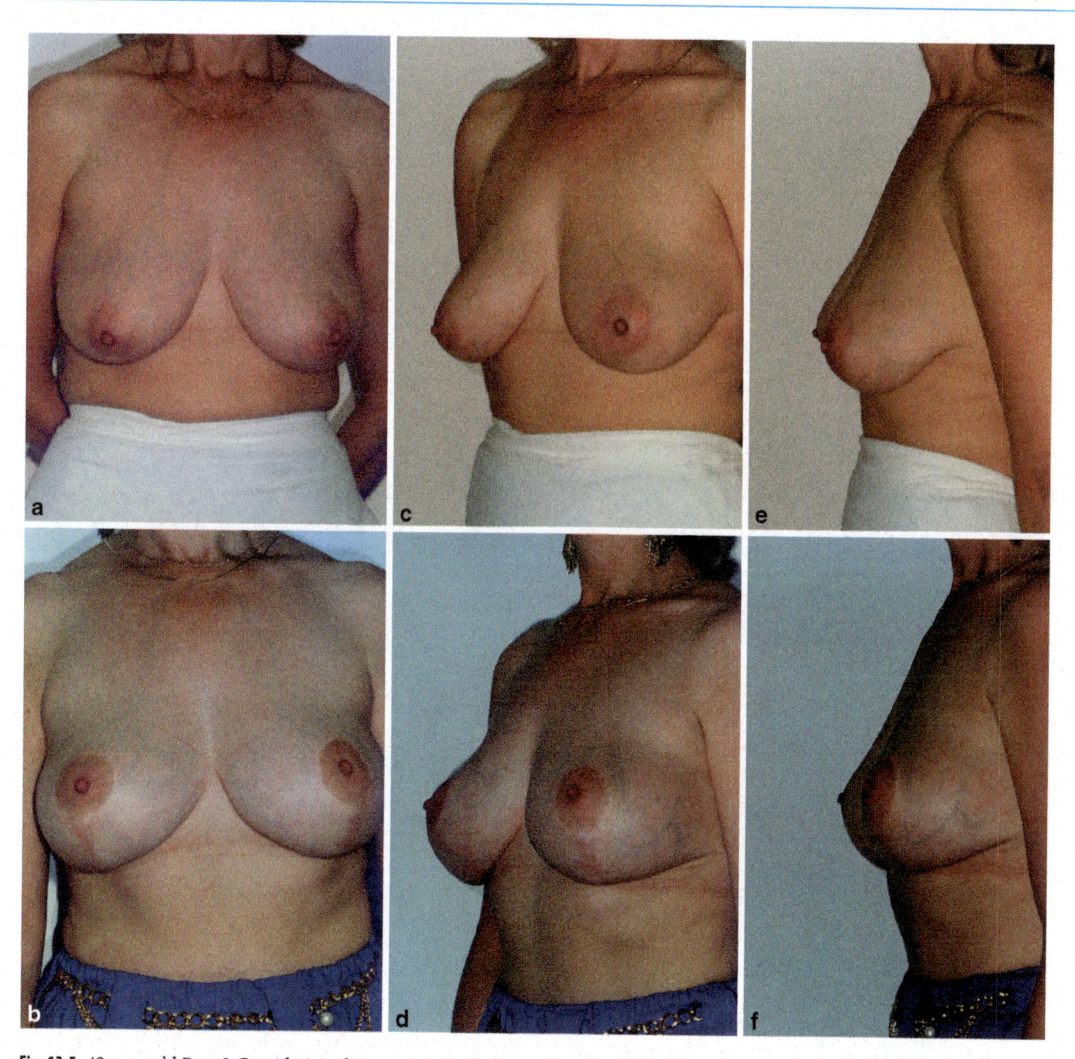

Fig. 13.5 42-year-old Para 2 Gravida 2 underwent a vertical incision mastopexy. Inferior pedicled flap was used as a biological implant as outlined in the text. 1 year post op photograph is presented. (**a**) Front view pre op; (**b**) front view 1 year post op; (**c**) oblique view pre op; (**d**) oblique view 1 year post op; (**e**) lateral view pre op; (**f**) lateral view 1 year post op

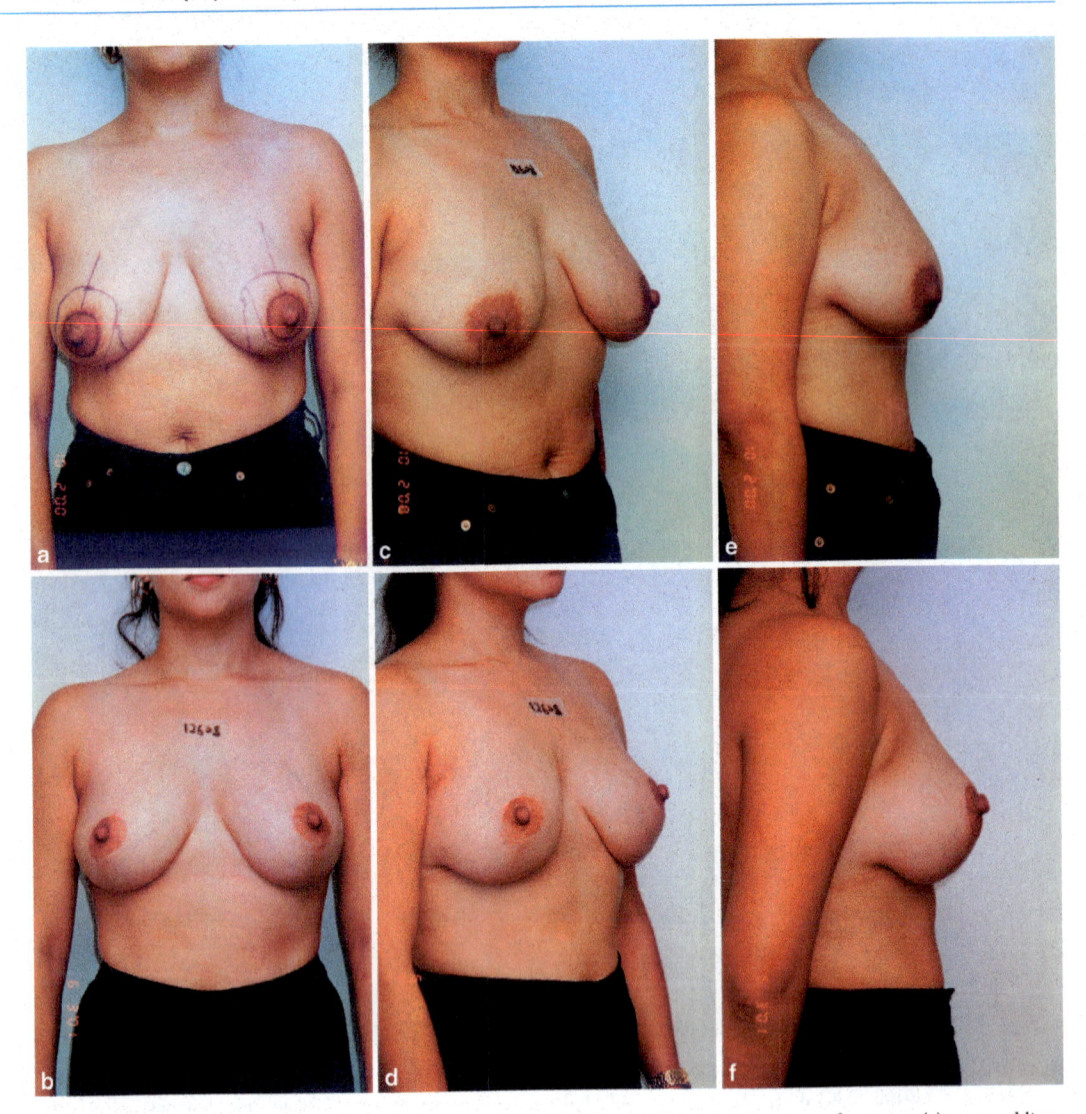

Fig. 13.6 This 27-year-old mother of three underwent a vertical mastopexy. NAC mobilized on a superior pedicle. An inferiorly pedicled dermo glandular flap was used to enhance NAC projection. She is shown 14 months after surgery. (**a**) Pre op front view; (**b**) 14 months post op front view; (**c**) pre op oblique view; (**d**) 14 months post op oblique view; (**e**) pre op lateral view; (**f**) 14 months post op lateral view

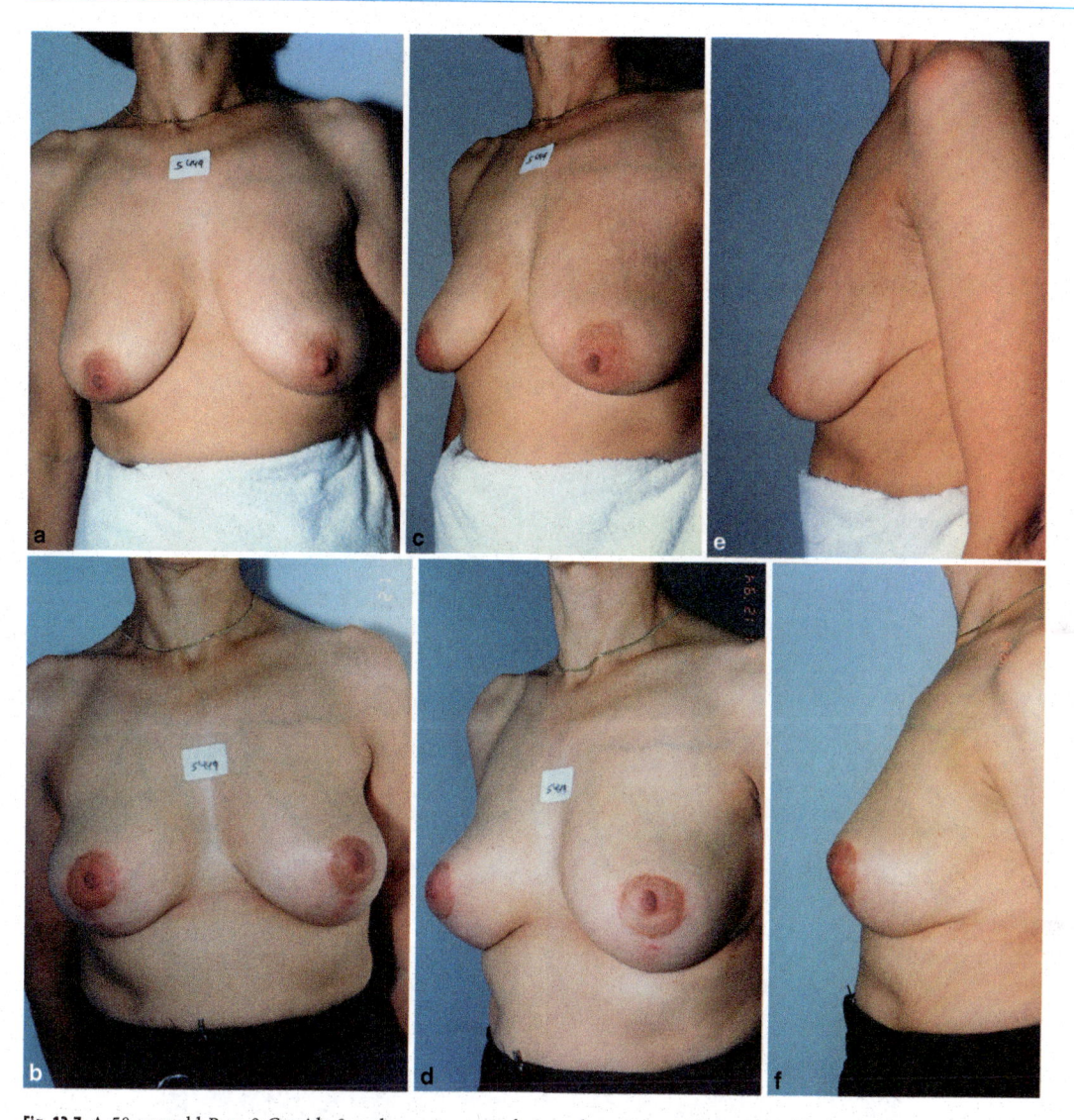

Fig. 13.7 A 50-year-old Para 0 Gravida 0 underwent a vertical incision mastopexy. NAC was mobilized as a supero-lateral pedicled flap. Inferior dermo-glandular flap was used as a biological projection and volume enhancer. Post operative photos are shown 1 year after surgery. (**a**) Pre op front view; (**b**) 1 year post op; (**c**) pre op oblique view; (**d**) 1 year oblique op; (**e**) pre op lateral view; (**f**) 1 year lateral op

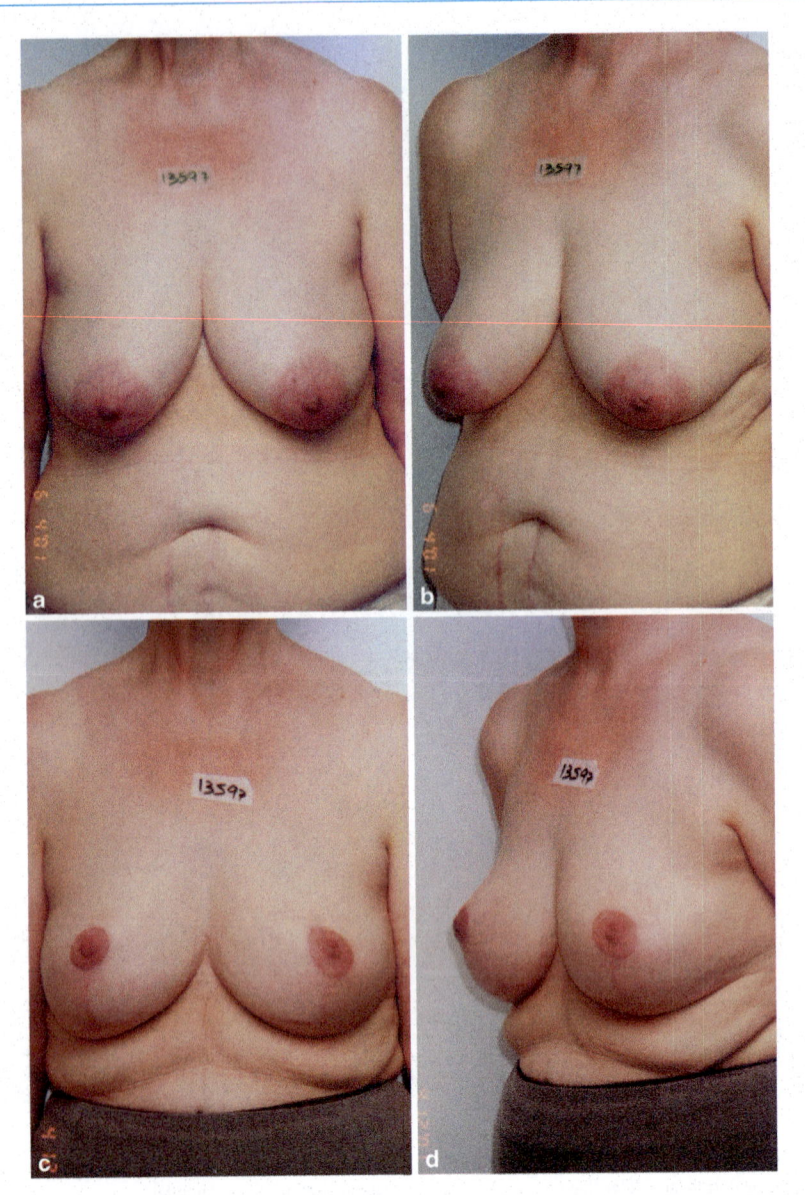

Fig. 13.8 This 65-year-old patient had a mastopexy with a short horizontal sub mammary scar. NAC was mobilized as an inferior pedicle. A superior dermo glandular flap was used as a biological prosthesis to increase NAC projection. A dermal graft was harvested from the superior dermo glandular flap for naso labial fold correction, which was accomplished at the same surgical session. The patient is shown 18 months after surgery. A modest upper pole deficiency correction was accomplished by folding the superior dermo glandular flap upon itself in the sagital axis. This folding was a consequence of the approximation of the medial and lateral flaps caudal to the NAC. (**a**) Pre op front view; (**b**) 18 months post op front view; (**c**) pre op oblique view; (**d**) 18 months post op oblique view;

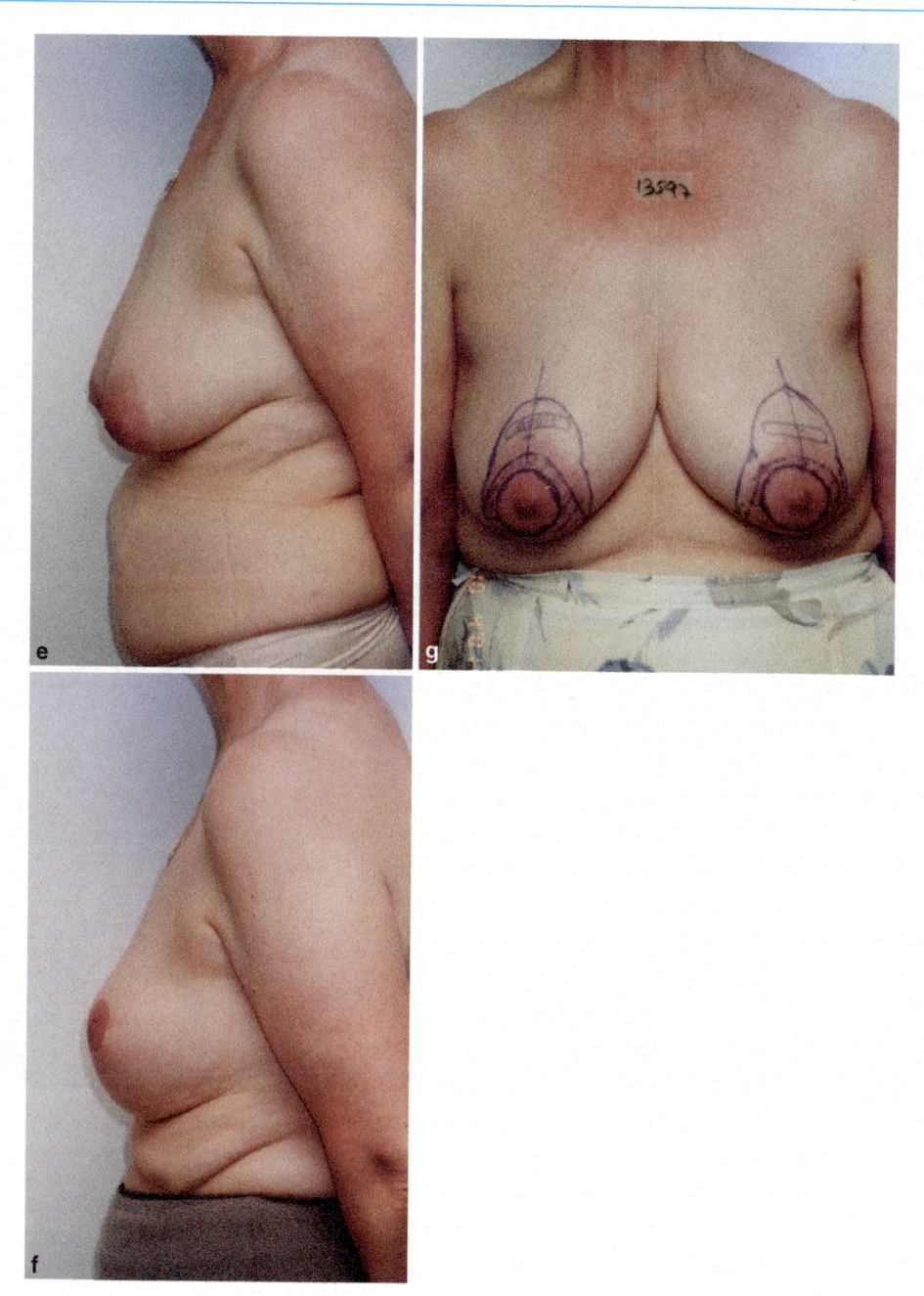

Fig. 13.8 (*continued*) (**e**) pre op lateral view; (**f**) 18 months post op lateral view; (**g**) pre op front view marked for surgery

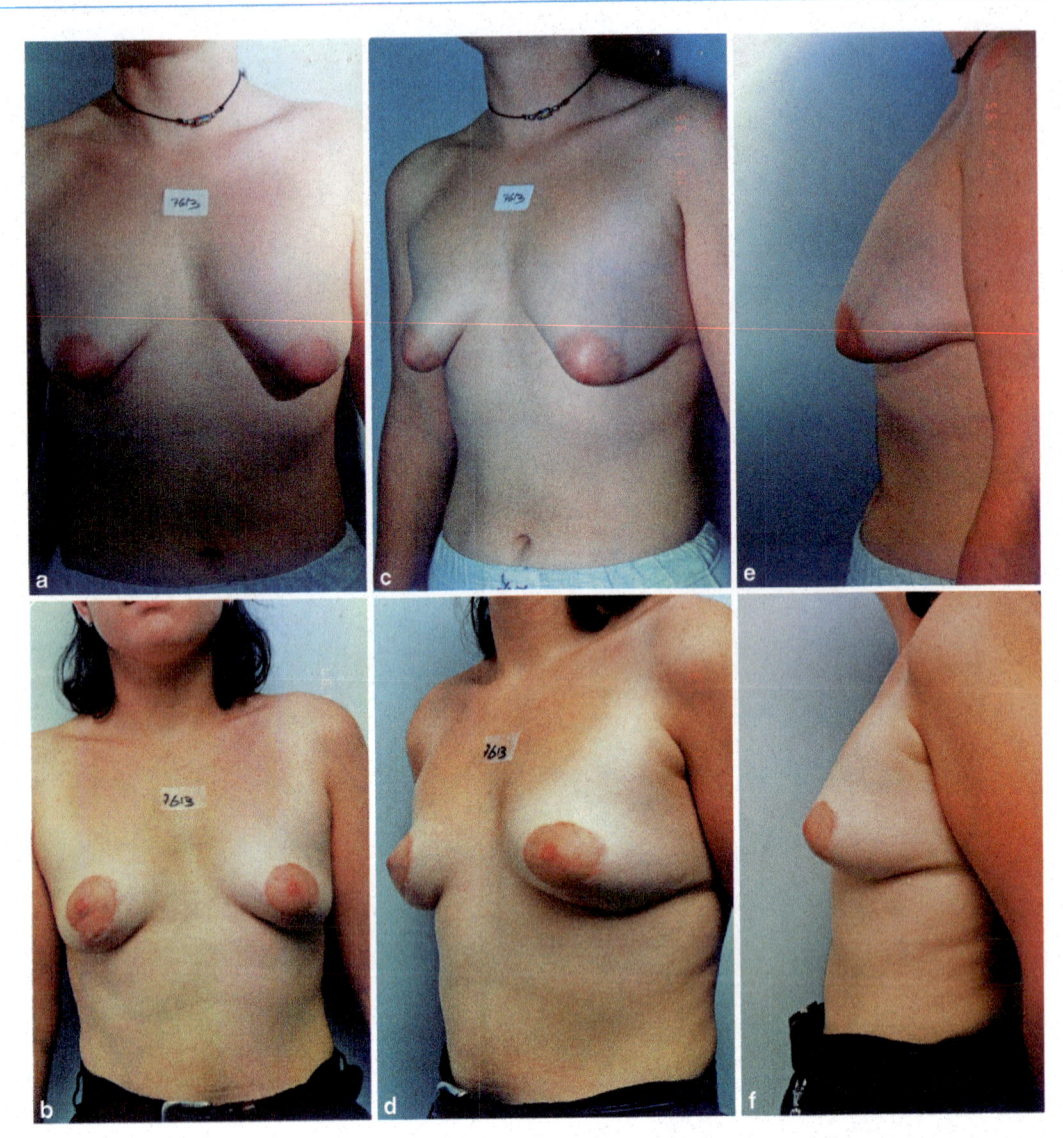

Fig. 13.9 Twenty-year-old woman underwent breast remodeling surgery. The NAC was mobilized on an inferior pedicle. The superior pedicled dermo glandular flap was used as a projection enhancer. Fifty gram reduction was performed on the left to address the asymmetry. Post op photos were obtained 16 months after surgery. (**a**) Pre op front view; (**b**) 16 months post op front view; (**c**) pre op oblique view; (**d**) 16 months post op oblique view; (**e**) pre op lateral view; (**f**) 16 months post op lateral view

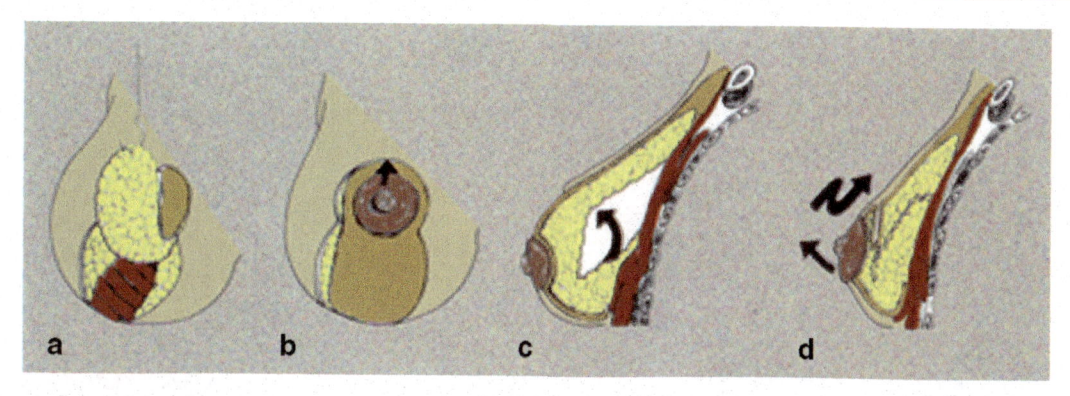

Fig. 13.10 (a–d) Extended superior pedicle: This variation is useful in secondary cases that were primarily operated through a sub mammary incision, as the old scar often severs the pedicle of the inferiorly pedicled dermo glandular flap thus compromising its vascular supply. Continuation of the flap into the infra areola area is folded upon itself behind the nipple–areola complex to increase projection. The superior NAC supporting pedicle is folded or transposed to allow positioning of the nipple at the appropriate level. The sub areolar extension is used as a volume enhancer.

13.3.2
Vertical Mastopexy with a Short Inframammary Scar

This skin incision is employed when the vertical scar caudal end is long, thus producing a "dog ear" effect. The short horizontal component is a worthwhile price to pay for the improved contour in the submammary fold area [31]. The incision resembles a "fish tail" in the caudal end of the vertical scar (Fig. 13.12). The breast tissue flap arrangement within the breast follows the same guidelines as previously outlined.

13.3.3
Wise Pattern (Key Hole) Incision

This approach is reserved for patients with extremely wide breast base on the chest wall, patients who require attention to axillary breast tail, and patients with large breast and severe ptosis. Flap utilization follows the guidelines previously outlined (Fig. 13.13).

13.4
Materials and Methods

Between 1992 and 2006, 132 patients underwent breast elevation by a single surgeon using this technique. This cohort excludes the surgeon's experience in breast reduction, mastopexy with simultaneous insertion of breast implants, and obviously minor ptosis corrected by insertion of breast implant alone. This cohort included 90 patients who had bilateral mastopexy, 20 patients who had a small (less then 100 g or less then 100 cc liposuction per breast) (Fig. 3.14) breast reduction and simultaneous mastopexy, and 22 patients who had a unilateral mastopexy as part of reconstruction after a contra lateral mastectomy. Two patients underwent mastopexy with augmentation using axillary tissue excess. This approach was employed to correct excess contour in that area (Fig. 13.15).

The patients were all females of 16–78 years of age. Follow up ranged from 8 months to 13 years, with a mean of 4.8.

Associated procedures included abdominoplasty [12], liposuction [9], and other procedures [7]

13.5
Complications

Complications were recorded in 12 patients and included the following:

Asymmetry in four patients, two requiring revision under local anesthesia on an ambulatory basis (Table 13.1). Hypertrophic scars occurred in three patients, two associated with MAC asymmetry. One of these patients required surgical revision and low dose radiotherapy (Fig. 13.16). The others were treated conservatively with silicone sheathing, intralesional cortisone injections and prolonged emotional support. Inverted nipples occurred in two patients early in the series. It was attributed to inappropriate pedicle selection. One was of no concern to the patient and the other was treated with a Niplet device. Hematoma and seroma were not recorded in this series. Flap loss of clinical significance was not detected either. There was no nipple loss. One case of areola partial epidermolysis occurred in a smoker, which healed spontaneously.

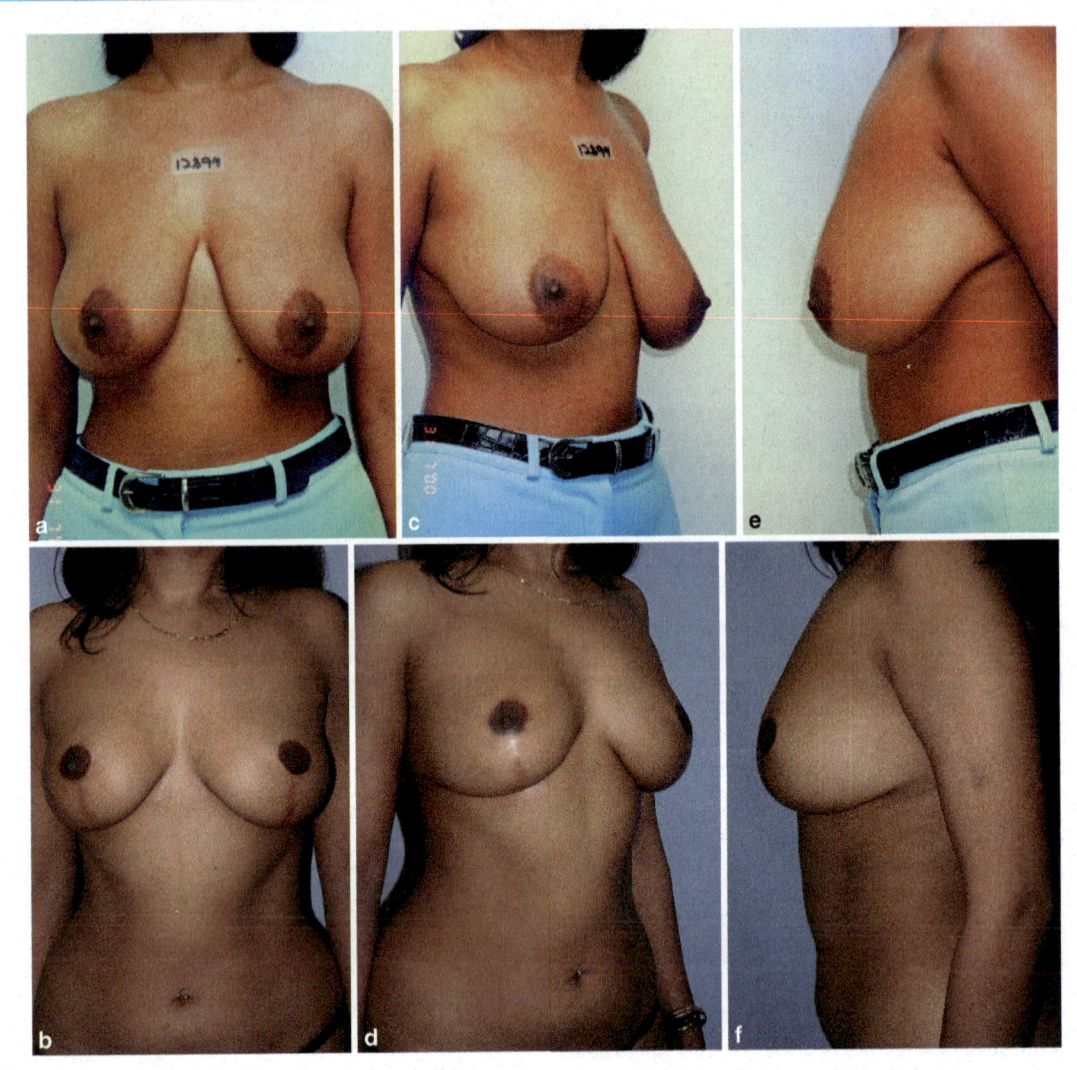

Fig. 13.11 A 27-year-old patient underwent mastopexy with reduction of 260 g on the right and 270 g on the left. A vertical mastopexy incision with a short horizontal submammary component was employed. Nipple–areola complex was mobilizes on a supero-medial pedicle. A small inferior dermoglandular pedicle was used as a biological implant behind the NAC. Post op photos were taken 7 years after surgery. (**a**) Pre op front view; (**b**) 7 years post op front view; (**c**) pre op left oblique view; (**d**) 7 years post op left oblique l view; (**e**) pre op right lateral view; (**f**) 7 years post op right lateral view

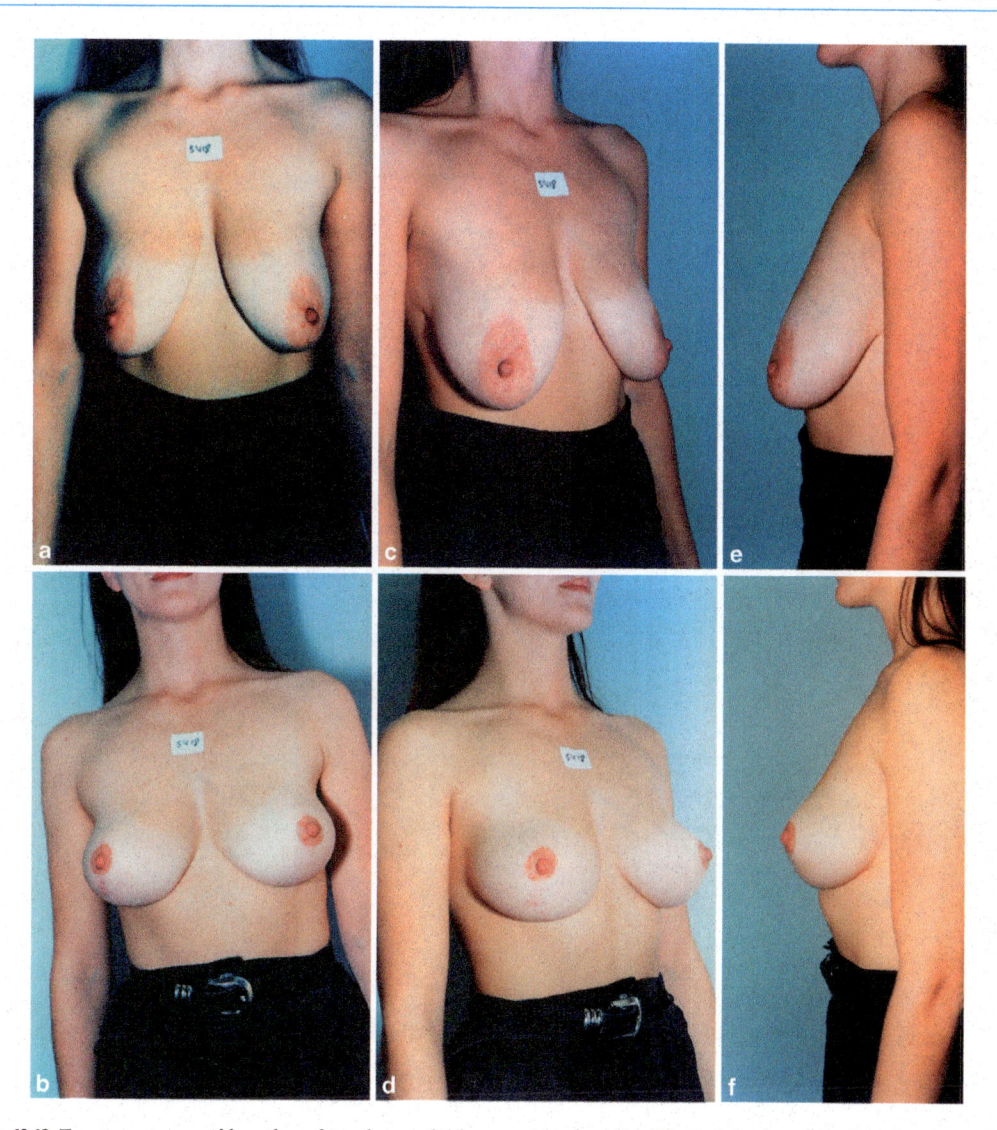

Fig. 13.12 Twenty-seven-year-old mother of two breasts fed her two children for 2 years each. Her mastopexy was done through a vertical mastopexy incision with a short horizontal submammary component. Areola diameter was reduced, NAC was mobilizes as a superiorly pedicled flap, inferior dermo glandular flap was used as a biological implant. one year post op photos are shown. (**a**) Pre op front view; (**b**) 1 year post op view; (**c**) pre op oblique view; (**d**) 1 year post op view; (**e**) pre op lateral view; (**f**) 1 year post op view

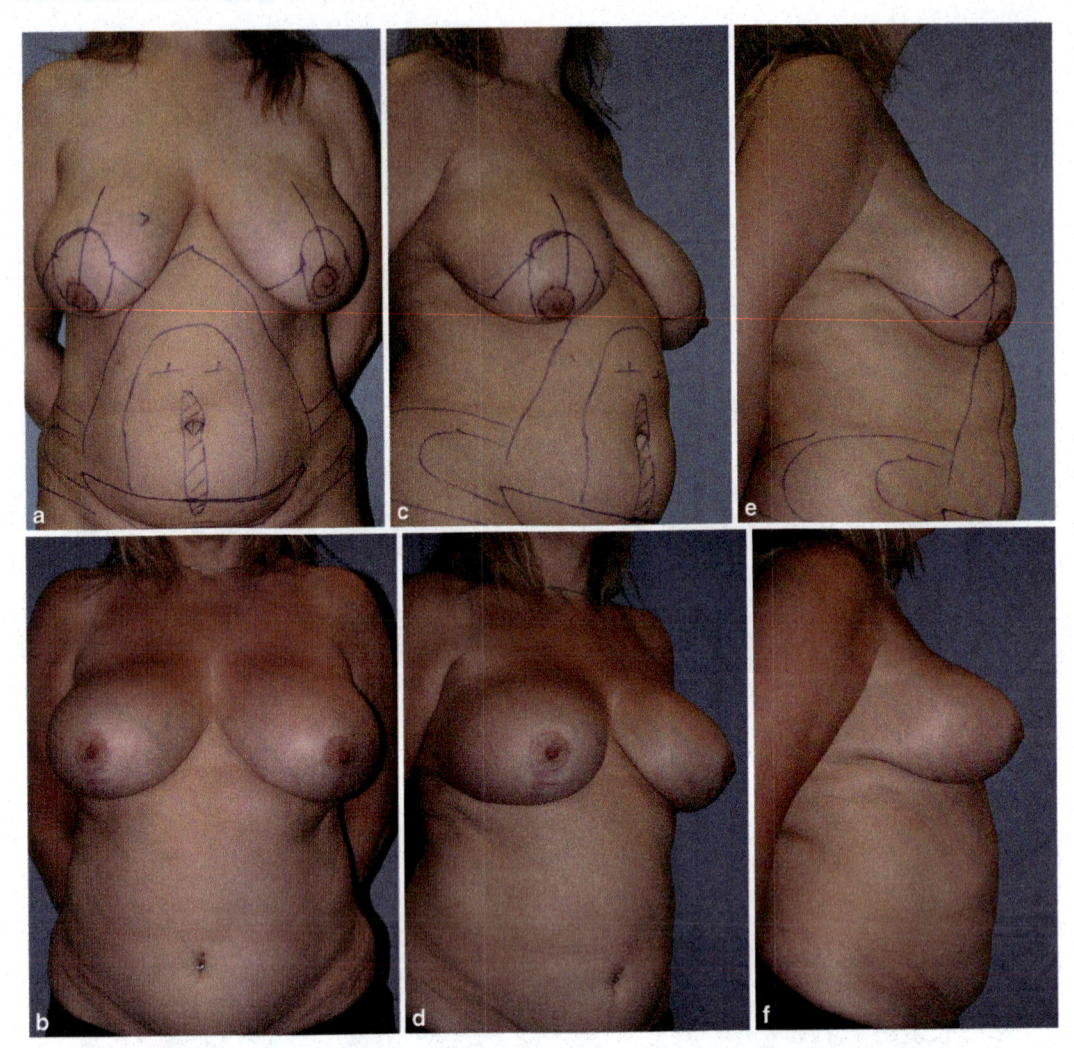

Fig. 13.13 This patient underwent Mastopexy through a Wise pattern incision. This approach was selected because of the severe ptosis she was presented with. NAC was mobilized on a supero lateral pedicle. A large dermo inferiorly pedicled glandular flap was used as a biological implant placed in a pocket that was dissected in the subglandular plan. The patient had liposuction and abdominoplasty dome at the same surgical session. Post op photos were taken 1 year after surgery. (**a**) Pre op front view; (**b**) 1 year post op front view; (**c**) pre op oblique view; (**d**) 1 year post op oblique view; (**e**) pre op lateral view; (**f**) 1 year post op lateral view

13.5 Complications   89

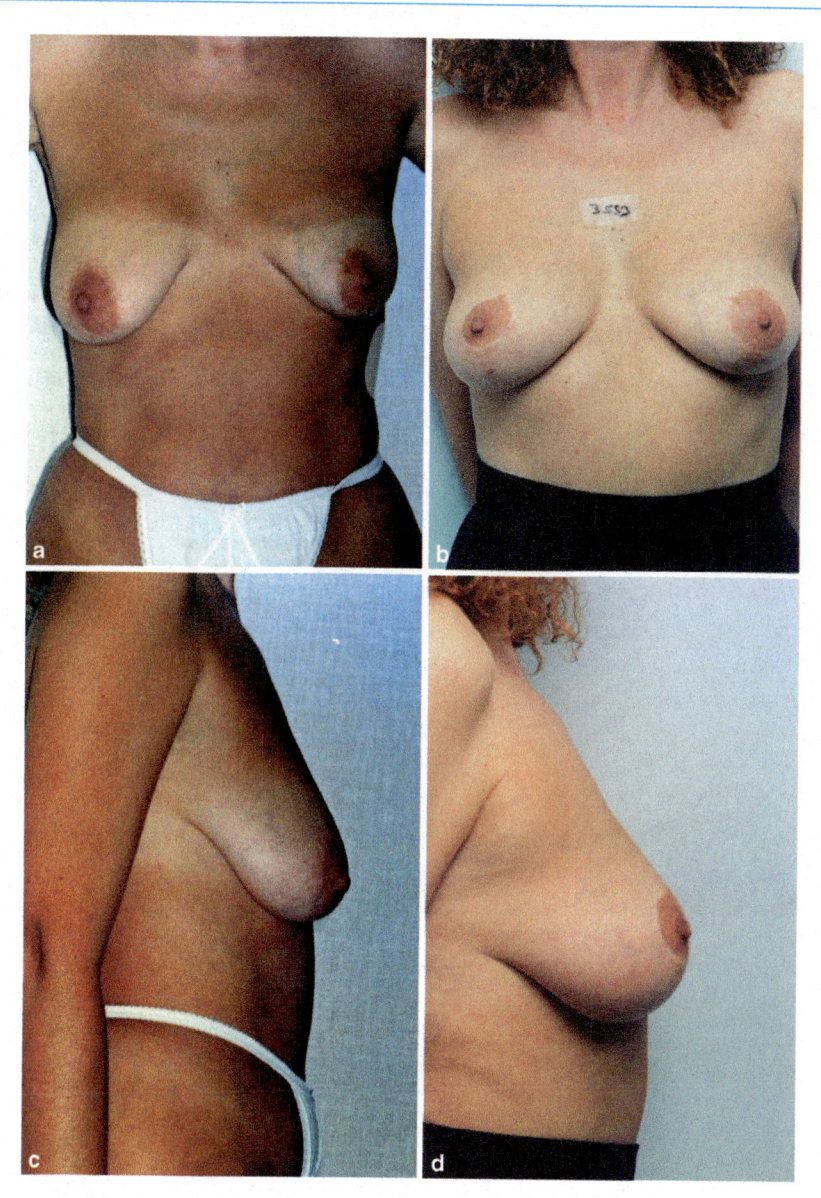

Fig. 13.14 This 36-year-old Para 6 Gravida 3 patient presented with a substantial asymmetry of her breasts. The mastopexy was done through a vertical incision. Eighty gram reduction was performed on the right breast. She is shown 2 year after surgery and there is some weight gain. (**a**) Pre op front view; (**b**) 2 years post op front view; (**c**) pre op lateral view; (**d**) 2 years post op lateral view

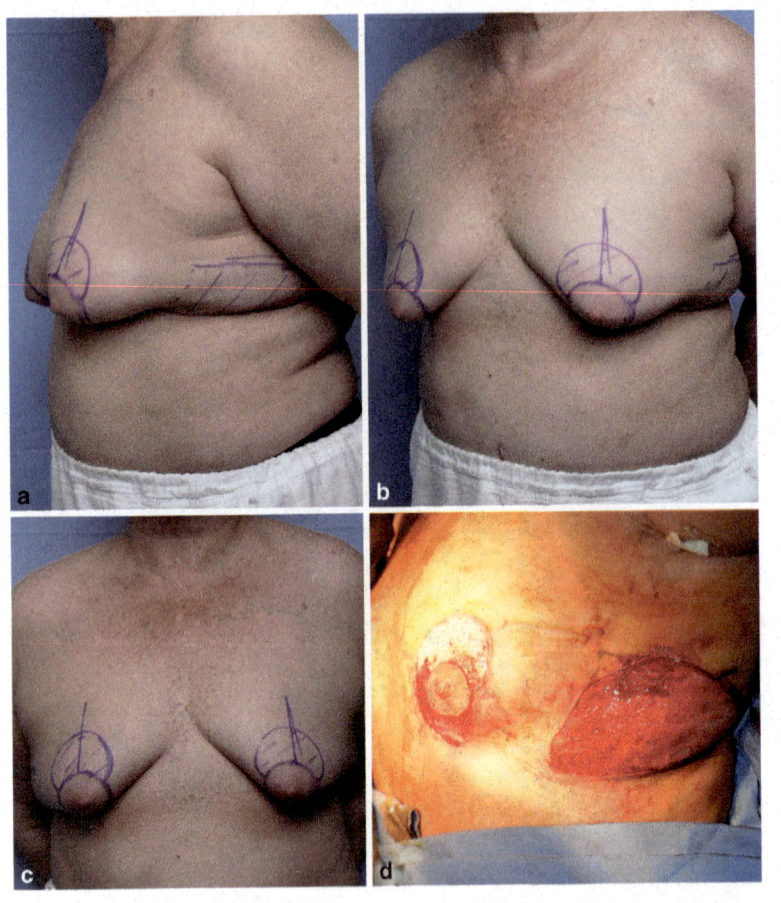

Fig. 13.15 This 68-year-old patient represents utilization of a long axillary excess for an additional volume during a short scar mastopexy. (**a–c**) Pre-operative views. Small breasts with NAC present close to the lower pole of the breasts. Axillary excess is evident and marked. (**d–e**) Intra operative views outlining the NAC, which is mobilized on an inferior dermo-glandular flap. The axillary excess is deepithelialized and mobilized as an anterior pedicled flap and used as extra volume for the breast

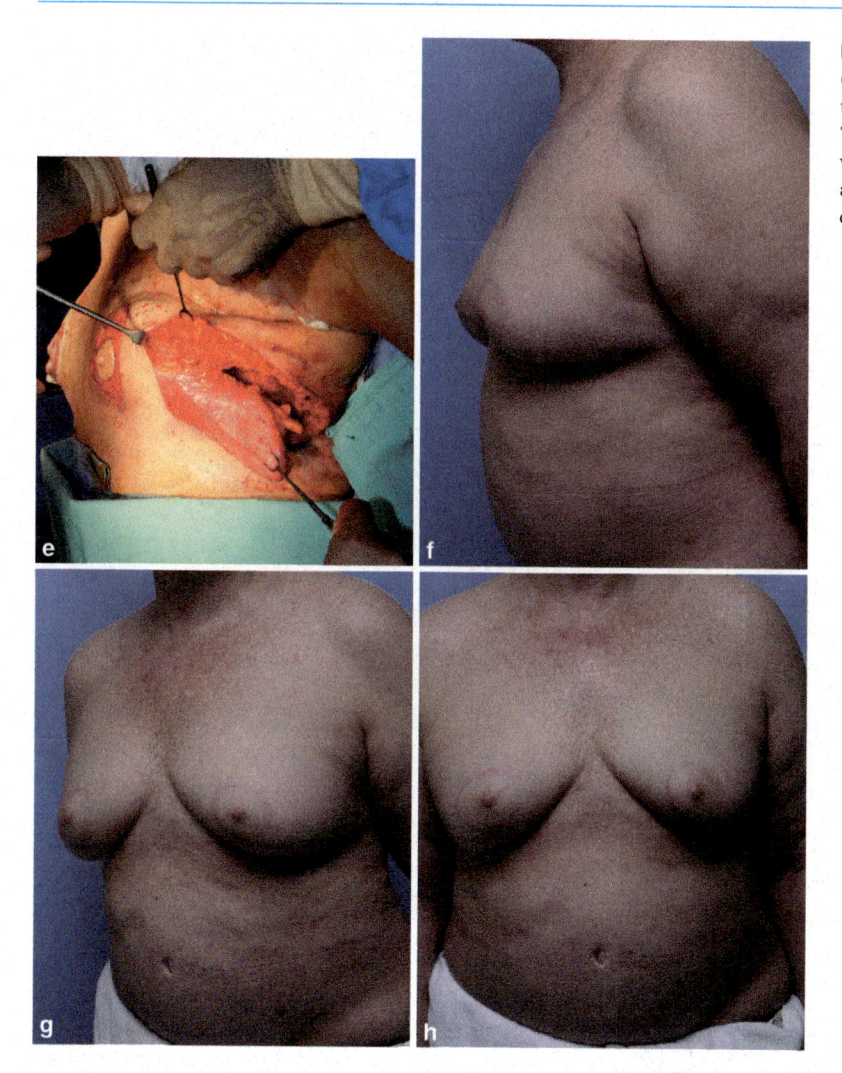

Fig. 13.15 *(continued)* (**f–h**) Post operative views taken 1 year after surgery. The improved shape and volume of the breasts as well as the flat axillary contour is evident

Table 13.1 Complications

Complications (n = 13)		Management
Asymmetry	3	1 revisions
Slow wound healing	3	Dressings only
Inverted nipple	2	1 niplet
Hematoma	0	
Seroma	0	
Hypertrophic scar	3	Conservative=2, Surgical revision=1
Nipple loss	0	
Flap loss	0	
Recurrent ptosis	2	Surgical revision=1

13.6 Discussion

The increasing popularity of short scar techniques supports the observation that patients are predominantly concern by scar [10, 35].

The periareolar approach offers the advantage of a scar position at an interphase of color and texture at the perimeter of the areola. Several studies compared the periareolar incision to other surgical incision groups of patients. Rorich et al. [36] surveyed the preference of American Board certified plastic surgeons. The survey indicated that the periareolar incision group reported significantly greater frequency of revision compared to short scar and inverted T incision groups. These problems include widening, scar hypertrophy, areolar widening and distortion, breast and areolar flattening,

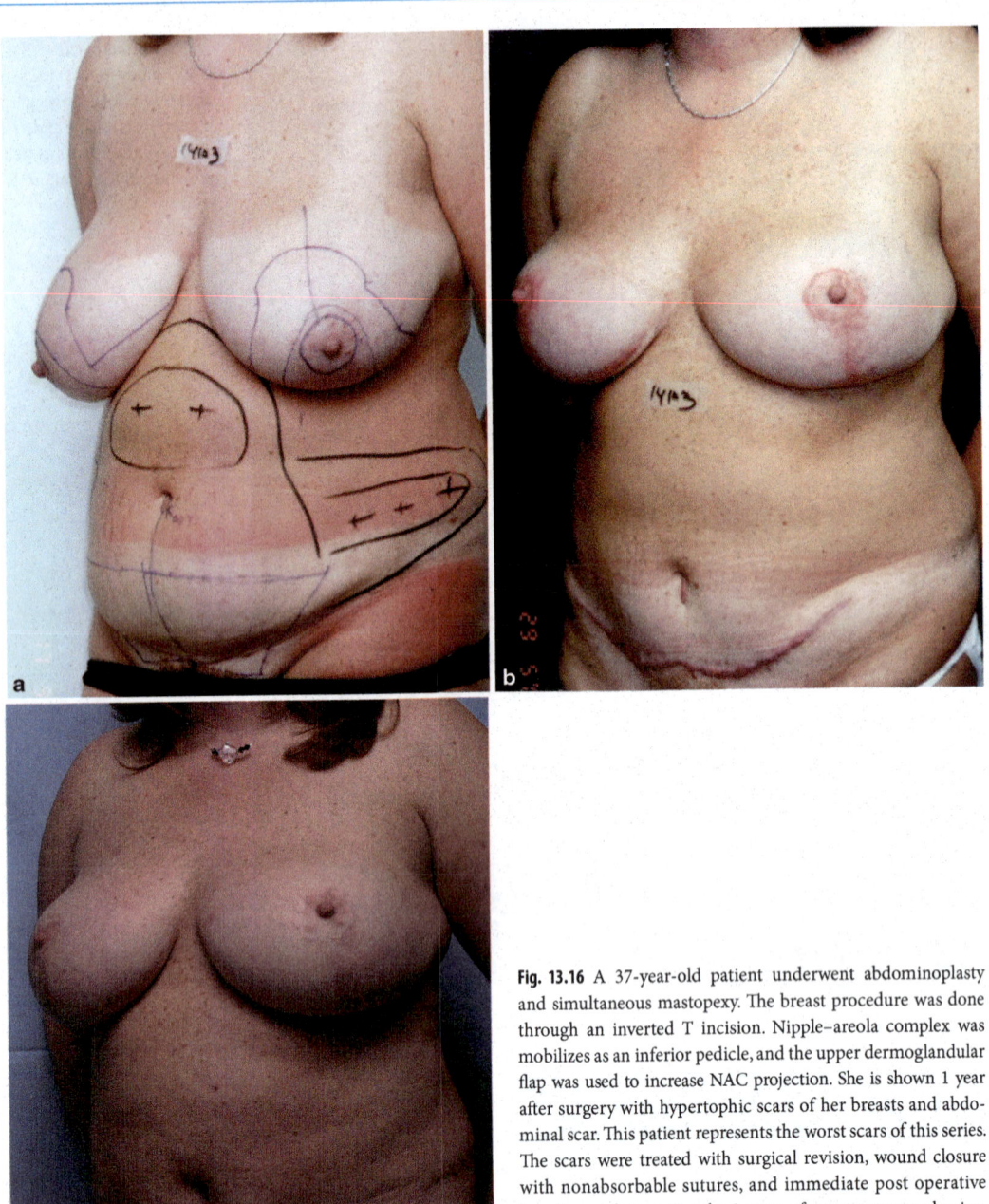

Fig. 13.16 A 37-year-old patient underwent abdominoplasty and simultaneous mastopexy. The breast procedure was done through an inverted T incision. Nipple–areola complex was mobilizes as an inferior pedicle, and the upper dermoglandular flap was used to increase NAC projection. She is shown 1 year after surgery with hypertophic scars of her breasts and abdominal scar. This patient represents the worst scars of this series. The scars were treated with surgical revision, wound closure with nonabsorbable sutures, and immediate post operative low dose radiation. Results 3 years after surgery are pleasing. (**a**) Pre op view; (**b**) 1 year post op – hypertrophic scars are evident; (**c**) 3 year post op, after scar revision and low dose radiation therapy

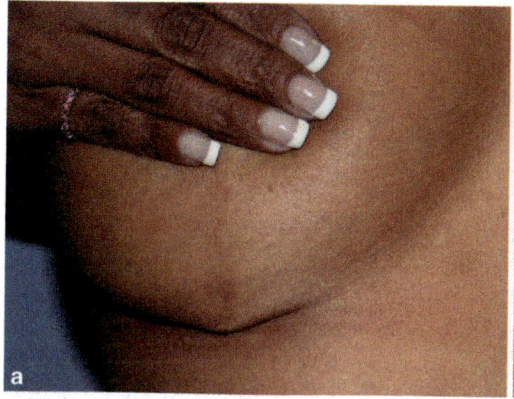

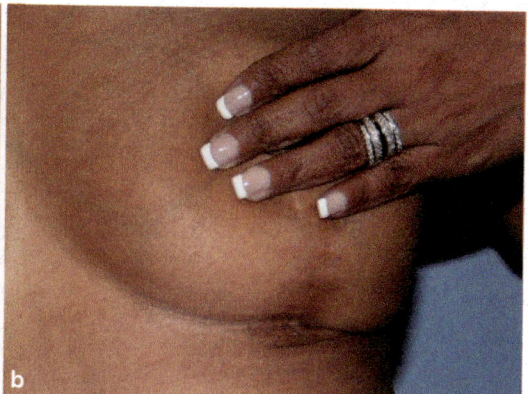

Fig. 13.17 Consequences of overstretching the vertical mastopexy incision technique to its limits and beyond are demonstrated by this patient shown here 8 years after surgery. On the right (**a**) a small skin excess (dog ear) never settled. On the left (**b**) the scar ends a few millimeters below the submammary fold. This outcome occurred in spite of an original design of the wound that ended 10 mm above the original submammary fold. It was attributed to a cephalad migration of the fold after surgery. This result was of no concern to the patient who declined an offer of scar revision

suture complications, and recurrent ptosis, all leading to secondary procedures of scar revisions. These findings were supported by others [7, 9, 14–20, 23, 36, 37].

The short scar group reported a greater frequency of asymmetry and NAC asymmetry compared with the periareolar group [36]. Other problems reported with short scar technique included suture complications, hypertrophy of scars, delayed healing, seroma, and need for revision. Average complication rate appears lower than in the periareolar group.

The inverted T incision remains the most popular technique employed by plastic surgeons in the USA. However, this technique is associated with the highest incidence of post operative glandular ptosis (bottoming out), particularly when inferior pedicle is employed. Average complication rate reported with this technique is 14%. Most reported problems with this technique are scar related.

Utilization of breast tissue to increase breast projection and breast tissue rearrangement has been employed by Fayman et al. [32] and others in various variations [38–45]. This concept is appealing for many reasons. It offers some advantages of the breast implant without the inherent disadvantage associated with the utilization of a foreign body. Indeed, the available material is limited by the amount of breast tissue at hand. However, within these limitations the resources can be put to good use.

There is no consensus among plastic surgeons with regards to the sustainability of the correction when breast tissue is used for breast sculpting. The author's experience is based on long-term follow up on cases such as the one presented in Fig. 13.3. This experience indicates that the correction is long term. As for the correction of upper pole emptiness, the limiting factor is the length of the inferiorly pedicled dermo glandular flap used for the task. If the flap is sufficiently long to reach the upper chest, the correction is adequate and sustainable.

Another lesson learnt over the years is the limitations of the vertical scars. The vertical mastopexy is a useful technique for the appropriately selected patients. A long vertical scar that traverses the submammary fold tends to produce a less than optimal scar (Fig. 13.17). In addition, the vertical incision approach offers a limited ability to correct ptosis as evident by the result presented in Fig. 13.18. In the author's view, a short submammary incision well concealed in the submammary fold is preferable to a suboptimally corrected ptosis.

13.7 Conclusion

Utilization of breast tissue as a biological implant is a versatile technique that can be adapted to a wide spectrum of surgical scenarios and has the potential to offer an easy solution to many clinical situations. The author recommends adding this technique as a valuable adjunct to the breast surgeon repertoire.

Dedication and Acknowledgments

This work is dedicated with love to my wife, Mirry, the wind beneath my wings. The author gratefully acknowledges the Medical art work skillfully performed by Dr. Estelle Potgieter and Ms. Dana Fayman.

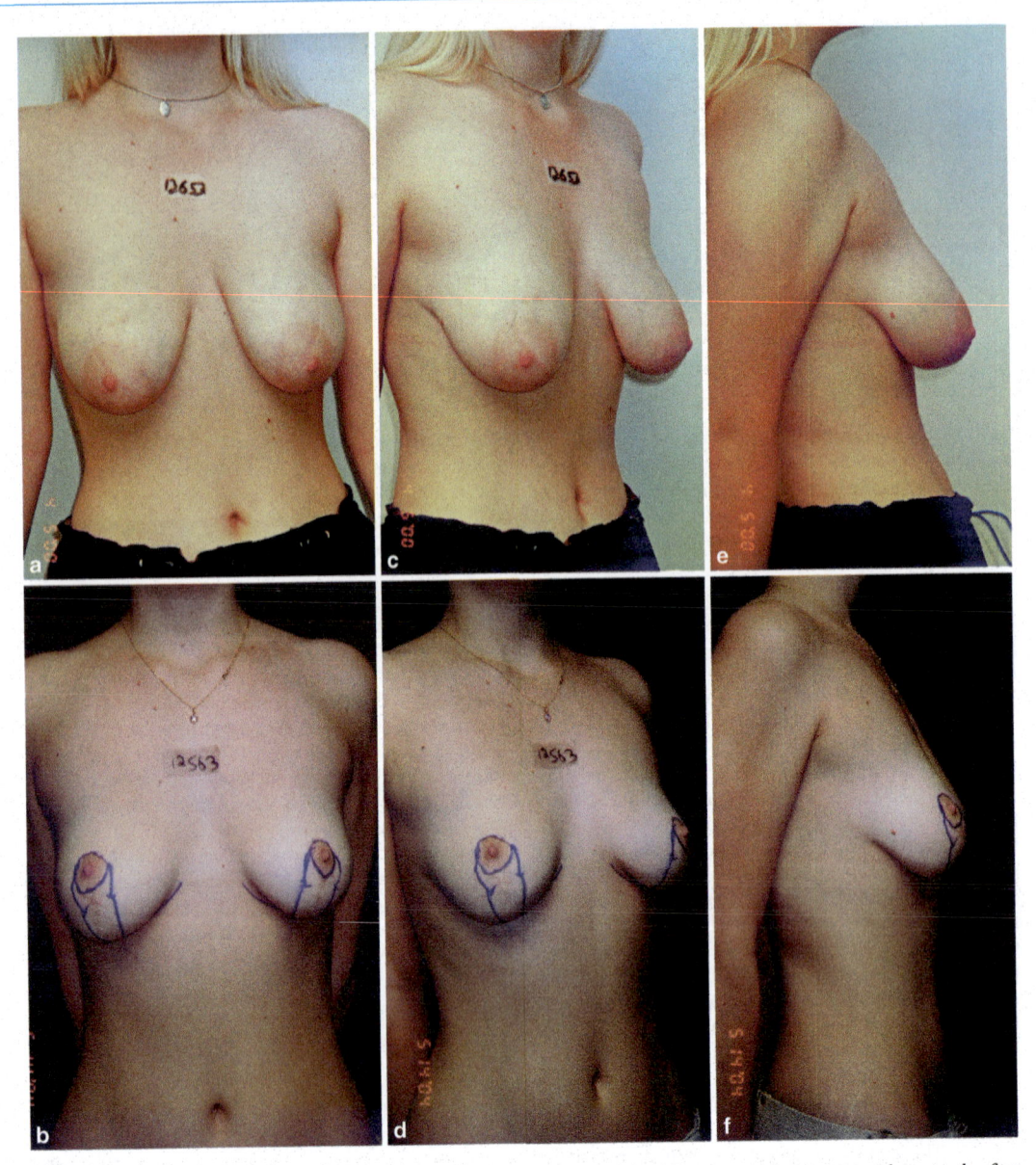

Fig. 13.18 A 23-year-old patient presented for mastopexy through a short scar. A vertical mastopexy approach was selected. The inferior pedicle was used as a biological implant behind the NAC. Four years after surgery she requested breast augmentation. Examination of the patient at this stage revealed bilateral mild ptosis. This patient was probably a poor candidate for a vertical mastopexy alone in the first place. She would have probably done better with a short submammary incision, which she refused to accept. (**a**) Pre op front view; (**b**) 4 years post op front view; (**c**) pre op oblique view; (**d**) 4 years post op oblique view; (**e**) pre op lateral view; (**f**) 4 years post op lateral view

References

1. Regnault P: Breast ptosis: Definition and treatment. Clin Plast Surg 1976;3(2):193–203
2. Brink R: Management of true ptosis of the breast. Plast Reconstr Surg 1993;91(4):657–662
3. Spear S, Mijidian A: Reduction mammaplasty and mastopexy: general considerations. In: Spear SL (ed), Surgery of the Breast: Principles and Art. Philadelphia, Lippincott-Raven 1998, p 673
4. Rohrich RJ, Beran SJ, Restifo RJ, Copit SE: Aesthetic management of the breast following explantation: evaluation and mastopexy options. Plast Reconstr Surg 1998;101(3):827–837
5. Elliott FL: Circumareolar mastopexy with augmentation. Clin Plast Surg 2002;29(3):337–347
6. Bartels RJ, Strickland DM, Douglas WM: A new mastopexy operation for mild or moderate ptosis. Plast Reconstr Surg 1976;57(6):687–691
7. Spear SL, Kassan M, Little JW: Guidelines in concentric mastopexy. Plast Reconstr Surg 1990;85(6):961–966
8. Puckett CL, Meyer VH, Reinisch JF: Crescent mastopexy and augmentation. Plast Reconstr Surg 1985;75(4):533–543
9. Erol OO, Spira M: A mastopexy technique for mild to moderate ptosis. Plast Reconstr Surg 1980;65(5):603–609
10. Fayman MS, Potgieter E, Becker PJ: Outcome study: periareolar mammaplasty patients' perspective. Plast Reconstr Surg 2003;111(2):676–684
11. Graf R, Biggs TM: In search of better shape in mastopexy and reduction-mammaplasty. Plast Reconstr Surg 2002;110(1):309–317
12. Wise RJ: A preliminary report on a method of planning the mammaplasty. Plast Reconstr Surg 1956;17(5):367–375
13. Andrews JM, Yshizuki MM, Ramos RR: An areolar approach to reduction mammaplasty. Br J Plast Surg 1975;28(3):166–170
14. Gruber RP, Jones HW: The donut mastopexy: indications and complications. Plast Reconstr Surg 1980;65(1):34–38
15. Hinderer UT: Circumareolar dermo-glandular plication: a new concept for correction of breast ptosis. Aesthetic Plast Surg 2001;25(6):404–420
16. Benelli L: Periareolar mammaplasty – round block technique. Rev Soc Bras Cir Plast 1990;5:44
17. Benelli L: Periareolar Benelli mastopexy and reduction: the round block. In: Spear SL (ed), Surgery of the Breast: Principles and Art. Philadelphia, Lippincott-Raven 1998
18. Goes JCS: Periareolar mammaplasty: double skin technique with application of polyglactin or mixed mesh. Plast Reconstr Surg 1996;97(5):959–968
19. Goes JCS: Periareolar mammaplasty: double skin technique with application of mesh support. Clin Plast Surg 2002;29(3):349–364
20. Qiao Q, Sun J, Liu C, Liu Z, Zhao R: Reduction mammaplasty and correction of ptosis: dermal bra technique. Plast Reconstr Surg 2003;111(3):1122–1130
21. Gulyas, G. Mammaplasty with a periareolar dermal cloak for glandular support. Aesthetic Plast Surg 1999;23(3):164–169
22. Hammond DC: Short scar periareolar inferior pedicle reduction (SPAIR) mammaplasty. Plast Reconstr Surg 1999;103(3):890–901
23. Becker H: Subareolar mastopexy: update. Aesthetic Surg J 2003;23:357
24. Lassus C: A technique for breast reduction. Int Surg 1970;53(1):69–72
25. Lassus C: Update on vertical mammaplasty. Plast Reconstr Surg 1999;104(7):2289–2298
26. Peixoto G: Reduction mammaplasty: a personal technique. Plast Reconstr Surg 1980;65(2):217–226
27. Lejour M, Abboud M, Declety A, Kertesz P: Reduction des cicatrices de plastie mammaire de l'ancre courte Ã la verticale. Ann Chir Plast Esthet 1990;35(5):369–379
28. Lejour M, Abboud M: Vertical mammaplasty without infer-mammary scar and with breast liposuction. Perspect Plast Surg 1990;4:67
29. Lejour M: Vertical mammaplasty: update and appraisal of late results. Plast Reconstr Surg 1999;104(3):771–781
30. Chiari A Jr: The L short-scar mammaplasty: a new approach. Plast Reconstr Surg 1992;90(2):233–246
31. Marchac D, de Olarte G: Reduction mammaplasty and correction of ptosis with a short inframammary scar. Plast Reconstr Surg 1982;69(1):45–55
32. Fayman MS: Short scar mastopexy with flap transposition. Aesthetic Plast Sur 1998;22(2):135–141
33. Hall-Findlay E: Pedicles in vertical reduction and mastopexy. Clin Plast Surg 2002;29(3):379–391
34. Hall-Findlay EJ: A simplified vertical reduction mammaplasty: shortening the learning curve. Plast Reconstr Surg 1999;104(3):748–759
35. Caldeira AM, Lucas A, Grigalek G: Mastoplasty: the triple-flap interposition technique. Aesthetic Plast Surg 1999;23(1):51–60
36. Rohrich RJ, Cosman AA, Brown SA, Reisch J: Mastopexy preference: a survey of board-certified plastic surgeons. Plast Reconstr Surg 2006;118(7):1631–1638
37. Gryskiewicz JM, Hatfield AS: Zigzag wavy-line periareolar incision. Plast Reconstr Surg 2002;110(7):1778–1783
38. Kwei S, Borud LJ, Lee BT: Mastopexy with autologous augmentation after massive weight loss: the intercostal artery perforator (ICAP) flap. Ann Plast Surg 2006;57(4):361–365

39. Voigt M, Andree C: Breast shaping by an isolated tissue flap. Aesthetic Plast Surg 2006;30(5):527–534
40. Hurwitz DJ, Agha-Mohammadi S: Postbariatric surgery breast reshaping: the spiral flap. Ann Plast Surg 2006;56(5): 481–486; discussion 486
41. Ritz M, Silfen R, Southwick G: Fascial suspension mastopexy. Plast Reconstr Surg 2006;117(1):86–94
42. Flowers RS, Smith EM Jr: "Flip-flap" mastopexy. Aesthetic Plast Surg 1998;22(6):425–429
43. Weiss PR, Ship AG: Restoration of breast contour with autologous tissue after removal of implants. Ann Plast Surg 1995;34(3):236–241
44. Svedman P: Correction of breast ptosis utilizing a "fold over" de-epithelialized lower thoracic fasciocutaneous flap. Aesthetic Plast Surg 1991;15(1):43–47
45. Ship AG, Weiss PR, Engler AM: Dual-pedicle dermo-parenchymal mastopexy. Plast Reconstr Surg 1989;83(2): 281–290

CHAPTER 14

Double Flap Technique: An Alternative Mastopexy Approach

Andreas Foustanos

14.1 Introduction

If we review the history of mammaplasty, we see that several techniques have been described. Although the subsequent reduction mammaplasties were probably performed by Dieffenbach (1848), Morestin (1909), and Villarde (1911), the first publication was made by Lexer (1921) describing a technique with nipple areola complex transposition using an inverted T scar [1–4]. The superiorly based dermal pedicle, the vertical bipedicle dermal flap, the inferior pyramidal free nipple graft, the concentric mastopexy techniques, and Benelli modifications of the old "donut" mastopexy are some of the techniques described previously [5–11]. Pitanguy [12] described the inverted-T incision with a superior pedicle carrying the areola. Strombeck [13] used a horizontal bipedicle cutaneous flap; Mckissock [14] described a vertical bipedicle flap. Courtiss and Goldwyn [15] used an inferior pedicle. Lassus [16], Lejour [17], Peixoto [18], Hallfindlay [19], Skoog [20], Qun Qiao et al. [21], and Hinderer [22] described other techniques. Goes [23] used a large sheet of mesh, placed over the entire upper pole. Flowers and Smith [24] described the "flip-flap" mastopexy technique. Hammond described the short scar periareolar inferior pedicle reduction mammaplasty [25]. Ali Eed [26] described a technique creating a cone; the nipple areola complex is carried on a subcutaneous inferior pedicle. Some surgeons proposed the L-shaped or J-shaped incision [27–29]. Cerqueira [30] described breast fixation with a dermoglandular upper pedicle flap under the pectoralis muscle. Marchac and de Olarle [31] introduced the concept of upper glandular plication and suspension to the pectoralis fascia. Ribeiro [32] mobilized a chest wall-based flap into the upper pole. Daniel [33] suggested the passage of the flap under an elevated loop of pectoral muscle. Regardless of the degree of ptosis, the theme of a mastopexy is to get long-term maintenance of upper pole volume, to contour the gland, to reposition the nipple areola complex preserving its vascular supply, and to resect the redundant skin. A reasonable solution to the upper pole deficiency is to relocate and secure tissue from the caudal breast into the upper chest.

The author's experience showed that there is not only one perfect technique. It is important for the plastic surgeon to improve the technique that he uses. Our goal towards achieving an ideal breast through mastopexy led us to a combination of superior and inferior breast flap approach. It is a modification of Pitanguy's mammaplasty technique of the superior pole. The concept of internal suspension to support the breast is not new [34–37]. However, advantages of this approach are that it fills out the deficient upper breast, it maintains the vascular supply to the breast tissue and the nipple areola complex, it places the nipple areola complex in an acceptable position, it preserves normal sensation, it allows a more comfortable closure, and it avoids exaggerated scar tension. It is a safe and versatile technique suitable for all degrees of breast ptosis. It produces excellent aesthetic and long lasting results and it is an easy procedure to learn.

14.2 Technique

14.2.1 Marking

General anesthesia is administered to the patient. Each breast is infiltrated with 100–150 ml of xylocaine–adrenalin–saline solution. The back of the patient is elevated in 45° and the skin markings are made. We mark the skin as we do in Pitanguy's technique for breast mammaplasty (Fig. 14.1). The desired areola height (point A) is marked on the mid-clavicular line at a level just below the projection of the submammary sulcus using the index finger. The breast is lifted manually to estimate points B and C. A measure compass is used to ensure symmetrical positioning of these points. The width of the keyhole is determined by the grade of breast ptosis, the size of the breasts, the amount of the

M.A. Shiffman (ed.), *Mastopexy and Breast Reduction: Principles and Practice*,
© Springer-Verlag Berlin Heidelberg 2009

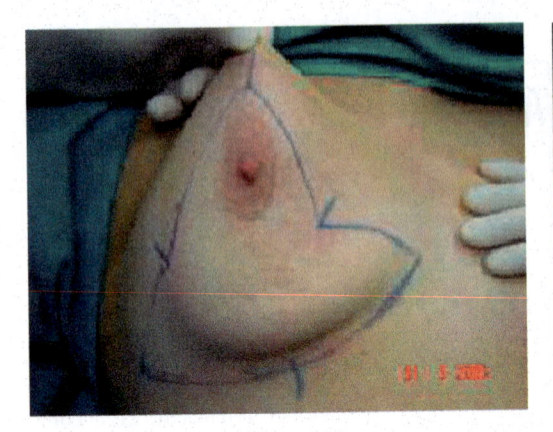

Fig. 14.1 The marking technique is the same as in Pitanguy's mammaplasty technique

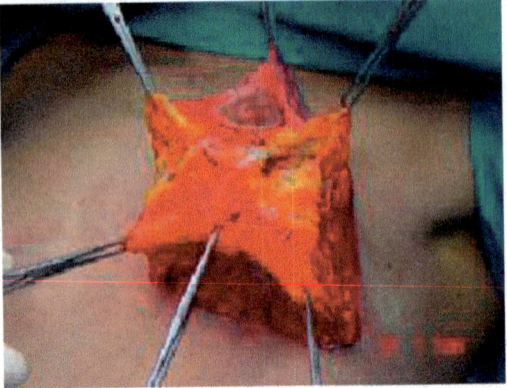

Fig. 14.2 Starting below the nipple areola complex, the inferior pedicle is dissected through the breast to the pectoral fascia. In this way the nipple areola complex is mobilized as a superior pedicled

skin to be reduced, and the patient's build. Then, lines AB and AC are drawn. The breast is lifted manually and a curved line of the submammary sulcus is drawn. Point D at the medial extremity of the submammary sulcus and point E at the lateral extremity of the submammary sulcus are marked. Lines CD and BE are marked in a curved way depending on the shape of the breast. The DE line is also completed. The opposite breast is marked in the same way and a measuring compass is used to ensure symmetry. A circular cookie cutter instrument is used to mark the nipple areola complex. This marking system allows flexibility in surgical closure of the wound and is easily adapted to many different degree of ptosis.

14.2.2
Operative Technique

The hands of the assistant are used as a tourniquet to the breast to improve tissue density and facilitate peeling of the epithelium. Two forceps are placed at the upper end of the incision, which corresponds to point A, and the skin is deepithelialized inside the incision markings. The skin flap results in an area of deepithelialization that corresponds to the triangle between points A, B, C. With a forceps applied at point A, the breast is lifted up and the skin is resected with its dermis. This full-thickness skin flap corresponds to the area between points B, C, D, E. Starting below the nipple areola complex, the inferior pedicle is dissected through the breast to the pectoral fascia. In this way the nipple areola complex is mobilized as a superior pedicled flap (Fig. 14.2). The inferior pedicle is a block of parenchyma of the lower pole of the breast. On all four sides of the flap, dissection is carried down to the pectoral fascia so that the block of tissue is totally mobile. The inferior flap is based only on the thoracic wall vasculature. The size of this flap depends on the size of the breast. With dissection, a large pocket is created beneath the superior pedicled flap. The inferior pedicle is fixed to the chest wall with absorbable sutures (Vicryl 3-0) (Fig. 14.3). These sutures do not threaten the blood supply. Tissue from the pedicle border can be resected in order to achieve a better shape. After finishing the montage, temporary sutures of nylon 2-0 are placed to the horizontal incision line starting from the lateral points of D and E to the middle of the submammary sulcus.

To facilitate closure, the assistant holds up the upper part of the breast and points B and C are stitched to the middle of the submammary sulcus with a nylon 2-0 suture, allowing the shape and symmetry of the new breast to be checked. Any further tidying of the wound markings can be performed at this stage. Two sutures of Vicryl 3-0 are placed just below the areola to the vertical line while the assistant is lifting the nipple areola complex (NAC) in a superior position. Then, 2–3 temporary sutures of nylon 2-0 are placed to the vertical line, burying the NAC temporarily inside the wound. The opposite breast is operated on in the same manner. The position of the NAC is now marked. It will be centered on or closed to point A. The NAC is secured at the most superior portion of the deepithelialized skin using interrupted U-sutures (nylon 4-0) which pass only through the dermis of the skin, thus avoiding suture marks in the skin surrounding the pigmented areola. Using a measuring compass, symmetry of the two NACs is achieved. The skin is closed with buried 3-0 Vicryl in the dermis and nylon 4-0 sutures in a mattress manner. It is important that the horizontal incision lines must not cross the midline. Micropore

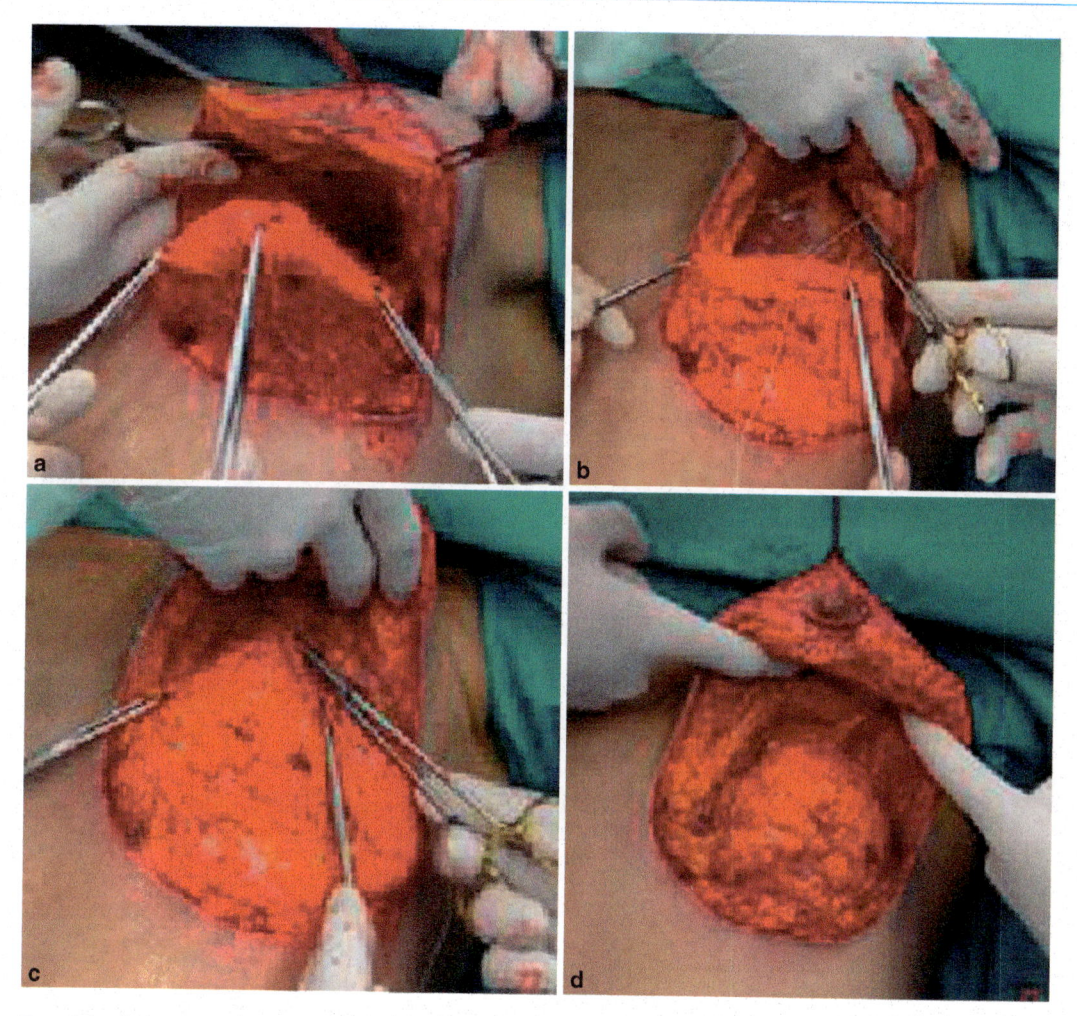

Fig. 14.3 (a–d) The inferior pedicle is a block of parenchyma of the lower pole of the breast. Dissection is carried down to the pectoral fascia so that the block of tissue is totally mobile. The inferior pedicle is fixed to the chest wall with absorbable sutures (Vicryl 2-0)

paper tapes are placed along the incisions lines. Suction-drains are not used. The patient is discharged from the hospital in 24 h.

14.3 Complications

One hundred ten patients with various degrees of breast ptosis underwent breast lifting (mastopexy) using this approach. Patient ages ranged from 18 to 70 years, with the highest proportion of patients between 35 and 45 years of age. The mean follow-up period was 5 years.

The majority of the patients were pleased with their outcomes. Results were judged to be pleasing by the surgeon in all cases (Fig. 14.4). The breasts were natural in their shape and appearance. Well vascularized skin flaps prevent necrosis and preserve sensation to the NAC. Fixation of the breasts to the chest wall was safe. Seroma and hematoma were avoided with vigorous hemostasis during surgery. Steatonecrosis or similar complications did not occur. There were no cases requiring secondary skin resection. No patients required blood transfusions.

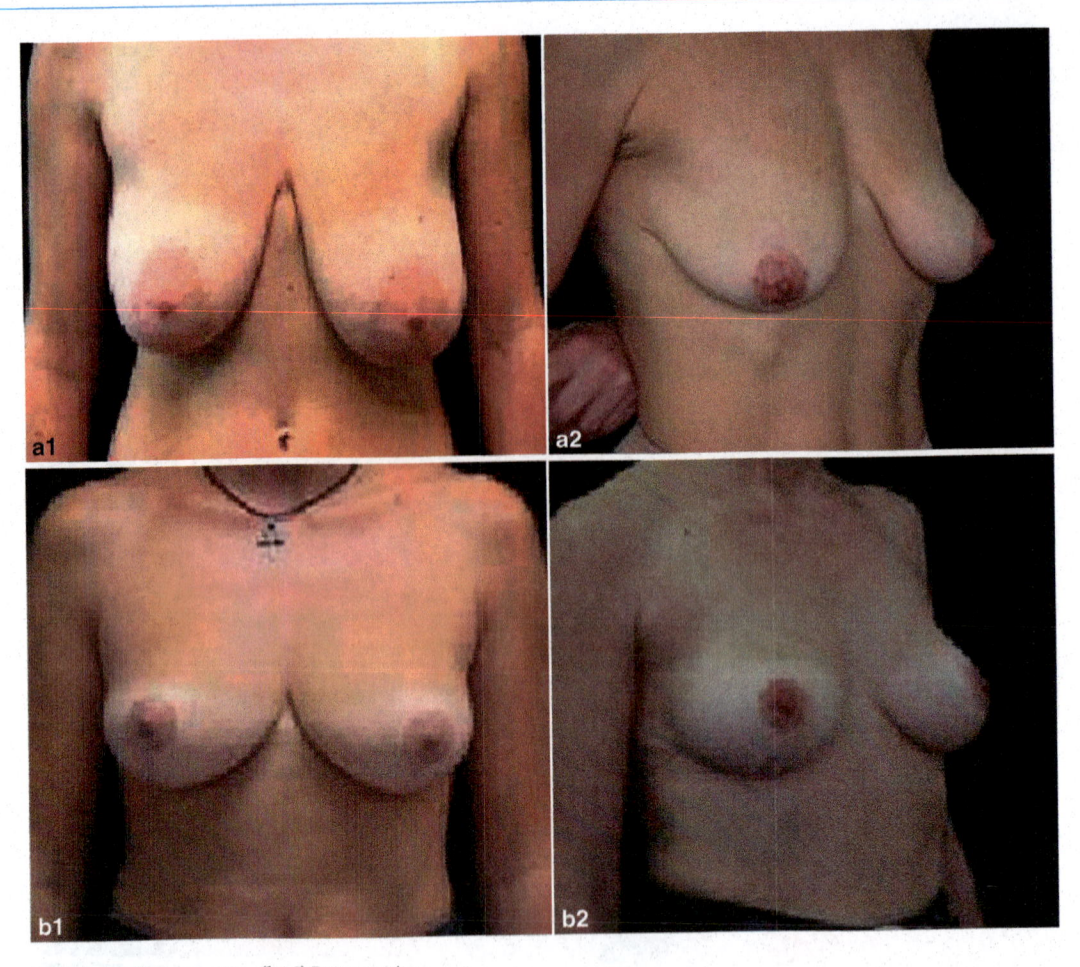

Fig. 14.4 (*a1,2*) Preoperative. (*b1,2*) Postoperative

Asymmetry and NAC epidermolysis were not specific problems.
Complications included the following:
1. Hypertrophic scar in three patients requiring hydrocortisone and prolonged use of silicone sheathing and pressure brassiere for 14 months.
2. Temporary decrease in nipple sensation, which was reported to return to the normal preoperative level within 3 months in two patients.

14.4 Discussion

Numerous plastic surgeons have described several mastopexy techniques. Changes in mastopexy techniques led to a better understanding of the three-dimensional shape of the breast and the interplay of the soft tissue dynamics.

With previous techniques, the authors observed that breast descent and loss of upper pole fullness were too common. The cause or recurrence of breast ptosis following mastopexy is faulty structural design in the operations in common use today. Each relies on the elastic skin and the dermis to suspend the breast and hold it in an unnatural position. Gravity and the thrust of the lower breast bulk ultimately exert their effect on the supporting skin and ptotic and sagging breasts typically recur with time, with the nipple relocating too high on the breast. In several techniques that have been described, the breast ended up with no projection or shape. Even though contour and position early after surgery are often good, the breasts progressively sag until they have a shape and position not very different from those prior to surgery. Many of these techniques do not relocate the mastopexy, taking breast mass from the caudal pole to fill out the deficient upper breast. The dermal or skin brassiere mastopexies, supported mainly by distensible skin flaps, deteriorate rapidly over ensuing months.

The techniques that utilize only a vertical scar that extended to the inframammary crease [16–19, 38] have the disadvantage of skin redundancy at the level of this crease. Skin based vertical scar mammaplasties resulted in wound closure under tension and therefore presented difficulties with the vertical component of the wound healing. Periareolar incision techniques allow the excess skin to be resected; however, the breast shape is not good and has only moderate areolar projection [5, 23, 39]. Periareolar mammaplasties usually resulted in widening of the periareolar scar, flattening of the breast contour, and early recurrence of the ptosis.

The author's experience showed that there is not only one perfect technique. The goal towards achieving an ideal breast through mastopexy led the author to a combination of superior and inferior breast flap approach. It is a modification of Pitanguy's mammaplasty technique of superior pole. The description of the inferior chest wall-based flap is for achieving a desirable shape that can be maintained over a long period of time. In this approach, the inferior flap is based only on the thoracic wall vasculature, completely detached from surrounding structures, maintaining a good volume. The upper flap of the breast covers the inferior flap. The physiological basis for this operation is utilization of the breast tissue as a biological implant to increase the breast projection. A flap support behind the NAC seems to reduce the risk of retracted nipple as a result of a drag inflicted by the weight of a folded superior flap previously seen more often. Follow-up for 10 years proves the stability of the result. By transposing lower breast tissue into the upper breast, most unwanted long-term side effects of mastopexy are avoidable. This approach diminishes caudal bulk while simultaneously correcting the deficiency of fullness in the upper pole of the breasts. The nipples retain their proper central breast mass location and do not redirect or migrate superiorly on the breast.

The concept of internal suspension to support the breast is not new [34–37]. However, the author's mastopexy approach satisfies the objectives of relocating the breast tissue superiorly while simultaneously reducing tension on the skin flaps allowing faster and less complicated healing. It ensures safe transposition of the NAC, nonrecurrence of ptosis, and aesthetically pleasing results. The flexibility during the operation suggests that the procedure is safe and appropriate for all sized ptotic breasts.

14.5
Conclusions

Mastopexy surgery has been modified in the past few years, as plastic surgeons worked to improve and maintain the breast shape and especially the "bottoming out" of the gland in the late postoperative period. The concept of internal suspension to support the breast is not new; however, in the author's approach the suspension achieves true permanent lifting in the mammary tissues utilizing a combination of superior and inferior breast flap. An inferior mobile, chest wall-based flap of breast tissue is created. This inferior breast tissue flap is transposed up and beneath the upper breast and behind the NAC with sutures anchoring to the pectoralis fascia. There is minimal breast descent when performing this approach, providing excellent long term aesthetic outcome.

References

1. Dieffenbach JF: Die extirpation der bruestdruese. In: Dieffenbach JF (ed), Die Operative Chirurgie. Brockhaus, Leipzig 1848, pp 359–373
2. Morestin H: Hypertophie mammaire unilaterale corrige par la resection discoide. Bull Mem Soc Chir Paris 1909;35:996
3. Villarde I: 1911-as mentioned in Dartigues L: Traitement chirurgical du prolapsus mammaire. Arch Franco-Belg Chir 1925;28:313
4. Lexer E: Correccion de los pechos pendulos (Mastoptose) por medio de la implantacion de grasa. Guipuzcoa Medica 1921;63:213
5. Strombeck JO: Mammaplasty: report of a new technique based on the two pedicle procedure. Br J Plast Surg 1961;13:79–90
6. Skoog T: A technique of breast reduction: transposition of the nipple on a cutaneous vascular pedicle. Acta Chir Scand 1963;126:453–465
7. Pitanguy I: Surgical treatment of breast hypertrophy. Br J Plast Surg 1967;20(1):78–85
8. McKissock PK: Reduction mammaplasty with a vertical dermal flap. Plast Reconstr Surg 1972;49(3):245–252
9. Skoog T: Plastic Surgery: New Methods and Refinements. Stockholm, Almqvist & Wiksell 1974
10. Ribeiro L: A new technique for reduction mammaplasty. Plast Reconstr Surg 1975;55(3):330–334
11. Courtiss EH, Goldwyn RM: Reduction mammaplasty by the inferior pedicle technique: an alternative to free nipple and areola grafting for severe macromastia or extreme ptosis. Plast Reconstr Surg 1977;59(1):500–507
12. Peixoto G: Reduction mammaplasty: a personal technique. Plast Reconstr Surg 1980;65(2):217–226
13. Marconi F: The dermal pursestring suture: a new technique for a short inframammary scar in reduction mammaplasty and dermal mastopexy. Ann Plast Surg 1989;22(6):484–493
14. Parenteau JM, Regnault P: The Regnault B technique in mastopexy and breast reduction: a 12 year review. Aesthetic Plast Surg 1989;13(2):75–79
15. Marchac D, Olarte G: Reduction mammaplasty and correction of ptosis with a short inframammary scar. Plast Reconstr Surg 1982;69(1):45–55

16. Regnault P: Breast reduction and mastopexy, an old love story: B technique update. Aesthetic Plast Surg 1990;14(2):101–106
17. Krupp S: Mastopexy: modification of periwinkle shell operation. Ten years of experience. Aesthetic Plast Surg 1990;14(1):9–14
18. Benelli L: A new periareolar mammaplasty: the "round block" technique. Aesthetic Plast Surg 1990;14(2):93–100
19. Sampaio Goes JC: Periareolar mammaplasty with mixed mesh support: the double skin technique. Plast Surg 1992;2:575
20. Chiari A Jr: The L short-scar mammaplasty: a new approach. Plast Reconstr Surg 1992;90(2):233–246
21. Marconi F, Cavina C: Reduction mammaplasty and correction of ptosis: a personal technique. Plast Reconstr Surg 1993;91(6):1046–1056
22. Daniel MJB: Mammaplasty with pectoral muscle flap. Presented at the 64th American Annual Scientific Meeting of the American Society of Plastic and Reconstructive Surgery, Montreal 1995
23. Goes JC: Periareolar mammaplasty: double skin technique with application of polyglactin or mixed mesh. Plast Reconstr Surg 1996;97(5):959–968
24. Flowers RS, Smith EM Jr: "Flip-Flap" Mastopexy. Aesthetic Plast Surg 1998;22(6):425–429
25. Fayman MS: Short scar mastopexy with flap transposition. Aesthetic Plast Surg 1998;22(2):135–141
26. De Araujo Cerqeira A: Mammoplasty: Breast fixation with dermoglandular mono upper pedicle under the pectoralis muscle. Aesthetic Plast Surg 1998;22(4):276–283
27. Lejour M: Vertical mammaplasty: Early complications after 250 personal consecutive cases. Plast Reconstr Surg 1999;104(3):764–770
28. Lassus C: Update on vertical mammaplasty. Plast Reconstr Surg 1999;104(7):2289–2298
29. Hall-Findlay EJ: A simplified vertical reduction mammaplasty shortening the learning curve. Plast Reconstr Surg 1999;104(3):748–759
30. Eed MD: A new personal surgical procedure for breast reduction and lifting. Aesthetic Plast Surg 2000;24(3):206–211
31. Spear SL, Giese SY, Ducic I: Concentric mastopexy revised. Plast Reconstr Surg 2001;107(5):1294–1299
32. Hinderer U: Circumareolar dermo-glandular plication: a new concept for correction of breast ptosis. Aesthetic Plast Surg 2001;25(6):404–420
33. Hall-Findlay EJ: Pedicles in vertical breast reduction and mastopexy. Clin Plast Surg 2002;29(3):379–391
34. Hammond DC: The SPAIR mammaplasty. Clin Plast Surg 2002;29(3):411–421
35. Graf R, Reis de Araujo LR, Rippel R, Neto LG, Pace DT, Biggs T: Reduction mammaplasty and mastopexy using the vertical scar and thoracic wall flap technique. Aesthetic Plast Surg 2003;27(1):6–12
36. Qiao Q, Sun J, Liy C, Liu Z, Zhao R: Reduction mammaplasty and correction of ptosis: dermal bra technique. Plast Reconstr Surg 2003;111(3):1122–1130
37. Perez-Macias JM: Personal mastopexy technique for breast stabilisation: update. Br J Plast Surg 2004;57(2):178
38. Graf R, Biggs TM: In search of better shape in mastopexy and reduction mammoplasty. Plast Reconstr Surg 2002;110(1):309–317
39. Gasperoni C, Salgarello M, Gasperoni P: A personal technique: mammaplasty with J scar. Ann Plast Surg 2002;48(2):124–130

# The Triple-Flap Interposition Mammaplasty

Alberto Magno Lott Caldeira, Georg Bernhard Roth

15.1 Introduction

The history of reduction mammaplasty from 1980 until now can be seen as a period of refinements of existing techniques which mostly focused on the reduction of the final scar. These existing techniques were established in the late fifties to the late seventies, a period defined by Cardoso de Oliveira in Goldwyn's "Reduction mammaplasty" as the "period of safety" [1]. Many of these techniques share the principle of Lexer-Kraske [2, 3], that is, central wedge dissection in the lower half and approximation of the lateral poles to form the breast. Almost all techniques reinforced an element that was felt to be neglected before and is nowadays associated with Schwarzmann [4], that is, deepithelialization of the skin around the areola and avoidance of skin separation from the gland to respect the cutaneous–glandular unity.

However, less consideration has been given to what we believe to be the fundamental principle in reduction mammaplasty. To produce a long lasting aesthetically pleasing breast shape, the gland itself has to be altered into the desired form. Some breasts need to have reduction in their base to control the height and form of the conical projection. Thus, there may be need for dissection of the gland from the pectoralis fascia. Other breasts need a reduction in their axillary pole and have to be put into a more medial position, with the areola on the apex of the newly created cone. Consequently, it may be necessary to manipulate the lateral and medial poles.

To transform a pendulous breast into a conical-shaped breast, there has to be a method that is versatile enough to allow this transformation. The concept of glandular shaping goes back to Biesenberger [5]. However, in retrospect, the critical attention given to his approach focused on the complete dissection of the skin from the gland and the associated complications [6, 7]. Less attention was given to the merit of glandular shaping.

If the goal of the surgical procedure is to alter form and volume of the breast, then the focus has to be on the "nature" of the breasts. This includes analysis of skin quality, shape and projection of the breast, asymmetries, contour of the surrounding areas (such as the upper abdomen and lateral thorax), and content of the gland. The latter two points will raise the question of whether liposuction should be applied to improve the surrounding contours of the breast to allow for better projection and to reduce the volume of the breast where needed. In many of the patients, the authors choose to use liposuction as the first surgical step.

Many of the existing techniques can produce excellent results, depending on the surgeon's ability to analyze the preoperative situation and to find a safe surgical solution for the required improvement in shape and thereby reduction in volume. As many have pointed out, there is no one single technique for every patient. Consequently, the authors suggest viewing the triple-flap interposition technique more as an approach, a base to start from, as the formation of three flaps offers various variables that can change the breast shape.

15.2 History

The senior author's first mammaplasties were performed in 1984 using classical Pitanguy, the Arie-Pitanguy, and the lozenge procedures [6–11]. Critical observation of the results, being in dialogue with other surgeons throughout the world, as well as reading critical publications, led to the conclusion that in many cases the results of these procedures did not meet the patients' and surgeons' expectations, especially in the long run, and sometimes also in the immediate postoperative state [12–22]. The results were considered sometimes unfavorable because of the lack of a conical shape of the breasts, pointing out that most procedures produce a round shape. Moreover, there was consensus that many procedures do not provide adequate resection of the breast base and do not allow for a medialization of the breast. Most important was the observation that the operated breasts tended to resume their previous shape in the late postoperative stage [23–28].

The Triple-flap interposition technique was first published in English in 1995 [27]. From 1987 to 2007, the approach was used by the senior author in his private practice in 1,289 cases.

M.A. Shiffman (ed.), *Mastopexy and Breast Reduction: Principles and Practice*,
© Springer-Verlag Berlin Heidelberg 2009

15.3 Principles of the Triple-Flap Interposition Technique in Mammaplasty

The Triple-flap interposition technique relies on an upper pedicle to the areola and is defined by the creation of three glandular flaps in order to shape a conical breast using skin resections that result in minimal scarring. Glandular tissue is resected in a rhomboid or oblique manner while creating a central, lateral, and medial glandular flap.

The idea of the technique is to shape glandular tissue to create a conical shaped breast, and to allow for, whenever necessary, the reduction of the mammary base and the axillary pole as well as the medialization of the breast. The areola is placed on the apex of the cone supplied by an upper pedicle.

The interposition and suturing of the three glandular flaps promote the reformulation of the Cooper ligament system, thus resulting in a long-lasting conical breast configuration. Accordingly, the skin simply covers what has been shaped, free of traction or tension.

Skin glandular undermining takes place only in a limited area of the inferior hemisphere; the breast base is widely undermined from pectoral fascia, though care has to be taken not to injure the perforators of the internal and lateral thoracic arteries, which supply the glandular flaps.

Liposuction might be the first surgical step, depending on the contour of the lateral thorax and upper abdomen, as well as on the fat composition of the gland.

The triple-flap interposition is a mammaplasty technique that involves the following:

1. Shaping of glandular tissue to create a conical breast configuration
2. Relocating the areola on a superior pedicle on the apex of the cone
3. Skin undermining on the inferior hemisphere of the breast
4. Undermining of the breast base from the pectoralis fascia
5. Skin resection that results in minimal scarring

The goals of the triple-flap interposition technique in mammaplasty can be outlined as (1) shaping of conical, aesthetically pleasing breasts, thereby reducing breast volume and (2) the breast shape has to be stable, scars limited, and the procedure safe.

15.4 Triple-Flap Interposition Technique

15.4.1 Markings and Skin Incision

It is not necessary to adhere to one fixed pattern of skin incision with this technique. Types of skin incisions may vary depending on the skin condition and breast volume. Generally, the authors apply the lozenge [10], Peixoto's [23], and circumferential techniques [29, 30] (Fig. 15.1). Alternatively, the markings of other short scarring techniques [31, 32], for example, the vertical mammaplasty of Lejour, can be used [33].

After skin incision, deepithelialization is carried out carefully to safeguard the nipple–areola complex and the central flap, which will be formed later. Skin-glandular undermining of the inferior hemisphere begins on the decorticated area and extends to the axillary region when necessary. This undermining should be carried out between the glandular and the areolar tissue (Fig. 15.2).

The breast base is undermined from the pectoral fascia, and on reaching the parasternal region, this should be done in a careful manner to preserve the perforators (rami II, III, IV) of the internal thoracic artery. The breast tissue is raised and two vertical incisions converging downward are carried out to create the central vertical flap with a base pedicle adequate to its extension. This flap is irrigated by the II. Perforators of the internal thoracic artery [34] (Fig. 15.3).

Two glandular tissue flaps corresponding to the medial and lateral pillars of the breast are created posteriorly (Fig. 15.3). The medial horizontal flap is vascularized mostly by the III and IV perforators of the internal thoracic artery and the lateral horizontal flap is vascularized by the ramifications of the lateral thoracic artery and rami acromialis [34, 35] (Fig. 15.3).

After comparing the total breast volume bilaterally, the glandular tissue is resected in an oblique, rhomboid manner [8]. Alternatively, the base of the gland can be removed in a disc-like fashion [23]. Thus, if the breast has a large base, it is easier to narrow and/or reduce the height of the projection of the new breast cone. In addition, the combination of both types of resection may be applied to achieve the desired shape [36]. Following

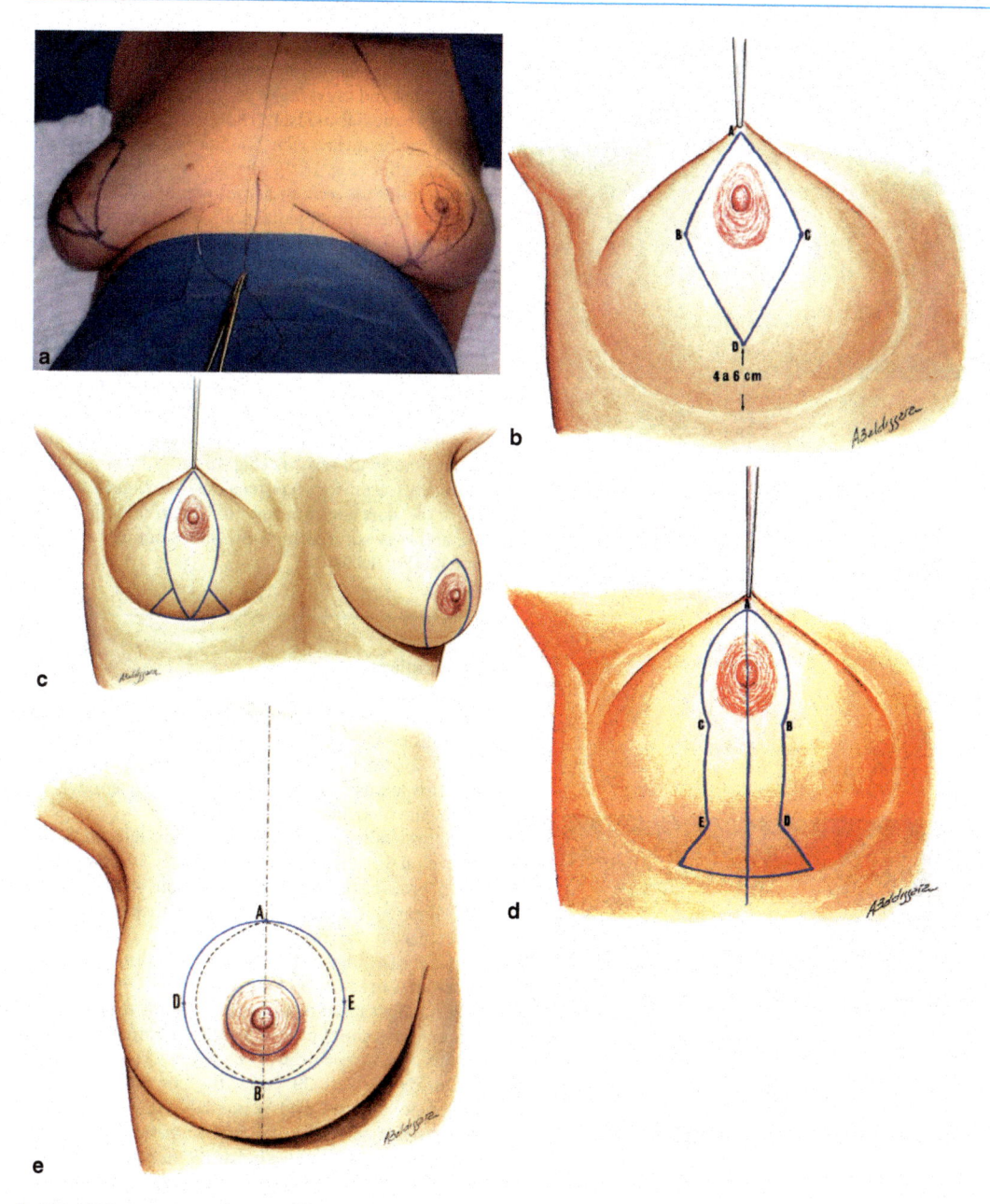

Fig. 15.1 (a) Preoperative marking. Note "dome-shaped" supra-areolar design. (b) Lozenge marking. Note that distance ACB equals the circumference of the areola. (c) Alternative markings. (d) Alternative markings. (e) Circumferential marking

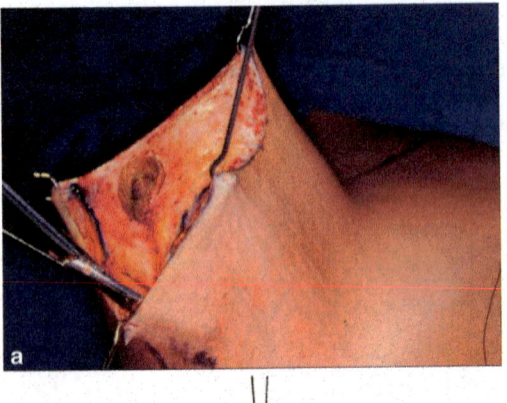

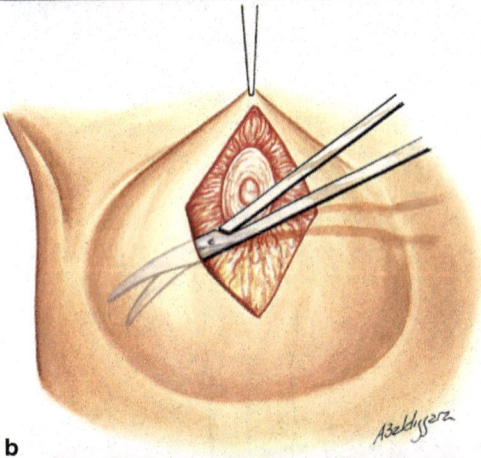

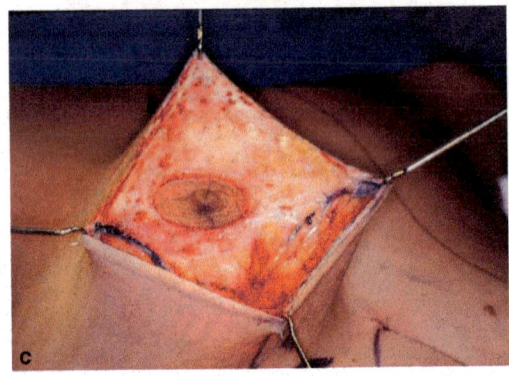

Fig. 15.2 (a) Intraoperative view. (b) Skin-glandular undermining. (c) After skin-glandular undermining

careful hemostasis, the breast is raised by a hook placed at the apex that remains throughout the shaping of the breast (Fig. 15.4).

The distal end of the central flap is sutured to the fascia pectorals using three 2-0 Vicryl or Prolene sutures. The adequate length of the flap will prevent downward traction of the areolar complex (Fig. 15.5). The main purpose of this flap is to provide projection of the areolar complex and prevent a flattened aspect (Fig. 15.6).

The two medial and lateral horizontal flaps are rotated toward the hemiclavicular line and are transposed one over the other (Fig. 15.7). The placement of these flaps will determine the contour of the lower breast hemisphere, shape the lateral and medial poles, and narrow the base. Moreover, this maneuver defines the new submammary fold, besides helping to correct important breast asymmetries.

Positioning of the medial and lateral flaps depends on the need to provide more volume to either of these segments. Generally, the medial flap is deeply secured to the base of the lateral flap that is rotated over the medial flap and sutured over its surface using 2-0 Vicryl or Prolene. Minor irregularities are corrected by trimming the fat tissue with scissors (Fig. 15.8).

Skin resection renders tension-free wound borders where the skin does not function as an outer brassiere. The areola is sutured by four Gillies sutures with 6-0 Prolene (Fig. 15.9).

15.5
Complications

During the initial development phase of this procedure, the authors observed three cases of partial steatonecrosis and one total steatonecrosis in the area of the central flap. This led us to always maintain a wide enough flap base while reducing the gland.

In three other cases, formation of nodules in the lateral region was observed, caused by partial steatonecrosis. Again, after limiting the manipulation of inferior and medial parts of the lateral flap, no further complication with regard to flap necrosis occurred.

In the early phase of using this procedure, there were 14 seromas in the area of the lateral pole. These seromas were mainly caused by liposuction of the thoracolateral region. On account of this, a second drainage was used for this region specifically.

During the last 20 years, the complications were limited to the so-called *minor* complications, such as hypertrophic scarring, especially in patients of African origin; the infection rate lies below 1.95%; partial skin dehiscence is below 1%, as well as hematomas is below 1%.

The occurrence of asymmetries in 18 patients in the later postoperative period was difficult to deal with. In 11 of these cases, a secondary reduction mammaplasty was undertaken to correct the asymmetry.

In 15 cases, the shape of the breast distorted 1 month postoperatively, because the lateral flap lost its internal fixation, causing the breast to shift laterally. All these cases were reoperated on, with satisfying results and no further complications.

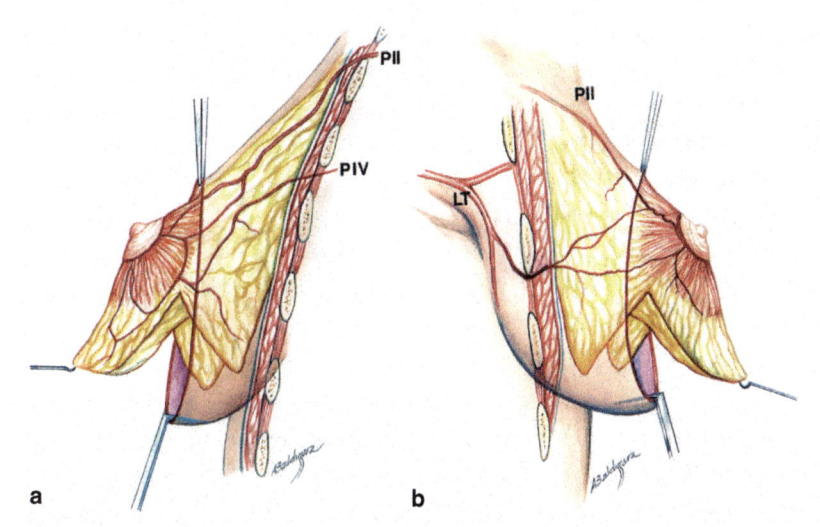

Fig. 15.3 (a) The skin surface area and the glandular tissue are considerably vascularized by the pII. It includes the upper portion of the breast, the nipple–areolar complex, and the subjacent antero-medial region. (b) Vascular network of the lateral artery

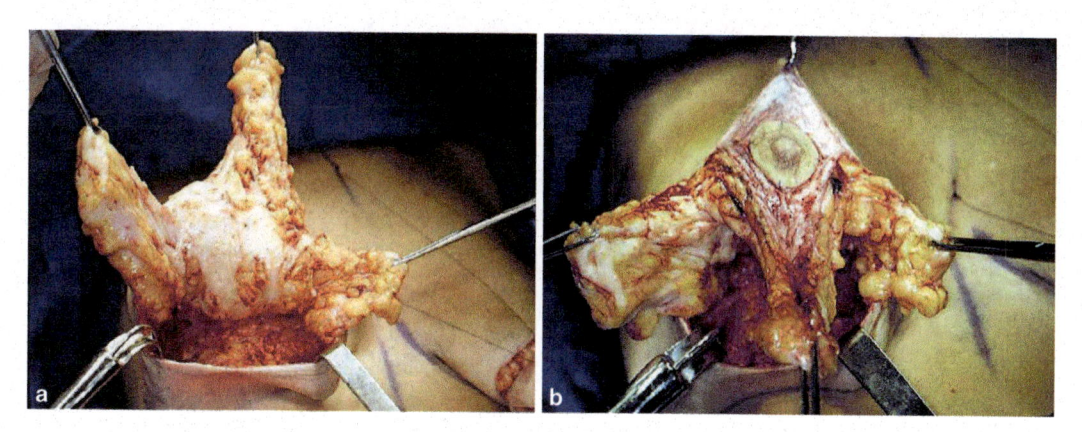

Fig. 15.4 (a) Central, medial, and lateral flaps. (b) Central, medial, and lateral flaps

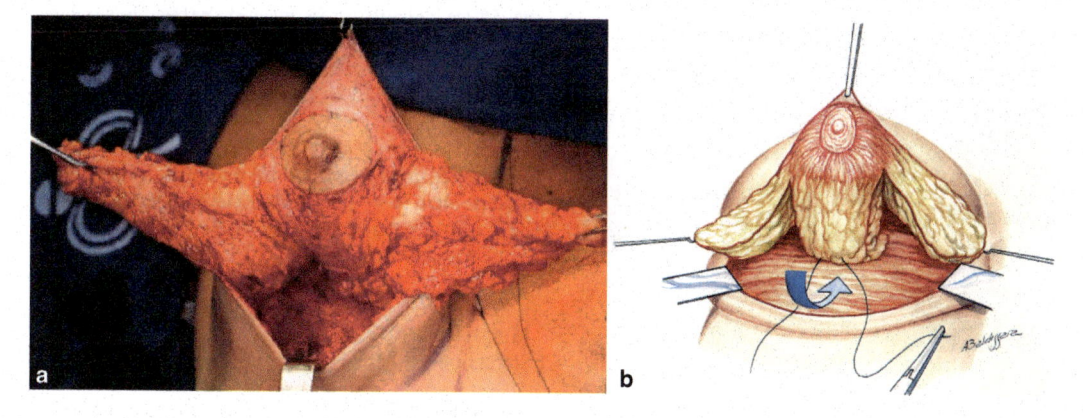

Fig. 15.5 (a) Positioning of the central flap. (b) Positioning of the central flap

Fig. 15.6 Resections of circumareolar skin have a truncating effect on breast contour

Fig. 15.8 (a) The breast shape is sustained even before being sutured to the skin. (b) The one-dimensional sector excisions from a cone, when carried out to an extreme, result in a shape of a spire

With regard to nipple sensitivity, the study the authors undertook in 1999 [36] showed a temporary decrease in 12% of the patients. In all these cases sensitivity recovered within 6 months.

15.6
Discussion

The goal of this technique is to provide a stable shape of the breast by forming a glandular cone. Consequently, the skin covers what has been shaped, without tension

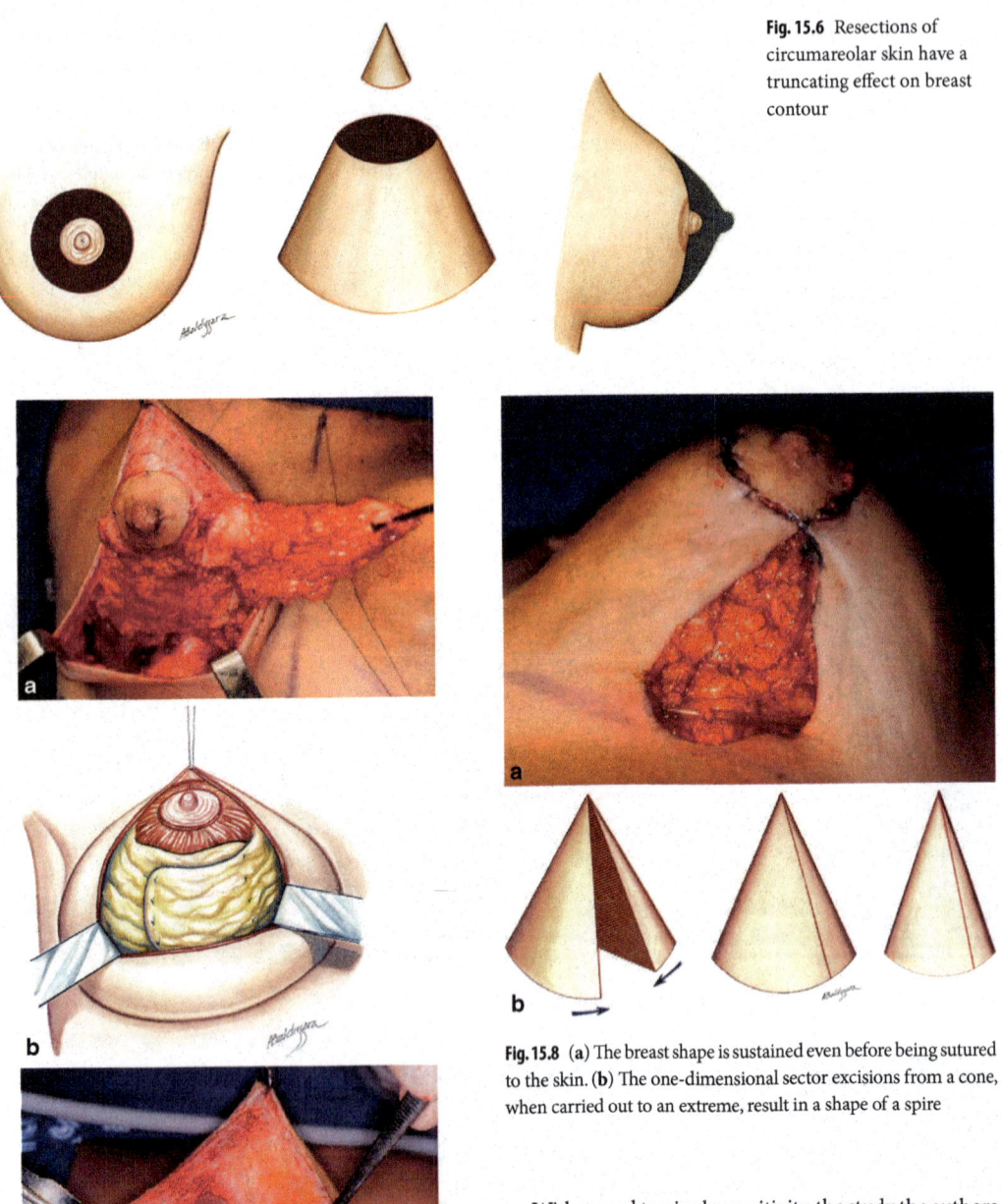

Fig. 15.7 Shaping the breast. (a) Interposition of lateral and medial flaps. (b) The interposition of the medial and lateral flaps sustains the breast and plays a crucial role in reshaping the gland. (c) Positioning of the lateral flap

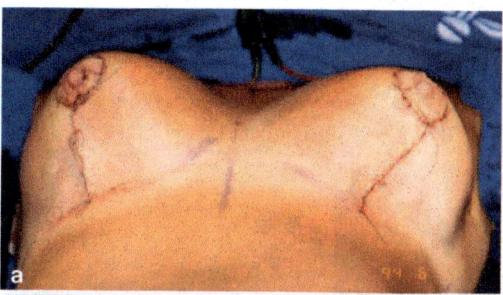

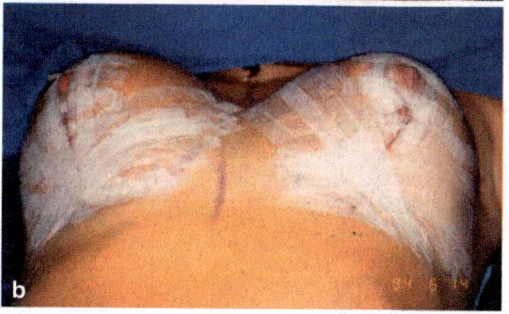

Fig. 15.9 (a) Completion of subcuticular and intradermal suturing. (b) During the first four postoperative weeks, the dressing substitutes a brassiere, which is recommended to be used only for 30 days after the operation

accommodating the ideal condition for the scar to heal. Postoperatively, the reshaped breasts proved to be stable and kept the desired conical shape in the long run (Figs. 15.10 and 15.11).

When used in narrow-based or slightly wide breasts, standard techniques generally produce good results. Many of these are Lexer-Kraske type methods that approximate the lateral and medial pillars after wedge dissection [2, 3, 6, 12, 33, 37–40]. However, they often do not yield a satisfactory and stable result when applied to large-based, pendulous breasts with inelastic skin [41, 42]. The reason for the breasts to relapse into their former ptotic shape is the fact that the nature of the shape has not been changed by these techniques. They have less volume, but the broad base and the glandular tissue have no "inner support" that prevents them from "falling down" [23, 43–45]. The authors believe that the forming of a narrow-based breast together with the interglandular suturing provides a stable shape. One reason for this is that the Cooper ligaments are reorganized, thus the gland is liberated from what could be called the "structural mammary memory."

Another reason is that interglandular scarring leads to a more fibrous content of the breast; the breast content will be firmer, especially in those cases where liposuction has been used to reduce the fat content of the gland. And most important, the formation of lateral and medial flaps which are rotated towards the hemiclavicular line and are transposed over each other creates an inner "brassiere," thereby giving the necessary inner support to prevent the breasts from relapsing into their former shape. One may argue that some of the heavy pendulous breasts have a substantial fat content and that the creation of a cone more or less consisting of fat tissue will not produce a long-lasting result. In these cases, we would extend the technique to a procedure that uses a strip of the pectoralis muscle to provide the "inner brassiere" [46]. Nevertheless, in our experience the indication for this procedure tends to be an exception in primary reduction mammaplasties, and is mostly applied to secondary reduction mammaplasties of breasts, which relapsed into their old ptotic shape and are dominated by a high fat content of the gland and inelastic skin.

The triple flap interposition technique involves glandular undermining from the pectoralis fascia. The axial blood supply of the flaps has to be respected, thus the gland is not dissected completely and parts of the upper inner and outer quadrants remain untouched. There is a tendency for large adipose breasts to atrophy in the postoperative period. This observation led the authors to reduce breast volume more conservatively in these breasts and perform a second intervention when necessary after 6 months. This second procedure could be liposuction alone depending on whether the breast shape proved to be stable or could be a secondary reduction mammaplasty using the triple flap interposition technique with or without the use of a pectoralis muscle flap.

Reports on liposuction as the sole procedure in the reduction of a hypertrophic breast are encouraging, though they lack large patient numbers [47, 48]. Nevertheless, in certain cases, liposuction alone achieves excellent results in breast reduction. It is evident that liposuction is not a tissue selective procedure with fat, glandular, and to a lesser extent supportive tissue being removed. It is thus possible to reduce a "glandular" breast as well, though in this case liposuction is more difficult and time consuming. Consequently, the authors do not limit liposuction to a breast with a high fat content per se.

The cutaneous–glandular undermining proposed by this technique allows complete visualization and manipulation of the various breast segments and consequently favors the treatment proposed. However, one has to avoid undermining the whole inferior hemisphere per se. Specifically, when the skin resection yields an inverted T scar, unnecessary wide undermining will cause skin necrosis in the conjunction area of the skin flaps. Consequently, the authors restrict the cutaneous–glandular undermining to an area that rarely exceeds the breast base. As a rule of thumb, undermining stops at approximately 1 cm away from the medial or lateral borders of the corresponding poles.

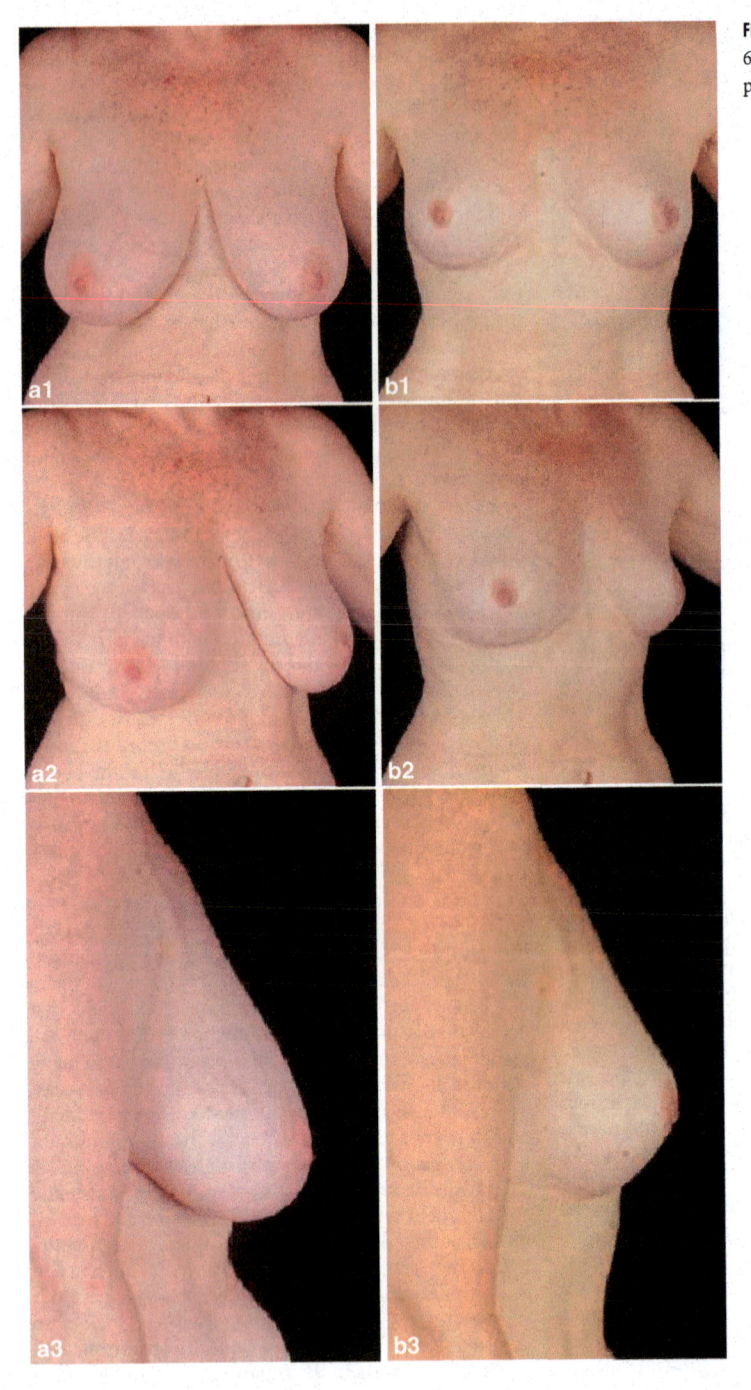

Fig. 15.10 (**a***1-3*) Preoperative 62-year-old patient. (**b***1-3*) Two years postoperative

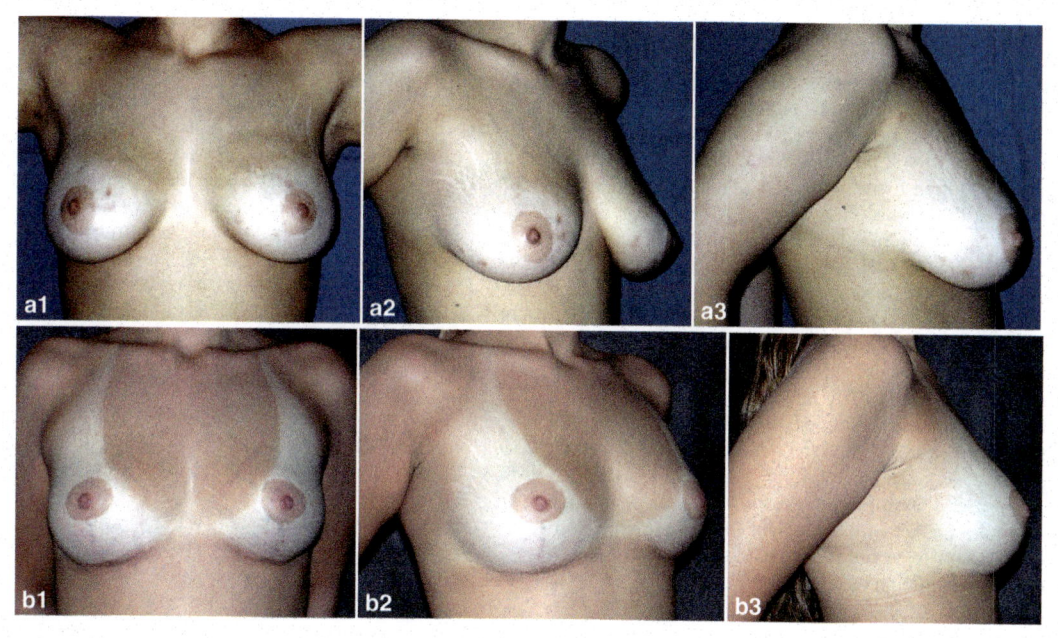

Fig. 15.11 (*a1–3*) Preoperative 19-year-old patient. (*b1–3*) nine years postoperatively

The use of a superior based flap to the areola has proved to be safe in this specific technique and corresponds to the experience of other authors who also rely on a superior based flap [48, 49]. The creation of the central flap that relies on the upper based flap for blood supply provides the volume that is needed in the central and upper part of conical-shaped breast. Thus, the fixation is not positioned superior to the future apex, but exactly under the future position of the areola. Plication of a central pedicle or flap to the pectoralis fascia alone does not provide sufficient long-lasting support for the glandular tissue, that is to say the breast will become ptotic again as the glandular tissue will slide, along the pectoralis fascia, downwards, as other authors have reported [8, 10, 22, 45, 50, 51]. Stability of the breast shape is granted largely by interpositioning the three flaps with one another and not by plicating glandular tissue to the pectoralis fascia.

After the cutaneous-glandular undermining in the lower half, dissection of the gland from the pectoralis fascia, and creation of conical shaped gland, the new submammary fold ideally lies 2–3 cm above the old. If not, there is need for further reshaping and reduction. The distance between the relocated areola and the new submammary fold should not exceed 6 cm. Underlying these statements is the observation that within the first two postoperative months, the breast descends by approximately 2–3 cm. Consequently, the distance between areola and submammary fold will enlarge as well. A distance of more than 8 cm is associated with a ptotic breast shape and thus the postoperative result would be less than ideal. The reason for the breast to descend, that is, the submammary fold to settle at a lower place, is subject to speculation. The superficial fascial system needs 2–3 months to reorganize its collagen fibers, settling at a point where the gravitational pull is offset by the suspension given by the newly reorganized superficial fascial system; this "suspension" is also influenced, among other factors, by the shape of the breast, its content, and skin quality. In other words, a multitude of factors play a role in the descending of the submammary fold. Therefore, the numbers described are the empirical answer to where the submammary fold settles and thus dictates the design of the breast intraoperatively.

Is the triple flap interposition technique easy to learn? In the authors' opinion, the technique is not more difficult to learn than other techniques. The creation of three flaps might sound complicated, but actually it only means that after dissection from the pectoralis fascia, the gland will be divided into three parts. A fixed, predetermined tissue excision pattern is advocated by many authors who often point out that residents will find it easier to adhere to fixed pattern during an operation [32, 36, 37]. However, it is exactly the "pattern" that often hinders the younger surgeon from really grasping the operation technique, as he or she just has to cut along the markings. With predetermined tissue excision patterns without skin undermining, the skin tends to be excised at an early operation state, that is, before the gland has been reshaped. In triple-flap interposition technique, skin excision takes place only after glandular shaping has taken place.

In cases of asymmetric breasts, it is easier to obtain a symmetric result with three flaps to shape the breast in comparison to techniques that use a wedge resection and approximation of two pillars.

15.7
Conclusions

The triple-flap method has proved to be safe as long as the blood supply of the glandular flaps is respected. The results accomplished are long lasting and render the desired, aesthetically pleasing, conical shaped breasts.

The Lexer-Kraske type methods reduce the volume but often fail to alter the nature of the breast form. As a consequence, they tend to resume to their former shape in the long run, in other words, they are often subject to bottoming out.

Reduction mammaplasty is about reshaping the gland into the desired form. Creating three glandular flaps to do this is suggested by the authors.

References

1. Psillakis JM, Cardoso de Oliveira M: History of reduction mammaplasty. In: Goldwyn RM (ed). Reduction Mammaplasty. Boston, Little, Brown and Company 1990, pp 1–15
2. Lexer E: Zur operation der mammahypertrophie und der hängebrust. Dtsch Med Wochenschr 1925;51:26
3. Kraske H: Die operation der atrophischen und hypertrophischen hängebrust. München Med Wochenschr 1923; 70:672–673
4. Schwarzmann E: Die technik der mammaplastik. Chirurgie 1930;2:932–943
5. Biesenberger H: Eine neue methode der mammaplastik. Zentralbl Chir 1928;55:2382–2387
6. Pitanguy I: Breast hypertrophy. In: Transactions of the International Society of Plastic Surgeons, Second Congress, London, Livingstone 1960, p 502
7. Pitanguy I: Mamaplastias. Estudo de 245 casos consecutivos e apresentação de técnica pessoal. Ver Brás Cir 1961; 42:201
8. Pitanguy I, Caldeira AML, Alexandrino A, Martinez JG: Mamaplastia redutora e mastopexia técnica Pitanguy vinte e cinco anos e experiência. Ver Brás Cir 1984;74:265
9. Ribeiro L: A new technique for reduction mammaplasty. Plast Reconstr Surg 1975;55(3):330–334
10. Ribeiro L: Redução mamária. In: Cirurgia Plástica da Mama Medsi, Rio de Janeiro 1989, p 185
11. Ribeiro L, Muzzy S, Accorsi JÁ: Mammaplastia redutora técnica circunferencial. Cir Plas Ibero Lat Am, 1992;18:249
12. Lassus C: An "all-season" mammaplasty. Aesthetic Plast Surg 1986;10(1):9–15
13. Lima JC: Our experience in breast reduction. VI Congress IPRS, Paris 1975
14. Maillard GF: A Z-mammaplasty with minimal scarring. Plast Reconstr Surg 1986;77(1):66–76
15. Marconi F: The dermal pursestring suture: new technique for a short inframammary scar in reduction mammaplasty and dermal mastopexy. Ann Plast Surg 1989;22(6):484–493
16. Marconi F, Cavina C: Reduction mammaplasty and correction of the ptosis. A personal technique. Plast Reconstr Surg 1993;91(6):1046–1056
17. Martins PD: Periareolar mammaplasty with flap transposition. Rev Soc Bras Cir Plast 1991;6:1
18. Mathes SJ, Nahai F, Hester TR: Avoiding the flat breast in reduction mammaplasty. Plast Reconstr Surg 1980;66(1):63–70
19. McKissock PK: Reduction mammaplasty with a vertical dermal flap. Plast Reconstr Surg 1972;49(3):245–252
20. McKissock PK: Avoiding the flat breast in reduction mammaplasty (discussion). Plast Reconstr Surg 1980;66(1):69
21. Nicolle FV, Chir M: Improved standards in reduction mammaplasty and mastopexy. Plast Reconstr Surg 1982; 69(3):453–459
22. Nicolle FV, Chir M: Reduction mammoplasty and mastopexy: a personal technique. Aesthetic Plast Surg 1984;8 (1):43–50
23. Peixoto G: Reduction mammaplasty: a personal technique. Plast Reconstr Surg 1980;65(2):217–226
24. Caldeira AML: New approach to breast surgery, personal technique. Annals 8th Internacional Congress on Senology, Rio de Janeiro, Brazil, May 12, 1994, p 1400
25. Caldeira AML: Nova abordagem de sustentação de mamoplastias. Comunication to the Jornada Paulista de Cirurgia Plástica. Brazilian Society Plastic Aesthetic and Reconstruction Surgery, São Paulo, Brazil, June 2, 1994
26. Caldeira AML: Nova abordagem de sustentação de mamoplastias redutoras. Comunication to the X Congresso Iberolatinoamericano de Cirurgia Plástica, Vina del Mar, Chile, Nov 17, 1994
27. Caldeira AML: Triple flap interposition technique. Comunication to the 11th Congress of the International

Confederation of Plastic, Reconstructive and Aesthetic Surgery, Yokohama, Japan, April 16, 1995, p 188

28. Candiani P, Campiglio GL, Signorini M: Personal experience with the central pedicle reduction mammaplasty. Rev Soc Bras Cir Plast 1991;6:11

29. Hinderer UT: Primera experiencia con una nueva tecnica de mastoplastia para ptosis ligeras. VI Reun Nac Soc Esp Cir Plast Rep Madrid 1969. Noticias Medicas y Tribuna Medica 1969;6:26

30. Bustus RA, Loureiro LEK: Mamaplastia redutora de retalho glandular triobulado de pedículo inferior por incisão periareolar. Trans XXIV Congr. Cir Plast. Gramado, APLUB 1985:484

31. Hollander E: Die operation de mammahyperthrophie und, der hangerbrust. Dtsche Med Wschr 1924;50:1.400

32. Lalaedrie JP, Mouly R: History of mammaplasty. Aesthetic Plast Surg 1978;2:167

33. Lejour M: Vertical mammaplasty and liposuction of the breast. Plast Reconstr Surg 1994;94(1):100–114

34. Bertelli JA, Pereira JFV: The inframammary island flap: anatomical basis. Ann Plast Surg 1994;32(3):315–320

35. Cardoso AD, Cardoso AD, Pessanha MC, Peralta JM: Three dermal pedicles for nipple-areola complex movement in reduction of gigantomastia. Ann Plast Surg 1984;12(5): 419–427

36. Caldeira AM, Lucas A, Grigalek G: Mastoplasty: The triple-flap interpostion technique. Aesthetic Plast Surg 1999; 23(1):51–60

37. Strombeck JO: Mammaplasty: report of a new technique based on the two-pedicle procedure. Br J Plast Surg 1961; 13:79–90

38. Wise RJ: A preliminary report on a method of planning the mammaplasty. Plast Reconstr Surg 1956;17:367–375

39. Thorek M: Possibilities in the reconstruction of the human form. NY Med J 1922;116:572

40. Skoog TA: Technique of breast reduction. Transposition of the nipple on a cutaneous vascular pedicle. Acta Chir Scand 1963;126:453–465

41. Williams G, Hoffman S: Mammoplasty for tubular breasts. Aesthetic Plast Surg 1981;5(1):51–56

42. Weiner DL, Aiache AE, Silver L, Tittiranonda T: A single dermal pedicle for nipple transposition in subcutaneous mastectomy, reduction mammaplasty, or mastopexy. Plast Reconstr Surg 1973;51(2):115–120

43. Hoffman S: Recurrent deformities following reduction mammaplasty and correction of breast asymmetry. Plast Reconstr Surg 1986;78(1):55–62

44. Hoffman S: Reduction mammaplasty: a medicolegal hazard? Aesthetic Plast Surg 1987;11(2):113–116

45. Pers M, Nielsen IM, Gerner N: Results following reduction mammaplasty as evaluated by the patients. Ann Plast Surg 1986;17(6):449–455

46. Caldeira AM, Lucas A: Pectoralis major muscle flap: a new support approach to mammaplasty, personal technique. Aesthetic Plast Surg 2000;24(1):58–70

47. Mellul SD, Dryden RM, Remigio DJ, Wulc AE: Breast reduction performed by liposuction. Dermatol Surg 2006; 32(9):1124–1133

48. Moskovitz MJ, Baxt SA, Jain AK, Hausman RE: Liposuction breast reduction: a prospective trial in African American women. Plast Reconstr Surg 2007;119(2):718–726

49. Hakme F: Técnica em "L"nas ptoses mamárias com confecção de retalhos cruzados. Rev Bras Cir 1983;73:87

50. de Souza Pinto EB, Ferraz de Almeida AE, Reyes MF: Dermoadipose and adenadipose flaps in mammoplasty. Aesthetic Plast Surg 1983;7(2):101–108

51. Rohrich RJ, Gosman AA, Brown SA, Reisch J: Mastopexy preferences: a survey of board-certified plastic surgeons. Plast Reconstr Surg 2006;118(7):1631–1638

"Flip-Flap" Mastopexy and Breast Reduction

Robert S. Flowers, Adil Ceydeli

16.1 Introduction

We all appreciate the importance of breasts in the aesthetics of the female body, which drives our vigilant search for better operations to improve their shape, design, and durability. Few of those described withstand the test of time. The "Flip-Flap Mastopexy" is, however, one that has done so, and remains our favorite among those that have withstood [1, 2].

The problem with mastopexy techniques that rely on the integrity of the dermis or skin flaps to hold and retain the breast in an elevated position is that the stretching of skin allows the breast to droop again in relatively few months. Most mastopexies and breast reduction operations leave heavy breast bulk to remain in the lower pole of the breast. The thrust of that bulk eventually causes "restretching" of the skin that is already "programmed" to expand and accommodate breast enlargement (Fig. 16.1). This manifests as recurrent ptosis, typically apparent within a year after mastopexy. Secondary skin resections temporarily restore breast contour, but regression rapidly recurs.

A similar outcome plagues breasts subjected to reduction mammaplasty, which results in ptosis of the caudal breast, while the nipple–areolar complex occupies a position above the center of the breast mass, pointing plaintively toward the sky (Fig. 16.2).

In this chapter we will show you how transposing ("flipping") a superiorly based "flap" of breast/fat tissue restores upper breast fullness, while at the same time preventing bottoming out. This operation is based on the principles of a classic inverted "T" skin excision design, using McKissock's vertical bipedicle [3]. The "flip-flap mastopexy" is simple, safe, reliable, and reproducible in correcting both breast ptosis and hypertrophy. It uses the breast and fatty tissue underneath a broadly beveled pedicle to achieve the superior pole fullness (as opposed to discarding it). Minimizing the breasts' lower pole mass further thwarts the bottoming-out, so common after other types of mastopexies and reductions, especially those embracing lower pedicles.

16.2 Technique

Mark the patient in an erect sitting or standing position. Place the nipple at mid-humerus level, or within 1 cm of the inframammary fold, centered at the breast meridian. Design an inverted "T" skin pattern to delineate the areas of skin and breast/fat tissue to be removed. Outline a broad pedicle (usually a minimum of 12 cm wide at its deepest level) to maintain good circulation to the distal "flip" flap (Fig. 16.3). This will also optimize nipple circulation.

In the case of the inverted "T" technique marking, make sure that the combined lengths of the caudal borders of the lateral flaps equate in length with the total width of the caudal marking. Designate on that line where the two flaps will meet. At that point the authors like to insert a 2-cm-high triangle, which makes a broader angled closure where the incisions come together (Fig. 16.4). This, of course, is optional, but reduces secondary healing at the stressed zone of suture line intersection.

Deepithelialize the skin of the keyhole area sparing the nipple–areolar complex in whatever manner you prefer. In huge breasted, especially thin-skinned persons, the authors like the "peeling orange" technique to decrease the operating room time and minimize vascular pedicle damage (Fig. 16.5) [4, 5]. Having deepithelialized the skin, proceed by making full thickness incisions on both sides of the bipedicle, beveling more widely (away from the pedicle) as the incisions move towards the pectoralis fascia (Fig. 16.3). To create and transpose a flap, first dissect a fairly extensive pocket at the level of the pectoralis fascia, extending up above the area of second rib. Carefully create the superiorly based breast-fatty tissue "flip-flap" by splitting the more superficial vertical bi-pedicle from its deeper part, which is then transposed to create upper breast fullness (Fig. 16.6). Applying traction and countertraction on either side of the pedicle using multiple skin hooks greatly facilitates this step (Fig. 16.7). Make sure that the base of this superiorly based flap is at least 1.5 cm thick. At no point should any proximal

M.A. Shiffman (ed.), *Mastopexy and Breast Reduction: Principles and Practice,*
© Springer-Verlag Berlin Heidelberg 2009

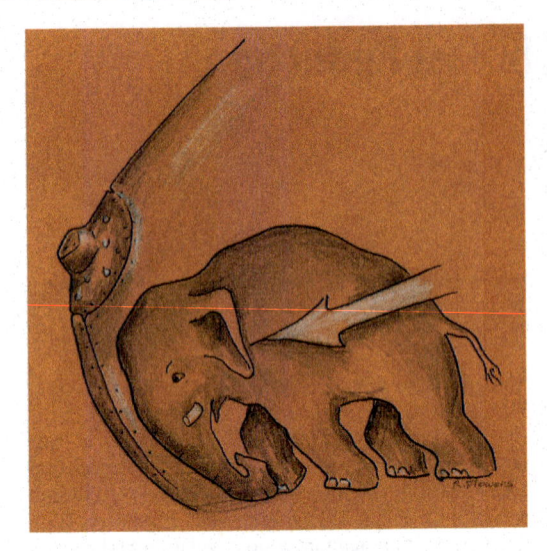

Fig. 16.1 The thrust of the remaining heavy lower pole breast bulk after mastopexies or breast reductions causes "restretching" of skin that is already "programmed" to expand

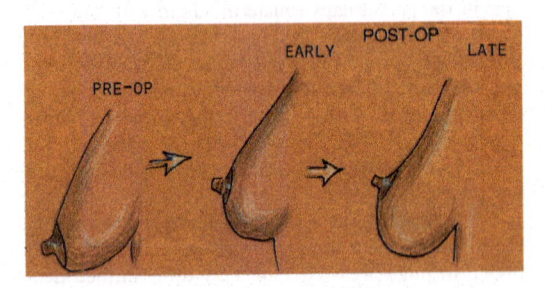

Fig. 16.2 Ptosis of the lower breast pole during the late postoperative period

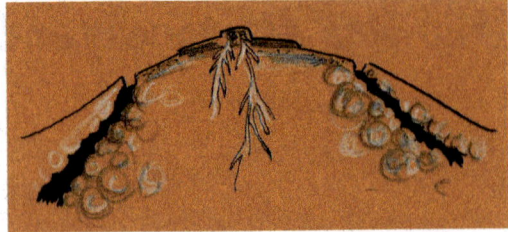

Fig. 16.3 Beveling during the dissection of the pedicle leaves a broad base for improved circulation to nipple–areola complex and "flip-flap"

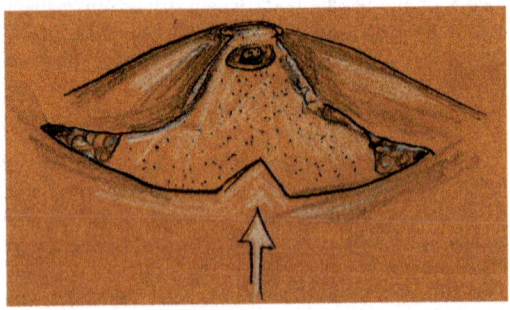

Fig. 16.4 Leaving a triangular shape skin island at the base of the pedicle facilitates a tension-free closure

part of the breast/fat flap be less thick or less wide than the more distal parts of the flap (Fig. 16.8). You may wish to taper the thickness of the flap as it progresses distally. This helps to retain a greater thickness of tissue at the base of the inferior pedicle, which provides most of the circulation to nipple–areola complex, and also reduces the amount of tissue at the distal end of the breast/fat flap, thereby decreasing its metabolic needs, minimizing the risk of distal flap necrosis. Then "flip" (transpose) the deep superiorly based breast/fat flap cephalad, turning it beneath itself, securing its distal end to the pectoralis fascia at the level of the second rib, with at least six 2-0 or 3-0 Vicryl sutures (Figs. 16.9 and 16.10). This transposition of the lower pole tissue bulk takes the unwanted weight off the bipedicle, moving it superiorly, and augmenting the usually deficient superior breast pole (Fig. 16.10).

This solves the bottoming-out phenomenon so common to breast lifts and reductions, and at the same time gives an internal deep support that counteracts the tendency of the breasts to sag with the passage of years (Figs. 16.11 and 16.12).

16.3
Complications

The authors have used the flip-flap mastopexy since 1977 on over 250 patients without any major complications. There was no instance of nipple/areola loss. In the first three patients where this technique was used, hard lumps occurred early in their recovery, indicating distal flap ischemia and tissue necrosis of the distal transposed fat/breast tissue. As the authors became more fastidious about following our own rules, leaving a wide superior base for the deep flap and with no increased thickness at any of the distal portion (Fig. 16.8), the incidence of transposed flap lumpiness disappeared.

Suction drains were used on two-thirds of the patients. Five percent of all the patients operated on had hematoma requiring evacuation, most of which occurred in the patients without suction drainage. All

16.3 Complications

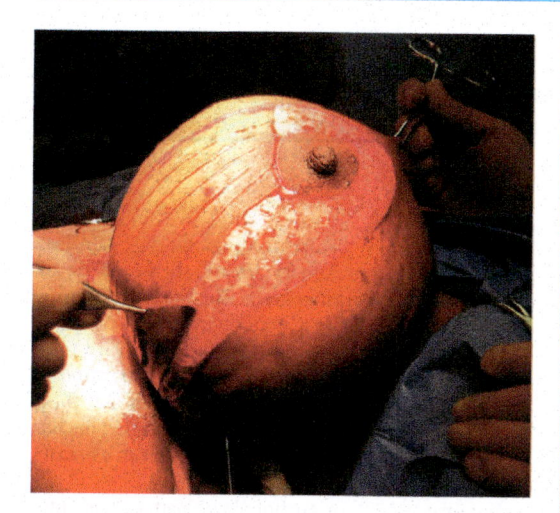

Fig. 16.5 The "peeling orange" deepithelialization technique

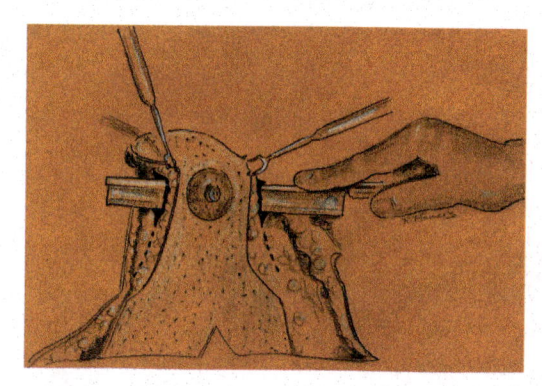

Fig. 16.6 Creation of the superiorly based breast-fatty tissue "flip-flap" by splitting the more superficial vertical bi-pedicle from its deeper part, which will be transposed to create upper breast fullness

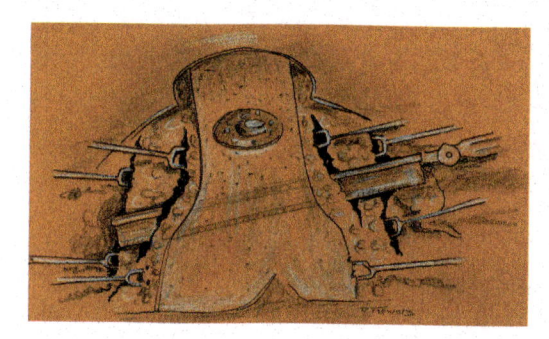

Fig. 16.7 Applying traction and counter-traction on either side of the pedicle using multiple skin hooks to facilitate the creation of superiorly based "flip-flap"

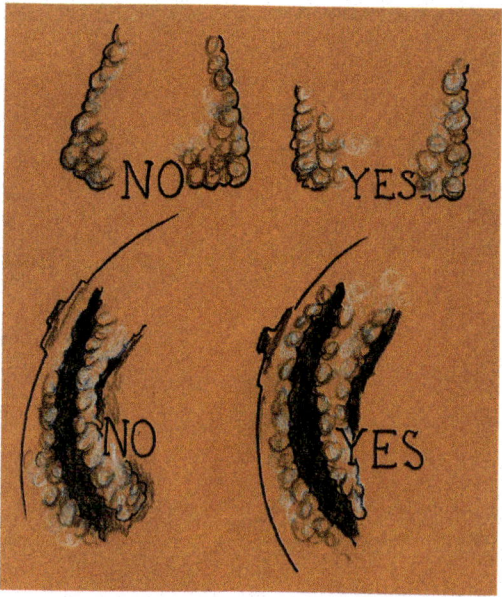

Fig. 16.8 At no point should any proximal part of the breast/fat flap ("flip-flap") be less thick or less wide than the more distal parts of the flap

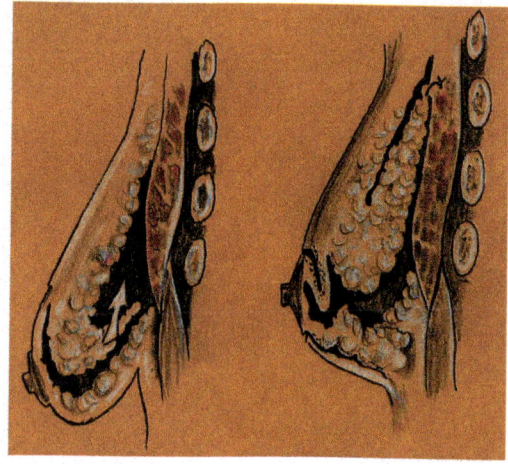

Fig. 16.9 Transposing the deep superiorly based breast/fat flap cephalad, beneath itself, and securing the distal end onto pectoralis fascia at the level of the second rib to create the superior pole fullness

the hematomas were small and none threatened the blood supply. No patients experienced deep vein thrombosis and none had any pulmonary embolus. Our recommendation is for suction drainage in all operated

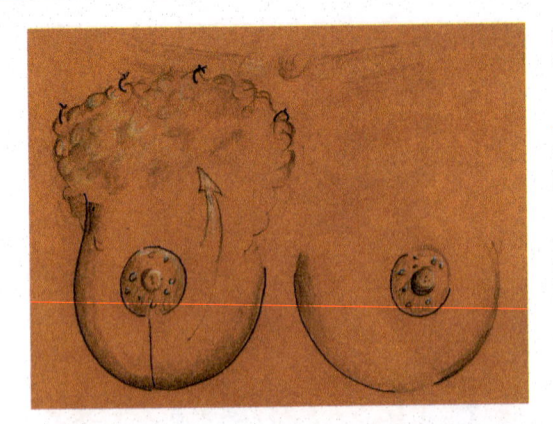

118   16 "Flip-Flap" Mastopexy and Breast Reduction

Fig. 16.10 The transposition of the lower pole tissue bulk takes the unwanted weight off the bipedicle, moving it superiorly, and augmenting the usually deficient superior breast pole, which solves the bottoming-out phenomenon so common to breast lifts and reductions

patients, but most importantly, for thorough intraoperative hemostasis.

16.4 Discussion

Aging, pregnancy, breast feeding, weight gain/loss, gravity, and retromammary breast augmentation all take their toll on breast contour. The breast's structural support systems (skin, Cooper's ligaments, and the breast itself) all progressively lose their elasticity, tone, and strength with time. The end result is droopy breasts with flat upper poles. When the breast is heavy, these changes are more dramatic and appear earlier in life. Pregnancy and breast feeding play a big role in a breast's early drooping and its severity.

The inverted "T" or anchor shape pattern and inferior pedicle-based mammaplasties are probably the most widely used technique, also enjoying as well the

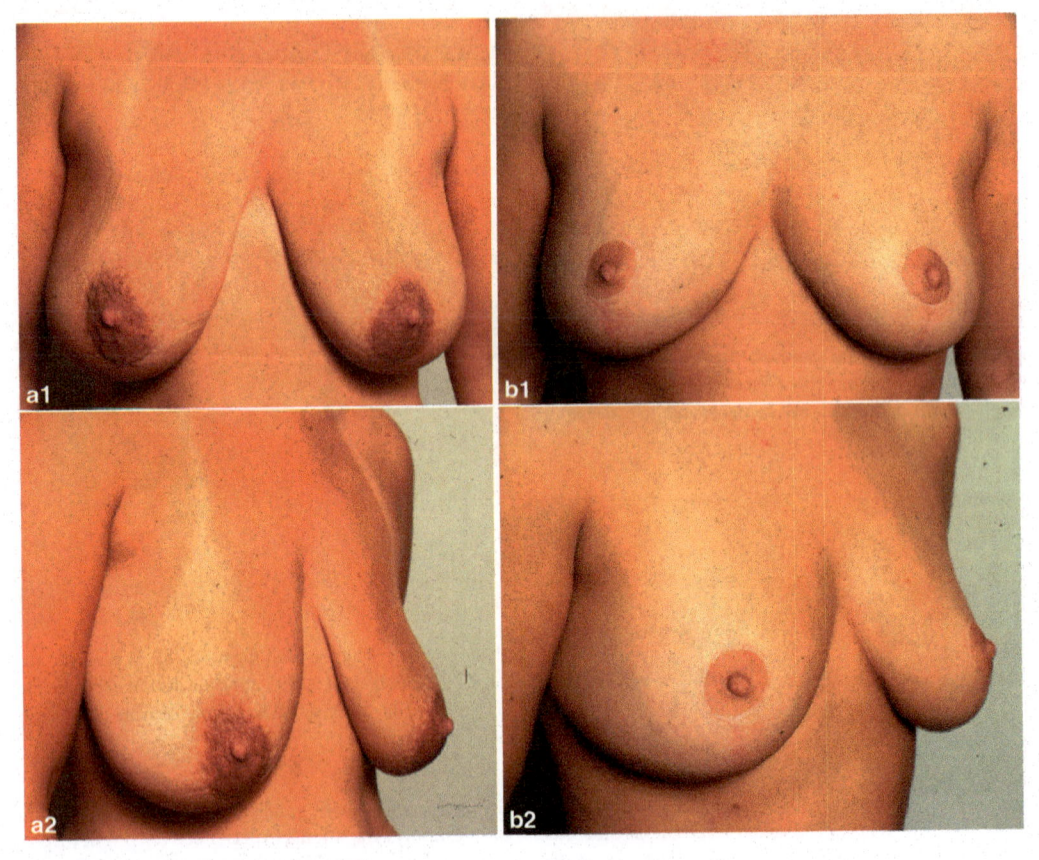

Fig. 16.11 (**a**1,2) Preoperative patient. (**b**1,2) Seven months after "flip-flap" mastopexy

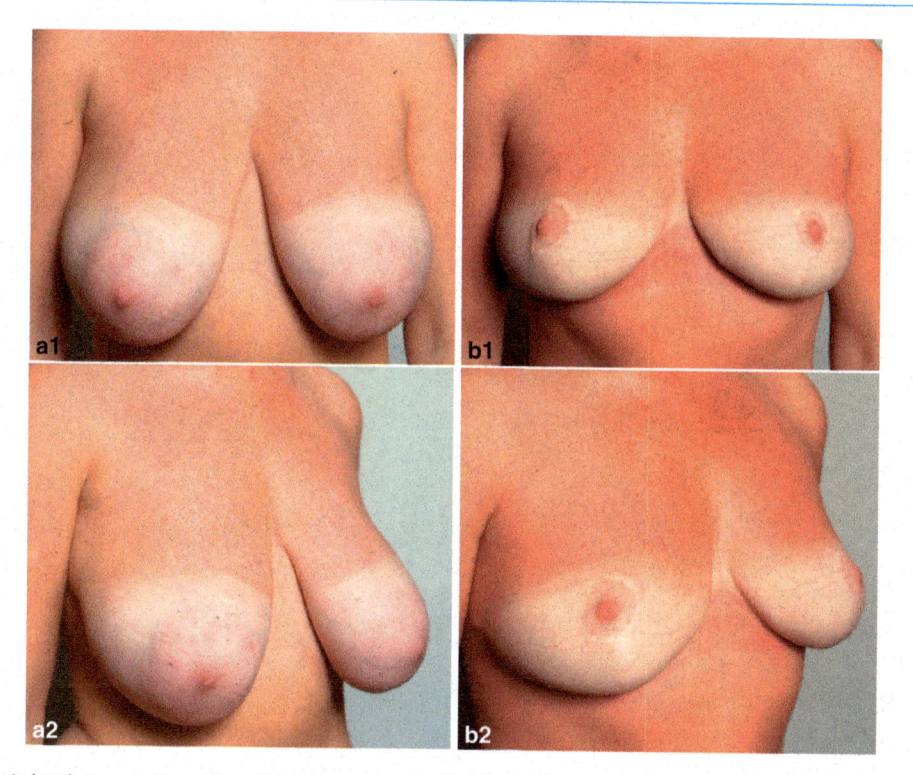

Fig. 16.12 (**a***1,2*) Preoperative patient. (**b***1,2*) Two years after "flip-flap" reduction mammaplasty. There is no tendency toward "bottoming-out".

likely honor of being the most uniformly successful operation to address breast ptosis in terms of being safe, reliable, and reproducible since it was first described more than 80 years ago in France [6]. Its major drawback, however, is the failure to address the superior pole deficiency and progressive bottoming-out. This often leaves a breast shaped much as it was preoperatively, except for now inappropriately high nipple complex, which points not anteriorly, but upwards.

The flip-flap mastopexy builds upon established concepts of breast surgery, departing radically with the "flipped-flap" that claims the superior pole, obviating the "bottoming-out."

The authors refer mainly to the Mckissock verticle bipedicle, and our established rule of maintaining the thickness of the pedicle is a minimum of 1.5–2 cm to assure adequate blood supply to the nipple–areolar complex. Instead of discarding the valuable breast tissue deep to the bipedicle, we use it to augment the superior pole, which, in turn, de-bulks the lower breast. Our other rule is keeping the base of superiorly based deep breast/fat flap as wide as possible, tapering its thickness distally to provide a robust circulation to the flap and to minimize the risk of flap ischemia and/or necrosis. The gradual decrease in the thickness of the flap distally leaves a wide base for the inferior aspect of the bipedicle, while transferring the unnecessary extra weight to superior pole to correct the upper pole deficiency.

References

1. Flowers RS, Smith EM Jr: "Flip-flap" mastopexy. Aesthetic Plast Surg 1998;22(6):425–429
2. Vogt T: Reduction mammaplasty – Vogt technique. In: Georgiade NG (ed). Aesthetic Breast Surgery. Baltimore, Williams & Wilkins 1983, pp 271–290
3. McKissock PK: Reduction mammaplasty with a vertical dermal flap. Plast Reconstr Surg 1972;49(3):245–252
4. Ceydeli A, Hunter JG: "Peeling orange" deepithelialization: a technique for rapid deepithelialization in reduction mammaplasty. Aesthetic Surg J 2004;24:580–581
5. Ceydeli A: Saving time and money in mammaplasty. Cosmetic Surgery Times 2006, April issue, pp 40–41
6. Lexer E: Correccion de los pechos pendulos (mastoptose) por medio de la implantacion de grasa. Guipuzcoa Medica 1921;63:213

L-Wing Superior Pedicle Vertical Scar Mammaplasty

Norbert Pallua, Erhan Demir

17.1 Introduction

The multitude of different techniques and modifications with regard to pedicle choice, scar position, and length or breast shaping reflects the challenge for every plastic surgeon to achieve an aesthetic shape with long-term stability and minimal scars in mammaplasty and mastopexy.

The past decade has been a witness to a paradigm shift in the treatment of macromastia and breast ptosis [1]. The wise pattern, inverted T inferior pedicle breast reconstruction with often clearly visible scars can no longer be accepted as the state of the art [2], as aesthetic improvement and scar reduction has become the new front line in breast reduction surgery [3]. Still, vertical scar techniques have not gained popularity in the United States as rapidly as in the Europe and South America. The development of the purely vertical incision mammaplasty was introduced by Lötsch [4] and Dartigues [5] for mastopexy surgery. It was reintroduced for breast reduction by Arié [6], modified by Lassus [7, 8], and extended by Marchac and De Olarte [9]. Further, Lejour [10, 11] popularized a technique derived from Lassus. She combined a superior pedicle for the areola and a central resection for the breast reduction associated with liposuction and wide skin undermining along the vertical scar. Over the past years there has been greater interest in short scar breast surgery, with increasing appreciation of the vertical techniques for reduction and mastopexy.

The L-wing superior pedicle vertical scar technique has become the standard mammaplasty technique in the authors' university hospital over the past 8 years.

17.2 Patient Selection

The L-wing vertical technique is applied to all reductions and mastopexy procedures regardless of the size. The authors do not believe that breast size is a limiting factor. We agree with Nahai [12] that the amount of excess skin, the skin quality, the relationship of the skin envelope to the breast tissue, and the distance the nipple has to be moved are far more important factors than breast size alone. The ideal patient has normal skin elasticity and adherence of the skin envelope to the underlying breast tissue, together with a moderate sized breast. In contrast, less ideal candidates have poor skin quality, a somewhat loose envelope where the skin adheres poorly to the underlying breast tissue, extreme ptosis, or breast hypertrophy. Still, the technique is especially suitable for larger resection weights, because it shortens the vertical scar while adding a well hidden short lateral horizontal inframammary scar component.

Smoking, diabetes, or overweight are not true contraindications for vertical scar mammaplasty, but patients are strongly encouraged for temporary nicotine reduction or abstinence, weight loss, and internal medicine consults prior to scheduled breast reduction surgery.

17.3 Surgical Technique

17.3.1 Basic Principle

The four cardinal elements of breast reduction applied to the L-wing technique are the following:
1. The nipple areola complex (NAC) is vascularized through a superior pedicle.
2. The breast parenchyma is removed centro-caudal below the pedicle.
3. Breast shaping occurs through medial and lateral pillar plication and is covered with a circumferential skin envelope with a short vertical scar and lateral L-shaped wing.

17.3.2 Photographs

Standardized photographic documentation, before and after breast reduction, provides documentation of each patient's outcome.

M.A. Shiffman (ed.), *Mastopexy and Breast Reduction: Principles and Practice*,
© Springer-Verlag Berlin Heidelberg 2009

17.3.3 Basic Marking

Preoperative markings are done with the patient in the standing position. The midsternal line, the submammary folds, and the mid-mammary line (breast axis) of each breast are marked. The breast axis line, passing through the nipple, is extended caudally beyond the submammary fold towards the epigastric region. The most cranial position of the future nipple site is determined on this axis between 19 and 23 cm from the suprasternal notch, depending on the submammary fold projection, the level of the forearm middle, and the breast volume (Fig. 17.1).

17.3.4 Nipple Areolar Complex Marking

From point A, a triangle is marked with the proportions of 5 cm caudally along the axis and then perpendicular to this 3–5 cm medial and lateral. This will fix the subsequent base of the superior-based pedicle of the NAC at 6–10 cm. The dome-shaped, curved periareolar line, as the line of resection, is marked symmetrically around the triangle. The breast shape is influenced by the angle of this triangle: larger angles will result in more conical breast shapes and in greater tension on the vertical scar.

An alternative method is the marking of a curved dome-shaped line starting from point A with a range of 7–8 cm on each site.

17.3.5 Marking of Resection Margins

Each breast is rotated upward medially and laterally to fix the vertical resection margins. This will add to a good conical projection and will avoid inferior skin redundancy. The distance between the medial boundary of the areola and the sternum must remain at at least 10 cm. The two lower ends of these lines are joined by an even curving line at a point fixed between 2 and 3 cm above the submammary fold (point F) (Fig. 17.1). The future vertical line is fixed at a height of 5–7 cm (line CD). From this point, the future horizontal section of the L-shaped scar is marked in a slightly concave curve lateral and caudal running towards the submammary fold (line DH). The corresponding vertical scar is fixed at 7–9 cm (line BE). The step of 2 cm is essential to facilitate the turnover of the flap to the lateral side into the horizontal L-shaped scar.

17.3.6 Positioning and Anesthesia

All breast reduction procedures are carried out under general anesthesia. The patient was positioned in a semi-seated position on the operating table. A single dose intravenously of a broad band antibiotic is administered in all patients.

17.3.7 Deepithelialization

Areola size is determined by pressure marking using a centered mammary ring with a diameter between 3.8 and 4.2 cm. The superior pedicle is deepithelialized, with an incision through the skin and subcutis according to the preoperative resection drawings.

17.3.8 Incisions and Resection

The skin is incised according to the previous markings. The lower boundary of the breast tissue dissection is 1–2 cm caudal beyond the natural submammary fold, with the skin remaining 2 cm above.

In the central region of the lower glandular base, mobilization of the corpus of the gland in a cranial direction up to the level of the second rib is then carried

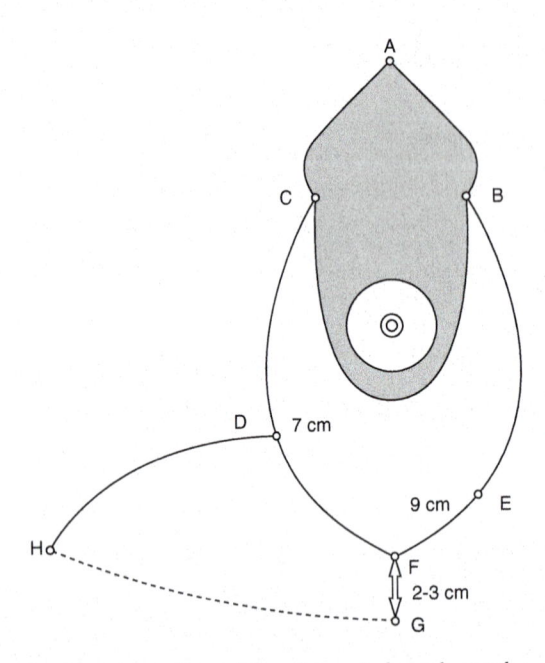

Fig. 17.1 Preoperative markings of new nipple areola complex (NAC) position and resection borders of breast tissue

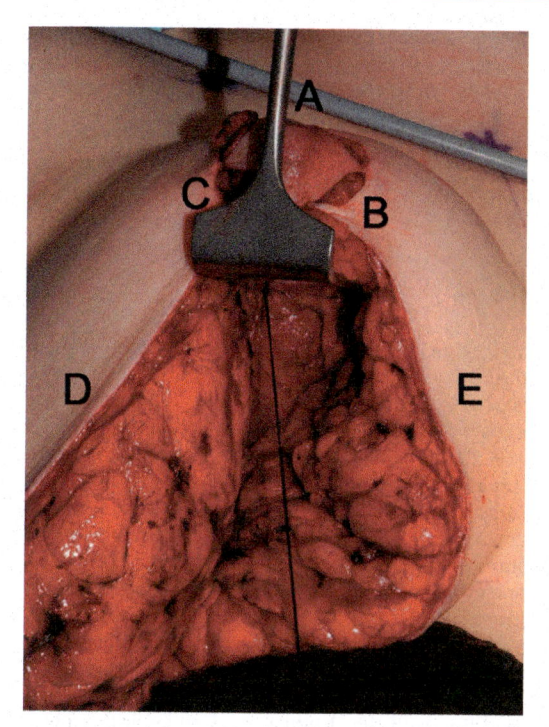

Fig. 17.2 Intraoperative following "en-bloc" centro-caudal resection of glandular tissue

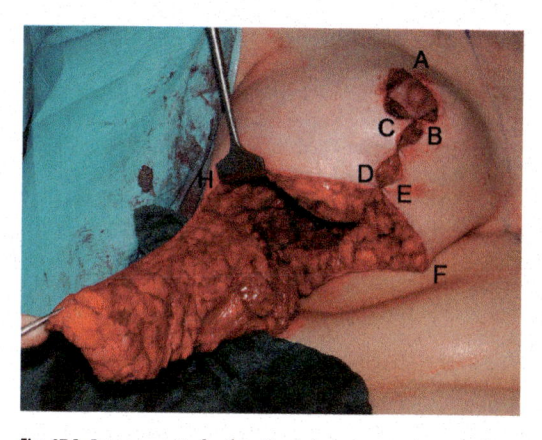

Fig. 17.3 Intraoperatively the glandular corpus along with its remaining medial and lateral pillar is modeled. Lateral rotation of the remaining skin flap is carried out following a wedge tissue excision at the medial caudal pillar. The skin envelope is then rotated laterally around the corpus of the gland

The remaining lateral glandular pillars will provide additional support for the newly formed gland.

The NAC pedicle is prepared cranially at an even thickness of 1.5–2 cm, remaining thicker superiorly. The skin-gland corpus is then excised in a wedge-shaped en bloc resection to the desired volume, centro-caudal of the areola (Fig. 17.2).

17.3.9
Breast Shaping

With a single suture, the uppermost pole of the areola is fixed to the most cranial point of the deepithelialized, dome-shaped resection figure (point A). To enhance desired projection and create sufficient upper pole fullness, a mastopexy suture is carried out at the level of the second intercostal space in younger patients. In older patients, this mastopexy suture will be placed more caudally at the third or fourth intercostal space in correlation with the anatomic proportions, and to achieve lesser projection.

The glandular corpus along with its remaining medial and lateral pillar is modeled with three to four craniocaudal gland-shaping sutures (Fig. 17.3). Base reduction is achieved in part by the glandular pillars pulled together with inverted sutures. These sutures need only to be strong enough to hold the breast together until the physiologic wound healing will take over. Only solid breast tissue, not fat, is approximated. Suction drains are placed bilaterally.

17.3.10
Management of the Skin

In the vertical technique, the skin envelope is sutured together in a pure vertical scar. In this modified technique, the authors first temporarily affix the 5–7 cm lateral side (distance CD) to the 7–9 cm medial side (distance BE) using staples. The lateral rotation of the remaining skin flap is made easier by the gathering effect to fix side BE 2 cm longer than side CD. At this point, a wedge tissue excision at the medial caudal pillar is carried out.

The skin envelope is then rotated laterally around the corpus of the gland (Fig. 17.4). Suturing along the line of the submammary fold forms the horizontal wing of the L-shaped scar. The cranial boundary of the skin pocket fixes the arched curve of the suture in the natural submammary fold and is incised correspondingly (line DH). The caudal boundary is excised to the principle of a dog-ear resection (Fig. 17.4). It is critical that breast shaping is performed through the design of glandular shaping sutures. The attempt to address desired breast shape with the skin envelope will lead to scar widening or hypertrophic scars.

out by epifascial preparation of the pectoralis major muscle. The width of the tunnel should not exceed 3–4 cm. The skin always remains attached to the breast.

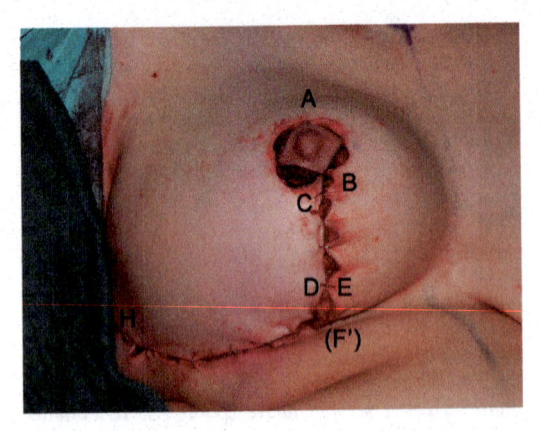

Fig. 17.4 Suturing along the line of the submammary fold forms the horizontal wing of the L-shaped scar. The cranial boundary of the skin pocket fixes the arched curve of the suture in the natural submammary fold and is incised correspondingly (line DH). The caudal boundary is excised to the principle of a dog-ear resection

17.3.11
Closure

Vertical and horizontal scars are closed in a bilayered fashion. Inverted corium sutures of absorbable 3-0 suture material follow by continuous cutaneous sutures with 3-0 or 2-0 nonresorbable suture material.

The areola is sutured with 5-0 single inverted corium absorbable sutures and then with continuous cutaneous sutures with 4-0 nonresorbable suture material.

17.3.12
Dressings

A soft sterile silicone-coated dressing is applied to cover the incisions. The patient must wear a modeling tape-type dressing for 7 days, and a sports-type brassiere must be kept on for 3 months, day and night.

17.4
Postoperative Care

The suction drains are removed on the first to second postoperative day. Single interrupted sutures will be removed on the third to fourth postoperative day. The periareolar cutaneous running sutures will be removed on the 12th to 14th day after surgery. The vertical and horizontal L-shaped wing scar will remain in place for up to 18 days post surgery.

Scar massage and treatment with ointments and soft silicone-sheet application immediately after suture removal is recommended.

Arm movements are not restricted but heavy exercise is not permitted up to 3 months after surgery. Patients can return to light work after suture removal, about 14 days after surgery.

17.5
Results

17.5.1
Measures

The authors have been performing this procedure more than 8 years now in 209 patients. A follow-up study in 2004 [13] has been carried out with 107 patients. The average reduction weight was 640 g per breast (range, 150–2,140 g). Average suprasternal notch to nipple distance (SSN:N) was 32 cm (range, 21–43 cm) before surgery. The distance shortened to an average length of 20 cm (range, 18–25 cm) after breast reduction. Vertical scar length was reduced from 13.5 cm before the operation to 6.8 cm immediately after the operation, with a final length of 8.3 cm in the postoperative examination. The average length for the lateral-horizontal L-wing hidden in the submammary fold was 10.9 cm. In patients with very broad breast base shapes and high reduction weights, base reduction with the glandular corpus modeled in a harmonic, aesthetic and projecting way was always possible.

17.5.2
Sensitivity and Breast Feeding

In relation to nipple–areola sensation, postoperative examination (average of 13 months) revealed that 81% of the patients in the low and medium reduction weight groups (below 800 g) experienced no reduction in sensation, while the remainder described slight reduced NAC sensation. In the high reduction weight group (above 800 g), 60% of the patients were found to experience no change in nipple areola sensation, although 40% described marked postoperative loss of sensibility, with two patients reporting a total loss of areola sensation.

The potential for lactation was not impaired, none of the breast feeding patients reported about problems.

17.6
Complications

17.6.1
Necrosis

Two patients who presented with gigantomastia (reduction weight of 2,000 g per side in one patient and 1,200 g in the second patient) developed bilateral partial NAC necrosis.

Among the remainder of the group, which consisted of three patients with resection weights ranging up to 1,200 g per side, there were no significant healing problems requiring secondary correction.

17.6.2
Hematoma

The en bloc resection technique lowered the incidence of hematoma formation requiring operative intervention from 5% to 3%. Those problems occured in the high reduction weight groups, which can always be treated as an small outpatient procedure.

17.6.3
Asymmetry and Bottoming Out

Inadequate consideration to the slightly curving horizontal suture of the running L-wing along the submammary fold was given by 3% of the patients. Appropriate correction was performed with a small procedure. A majority of 90% expressed great satisfaction with their outcome following surgery, and the remaining rated their results to be good without any signs of bottoming out.

17.6.4
Wound-Healing Problems

Very slight wound-healing problems in the region of the caudal vertical scar in the L wing transition zone occurred in 13%, although secondary healing with complete wound closure was achieved after an average period of 2 weeks.

17.7
Discussion

The authors' experience demonstrates the advantages of reduction mammaplasty with the vertical incision in terms of glandular shaping combined with scar minimization (Figs. 17.5 and 17.6). Cases of high reduction

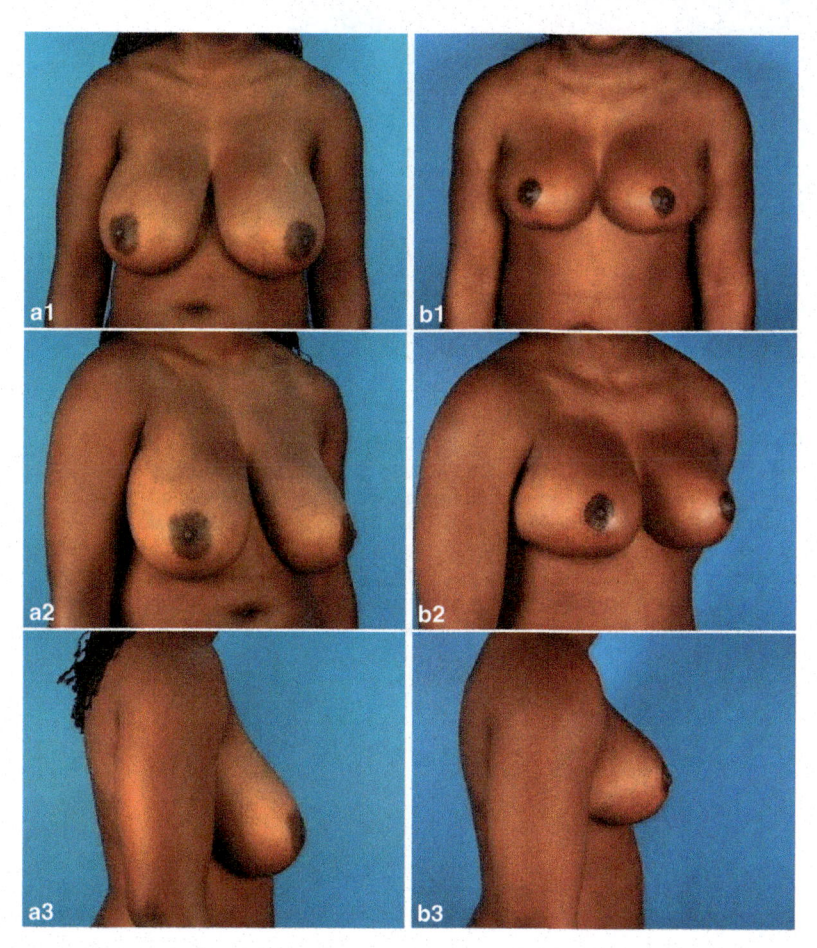

Fig. 17.5 (*a1-3*) Preoperative 24-year-old woman. (*b1-3*) Sixteen months postoperative after bilateral reduction mammoplasty. Volumes of resection were 505 g left breast and 490 g right breast

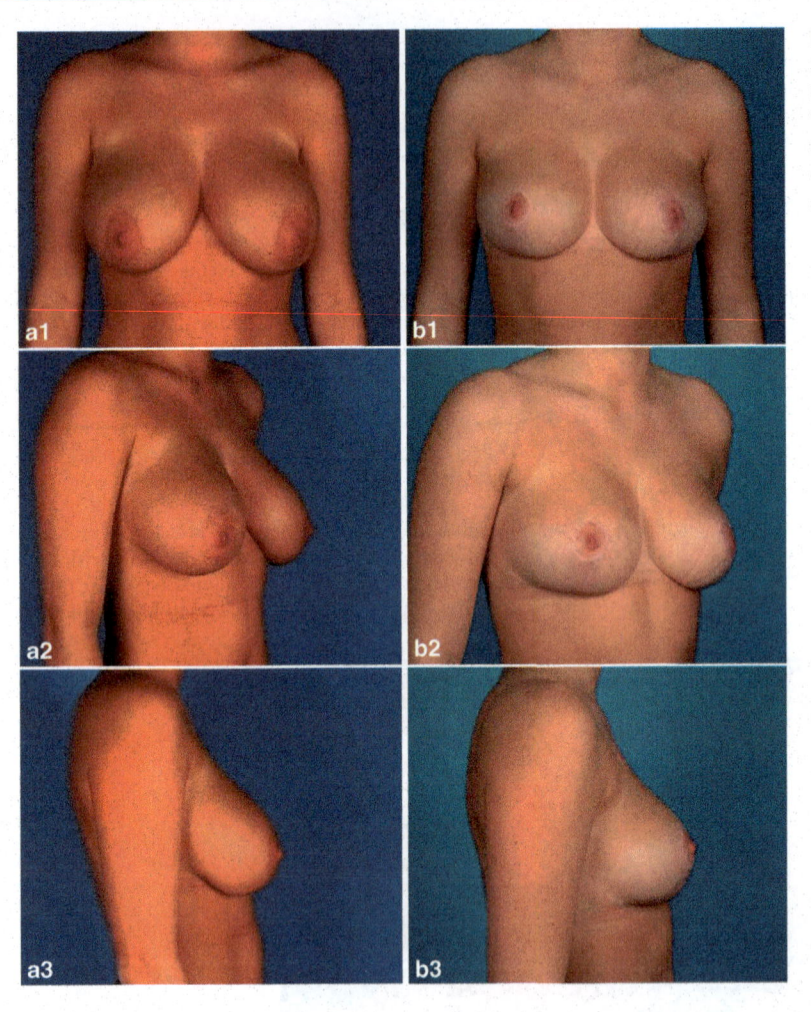

Fig. 17.6 (**a***1-3*) Preoperative 28-year-old woman with hypertrophic breasts. (**b***1-3*) Two years postoperatively following volume resections of 760 g from the right breast and 790 g from the left breast

weights are more frequently associated with wound-healing problems around the vertical scar, in addition to impaired breast shapes with sagging of the breast, and the necessity for later correction. The presented L-wing mammaplasty technique was inspired mainly by the idea from former vertical scar techniques. It combines the principle of vertical scar shortening [10] with an L-shaped scar wing [14]. The esteemed goals of aesthetic breast shape and projection together with scar minimization are confirmed by our patients [15]. Especially, the absence of scars in the visible part of the cleavage is appreciated by every patient. The lateral L-wing of the incision is well hidden in the submammary fold. The complication rates are low.

The method is suitable in the cases of high reduction weights (1,500–2,000 grams per side) or in adjunct mastopexy procedures. Experience with a superior vascular pedicle in relation to its effect on NAC sensation shows satisfactory results, with good preservation of sensibility for most patients.

17.8 Conclusions

The transformation of the pure vertical incision of the vertical technique to the L-shaped scar wing shortened the vertical scar, reduced the incidence of wound healing problems, and achieved aesthetic long-lasting breast shapes, even with high breast reduction weights. With a clear preoperative planning and a standardized surgical step-by-step operative procedure, the method is easy to teach and well reproducible. This technique would be useful to be added to the armamentarium of short-scar mammaplasty techniques of each plastic surgeon.

References

1. Hammond DC: Short scar periareolar inferior pedicle reduction. Plast Reconstr Surg 1999;103(3):890–901
2. Giovanoli P, Meuli-Simmen C, Meyer VE, Frey M: Which technique for which breast? A prospective study of different techniques of reduction mammaplasty. Br J Plast Surg 1999;52(1):52–59
3. Greuse M, Hamdi M, DeMay A: Breast sensitivity after vertical mammaplasty. Plast Reconstr Surg 2001;107(4):970–976
4. Lötsch F: Über hängebrustplastik. Zentralbl Chir 1923; 50:1241
5. Dartigues L: Chirurgie réparatrice. In: Lépine R (ed). Plastique et Esthétique de la Poitrine et de l'Abdomen. Paris 1924, pp 44–47
6. Arié G: Una nueva téchnica de mastoplasia. Rev Lat Am Cir Plast 1957;3:22
7. Lassus C: New refinements in vertical mammaplasty. Chir Plast 1981;6:81
8. Lassus C: Breast reduction: evolution of a technique – a single vertical scar. Aesthetic Plast Surg 1987;11(2): 107–112
9. Marchac D, de Olarte G: Reduction mammaplasty and correction of ptosis with a short inframammary scar. Plast Reconstr Surg 1982;69(1):45–55
10. Lejour M, Abboud M, Declety A, Kertesz P: Reduction des cicatrices de plastie mammaire: De l'ancre courte a la verticale. Ann Chir Plast Esthet 1990;35(5):369–379
11. Lejour M: Vertical mammaplasty and liposuction of the breast. Plast Reconstr Surg 1994;94(1):100–114
12. Nahai F: Breast reduction with no vertical scar. Aesthetic Plast Surg 2004;28(5):354
13. Pallua N: unpublished data
14. Meyer R, Kesselring UR: Reduction mammaplasty with an L-shaped suture line. Development of different techniques. Plast Reconstr Surg 1975;55(2): 139–148
15. Pallua N, Ermisch CZ: "I" becomes "L": modification of vertical mammaplasty. Plast Reconstr Surg 2003;111(6): 1860–1870

Fascial Suspension Mastopexy

Ram Silfen, Morris Ritz, Graeme Southwick

18.1
Introduction

Breast projection, preservation of the natural submammary fold, and breast shape still represent a challenge in aesthetic breast surgery. Various techniques have been suggested in the literature to achieve a pleasant, youthful breast shape, which would oppose the gravitational forces that create the continuous ptotic effect. Among these, different suspension sutures and breast parenchymal flaps have been suggested [1–5].

Factors contributing to the gravitational effect of the breast were discussed vastly in literature. Whilst much attention was given in the past to the skin envelope as a major contributor for durable projection, recent attention was shifted towards the internal arrangement of the breast as playing major role in this task. Latest techniques described especially by South American authors [1, 6] burrow a lower pole breast parenchymal flap underneath a bipedicled pectoralis major muscle flap. Although a more durable projection of the breast is obtained, these techniques were not supported world wide, because breast cancer screening was made difficult and compartments have been violated.

In view of the concept that a durable mastopexy procedure should rely rather on the internal rearrangement and relocation of the parenchymal breast tissue and less on its external skin envelope, removed due to its excess, and in order to overcome the above mentioned criticisms, we have developed the Fascial Suspension Mastopexy (FSM).

18.2
History

The history of mastopexy surgery reveals significant fluctuation in the approach for achieving a rejuvenated, well-projected, and less ptotic breast. While much of the history of mastopexy parallels that of breast reduction, various techniques in mastopexy that have been suggested lately obliged us to re-evaluate our breast reduction procedures and to assess more carefully their outcomes, especially in regard to their long-term results.

Breast reduction techniques have evolved in the last century dramatically. While older techniques tended to emphasize on the safety of the procedure using different vascular pedicles to transpose the nipple–areola complex, preservation of the sensation and refinement of the external scars, our better understanding of the anatomy, simple classification of the ptotic breast as well as improved assessment of the preoperative breast and critical analysis of patient outcomes have led us to make a step further in the thrive of achieving better aesthetic result as represented by a better projected and youthful breast.

While most of the essential technical elements of the mastopexy had been developed by the 1930s with the description of the use of periareolar deepithelialization to preserve the neurovascular supply of the NAC by Schwarzmann [7], further advancement in mastopexy was achieved by Gonzalez-Ulloa [8] who first advocated mastopexy with augmentation for ptotic and hypoplastic/atrophic breast. Further landmarks in the development of mastopxy were the use of the dermal mastopexy [9] and B mammoplasty [10].

After the first description by Lassus [11] and the introduction of the vertical scar approach for breast reduction, true progress in the breast appearance was possible as the concept of using breast autologous tissue to mold and reshape the breast in the effort of achieving long-lasting breast fullness was developed. From that time and on, our understanding that skin envelope alone does not provide the sufficient resistance to the gravitational forces led us to develop new procedures that would create an internal reorganization of the breast parenchyma, so that in engineer-like design the structure would have the adequate support to resist these forces.

Different procedures that reorganized the breast parenchyma were suggested and embraced by many plastic surgeons. These consisted of using combination of vertical mammaplasty and liposuction to improve the lateral edges of the breast [12], procedures that used different autologous dermo-parenchymal flaps [13–16], procedures that supported the breast parenchyma using distant autologous tissues [17] and non-autologous tissue description of Marlex mesh to lift the breast parenchyma [18], and finally procedures that identified and used breast parenchymal excess and utilized it, by placing it deep to a strip of pectoralis muscle, in breast upper pole to improve shape and maximize longevity of the lift.

M.A. Shiffman (ed.), *Mastopexy and Breast Reduction: Principles and Practice*,
© Springer-Verlag Berlin Heidelberg 2009

18.3 Technique

FSM can be performed using autologous tissue alone either with Wise (Fig. 18.1) or vertical pattern (Fig. 18.2). The procedure can be combined with augmentation or can be performed at the same time of breast prosthesis removal.

18.3.1 Operative Technique for Wise Pattern Mastopexy

The markings for breast mastopexy are done with the patient in an upright, symmetrically equal position. The nipple is marked for a wise pattern from the suprasternal notch to the NAC, a measurement of between 18 and 22 cm, but is a combination measuring from the suprasternal notch as well as the mid-humeral level, in particular, in relation to the inframammary fold. The marking should be at the level of the inframammary fold.

The nipple is marked in the mid-clavicular line, approximating to where it was initially. The nipple areolar measurement is marked as an oval marking wider than the higher measurement $6 \times 4 \text{ cm}^2$. The two lateral arms of the wise are measured between 5 and 7 cm and the inframammary extension is drawn in the inframammary fold with a particular fold, with a slight circular curve medially and laterally to encompass the curvature of the new breast shape.

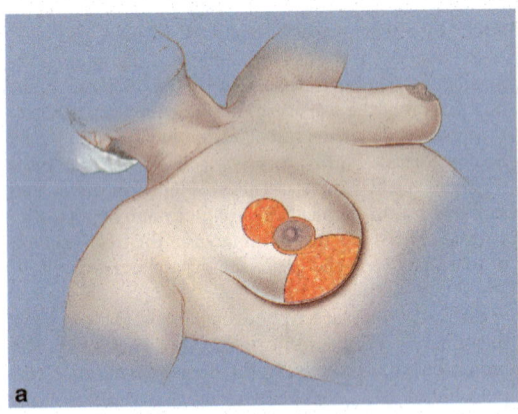

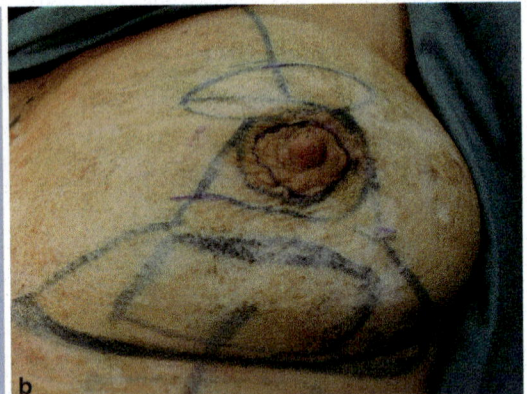

Fig. 18.1 Breast mastopexy markings as for wise pattern

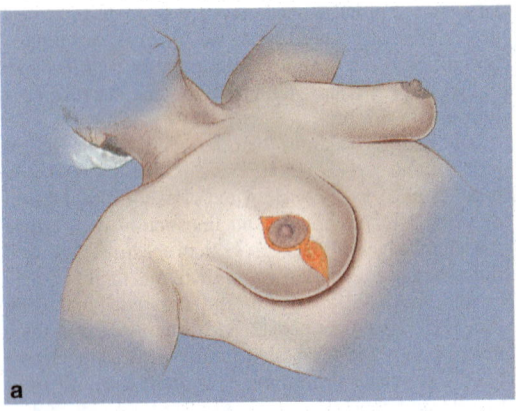

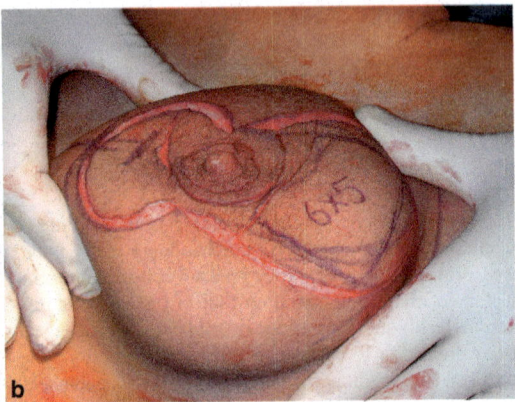

Fig. 18.2 Breast mastopexy designed as for vertical pattern

The nipple is marked as a superomedial pedicle to be raised on the medial inframammary leg and can include some of the new areolar incision. The pedicle length is usually marked not longer than 8 cm and can be made fairly broad.

Below the nipple, between the nipple and the inframammary incision, a flap is drawn for the mastopexy, measuring 5×5 cm^2 or 5×6 cm^2 on the skin (Fig. 18.3), and this will allow a small deepithelialized paddle below the flap (Fig. 18.4) for the closure of the inverted T, so that it is closed with sufficient tissue beneath it to allow good breast projection. With the patient standing upright, three points are marked on the skin where the lower thoracic breast parenchymal flap will be anchored to the prepectoral fascia with permanent sutures.

The incisions are made as per breast reduction, raising it as with a superomedial pedicle, removing skin and some breast tissue medially and laterally, and raising the inferior thoracic flap directly perpendicular to the chest wall, so that it is incised from inferiorly down to the prepectoral fascia and to the two lateral sides of the prepectoral fascia (Fig. 18.5). The superior dissection is taken a little more superiorly under the nipple but onto the prepectoral fascia. The prepectoral fascia is then exposed by dissecting the breast tissue superiorly off the prepectoral fascia to a point where the flap would be proposed in order to give enough superior fullness. At this point the prepectoral fascia is incised inferiorly and superiorly to create a bipedicled flap going from side to side in a slightly oblique fashion, higher laterally than medially following the pectoral muscle fibres (Fig. 18.6).

The prepectoral fascial flap is 3–4 cm in width and is raised carefully using a scissor with a cutting action, as this is not a very easy natural plane and does require dissection. This should be done meticulously; bleeding is possible on the muscle itself, but this is easily controlled and this flap needs to be raised wide enough to allow passage of the breast parenchymal flap to fit snugly. The breast parenchymal flap is then passed through and under the prepectoral fascial flap (Fig. 18.7) and the deepithelialized section is sutured superiorly to the prepectoral fascia superiorly with a long absorbable or permanent suture (Fig. 18.8). A 3-0 PDS suture is used to anchor the flap in three locations: superiorly, superomedially, and supero- laterally. The flap is anchored according to the preoperative skin markings, which are

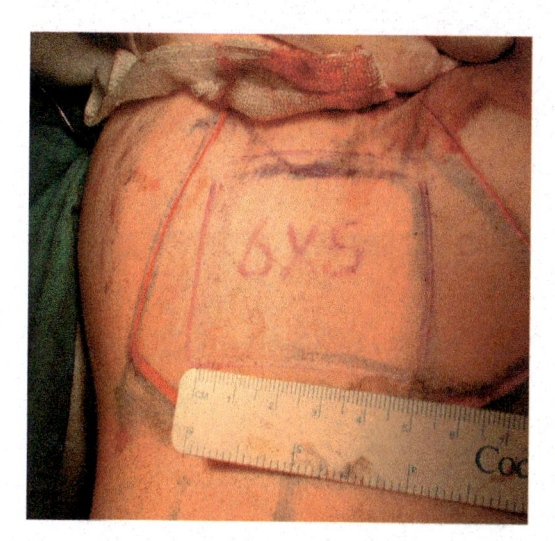

Fig. 18.3 Lower thoracic flap design. Note: different sized flaps can be performed according to tissue availability and breast projection needed

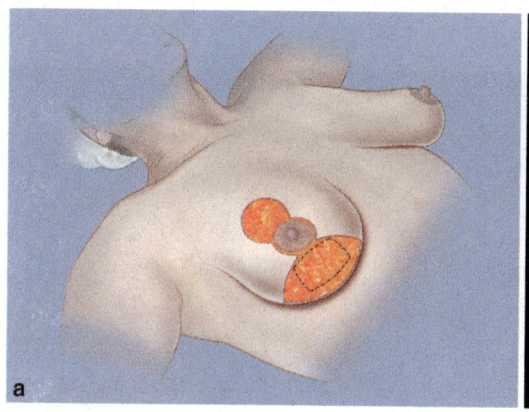

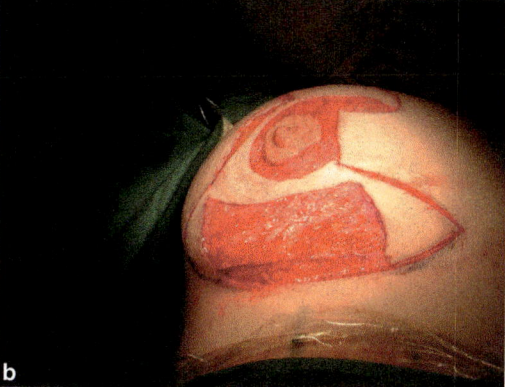

Fig. 18.4 (a,b) Lower thoracic flap and supero-medial pedicle after deepithelialization

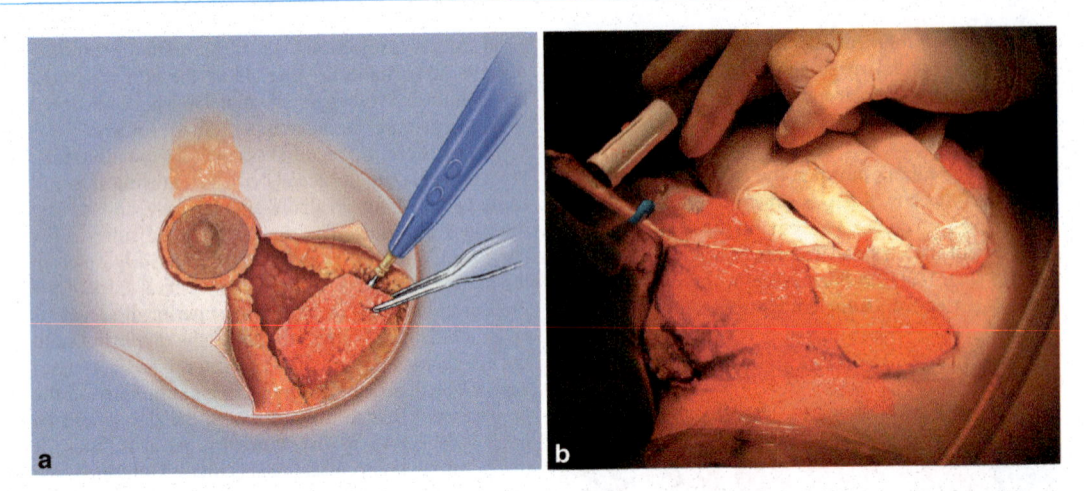

Fig. 18.5 (a,b) Lower thoracic flap harvesting

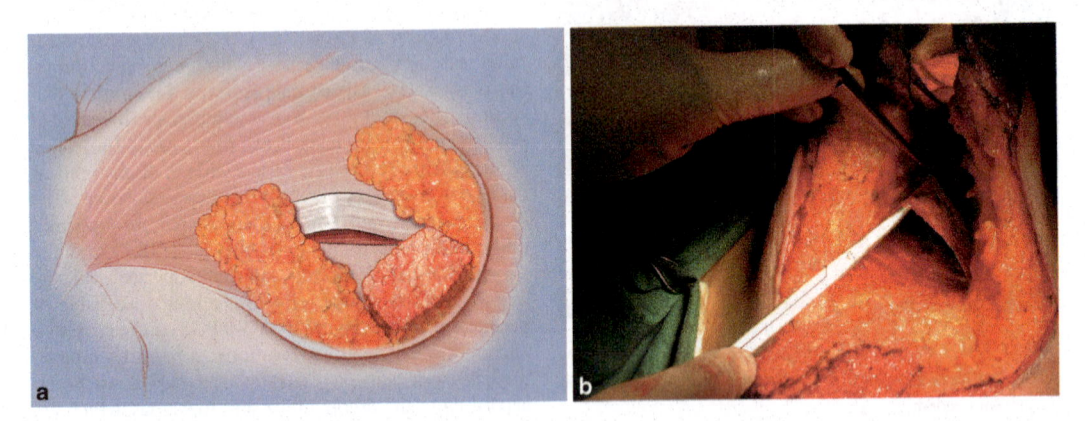

Fig. 18.6 (a,b) Bipedicled prepectoral fascia flap. The flap is usually 3 cm wide and 5 cm long in order to allow smooth tunneling of the lower thoracic breast parenchymal flap underneath it

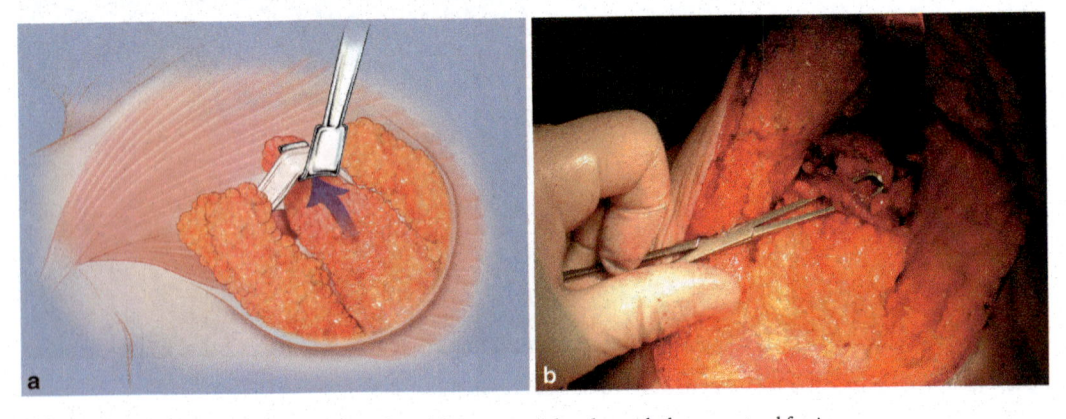

Fig. 18.7 (a,b) The lower thoracic breast parenchymal flap is tunneled underneath the prepectoral fascia

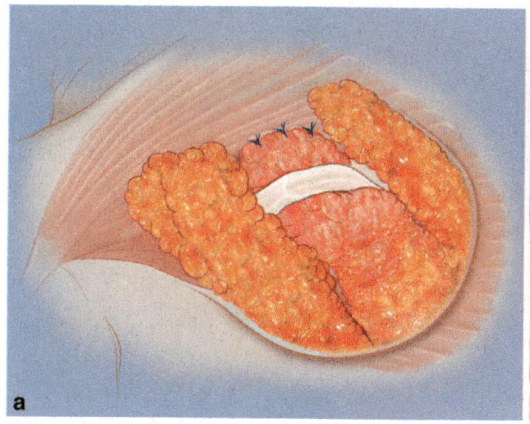

Fig. 18.8 (a,b) The lower thoracic breast parenchymal flap is secured both to the harvested bipedicled prepectoral fascia and to the prepectoral fascia superiorly to the flap. This is performed according to the preoperative marking and is usually at the level of the second or third intercostal space. The deepithelialized lower thoracic flap is attached with permanent sutures superomedially, superiorly, and supero-laterally

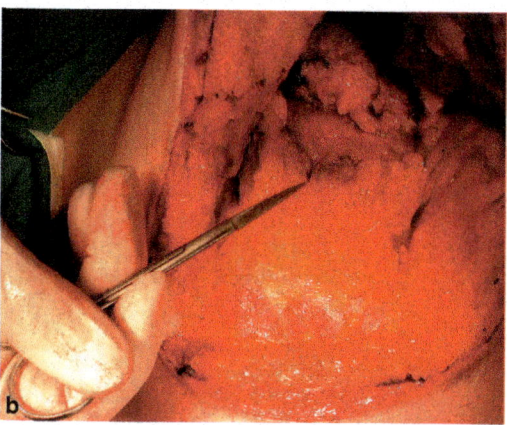

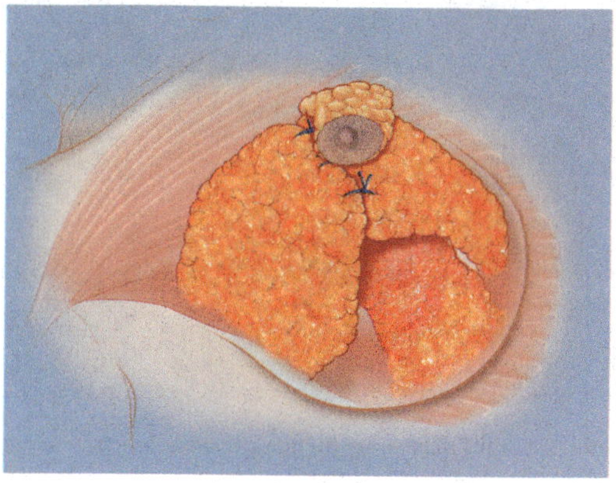

Fig. 18.9 Once the lower thoracic breast parenchymal flap is secured in place, the medial and lateral pillars of the breast are sutured together on top of it. Lateral stitches are added in order to obtain a better contour of the lateral breast

usually at the level of the second or third intercostal spaces. An additional suture is placed between the breast parenchymal flap and onto the prepectoral fascial flap in order to attach and to stabilize the parenchymal flap.

The breast is then closed bringing the two side walls together (Fig. 18.9), suturing the NAC into position, and then closing the inframammary fold (Fig. 18.10). The authors prefer to use lateral breast sutures to create an enhanced pleasing lateral breast fold. These are made between the breast parenchyma and the chest wall.

Drains are positioned and the wounds are then closed with a subcuticular closure (Fig. 18.11).

18.3.2
Operative Technique for Vertical Breast Mastopexy

The markings for the vertical mammaplasty correction are done placing the superior edge of the NAC about 2 cm from the inframammary fold with a nipple areolar measurement of around 5 cm in diameter, creating an incision for the areola of about 14–16 cm in a sloped direction, as per the Hall-Findley technique. The two vertical limbs are continued down below the nipple areolar complex to be approximately 2 cm above the inframammary fold and then connected together.

The medial and lateral wedges of tissue are drawn for debulking and liposuction to create a better breast shape. The nipple is marked as a superomedial or medial pedicle, and below the nipple areolar complex an inferior breast parenchymal breast flap is designed approximately 5×5 cm^2. Once again the skin is incised, the flaps are deepithelized and the breast tissue that is required just above the nipple areolar complex and the medial and lateral wedges are removed in the superior part to allow the nipple to fit in correctly. A small amount of breast tissue is removed and the medial and lateral inferior edges are debulked and liposuction is used to create a good breast shape.

The inferior parenchymal flap is raised approximately 5×5 cm^2 incising vertically and perpendicularly to the

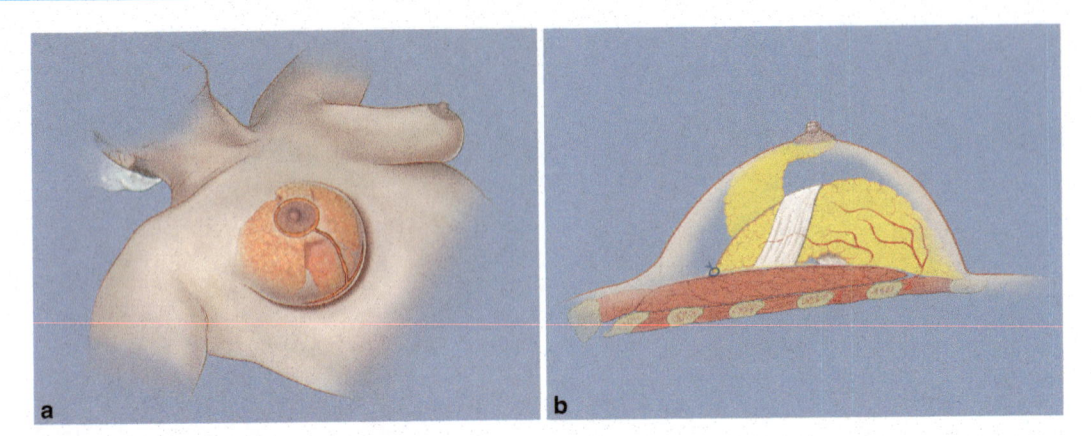

Fig. 18.10 (a,b) Breast closure in layers

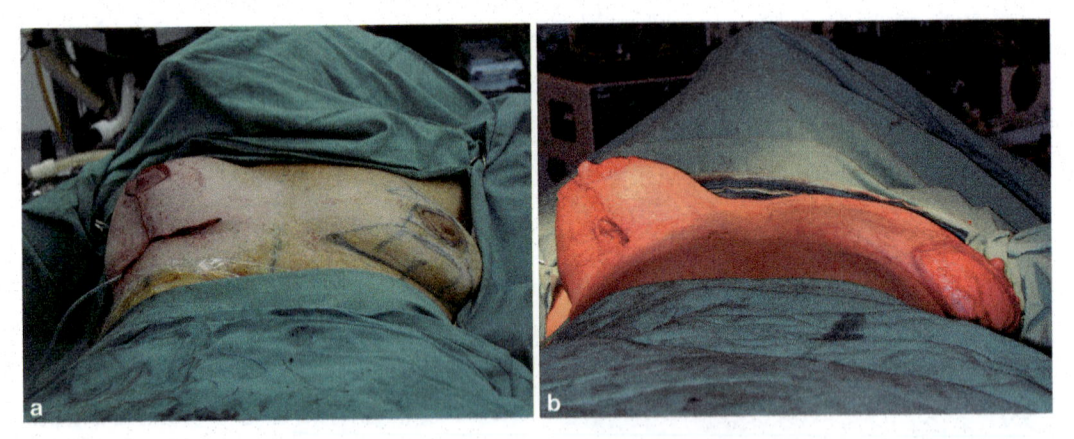

Fig. 18.11 (a) Immediate postoperative image of wise pattern FSM performed on the right breast. (b) Immediate postoperative image of vertical pattern FSM performed on the right breast. Note the significant breast projection obtained

chest wall inferiorly and then the lateral sides followed superiorly with some slight undermining of the nipple until the prepectoral fascia. The prepectoral fascia is dissected to the point of suspension. The parenchymal flap and suspension is as for the wise pattern described earlier (Fig. 18.11).

18.3.3
Operative Technique for Combined Subfascial Mastopexy and Augmentation

The procedure is as described in Sects. 18.3.1 and 18.3.2. Once the chest wall flap is inserted underneath the prepectoral fascia, augmentation with breast prosthesis begins. The subpectoral muscle pocket is developed at the level of the inframammary crease and the breast prosthesis is inserted under the muscle in a dual plane technique (Fig. 18.12). The pocket is closed in layers (Fig. 18.12). A lateral incision (4–5 cm) is normally used to insert the prosthesis. This lateral incision serves to preserve the blood supply to the lower thoracic flaps, which is nourished by vertical perforators from the prepectoral fascia (Fig. 18.13). In combined procedure, we tend to avoid using large breast prosthesis (not more than 300 ml based on case by case) as we feel that these would create unnecessary pressure on the lower thoracic flap's blood supply.

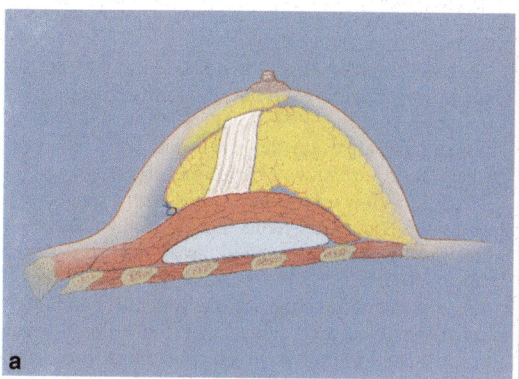

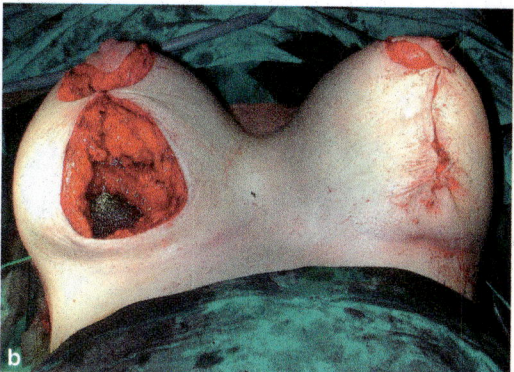

Fig. 18.12 (a,b) Breast prosthesis is inserted under the muscle in a dual plane technique. Using the combined FSM and augmentation approach, significant projection is obtained

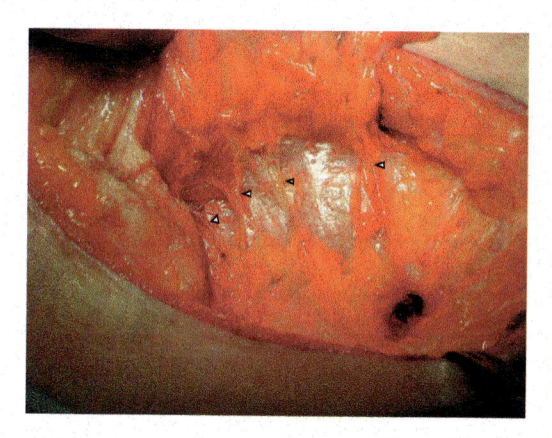

Fig. 18.13 Vertical perforators (*marked with arrows*) nourishing the lower thoracic flap

18.3.4
Operative Technique for Combined Subfascial Mastopexy and Explantation of Breast Prosthesis

FSM can be performed at the same time of breast prosthesis removal (Fig. 18.14). Following breast prosthesis explantation and pocket closure using absorbable sutures, careful dissection of the lower thoracic flap is performed. The authors have performed the FSM procedure only in the cases of breast prosthesis that were inserted under the pectoralis muscle and not for submammary positioning. The authors have found that the lower thoracic flap is often much thinner and frail in these occasions. Therefore, care should be taken to preserve as many perforators as possible to keep the flap base not less than $5 \times 5\,cm^2$. Using magnifying loupes does help in achieving this goal. Otherwise, the procedure is performed as described previously.

18.4
Complications

Between December 2001 and December 2006, 54 patients underwent fascial suspension mastopexy (FSM). Seventeen women had grade 1 ptosis (31%), 32 had grade 2 ptosis (60%), 3 had grade 3 ptosis (5%) and 2 had pseudoptosis (4%). Out of the 54 patients, 47 patients (88%) underwent FSM only, 4 patients (7%) underwent FSM combined with breast augmentation (with breast prosthesis less than 300 g), 3 patients (5%) underwent FSM following immediate breast prosthesis removal. Out of the 54 patients, 9 (17%) underwent the procedure through an inverted T approach, while 45 patients (83%) underwent FSM through vertical mammaplasty approach. Three patients (5%) underwent combined procedures: one patient underwent a concomitant abdominoplasty and two patients underwent liposuction to the thighs and to the neck area, respectively.

Complications (Table 18.1) were divided into mild, moderate, and severe. Among the mild complications, we had one patient with immediate post-operative hematoma. One patient underwent localized infection that was treated conservatively. Sensation changes were reported by ten patients who underwent the procedure using the inverted T approach and by four patients who underwent the procedure through a vertical mammaplasty incision. Two patients who underwent combined procedure had mild postoperative asymmetry. These patients had significant asymmetry preoperatively. Fat necrosis was observed in two patients but required no further procedure.

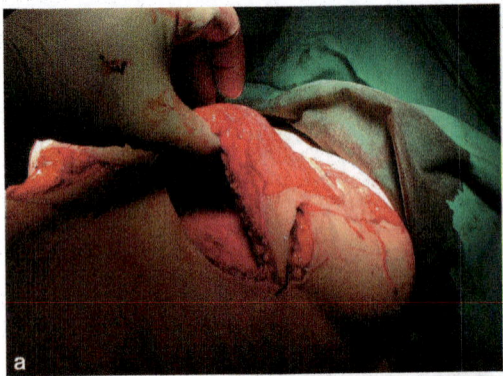

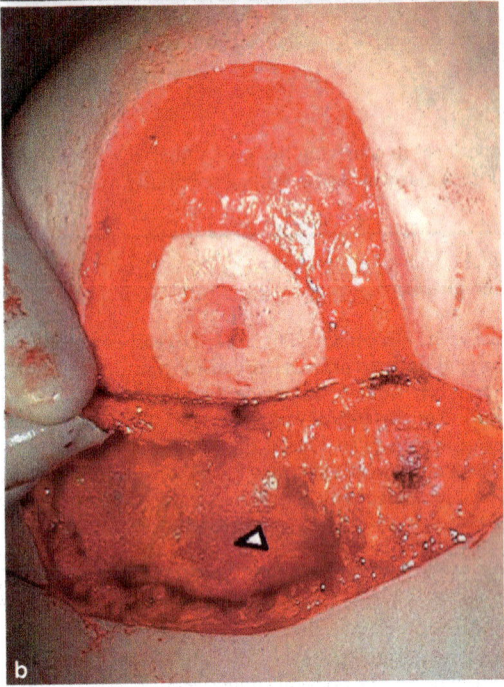

Fig. 18.14 Autologous FSM performed immediately after (**a**) breast prosthesis explantation. (**b**) The submuscular pocket is marked with an arrow

Among the moderate complications, one patient suffered from partial nipple necrosis that settled without a secondary procedure. Scar problems (mainly skin excess at the lower breast pole) were observed in three patients who underwent vertical mammaplasty approach and in one patient who underwent an inverted T approach. These patients underwent secondary local procedure to correct the scar.

Among the severe complications, we had one patient who had complete unilateral nipple necrosis. This patient, who was a smoker, underwent combined FSM and breast augmentation.

Average time for surgery was 2.5 h. Most patients (49 patients) were admitted to hospital for a one night after care. Average time of hospitalization was 1.5 days. Average time for drain tubes removal was 1 day post surgery. No transfusion of blood was necessary.

Average follow up was for 2 years, with a longest follow up of 5 years. All patients had an excellent aesthetic outcome, resulting in a good breast projection and shape contour.

For the aesthetic rating scale, preoperative and postoperative photographs taken after more than 1 year were evaluated. On the scale of 1 (poor) to 4 (excellent), overall ptosis correction was rated as 3.4, asymmetry correction as 3.4, postoperative breast symmetry as 3.2, scar quality as 3.3, breast shape as 3.1, nipple/areola size as 2.9, and overall result as 3.

18.5 Discussion

Correction of breast ptosis is regularly sort by patients, but many techniques of mastopexy have been disappointing in their long-term results and associated breast scarring. The popularity of mastopexy is born out by the constant increase in reported procedures. The American Society of Plastic Surgeons member statistics between 2000 and 2006 reports a significant increase of 96% in the number of mastopexies performed [19]. In addition, it seems that there is a significant increase in older patients (age group 35–50 years) seeking mastopexy. The increased number of procedures could be due to several factors such as our better knowledge of breast cancer and screening, as well as the fact that the general trend today is towards more conservative procedures (lumpectomies and skin sparing techniques) than the past radical procedures. In addition, the public has an opinion regarding the desired breast shape and superior fullness.

While much of the history of mastopexy parallels that of breast reduction, the latest described techniques rely more on parenchymal shaping than on skin tightening. Most modern techniques aim to oppose the natural attenuating process of Cooper's ligament and dermis laxity that cause the inevitable ptotic breast appearance [20–26]. The steps that need to be fulfilled include elevation and reshaping of the breast parenchyma with the transposition of the attached NAC and the removal of the redundant skin and redraping of the skin envelope.

In our institute, we have previously performed several mastopexies according to Graf and Biggs [1], who suggested the inferior thoracic flap to improve breast projection and upper pole fullness. Follow up of patients undergoing this technique showed that a better and

Table 18.1 Fascial suspension mastopexy (FSM) complications*

	Vertical mammoplasty	Inverted T	Combined procedure Augmentation + FSM
Mild			
Bleeding	–	–	1
Infection	–	1	–
Sensation changes	4	10	–
Asymmetry	–	–	2
Fat necrosis	1	1	–
Mild			
Partial nipple necrosis	–	1	–
Scar problems	3	1	–
Severe			
Complete nipple necrosis	–	–	1

*Represented by number of patients

more durable breast suspension can be achieved. We were concerned, however, as to the several aspects of the technique: First, disruption of normal breast architecture, that is, burying breast parenchyma under a bulk of pectoralis muscle, may represent a serious obstacle in breast cancer screening. Second, since pectoralis muscle remained functional, we have noticed "pulling" of breast parenchyma as a result of muscle contracture. In addition, the technique was painful and relatively bloodier.

The authors were searching for a solution that would overcome these problems, and at the same time allow a durable autologous suspension, that is, not relying entirely on either absorbed or nonabsorbed sutures. Pectoralis fascia or a superficial fascial system suspension as described by Lockwood [4] was described on several occasions for breast parenchyma suspension and was suggested to have longer-lasting contour results. Using exclusively the pectoralis muscle fascia allowed us to achieve a better durable autologous breast parenchymal suspension, and at the same time, to avoid the harvesting of a pectoralis muscle strip with all its drawbacks.

The authors' technique takes into consideration the above and adds to the mastopexy molding and reshaping of the breast parenchyma to obtain maximal projection and fullness where the breast needs it most. The technique is based on two concepts: the first is that the breast's internal arrangement is crucial in achieving maximal tissue stability, and we are therefore of the opinion that it is not the skin incision or the skin envelope that are important in achieving the final breast shape, but rather the internal rearrangement of the breast tissue. The solution is, therefore, to reshape the breast parenchyma according to the problem that the surgeon has to address. For example, in a pseudoptotic breast, the breast parenchyma fullness of the lower pole may be utilized to enhance the projection of the breast in its middle portion and hence at the same time reduce the lower pole fullness. The second concept is that all viable tissue of breast parenchyma should be utilized, as in other preservation techniques, in order to get the necessary breast fullness. Breast parenchyma changes its composition with time to a less solid parenchyma with an increase of the adipose component. The breast tissue should be preserved as much as possible. This will maintain breast volume, and is used behind the NAC for obtaining also breast projection, upper pole fullness, and improved shape. At the same time, it narrows the often broadened breast and improves the contouring of the inframammary sulcus. In our technique, parenchymal breast tissue acts as autologous breast prosthesis; it may fill the breast "gaps" and it creates the necessary projection by correcting breast ptosis. All implant complications (introduction of foreign body, capsule formation, infections) are avoided.

In addition, our technique is based on the suspension of the inferior flap by the prepectoral fascia. The fascia represents a natural, durable, elastic way of suspending the breast parenchymal flap. The advantages of using such suspension are numerous; since the fascia is

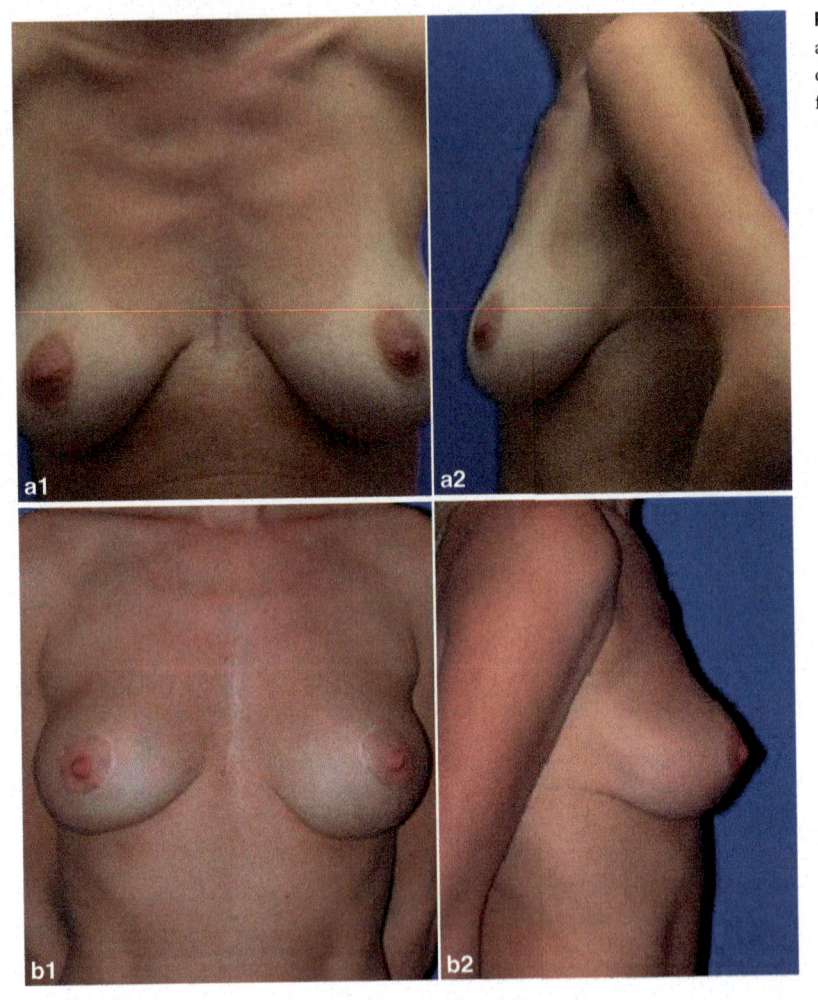

Fig. 18.15 FSM performed in a vertical pattern. (*a1,2*) Preoperative. (*b1,2*) Two year follow up

prepectoral and natural anatomical planes are not disrupted, screening of the breast in the future is made more amenable. Furthermore, surgery is made simple, consumes less time, and is less bloody. Postoperative sequelae such as contraction of the parenchymal flap by the pectoralis muscle contraction are avoided.

The authors found that fascial suspension mastopexy represents a very versatile procedure. Although performed by our team only as a bipedicled pectoralis fascia strip, the technique may be performed in various other modes. For example, instead of using the fascia in a bipedicled pattern, the fascia could be molded in various other ways to achieve breast parenchymal suspension where such suspension is needed. Hence, for upper pole fullness, the design of the flap could be more superior, allowing more medial breast tissue to be pulled towards the upper pole and the prepectoral fascia could be used as such to hold the parenchyma suspending.

The authors have performed the technique using superiorly based pedicles (superior, superomedial, and superolateral). The technique was performed both in a vertical (Fig. 18.15) and a Wise pattern (Fig. 18.16) technique.

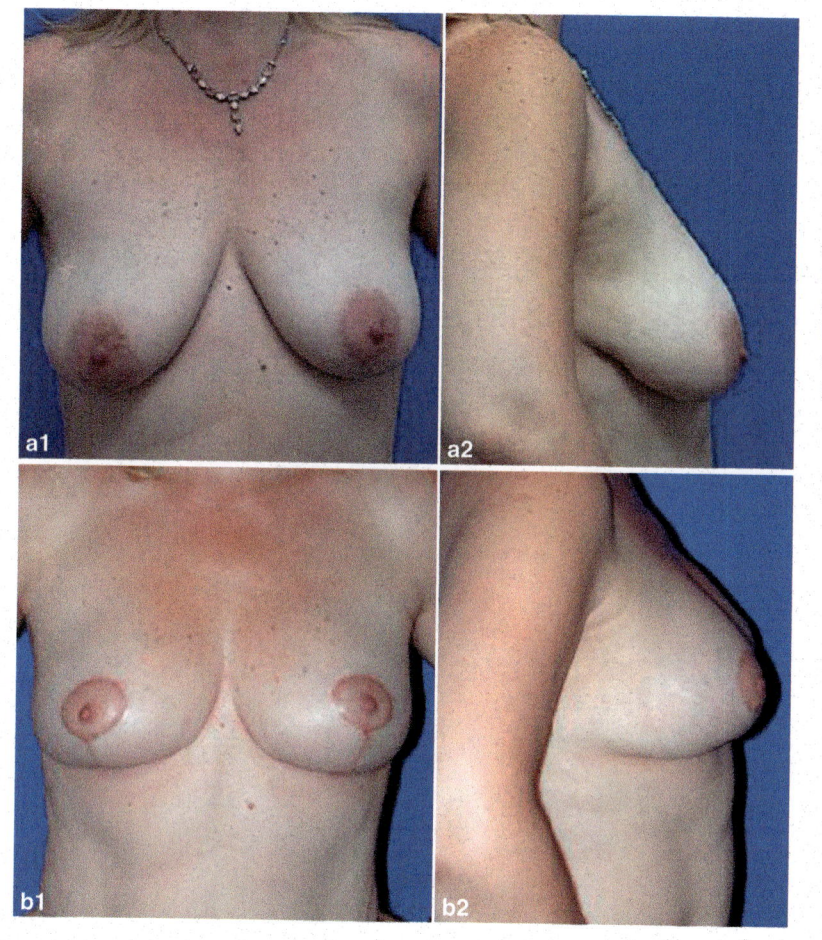

Fig. 18.16 A wise pattern FSM. (**a**) Preoperative 35-years-old patient. (**b**) Twelve months postoperative after bilateral vertical breast reduction (right breast, 100 g; left breast, 80 g) with supero-medial NAC pedicle and bilateral FSM. Note significant improvement in breast projection, contour, and shape as well as upper pole fullness

In addition, FSM was performed in patients who underwent combined procedures where breast prosthesis was inserted at the time of FSM (Fig. 18.17), and in cases where patients wished to remove the breast prosthesis and replace them with autologous tissue (Fig. 18.18). The authors believe that the best aesthetic result could be obtained using the supero-medial pedicle, because this resulted in a well defined medial fullness and at the same time helped to define the lateral breast contour with lateral breast fold sutures. In addition, the technique is suitable in cases of breast asymmetry (Fig. 18.19). In these cases, asymmetrical flaps and flaps from lateral and medial breast parenchyma are raised and the flaps are suspended with a fascial sling.

The lower thoracic flap described by Graf et al. [6] represents a real improvement in mastopexy results. While actually acting as an inferior pedicle flap as performed in a routine breast reduction, we noted clinically the evidence of different vertical perforators supplying the flap (Fig. 18.13). Furthermore, by examining the flap using ultrasound at a 1 year follow up, we were able to ascertain its long-term viability (Fig. 18.20). This flap, in our opinion, is crucial for obtaining better durable mastopexy results, as we felt that this can be achieved only

140   18 Fascial Suspension Mastopexy

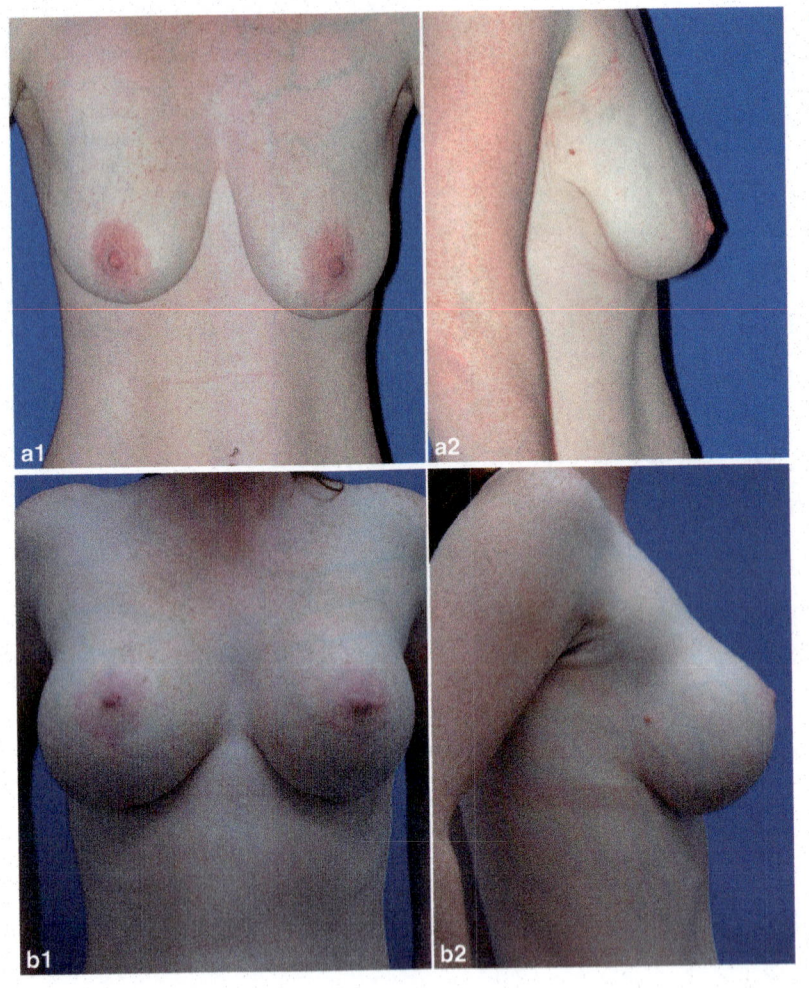

Fig. 18.17 Combined FSM (vertical pattern) with breast augmentation using breast prosthesis of 250 cc. 36-years-old patient reoperative views (1a-1b) showing bilateral ptotic breasts as well as mild asymmetry. 12 months postoperative views (b1-b2)

by a true rearrangement of the breast tissue. The history of mastopexy shows that different local flaps, suspension stitches, and breast skin excision do not obtain a durable projected breast. Furthermore, our experience in other anatomical areas show the importance of rearrangement of underlying tissues and the correct skin redraping over them for obtaining tensionless closure and longstanding results.

The advantages of our technique are that it can be performed either as a vertical mammaplasty or in a wise pattern modality. This provides a significant versatility to the technique performed. The technique is simple to perform. Learning curve is short. Surgery time is not much longer (average surgery duration was 2.5 h). Since the pectoralis muscle is not harvested, pain is reduced and bleeding is avoided. We have noticed that the lower

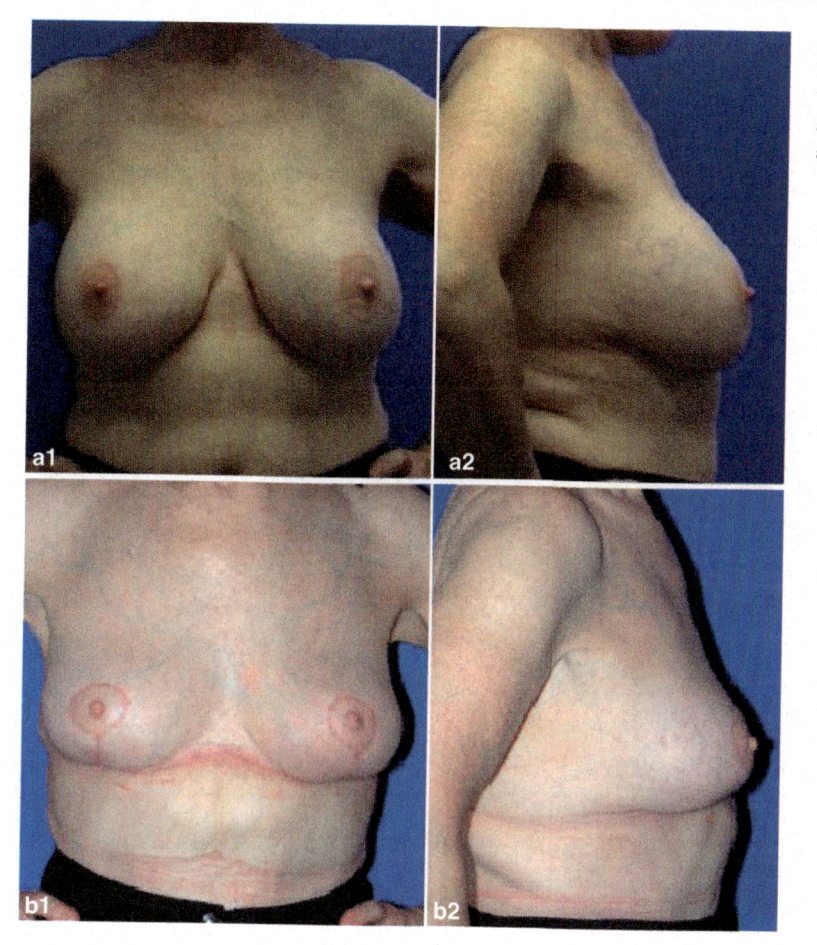

Fig. 18.18 (**a**1,2) Preoperative 54-year-old patient. (**b**1,2) Twelve months postoperative after breast prosthesis removal and immediate FSM

thoracic flap described by Graf et al. [6] is a mobile flap, and can sometimes reach the upper middle breast area. Hence, upper pole fullness is sometimes visible in addition to the improved breast projection. Also, using the pectoralis fascia and not the muscle represents an advantage if breast cancer screening is considered, since derangement of entire breast parenchyma and interference of major tissue planes are avoided.

The main disadvantage of the technique is harvesting of the pectoralis muscle fascia strip. Since there is no natural anatomical plane, separating the fascia from its underlying muscle can be sometimes fastidious. Hence, harvesting of the fascia should be performed meticulously. This is not a real obstacle, as only a relatively small strip of bipedicled fascia is harvested.

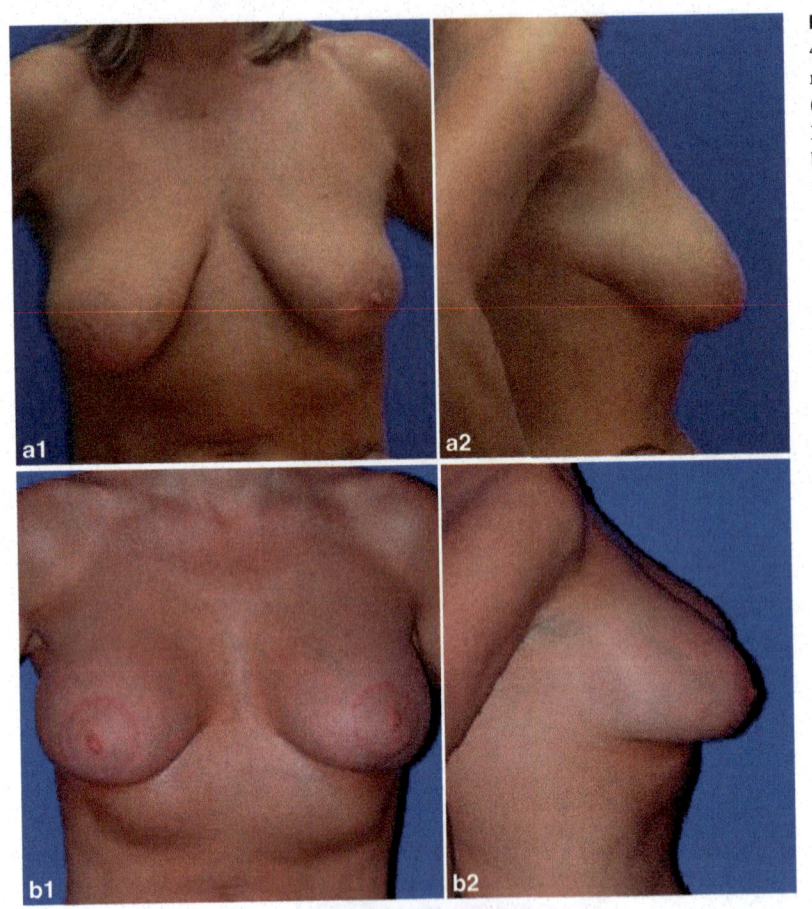

Fig. 18.19 (**a***1,2*) Preoperative 44-year-old patient with mild breast asymmetry. (**b***1,2*) Sixteen months after FSM performed without breast prosthesis

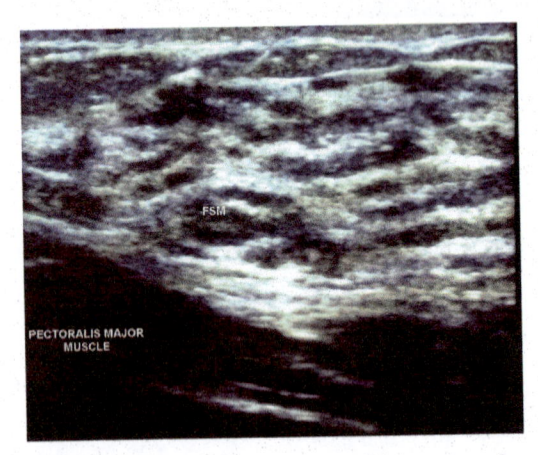

Fig. 18.20 Ultrasound performed at 1 year follow up shows flap viability

18.6 Conclusions

Mastopexy techniques have changed significantly in the last decades. Repositioning of the skin envelope is no longer considered sufficient in obtaining durable results. To achieve long-standing projected breast, it is necessary to reshape the underlying breast parenchyma and to restructure the breast so as to oppose the gravitational forces acting continuously on the breast tissue.

FSM offers both restoration of underlying breast structure as well as creation of autologous support. The technique is suitable for different types of breast ptosis (grade 1–3), versatile, simple to perform, and allows good breast cancer screening. It does not violate major tissue planes, for example, by putting breast tissue behind the muscle. The technique presents a better long-standing breast contour shape and achieves a well rejuvenated and projected breast.

References

1. Graf R, Biggs TM: In search of better shape in mastopexy and reduction mammoplasty. Plast Reconstr Surg 2002;110(1):309–317
2. Hinderer UT: Circumareolar dermo-glandular plication: a new concept for correction of breast ptosis. Aesthetic Plast Surg 2001;25(6):404–420
3. Caldeira AM, Lucas A: Pectoralis major muscle flap: a new support approach to mammaplasty, personal technique. Aesthetic Plast Surg 2000;24(1):58–70
4. Lockwood T: Reduction mammaplasty and mastopexy with superficial fascial system suspension. Plast Reconstr Surg 1999;103(5):1411–1420
5. Frey M: A new technique of reduction mammaplasty: dermis suspension and elimination of medial scars. Br J Plast Surg 1999;52(1):45–51
6. Graf R, Reis de Araujo LR, Rippel R, Neto LG, Pace DT, Biggs T: Reduction mammaplasty and mastopexy using the vertical scar and thoracic wall flap technique. Aesthetic Plast Surg 2003;27(1):6–12
7. Schwarzmann E: Avoidance of nipple necrosis by preservation of corium in one-stage plastic surgery of the breast. Rev Chir Struct 1937;7:206–209
8. Gonzales-Ulloa M: Correction of hypotrophy of the breast by means of exogenous material. Plast Reconstr Surg 1960;25:15–26
9. Goulian D Jr: Dermal mastopexy. Plast Reconstr Surg 1971;47(2):105–110
10. Regnault P: Breast ptosis. Definition and treatment. Clin Plast Surg 1976;3(2):193–203
11. Lassus C: A technique for breast reduction. Int Surg 1970;53(1):69–72
12. Lejour M: Vertical mammaplasty and liposuction of the breast. Plast Reconstr Surg 1994;94(1):100–114
13. Weiss PR, Ship AG: Restoration of breast contour with autologous tissue after removal of implants. Ann Plast Surg 1995;34(3):236–241
14. Muti E: Personal approach to surgical correction of the extremely hypoplastic tuberous breast. Aesthetic Plast Surg 1996;20(5):385–390
15. Flowers RS, Smith EM Jr: "Flip-flap" mastopexy. Aesthetic Plast Surg 1998;22(6):425–429
16. Hall-Findlay EJ: A simplified vertical reduction mammaplasty: shortening the learning curve. Plast Reconstr Surg 1999;104(3):748–759
17. Lewis GK: A method of mastopexy with fascia lata transplants. J Int Coll Surg 1956;26(3):346–353
18. Johnson GW: Central core reduction mammoplasties and Marlex suspension of breast tissue. Aesthetic Plast Surg 1981;5(1):77–84
19. http://www.plasticsurgery.org/media/Press_Kits/Procedural-Statistics-Press-Kit-Index.cfm
20. Persoff MM: Vertical mastopexy with expansion augmentation. Aesthetic Plast Surg 2003;27(1):13–19
21. Hammond DC: The SPAIR mammaplasty. Clin Plast Surg 2002;29(3):411–421
22. Hall-Findlay EJ: Pedicles in vertical breast reduction and mastopexy. Clin Plast Surg 2002;29(3):379–391
23. Lejour M: Vertical mammaplasty: early complications after 250 personal consecutive cases. Plast Reconstr Surg 1999;104(3):764–770
24. Hagerty RC: External mastopexy with imbrication following explantation. Plast Reconstr Surg 1999;103(3):976–979
25. Fayman MS. Short scar mastopexy with flap transposition. Aesthetic Plast Surg 1998;22(2):135–141
26. Goes JC: Periareolar mammaplasty: double skin technique with application of polyglactine or mixed mesh. Plast Reconstr Surg 1996;97(5):959–968

Internal Mastopexy

J. Dan Metcalf M.D.

19.1 Introduction

A variety of mastopexy and nipple-lift procedures have been performed successfully, but often associated with the problem of undesirable scarring. The author has developed a procedure to elevate the breast or nipple–areolar complex by plicating the anterior superior fibrous capsule in patients who have had previous breast augmentation.

19.2 History

Internal mastopexy was first performed by the author in 1989 on a patient with asymmetrical nipples with one lower than the other. At that time, long-lasting absorbable suture (0-PDS) was used. Although this was initially done with a "Z" suture and later with a purse string suture, it is now done with a simple continuous interlocking suture of 0-Ethibond or braided nylon.

19.3 Patient Selection

1. The patient must have an implant in a submammary or subfascial position. The procedure has been performed on submuscular augmented patients, but the results are not consistent.
2. The procedure should not be performed in patients with "diseased" capsules. This would consist of a calcified capsule or a very thick capsule with contracture.
3. The patient must have implants for at least 9 months to ensure adequate capsule to work with. Some patients form very thin and almost nonexistent capsules and results may not be satisfactory in this group of patients.

19.4 Technique

The patient is evaluated in a sitting position by obtaining measurement from the suprasternal notch to the mid-nipple and from the nipple to the inframammary fold. The objective is to make the distances from the suprasternal notch to nipple and from the nipple to inframammary folds equal on both sides. The procedure is performed through an inframammary or areolar incision, using the original scar if present.

The implant is removed and the anterior superior capsule is plicated (Fig. 19.1). First an anchor suture is placed in the medial aspect of the anterior superior capsule. A continuous suture, locking every other suture, is then used to plicate the anterior superior capsule. The bites are taken at about 1 cm apart, and as they are continued across the anterior superior capsule, the

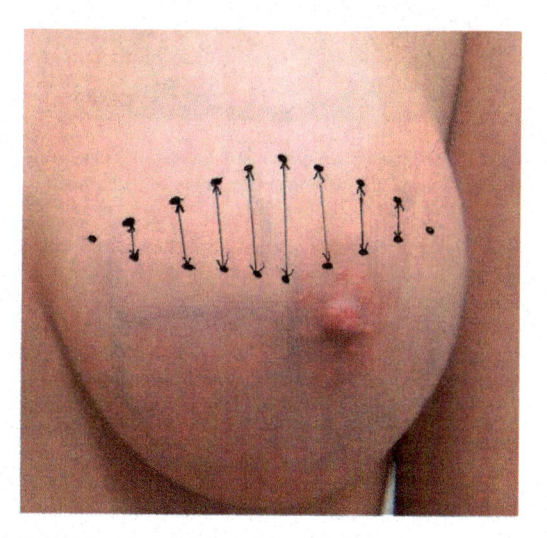

Fig. 19.1 Position of the interlocking continuous suture of the anterior capsule shown on the breast skin

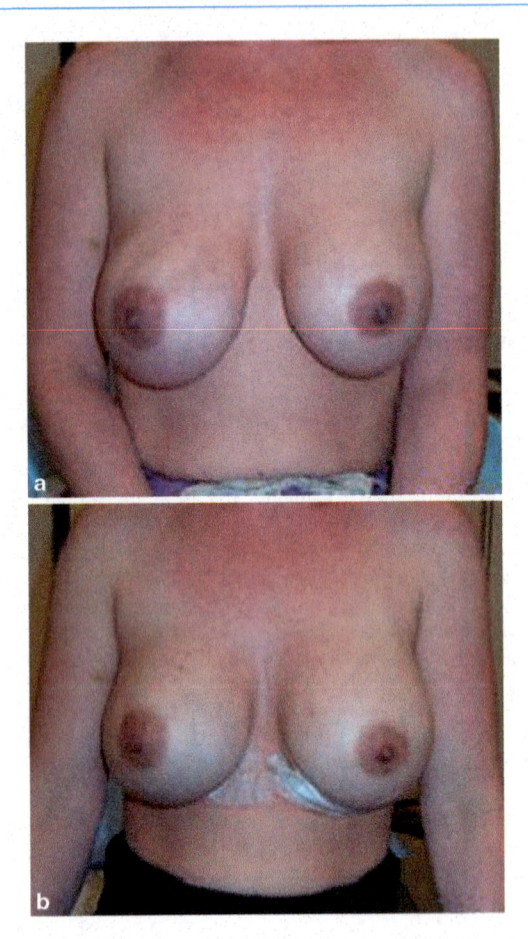

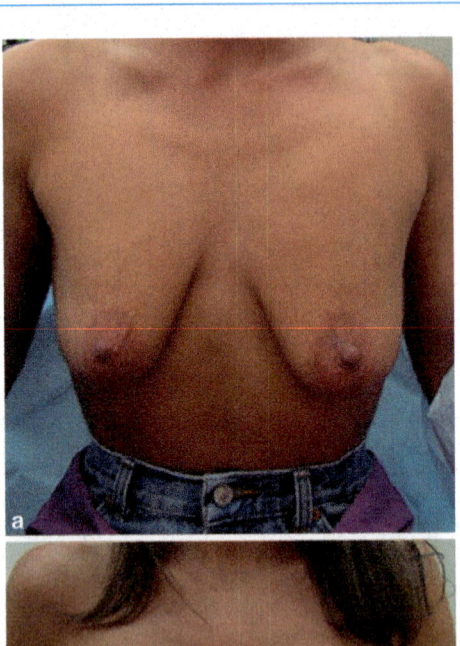

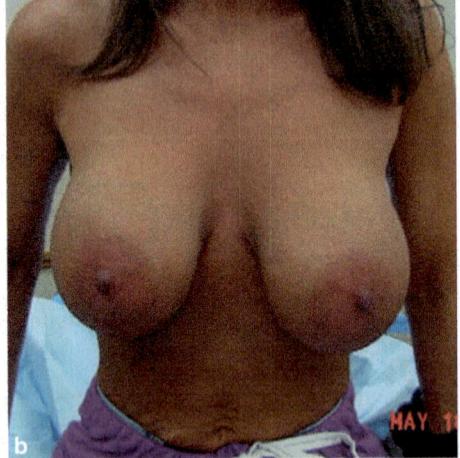

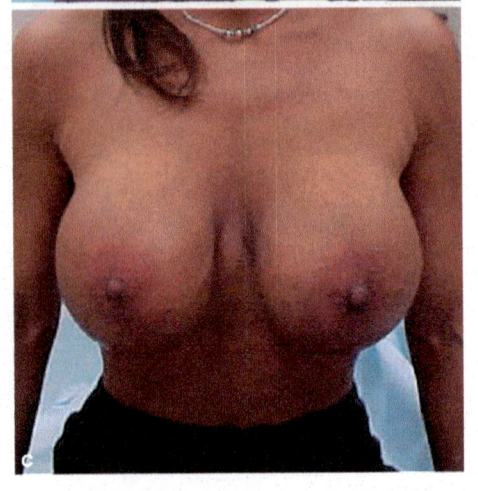

Fig. 19.2 (a) Preoperative patient with ptosis of right breast. (b) Postoperative following internal mastopexy

bites are progressively widened until they are approximately 3–4 cm at the mid-nipple level (vertical line traversing the nipple.)

After the suture has passed the mid-line, the bites are then progressively decreased until the anchor suture is taken at the lateral aspect of the anterior superior capsule. This is tied securely and then three or four interrupted sutures are taken to reinforce the plication without doing any further plication.

Since this procedure results in an implant pocket with decreased volume, an open capsulotomy is usually necessary to accommodate the decreased volume of the implant pocket. The preferred location of the

Fig. 19.3 (a) Preoperative patient prior to breast augmentation (b) Following breast augmentation ptosis occurred on the left side. (c) One year postoperative after internal mastopexy

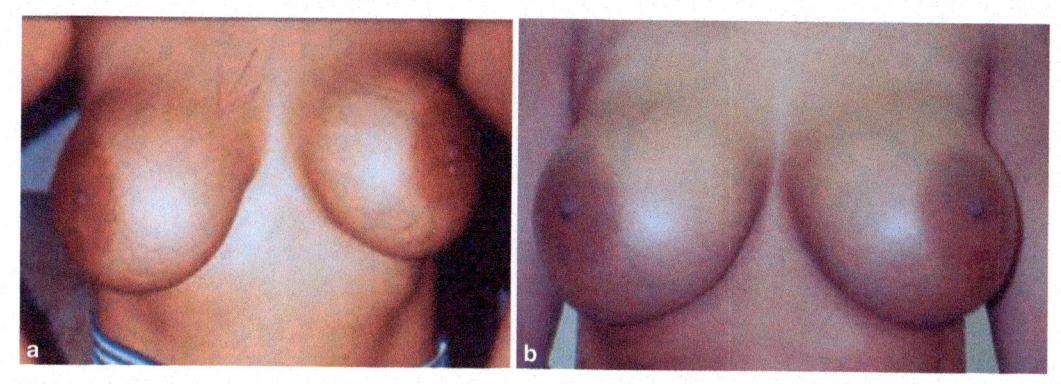

Fig. 19.4 (a) Preoperative patient with ptosis of right breast. (b) Postoperative following internal mastopexy

capsulotomy would be inferior and anterior-inferior to allow the implant to sit in the lower portion of the pocket, which allows the lifting of the nipple–areolar complex. If the distance between the nipple and the inframammary fold is greater on one side than the other, the same plication can be used in a similar manner, plicating the anterior-inferior capsule and decreasing the distance between the nipple and the inframammary fold. Following the procedure, an implant sizer is placed and adjustments are made since there may be minor areas of irregularity of the anterior capsule. The permanent implant is then placed and the incision is closed.

19.5
Complications

One would perhaps expect a higher incidence of capsular contracture, but this has not been experienced by the author. Recurrence of the ptosis will be a complication if the proper support is not used following surgery. This would probably be no more than in any augmented breast, as the capsule is usually very strong and supportive. Ptosis would tend to recur more in women who do not have good supportive capsules. In thinner women, the sutures of internal mastopexy may be palpable, but this usually resolves with healing.

19.6
Discussion

Anterior fibrous capsule plication is limited to patients who have had prior submammary or subfascial augmentation, who have adequate skin and subcutaneous tissue thickness, and require nipple–areolar complex elevation less than 3 cm. The procedure does not include extra incisions, which are necessary for routine mastopexy or nipple lift. The operation is relatively simple and can be performed through a prior scar in the areola or inframammary fold.

19.7
Conclusions

In carefully selected patients, internal mastopexy can be performed to improve ptosis without conventional mastopexy scars (Fig. 19.2–19.4).

Combined Mastopexy/Augmentation

Alan A. Parsa, Natalie N. Parsa, Fereydoun D. Parsa

20.1
Introduction

In all cultures, beautiful breasts are evocative of femininity and sensuality. In the context of modern Western world, breasts have gained a considerable social and psychological importance as witnessed daily in social encounters as well as in the media and on the movie screens.

Representation of breasts in fine arts reached its golden age in the era of classic Greece, where it assumed an importance that surpassed other secondary sexual organs. Centuries later, renaissance artists, heirs to Greek and Roman cultures, played a major role in disseminating classic images of beautiful breasts in paintings and sculptures. Perhaps one of the best examples of such a representation is Leonardo da Vinci's "Leda and the Swan" (Fig. 20.1). "Flora" (Fig. 20.2) is another example and was painted by Leonardo's most favorite student Francesco Melzi (1493–1570) circa 1515. Melzi was most close to Leonardo and was at his bedside when he died in France in 1519 at the court of Francis I. It is strongly hypothesized that Leonardo may have begun Flora in Florence and left it unfinished as he often did with many of his other paintings. It is also assumed that the model for Flora is actually the wealthy Florentine lady Mona Lisa Gioconda, whom Leonardo immortalized in the painting by the same name. The great value we attach to these two renaissance paintings, one by Leonardo and the other by his favorite student Francesco Melzi as well as to other paintings such as the "Birth of Venus" (Fig. 20.3) by Sandro Botticelli (1445–1510), and some three centuries later, the "Turkish Bath" (Fig. 20.4) by Ingres (1780–1867), are eloquent testimonies to the important role that feminine beauty and depiction of breasts play in Western societies. One may say – at least as it relates to the Western world – that our perception of what constitutes beautiful and sensuous breasts have not changed for the past 2,500 years.

In contrast to breast reduction that is often performed for functional purposes to alleviate symptoms of discomfort and pain, mastopexy combined with breast augmentation is done for aesthetic reasons and, therefore, the appearance of the external scars is very significant for patient satisfaction. The evolution of mastopexy has hinged during the past three decades on a constant desire to reduce and improve the extent and the quality of the resulting scars.

Modern era of mastopexy began in 1976 when Bartels [1] first described concentric mastopexy in an attempt to avoid the usual Wise pattern [2] of inverted-T scars. These original circumareolar procedures were often complicated by poorly shaped breasts, wide or thick scars, and enlarged areola, and have not gain full acceptance [3]. One may assume that the loss of popularity of circumareolar mastopexy may be as much due to poor patient selection and the method of wound closure as to the operation itself. The so-called crescent mastopexy whereby a crescent-shaped segment of skin is removed from the upper aspect of the areola does not correct breast ptosis or the breast shape to any noticeable degree and is no longer performed by the majority of surgeons.

Peled in 1985 [3] and Benelli in 1990 [4] improved the technique of circumareolar mastopexy by the addition of purse string sutures that bears their names. Later, in 1990, Spear et al. [5] described certain rules to mark the patient having concentric circle mastopexy that would produce better aesthetic results. In 1990, Lejour [6] popularized the vertical scar that had been previously introduced by Lassus [7] for more advanced cases of breast ptosis.

Finally in 2001, Tebbetts [8] introduced the concept of dual plane mastopexy/augmentation (that avoids any added scar) to that of standard breast augmentation incision for correction of mild to moderate degrees of glandular ptosis and breast hypoplasia. Table 20.1 shows the chronological evolution of these various techniques and Fig. 20.5 depicts the appearance of external scars from various surgical approaches.

20.2
Initial Consultation

Combined mastopexy/breast augmentation is among the most challenging procedures in aesthetic surgery and perhaps has the highest incidence of patient dissatisfaction, not because of poor aesthetic outcome, but because of poor communication between patient and surgeon. At times, patients themselves have not made up

M.A. Shiffman (ed.), *Mastopexy and Breast Reduction: Principles and Practice,*
© Springer-Verlag Berlin Heidelberg 2009

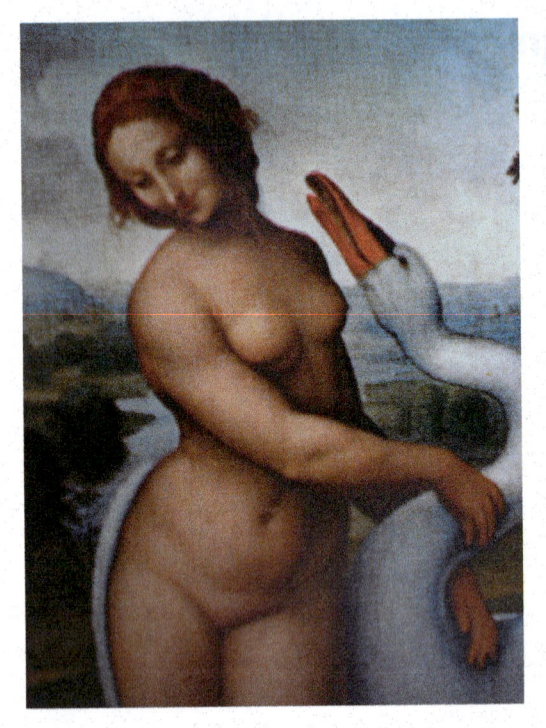

Fig. 20.1 Leda and the Swan by Leonardo da Vinci (c. 1513)

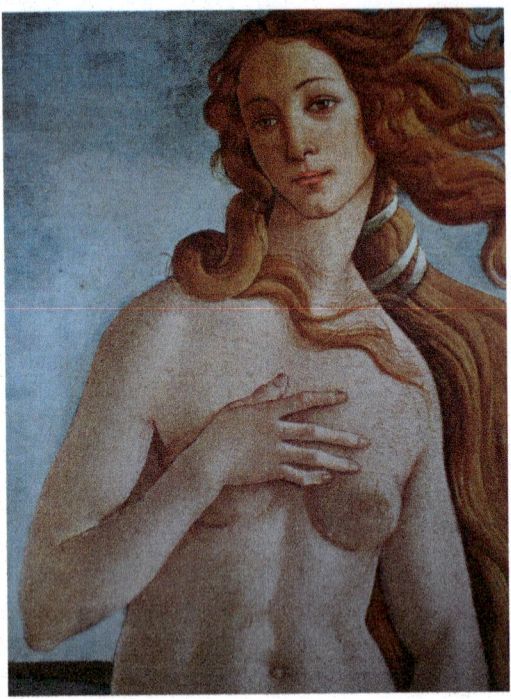

Fig. 20.3 Birth of Venus by Sandro Botticelli (c. 1482)

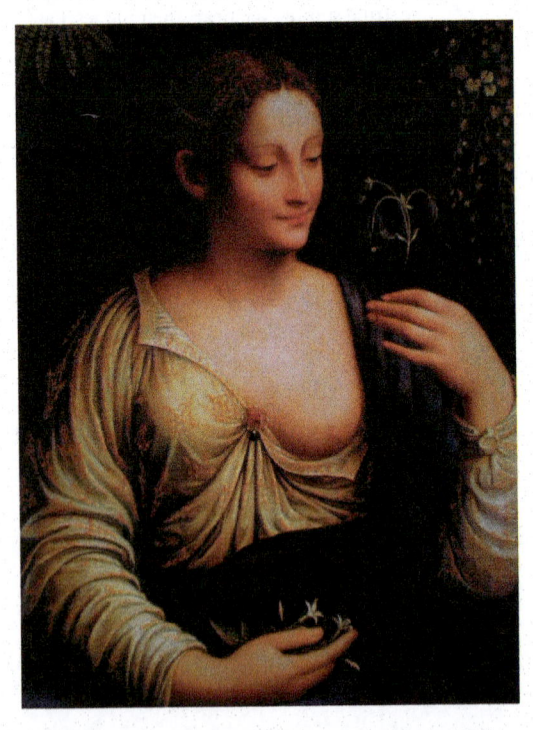

Fig. 20.2 Flora by da Vinci's student Fancesco Melzi (c. 1515)

their minds as to what they truly wish or change their thoughts in the course of preoperative consultation and office visits. And a few change their minds after the operation, regretting for the choice they have made.

Mastopexy/augmentation also carries a high incidence of complications when performed in a single stage [5, 9] and therefore the authors advise all patients with moderate to severe degree of ptosis to consider staging the operation with mastopexy as the initial procedure followed by breast augmentation 3–6 months later. It has been our experience that some patients are most satisfied with the mastopexy alone and do not request breast augmentation at a later date. In those patients who opt for breast enlargement after completion of mastopexy, the augmentation procedure would be performed under much better circumstances of healed wounds, with more predictable outcome and more satisfactory external scars. This approach has yielded the best aesthetic results with the highest degree of patient satisfaction. Unfortunately, the majority of patients do not accept a two-stage approach for reasons of time and budget.

There is no single operation or technique that satisfies all degrees of sagging breasts associated with hypoplasia. In contrast to breast reduction where patient satisfaction is very high even when extensive scars are present, mastopexy/augmentation patients often have unrealistic expectations and frequently become dissatisfied

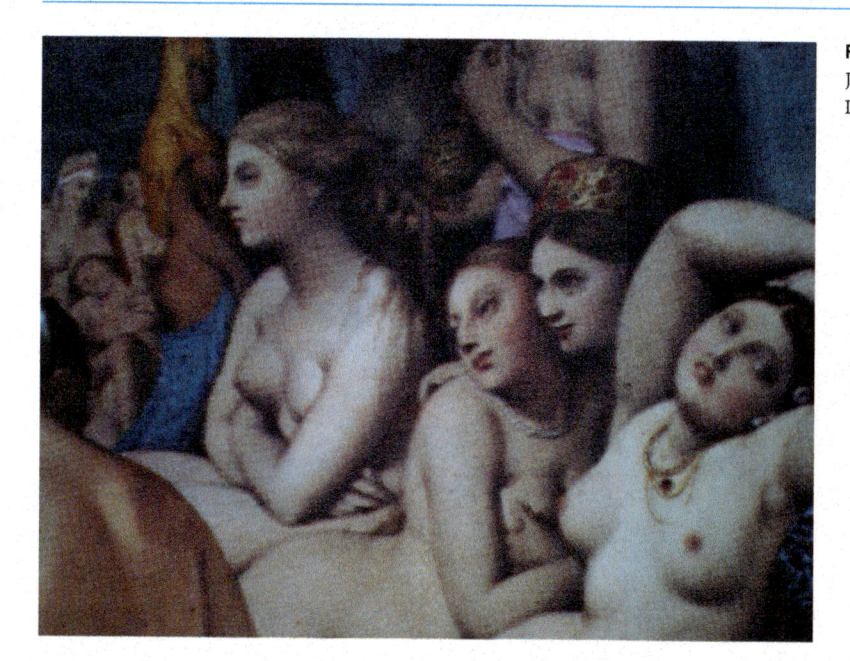

Fig. 20.4 Turkish Bath by Jean Auguste Dominique Ingres (1862)

Table 20.1 Chronological evolution of the various techniques

1950s	Wise's inverted-T pattern
1970s	Bartels: Concentric circles
1980s	Peled-Benelli: modified concentric circles
1990s	Lassus-Lejour: vertical scar
2000s	Tebbetts: dual plane

even when the outcome is judged most satisfactory by the operating surgeon as well as by other observers. For this reason, good communication and a clear understanding must be established regarding the patient's goals and desires and what realistically may be delivered.

Patients often confuse the terms "breast lift" with breast enlargement and expect a noticeable increase in breast volume with mastopexy alone. Many patients are also under the assumption that breast implants will automatically lift the breasts and correct all degrees of ptosis. Prior to the initial office visit, relatively few patients understand the nature of their problems or the necessity of combining mastopexy with augmentation in order to obtain the desired goals.

To minimize patient's confusion regarding the differences between breast "lift" and breast "enlargement," the authors devised the following approach in patients who could be candidates for either mastopexy, augmentation, or combined mastopexy with breast augmentation. The authors refer to this simple scheme as "paperpexy" [9], that is, mastopexy performed with paper tape. This simple and quick step consists of applying paper tape (1 or 2 in. wide) to the breasts (Fig. 20.6). The patient is sent home with the tapes in place and has ample opportunity to examine her breasts and to report back her impressions on whether or not she wishes mastopexy only, augmentation only, or a combination of both. It is not unusual that patients who initially request breast "lift" eventually undergo breast augmentation and those who think that breast implant would correct their condition ultimately have mastopexy or a combination of mastopexy and breast augmentation.

20.3 Preoperative Planning

Breasts have three main features that must be considered at the time of preoperative planning. These are skin elasticity, thickness of subcutaneous fat and breast tissue, and finally the degree of ptosis. The authors use the term "soft tissue support" to describe the combined qualities of skin elasticity and subcutaneous tissue thickness. When breasts are described as lacking good tissue support, this usually signifies one and often more than one of the following conditions: presence of striae, paucity of subcutaneous tissue (fat and breast parenchyma), older patients, multiple pregnancies, and a history of breastfeeding. One important objective factor is

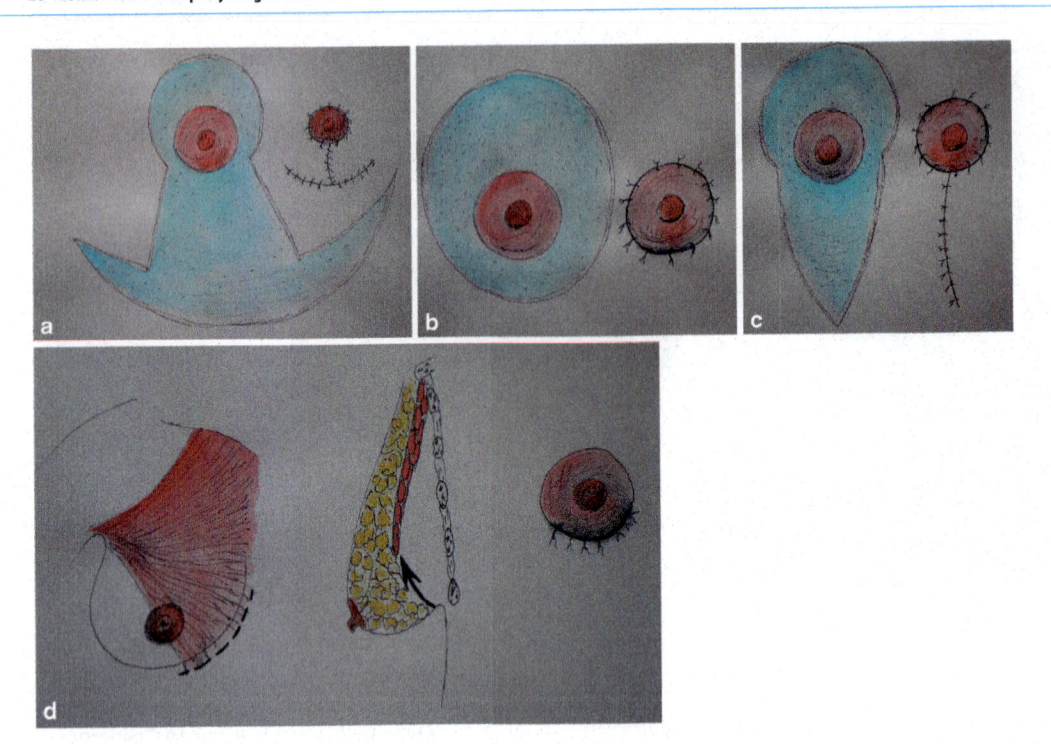

Fig. 20.5 (**a**) Wise pattern incisions with resulting inverted-T scar. (**b**) Circumareolar scar. (**c**) Vertical mastopexy scar. (**d**) Dual Plane mastopexy/augmentation for correction of mild to moderate ptosis with resulting scar

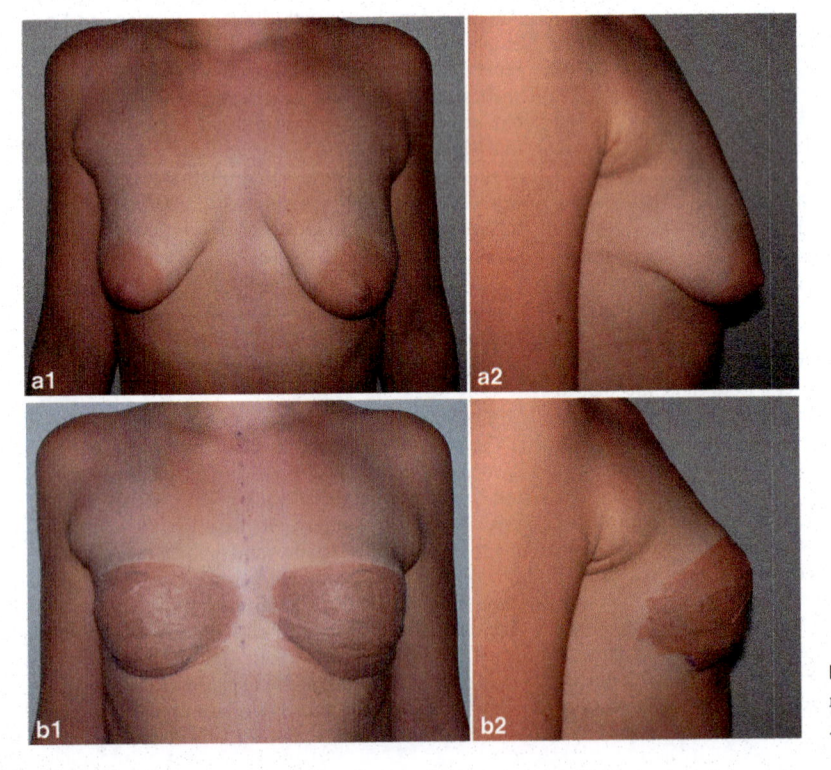

Fig. 20.6 (**a1,2**) Patient with moderate ptosis. (**b1,2**) After "paperpexy"

the measurement of the thickness of the supporting soft tissue. This is done using the caliper pinch test (Fig. 20.7). Patients whose thickness measure less than 2 cm are considered as possessing poor soft tissue support, particularly if this is associated with diminished skin elasticity.

Since there are no tests that objectively measure or document one of the major elements of soft tissue support such as skin elasticity, this must be based on the surgeon's experience and personal judgment [10, 11]. Even with good experience, it is not possible to predict with any certainty the outcome and particularly the duration of mastopexy result, as soft tissue support will eventually attenuate and stretch in time due to gravity, aging, pregnancy, weight fluctuation, as well as other factors.

The authors have modified Regnault's classic description of breast ptosis and use the one that is outlined in Table 20.2 and Fig. 20.8. The position of the nipple as it relates to the inframammary fold (IMF) as well as the degree of glandular ptosis as it relates to the IMF are the criteria used in this classification that we proposed in 2006 [9]. The simpler term of "breast nadir" refers to the "lowest contour of the breast."

In mild ptosis, nipple is located at or less than 2 cm above the IMF and the breast nadir is situated below the IMF but no more than 1 cm below the fold.

In moderate ptosis, nipple is located at, above, or below the IMF and the breast nadir is situated between 1 and 3 cm below the IMF.

In severe ptosis, the breast nadir is located more than 3 cm below the IMF and/or the nipple is located below the breast parenchyma and becomes the breast nadir.

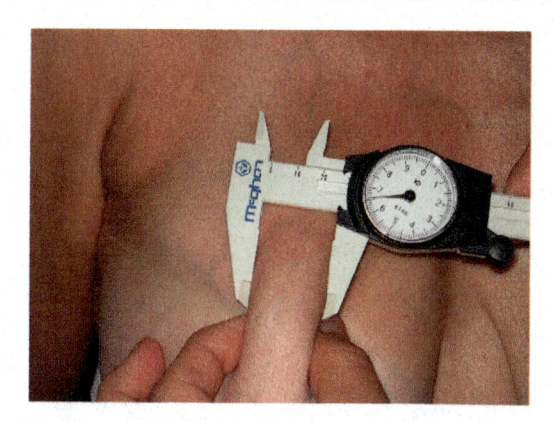

Fig. 20.7 Thickness of subcutaneous tissue is measured by caliper pinch test

Table 20.2 Modified Regnault's classification of breast ptosis

Mild ptosis	Nipple located at or less than 2 cm above the inframammary fold (IMF) and the breast nadir situated below the IMF but no more than 1 cm below the fold (Fig. 20.14a)
Moderate ptosis	Nipple located at, above, or below the IMF and the breast nadir situated between 1 and 3 cm below the IMF (Fig. 20.14b)
Severe ptosis	The breast nadir is >3 cm below the IMF and/or nipple is below breast nadir (Fig. 20.14c and d)

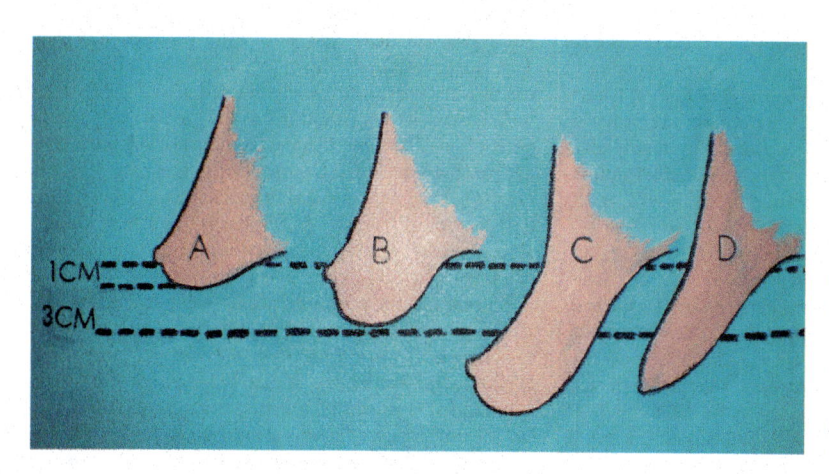

Fig. 20.8 Classification of breast ptosis into three categories of mild (**a**), moderate (**b**), and severe (**c** and **d**) based on nipple position, breast nadir and the inframammary fold

20.4 Operative Techniques and Choice of Implants

Because there is great variation in the anatomy of each breast as well as in its degree of ptosis and hypoplasia, it is important to evaluate and document such differences and select the procedure that corresponds best to patient's anatomy as well as to her wishes.

All patients who present with moderate to severe ptosis or whenever skin resection is contemplated should be offered the option of a two-stage operation consisting of mastopexy as the first stage and breast augmentation some 3–6 months later as the second stage. This approach is particularly indicated in ambivalent patients with reasonable and adequate breast volume, as a relatively good percentage of them are ultimately satisfied with mastopexy alone.

Implant selection is often dependent on surgeon's experience and judgment as well as on patient's preference, and for this reason it varies greatly. The impact of publicity by implant manufacturers as well as by testimonials posted on the internet cannot be underestimated in patients' choices.

With the reintroduction of silicone gel implants in addition to the already existing array of saline implants, there are currently a wide variety of prostheses to choose from. The authors' preference has been with the textured anatomic contoured saline prostheses such as Allergan's style 468 (Natrelle), and have only recently begun utilizing gel-filled implants. Short-term experience has been very good with these implants as well.

The selection of the size of implants is based primarily on patient's wishes as long as she understands the importance of following certain parameters. The most important objective parameter has been the base dimension of the breast that in average ranges from 10 to 13 cm. This is measured using calipers from medial aspect of the IMF to an imaginary anterior axillary line (Fig. 20.9).

Implants are selected according to chest wall's base dimension and may be +1 to −1 cm larger or smaller in diameter than the chest wall's measurements. Charts indicating the dimensions of the implants are provided by the manufacturers and are most helpful in size selection. The height as well the projection of the implants must also be taken into consideration as well as the adjusting for any volume difference between the two breasts. Such differences are often due to musculo-skeletal asymmetry as much as to breast parenchyma volume. This is particularly important when the smaller breast is located on the side of the chest wall that has more musculo-skeletal projection. In these instances, one may have to select an implant with larger volume but with lesser projection to compensate for the differences. All patients and in particular thin patients with paucity of soft tissue coverage must also be informed that obtaining completely natural breasts is an unrealistic goal and cannot be achieved with prostheses.

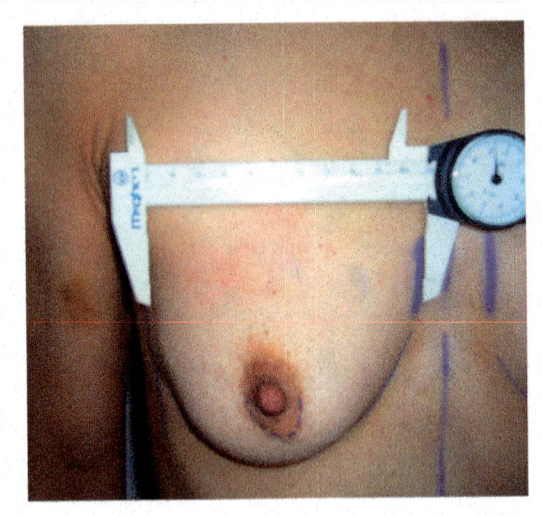

Fig. 20.9 Measurement of base dimension with calipers

Mastopexy/augmentation procedures are divided into three general categories: operations designed to augment and correct mild ptosis, procedures to augment and correct moderate ptosis, and procedures that enlarge and correct severe ptosis.

20.5 Operative Technique: Mild Ptosis

In women who have mild ptosis, nipples are situated at or less than 2 cm above the level of the IMF, with the lowest contour of breast (breast nadir) situated not more than 1 cm below the IMF (Table 20.2, Fig. 20.8). In these patients, Type I dissection and subpectoral breast augmentation is recommended (Fig. 20.10) if there is good skin elasticity and soft tissue support [8, 9]. In Type I dissection, the fibers of origin of the pectoralis major muscle are completely divided across the IMF as well as across the distal third of the parasternal region, with no dissection in the retromammary plane. This approach corrects mild ptosis in the majority of cases (Fig. 20.10), where the distance from the nipple to the IMF is typically less than centimeters and the existing skin excess is readily compensated for by the volume of implants (Fig. 20.11).

In rare instances of mild ptosis where nipple to IMF distance measures more than 6 cm or when the skin envelope is inelastic with poor soft tissue support, Type II or uncommonly Type III dual plane dissection is recommended (Fig. 20.12), utilizing the same technique as for the correction of moderate ptosis.

Subglandular rather than subpectoral breast augmentation, although not favored by us, is also an option in certain patients who possess good soft tissue support.

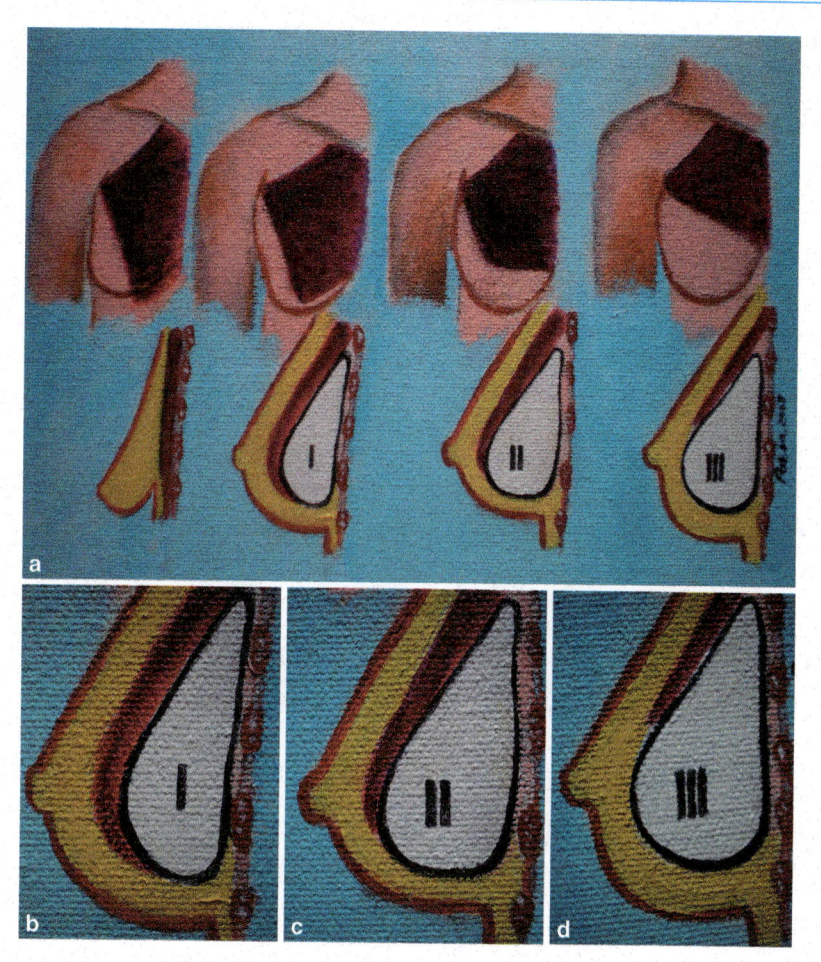

Fig. 20.10 (**a**) Three different types of subpectoral dissection. In Type I dissection, fibers of origin of pectoralis major muscle are completely detached from the ribs and the lower one third of the sternum. In types II and III dissection, the fibers of origin of pectoralis major muscle are completely detached from the ribs and additionally the planes between pectoralis fascia and breast parenchyma are separated without detaching the parasternal muscles. (**b**) Type I dissection: the fibers of origin of pectoralis major muscle have been detached from the ribs and lower sternum with no subglandular plane dissection. (**c**) Type II dissection: the fibers of origin of pectoralis major muscle have been detached and there is limited subglandular dissection to about the lower level of areola. About 1/3 of the implant is subglandular and 2/3 subpectoral. (**d**) Type III dissection: The fibers of origin of pectoralis major muscle have been detached from the ribs and there is extensive subglandular dissection to about the upper level of areola. About the lower half of the implant is subglandular and upper half subpectoral

20.6 Operative Technique: Moderate Ptosis

In women with moderate ptosis, nipple is located either at, slightly above, or below the IMF, with the lowest contour of breast (breast nadir) situated between 1 and 3 cm below the IMF (Table 20.2, Fig. 20.8). In these situations, the nipple to IMF distance typically measures more than 6 cm in most patients. In Type II dual plane dissection, the fibers of origin of the pectoralis major muscle are divided along the IMF to the medial aspect of the IMF, with no parasternal division of the muscular fibers. In addition, the retromammary plane is also dissected free from the pectoralis muscle to approximately 2–6 cm above the IMF or to about the inferior border of the areola as estimated in supine position. In type III dissection, the retromammary plane is dissected free from the pectoralis muscle from

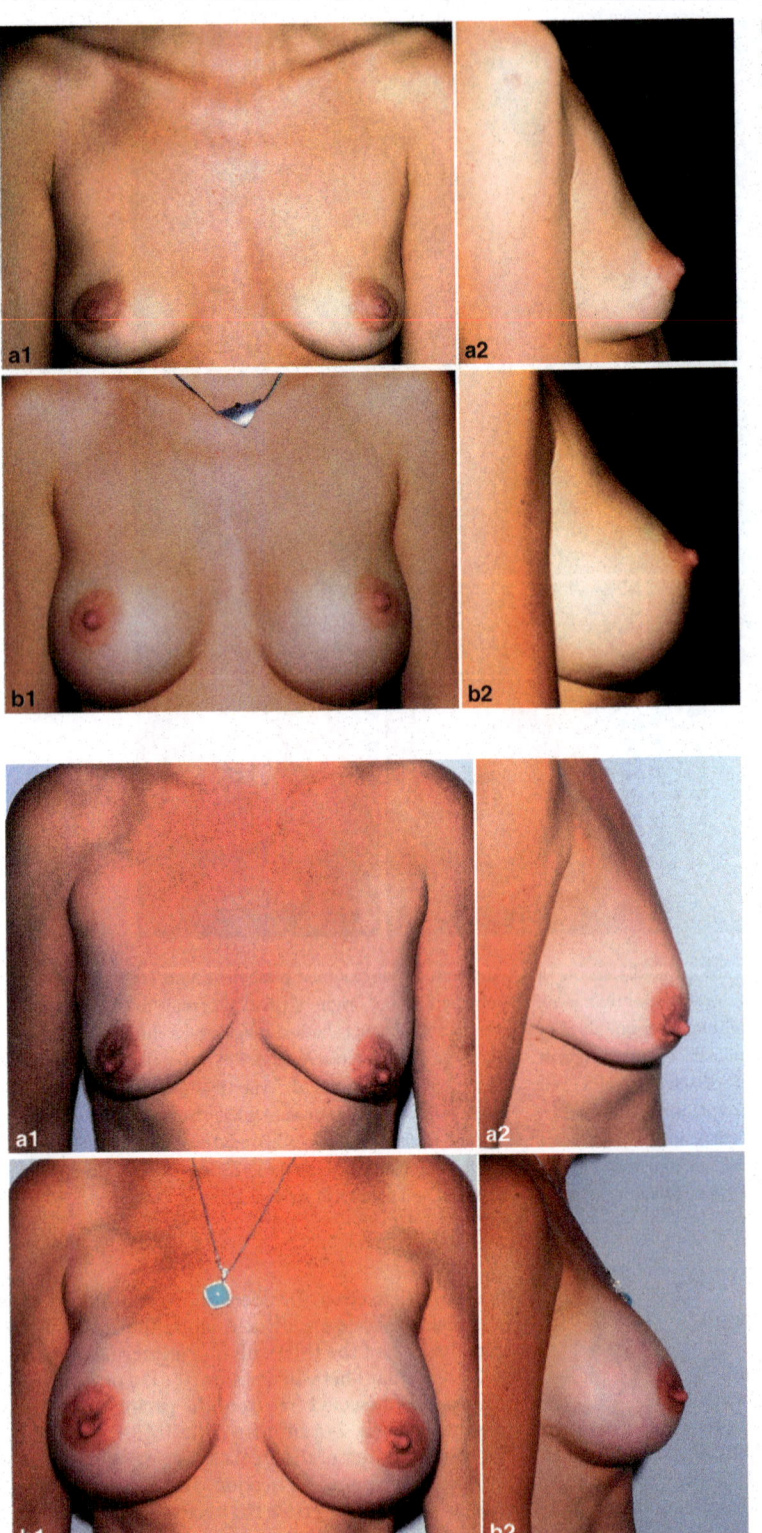

Fig. 20.11 (**a***1,2*) Patient with mild ptosis with the breast nadir 1 cm below the IMF. (**b***1,2*) Postoperative after Type I dissection through areolar incision

Fig. 20.12 (**a***1,2*) Patient with mild ptosis with breast nadir 1 cm below the IMF. (**b***1,2*) Postoperative after Type II dissection through areolar incision

6 to 12 cm above the IMF or to about the superior border of the areola. The parasternal muscle fibers may be partially divided in their most lateral portion, maintaining their most medial attachments intact only if deemed necessary for reduction of space between the breasts. Otherwise they are left undisturbed. Full division of the pectoralis muscle fibers at the parasternal level must be avoided, as it may result in the formation of a visible horizontal traction band across the breast, which is most visible during muscle contraction ptosis (Fig. 20.13).

During instances when one suspects preoperatively that Type III dual plane dissection may be insufficient in correcting the patient's moderate ptosis, implants are inserted at the completion of the dual plane dissection and patient is examined in a sitting position. If there still remains residual ptosis, the next step would consist in circumareolar removal of the excess skin. If this proves insufficient, any remaining skin excess is removed through a vertical approach.

20.7
Operative Technique: Severe Ptosis

In severe ptosis, the lowest contour of breast (breast nadir) is >3 cm below the IMF and/or nipple is situated below the breast nadir (Table 20.2, Fig. 20.8). When good tissue support and good skin elasticity are present and ptosis is not significant, with the breast nadir located at about 3–6 cm below the IMF, Type III dissection and circumareolar mastopexy often corrects the condition (Fig. 20.14). Once implants are inserted and patient is placed in a sitting position, breasts are examined for any residual ptosis, and if necessary, more skin is removed through vertical incisions (Fig. 20.15). In cases of more advanced ptosis (breast nadir at more than 6 cm below the IMF), particularly, when combined with poor soft tissue support, one may consider further skin excision from within the IMF, resulting in an anchor-shaped scar. In such situations, the horizontal limb is not added until the implant has been inserted and the patient has been

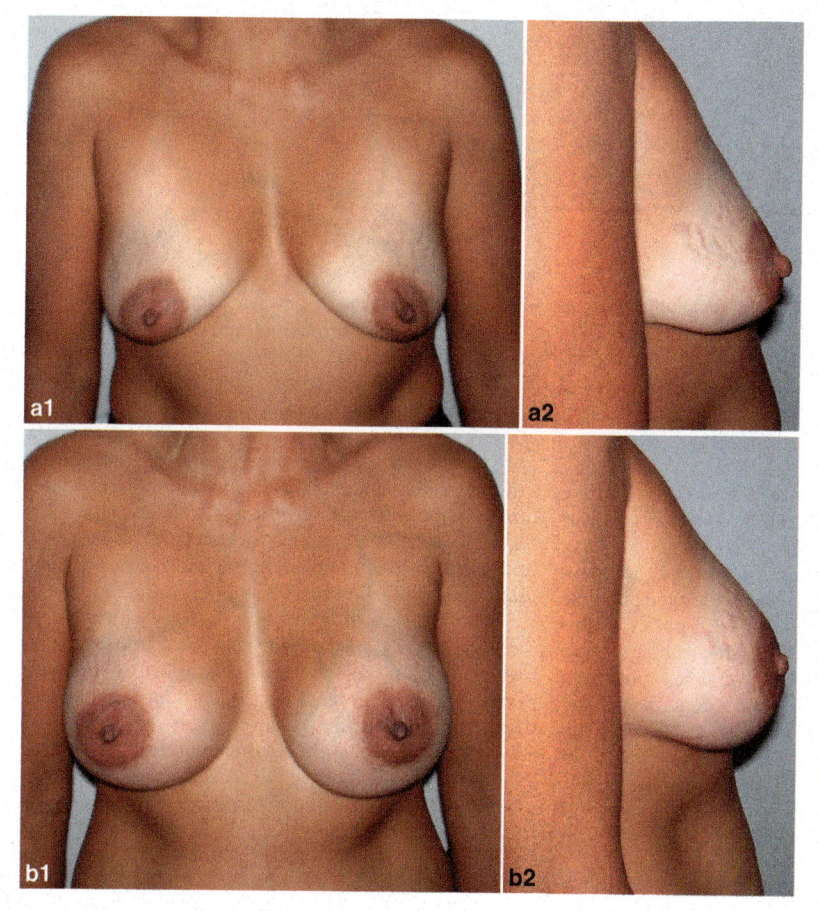

Fig. 20.13 (a1,2) Patient with moderate ptosis. (b1,2) Postoperative after Type II dissection through areolar incision

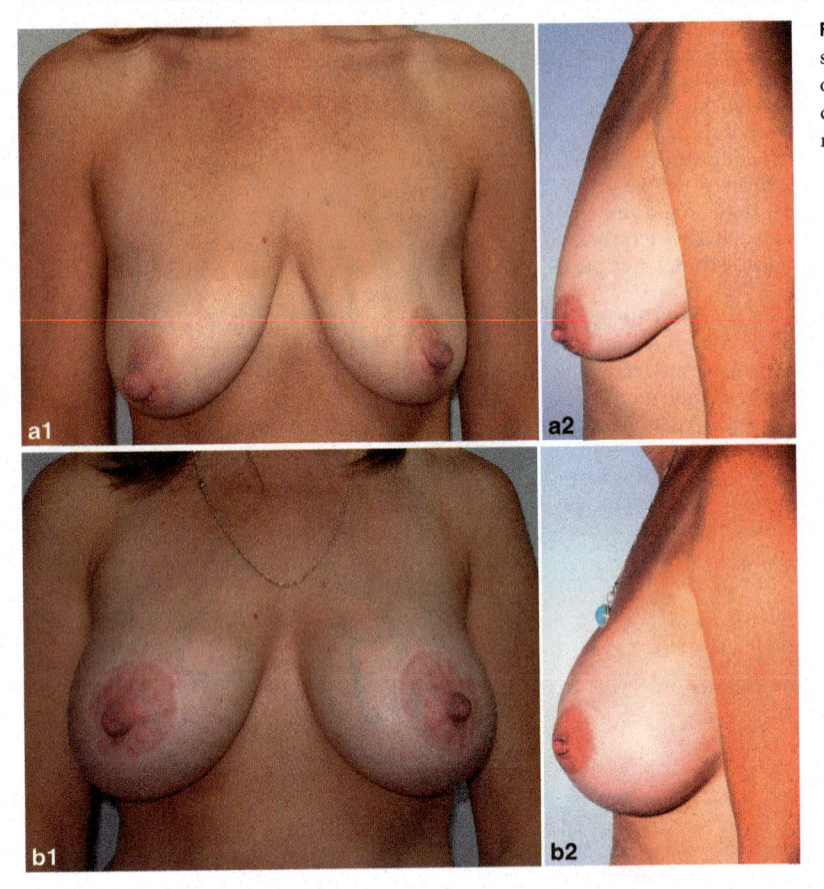

Fig. 20.14 (*a1,2*) Patient with severe ptosis. (*b1,2*) Postoperative after Type III dissection and circumareolar mastopexy

20.8 Complications

placed in a sitting position and any residual ptosis has been properly assessed.

Capsular contracture is the most common complication after implant insertion and there is no evidence that combined mastopexy/augmentation increases the risk. Main measures to optimize healing and therefore minimize capsular contracture include adherence to rigid principles of gentle tissue handling, with minimal use of electrocautery, and the use of no-touch sterile technique when manipulating the implants. Close drainage postoperatively also minimizes fluid collection around the implants and therefore reduces risks of infection and capsular contracture. The use of sleeves in order to avoid implant contact with skin is also a good measure during implant insertion. An extensive meta-analysis has shown that textured implants inserted under muscle also significantly reduce the incidence of capsular contracture [1, 2]. The authors' experience with subpectoral insertion of implants parallels these findings.

Hypertrophic and keloid scars (Fig. 20.16) may be minimized by utilizing a two-stage technique, with mastopexy as the first stage followed by augmentation about 3–6 months later. In one-stage operations, the wounds must be closed under the least tension to prevent abnormal healing with pathologic scar formation. Taping the incisions with micropore paper tape (such as 3M) for 6 months is helpful in obtaining superior scars and there has been no keloid formation with this simple approach.

Wound dehiscence and skin necrosis with pending implant extrusion is rare but may occur under tension when the skin is closed, particularly in patients with poor soft tissue support (Fig. 20.17). Superficial wound separations secondary to skin necrosis respond well to local wound care with debridement and the use of topical antibiotics such as silver sulfadiazine. However, in cases of major wound dehiscence and in particular with exposed implant, explantation is warranted.

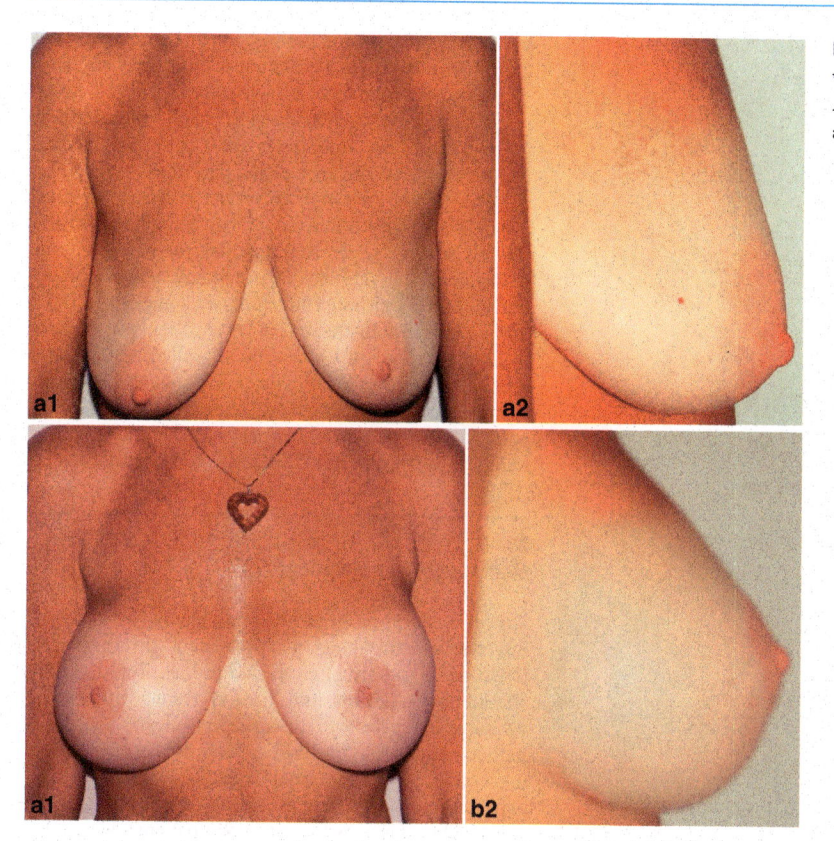

Fig. 20.15 (**a1,2**) Patient with severe ptosis. (**b1,2**) After Type III dissection and vertical mastopexy

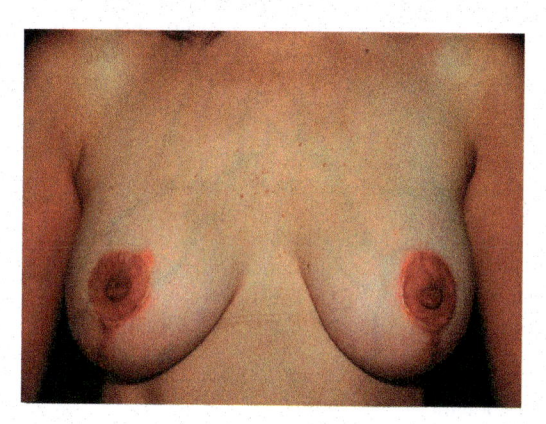

Fig. 20.16 Hypertrophic scars after vertical mastopexy/augmentation

Implant malposition, breast asymmetry, and breast deformities constitute the worst complications after mastopexy/augmentation procedures. Figure 20.18 shows such an extreme case of malposition not only of the implants but also of the nipples, as well as poor breast contour due to improper planning and execution of the operation. The hypertrophic scarring is likely due to skin approximation under excessive tension. Reportedly, this patient developed skin discoloration and eventual necrosis within a few days after surgery. This resulted in wound separation within a week. Wounds eventually healed by secondary intention and hypertrophic scar formation after 8 weeks of wound care. This patient did not develop implant infection or implant extrusion that commonly occurs after a major wound dehiscence. It is likely that proper planning with conservative skin excision could have avoided skin necrosis and wound dehiscence.

When there is doubt as to whether or not a patient may require mastopexy through external incisions, we recommend marking the breasts initially for augmentation and type II or type III dissection. The authors' preference is an inferior areolar incision. Only after implants have been inserted and patient has been placed in a sitting position, one may proceed to the next step that consists of circumareolar mastopexy if there is residual ptosis. Furthermore, if one plans a circumareolar mastopexy and one is in doubt as to whether or not vertical mastopexy may be required, on should proceed with Type III dissection and circumareolar mastopexy, and

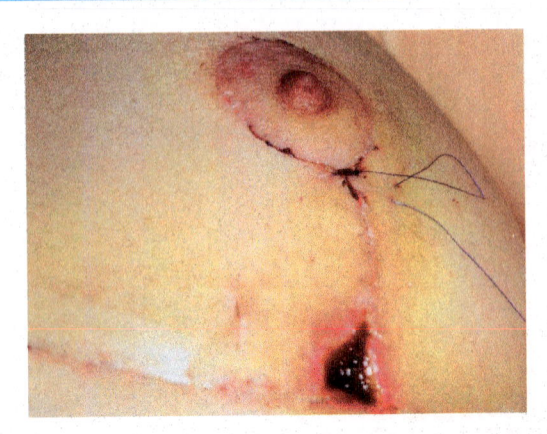

Fig. 20.17 Skin necrosis with limited wound separation but not implant exposure after Wise-pattern mastopexy/augmentation

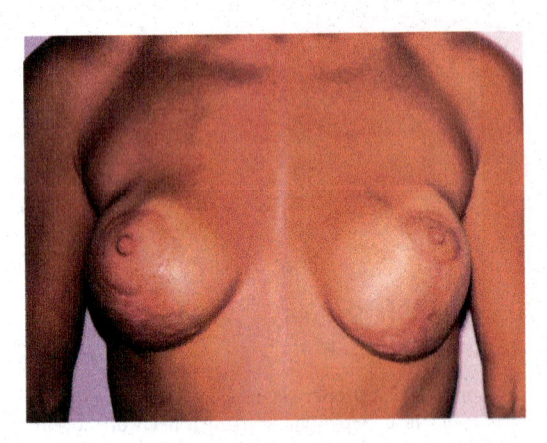

Fig. 20.18 An extreme case of malposition of not only the implants but also of the nipples as well as poor breast contour due to improper planning and execution of the operation. Note the hypertrophic scarring

only after implant insertion and placement of the patient in a sitting position, one may proceed with vertical mastopexy, if necessary. Similarly, when one is in doubt as to the necessity of Wise pattern skin excision, one should proceed with Type III dissection and vertical mastopexy, and only after implants have been inserted, one may plan further skin removal through the inframammary crease. We refer to this concept as "one step behind" approach.

20.9
Psychological Considerations

As in all aesthetic procedures, patients seeking mastopexy/augmentation have a higher likelihood of impaired body image than the general population. Miscommunication between the patient and her surgeon are frequent in situations when two operations such as mastopexy and augmentation are combined, and we recommend more than one preoperative visit in order to clarify all concerns. Many patients are ambivalent and not certain of their choices and need guidance before final decision is made.

Patients with moderate to severe ptosis who request "scarless" operations may be difficult to be satisfied, and it is advisable to see these individuals on more than one occasion or preferably refer them to colleagues for a second and third opinion. Unfortunately, some of the information that clutters the internet give patients false hopes of easy success and must be dispelled accordingly. Finally, we advise operating in two stages whenever circumareolar or more extensive external scars are anticipated. Mastopexies would be performed in the first stage followed by implant insertion some 3–6 months later.

20.10
Medicolegal Considerations

An increasing number of patients regularly search the internet before making an appointment with their plastic surgeon and are often misled in believing that they should obtain optimal and "natural" results without any visible scar. It behooves the surgeon to clearly explain to patients and document in her records the rational for placement of any external scars as well as realistic expectations and potential side effects and complications. When faced with unrealistic patients, we advise referring them to other surgeons for their opinion.

Some patients do not seem unrealistic but are most ambivalent as to their own wishes. This is particularly the case when a patient seeks mastopexy but is unsure about breast augmentation. To minimize misunderstandings in such situations, we recommend the routine use of paper tape, a step we refer to as "paperpexy," to accomplish a temporary lift (Fig. 20.9–20.12).

With good communication between patient and surgeon and clear understanding of the location of the scars as well the possibility of pathologic cicatrix, combined mastopexy/augmentation remains one of the most rewarding operations with very high patient satisfaction.

References

1. Bartels RJ, Strickland DM, Douglas WM: A new mastopexy operation for mild or moderate breast ptosis. Plast Reconstr Surg 1976;57(6):687–691
2. Wise RJ: A preliminary report on a method of planning the mammaplasty. Plast Reconstr Surg 1956;17(5):367–375
3. Peled IJ, Zagher U, Wexler MR: Purse-string suture for reduction and closure of skin defects. Ann Plast Surg 1985;14(5):465–469

4. Benelli L: A new periareolar mammaplasty: the "round block" technique. Aesthetic Plast Surg 1990;14(2):93–100
5. Spear SL, Kassan M, Little JW: Guidelines in concentric mastopexy. Plast Reconstr Surg 1990;85(6):961–966
6. Lejour M, Abboud M: Vertical mammaplasty without inframammary scar and breast liposuction. Perspect Plast Surg 1990;4:67
7. Lassus C: Breast reduction: evolution of a technique – a single vertical scar. Aesthetic Plast Surg 1987;11(2):107–112
8. Tebbetts JB: Dual plane breast augmentation: optimizing implant-soft-tissue relationships in a wide range of breast types. Plast Reconstr Surg 2001;107(5):1255–1272
9. Parsa FD, Parsa AA: Breast ptosis: to augment, to lift, or to do both? Plast Reconstr Surg 2006;117(6):2101–2102
10. Elliott LF: Circumareolar mastopexy with augmentation. Clin Plast Surg 2002;29(3):337–347
11. Parsa FD, Brickman M, Parsa AA: Breast augmentation/mastopexy. Plast Reconstr Surg 2005;115(5):1428–1429
12. Barnsley GP, Sigurdson LJ, Barnsley SE: Textured surface breast implants in the prevention of capsular contracture among breast augmentation patients: a meta-analysis of randomized controlled trials. Plast Reconstr Surg 2006;117(7):2182–2190

Breast Augmentation and Mastopexy: How to Select and Perform the Techniques Minimizing Complications

Lázaro Cárdenas-Camarena

21.1 Introduction

The female breast forms one of the most attractive esthetic areas of the female anatomy. A beautiful breast is synonymous with sensuality. For that reason, there are multiple and varied surgical procedures for improving it [1–6]. Because of the mammary gland's own characteristics and the current tendency toward thin and stylized figures, the combination of hypoplasia and mammary ptosis is common in a single patient. This combination of alterations in the mammary gland is secondary primarily to pregnancies or significant variations in weight. Growth of the mammary gland during pregnancy and lactation stretches the breast's supporting tissues. This stretching results in a certain degree of damage to them, which causes the glands to lose support following pregnancy [7]. Adding to this factor, the weight loss that many patients experience, ptosis, and mammary hypoplasia are even greater. This alteration is also common in patients who, not being pregnant, have suffered significant changes in body weight. All of this causes the combination of ptosis and hypoplasia in a single patient to become more and more frequent.

In spite of it being a common combination of pathologies, the medical literature expounds very little on the subject, and scientific studies have only recently begun appearing more consistently [8, 9]. The relevant thing about the combination of these two procedures at the same surgical time is that opinions regarding the benefit or difficulty and incidence of complications are quite diverse. While some authors say that performing mastopexy and augmentation is a procedure that gives very good results, and that the incidence of complications is low [10–12], other studies state that it is a high-risk procedure with a greater number of complications than if the two surgeries were performed separately [8, 9, 13–15]. The authors who report a greater incidence of complications even warn that in some cases these complications can be severe and deforming [15]. Persoff reports that combining both procedures is difficult and entails many complications [14], while Spear emphasizes that it is a complicated procedure with unpredictable results [9, 15]. The author agrees with Spear [15] that the combination of mastopexy and mammary augmentation is not as simple a procedure as performing mammary augmentation or mastopexy separately. Placing the implant and performing the lifting entails many factors that should be taken into account and that do not appear in the separate procedures. All these factors have been amply commented on by Spear himself in his studies on the topic [8, 9, 15]. Therefore, when performing both procedures, the care and precautions taken to avoid complications should be fully exercised, one of them being the proper choice of the surgical technique to be employed. The authors who report good results with augmentation and mastopexy state that one of the most important points is proper selection of the surgical technique [10–13, 15, 16].

Although it is true that managing mammary hypoplasia or mammary ptosis individually is simpler than handling them together [15], our experience has demonstrated to us that by following certain premises, the procedure is feasible to perform with reduced number of complications [17]. The author recommend a methodology for selecting the best option from among the different surgical techniques for obtaining the best results and for maximum avoidance of complications.

21.2 Marking

To select the surgical procedure to be employed, it is of vital importance to do an examination and take detailed measurements of the breast to be treated. In this examination, we must determine the excess tissue both above and below the nipple–areolar complex (NAC), because this is going to be the main factor that decides the surgical technique. All patients are marked preoperatively in a sitting position. Four points or basic areas are delimited,

M.A. Shiffman (ed.), *Mastopexy and Breast Reduction: Principles and Practice*,
© Springer-Verlag Berlin Heidelberg 2009

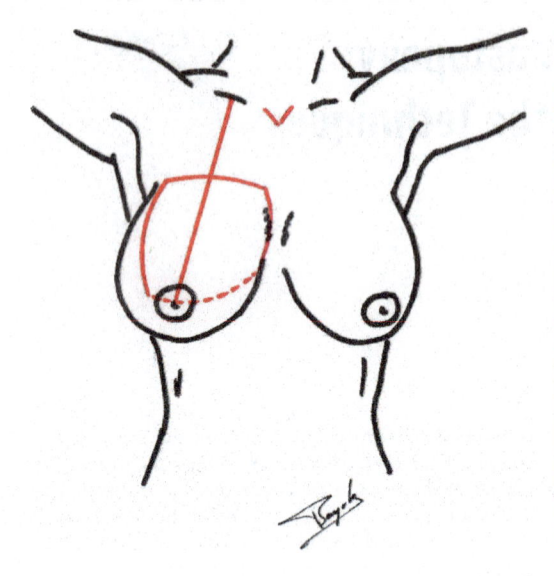

Fig. 21.1 Areas of the mammary gland that need to be delimited, which are necessary to design any of the surgical techniques

Table 21.1 Measurements, analyses, and characteristics of the mammary gland

Marking areas	Breast measurements	Variables or asymmetries
Inframammary crease	Distance from the suprasternal notch to the nipple	Shape
Midclavicular line	Distance from the nipple to the inframammary crease	Size
Suprasternal notch	Height of the mammary gland	Position of the inframammary crease
Mammary gland base	Width of the mammary gland	Degree of ptosis

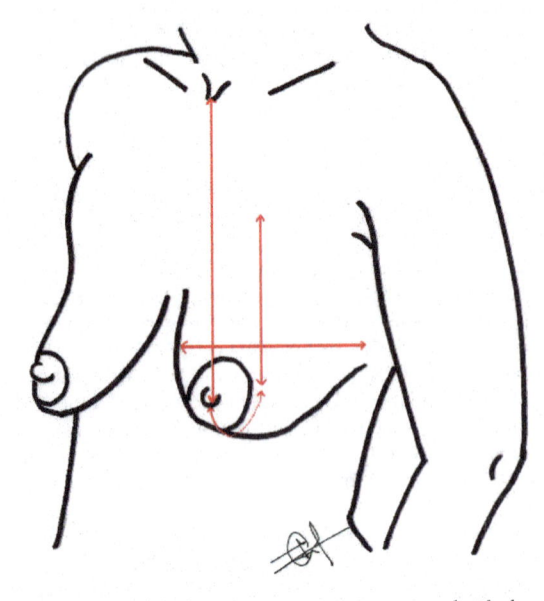

Fig. 21.2 Four breast's measurements are necessary to decide the surgical technique. (1) Distance from the suprasternal notch to the nipple, (2) distance from the nipple to the inframammary crease, (3) width of the breast base, (4) height of the breast base

which are necessary for using any of the surgical techniques: inframammary crease, midclavicular line, suprasternal notch, and base of the mammary gland in its normal position (Fig. 21.1). With these four points indicated, it is possible to take four measurements that are necessary to perform the surgical technique, as well as to decide which technique to use: the distance from the suprasternal notch to the nipple, the distance from the nipple to the inframammary crease, the width of the breast base, and the height of the breast base (Fig. 21.2). Characteristics of the mammary glands, such as shape, asymmetry in the crease's location, asymmetry in the size and degree of the ptosis, are all evaluated and recorded. These measurements, points, and characteristics of the breast are shown in Table 21.1. The new location of the NAC is indicated on the midclavicular line, taking into account the average normal distance from the suprasternal notch and the forward projection of the mammary crease, as described by Pitanguy (Fig. 21.3) [3, 4].

21.3
Selection of the Surgical Technique

With these points and areas marked and the measurements taken, the surgical procedure to be employed is then selected, depending basically on the distance from the NAC to the inframammary crease (the amount of excess tissue in the inferior pole) and the distance to which the NAC needs to be lifted. These two variables will be the determining points for selecting the surgical procedure.

Trying to lift an NAC in a periareolar fashion with ptosis greater than 5 cm will generally produce a long-term, inadequate aesthetic result and a greater incidence of short-term complications because of the closure with tension that would be produced [10–12, 16]. For that reason, the selection of the surgical technique when performing mastopexy with augmentation is the single most important factor for obtaining good mid- and long-term aesthetic results and for minimizing short-term

21.3 Selection of the Surgical Technique

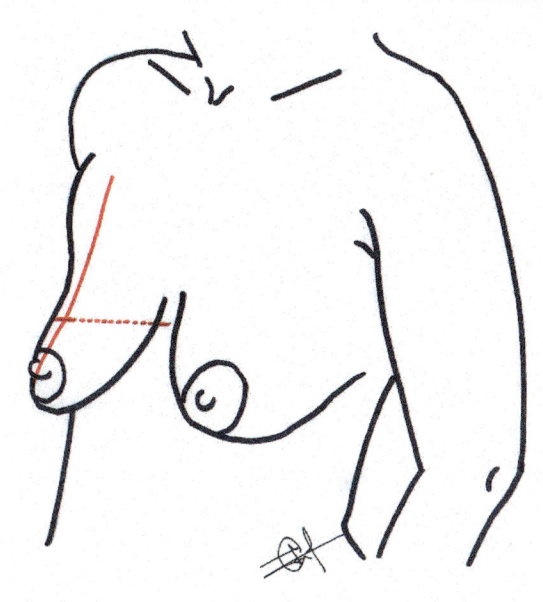

Fig. 21.3 New location of the nipple–areola complex (NAC) indicated on the midclavicular line

complications. Likewise, the type of pexy to be performed involves certain criteria that we should follow in order to achieve the desired result. A pexy where only lifting the NAC is going to be done has a different approach than a periareolar pexy or an inverted T pexy. Each of the approaches has its own indications and reasons. Likewise, a ptotic breast with an inferior pole deficit, and which only needs elevation of the NAC, almost invariably will require an anatomical implant with downward displacement of the inframammary crease to compensate for this problem. Therefore, the selection of the surgical technique implicitly involves specific steps to be taken. This is important because choosing a proper surgical technique, besides providing aesthetic improvement, greatly minimizes complications.

With all the marks done, it is possible to decide the surgical technique to be utilized. The amount of NAC ptosis will tell us how far it must migrate, and the distance from the NAC to the inframammary crease will tell us how much tissue should be managed in the inferior portion. These determinations will tell us the technique to be used and will be an orienting factor when the technique is employed. If there is little ptosis of the NAC (less than 3 cm), and the distance from the NAC to the inframammary fold is short (less than 5 cm), the surgical procedure to be performed is only an upward migration of the NAC. If there is a significant excess of tissue in the inferior portion of the breast (more than 5 cm from the NAC to the inframammary crease), it indicates that the excess produced by the ptosis must be managed; therefore, the isolated upward displacement of the NAC is totally inadequate. In these cases, one must choose between a periareolar technique or an inverted T technique. The choice of either of these two techniques will depend on the distance between the NAC and the inframammary crease and on the existing ptosis. If there is significant ptosis (more than 4–5 cm), the excess from the inferior portion of the NAC to the inframammary crease will also be large (more than 7 cm), and therefore, the technique will be the one that significantly corrects the mammary tissue in the superior mammary pole, as well as in the inferior. The choice in these cases will indisputably be an inverted T technique. The author prefers to use the inverted T technique instead of the vertical technique for two reasons. The first is that we obtain a more aesthetic result compensating for the excess skin laterally in the inframammary crease. The second reason is that if the necessary compensation were only vertical, the correction of that breast would be achieved with a periareolar technique instead of a vertical one. Therefore, the periareolar technique is the proper one for small ptosis (less than 3 cm), which entails little excess sub-mammary tissue (the distance from the NAC to the inframammary crease being between 5 and 7 cm), leaving the upper migration of the NAC only in cases in which the distance to migrate is minimal (less than 3 cm), and which at the same time involves a very short distance to the inframammary crease, which will have to be increased with the corresponding inferior dissection, so that the implant will remain in a lower position. All these indications are described on Table 21.2.

Table 21.2 Determination of the surgical technique to be used

Distance from the NAC to the inframammary crease	NAC ptosis	General mammary gland characteristics	Surgical technique to be used
Less than 5 cm	Less than 2–3 cm	Low position of the NAC but with no skin excess at the inferior pole of the breast	Upward displacement of the NAC
Greater than 5 cm	Less than 3 cm	Little excess skin above and below the NAC	Periareolar pexy
Greater than 5 cm	Greater than 3 cm	Much excess skin both above and below the NAC	Inverted T pexy

21.4
Surgical Technique

Surgery is performed after sedation and local anesthesia. The anesthetic solution to be infiltrated is prepared using 250 ml of 0.9% saline solution, 100 ml of 1% lidocaine, and 1 ml of adrenaline 1:100,000. Depending on the breast size, between 125 and 150 ml of the prepared solution is infiltrated into each breast. The intercostal nerves are blocked with the same solution. Two reference sutures are placed, which will be used to confirm the location of the NAC and its symmetry. These sutures are placed in the suprasternal notch and the xyphoid process of the sternum. Most patients are ambulatory, leaving the hospital within 12 h after surgery.

21.5
Lifting the Nipple–Areola Complex

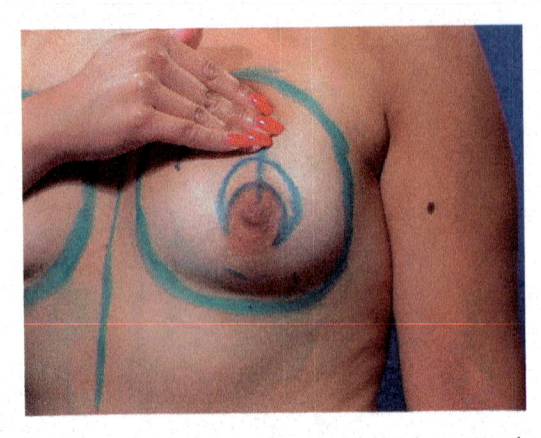

Fig. 21.4 Patient who needs minimal lifting of the NAC, with deficit of mammary tissue in the inferior pole of the breast requiring reposition of the inframammary crease. In these cases, the ideal implant is anatomical shape

The first point for any of the surgical techniques is the circumferential cut of the desired size around the NAC. The usual measurement is 4.2 cm. The implant is placed through a supra-areolar incision, with transglandular dissection extending to the pectoral fascia. The supra-areolar approach is preferred because the NAC is going to be moved upward, and there is often no need to make an infra-areolar cut. Another reason for preferring this approach is that it provides greater covering of the implant, as in most of these cases, the inferior pole of the breast is hypotrophic with minimal glandular tissue. On reaching the pectoral fascia, dissection continues toward the inframammary crease on a subglandular plane. This dissection should reach the edge of the inframammary crease that has been marked preoperatively. A large majority of patients who require minimum upward displacement of the NAC need a repositioning of the inframammary crease, as the original distance is very short, exhibiting a high crease (Fig. 21.4). In these cases, there is a deficit of mammary tissue in the inferior pole of the breast, which must be compensated by the implant. When this deficit exists, the ideal implant is of anatomical shape, whose characteristics compensate for this problem very satisfactorily. Subglandular dissection ends at the inframammary crease. Most of the author's cases involve dual plane implant placement, as described by Tebbets [18]. Therefore, at the inframammary crease level, the major pectoral muscle is incised and separated from its costal insertion. This disinsertion also takes place in its inferomedial portion at the sternum level. The disinsertion should not go beyond the inferior portion of the major pectoral muscle; otherwise, there is the risk of a significant upward displacement of the muscle, with the consequent deterioration of the aesthetic result. This is because the disinserted pectoral muscle, being very high, produces a constrictive band that squeezes the implant in half, creating the unaesthetic appearance of a gland cut in half. The submuscular dissection will include sufficient space for the size of the implant that is to be placed. The only instance the implant is preferred to be placed into a totally subglandular plane instead of a dual plane as described by Tebbets is when it is necessary to cut the mammary gland at its base to permit amplification, as in the case of tuberous breasts (Fig. 21.5). In all other patients, dual plane placement is used in which approximately 30% of the implant – the inferior part – remains subglandular and the rest is in a submuscular plane. A counter-opening drain is placed laterally, which is removed within 24–48 h postoperatively, depending on bleeding. The supra-areolar approach for implant placing is closed in planes, using Monocryl 2-0, without suturing the muscular plane. Closure of the planes should reach the dermis to allow correct design of the pexy. Having placed the implant, the cutaneous resection is designed. It is of primary importance to rely on the preoperative markings, principally for the new location of the center of the NAC. This new NAC location is confirmed, in case of doubt, by placing the patient in a semi-seated position. To achieve symmetry in the location of both NACs, the two sutures that were placed in the supraclavicular notch and the xyphoid process at the start of surgery are used (Fig. 21.6). These two sutures will form a medial-based triangle that will extend from one breast to the other, verifying the position of the new NAC

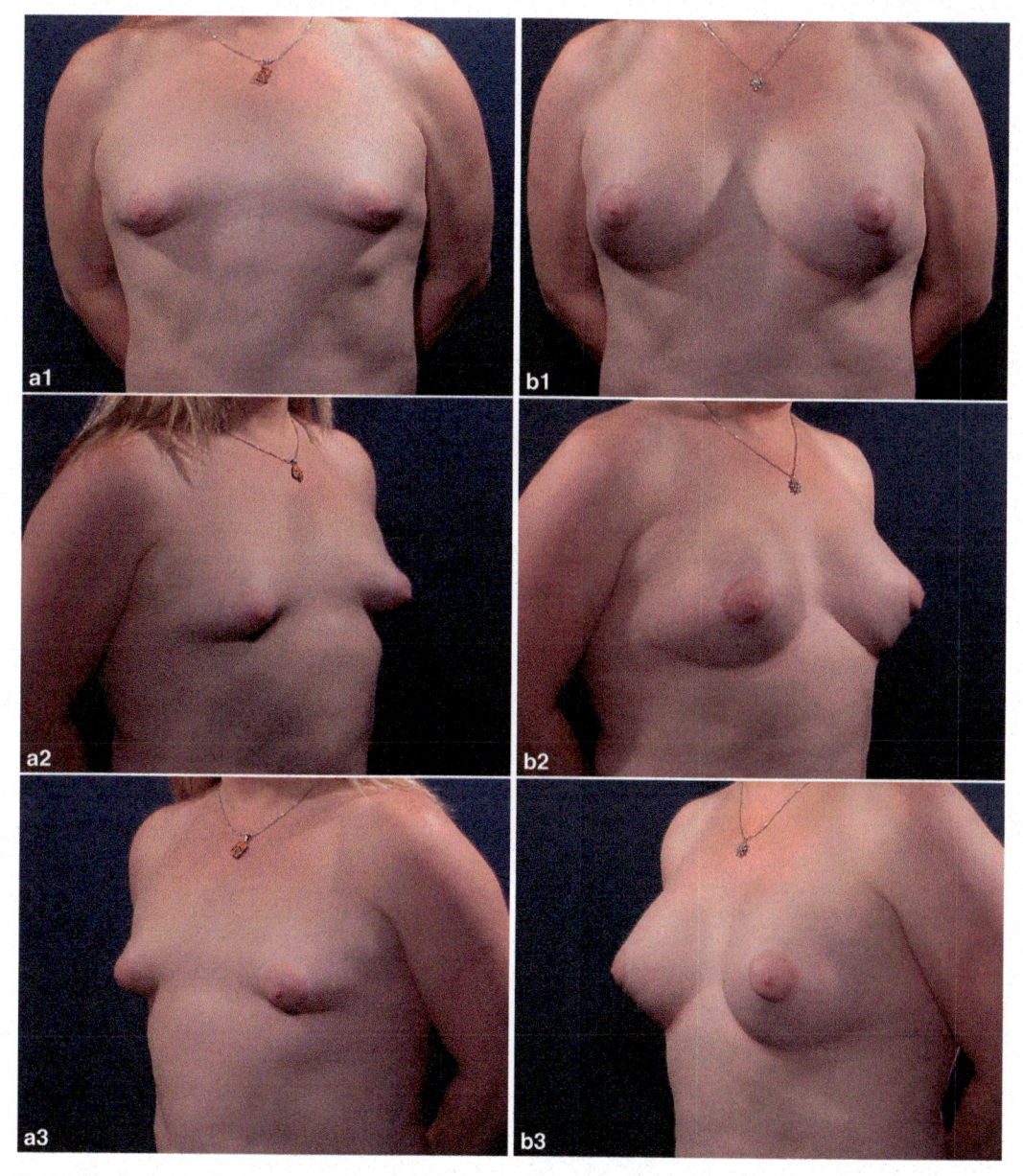

Fig. 21.5 (**a***1-3*) Patient with tuberous breasts. (**b***1-3*) Two years after lifting of the NAC, reposition of the inframammary crease, and subglandular 450 ml anatomical implants (Inamed Breast Implants, McGhan 410 FF Model)

design. Once the central position of the new NAC is confirmed, a half-moon is delimited, which includes, as an upper limit, the highest part of the new NAC, and as a lower limit, the previously delimited areola, removing all excess skin from the areola. In special cases where the NAC is not going to be reduced in size to the 4.2 cm indicated previously, the half-moon's inferior edge will include the inferior edge of the areola

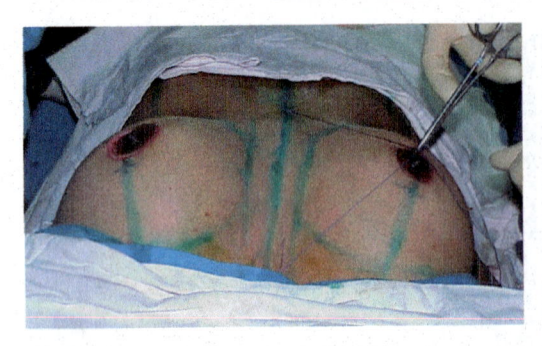

Fig. 21.6 NAC's position verification using two sutures, placed in the supraclavicular notch and the xyphoid process

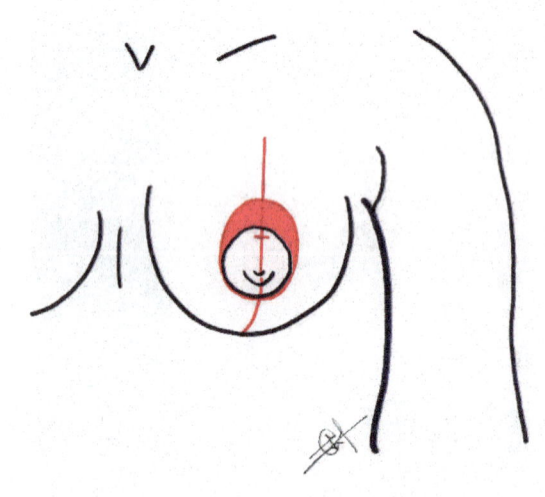

Fig. 21.7 When the NAC's lifting can produce some distortion of the NAC or widening of the scar, the author prefers to use a complete incision all around the NAC instead of only the upper half moon

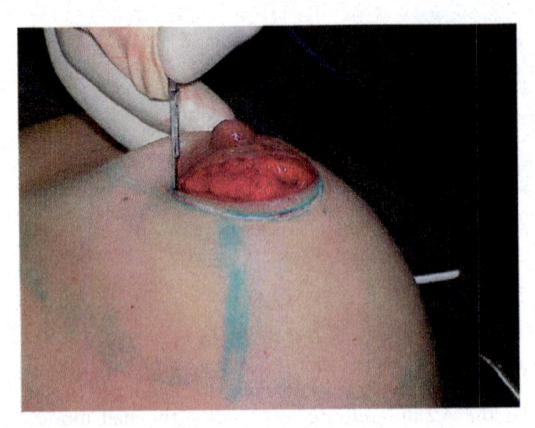

Fig. 21.8 In cases of minimal NAC lift, the upper half moon resection is the best choice

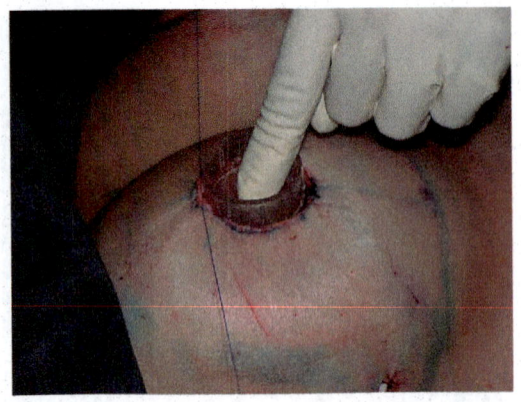

Fig. 21.9 Benelli's round block procedure to prevent NAC and scar widening

(Fig. 21.7). The design and position of the half-moons designed on the submammary glands are again verified by the sutures. The area within the half-moon is excised (Fig. 21.8). On the one hand, if the larger portion of the half-moon, which corresponds to the superior portion, does not exceed 1.5 cm, and if the skin was not removed from the inferior portion, closure will be done directly with interrupted subdermal Monocryl 3-0 sutures, and the skin will be closed with continuous intradermal Monocryl 3-0 sutures. On the other hand, if the amount of skin in the half-moon is greater than 1.5 cm, or skin from the inferior portion was resected to reduce the size of the areola, closing should be done using a round block Prolene 3-0 suture, as described by Benelli (Fig. 21.9) [19]. This closing prevents scars widening the new NAC with the passage of time, which happened to the author in the first patients operated on with this procedure. Closure limits in round block are realized by using the 3.8 cm areola marker in order to place the previously cut 4.2 cm NAC. This is another action that helps avoid tension and helps prevent the NAC from increasing in diameter over the long term. Having placed the round block periareolar suture, the NAC is distributed with interrupted Monocryl 3-0 sutures, and closing is done with continuous intradermal Monocryl 3-0 sutures. In every case, when the implant has been placed in a dual plane, a supramammary compress dressing is applied to avoid implant displacement in the immediate postoperative period due to muscular contracture produced by surgical manipulation. Postoperative therapeutic ultrasound is recommended every third day following the fourth postoperative day, for approximately three weeks, to improve postoperative evolution (Fig. 21.10) [20].

21.5 Lifting the Nipple–Areola Complex

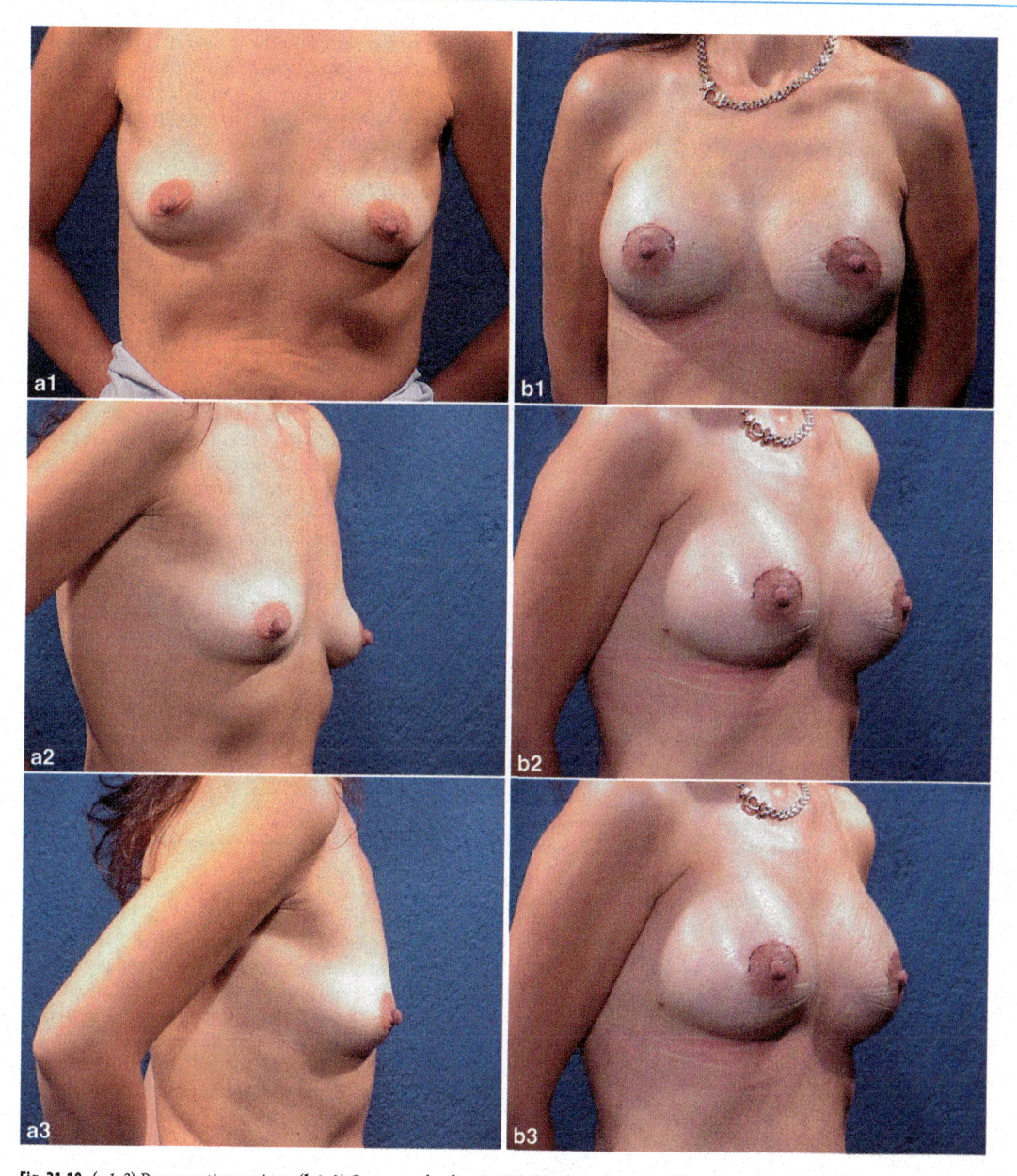

Fig. 21.10 (*a1-3*) Preoperative patient. (**b***1-3*) One month after NAC lift with an upper half moon incision. Anatomical implants 320 and 280 ml were used on the right and left breast, respectively, to correct asymmetry

21.6 Periareolar Pexy

The beginning of the technique is similar to the one explained in lifting the NAC, except that here an infra-areolar approach is preferred. That way, superior vascularity of the NAC is maintained and the amount of mammary tissue in the inferior pole is sufficient to cover the implant. Design of the areola, dissection, placement plane of the implant, and closing by planes are those described in the technique for lifting the NAC. Once the implant is placed, the cutaneous resection is designed to perform the periareolar pexy. The superior and inferior edges must be marked, which will form the resection of the skin, and the design of the periareolar circumference is made over these marks. These two points will be placed over the midclavicular line that was indicated preoperatively. To mark the superior edge of the circumference, the center of the new NAC location that was indicated preoperatively is used. The superior edge will be marked 3 cm above this point. This 3 cm corresponds to the 2 cm that form the radius of the new areola, plus one additional centimeter to compensate for downward skin displacement when the periareolar design is closed. To mark the inferior edge of the circumference, the location of the inframammary crease is taken as a reference. In these cases, the inframammary crease does not need to be displaced, since what indicates the use of this surgical technique is precisely a distance greater than 5 cm. Depending on the implant size, the distance from the inframammary crease to the inferior edge of the circumference will be 5–7 cm (Fig. 21.11). The larger the breast size, the greater the distance will be. In most cases, the distance is 6 cm. Once the superior and inferior points are delimited, the periareolar circle is drawn, making it as symmetrical as possible. The skin between the areola mark and the circumference is then deepithelialized (Fig. 21.12). When the author began, dermal detachment completely around the circumference was performed but is no longer used. This decreases the devascularization of the NAC, and at the same time prevents the cutaneous defect from worsening. Periareolar closing is done using Benelli's round block technique [19], similar to the technique for lifting the NAC (Fig. 21.13).

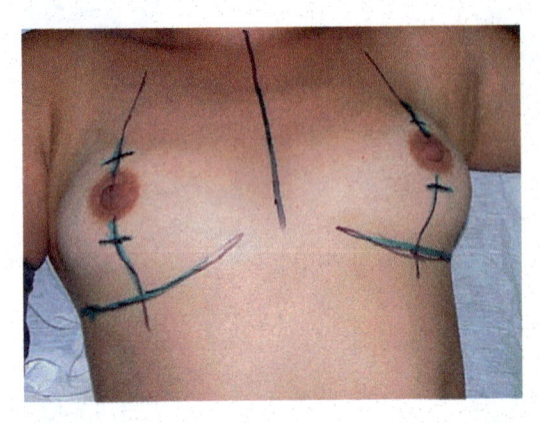

Fig. 21.11 Determination of the marks necessary to design the periareolar pexy. The superior edge of the circumference will be marked 3 cm above the center of the new NAC location. The inferior edge will be marked 5–7 cm above the inframammary crease. This distance can vary depending on the implant size

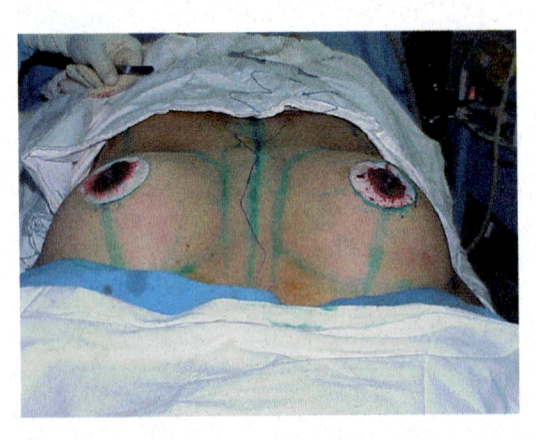

Fig. 21.12 The skin between the areola mark and the circumference is then deepithelialized to permit the closure

21.7 Inverted T Pexy

When the surgical indication is an inverted T technique, the procedure manipulations are substantially modified. In these cases, implant placement is through the inframammary crease. Using this approach, the retropectoral space is reached, and dissection of the major pectoral muscle is similar to that used in lifting the NAC. With the implant and drain placed, closing follows, using Monocryl 2-0 and 3-0, without closing the skin. Pexy design entails specific steps for achieving the desired surgical result. The first step consists of choosing a point on the midclavicular line at 8 cm below the center of the new NAC that was preoperatively marked. This 8 cm corresponds to 2 cm of radius of the new areola plus 6 cm from the edge of the new NAC to the inframammary crease. Pinching is done at this level to determine precisely how much skin is to be resected (Fig. 21.14). The pinched amount can vary from 4 to 12 cm, depending on the excess skin in the inferior pole of the breast and the amount of tissue to be resected. This amount will constitute the bases of two triangles

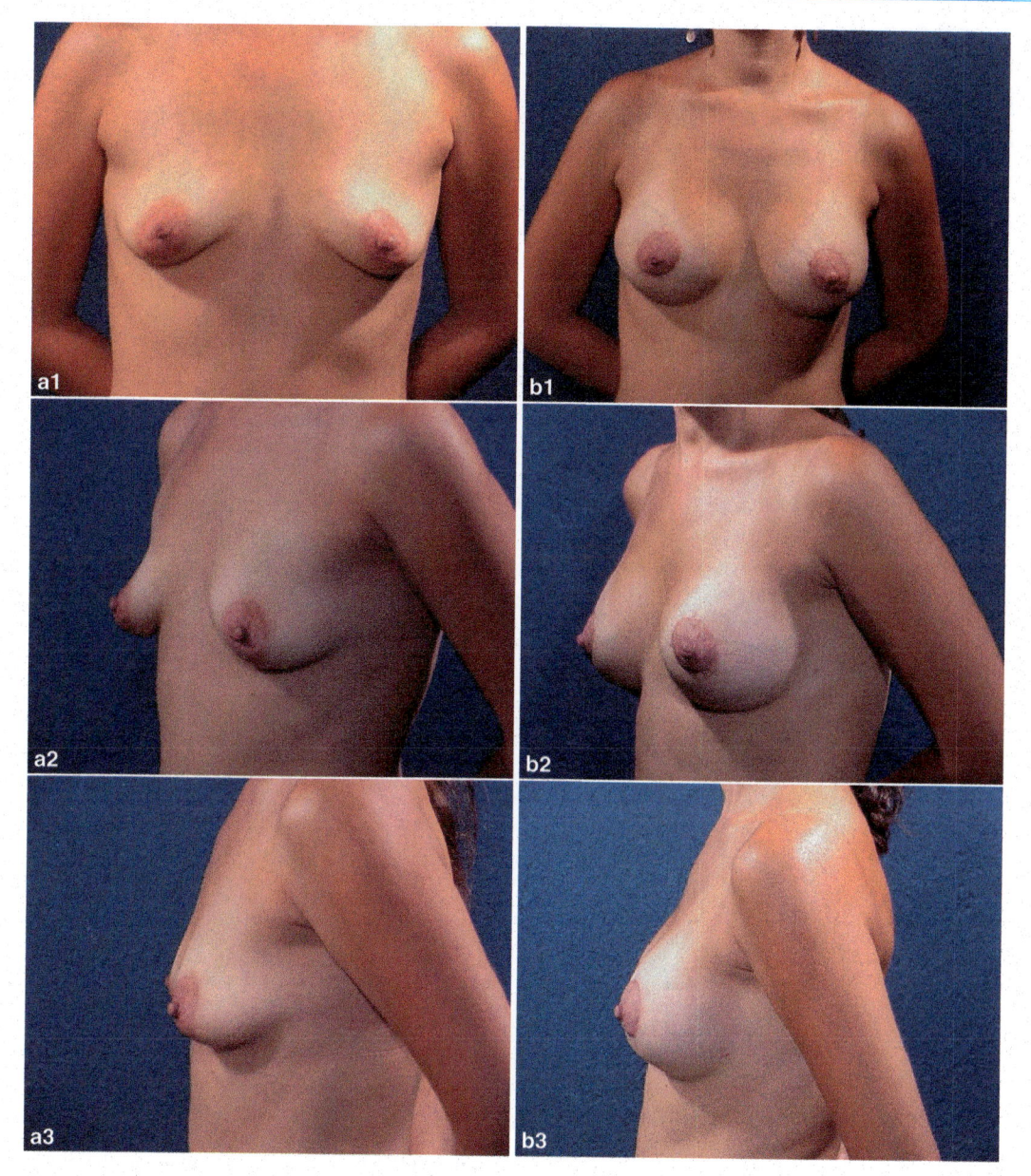

Fig. 21.13 (*a1-3*) Preoperative patient. (*b1-3*) One year after periareolar pexy. Round implants 330 cc implants were used

that will form a rhomboid in the design of the skin to be resected, where the vertex of each triangle will correspond to the new NAC and the inframammary crease. After delimiting this area and indicating the diameter of the new areola, tissue within the rhomboid is resected (Fig. 21.15). Half of the upper triangle is exclusively deepithelialized, while in the rest of the triangles subcutaneous cellular tissue is removed as far as the preglandular fascia. This tissue is removed to permit closing with less tension, eliminating tissue from the inferior pole of the breast, thus decreasing the risk of short-term pseudoptosis and forming two pillars that permit us to

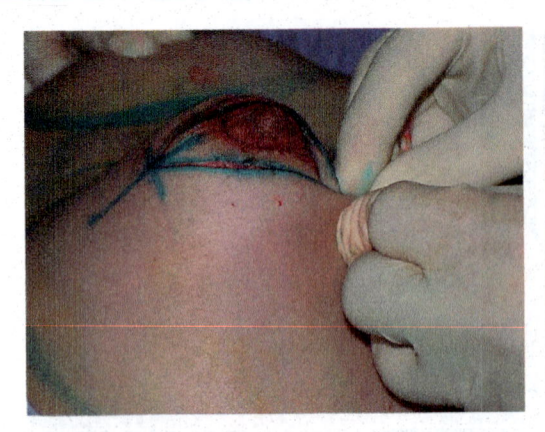

Fig. 21.14 It is necessary after implant placement to use the pinch test to determine precisely how much skin needs to be eliminated

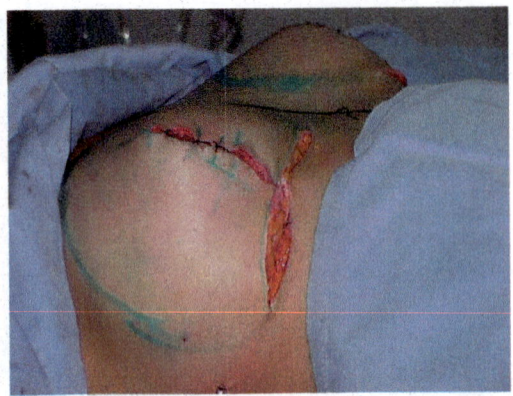

Fig. 21.16 The upper portion of the areola is then overlapped with temporary cutaneous external stitches and the rest of the breast is closed

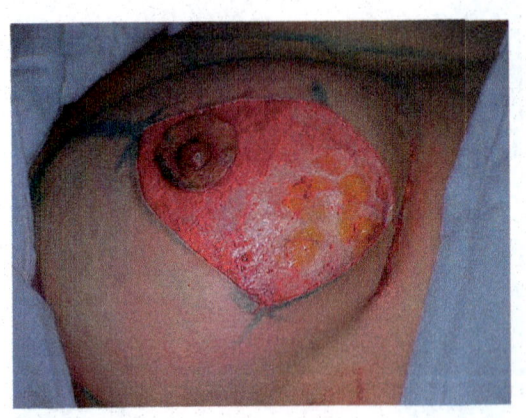

Fig. 21.15 With the pinch test done, a rhomboid can be formed and tissue within the rhomboid is resected

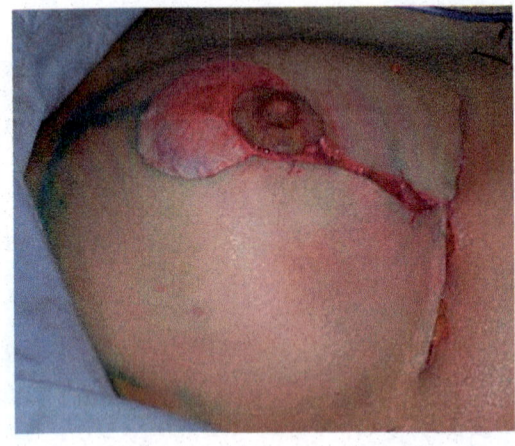

Fig. 21.17 The overlap stitches are removed from the areola to free it, the skin is deepithelialized, and the NAC is moved upward

perform the mastopexy and closure. With the tissue removed, the pillars of the inferior portion of the areola are closed, using Monocryl 2-0 and 3-0. This closure extends only up to the 8 cm that correspond to the upper triangle, since the lower triangle corresponds to tissue that will be resected when the pexy is completed. The upper portion of the areola is then overlapped, with the temporary cutaneous external stitches following the lines of the upper triangle. The inferior closing stitch that corresponds to the 8 cm from the center of the new NAC is carried to the inframammary crease, thereby producing two excess amounts of tissue toward either side, which will be horizontally resected along the line of the inframammary crease (Fig. 21.16). Removal of this tissue will give form to the new breast. With the new breast formed, the same procedures are performed on the contralateral breast, so that the two will be in harmony. The next step consists of using the areola marker to draw the new location of the NAC, which is done on the point marked preoperatively, and symmetry is confirmed with the reference sutures that were placed at the beginning of the surgery. If necessary, to confirm the position and symmetry, the patient is placed in a semi-seated position. The cutaneous resection is marked with a 3.8 cm diameter and the skin is deepithelialized. The overlap stitches are removed from the areola to free it and move it upward (Fig. 21.17). This is not usually a major problem if the dermis is cut in the lateral portions to the midpoint of the circumference of the new NAC, and the inferior portion of the areola is somewhat freed. Once it is moved upward, the areola, as well as the horizontal and vertical incisions, is closed by planes. The areola is distributed with interrupted Monocryl 3-0 stitches and closure with continuous intradermal suturing using Monocryl 3-0. In these cases, in addition to leaving a drain in the subpectoral plane at implant level, another one is left in the subcutaneous plane at the level of the inframammary crease (Fig. 21.18).

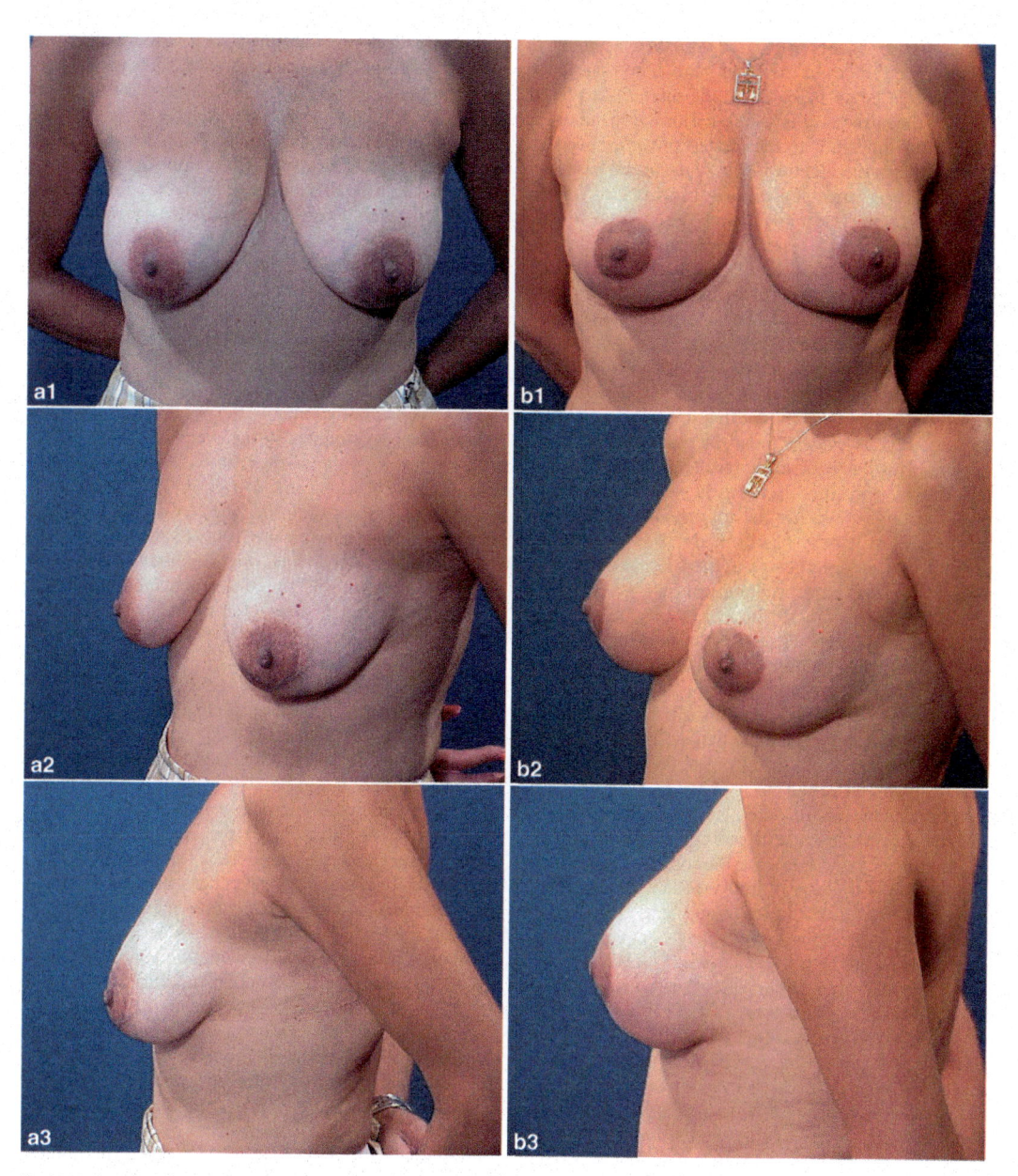

Fig. 21.18 (**a***1-3*) Preoperative. (**b***1-3*) Six months after "T" inverted pexy and 230 ml round implants

21.8
Important Considerations

The most important thing to point out is that proper performance of the technique is one of the most significant factors in avoiding early complications or undesirable results over the long term. In cases where the NAC is only going to migrate upward or a periareolar technique is going to be employed, implant placement is through the areola. On the other hand, if an inverted T technique is going to be used, the implant is placed through the inframammary crease. This is done in order to leave the implant with the greatest possible covering. Marking the width and the height of the breast base is of primary importance for placing the implant in the proper position. The implant should be placed in that location, except in the cases in which the inframammary crease has had to be displaced downward, as it happened in patients in whom the distance from the NAC to the original inframammary crease is very short. In all patients, the dual implant placement plane is preferred, as described by Tebbetts [18], except in tuberous breasts, where placement is sub-glandular.

It is important to point out that it is not advisable to try to correct an evident ptosis by placing a very large implant. This behavior often results in an undesirable breast size, and the problem is seldom corrected. Likewise, one should not fall into the error of having planned a breast pexy based on the examination and preoperative measurements and then decide not to do it after placing the implant. Frequently, after placing the implant and observing the patient in a supine position, the problem gives the false impression of having been corrected. This is because the volume of the implant projects the breast out at its inferior pole and at the same time lifts the gland, the NAC thus appearing more elevated. However, by placing the patient in a sitting position, the mammary tissue in front of the implant shows the ptosis just as it had been observed preoperatively. Not taking into account the details pointed out above will cause a very unaesthetic postoperative deformity of the mammary gland known as "Snoopy Deformity."

Selection of the type of implant to be used is of primary importance to the technique. It is obvious that financial considerations oblige many of our patients to choose round implants over anatomical ones, even when the latter are ideal in certain cases. Anatomical implants have two primary characteristics that should be considered in this type of surgical combination. First, they offer greater volume in the inferior portion, which addresses one of the basic deficiencies in many of these patients. Such is the case of patients who have a very high inframammary crease, or in other words, a very short distance between the NAC and the crease. These patients are undoubtedly going to require a downward migration of the crease and therefore, a greater compensatory filling of that area. This compensation is achieved precisely by using anatomical implants. The principal patients who will require this type of implant are those who are going to have only the NAC moved upward, that is, those who need a minimum periareolar pexy and have the deficiency mentioned earlier. A second advantage of anatomical implants is the possibility of combining the three necessary dimensions that exist in any volumetric body such as the breast to achieve a harmonious result. The use of anatomical implants in the indicated cases produced more satisfactory results than those the round implants would have given. Round implants undoubtedly have their advantages and indications, too, for mastopexy with implant placement. Patients with a significant deficit in the superior pole of the breast, which is very common in this type of patient, will have a more pleasing result than with anatomical implants, since what they are looking for is increased volume, where they have had a deficit for years. Therefore, the type of implant will depend on each patient's characteristics and the surgeon's indications, although in many cases, each patient's personal preferences are a primary factor in the decision.

It is important to point out the necessary changes the author has implemented in the evolution of the different surgical techniques over time. These changes are due to modifications made necessary by inadequate results or a desire to improve the results. Initially, with upward migration of the NAC, only the half-moon portion drawn over the NAC was deepithelialized. With time, however, it was found that cutaneous support alone was inadequate, causing scar widening and resulting in ptosis relapse (Fig. 21.19). This technique is used only in minimal migrations of less than 1.5 cm. When the migration is between 1.5 and 3 cm, the same half-moon resection is done, but the incision is completely on the areola, and the round block periareolar closure is used. With this modification long-term results have improved. Initially, and because of reports in the literature [10], a complete incision of the dermis was made after having deepithelialized the area to be resected. This incision was made to detach the periareolar skin and facilitate closing. However, this incision enlarged the area more, and at the same time reduced the vascularity of the NAC. For that reason, the dermis is no longer incised and there have been no serious complications except in the early cases. Another modification that has not been used is absorbable material in the round block suturing with the periareolar pexy technique. Although it might be a basic premise of that technique, one would think that after 3 or 4 months of support with absorbable sutures in various planes, the problem of tension over the areola would disappear, but it is not so. On several occasions it was necessary to remove the nonabsorbable Prolene suturing because the patients could feel it or there was a very disagreeable effect of conges-

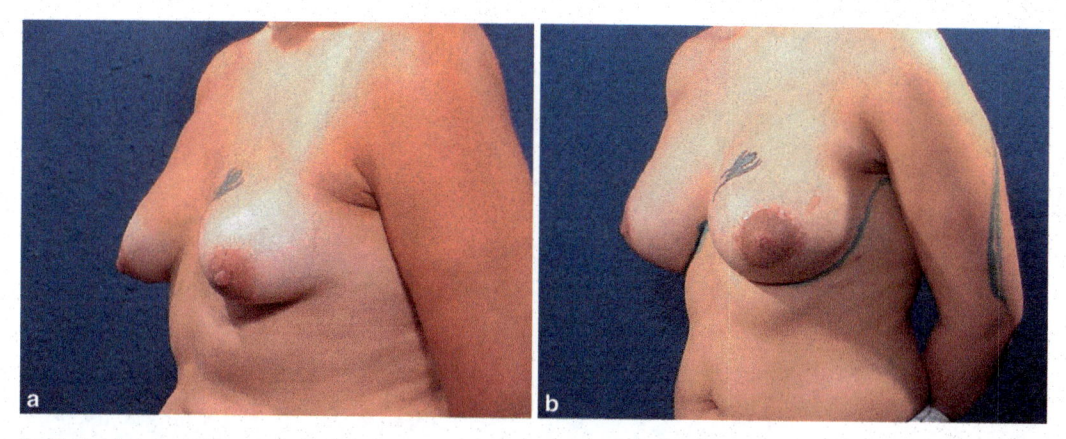

Fig. 21.19 (a) Patient with ptosis relapse and scar widening because NAC lift was used instead of a complete NAC periareolar closure. (b) Six years after pexy and 390 ml FM anatomical implants placement

tion of the NAC that was produced. This also led to the use of Monocryl and PDS for the round block suturing, to allow absorption to eliminate this effect. Tension will always exist, however, and using nonabsorbable material or removing the absorbable stitching will invariably result in areola widening and residual ptosis over the middle and long term.

Another important factor in the surgical technique is the proper approach to implant's introduction, always seeking the best possible coverage and avoiding maximum tension where tissue extrusion is most probable. Thus, placing an implant via the transareolar route when periareolar pexy is to be performed is as important as placing it by the inframammary route in the case of inverted T pexy. It is very risky to approach the breast by the midline to place an implant in inverted T pexy, since it is the area of greatest postoperative tension. Likewise, the implant should always be placed before removing any tissue to perform the pexy. To do otherwise is to face more possibilities of failure than success. Simple details like those mentioned here are of vital importance for ensuring the success of the surgery and for maximum avoidance of complications.

21.9 Avoiding Complications

The author's experience supports what a lot of authors have reported about complications. The author's incidence of complications has been strictly a very low percent of minor problems. Most of the reports on pexy with implants speak of techniques and results, but few speak of complications [8]. If we analyze carefully the reasons for these complications and correlate them with the surgical technique, we can detail how to achieve maximum avoidance of the complications and poor results.

One of the principal causes of complications, second to the choice of surgical technique, is the increased undermining involved in doing both procedures [8]. The author recommends undermining enough only to be able to place the implant. Flaps are not raised in doing the different pexies. In the case of NAC lifting or with periareolar pexy, deepithelialization is only used without doing more cutaneous undermining of the areola edges. In the inverted T technique, there is no undermining except what is necessary to place the implant. Pexy is achieved with approximation of the lateral and medial breast pillars, without the need of any undermining at all. Since there is only undermining for placing an implant, the risk of greater infection or tissue necrosis from tissue devascularization [8, 9] is also decreased (Fig. 21.20), and one avoids affecting NAC sensitivity excessively, as the undermining is similar to that for placing an implant. Another high-risk factor is the larger number of incisions over the implant area [8, 9]. This problem is solved by not incising on the vertical midline of the breast. The implant will always be placed by a periareolar approach or by the inframammary crease, without opening the midline for any reason at all. With this premise, there will always be breast tissue covering the placed implant, which is very important. The same thing happens if the supra-areolar approach is used to place an implant in case only elevation of the NAC is required. Because of the deficiency of breast tissue in the inferior pole in this type of patient, this approach allows leaving a larger amount of tissue covering the implant. Another known problem with this type of surgical combination is greater tension

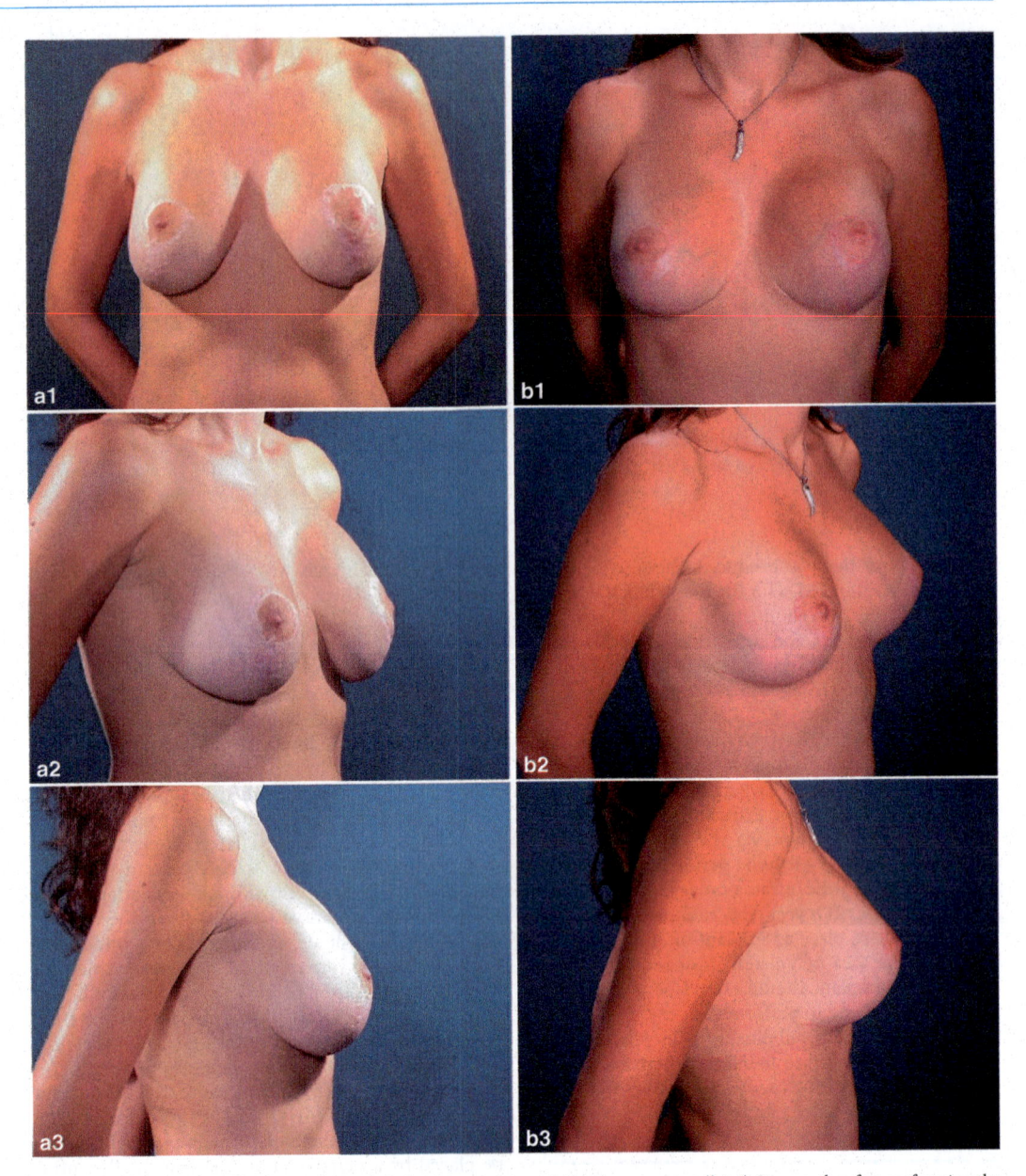

Fig. 21.20 (*a1-3*) Patient had an inverted "T" pexy and implants placed by another surgeon with poor results. She had ptosis relapse, NAC partial necrosis, scar widening, and NAC asymmetry. (*b1-3*) Six months after performing the same technique and putting in smaller implants

from the pressure the implant exerts on the soft tissues, which can also cause major tissue devascularization. This problem is more frequent when placing the subglandular implant, as well as when using very large implants [8]. The problem has been resolved in two ways. The first is by placing implants in a dual plane, as described by Tebbetts [18]. If this technique is used, the implant will always be covered by muscle in the vertical portion of the inverted T, in addition to the glandular covering already mentioned. The only indications in our cases for placing them subglandularly is in tuberous breasts, but in these cases, the pexy will never be vertical, rather periareolar. The second factor for avoiding tension consists of an elementary concept when performing any pexy, but which is often ignored. We never remove tissue for the pexy until the implant has been placed. This way, the tissue to be eliminated in any of the pexies is selected by pinching or tensing the skin after implant placement to calculate how much tissue it is possible to eliminate. So tissue should never be removed before placing the implant. This precaution will cause a closing tension similar to that of a pexy or breast reduction; therefore, the incidence of hypertrophic scars from tension will be similar to that of any of the surgeries mentioned. Taking this premise into account, the implant's size is not influential, since if it is large, there will be less tissue resection than if a small implant is used.

In addition to the problems of vascularity, tension, and undermining, which are commonly produced if the above guidelines are not followed, errors are frequently made in the surgical technique that affects the aesthetic result. It has been pointed out that there is a major risk of malpositioning the NAC by moving it at the same time the implant is placed [8, 9]. In these cases, marking the new position of the NAC preoperatively, placing the implant before performing the pexy, and using reference threads in the suprasternal notch and xyphoid appendix all help to achieve a proper location and symmetry. Also to be stressed is the importance of placing the patient in a sitting position when in doubt. Marking the area of the base of the breast preoperatively is a primary factor in avoiding malpositioning of the implant. Displacement of the implant with the consequent malpositioning of the NAC can be due to improper placement trans-operatively or capsular contracture in the postoperative period. Although these complications are inherent in placing implants, they are not so in a combination of pexy with implants.

Complications are very rare in the author's experience, since a very scrupulous protocol is followed in choosing the technique and in performing the surgery. To avoid the double contour that is observed in patients with a deficiency in the inferior pole of the breast, as would be the case with tuberous breasts, an anatomical implant is recommended. In cases of a 1.5 cm upward migration of the NAC, complete periareolar incision is always performed and closed with the round block technique. This has avoided hypertrophic scars and ptosis relapse. Likewise, round block suturing should always be done with permanent sutures, not very thick (Prolene 2-0). Using permanent sutures avoids long-term widening of the areola, and if they are not too thick, it prevents them from being very palpable in the periareolar area. To avoid ptosis relapse, it is very important not to modify the new location that has been decided for the new NAC before surgery. Otherwise, errors in positioning will be common. Flattening of the breast will be greater in cases in which a significant amount of tissue is removed during the periareolar pexy. When the amount of resected tissue is very significant, the main problem could be that the proper technique was inverted T, and not periareolar. Erythema and cysts in the periareolar suture line has been avoided by placing the round block suture deeper into the dermis, thus avoiding introducing epidermal tissue into the suture line. Scar thickness is inherent in any surgical procedure and not an exclusive side effect of combining both procedures.

Performing both procedures is not only feasible, but also recommendable for resolving both problems at the same surgical time. It is true that the combination of both procedures is more laborious and detailed than either of the two done separately [8, 9, 11, 13, 15], and so the author's recommendations are focused on three aspects: follow the parameters for properly choosing the technique to be used [6, 10–12], perform the surgery correctly [6, 10–12], and know the reason for the complications and how to maximize avoidance of them. With this in mind, mastopexy with implants at the same surgical time should be considered totally feasible, without major complications from having combined the two procedures at the same surgical time.

References

1. Baroudi R, Lewis JR: The augmentation-reduction mammaplasty. Clin Plast Surg 1976;3(2):301–308
2. McKissock PK: Reduction mammaplasty with a vertical dermal flap. Plast Reconstr Surg 1972;49(3):245–252
3. Pitanguy I: Mammaplasty. Study of 245 consecutive cases and presentation of a personal technique. Rev Bras Cir 1961;42:201–220
4. Pitanguy I: A new technique of plastic surgery of the breast. Study of 245 consecutive cases and presentation of a personal technique. Ann Chir Plast 1962;7:199–208
5. Pontes R: Reduction mammaplasty – variations I and II. Ann Plast Surg 1981;6(6):437–447
6. Rohrich RJ, Gosman AA, Brown SA, Tonadapu P, Foster B: Current preferences for breast reduction techniques: a survey of board-certified plastic surgeons 2002. Plast Reconstr Surg 2004;114(4):1724–1733
7. Goldwyn RM: Plastic and Reconstructive Surgery of the Breast. Little, Brown and Company, Boston 1979
8. Spear SL, Pelletiere CV, Menon N: One-stage augmentation combined with mastopexy: aesthetic results and patient satisfaction. Aesthetic Plast Surg 2004;28(5):259–267
9. Spear SL, Low M, Ducic I: Revision augmentation mastopexy: indications, operations, and outcomes. Ann Plast Surg 2003;51(6):540–546

10. de la Fuente A, Martin del Yerro JL: Periareolar mastopexy with mammary implants. Aesthetic Plast Surg 1992;16(4):337–341
11. Elliott LF: Circumareolar mastopexy with augmentation. Clin Plast Surg 2002;29(3):337–347
12. Karnes J, Morrison W, Salisbury M, Schaeferle M, Beckham P, Ersek RA: Simultaneous breast augmentation and lift. Aesthetic Plast Surg 2000;24(2):148–154
13. Baran CN, Peker F, Ortak T, Sensoz O, Baran NK: Unsatisfactory results of periareolar mastopexy with or without augmentation and reduction mammoplasty: enlarged areola with flattened nipple. Aesthetic Plast Surg 2001;25(4):286–289
14. Persoff MM: Vertical mastopexy with expansion augmentation. Aesthetic Plast Surg 2003;27(1):13–19
15. Spear SL: Augmentation/mastopexy: "surgeon, beware". Plast Reconstr Surg 2003;112(3):905–906
16. Puckett CL, Meyer VH, Reinisch JF: Crescent mastopexy and augmentation. Plast Reconstr Surg 1985;75(4):533–543
17. Cardenas-Camarena L, Ramírez-Macias R: Augmentation/mastopexy: how to select and perform the proper technique. Aesthetic Plast Surg 2006;30(1):21–33
18. Tebbetts JB: Dual plane breast augmentation: optimizing implant-soft-tissue relationships in a wide range of breast types. Plast Reconstr Surg 2001;107(5):1255–1272
19. Benelli L: A new periareolar mammaplasty: the "round block" technique. Aesthetic Plast Surg 1990;14(2):93–100
20. Planas J, Cervelli V, Planas G: Five-year experience on ultrasonic treatment of breast contractures. Aesthetic Plast Surg 2001;25(2):89–93

Vaser®-Assisted Breast Reduction and Mastopexy

Maurice P. Sherman

22.1
Introduction

Modern body contouring procedures date back to the late 1970s when Europeans such as Fischer [1, 2] and others described a selective localized fat removal procedure using suction cannulas. Scuderi, in 1987, first reported the use of ultrasonic energy for lipoplasty. The first generation of ultrasonic devices was a SMEI device, which utilized a 4–6 mm solid probe. Lysonex, in 1996, developed a second generation ultrasonic device, which had a golf tee shape at the end of a 5 mm cannula, with a 2 mm lumen for simultaneous aspiration. Finally, in 2002, a third generation ultrasonic device marketed by Sound Surgical Technologies, termed the Vaser® System, became available and was marketed as Liposelection® due to its selectivity in emulsifying adipose tissue.

This new technology was initially applied to body fat to emulsify only fat cells while sparing the supported vascular and connective tissue components of the cutaneous network. Over the past decades, Zocchi [3, 4], Benelli [5], and Di Giuseppe [6, 7] have applied this technology to the breast tissue to achieve breast reduction and correction of mild to moderate ptosis. The author has expanded its use in mastopexy techniques due to the tightening or contraction effect that has also occurred, along with the preservation of vascularity in the reduction of breast tissue without the need for creating large surgical resections and incisional flaps with their inherent potential devascularized tissue and delayed healing.

22.2
Vaser Technology

Vaser technology has been well described in numerous articles on the specifics behind Vaser that have been well outlined by Cimino [8], the founder and chief scientist of Sound Surgical Technologies. The author has also used the guidelines supplied by Alberto Di Giuseppe and his articles on Vaser-assisted liposuction for breast reduction [9–11].

22.3
Patient Selection

The ideal candidate for any Vaser-assisted liposuction technique of the breast is a breast with significant fatty parenchyma. With involutional changes in the post menopausal breast, between 60 and 70% of women are candidates for reduction and tightening with Vaser UAL alone or in combination with surgical resection. Initial screening should include a mammogram to evaluate the nature and consistency of breast tissue and the presence of any abnormalities that might necessitate further studies or biopsies. Patients with a personal history or strong family history of breast cancer probably should not receive Vaser nor should patients with breast tissue of a primarily glandular nature.

22.4
Surgical Technique

Whether intravenous (IV) sedation or general anesthesia is utilized, tumescent infiltration of Klein's solution is needed to induce vasoconstriction and allow transmission of ultrasonic energy to emulsify adipose cells. Usually 500–1,000 ml solution per side is infiltrated to achieve good tumescence. Stab incisions are made in the anterior axillary line and 2 cm below the inframammary crease. Periareolar incisions are also made to gain access to the superficial plane to promote skin contraction. Work is done on a criss-cross manner and all quadrants of the breast can be approached as needed. The periareolar cone, where the glandular tissue is concentrated, is preserved. A 3.7 mm, three-ring probe set at 60–70% power setting is used for parenchymal emulsification. Ten to fifteen minutes of energy application usually results in 300–500 ml of fat aspiration. For skin retraction, Vaser stimulation is superficial. Subdermal layers are treated initially with a 2.9-mm probe at 50% power settings using the periareolar incision sites. Fibrosis that follows the thermal insult from the probe passage produces a significant degree of skin retraction in the healing

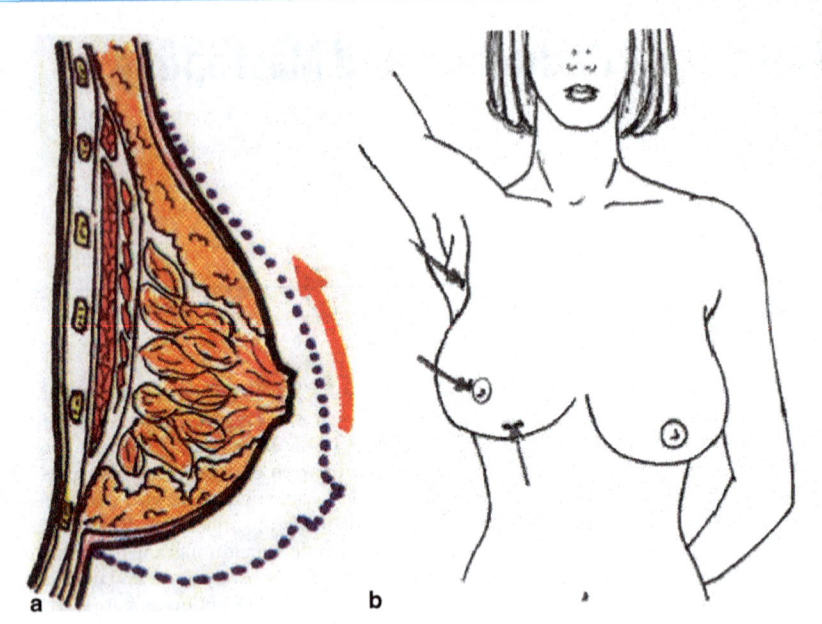

Fig. 22.1 (a) By thinning the lower pole, the breast cone naturally rotates upward. (b) With the thinned lower pole, the axillary, submammary, and periareolar incision lines rotate upward

period, which contributes to the correction of ptosis and enhanced redraping of the breast skin.

Postoperative care consists of drains only if a mastopexy with breast resection is performed. For liposuction only, incision sites are left open for drainage. Foam tape is used to support the breast and enhance compression. Additionally, a compression garment with ace wrapping is used for 1 week. The patient is instructed to use a support bra 24 h a day for 7 days a week for the next 3 months (Figs. 22.1 and 22.2)

Over the past 5 years, the author has used Vaser breast liposuction techniques to provide improved aesthetic results in vertical mastopexy with and without augmentation and to minimize surgical breast tissue with the horizontal mastopexy- reduction technique of Passot.

22.5
Vaser-Assisted Vertical Mastopexy

In vertical mastopexies, the Vaser-stimulated degree of retraction and fibrosis produces a greater degree of lift and redraping as well as improved longevity of the lift (Figs. 22.3 and 22.4). This is especially true for the combined vertical mastopexy with augmentation. Addition-ally, the reduction in ptotic breast volume improves the mastopexy closure by reducing tension on the vertical wound closure, leading to a reduction in wound healing problems and a more aesthetic scar production.

Initially, the Vaser liposuction is completed on each breast, with limitation of volume reduction to the inferior pole and superficial liposuction of the superior anterior aspect of the breast to aid in the lift. A standard Lejour vertical mastopexy is performed with or without augmentation. The author prefers the submuscular augmentation position, using either saline or silicone gel implants. Induration of the lower pole is noticeable for several months, but leads to a firmer, more fibrotic connective tissue support of the lower pole and helps to eliminate recurrent ptosis or "bottoming out." Potentially, in selected patients, use of more conservative techniques (i.e., crescent mastopexy or periareolar mastopexy) combined with Vaser application may provide for an aesthetic breast shape and lift with reduction of surgical scarring.

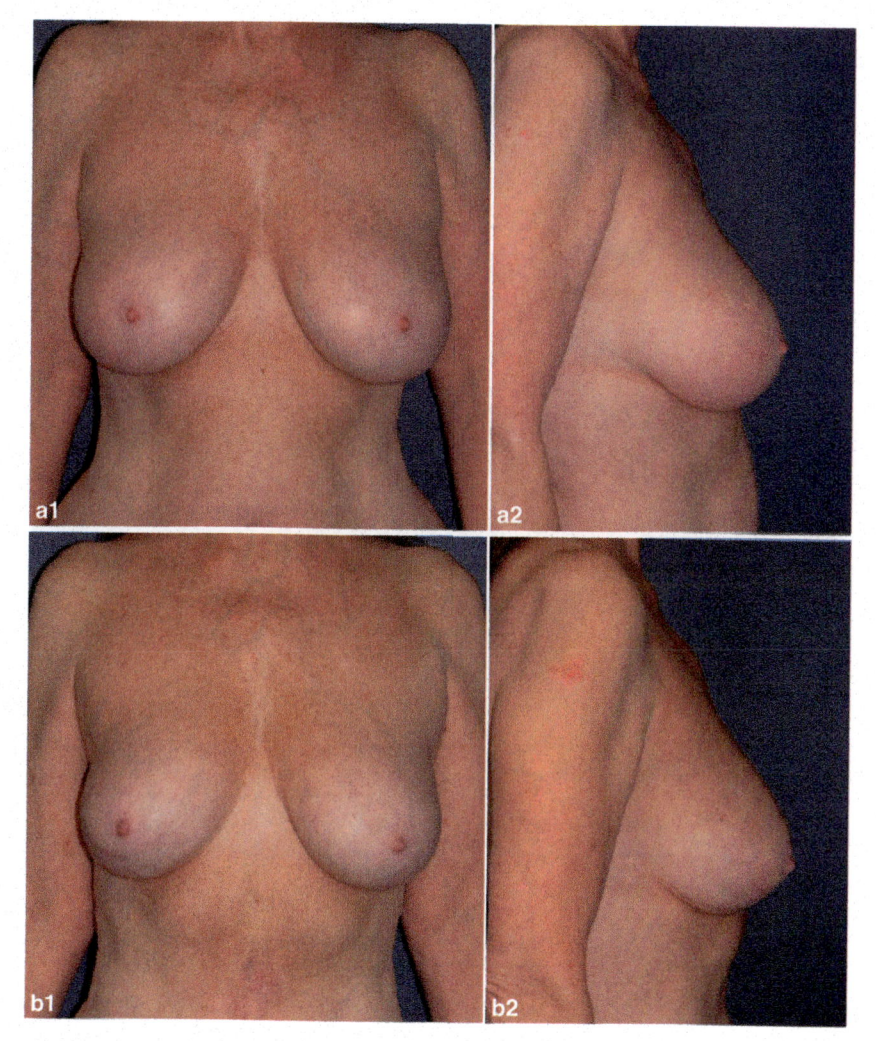

Fig. 22.2 Vaser breast liposuction. (*a1,2*) Preoperative. (*b1,2*) Six months postoperative

22.6
Vaser-Assisted Horizontal Mastopexy

Over the past 6 years, the author has used Vaser liposuction to enhance safety and results in a reduction-mastopexy technique first described by Passot in 1925 [12], also called "the apron technique" by Yousif in 1992 [13] and which the author refers to as a horizontal mastopexy-reduction with elimination of the vertical scar (Figs. 22.5–22.10).

Indications are patients with combined enlargement and severe ptosis of breasts. Initial preoperative markings place the new nipple site at the level of the inframammary crease (IMC). The nipple areolar complex (NAC) is

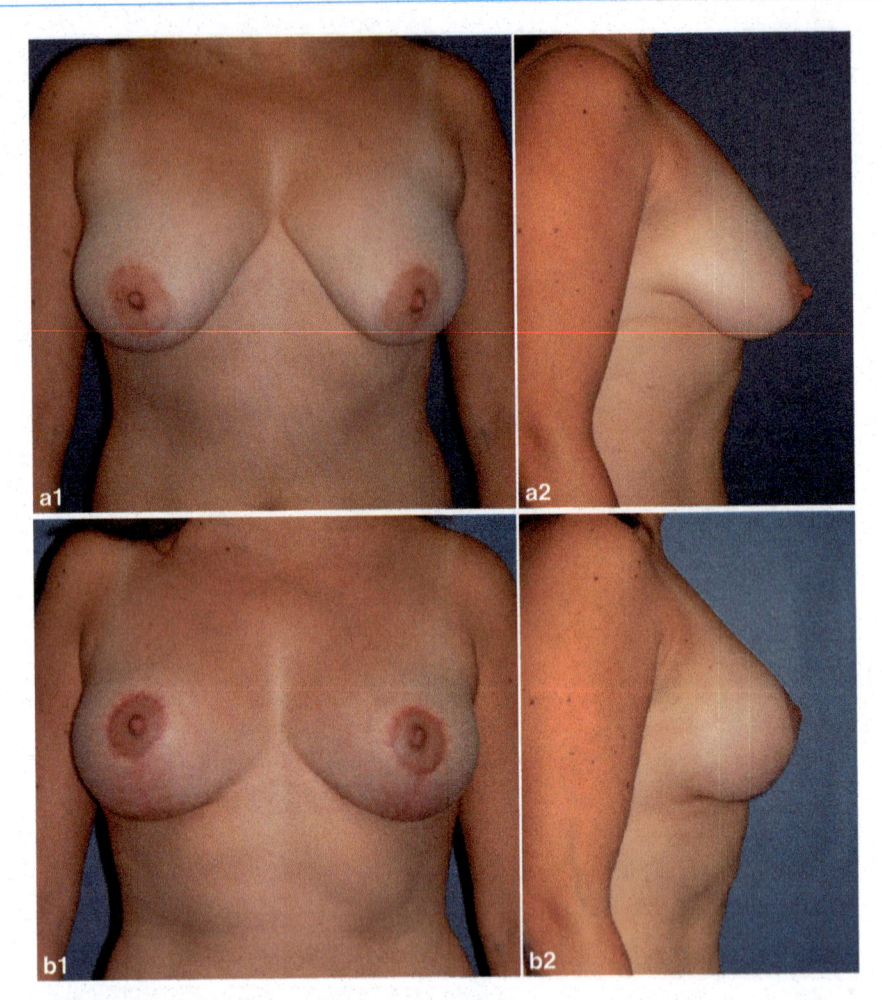

Fig. 22.3 Vertical mastopexy with Vaser liposuction breast reduction. (**a**1,2) Preoperative. (**b**1,2) Two months postoperative

retained on a vascularized inferior/medial pedicle, with major reduction of breast tissue being done in the lateral and medial aspects using Vaser liposuction techniques. This central deepithelialized breast mound with NAC is tucked underneath the superior skin flap or apron and brought out through a new circular opening in the apron flap, much like an umbilicus is recreated in an abdominoplasty. The periareolar closure is under no tension and heals with an excellent inconspicuous scar. The apron flap is closed at the IMC in a horizontal closure, eliminating trifurcation wound healing problems seen in the Wise anchor incision. The breast mound is recreated using sutures molding the lateral and medial edges of the breast pedicle. Surgical resection of breast tissue is

22.6 Vaser-Assisted Horizontal Mastopexy   183

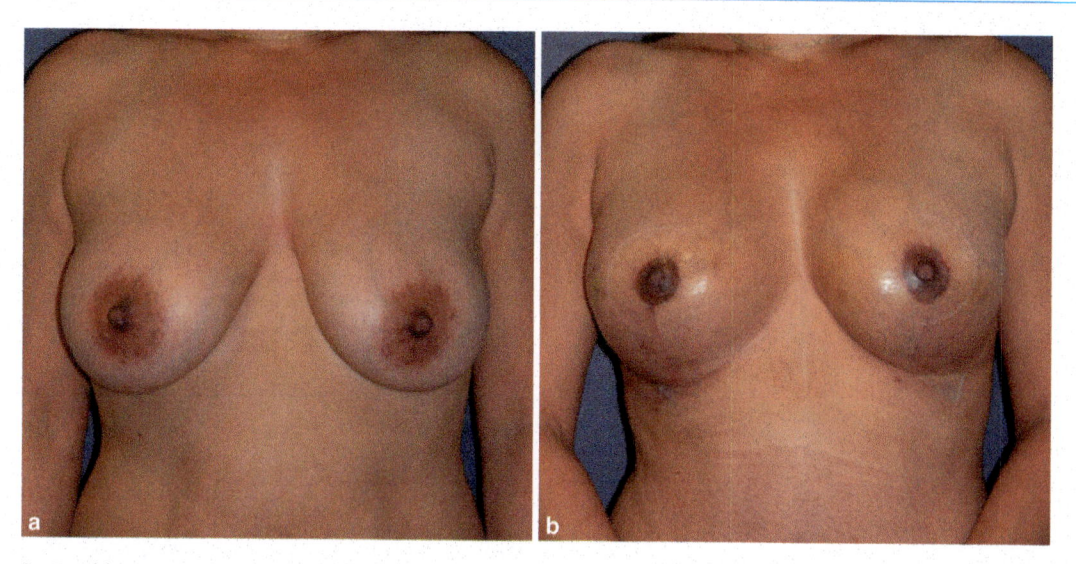

Fig. 22.4 (a) Preoperative patient with prior breast augmentation. (b) One month postoperative following vertical mastopexy with Vaser liposuction/reduction of inferior pole

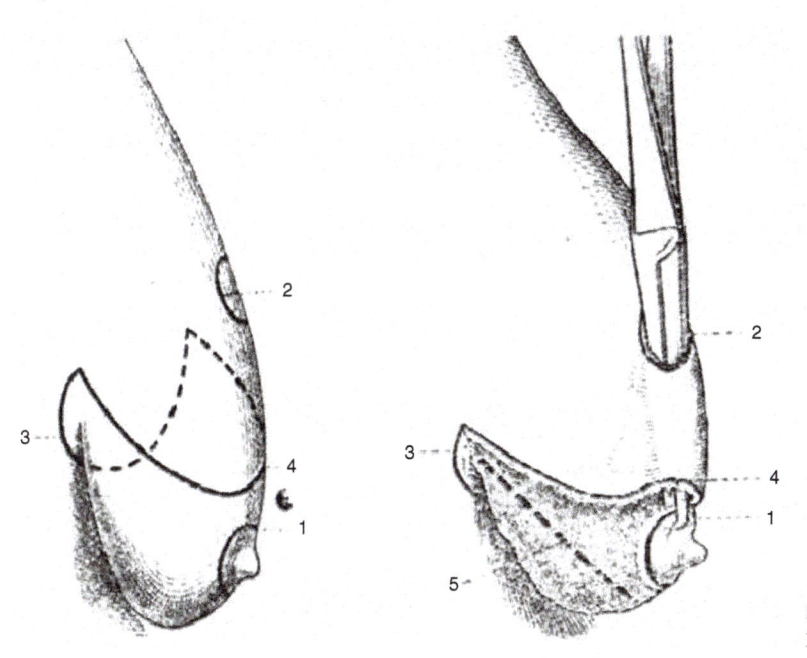

Fig. 22.5 Passot's 1925 Illustration

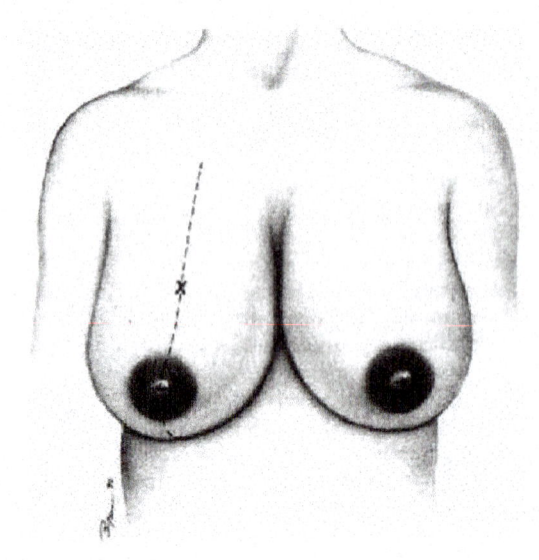

Fig. 22.6 The new nipple site is marked at the new level of the inframammary crease

minimized by using Vaser liposuction for reduction of excess tissue. The Vaser technique also creates fibrosis of the mound, which helps preserve the breast shape and avoids potential devascularization and sensory injury to the breast tissue. The potential for hematoma formation is also minimized.

Forty two cases have been performed in the past 5 years, with two cases of superficial necrosis of the inferior skin flap that healed with conservative care and did not need grafting. Nipple sensitivity and erectile function has been normal in all cases. Patients have been temporarily concerned about decreased breast volume and were counseled regarding the availability of breast augmentation through transaxillary, subpectoral approach in 6–9 months postoperatively, but no patients have requested this additional surgery (Figs. 22.11 and 22.12).

22.7
Complications

No major complications have occurred in the authors experience with Vaser breast techniques (Fig. 22.13). However, practitioners must learn how to work in the superficial and subdermal layer to obtain good redraping and skin retraction, while avoiding skin burns or necrosis. Thus experience at Vaser body contouring procedures is necessary. Hematoma formation can follow any surgical resection and must be recognized and evacuated. Mastitis, an inflammatory breast parenchymal response, can be treated with anti-inflammatories and antibiotics. Seroma formation needs

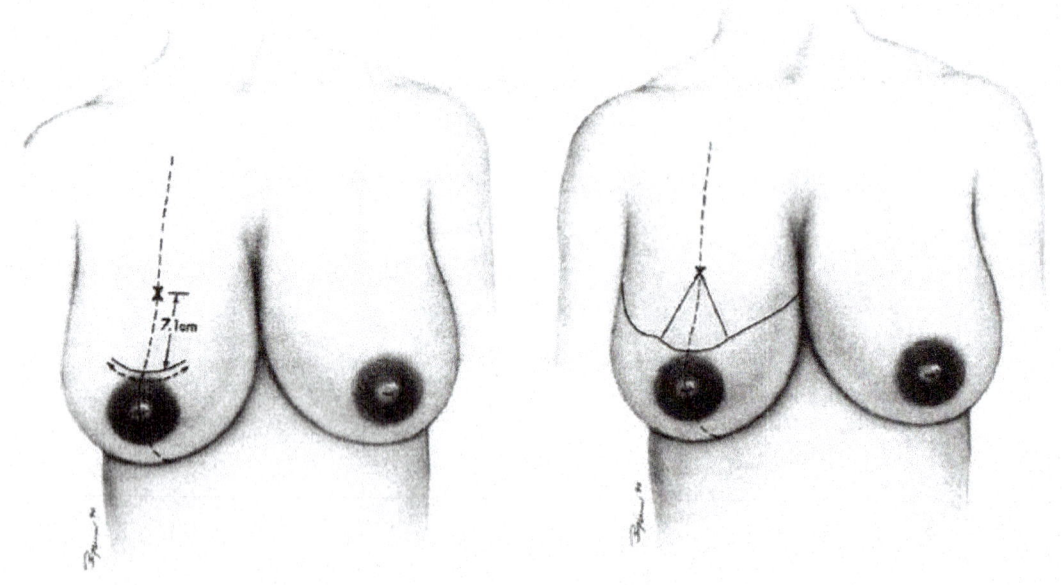

Fig. 22.7 *Left*: The skin space between the new nipple site and the inferior excision is 5.5–7 cm. *Right*: The lines are extended medially and laterally to meet the inframammary line

22.7 Complications 185

Fig. 22.8 (a) Conversion to a Wise pattern is easily performed if desired. (b) The new areolar site is kept at 2.5 cm, allowing for tension free closure

Fig. 22.9 (a) The breast mound flap is shaped with internal sutures. (b) The apron skin flap is kept at 1.5 cm thickness to permit adequate blood supply to the skin flap

Fig. 22.10 (a) Breast shaping sutures. (b) Closure with midline gathering

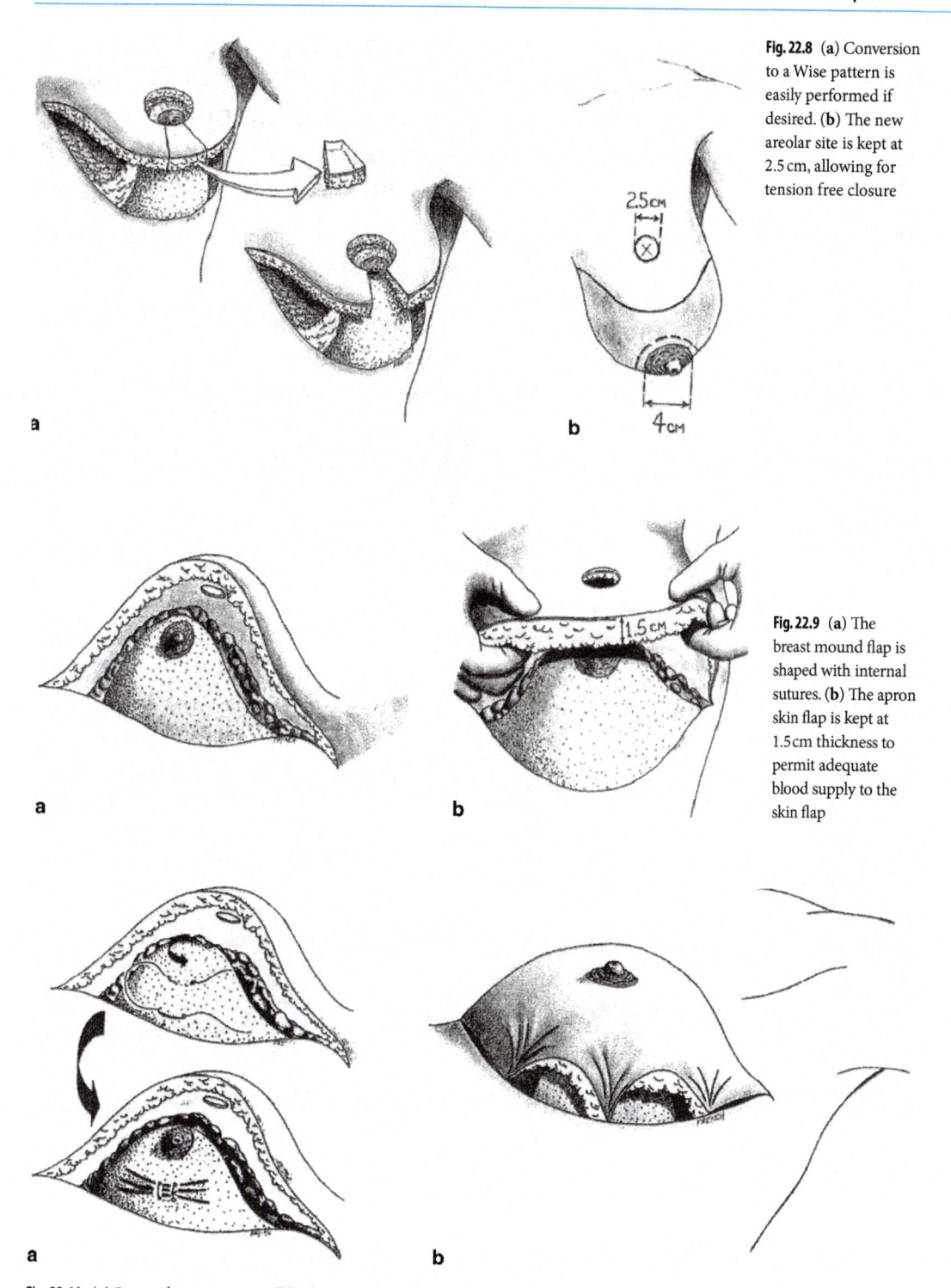

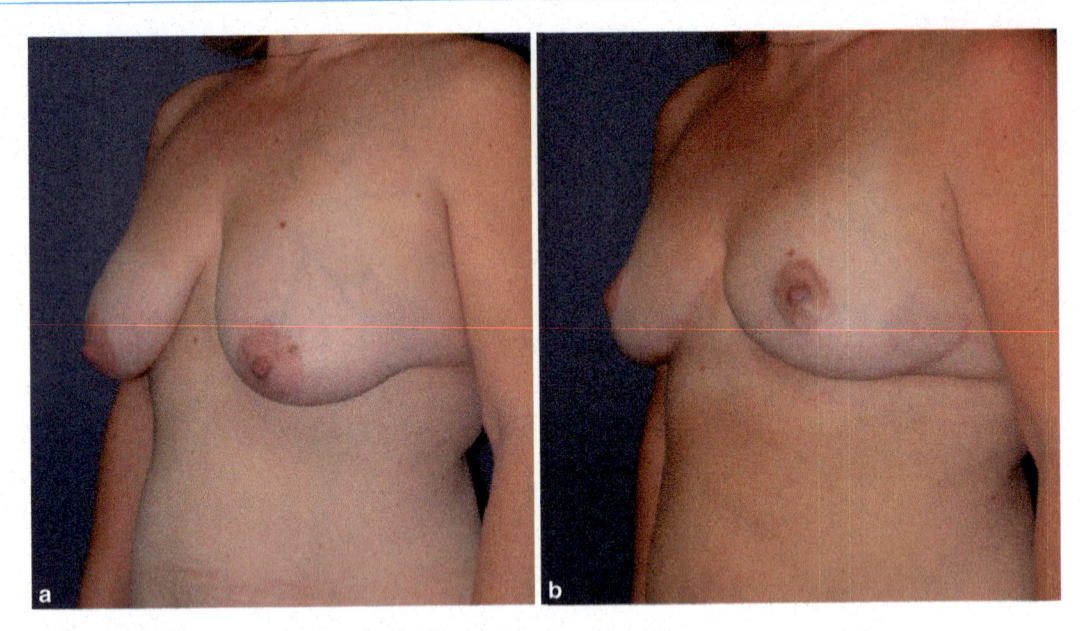

Fig. 22.11 Horizontal mastopexy. (**a**) Preoperative. (**b**) Seven months postoperative

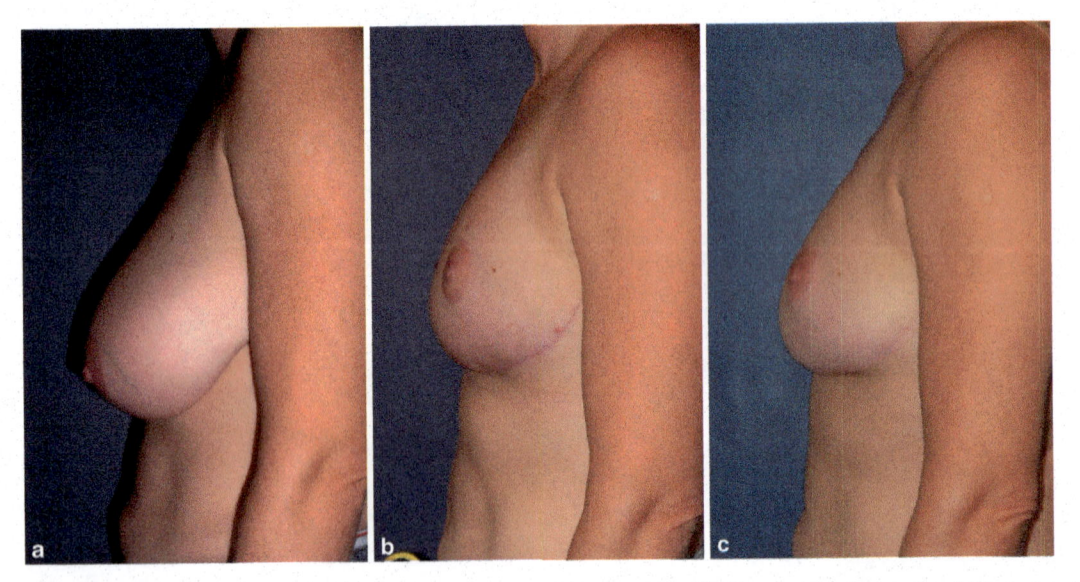

Fig. 22.12 Horizontal mastopexy with Vaser liposuction/reduction. (**a**) Preoperative. (**b**) Three months postoperative. (**c**) One year postoperative

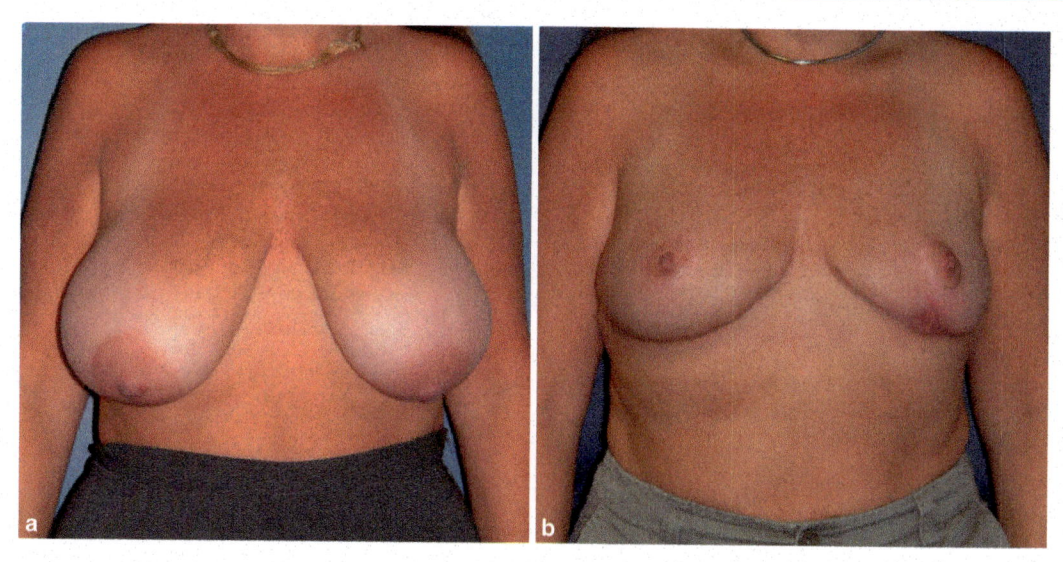

Fig. 22.13 Horizontal mastopexy. (**a**) Preoperative. (**b**) Three months postoperative with left inferior breast delayed healing

22.8
Conclusions

The use of Vaser ultrasound-assisted liposuction (UAL) in breast surgery can be a safe and effective technique when applied to appropriately selected cases and performed by a surgeon with expertise in Vaser body contouring. The selectivity of the UAL enables emulsification of the fatty component of the breast parenchyma, while sparing the glandular, vascular, and connective tissue network. Furthermore, long-term mammographic studies have revealed no alteration of morphology of breast parenchyma resulting from Vaser usage. Additional advantages consist of the volume reduction without the need for extensive surgical resection, and skin and gland contraction and redraping that assists in the breast lifting and shaping of the breast mound. Thus, a correction of a ptotic breast may be achieved without visible scarring

to be evacuated and treated with steroids and drainage. Loss of sensation and prolonged breast pain may rarely be seen and has always been transitory, resolving in 3–4 months.

or may compliment the use of more conservative surgical mastopexy techniques. In more aggressive surgical techniques such as the vertical and horizontal mastopexies, safer reduction of breast tissue and prolongation of the effective lifting are expected benefits of using the Vaser technology in cosmetic breast surgery.

References

1. Fischer G: Surgical treatment of cellulitis. Third International Congress of International Academy of Cosmetic Surgery, Rome, May 31, 1975
2. Fischer G: First surgical treatment for modeling body's cellulite with three 5 mm incisions. Bull Int Acad Cosm Surg 1976;2:35–37
3. Zocchi ML: Clinical aspects of ultrasonic liposculpture. Perspect Plastic Surg 1993;7:153–174
4. Zocchi ML: Ultrasonic assisted lipoplasty. Clin Plastic Surgery 1996;23(4):575–598
5. Benelli L: Technique de plastie mammaire: le "round bloc." Rev Fr Chir Esthet 1988;50:7
6. Di Giuseppe A, Santoli M: Ultrasound assisted breast reduction and mastopexy. Aesthetic Surgery J 2001;21: 493–506

7. Di Giuseppe A: Mammoplasty reduction and mastopexy utilizing ultrasound liposuction. Mammographic study preoperative. 46th National Congress of Italian Society of Plastic Reconstructive and Aesthetic Surgery. Venice, Italy, June 9–12, 1997
8. Cimino WW: Ultrasonic surgery: power quantification and efficiency optimization. Aesthetic Surg J 2001;21(3): 233–240
9. Di Giuseppe A: Ultrasonically assisted breast reduction and mastopexy. Int J Cosm Surg Aesthet Derm 2001;3(1):23–29
10. Di Giuseppe A: Ultrasound assisted breast reduction and mastopexy. Aesthet Surg J 2001;21(6):493–506
11. Di Giuseppe A: Breast reduction with ultrasound assisted lipoplasty. Plast Reconstr Surg 2003;112(1):71–82
12. Passot R: La correction esthetique du prolapsus mammarie par le procede de la transposition du mamelon. La Presse Medicale 1925;33:317
13. Yousif NJ, Larson Dl, Sanger JR, Matloub HS: Elimination of the vertical scar in reduction mammoplasty. Plast Reconstr Surg 1992;89(3):459–467

Periareolar Mammaplasty for the Treatment of Gynecomastia with Breast Ptosis

Marco Túlio Rodrigues da Cunha, José Fernando Borges Bento, Antonio Roberto Bozola

23.1 Introduction

Gynecomastia, or enlargement of the male breast, may lead to serious psychological disturbances. The most common patient complaint is his embarrassment of his body image.

Simon et al. [1], in 1973, described a clinical classification after analysis of 77 cases of gynecomastia: Grade 1, small, visible breast enlargement without skin redundancy; Grade 2A, moderate breast enlargement without skin redundancy; Grade 2B, moderate enlargement with skin redundancy; Grade 3, marked breast enlargement with marked skin redundancy.

The first description of a surgical treatment was made by Paulus of Aegina [2] (AD 635–690) using a semilunar inframammary incision. Dufourmental [3], in 1928, described an infra-areolar marginal incision, divulged by Webster [4], in 1946. The transareolar mammary incision was published by Pitanguy [5], in 1966.

Many surgical difficulties are found in Group 2B and 3, where excess skin is present. Some authors describe excess skin resection using a "half-moon" located at the borders of areola [6], others utilize vertical [7, 8], transverse [2], or oblique [9] skin ellipses.

Free graft [10], as well as superior pedicle [7] and bipedicle flaps [2], is employed to elevate the nipple–areola complex in large gynecomastia. Joseph [11], in 1925, published a method of female mammaplasty, in two stages, where the nipple–areola complex is transplanted by means of an inferior pedicle flap.

Andrews et al. [12], in 1975, described a periareolar approach for breast reduction. Ribeiro [13], in 1975, used an inferior pedicle flap with the aim of projecting the mammary cone and stabilizing its shape. Davidson [14], in 1979, removed excess skin in concentric circles, limiting the final scar to a circle at the perip-hery of the areola. Benelli [15], in 1988, presented a permanent periareolar circling to avoid late widening of the nipple–areola complex. Martins [16], in 1991, described a periareolar mammaplasty with flap transposition.

Kornstein and Cinelli [17], in 1992, reported an inferior pedicle flap associated with a superiorly based chest wall flap to reposition the nipple–areola complex, resulting in a periareolar and inframammary scar. The authors reported in 1993 [18] the use of the periareolar mammaplasty, with an inferior pedicle flap including the nipple–areola complex, to correct a male breast ptosis.

The aim of the present work is to evaluate the use of the periareolar skin approach associated with inferior or superior pedicle flaps that include the nipple–areola complex.

23.2 Technique

The criteria adopted for patient selection were breast ptosis, massive gynecomastia, and skin excess.

Skin markings (Fig. 23.1) are performed using a longitudinal line dividing the breast into two equal halves (meridian), as well as the inframammary crease. The breast meridian is marked:

- Point A, 17–19 cm from the sternal notch, however until 25 cm in special cases
- Point B, 4–6 cm proximally to the inframammary crease
- Point C, half the distance between points A and B.

A transverse line perpendicular to the breast meridian is marked passing on Point C (line C). On line C, the points D and E are marked by means of bidigital pinching, bringing them near, equidistant from the breast meridian. Excessive tension should be avoided in this procedure. The diameter of periareolar skin, to be removed, should not exceed twice the diameter of the areola. The points A, D, B, and E are joined, obtaining an oval-shaped form. The new areola is marked with 3 cm diameter.

The surgery is performed under general anesthesia. The excess skin marked is removed in its total thickness. The infra areolar area is carefully deepithelialized, preventing injuries in the pedicle of the flap. An inferior

M.A. Shiffman (ed.), *Mastopexy and Breast Reduction: Principles and Practice*,
© Springer-Verlag Berlin Heidelberg 2009

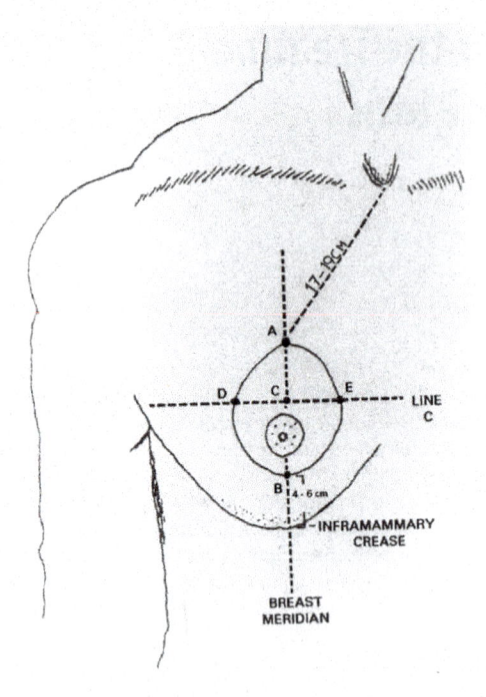

Fig. 23.1 Oval-shaped preoperative skin markings around the areola

pedicle is made embodying the nipple–areola complex (used in 8 of 15 cases) or a superior pedicle is used (in 7 cases). The flap thickness is reduced to that of the patient's subcutaneous tissue and its width to approximately 5 cm. The flap is freed from the remnant skin that covers it anteriorly, undermining it until next to the inframammary crease in inferior pedicle cases. In the superior pedicle cases, after skin removal a hemicircular incision is made distal to nipple–areola complex. The excess adipoglandular tissues are easily removed next to the flap, inside and outside the area of skin resection. Hemostasis is carefully made under direct vision. The tip of the flap is fixed to the anterior pectoral fascia with four cardinal sutures, 17–19 cm from the sternal notch, in the breast meridian. The superior pedicle nipple–areola complex does not need to be sutured to pectoral fascia or to be freed from remnant proximal skin. A permanent periareolar circling is made using 5-0 monofilament nylon, "closing" the purse until it is 3 cm in diameter. A catheter for suction drainage is placed through an inframammary stab.

"U" sutures unite the areola to the periareolar "purse string" skin. An occlusive, lightly compressive dressing is applied.

23.3
Postoperative Care

1. Suction drainage is maintained for 2–5 days.
2. The sutures are removed on the seventh to twelfth postoperative day.
3. Compressive dressing is kept for 2 weeks.

23.4
Complications

1. Postoperative bleeding: 1 case
2. Seroma: 2 cases
3. Areola enlargement: 1 case
4. Infection: 1 case
5. Bulging in the inferior pole of the breast: 2 cases
6. One patient with skin hypoesthesia that lasted for 30 days.

23.5
Discussion

Most of the difficulties in the surgical treatment of the gynecomastia are due to the restricted size of the incision that prejudices the illumination of the operative field and the hemostasis. The transareolar mammary [5] and infra-areolar marginal incisions [3, 4] are not always efficient to correct gynecomastia with marked skin redundancy and to elevate the nipple–areola complex. Skin resections by means of "inverted T" technique [11], vertical [7, 8], and transverse [9] skin ellipses result in long scars and can leave the breast cone like. The illness stigma is replaced by a scar stigma, especially in patients with hairless chest wall.

The authors used the periareolar mammaplasty with skin markings similar to those described by Martins [16], in 1991, associated with an inferior pedicle flap including the nipple–areola complex. Fixing the flap to the anterior pectoral fascia did not significantly reduce the areola mobility due to its contact with the flap pedicle and not directly with the fascia.

One of the greatest disappointments of the periareolar mammaplasties in female patients is due to the "flattening" of the breast cone. This is one of the most desired events in gynecomastia operation.

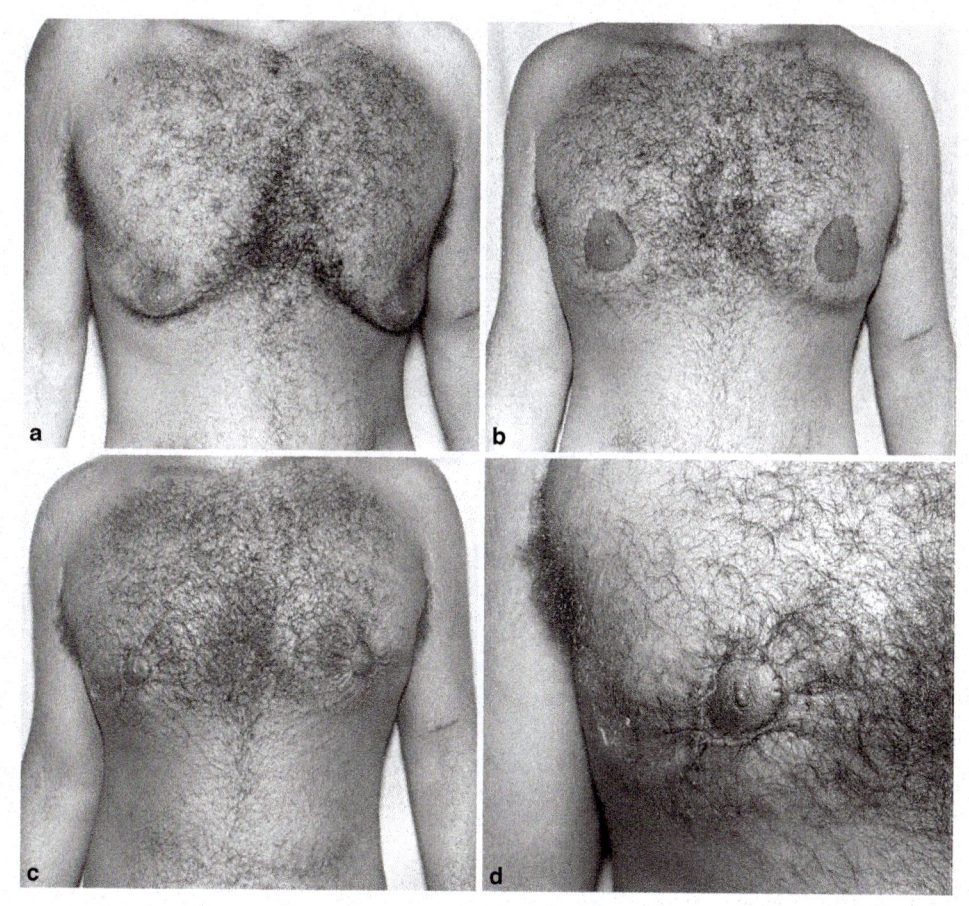

Fig. 23.2 (a) Preoperative patient. (b) Two years postoperatively after inferior pedicle technique showing bilateral widening of the nipple–areola complex and excess adipoglandular tissue at the distal part of the left breast. (c) Twelfth postoperative day after second stage correction. This result was considered final and stable after 6 month follow-up. (d) Close-up of right areola on the twelfth postoperative day

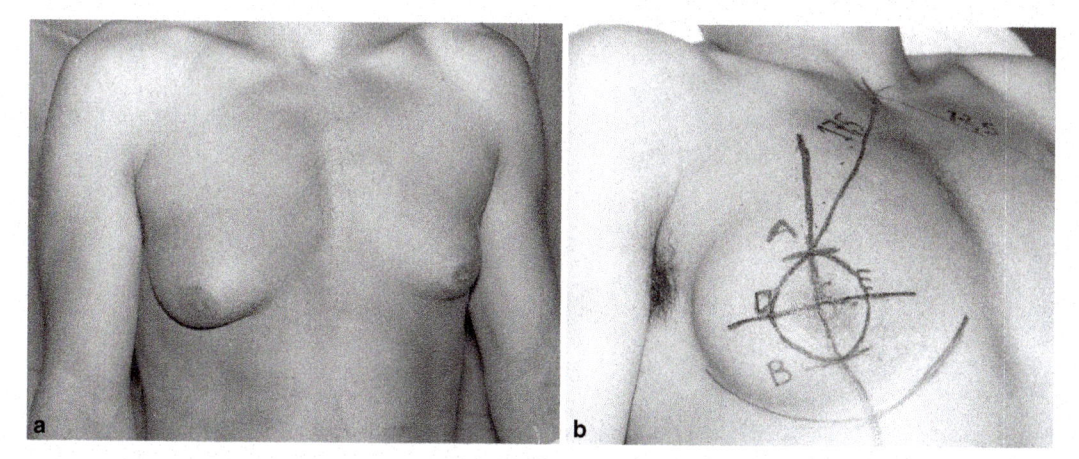

Fig. 23.3 (a) Preoperative patient with gynecomastia. (b) Skin markings on right breast for inferior pedicle technique

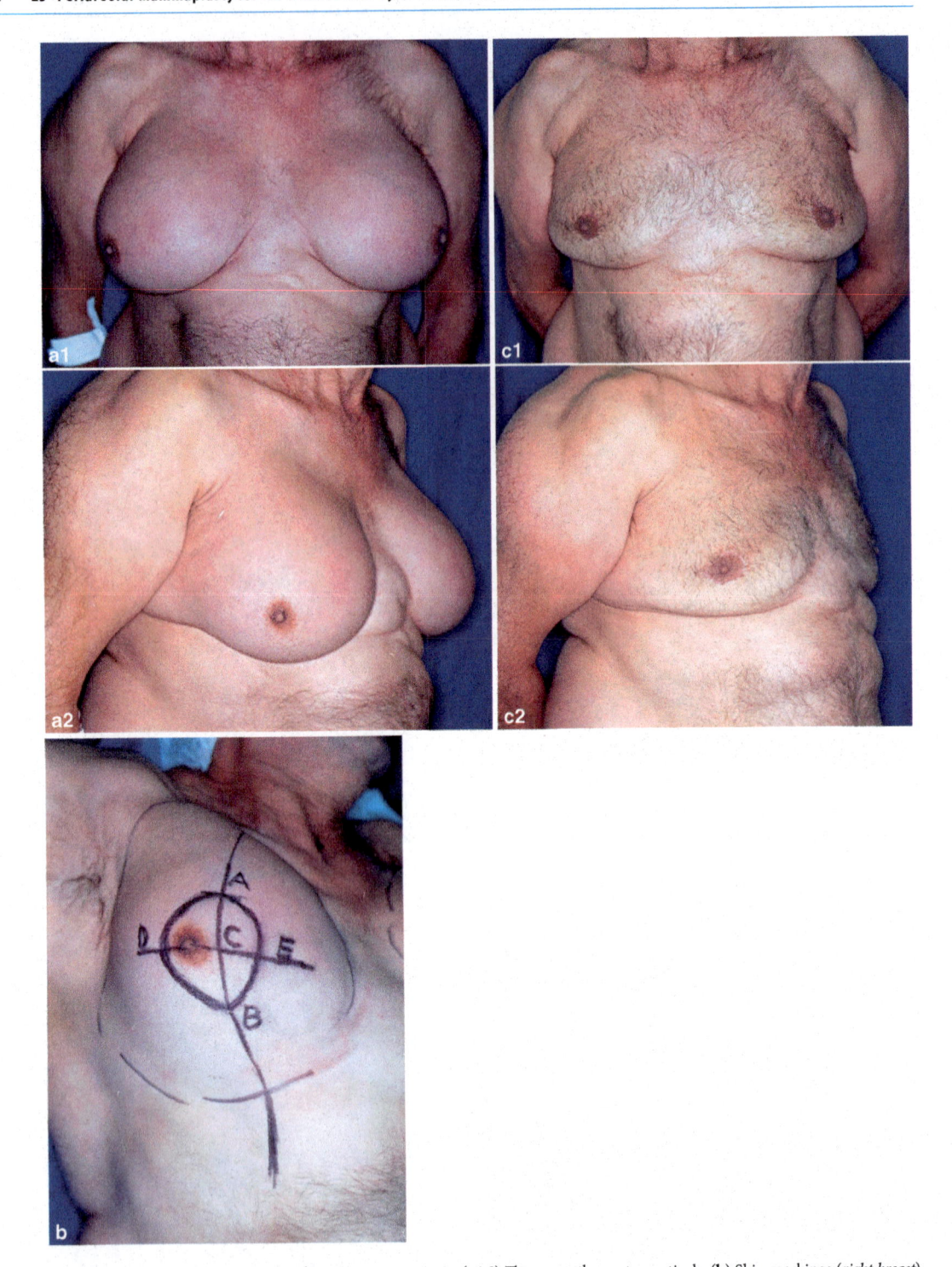

Fig. 23.4 (**a1,2**) Preoperative patient with severe gynecomastia. (**c1,2**) Three months postoperatively. (**b**) Skin markings (*right breast*) for superior pedicle technique, keeping more medial toward the breast meridian to keep the nipple–areola complex medially

The authors believe that the widening of the nipple–areola complex resulted from a small undermining of the remnant skin and tension in the suture by insufficient "closure" of the permanent periareolar circling. When there is marked tension in the suture, the purse string should be "closed" approximately 20% more than the desired areolar diameter. In our hands, this procedure was not always effective. It is important that the diameter of the skin that will be removed does not exceed twice that of the new areola. The patient should be advised about the possibility of a second-stage procedure. The redundant adipoglandular tissue in the inferior pole of the breast is credited to the fear of thinning excessively at the base of the flap.

The use of 2-0 monofilament nylon suture in the periareolar purse string in our first cases led to the extrusion of the suture material and infection in one case. This problem was solved with the use of 5-0 monofilament nylon and performing a tensionless purse string.

Marking of the point B, 4 cm proximally to the inframammary crease, seemed to limit its elevation up to the desired position of nipple–areola complex in some cases. Its marking of 1–2 cm higher would be better to adequately bring the purse string to the new position of the areola.

The use of the periareolar skin resection associated with inferior or superior pedicle flaps gave a high index of satisfaction to our patients and would be another option in well-selected cases (Figs. 23.2–23.4).

References

1. Simon BE, Hoffman S, Kahn S: Classification and surgical correction of gynecomastia. Plast Reconstr Surg 1973;51(1):48–52
2. Ward CM, Khalid K: Surgical treatment of grade III gynaecomastia. Ann Roy Coll Surg Engl 1989;71(4):226–228
3. Dufourmental L: L'incision aréolaire dans la chirurgie du sein. Bull Mem Soc Chir Paris 1928;20:9
4. Webster JP: Mastectomy for gynecomastia through semicircular intra-areolar incisions. Ann Surg 1946;124:557
5. Pitanguy I: Transareolar incision for gynecomastia. Plast Reconstr Surg 1966;38(5):414–419
6. Letterman G, Schurter M: Surgical correction of massive gynecomastia. Plast Reconstr Surg 1972;49(3):259–262
7. Hrinakova MF: Reduction mammaplasty in serious gynecomastias using a single superiorly based flap. Transaction of the VIII International Congress of Plastic Surgery, Montreal, Canada 1983, p 535
8. Pers M, Breteville-Jensen G: Reduction mammaplasty based on vertical vascular pedicle and "tennis ball" assembly. Scand J Plast Reconstr Surg 1972;6(1):61–68
9. Dufourmental C, Mouly R: Plastie mamaire par la methode oblique. Ann Chir Plast 1961;6:45
10. Wray RC, Hoopes J, Davis GM: Correction of extreme gynaecomastia. Br J Plast Surg 1974;27(1):39–41
11. Sinder R: Mamaplastia redutora – histórico. In: Cirurgia Plástica da Mama, Rio de Janeiro, MEDSI, 1989, chap 1, pp 1–35
12. Andrews JU, Yshizuki MM, Martins DM, Ramos RR: An areolar approach to reduction mammaplasty. Br J Plast Surg 1975;28(3):166–170
13. Ribeiro L: A new technique for reduction mammaplasty. Plast Reconstr Surg 1975;55(3):330–334
14. Davidson BA: Concentric circle operation for massive gynecomastia to excise the redundant skin. Plast Reconstr Surg 1979;63(3):350–354
15. Benelli L: Technique de plastie mammaire: le round block. Rev Fr Chir Esthet 1988;13:7–11
16. Martins PA: Mamaplastia periareolar com transposição de retalhos. Rev Bras Cir Plast 1991;6:8–10
17. Kornstein AN, Cinelli PB: Inferior pedicle reduction technique for larger forms of gynecomastia. Aesthetic Plast Surg 1992;16(4):331–335
18. Cunha MTR, Bento JFB: Periareolar mammaplasty for treating gynecomastia with breast ptosis. Prior note. Rev Soc Bras Cir Plast Est Reconstr 1993;8(1–3):125–130

Mastopexy Complications

Melvin A. Shiffman

24.1 Introduction

Each form of mastopexy has its own types of complications. Some general principles from many years of past experience are presented to help the surgeon minimize and possibly avoid the complications.

24.2 Complications

24.2.1 Asymmetry

Most patients have some asymmetry before surgery and should be specifically discussed with the patient. Correction of the asymmetry can be performed at the time of surgery. Sometime there is postoperative asymmetry from the procedure because of improper marking, not following the original markings, or because there is uneven healing and scarring from the procedure.

24.2.2 Bleeding, Hematoma

As with any surgical procedure, hemostasis at the time of surgery is important. However, postoperative bleeding is usually due to causes other than missing bleeders at the time of surgery. Clots can be dislodged by hypertension, coughing, or too much motion of the implant, especially with textured implants. Medications should be considered, especially aspirin and nonsteroidal anti-inflammatory drugs (NSAIDS). The use of Toradol after cosmetic procedures is a breach to the standard of care, as it is a drug that inhibit platelet reaction and cause bleeding.

Hematoma should be treated immediately by evacuation and coagulation of active bleeders, as distention of the tissues from the hematoma may result in tissue necrosis, especially of the nipple–areolar complex.

24.2.3 Bottoming Out

Most mastopexies do not fix the breast to the chest wall by sutures and, therefore, the weight of the breast can cause inferior migration, with "bottoming out" as the result (Fig. 24.1). This will usually require fixation of the breast to the underlying pectoralis major fascia, with permanent sutures to hold the breast in a high enough position and prevent future downward migration.

24.2.4 Flattening of the Breast

The periareolar mastopexy is very prone to flattening of the breast and patients should be forewarned of this possible problem.

24.2.5 Infection

Possible infection can occur with any surgical procedure. With the inset of fever and/or erythema, the surgeon should always be aware of the possible inflammation vs infection. Usually the patient is on antibiotics after surgery and a decision has to be made as to whether to increase the dose of medication or start a different antibiotic. If there is drainage, then culture and sensitivity should be done and appropriate antibiotic should be utilized when the particular offending germ or germs is known.

An abscess must be drained surgically and the cavity must be irrigated with saline. A drain (penrose or suction catheter) is usually necessary. If an implant is present, the implant should be removed if the pocket is involved, and the implant should be replaced at least 3 months after complete healing has occurred.

M.A. Shiffman (ed.), *Mastopexy and Breast Reduction: Principles and Practice*,
© Springer-Verlag Berlin Heidelberg 2009

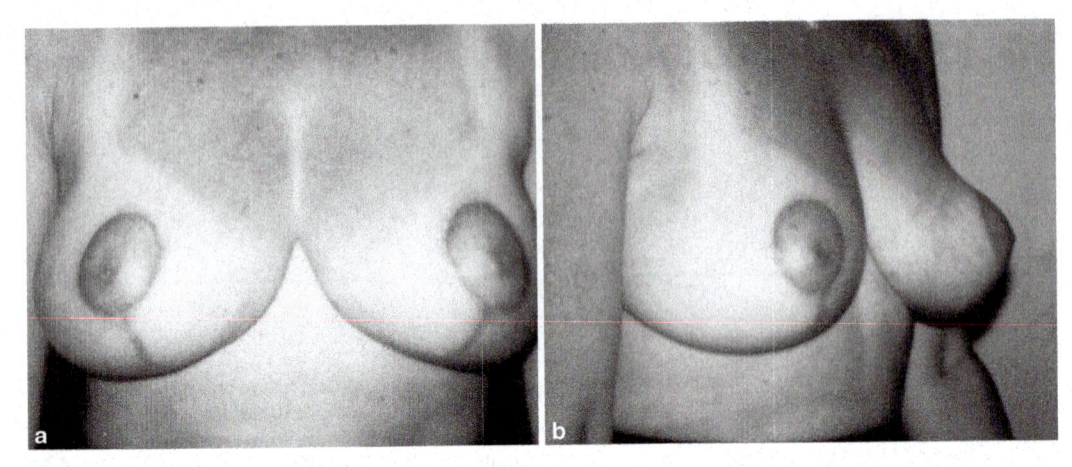

Fig. 24.1 Bottoming out after modified Arie Pitanguy mastopexy

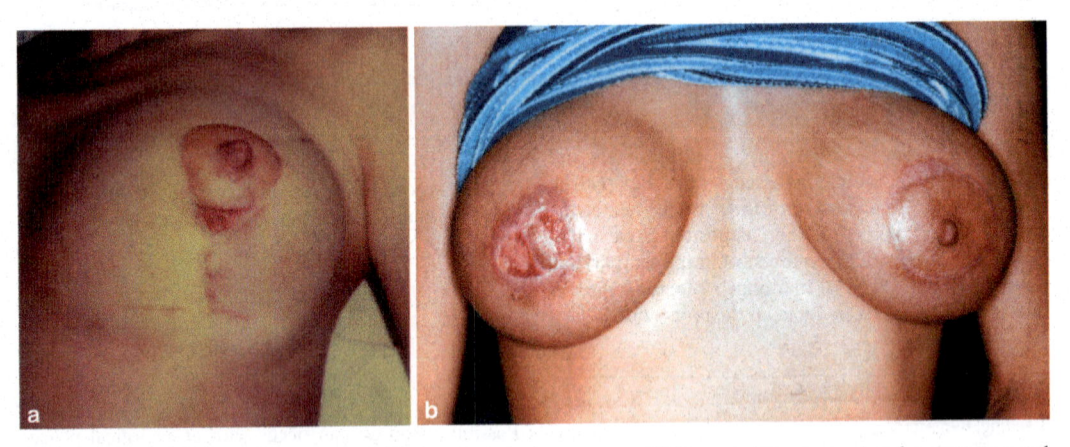

Fig. 24.2 Necrosis. (**a**) Necrosis following modified Arie Pitanguy mastopexy. (**b**) Necrosis following periareolar mastopexy and breast augmentation

24.2.6
Necrosis

Necrosis, especially of the nipple–areolar complex, is unusual but can occur when the blood supply has been compromised (usually from prior breast surgery) or when there is infection or hematoma (Fig. 24.2). Tight closure of the skin can result in necrosis if the vessels become stretched and thrombose, causing interrupted blood supply. There is a slightly increased incidence of necrosis when breast augmentation is concomitantly used at the time of mastopexy.

24.2.7
Pleating

The effect of closing the periareolar type of mastopexy is prone to a "pleating effect," because the larger outer rim is attached to a shorter inner rim and the discrepancy results in pleating (Fig. 24.3). This usually resolves without treatment in 6–12 months. However, when the pleating persists, the excess tissue may need to be excised, taking care not to disrupt the circumareolar purse string suture that holds the scar from spreading.

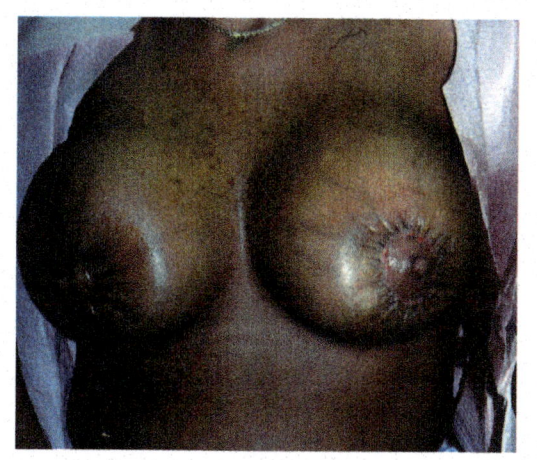

Fig. 24.3 Pleating following periareolar mastopexy

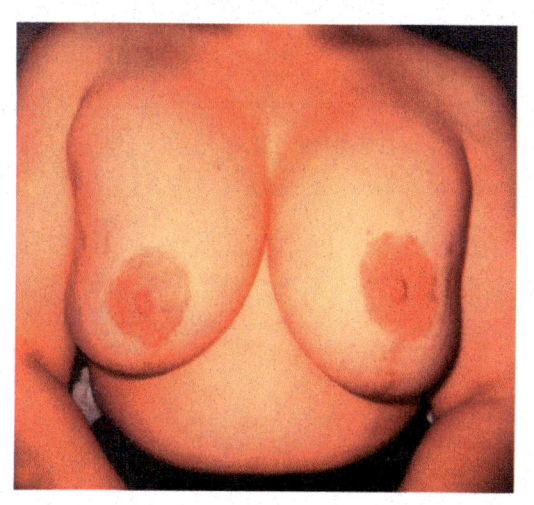

Fig. 24.4 Poor implant position following mastopexy

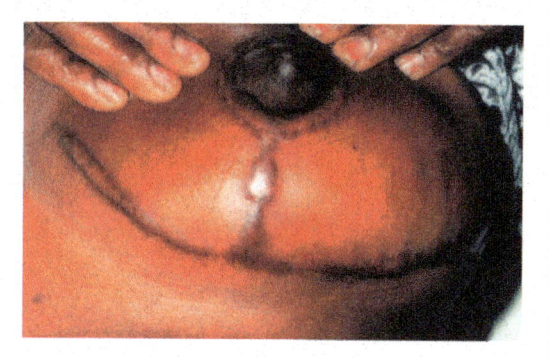

Fig. 24.5 Thickened scar following mastopexy

24.2.8
Poor Implant Position

If a breast augmentation is performed along with mastopexy, it is possible to place the implant in the proper position, as the pocket is determined preoperatively with marking prior to the breast lift (Fig. 24.4). This pocket position may need to be adjusted following the mastopexy and before the implant is placed or after the implant is in the pocket and the patient examined in a sitting position.

24.2.9
Recurrent Breast Ptosis

Recurrent breast ptosis is usually a problem of loose skin and gravity. Without fixation of the breast to the underlying pectoral major fascia by permanent sutures, the breast may descend postoperatively either within months or years.

24.2.10
Scar

Any surgical scar can become hypertrophic or keloid (Fig. 24.5). Tight skin closure may result in the widening of the scar, except with the purse string suture(s) of the periareolar mastopexy. The hypertrophic scar may resolve without treatment, while the keloid scar may become a difficult problem to treat, as it tends to recur in 80% of patients after treatment.

Kenalog (10–20 mg) injection diluted with 5-fluorouracil, 50 mg, seems to work fairly well for hypertrophic scars and keloids, but requires reinjection every few weeks. One must be careful while injecting into the center of the scar to prevent leakage into the deeper fatty tissues, which results in steroid fat atrophy. If steroid fat atrophy occurs, then tumescence with saline solution, which may be repeated in 30 days, will usually resolve the problem.

24.3
Discussion

It would behoove the surgeon performing mastopexy to learn how to avoid and to treat the various possible complications.

Part IV
Combined Mastopexy and Breast Reduction

Boustos' Technique of Periareolar Mastopexy and Breast Reduction

Jacques Faivre

25.1 Introduction

Boustos' periareolar technique for ptosis and moderate breast hypertrophy constitutes an important advancement in the cosmetic surgery of the breast. The technique provides excellent aesthetic results.

25.2 Periareolar Techniques

To understand Boustos' technique, it is necessary to discuss the periareolar techniques; there are three practical techniques:
1. Faivre Technique
2. Benelli Technique
3. Ribeiro Technique

25.2.1 Faivre Technique

This technique is an ideal method to limit the characteristics of the scar, resulting in a scar of good quality. The author, in 1975, published his modified technique to prevent secondary expansion of the areola. The precautions considered were the following:
1. Not removing a large area of subcutaneous tissue
2. Plication of the inferior pole of the gland without glandular incision, thereby, respecting the inferior anastomotic arcade of vessels
3. Deepithelialization

This technique is valuable to address minimal ptosis for an areola of 5 cm in diameter and deepithelialization of not more than 8 cm in vertical length. More than this, the areolar spread is inevitable. Without all this, the stability of the conoïd breast cannot last more than the 3 to 5 years following the intervention.

25.2.2 Benelli Technique

A principle to be aware of is to deepithelialize a wide area to relieve the cutaneous ptosis or the breast hypertrophy (Fig. 25.1). The unseemly skin that results is corrected using a purse string suture that is tightened, called the "round block." This suture will cause the inconvenience of a flattened breast. Benelli proposed a technique in which two or three areas of the inferior pole of the gland are tied down to the sternal periosteum. This technique is very inconvenient.

25.2.2.1 Limits

There are limitations to the use of the periareolar suture. To obtain a good periareolar scar, the following relationships should be respected: (1) deepithelialization of the areola is at 5 cm, with a maximum of 10 cm in the wide axis. (2) Deepithelialization at 2 cm supplementally gives an uncertain quality of the scar. (3) At more than 12 cm of the wide axis of deepithelialization, the suture is not reliable, the scar is of poor quality, and elongation of the areolar diameter is inevitable.

25.2.2.2 Inconveniences

Incising the Gland

At the inferior pole, there is a risk of compromising with the vascularity of the gland that is free and without skin attachment. The inferior pole of the breast gland has an anastomotic arcade, which is the point of the three vascular pedicles: external, internal, and posterior inferior. The portion of the gland that is deprived of its

M.A. Shiffman (ed.), *Mastopexy and Breast Reduction: Principles and Practice*,
© Springer-Verlag Berlin Heidelberg 2009

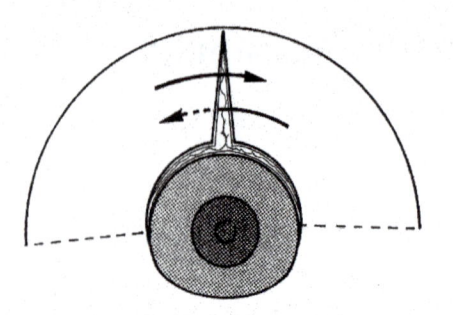

Fig. 25.1 Crossing of the gland sections with vertical sectioning. External gland piece attached to sternal periosteum and internal gland piece crossing over the external piece

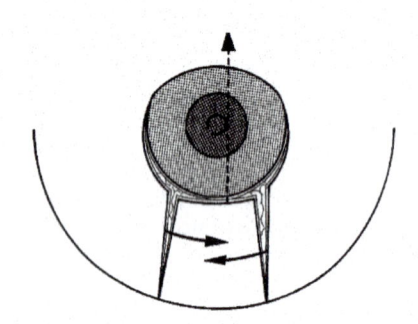

Fig. 25.2 The cut medial piece to the posterior pedicle raises the deep face of the gland. Two other sections are sutured. The detachment under the skin is important to pass a horizontal loop of the areola

attachments risks compromise with the inferior anastomosis (Fig. 25.2).

Breast Form

The procedure is not aesthetic. The breast takes a flat appearance like a "tomato," which is the result of poor plastic surgery.

Stability of the Breast

The breast gland is free from its attachments in 2/3 of the superior circumference and remains attached only between 10 and 12 o'clock. The gland-to-gland or gland-to-periosteum sutures that serve to remodel the breast are not reliable for the long term. Benelli feels that the connections of the scar secondary to the detachment support the gland, but experiences prove that this is uncertain and often illusory. The lifting of the breast by superior dermal attachment often poses problems.

25.2.3
Ribeiro Technique

This procedure is for ptosis and moderate hypertrophy with ptosis. The projection of the breast is assured by the incision and vertical lift of a quadrilateral gland pedicle at the posterior inferior base respecting the anastomotic arcade between the different vascular systems. The two glandular portions, external and internal, are flaps to remodel the gland.

The inconveniences of the technique are the following:
1. Frequent difficulty in lifting the nipple–areolar complex
2. Poor modeling of the gland
3. As with the Benelli technique, the intercutaneous glandular detachments that are necessary compromise with the long-term stability of the breast.

25.3
Boustos Technique

The principles are as follows:
1. Removing the excess skin and cutaneous glandular detachment
2. The excess gland is removed at the superior pole and at the posterior surface of the gland, without going past the fourth intercostal space to respect the posterior inferior vascularity of the gland and areola
3. Lifting the nipple–areola complex assures a graceful vertical median pedicle
4. The stability of the remodeled gland is from placing a piece of Dacron or Vicryl that constitutes deep breast support

25.3.1
Description of the Technique

25.3.1.1
Plan

Plan a straight line xy (Fig. 25.3) to the middle of the clavicle, around the top of the areola and up to the middle of the inframammary fold. Mark two points on the right (Fig. 25.4):
1. Point a is situated between 17 and 21 cm from the mid clavicle
2. Point b is situated between 6 and 8 cm from the inframammary fold

25.3 Boustos Technique

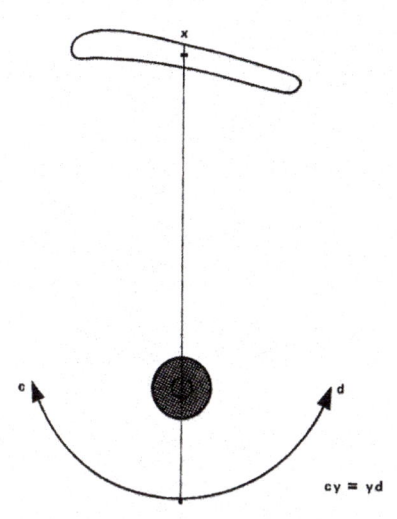

Fig. 25.3 Plan the vertical part from the mid clavicle towards the middle of the inframammary fold and loop to the top of the areola

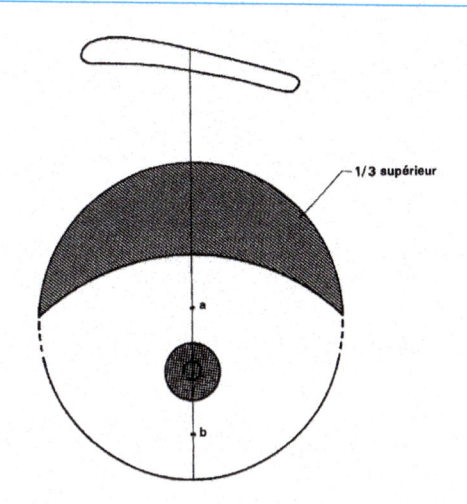

Fig. 25.5 The external limits of the gland and ½ superior part of the gland

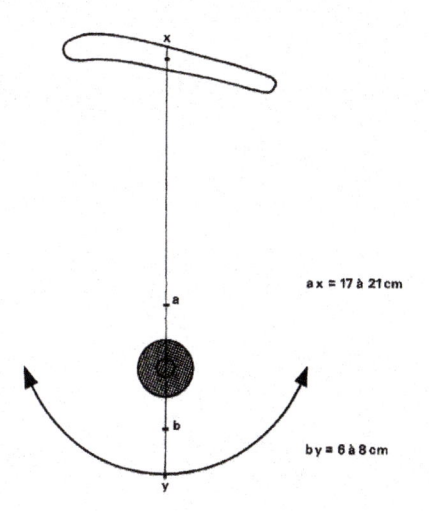

Fig. 25.4 Limit the cut of the new areola and the zone of deepithelialization fixed at points a and b on the vertical axis xy, a is between 17 and 21 cm to point x and b is between 6 and 8 cm from point y

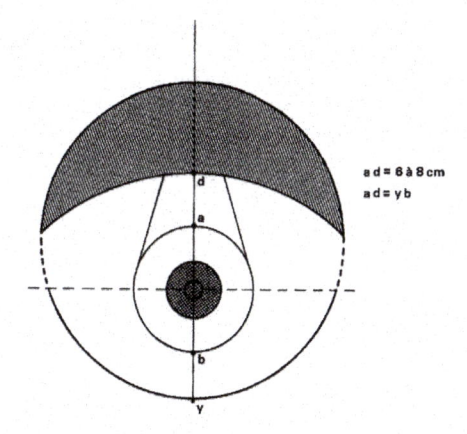

Fig. 25.6 Plan the medial piece that permits lifting of the nipple areola complex

The two points reunite at the arc defining the zone of periareolar deepithelialization. The limits of the new areola define, in general, a diameter of 4 cm.

25.3.1.2
Afterwards

1. Locate the external limits around the perimeter of the gland (Figs. 25.5 and 25.6).
2. Define the superior 1/3rd of the gland that is superficial or is attached between the gland and the skin.
3. Mark a horizontal at the apex of the areola, which will limit the gland.
4. Mark at the midline a quadrilateral at the wider inferior base of the top.
5. Laterally, the internal and external triangles whose angles correspond to the base of the mid quadrilateral are defined.

25.3.1.3
Infiltration

The fat cells are infiltrated to facilitate the inter-cutaneoglandular tissues. This infiltration is on practically the whole surface of the conoid breast, except the level of the superior 1/3 or the attachments of skin to gland.

25.3.1.4
Detachment of the Inter-Cutaneo-Glandular Tissues

Large detachment of the inter-cutaneous gland tissue should not go beyond the gland limits. At the inferior limit of the gland, a beveled cut is made to reach the plane of the pectoralis major muscle. When this is attained, the gland is detached at the deep base as far as the superior limit. The principal artery, a branch to the internal mammary, is at the second intercostal space and, not as often, at the third intercostal space, which should be preserved intact.

25.3.1.5
Retroglandular Detachment

The detachment of the retroglandular portion of the breast gland starts at the level of union of the superior 1/3rd and middle 1/3rd, descending to the avascular space of Chassaignac as far as the level of the areola. It should not go beyond the fourth intercostal space.

25.3.1.6
Gland Resection

In this way the gland is freed from the deep face, and the superficial face can be exteriorized to be examined. First, the incision of the medial gland in the inferior base follows the defined limits of the skin. The glandular resection starts at the superior limit, removing the two lateral triangles contiguous with the medial part, descending to the posterior gland and stopping at the level of the fourth intercostal space (Figs. 25.7, 25.8).

25.3.1.7
Repair of the Conoid Breast

The middle of the gland is fixed to the pectoral major muscle and to the deep superior 1/3rd of the detached gland. A lateral suture on the pieces of the lateral internal and the lateral external gland in this way will lift the gland. The inferior pole of the gland at a distance of 6–8 cm corresponding to the distance already marked is made fast at several points of the breast gland to the muscle aponeurosis of the abdomen (Figs. 25.9–25.12). The glandular cone is thus restored. If the projection of the nipple–areola complex is judged insufficient, an external plication can augment the projection.

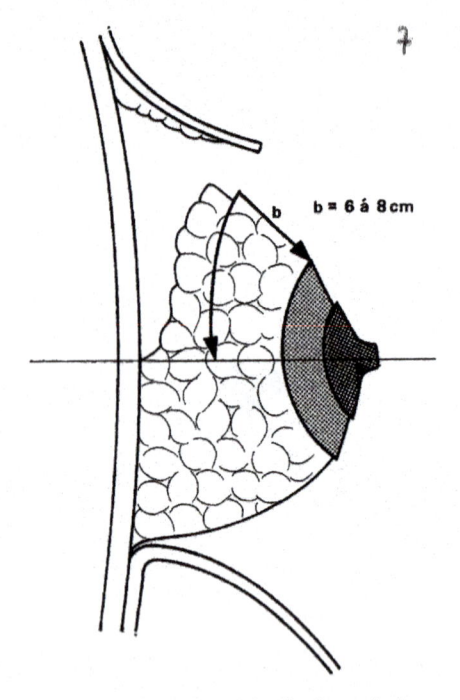

Fig. 25.7 Resection at the face of the gland completely preserving the vascularization of the gland (external, internal, posterior, and anastomotic arcade)

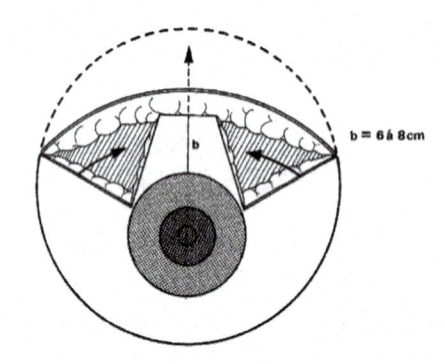

Fig. 25.8 The gland resection that descends to the deep face of the gland as far as, not past, the height of the fourth intercostal space

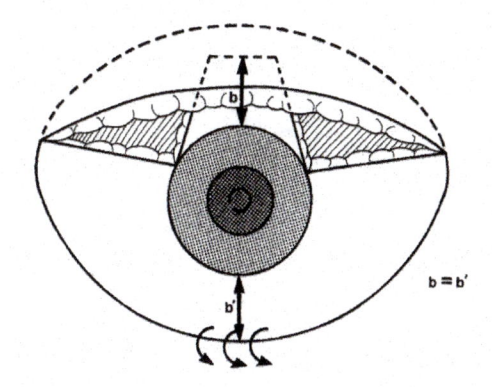

Fig. 25.9 The arrow indicates the lifting of the mid gland to the deep face of the 1/3rd superior part of the gland and the lateral part brought towards the mid part

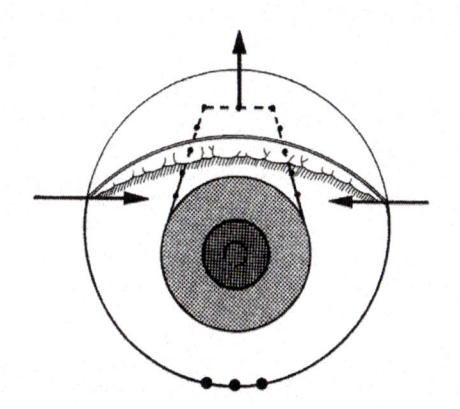

Fig. 25.10 The plan is to suture the gland at the level of the submammary fold to restore the fold

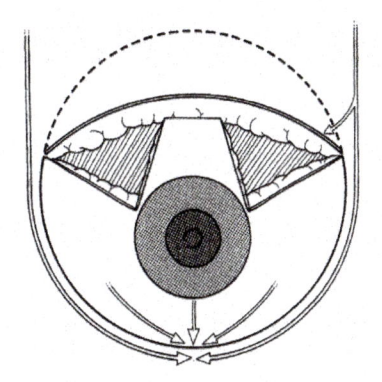

Fig. 25.11 Suturing of the conoid breast is finished. The superior part of the gland is placed at the deep face of the 1/3rd superior part not adherent to the skin

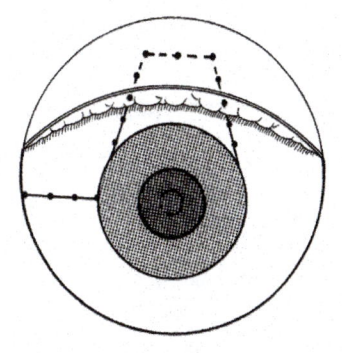

Fig. 25.12 It is necessary to give projection to the nipple–areolar complex. An external suture following the generation of the conoid breast may possibly be useful

25.3.1.8
Detachment of the Periareolar Dermal Strip

Later, the periareolar dermal strip is detached to the limits of the areolar dermis.

25.3.1.9
Placing a Patch of Dacron or Vicryl

The patch should be placed without excessive tension in a manner that the two superior edges correspond to the superior breast gland quadrants (Fig. 25.13). It needs to put in place three periareolar points under the dermal bandage before detachment, one medial and two lateral. It does not need points to be placed on the superior pole. The patch is to take up the slack of the breast without tension and the sutures are limited to the corresponding muscular external aponeurosis. No suture is placed at the level of the superior pole of the gland, allowing normal development in the case of pregnancy.

25.3.1.10
Drainage

Aspiration drainage is placed in the axillary region.

25.3.1.11
Suture

The areolar suture is then placed without difficulty. Points that are completely separated are closed with a continuous intradermal suture.

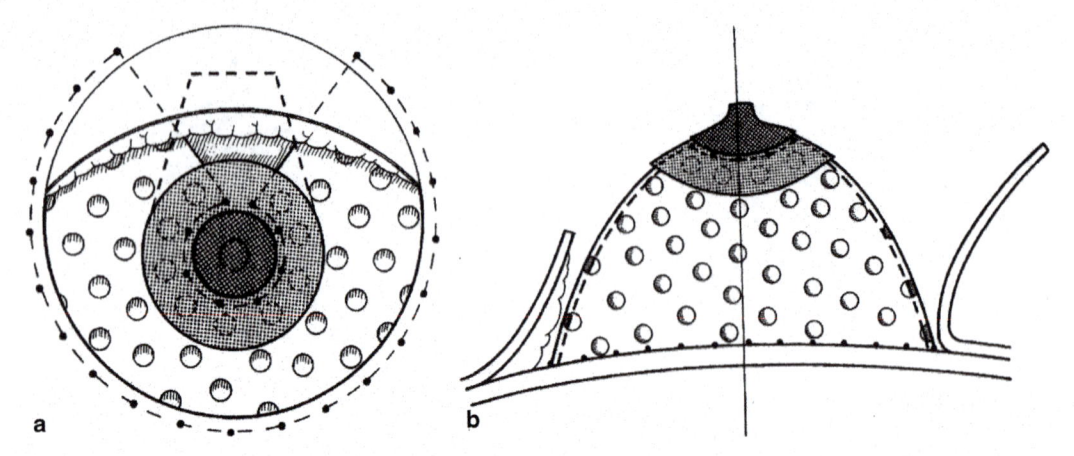

Fig. 25.13 Looking at the (**a**) face and (**b**) profile shows placement of a sheet of Dacron or Vicryl. This remains open to view the superior pole of the gland and to suture beneath the dermal strip, first removing contact with the areolar skin, and laterally at the muscle aponeurosis corresponding to the length of the base of the breast

25.3.1.12
Bandage

Bandage is important. The aim is to model the skin perfectly to restore the detached conoid breast gland. Adhesive bandages help to place, in this manner, the external side of the gland then the internal side. Finally, the superior pole is bandaged and kept in place for 15 days.

25.4
Advantages of the Technique

1. It does not risk areolar spreading.
2. The lift of the areolar complex is easily done.
3. It is an anatomic intervention that respects the vascularization of the deep part of the breast gland cut parts and the resected gland between the internal and external vascular pedicle at the superior pole of the gland.
4. The incised tissue of the geometric gland allows excellent remodeling of the gland and breast harmony is obtained.
5. The perpetual result is assured with the placement of a piece of Dacron or Vicryl that gives deep breast support. The risk of intolerance is about 1%.

25.5
Conclusions

This new intervention that is anatomic in concept brings an elegant solution to minimize the scar of the areola in all patients with ptosis and hypertrophy with ptosis, wherever the glandular excision does not surpass 500 g.

Dermal Purse String Reduction Mastopexy

Franco Marconi, Filippo Brighetti

26.1
Introduction

Despite the inventiveness, skill and efforts on the part of plastic surgeons to set up an ideal method for correction, reduction mammaplasty remains one of the most problematic and exciting chapters of plastic surgery. Many advances have been made since the time of Biesenberger, and patients can now be assured of good average results in terms of morphology, projection, symmetry, and residual scars. The ideal reduction mammaplasty still, however, does not exist and probably never will.

Every surgeon uses his or her own most suitable methods, and although the creators of new techniques tend to urge their colleagues to adopt these, perhaps this is a mistake, because the same clinical results will not necessarily be obtained from the hands of others. Thus, the main duty of the scientist should be to publish his achievements and submit his results for public approval and review.

The senior author carried out his first reduction mammaplasty using a personal technique in 1987. This technique was inspired by the impressive work of Marchac [1] and his correction method. The results were first published in 1989 [2] and then in 1993 [3] and since then the technique has not been modified.

The basic concepts of the purse string mammaplasty are (a) to create a support for the reduced gland to delay postoperative ptosis; (b) to drastically reduce the length of the inframammary scar. All surgical techniques attempt to delay postoperative ptosis; some methods also reduce the inframammary scar.

26.2
Surgical Technique

26.2.1
Preoperative Markings

The preoperative markings are the same as those described by Marchac and de Olarte [1], the ideal breast axis being 9–10 cm from the midsternal line. This axis is extended below the inframammary fold and used as a reference point when tracing the extent of the area for deepithelialization. This area is established by moving the breast laterally and medially and tracing on the breast the maximum lateral and medial points. A line is drawn between these points, over the top of the areola (at about 1/2 cm from the latter) and below, indicating the new inframammary fold at 3–5 cm from the natural one. The extent to which the fold is raised depended on the degree of breast ptosis and was directly proportional to this. The shape of the area traced is that of an arched gateway (Marchac) (Fig. 26.1).

26.2.2
Reduction Mammaplasty

The skin is deepithelialized from the previously traced cutaneous area, isolating the nipple–areola complex. If the latter is excessively large, it could be made smaller, keeping in mind that to obtain an areola with a diameter of 4–4.5 cm, it is always preferable to allow for a larger areolar area, even up to 6 cm (if possible), to avoid excessive tension when the areola is sutured to its new site. A dermal flap incision is made under the areola in the shape of an isosceles trapezoid with its widest base on the line aa_1. The flap is lifted and turned back (Fig. 26.2).

Glandular dissection is started from below, from the baseline. The gland and fat are separated from the skin along a superficial (subcutaneous) plane until the pectoralis major muscle is reached in correspondence with the natural inframammary fold. Stripping is continued upward and the entire breast is lifted away from the pectoralis major muscle (Fig. 26.3). Once the breast is released, a wedge-shaped resection was made, as described by Pitanguy [4], up to the tip of the breast. During this stage, a clinical assessment is made to determine the most hypertrophic quadrants and the parts of the gland to be eliminated (Fig. 26.4).

The breast unit is reformed by suturing the two hemispheres together and suspending them with absorbable sutures on the pectoralis major muscle (Fig. 26.5). Maintaining the dermal flap in a raised

M.A. Shiffman (ed.), *Mastopexy and Breast Reduction: Principles and Practice*,
© Springer-Verlag Berlin Heidelberg 2009

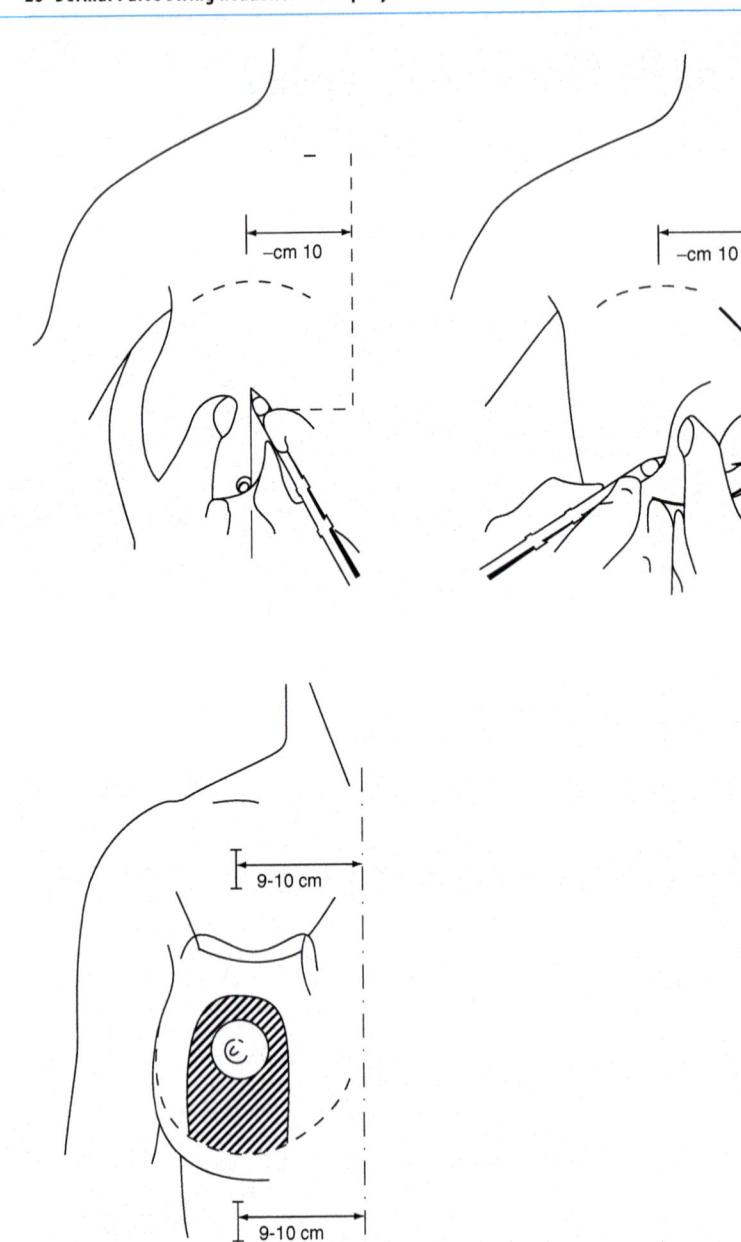

208 26 Dermal Purse String Reduction Mastopexy

Fig. 26.1 (*Above*) The ideal breast axis is found approximately 10 cm from the midsternal line. Lines are traced indicating the boundaries of the area to be stripped, which at the top surrounds the areola. (*Below*) The area within the broken lines represents the zone to be stripped. The new inframammary fold will fall approximately 3–5 cm from the natural inframammary fold

position, lateral and medial incisions (lines ab and a_1b_1) (Fig. 26.6) are made in the dermis where it joins the skin. Scissors is used to detach enough of the subdermis for the two dermal triangles and the gland below to slide toward the center without tension. The medial part of the gland is then sutured. The two strips of dermis are designed to facilitate suturing and to guarantee a better hold.

When gland suturing is completed, the flap of dermis previously prepared is turned back over the breast and sutured to the pectoralis major muscle 1 cm above the new inframammary fold (Fig. 26.7). Center of the

26.2 Surgical Technique

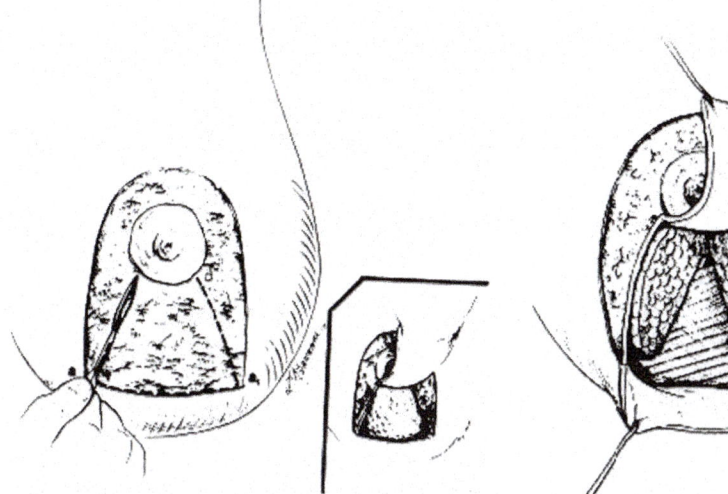

Fig. 26.2 (*Above*) Dermal flap incision is made under the areola in the shape of an isosceles trapezoid. (*Below*) The flap is lifted and turned back

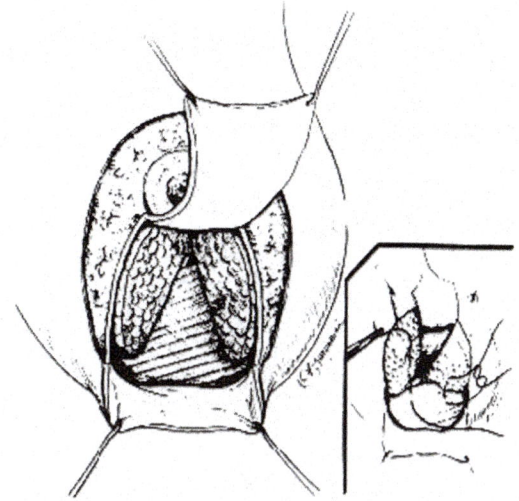

Fig. 26.4 (*Above*) A wedge-shaped resection is made in the breast. (i) The breast is suspended on the pectoralis major muscle

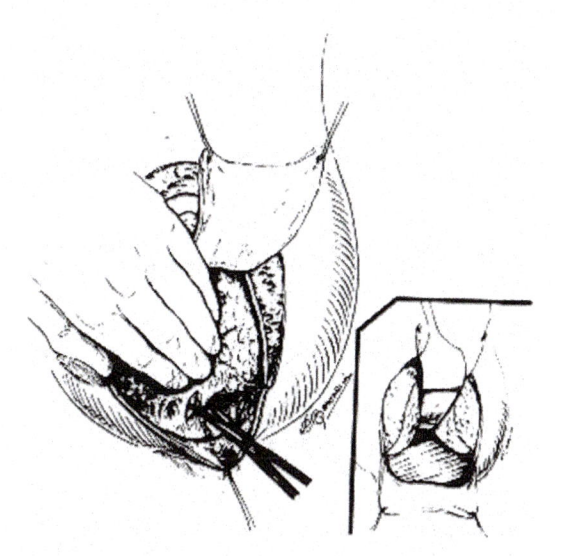

Fig. 26.3 (*Above*) Separation of the mammary gland and the fat from the skin down to the natural inframammary fold. (*Below*) The entire gland is lifted away from the pectoralis major muscle

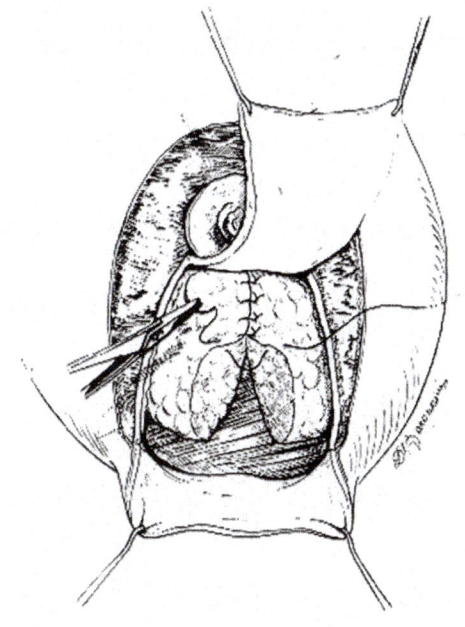

Fig. 26.5 The two hemispheres are sutured together

new inframammary fold is created by joining the two points aa$_1$ (3–5 cm above the natural fold). The resulting dog-ear is treated using the dermal purse string method (Fig. 26.8).

Vertical suturing is started from below, the point corresponding to the south areolar pole is found at approximately 5–6 cm from the new inframammary fold. The areola is then placed in its new position and any excess skin eliminated (Fig. 26.9). Subcutaneous and cutaneous suturing is completed. Jackson–Pratt suction drainages were always inserted and kept in place for an average of 3 days.

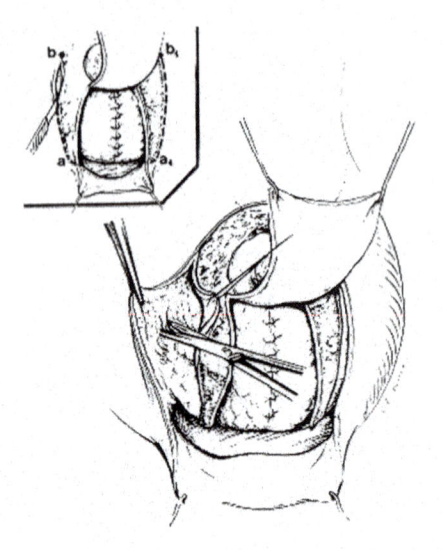

Fig. 26.6 (*Above*) Dermal incision along the lines ab and a_1b_1. (*Below*) Separation of the two dermal triangles from the breast skin and subdermal separation to permit the central suturing of the two dermal triangles

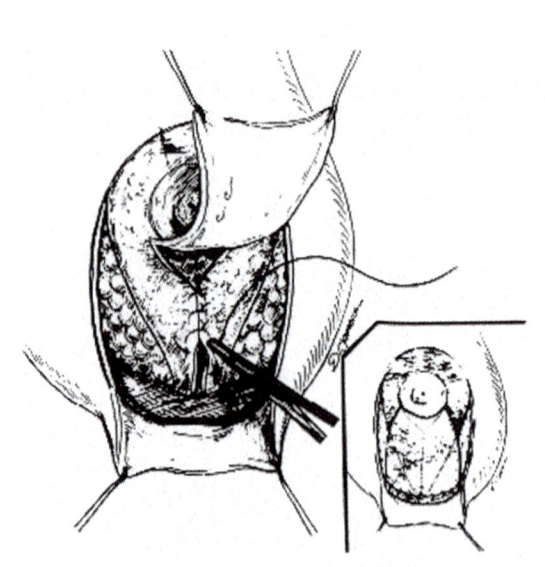

Fig. 26.7 (*Above*) The two dermal triangles are sutured together. (*Below*) The previously prepared dermal flap is sutured to the pectoralis major muscle approximately 1 cm from the point of the new inframammary fold. An outline of the two triangular flaps of dermis sutured together is shown beneath

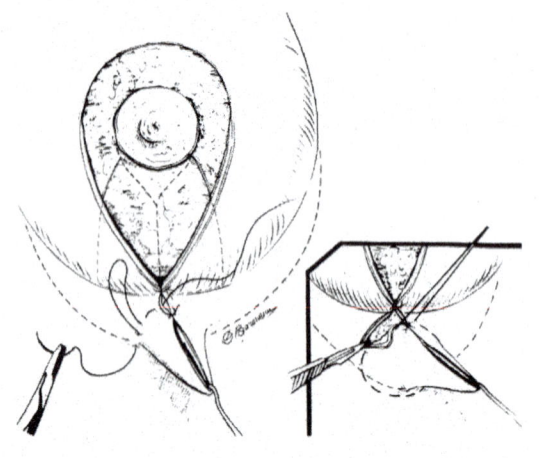

Fig. 26.8 (*Above*) Joining of points a and a_1 corresponding to the center of the new inframammary fold. (*Below*) Preparation of the purse string by excision of the lower dog-ear

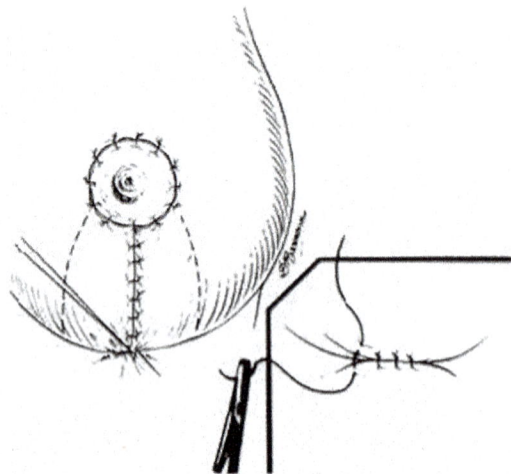

Fig. 26.9 (*Above*) When the purse string is complete, the vertical suturing is made with the areola in its new position. (*Below, right*) Detail of the scar at the inframammary fold

26.2.3
Mastopexy

Mastopexy involved a different surgical procedure. After stripping the epithelium from the area delimited by the preoperative drawing and after isolating the nipple-areola complex, a rectangular dermal flap incision is made under the areola. The bottom part of the flap is raised. As with reduction mammaplasty, the adipose-glandular tissue is separated from the skin along a subdermal plane, reaching the pectoralis major muscle at the natural inframammary fold. The entire gland is then lifted off the pectoralis major muscle and sutured in its new position with absorbable sutures (Fig. 26.10).

The dermal flap is placed over the breast and sutured 1 cm above the new inframammary fold. As with reduction mammaplasty, the tip of the new inframammary fold is created. Again, vertical suturing is started from below, and the southern areolar pole is 5–6 cm from the new fold. The dog-ear is treated in the same way as with reduction mammaplasty, and the areola is positioned in its new site (Fig. 26.11). Jackson–Pratt suction drainages are always inserted and kept in place for an average of 3 days.

26.3 Discussion

26.3.1 Postoperative Ptosis

The double dermal support provided by purse string mammaplasty provides a strong counter-measure to the force of gravity and tissues laxity. This is at least one of the theoretical assumptions. Basically, the gland is held by two dermal layers plus the skin. These three barriers should delay the sliding of the gland downwards.

The only way to verify this assumption is by follow-up. The first report [3] of 25 consecutive cases with a mean follow-up of 31.5 months described a 96% of minimal or moderate postoperative ptosis and only 4% of severe postoperative ptosis. These data encouraged the first author to continue with this method.

A new review has now been made of 40 cases with a mean follow-up of 84 months. The new data are certainly more significant and can probably be considered as a more realistic clinical assessment of the value of the technique. The results showed 70% of minimal or moderate ptosis and 30% of severe ptosis.

In terms of correction (of mammary ptosis), the technique appears to provide statistically reliable results and good patient satisfaction (Figs. 26.12 and 26.13).

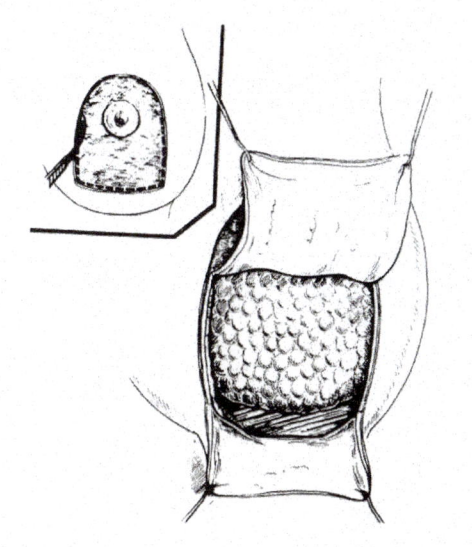

Fig. 26.10 (*Above*) Rectangular dermal flap incision beneath the areola. (*Below*) The flap is raised, and the entire gland is lifted off the pectoralis major muscle

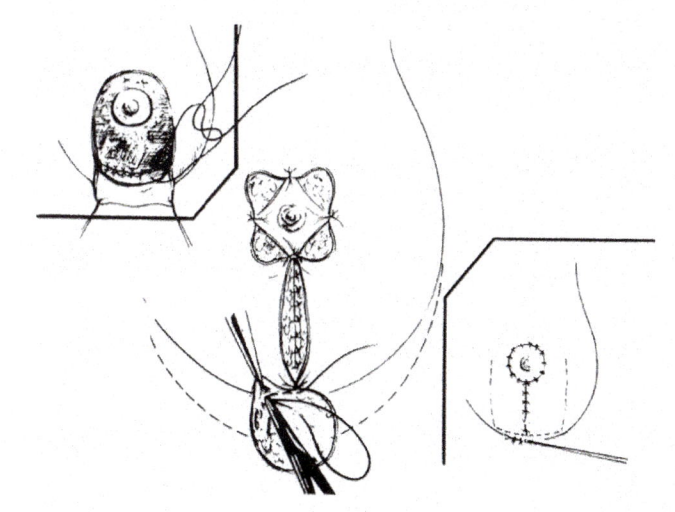

Fig. 26.11 (*Above*) The flap is sutured to the pectoralis major muscle 1 cm above the point of the new inframammary fold. (*Center*) The inframammary fold is made. Starting from the vertical suture, the nipple–areola complex is positioned. Then the dog-ear is dealt with. (*Below*) Suturing the dermal flap to the pectoralis major muscle beneath

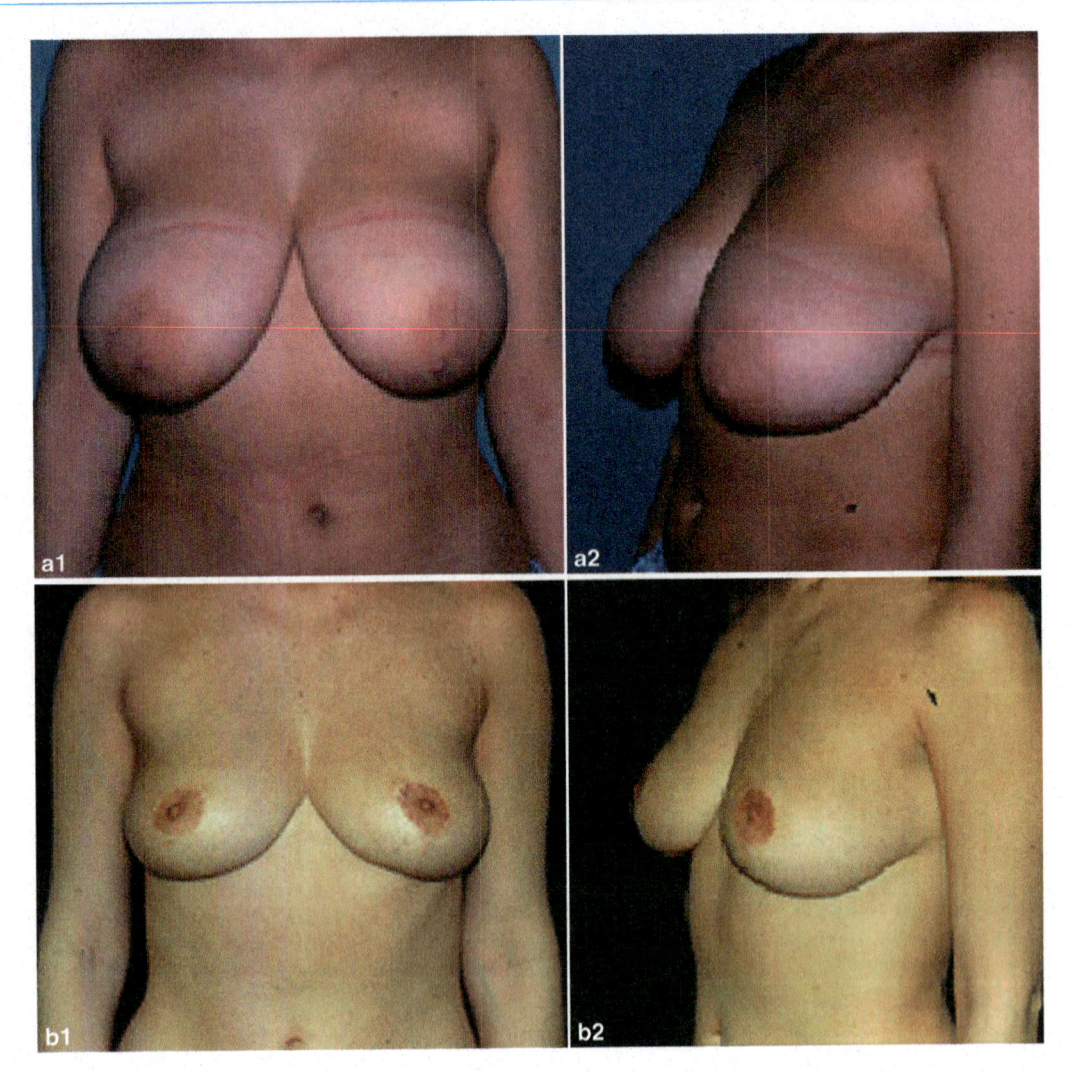

Fig. 26.12 (*a1,2*) Preoperative bilateral hypertrophy and mammary ptosis. (*b1,2*) Eight years postoperative

The 30% of severe postoperative ptosis can be considered as an acceptable value.

26.3.2
Scar

Purse string mammaplasty makes it possible to obtain a very short scar at the inframammary sulcus. The problems related to inframammary scars are well-known and plastic surgeons try to reduce these as much as possible. The first report [3] was also encouraging as regards the quality of the inframammary scar. This was very short, not longer than 4 cm, and located at the lower pole of the breast and usually hidden by the breast after a few months due to natural postoperative ptosis.

Although at the end of the operation the scar appears constricted, visible, and of poor quality, after some months it generally becomes less evident, the colour tends to be similar to that of the surrounding skin and the boundaries tend to merge.

The majority of complications refers to the purse string area. In the first report [3], 20% of the complications were related to this area. This new analysis shows a similar percentage of complications for this area. Diastasis of the purse string area is the most important complication

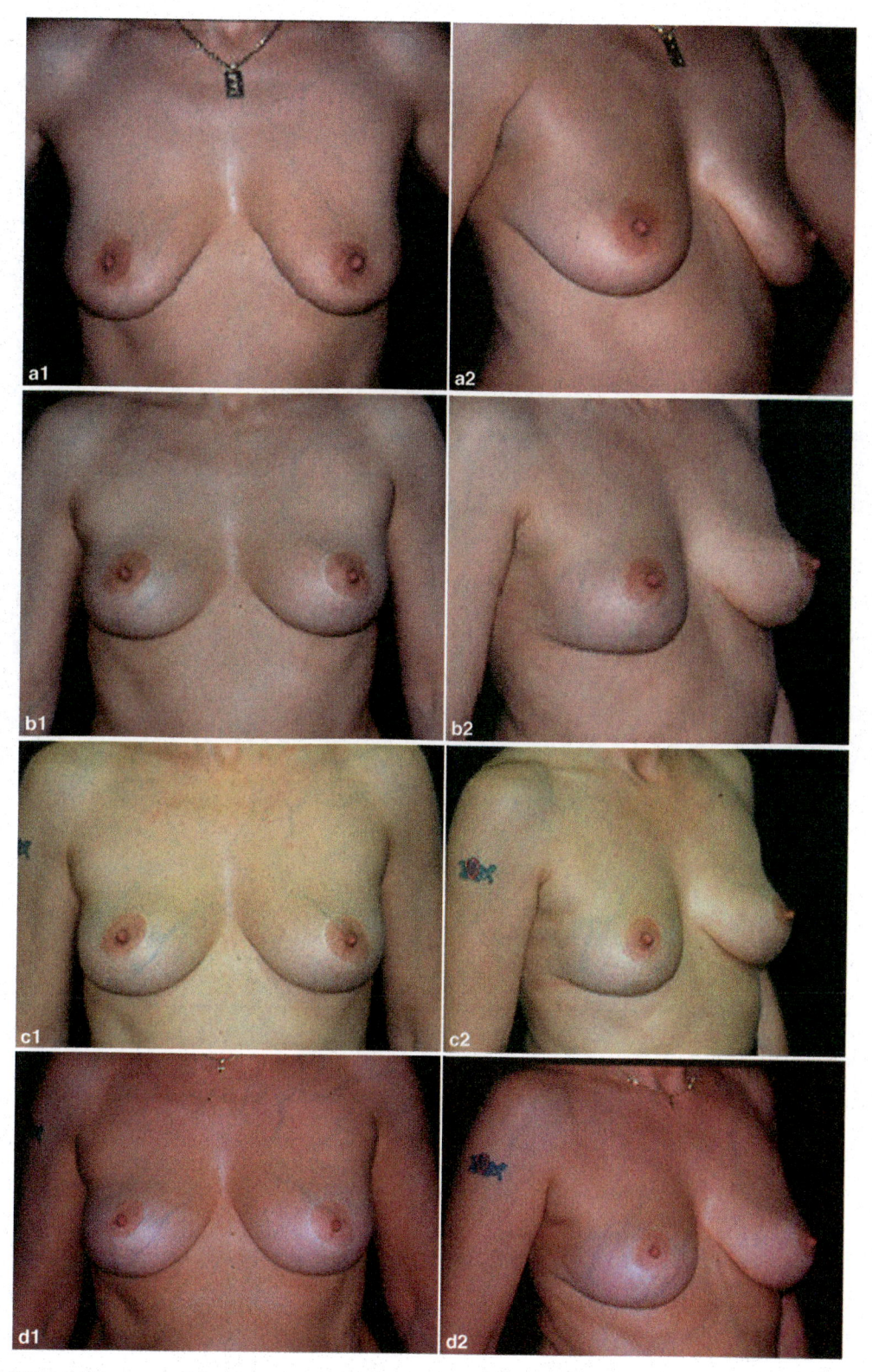

Fig. 26.13 (*a1,2*) Preoperative bilateral mammary ptosis. (*b1,2*) Two years postoperative. (*c1,2*) Six years postoperative. (**d**) Twelve years postoperative

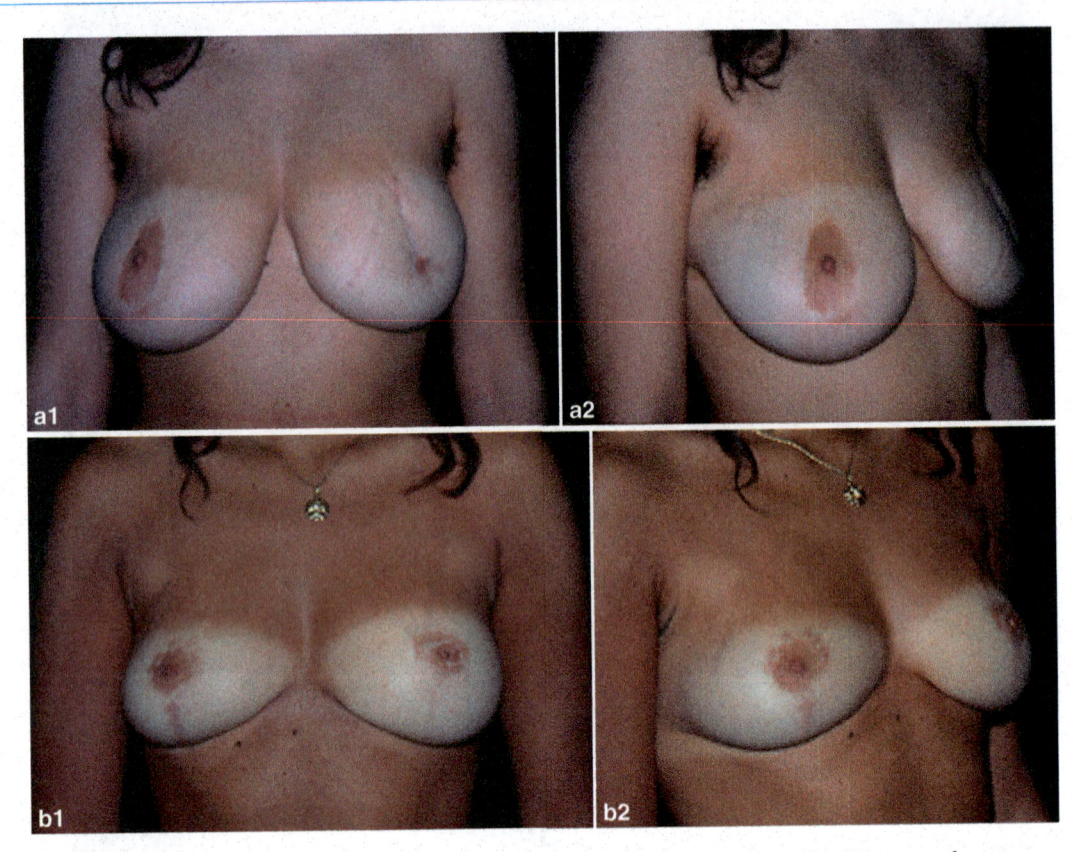

Fig. 26.14 Outcomes of breast reduction with nipple–areola complex necrosis. (**a***1,2*) Preoperative. (**b***1,2*) Two years after surgery

(15%) followed by hypertrophic scars or keloids, which are less common. Necrosis of the nipple areolar area may result in scar and loss of pigmentation (Fig. 26.14). for this reason, and with a follow-up that is worth-while, it must be defined as "another technique" in our hands.

26.4 Conclusions

As doctors and plastic surgeons, we have a debt of gratitude towards the surgeons of the past, each one of which has provided us with the seeds of knowledge and the fertility of inspiration to improve our surgical techniques. Certainly the embryo of every new surgical technique is to be found in the past and, inevitably, this new progress provides new stimulus for future developments.

Purse string mammaplasty, like other surgical techniques, is traveling along the road towards improved clinical results with breast reductions and pexies. We have not reached the destination but are merely a step along the way;

References

1. Marchac D, de Olarte G: Reduction mammaplasty and correction of ptosis with a short inframammary scar. Plast Reconstr Surg 1982;69(1):45–55
2. Marconi F: The dermal purse-string suture: a new technique for a short inframammary scar in reduction mammaplasty and dermal mastopexy. Ann Plast Surg 1989;22(6): 484–493
3. Marconi F, Cavina C: Reduction mammaplasty and correction of ptosis: a personal technique. Plast Reconstr Surg 1993;91(6):1046–1056
4. Pitanguy I: Surgical treatment of breast hypertrophy. Br J Plast Surg 1967;20(1):78–85

Breast Reduction/Mastopexy with Short Inverted T Scar

Toma T. Mugea

27.1 Introduction

Poor scars, breast size error, odd shape, and unequal breasts are the commonest causes of postoperative dissatisfaction. Women request this operation for functional reasons and are willing to accept complications, but would obviously like the best cosmetic outcome possible. There is a point at which reduced scar burden is not worth a trade for compromised breast shape and nipple areola complex (NAC) aesthetics.

Breast reduction is a common and continually evolving procedure. There are many surgical procedures for reduction mammaplasty [1]. Each presents particular advantages in terms of indications, vascular preservation, technique design, ease of realization, minimum scarring, maintenance of innervation, long-term results, etc.

Despite the aesthetic complications of poor scars, asymmetry of breast shape, and the NAC, this operation shows a high degree of long-term satisfaction of the patients [2, 3]. Because of the rich mammary vascularization and the importance of preserving the vascular integrity of the NAC [4], the great majority of breast reduction techniques have based their design on preserving the vascularization of this complex. It is also important to preserve the innervation of the NAC [5, 6], and the integrity and the continuity of the galactophorous ducts [7, 8]. Strömbeck [9] set a golden standard with his mammaplasty technique in 1960. A few years later, for small reductions and for mastopexies, Pitanguy [10] showed how to minimize the submammary scar and how to improve the shape of the reduced breast and the position of the NAC. Very large breasts were better managed by the technique of McKissock [11] in 1972. This replaced the widely performed Strombeck [9] technique. Soon thereafter, in 1977, an inferior pedicle technique was proposed by Robbins [12]. This technique became popular and it is still used for relieving breast hypertrophy and ptosis.

The author uses Robbins technique, with several technical variations that eliminate the main drawback of the original procedure: the long submammary scar. The modification includes a precise preoperative breast assessment using TTM chart [13], a precise planning and marking prior to surgery, and also several combined maneuvers based on the breast fascial and ligamentous anatomy. The primary indication of the procedure is mammary hyperplasia and/or ptosis of moderate to severe degree.

27.2 Breast Fascia and Sustaining Ligaments

Breast shape and contour are influenced by the volume of the breast parenchyma, the amount and location of the subcutaneous and intraparenchymal fat, the body contour of the chest wall, its muscular covering and thickness, and the tightness and elastic quality of the skin. The fascial attachments of the breast to the underlying chest wall also influence breast appearance.

The breast develops and is contained within supporting layers of superficial fascia. The superficial layer of this superficial fascia is the outer layer covering the breast parenchyma, located near the dermis and is not always distinct from it. More distinct is the superficial fascia's deep layer on the deep posterior surface of the breast. A loose areolar area is interposed between the deep layer of the superficial fascia and the superficial layer of the deep fascia that covers the outer layer of musculature chest wall. The retromammary space will allow the breast tissue to have a natural gliding over the chest. The superficial layer of the deep fascia overlays the outer surface of the pectorals major, the upper portion of the rectus abdominis, the medial serratus anterior, and the external oblique muscle in the lower central breast. This fascia is thinner over the muscular portions of the pectorals major and the serratus anterior [14].

Although the pectoral fascia is very thin, it is a dense tissue and its integrity can be carefully preserved during dissection. The connective tissue that supports structures of the breast (Cooper's ligaments) runs from the deep muscle fascia, through the breast parenchyma, to the dermis of the overlying skin (Fig. 27.1).

The attachments of these suspensory ligaments between the deep layer of the superficial fascia and the

M.A. Shiffman (ed.), *Mastopexy and Breast Reduction: Principles and Practice*,
© Springer-Verlag Berlin Heidelberg 2009

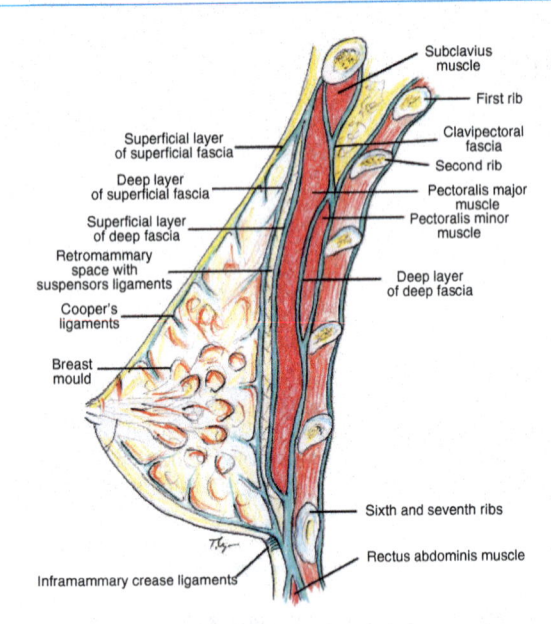

Fig. 27.1 Breast and pectoral fascias (after Nahai, [1] modified)

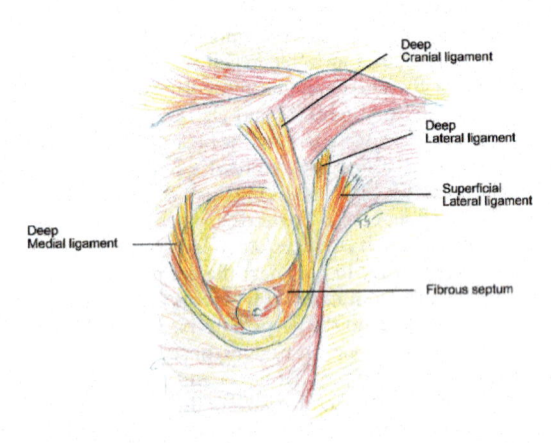

Fig. 27.2 Ligamentous suspension of the mammary gland (after Würinger, [17] modified)

deep muscular fascia are not tight and allow breast mobility. These attachments can be stretched and attenuated by weight changes, pregnancy, and aging, which can result in excess breast mobility over the chest and ptosis.

At the upper pole of the breast, near the second rib space, the pectoral fascia tightly connects with the superficial fascia of the breast and it is difficult to dissect it bluntly [15]. This is the meeting point of the three fascias, hanging from the clavicle. The superficial layer of the superficial fascia joins the deep layer of the superficial fascia (including the breast mound between them) and the superficial pectoralis fascia. At the upper and middle pectoral fascia, many thin fibers are found between the pectoral fascia and the deep layer of the superficial fascia of breast [16].

The breast suspensor ligaments described by Würinger [17] (Fig. 27.2) consists of a horizontal septum, which originates and emerges from the pectoral fascia at the level of the fourth intercostal space and traverses the entire breast from medial to lateral, heading toward the nipple. This is the central neurovascular pedicle of the breast. The horizontal septum divides the gland into a cranial and a caudal part that are delimitated from each other by loose connective tissue located above the horizontal septum [18]. At its borders, the septum curves upward into vertical ligaments, which attach the breast to the sternum and axilla, guiding vessels and nerves to the NAC also.

At the thoracic wall, the medial and lateral ligaments each have a deep and a superficial origin. This suspensory connective tissue not only connects the breast to the thoracic wall but also has superficial insertions into the skin medially, laterally, and caudally. These superficial ligaments determine the actual border of the breast. Medially, the superficial ligament is rather weak, but caudally it connects with the inframammary crease ligament [19–21]. Laterally, it fulfils a strong suspensory function by attaching to the axillary fascia along the midaxillary line.

The shaping effect of this suspensory connective tissue is being able to be demonstrated by increasing the upward tension on the medial and lateral ligaments, which result in a distinct lifting and shaping of the entire breast (Fig. 27.3). The medial and lateral ligaments merge into the superficial mammary fascia from an anterior direction. Thus, the ligamentous suspension also connects with Cooper's ligamenta suspensoria, which extends from the mammary fascia and inserts into the skin. So, even platysma contraction can produce a mild lifting effect on the breast mould through the breast suspensory ligaments connections (Fig. 27.4). Würinger [17] demonstrated that the breast is a well-structured organ and the courses of its main vessels and nerves as well as its ligamentous suspension are predictable and could be of value and relevance in clinical application [19].

In the normal growing phase, the breast can be considered to have a hemispheric shape, with the nipple in the middle in the most prominent point (Fig. 27.5). As the breast gains weight, because of the gravity and ligament tightening, the breast mound will descend in the vertical meridian of the lower two-thirds of the breast, together with the NAC.

Age, gravity, breast volume, and decreased elasticity contribute to a gradual lowering of the breast landmarks over time, as a woman gets older and experiences normal physiologic changes. The extent of this descent depends primarily on the volume of the breast and the elasticity of the tissues. The breast mound and central

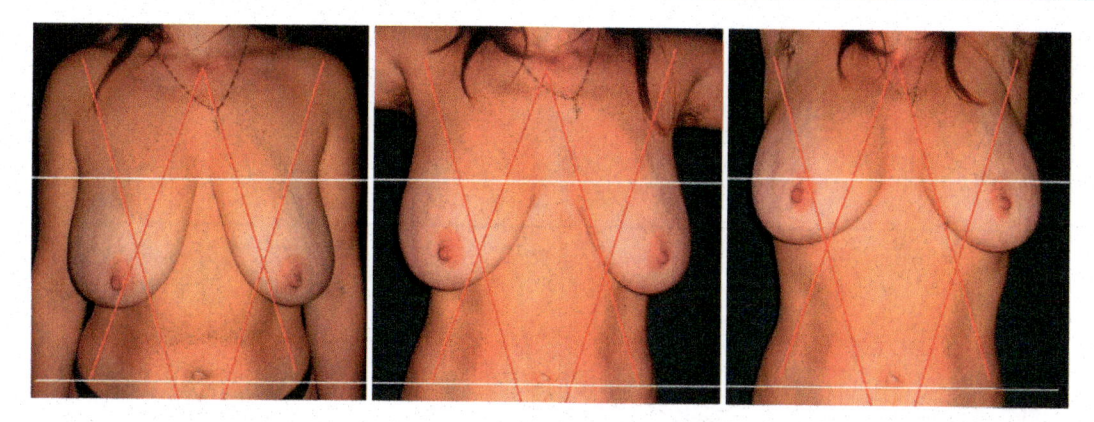

Fig. 27.3 The lifting effect of the breast suspensory ligaments tightening during arm elevation

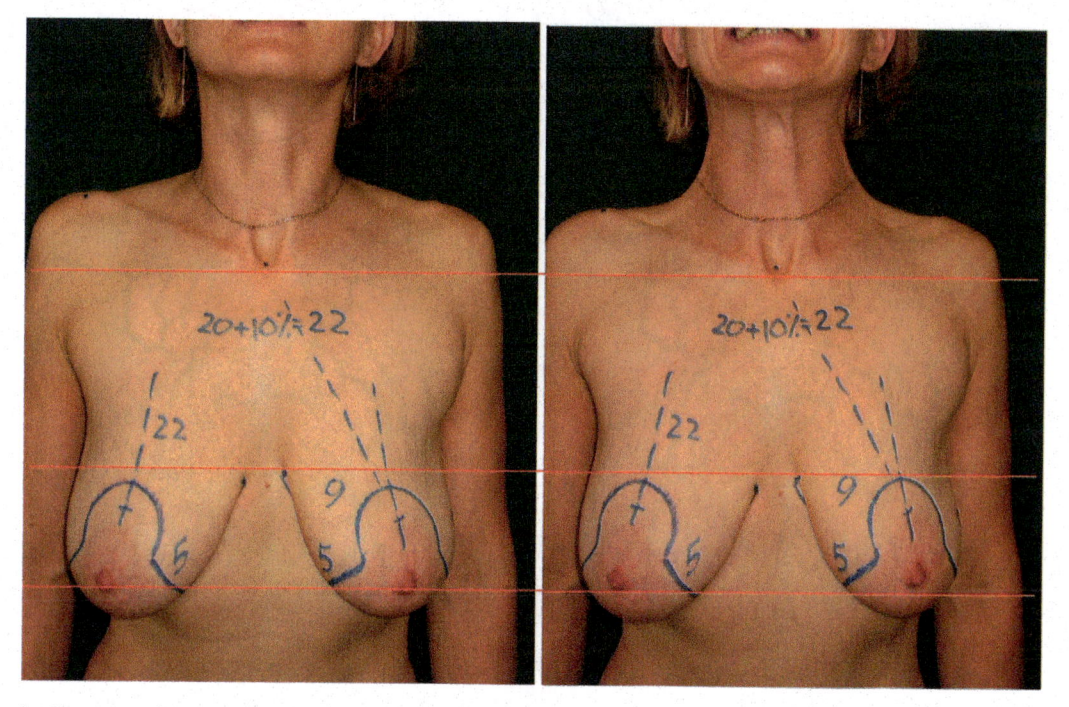

Fig. 27.4 Breast skin vertical gliding of 1 cm, just during platysma (subcutaneous musculoaponeurotic system or SMAS) contraction

pedicle will change the position according to ptosis gravity (Fig. 27.6).

In breast pseudoptosis, only the breast mound is hanging. The nipple and the inframammary fold are at the same level as in the normal situation (Fig. 27.7).

In glandular ptosis, the breast and inframammary fold glide over the chest.

In the true breast ptosis, the breast and nipple glide over the chest but the inframammary fold is at the same level [20, 21].

Botti [22] proposed a new classification scale of breast tissue and NAC ptosis according to the distance between these and the inframammary fold level. The breast ptosis degree is assessed by the distance between

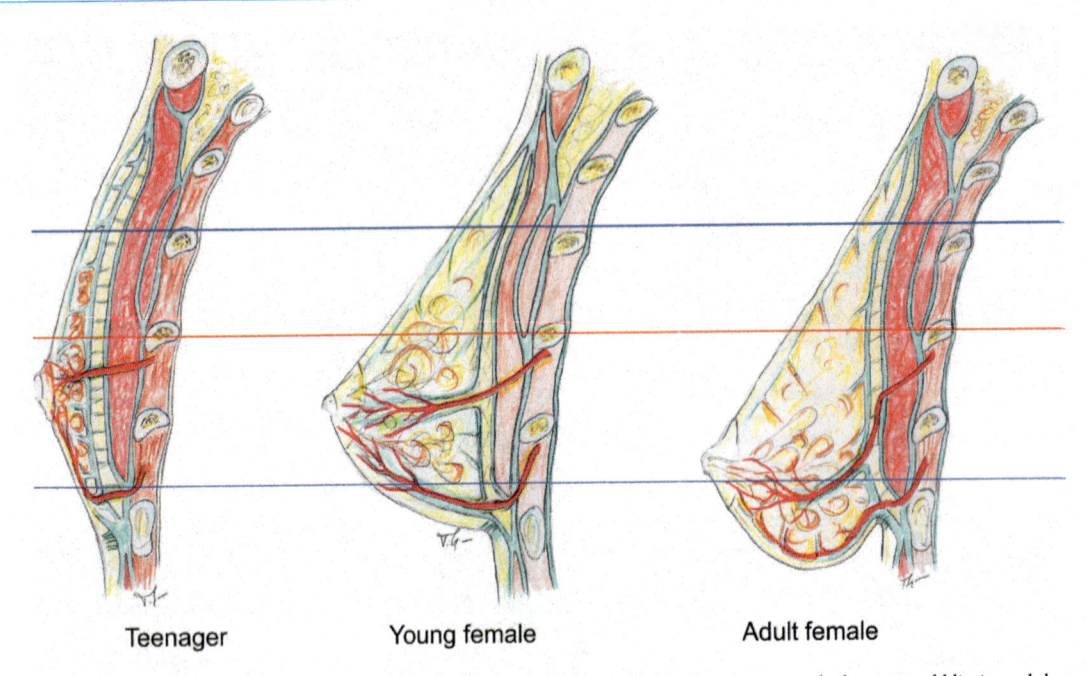

Fig. 27.5 Breast mould development and natural gliding on the chest wall. The blue lines represent the breast mould limits and the red one the initial nipple level. Breast central and inferior pedicles follow the breast mould in its descending movement

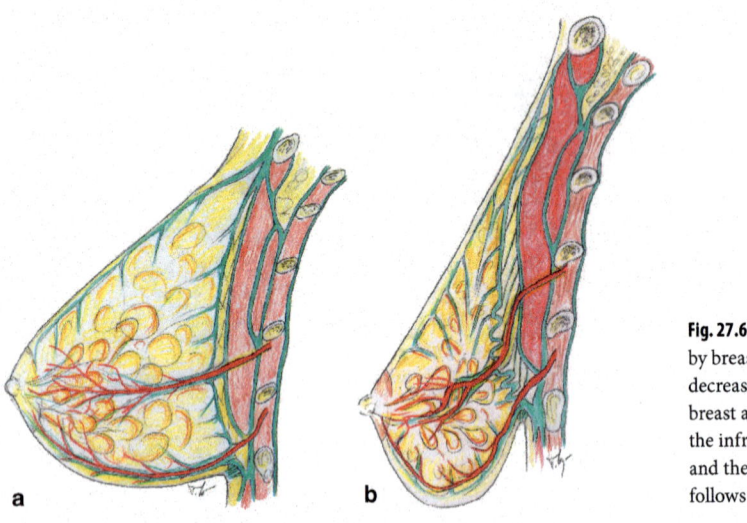

Fig. 27.6 (**a**) Breast hypertrophy followed by breast ptosis as the breast volume decreases. (**b**) In true breast ptosis, the breast and nipple glide over the chest, but the inframammary fold is at the same level and the central neurovascular pedicle follows the breast gliding over the chest

Pseudoptosis **True Breast Ptosis** **Glandular Ptosis**

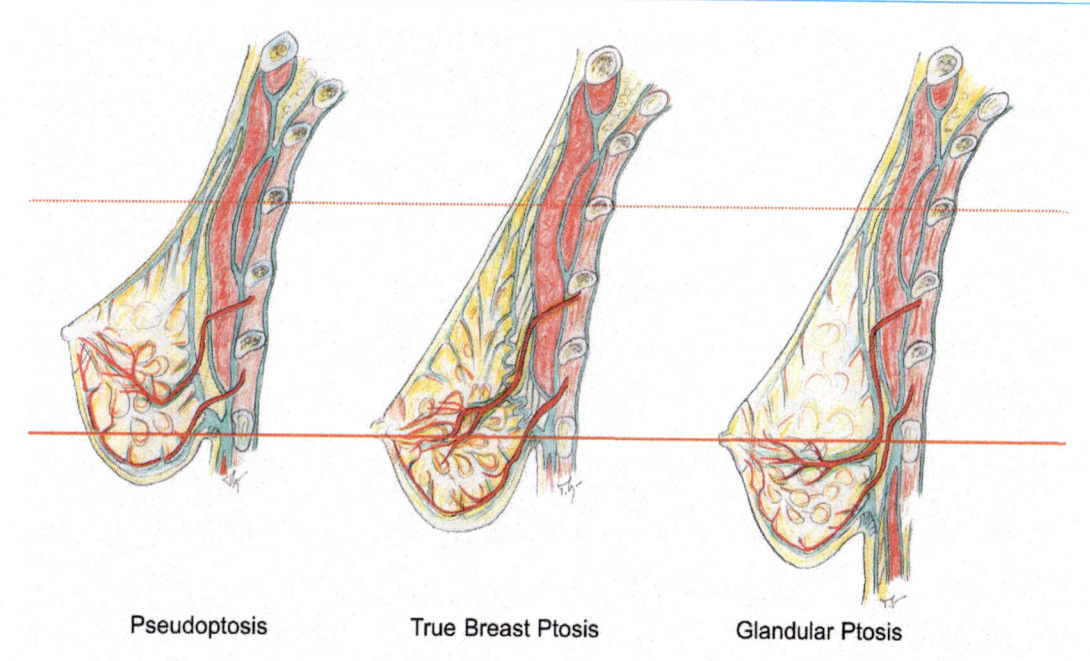

Fig. 27.7 The three types of breast ptosis, according to the nipple position and inframammary fold level [1]. The dotted line shows the breast upper pole level (anatomical landmark); the continuous line shows the sixth rib level, where normally is the inframammary fold level

the lower pole of the breast and the inframammary fold level (Fig. 27.8).

Nipple areola complex (NAC)	1st degree	0–1 cm
	2nd degree	1–2 cm
	3rd degree	2–4 cm
	4th degree	4 cm
Breast tissue	1st degree	0–1 cm
	2nd degree	1–2 cm
	3rd degree	2–4 cm
	4th degree	4 cm

According to Botti, the NAC/breast ptosis degree code could have different kinds of combinations between 1/1 and 4/4.

To better define the position of the NAC on the chest wall, two inverted triangles are used that are specific for the trunk as landmarks: the Acromion Pubic Triangle (AcAcPb), defined by the lines between the acromion apophysis of scapula bone and the superior edge of the pubic bone, and the Spino Manubrial Triangle (SpSpMn), defined by the lines between the manubrium (sternal notch) and the Antero Superior Iliac Spine points (Fig. 27.9).

Considering the natural evolution with aging, normal nipple positions is downward gliding on the external margins of the "inverted triangles," corresponding to a high position in young teenagers and to a low position in elder female patients. The aesthetic perfect position was found to be in the upper part of the triangles, close to the junction point of the external margins.

27.3 Surgical Plan

The entire procedure is designed before surgery, with the patient sitting and arms placed to the sides. The following clue points and lines are marked: manubrium, acromion, supero-anterior iliac spine, pubis, and the inframammary fold with its medial and lateral end point. After marking these reference points, the length of the inframammary fold is determined and the middle point of the fold marked with a small triangle.

To obtain a proportional breast in terms of position, volume, and shape of the body, the distance from manubrium to the new nipple position and also the breast circumference should be equal to the length of the

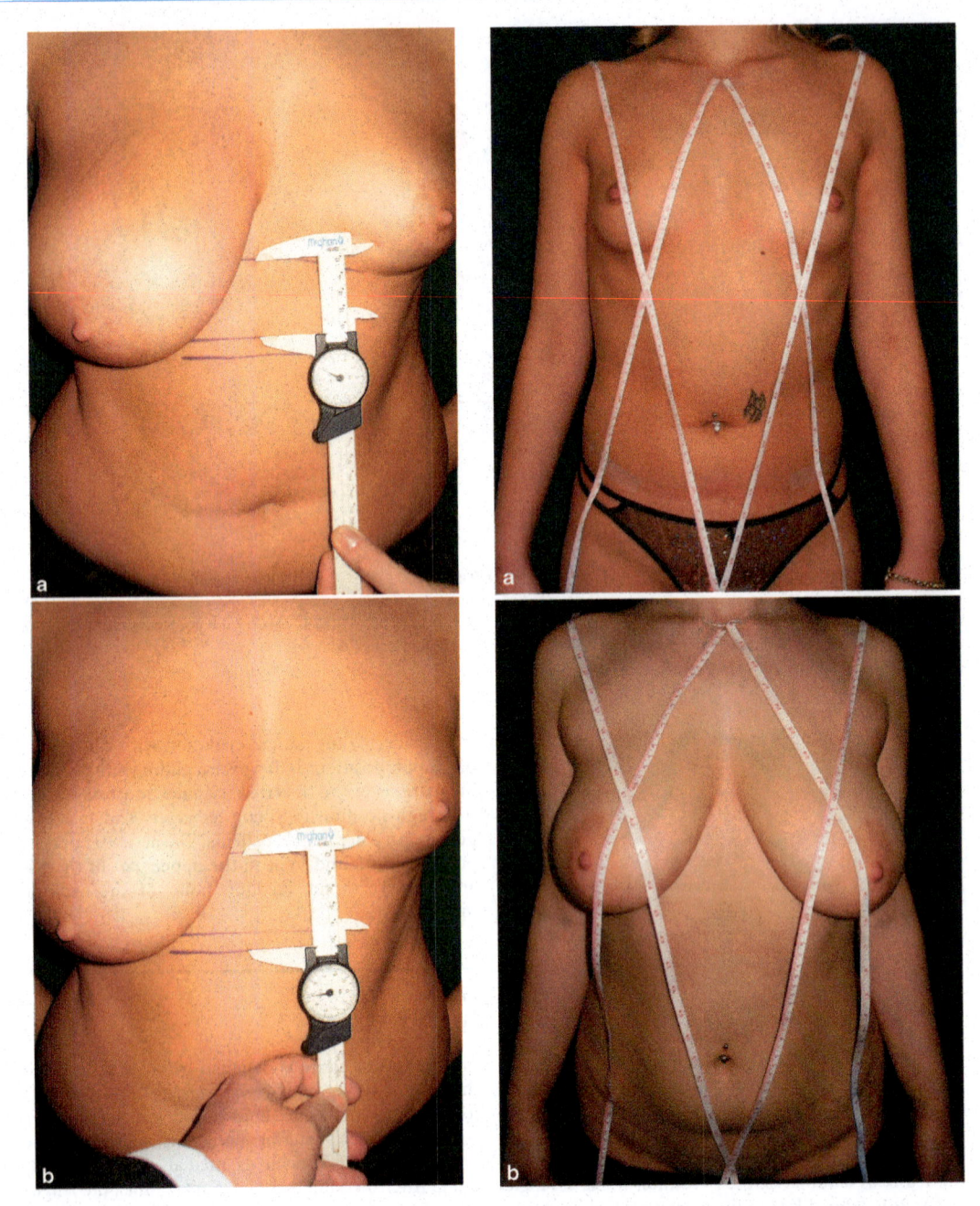

Fig. 27.8 Patient with right breast ptosis NAC 3/Breast 4.

Fig. 27.9 (**a**) Normal nipple position related to the inverted triangles in a young female. (**b**) Nipple position in a mature female with breast ptosis

patient's actual inframammary fold. This is the key to breast reduction.

During breast reduction, a significant part of the mammary gland is removed and the remaining skin envelope will have a smaller weight to support and retract. This is called the *coil spring rule* in breast surgery [23], and to compensate, 10% is added to the distance calculated for the new manubrium–nipple length. If not, the NAC will have a higher location than that planned. The same 10% value should be added in the case of breast ptosis according to the "pendulum rule" [23] (Fig. 27.10).

As the upper pole of the breast is flat at the time of marking, when the breast cone is filled, the nipple's new position with breast tissue behind it will be pushed forward like a pendulum and the manubrium–nipple distance will become shorter (from an aesthetic point of view), with the nipple situated in a higher position than

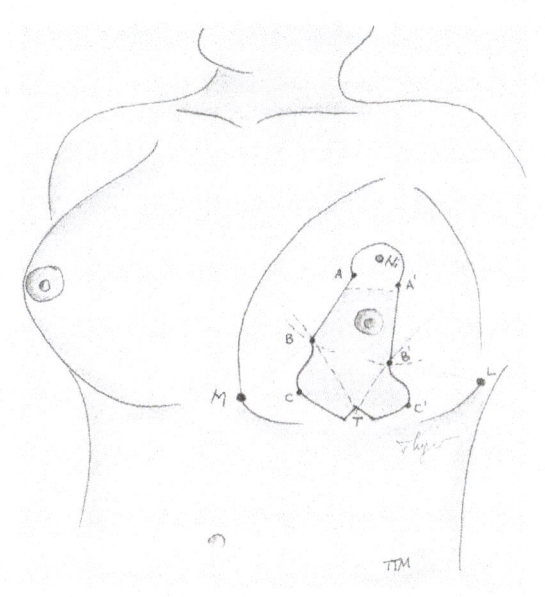

Fig. 27.11 The markings of the deepithelialized area and skin reduction

desired. To correct this, 10% extra length is added to the calculated manubrium–nipple distance for the new nipple position.

Patient's body and actual parameters of the breast are introduced into the TTM program and the computer listed in red color the ideal dimensions of the patient's breast for it to be aesthetic. In this specific case, the Breast Golden Number is 20 cm (computer suggestion is 20.34 cm).

To determine the correct position of the NAC from the sternal notch, we take 20 cm and add 10% of it (2 cm), according to the pendulum rule. Around this point, the Wise pattern key hole is used and an oval from A to A' (corresponding to the new NAC) and the vertical lines of T (corresponding to the lateral and medial cutaneo-glandular flaps AB and A'B') are drawn (Figs. 27.11–27.13).

The new areola diameter is usually 5 cm. In the aesthetic breast, the length of vertical line of T together with areola half diameter should be equal to the Breast Golden Number divided by 3. In this case, this will be 22 ÷ 3 = 7.3 cm. This means that the vertical scar will have 5 cm length (7.5−2.5 cm = 5 cm).

The opening angle of these lines will vary until they meet the dotted lines MT and LT, which represent medial and lateral branches of the inframammary fold. These lines are measured from the medial (M) and lateral (L) end points of the inframammary fold to point T.

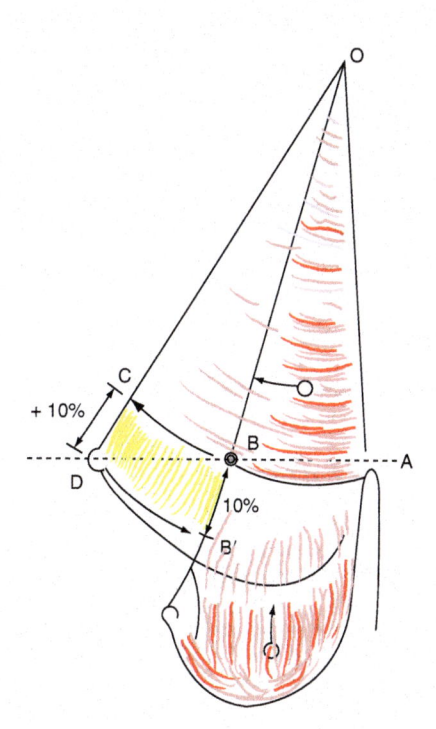

Fig. 27.10 "Pendulum rule" in breast surgery. In mastopexy and breast reduction, the bottom of the breast is pushed upward and, as a result, the upper pole is pushed forward together with the NAC. O = the midclavicular point, A = the inframammary fold level, B = the new position for NAC without correction, C = the NAC achieved position, after the operation without position correction, D = the correct position of the NAC, maintained at the aesthetic planed level, The distance OD is 10% longer that OC

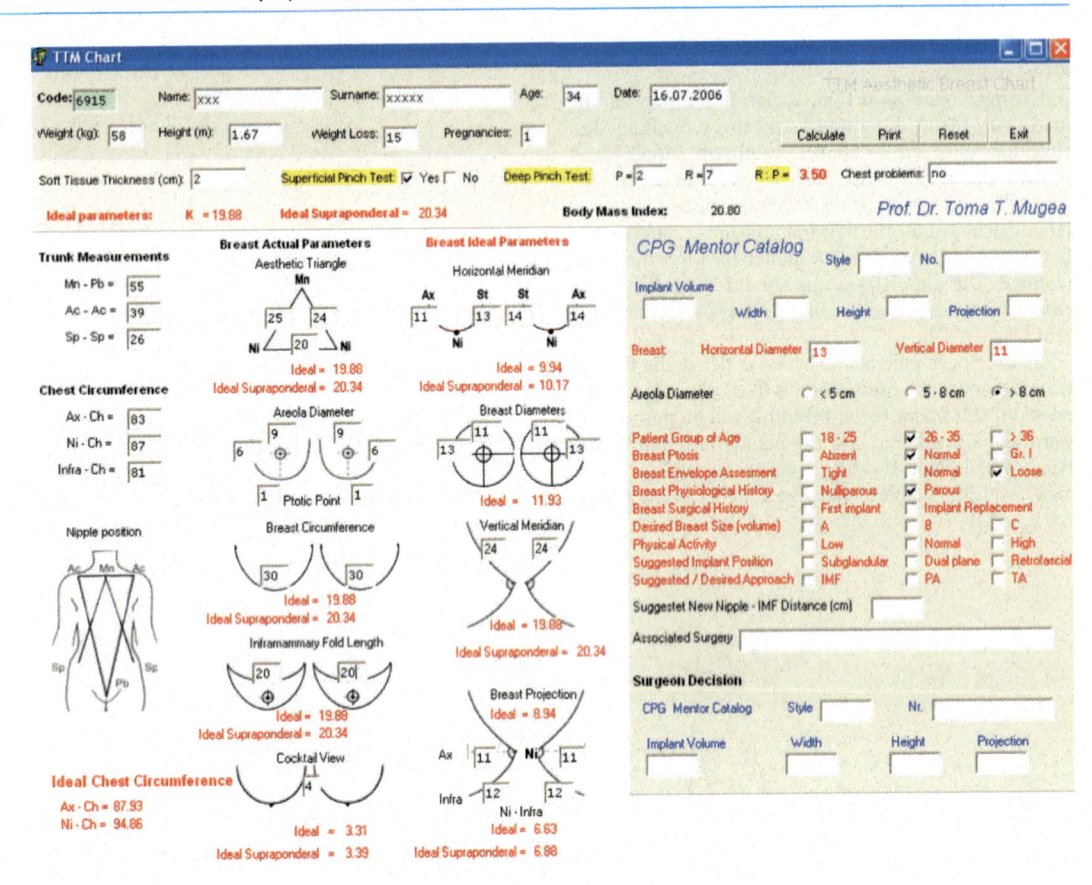

Fig. 27.12 TTM computer program with breast's actual dimensions and the ideal parameters (*in red*)

To obtain a short horizontal T scar branch, we glide M and L points to the breast vertical meridian, M becoming C and L becoming C′, until two equilateral triangles appear, TBC and TB′C′ respectively. The length of CB line is equal to that of CT and the length of C′B′ line is equal to that of C′T. The TBB′ points will be stitched together. The lines CB and C′B′ should have an "S" shape (as the third rule of breast aesthetic surgery) to match with the length of the horizontal lines of "T."

Once the surgical resection pattern is laid out, the base of the vascular pedicle for the NAC will be in fact all the line CTC′.

27.4
Surgical Procedure

The surgical procedure is performed under general anaesthesia, in the supine position, and with the arms extended at the elbow. The skin surrounding the new areola and the pedicle is deepithelialized (Fig. 27.14). Two incisions are made along lines ABC and A′B′C′ deep to the retroglandular areolar tissue (Fig. 27.15). Attention must be paid to keep the skin, superficial fascia, and glandular tissue at the same level of incision, avoiding dermo-cutaneous elevation from the breast tissues. The dermal incision is done preserving 2–3 mm margin close to the skin flap. This will help in wound closure, with a good dermal suture bite (the skin tension will decrease in the upper dermis, improving the healing and scar appearance).

Because there is a small amount of glandular tissue in the upper pole of the breast, usually there is no need for excision. In this area only the skin is excised and all the fatty tissues are kept in place. The glandular tissue to be excised is mainly located in the central and lateral quadrant of the breast. From the top of the dermo-glandular flap, including the NAC, the dissection progresses in a caudal direction along the loose layer of the fourth intercostal space by blunt preparation. Here, the retromammary space changes its direction and merges into a layer of loose connective tissue in a vertical plane, heading toward the nipple [19].

27.4 Surgical Procedure 223

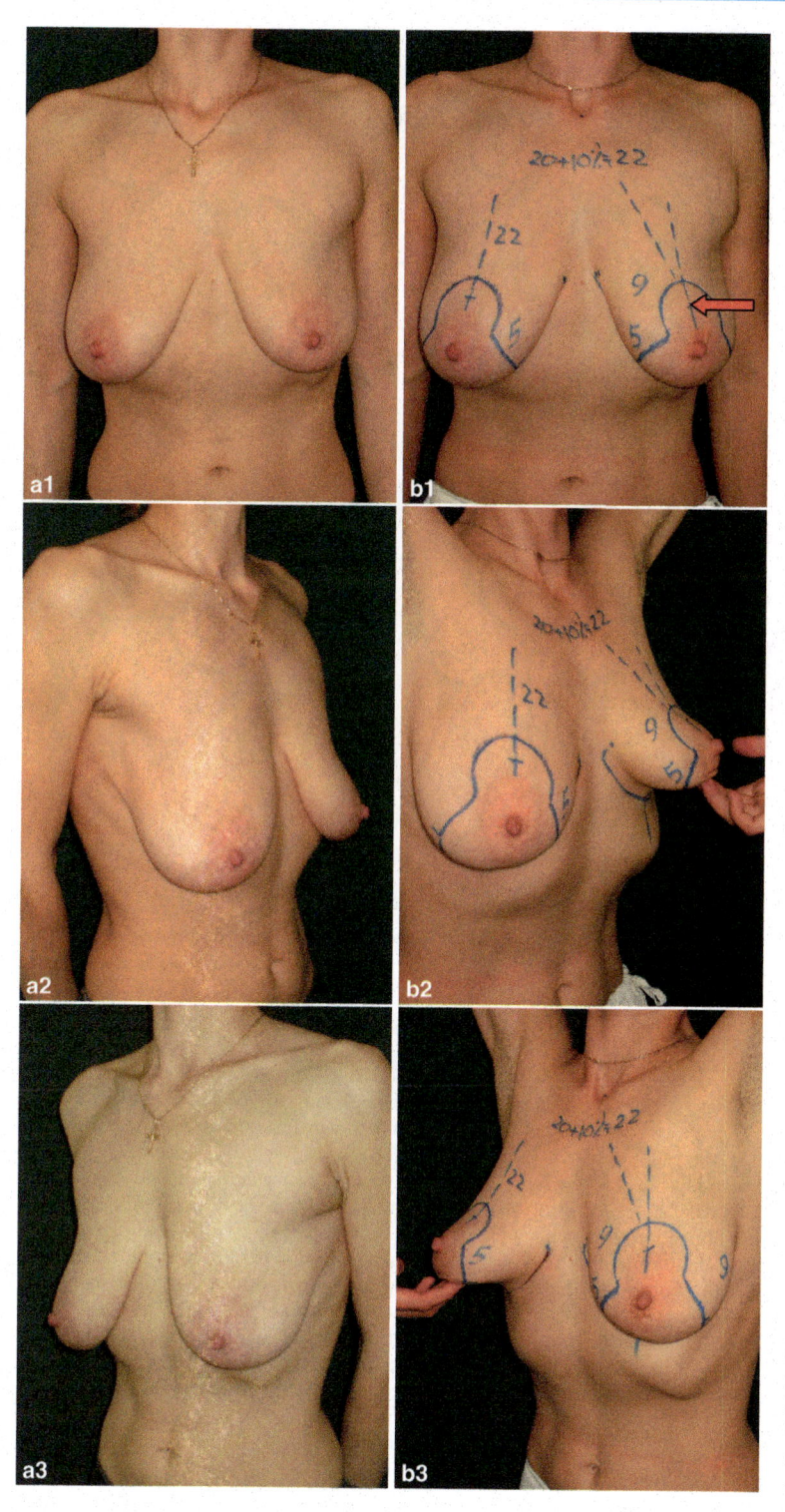

Fig. 27.13 (*a1-3*) Preoperative view with a severe breast ptosis case. (*b1-3*) Preoperative marking according to the suggested breast dimensions, based on 20 cm as the breast golden number. The new position of the NAC will be located at the meeting point between the midclavicular to nipple line and the inverted triangles (*red arrow*)

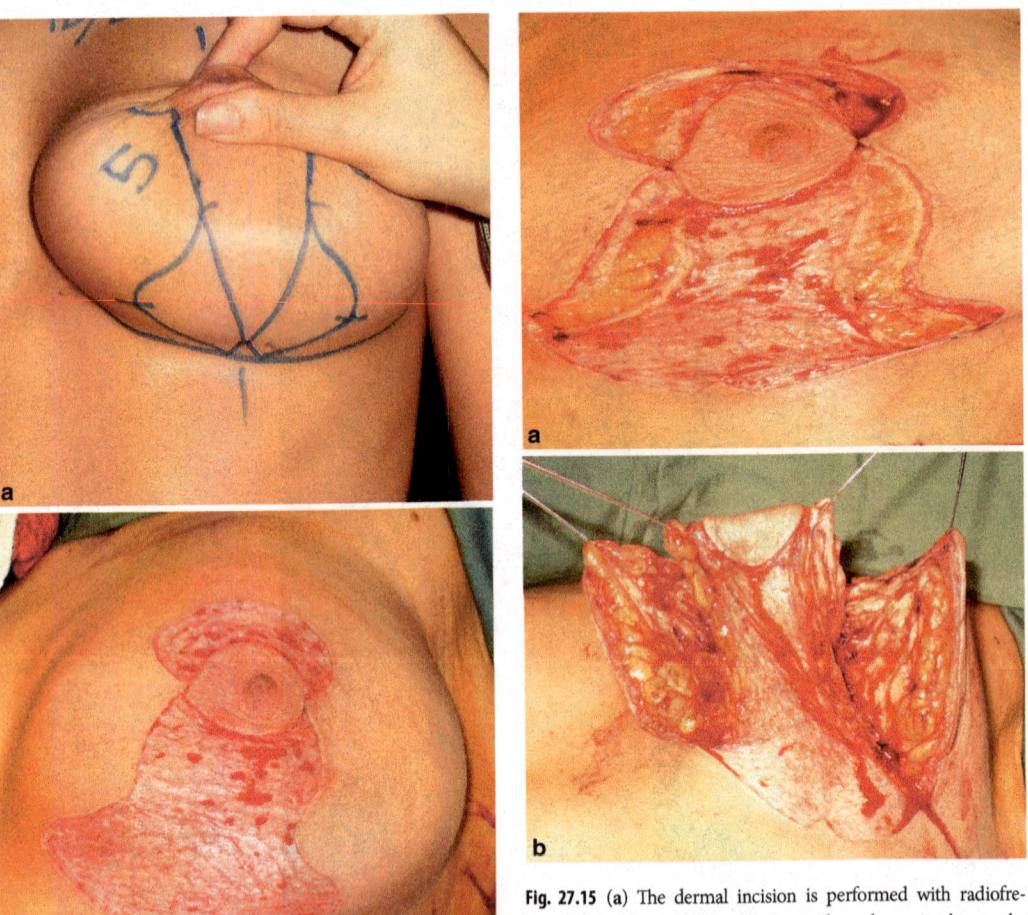

Fig. 27.14 (a,b) Skin deepithelialization on the marked area. The pedicle flap width corresponds to the horizontal T branch length

Fig. 27.15 (a) The dermal incision is performed with radiofrequency needle point, preserving 2 mm dermal margin close to the skin. (b) Vertical incisions deep to the retroglandular areolar tissue

The caudal part of the gland together with the horizontal septum is left intact. The glandular excess from the central area is excised, preserving at least 2 cm of tissue behind the NAC. The connection between the nipple and the thoracic wall is maintained by the horizontal breast septum (Fig. 27.16) and its attached neurovascular layers [17, 19].

To obtain a good breast projection and to avoid the ptosis of the breast tissue, several reverse sutures are used with 2/0 Vicryl, deep in the lateral and medial pillars tissue. This will include the medial and lateral suspensor ligaments of the breast sutured in front of the dermoglandular pedicle of the NAC (Figs. 27.17 and 27.18).

The next layer is a reverse dermo-hypodermic suture that includes the anterior layer of the superficial fascia of the breast [24] with 2/0 Vicryl. This suture technique allows minimal tension skin repair, with more predictable scarring, using the 2–3 marginal deepithelialized area left close to the skin flap margin (Fig. 27.19).

The skin suture is performed using intracuticular running suture with 5/0 PDS. The whole incision length is taped with SteriStrips changed every 5 days,

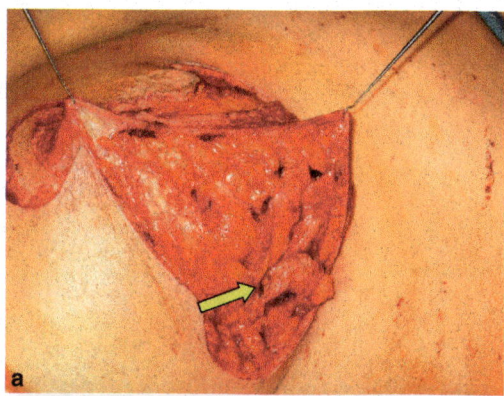

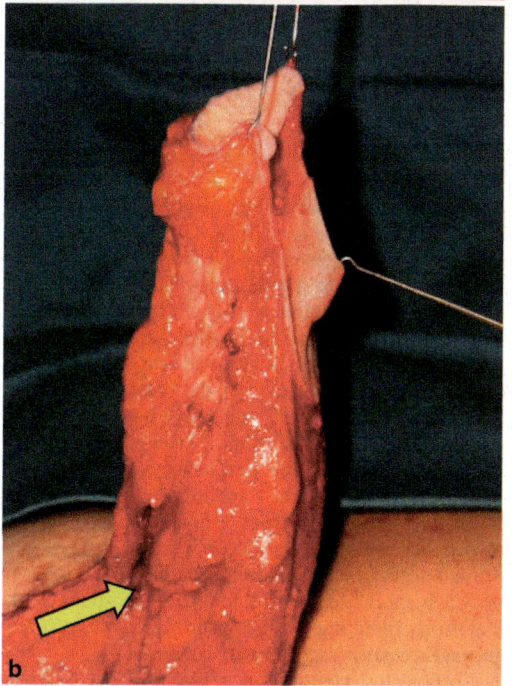

Fig. 27.16 The central breast pedicle and fibrous septum

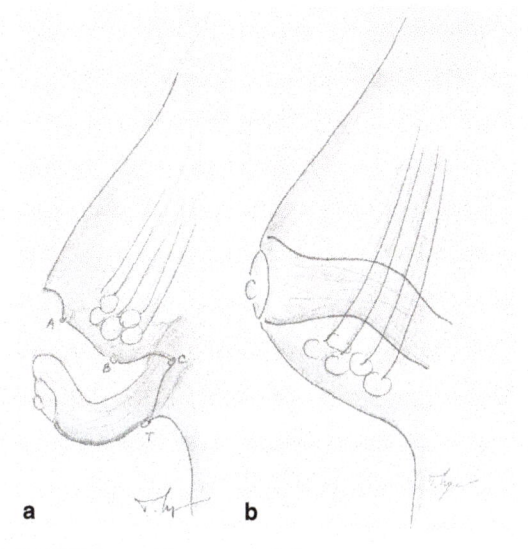

Fig. 27.17 Internal brassiere, made by suturing the medial and lateral pillars, including the medial and lateral suspensory ligaments, in front of the NAC dermoglandular pedicle

for 3–6 weeks. Patients are asked to wear a brassiere for 6 weeks.

27.5
Clinical Cases

In the author's series of 250 cases with the short inverted "T" scar breast reduction or mastopexy, the aesthetic results were considered good to excellent in all cases at 6 and 12 months, and the contour results were stable in long-term follow-up (Fig. 27.20). Complications that occurred in 4 cases (1.6%) included minor wound breakdown at the base of the vertical scar. No infection and no necrosis of the NAC occurred. The NAC sensibility at 3 month was similar to that before surgery in 223 cases (89%). NAC hypopigmentation was not observed.

27.6
Conclusions

Reduction mammaplasty involves much judgement by the surgeon to meet the patient's desired outcome. The preoperative markings, the techniques used, and the nature of the patient's tissues will affect the result. Poor scars, breast size error, odd shape, and unequal breasts are the commonest causes of postoperative dissatisfaction. Patients requiring primary correction of ptosis often seek improvement of their aesthetic appearance and are more worried about scars than patients with large breasts [2, 25].

The inverted T method is the most commonly used technique [9–12, 26–28]. It is regarded as predictable and reliable in outcome and can be used in a complete

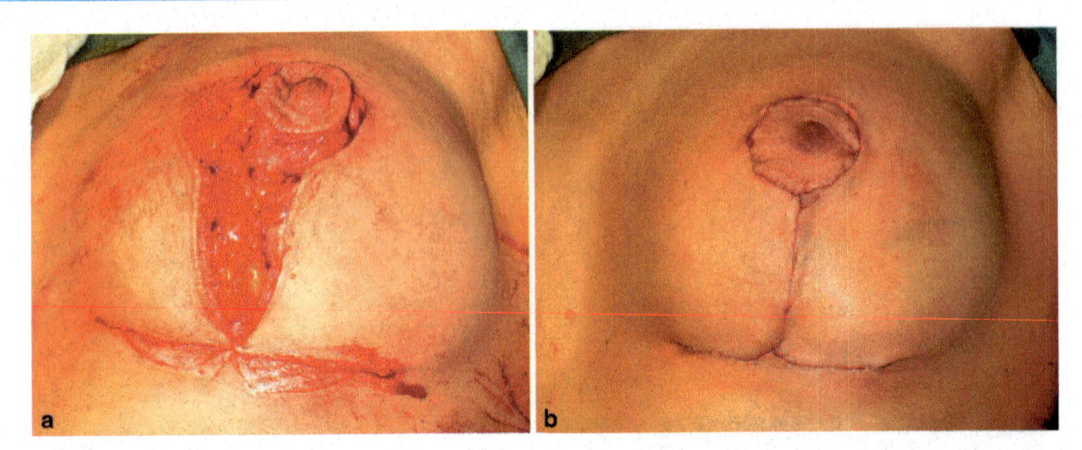

Fig. 27.18 Intraoperative view with breast lateral and medial pillars sutured in front of the NAC dermoglandular pedicle (a), and reverse dermohypodermic stitch (b)

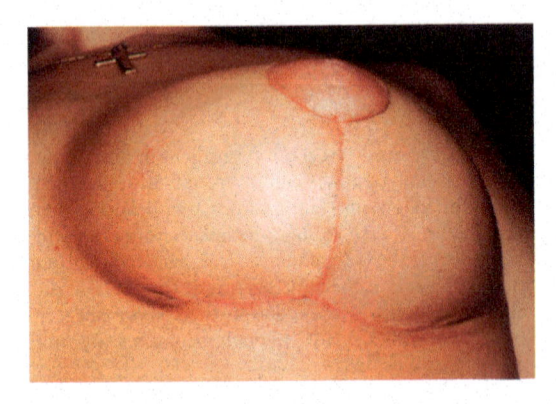

Fig. 27.19 Short inverted "T" scar appearance 6 months later

range of sizes and is easy to learn. The short inverted T scar procedure with inferior pedicle is indicated when the degree of ptosis increases to grade II or grade III and mild to moderate macromastia is present.

The skin is reduced and distributed to the required size and shape at the same time with parenchyma that fills this new skin envelope. The horizontal branch of the inverted "T" scar is shorter and situated just above the inframammary fold line, being very well hidden.

This technique provides a stable and long-lasting suspension along an exactly defined line, using the glandular and fascial structures of the breast as one unit. Simple cutaneous flaps are not used without dermoglandular support. Nipple sensibility, lactation, and vascularization are preserved by the inferior pedicle, including NAC neurovascular pedicle and inferior breast mould.

Although, the technique is suitable for the majority of patients, problems can occur when there is a mild ptosis and the breast tissue is very firm. The inferior pedicle is short and does not fold enough behind to lateral flaps, generating tension in the NAC, with a droopy appearance when the pillars are sutured.

An objective comparison of the result of different techniques of reduction mammaplasty is extremely difficult, but to provide the basis for a critical analysis of the results, the TTM chart is proposed.

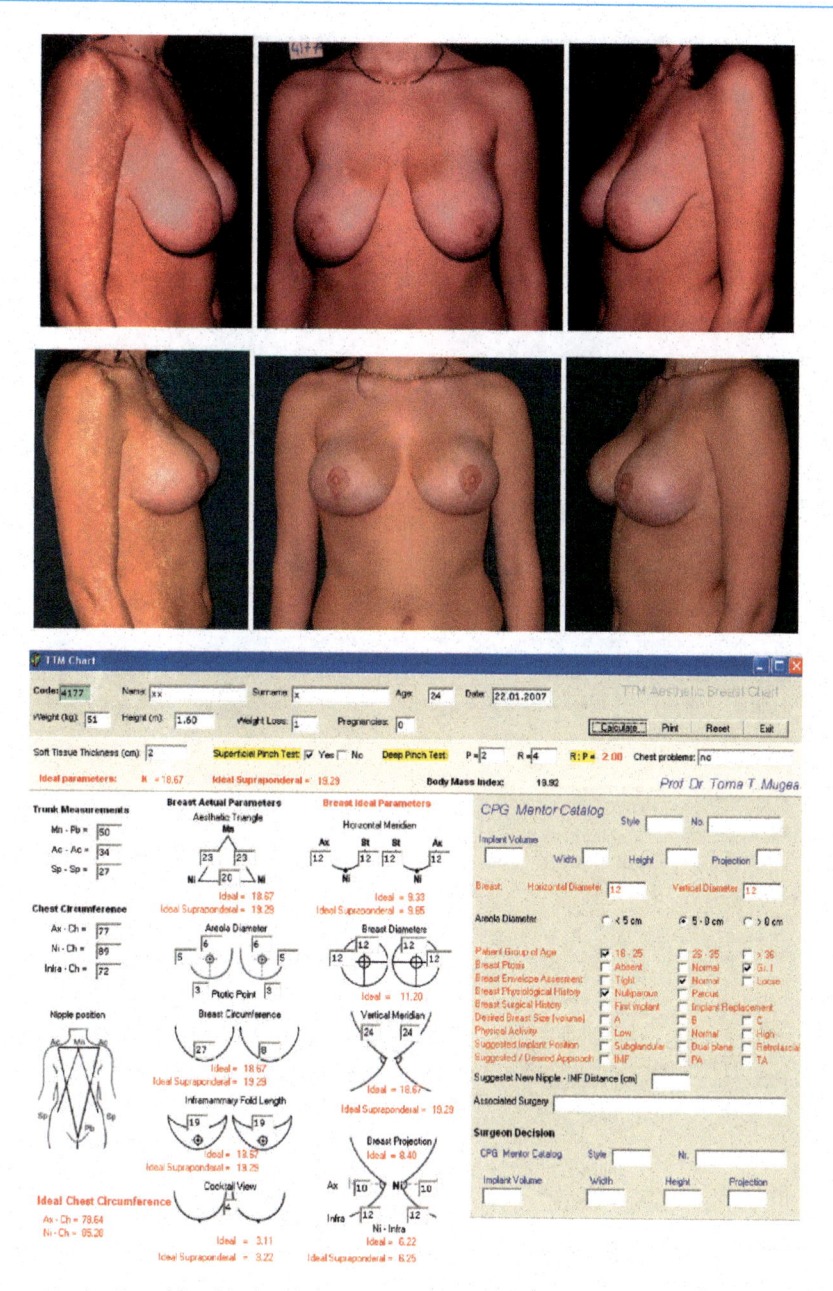

Fig. 27.20 Case nr. 1: preoperative (above) and postoperative view (below). TTM Computer Program with breast actual dimensions and the ideal parameters (in red).

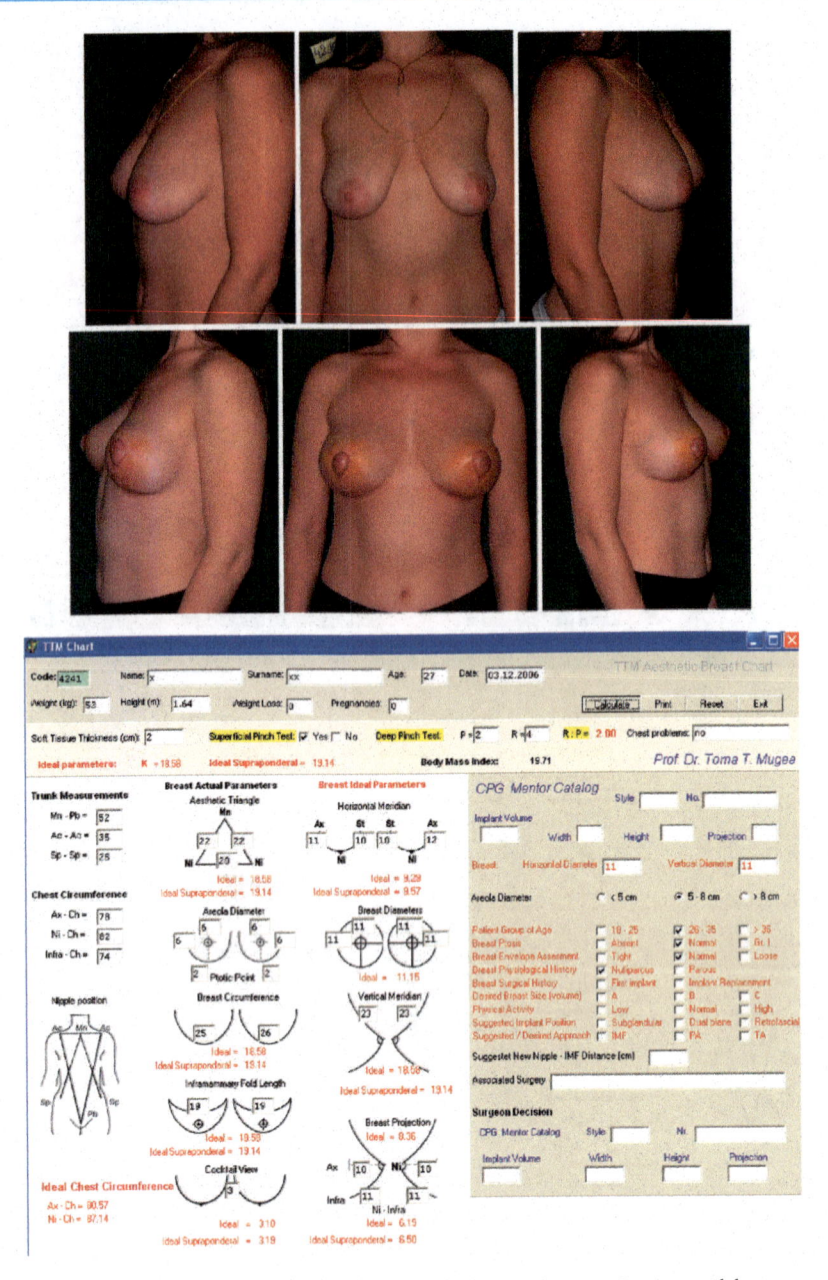

Fig. 27.21 Case nr. 2: Preoperative (above) and postoperative view (below). TTM Computer Program with breast actual dimensions and the ideal parameters (in red).

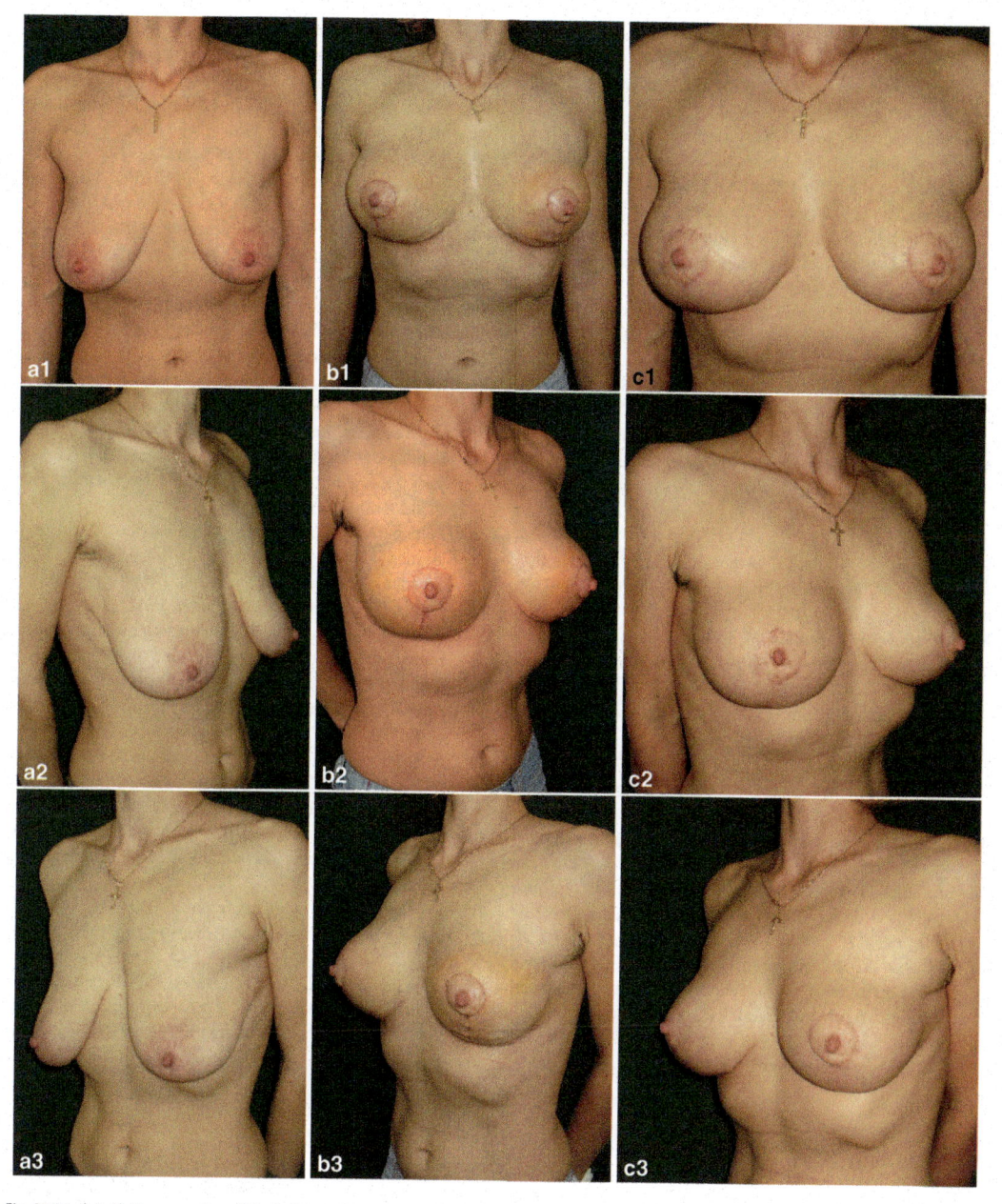

Fig. 27.22 (**a***1-3*) Preoperative. (**b***1-3*) Seven days postoperative. (**c***1-3*) Six months postoperative. According to Botti classification the degree of ptosis is NAC 4/Breast 4

References

1. Regnault P: Breast ptosis. Definition and treatment. Clin Plast Surg 1976;3(2):193–203
2. Shakespeare V, Popstle K: A qualitative study of patients' views on the effects of breast-reduction surgery: a 2-year follow-up survey. Br J Plast Surg 1999;52(3):198–204
3. Blomqvist L, Eriksson A, Brandberg Y: Reduction mammaplasty provides long-term improvement in health status and quality of life. Plast Reconstr Surg 2000;106 (5):991–997
4. Nakajima H, Imanishi N, Aiso S: Arterial anatomy of the nipple-areola complex. Plast Reconstr Surg 1995; 96(4):439–450
5. Sarhadi NS, Shaw Dunn J, Lee FD, Soutar DS: An anatomical study of the nerve supply of the breast, including the nipple and areola. Br J Plast Surg 1996;49(3):156–164
6. Hamdi M, Greuse M, Nemec E, Deprez C, DeMey A: Breast sensation after superior pedicle versus inferior pedicle mammaplasty: anatomical and histological evaluation. Br J Plast Surg 2001;54(1):43–46
7. Marshall DR, Callan PP, Nicholson W: Breastfeeding after reduction mammaplasty. Br J Plast Surg 1994;47(3): 167–169
8. Brzozowski D, Niessen M, Evans B, Hurst LN: Breastfeeding after inferior pedicle reduction mammaplasty. Plasr Rec Surg 2000;105(2):530–534
9. Strombeck JO: Mammaplasty: report of a new technique based on the two-pedicle procedure. Br J Plast Surg 1960;13:79–90
10. Pitanguy I: Surgical treatment of breast hypertrophy. Br J Plast Surg 1967;20(1):78–85
11. McKissock PK: Reduction mammaplasty with a vertical dermal flap. Plast Reconstr Surg 1972;49(3):245–252
12. Robbins TH: A reduction mammaplasty with areolar-nipple based on an inferior dermal pedicle. Plast Reconstr Surg 1977;59(1):64–67
13. Mugea TT: A new system for breast assessment using TTM chart. The 17th International Congress of the French Society of Aesthetic Surgery, Paris 19–21 May, 2001
14. Nahai F: The Art of Aesthetic Surgery: Principles and Techniques, Quality Medical Publishing, Inc. 2005, p 1799
15. Graf RM, Bernades A, Auerswald A, Damasio RC: Subfascial endoscopic transaxillary augmentation mammaplasty. Aesthetic Plast Surg 2000;24(3):216–220
16. Jinde L, Jianliang S, Xiaoping C, Xiaoyan T, Jiaging L, Qun M, Bo L: Anatomy and clinical significance of pectoral fascia. Plast Reconstr Surg 2006;118(7):1557–1560
17. Wuringer E, Mader N, Posch E, Holle J: Nerve and vessel supplying ligamentous suspension of the mammary gland. Plast Reconstr Surg 1998;101(6):1486–1493
18. Bayati S, Seckel BR: Inframammary crease ligament. Plast Reconstr Surg 1995;95(3):501–508
19. Würinger E: Refinement of the central pedicle breast reduction by application of the ligamentous suspension. Plast Reconstr Surg 1999;103(5):1400–1410
20. Nava M, Quattrone P, Riggio E: Focus on the breast fascial system: a new approach for inframammary fold reconstruction. Plast Reconstr Surg 1998;102(4):1034–1045
21. Muntan CD, Sundine MJ, Rink RD, Acland RD: Inframammary fold: a histologic reappraisal. Plast Reconstr Surg 2000;105(2):549–556
22. Botti G: Mastoplastiche Estetiche: Atlante di Chirurgia Plastica Pratica, S.E.E. Societe Editrice Europa di Nicodemo Maggiulli & C snc, Firenze, Italy 2004, p 251
23. Mugea TT: Rules in breast aesthetic surgery. The 4th International Congress of Romanian Aesthetic Surgery Society, Bucharest, Romania, October 3–5th, 2002
24. Lockwood T: Reductiom mammaplasty and mastopexy with superficial fascial system suspension. Plast Reconstr Surg 1999;103(5):1411–1420
25. Faria FS, Guthrie E, Bradbury E, Brian AN: Psychosocial outcome and patient satisfaction following breast reduction surgery. Br J Plast Surg 1999;52(6):448–452
26. Hidalgo DA, Elliot LF, Palumbo S, Casas L, Hammond D: Current trends in breast reduction. Plast Reconstr Surg 1999;104(3):806–815
27. Hidalgo DA: Improving safety and aesthetics in inverted T scar breast reduction. Plast Reconstr Surg 1999; 103(3): 887–889
28. Giovanoli P, Meuli-Simmen C, Meyer VE, Frey M: Which technique for which breast? A prospective study of different techniques of reduction mammaplasty. Br J Plast Surg 1999;52(1):52–59

Regnault B Mastopexy: A Versatile Approach to Breast Lifting and Reduction

Howard A. Tobin

28.1
Introduction

Mastopexy remains a challenging operation for most surgeons. In some ways, patients and surgeons alike are fighting a losing battle, in which they are trying to uplift a sagging breast that is usually the result of a lack of tensile strength in the skin. Since it is only the skin that supports the breast, recurrent skin stretch is the rule rather than the exception. Although women with pseudoptosis or mild ptosis may be satisfied with breast augmentation alone, mastopexy is often indicated to obtain the desired "lift" when there is more significant ptosis. The disadvantage of choosing mastopexy over augmentation alone is the resulting scars on the breasts. Classic mastopexy produces a scar around the areola as well as a vertical scar extending from the areola down to a transverse scar in the fold beneath the breasts.

A number of techniques have been developed over the years in an effort to minimize the extent of scarring. In 1976, Regnault [1] published the B Mastopexy technique that unites the vertical and horizontal scars into a single curving incision, thus eliminating the medial scar. This technique also may be used in breast reductions. This technique has been the preferred technique in the author's hands for over 15 years. The advantage of this procedure is that a long inframammary incision is avoided and is replaced by a much shorter lateral continuation of the vertical incision. Since there are no specific markings to guide the surgeon, the procedure requires more experience and judgment than the more standard cookie cutter techniques using anchor-shaped incisions.

Conceptually, the operation can be viewed as creating a laterally based rotation flap that is advanced around and under the breast to provide tightening and lifting.

28.2
Surgical Technique

Patients undergo extensive consultation related to risks, limitations, and benefits of mastopexy with or without simultaneous augmentation. Patients are always advised that mastopexy procedures often fall short of ideal expectations. This is stressed to attempt to discourage patients with unrealistic expectations. Detailed before and after photos are reviewed. These pictures were selected to clearly show the nature and extent of the incisions as well as the resulting scars. Patients are educated that scars "look bad before they look good" and that may take up to a year for scar maturation and final breast contour. Since most mastopexy patients also undergo simultaneous augmentation at our Center, the limitations and the risks of augmentation are discussed thoroughly, including the alternative of staged procedures.

Patients who undergo simultaneous augmentation have the implants inserted endoscopically beneath the muscle through a transaxillary incision. The two procedures are accomplished simultaneously. A major advantage of this technique is that there is no continuity between the implant pocket and the mastopexy itself. Therefore, if there is an infection at the mastopexy site, it is far less likely to reach the implant. In spite of the recent release of gel-filled implants, the author continues to prefer and recommend saline-filled implants, although patients do have the option of choosing gel. In either case, the technique is the same.

It is recognized that it will take months for the breasts to fully settle and take on a pleasing shape. Therefore, patients are shown photographs of various stages of healing to help reassure them during their postoperative course, as the breasts will usually look quite distorted initially.

Preoperative markings are performed with the patient in the standing position. The distance from the suprasternal notch to the nipple is measured and documented. The inframammary fold is identified and marked on the anterior breast as an indication of the level to which the nipple is to be elevated (Fig. 28.1). The medial aspect of the new position of the areola is marked at approximately 10–11 cm from the midline along the mid breast (Fig. 28.2). A 38 mm diameter line is marked around the nipple corresponding to the new preserved areola. An estimate of the incisions is outlined recognizing that this will be modified in surgery. The estimate must take into

M.A. Shiffman (ed.), *Mastopexy and Breast Reduction: Principles and Practice*,
© Springer-Verlag Berlin Heidelberg 2009

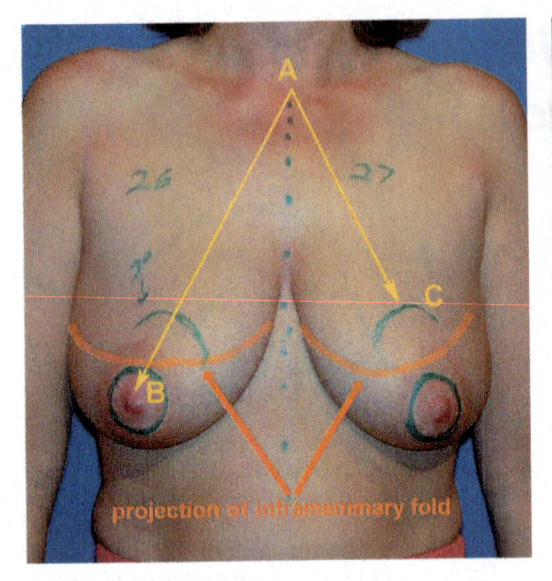

Fig. 28.1 The inframammary fold is identified and marked on the anterior breast as an indication of the level to which the nipple is to be elevated

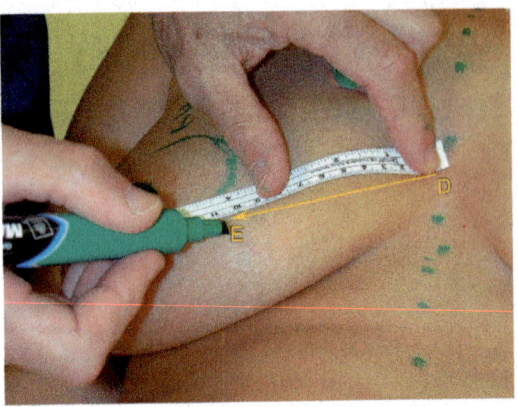

Fig. 28.2 The medial aspect of the new position of the areola is marked approximately 10–11 cm from the midline along the mid breast

account that usually implants will be used, which will reduce the amount of skin excision. Photographs are taken to be used for reference in the operating room. The patient is then brought for surgery.

During surgery, under general anesthesia, the patient is placed in the supine position on the operating table and a freehand "B type pattern" is drawn (Fig. 28.3). Using the initial landmarks, a semicircular pattern is made around the nipple. The upper portion of this semicircle represents the amount by which the nipple–areolar complex will be elevated. The medial extent of the semicircle represents the distance that will be created between the nipple–areolar complex and the medial limit of the breast, near the sternum. The vertical and horizontal component of the mastopexy is created using a tapering curvilinear incision from the lower portion of the areola to the lateral breast crease. This results in vertical closure that will be about 5–7 cm from the bottom of the areola to the inframammary fold. The medial component of the usual inframammary incision is thus eliminated. A simple maneuver is performed to assess closure tension by infolding the breast over the index finger (Fig. 28.4). One must allow for the added volume that will result when implants are used.

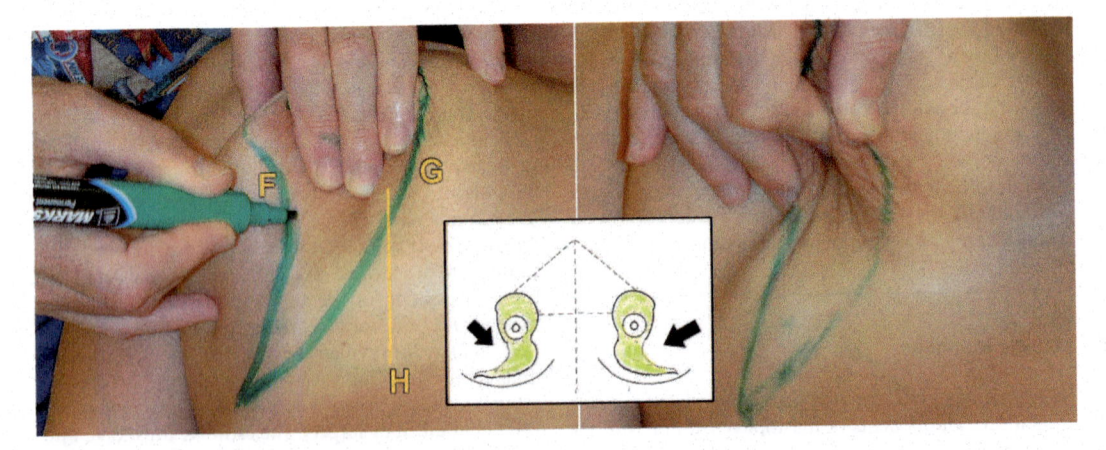

Fig. 28.3 The patient is placed in the supine position on the operating table and a freehand "B type pattern" is drawn

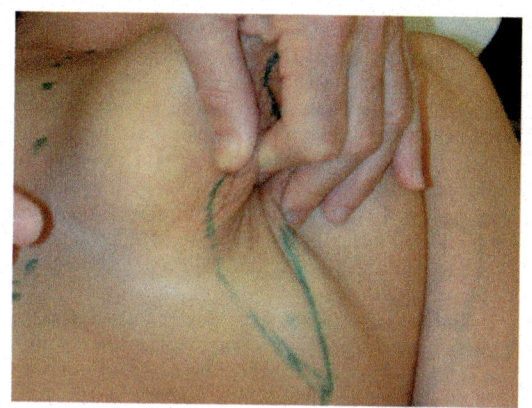

Fig. 28.4 Assess closure tension by infolding the breast over the index finger

A modified tumescent infiltration consisting of 100 ml of normal saline, 25 ml of 1% lidocaine plain, and 0.25 ml of 1:1,000 adrenaline is injected into the dermis in the area to be de-epithelialized as planned using a 20 gauge 1 in. needle (Fig. 28.5). If simultaneous breast augmentation is to be performed, an additional solution of 250 ml of normal saline, 50 ml of 1% lidocaine plain, and 0.5 ml of 1:1,000 adrenalin is injected using a 20 gauge 3½ in. needle. This is injected above and below the pectoralis muscle and around the circumference of the breast, as well as in the axilla. To facilitate the submuscular injection, the muscle is gently grasped and elevated to help position the needle into the correct plane. Great care must be taken to make the plane of infiltration parallel to the ribcage to avoid inadvertent penetration of the pleura.

Subepithelial undermining is carried out using a sharp razor scalpel following injection of the tumescent fluid. During this process, deepithelialization of the skin edges is continued at 3–4 mm to allow closure of the skin without tension. Deepithelialization is typically performed after implant sizers are inserted when simultaneous augmentation is accomplished, and the amount of skin to be removed can be estimated only after the sizers are in place.

When the patient has elected to undergo simultaneous submuscular breast augmentation, a transaxillary endoscopic approach to place the implant is preferred. The endoscope is used to aid in visualization as the pectoralis major muscle is divided from the sternum and ribs. After developing a pocket, implant sizers are used to ensure best possible symmetry. At this point, final markings are made and deepithelialization is performed. During dermal closure, the sizer can then be displaced up into the pocket or partially deflated to allow approximation with minimal tension. If the clo-

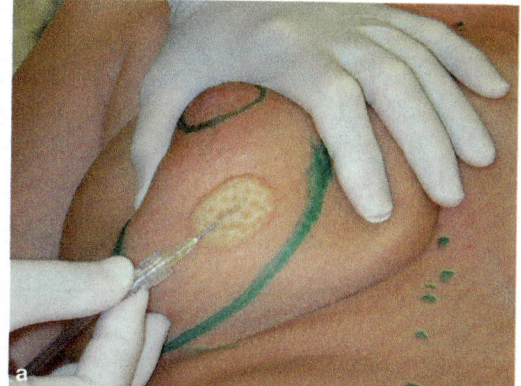

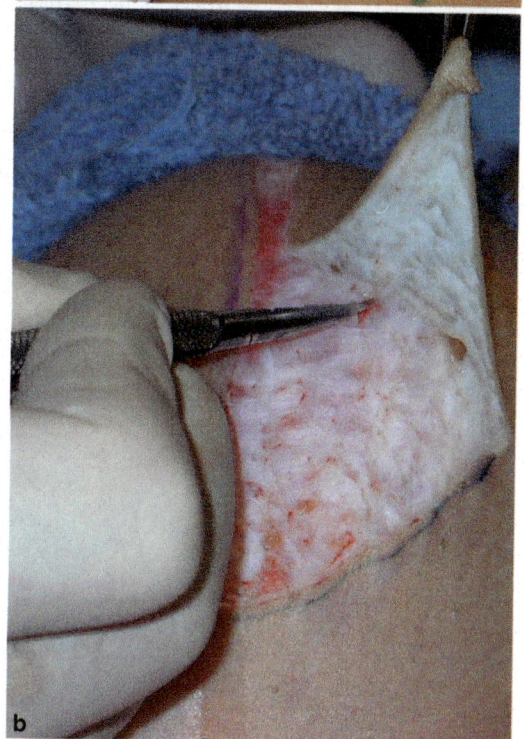

Fig. 28.5 (a) A modified tumescent solution is injected into the dermis in the area to be de-epithelialized as planned using a 20 gauge 1 in. needle. (b) Scalpel de-epithelialization is performed

sure demonstrates too much tension, this can be corrected by inserting a smaller implant or by reducing the final fill volume. Fine cannula liposuction of the breast tissue may also be performed to reduce the breast volume and to aid in closure in certain cases.

A tension-free closure is critical for optimal healing and for avoiding the formation of wide scars. The dermis

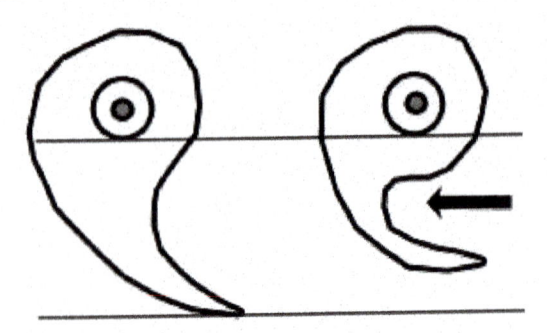

Fig. 28.6 The lateral flap is rotated down and medially to create the curvilinear scar that results. Adjustment of this rotation determines the length of the distance between the inferior margin of the areola and the inframammary crease. The more of the flap that is rotated around the areola, the shorter this distance will be to the inframammary fold

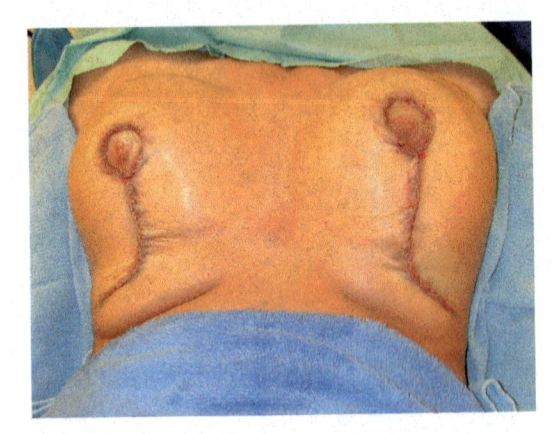

Fig. 28.7 After dermal closure, 5-0 or 6-0 plain catgut is used to approximate the areola to the adjacent skin edge and the lower skin incisions in a continuous fashion

is used to provide the initial closure. Subepithelial undermining at the edge of the incision allows the performance of a dermal closure to avoid any tension on the skin. During dermal closure, the nipple is brought into its new position based on the pedicle of dermis. The lateral flap is rotated down and medially to create the curvilinear scar that results. Adjustment of this rotation determines the length of the distance between the inferior margin of the areola and the inframammary crease. The more of the flap that is rotated around the areola, the shorter this distance will be to the inframammary fold (Fig. 28.6). The deep dermis is approximated using 3-0 and 4-0 Monocryl in a simple interrupted fashion. The key suture is at the junction where the lateral flap meets the medial skin edge at the inferior margin of the areola, because this is the area of greatest tension. Subcutaneous dermal closure is performed with interrupted 4-0 Monocryl, avoiding any tension on the skin. Final adjustments prior to skin closure may include micro liposuction or additional deepithelialization if needed. After dermal closure, 5-0 or 6-0 plain catgut is used to approximate the areola to the adjacent skin edge and the lower skin incisions in a continuous fashion (Fig. 28.7).

Following the mastopexy closure, if combining breast augmentation, the sizers are replaced by the final implant, which is then filled to the desired amount. The axillary incision is closed with a simple interrupted layer of 6-0 plain catgut.

Postoperative care is minimal. The breast is supported with a porous soft elastic tape. The tape is removed in 7–10 days and may be reapplied to the incisions for an additional week, or the patient may simply elect to cover the incision with a preparation such as Scarguard®. A surgical bra is worn for comfort, and an underwire bra is avoided until the implants have settled into position. If the implants tend to rise, as may be the case with submuscular implants, an ace wrap may be used for a day or so after surgery. Patients' activity is not limited after surgery and they are encouraged to resume normal activity as soon as possible. Intravenous antibiotics are given immediately before surgery and continued orally for 2 days afterwards. Pain medication is prescribed as needed, but rarely is any type of narcotic required for more than 2 or 3 days.

28.3
Complications

Complications are infrequent following the B mastopexy, as the procedure does not completely penetrate the skin. It goes without saying that when combined with breast augmentation, all complications related to that procedure are possible. An unsatisfactory cosmetic result is always possible, but this is largely related to the experience of the surgeon. There is no question that there is a fairly steep learning curve to the operation. Wound separation can occur if the closure is too tight but it is important to include some degree of over correction, as there will be some skin stretching during healing. Thickened or widened scars are always possible; however, undermining with a good dermal closure minimizes this problem. Sensory disturbance should not occur, as the procedure is carried out above the dermis. Regnault has also described no increased incidence of hypertrophic scarring or loss of nipple sensation [1, 2], although it must be kept in mind that loss of nipple

Mastopexy/Reduction and Augmentation without Vertical Scar

Sid J. Mirrafati

29.1
Introduction

Breast lift or reduction is a common procedure frequently performed by a cosmetic breast surgeon. Breast reduction is a very satisfying procedure for the patients, as they do not have to carry such a massive weight and there is relief from the shoulder pain radiating to the arm or the lower back pain. The results are so satisfying that patients, for most part, do not complain about the scarring that is left behind from the breast reduction procedure. In the case of breast lift with augmentation, the patients are so happy with the new upright, fuller breast that they are not too concerned about the incisional scar.

As a cosmetic surgeon, we owe it to our patients to always strive for the best results with minimal incision. Cosmetic surgeons around the world have been introducing new techniques that would deliver results with minimal scarring. There have been several techniques that have been introduced for the full breast lift/reduction procedure that entail having a vertical scar running down from the areolar to the inframammary fold. The only scar that seems to bother the majority of the patients is the vertical scar and the scar on the sides when the inframammary scar is not kept under the breast, such as with the McKissock reduction and the Lejour technique.

The lift/reduction that the author utilizes avoids the vertical incisional scar and keeps the inframammary incisional scar invisible under the breast. This technique would not work for extremely large breast that would like to be moderately small or cup size "A," but would work for most other instances. If the patient adamantly does not want the vertical scar and there is too much skin or the surface area is too large, then the inferior part of the vertical scar that is mostly hidden by the inferior pole of the breast can be added. This technique would work great for ptotic breast that requires a full breast lift and an augmentation.

29.2
Consultation

During the consultation, it is important that you completely assess the patient and review all the available options, especially in a ptotic breast that the patient would like to have a moderately large implant. Generally in grade II ptosis, if the patient is willing to place a large implant and if the skin integrity is good with not much stretch marks, the patient can have a crescent lift with augmentation and can avoid the full lift, but in grade III ptosis, the patient would require a full breast lift no matter how big the implant size would be. The chest size is measured from the midline going 2 cm laterally to the anterior axillary line. One centimeter is reduced from this measurement and this would be the diameter of the implant that can be placed in. Even though the vertical scar is not done, the patients are still told about the other scars. Patients are told that the scar takes one year to be less visible. The scar will first look red, then turn dark, and eventually will be the color of the skin.

29.3
Surgical Procedure

Preoperative photos are taken in a straightforward position at 45° and 90° angles.

29.3.1
Marking

Preoperative markings are done (Fig. 29.1). The areolar is marked with a cookie cutter of 4 cm in diameter. The new nipple position is marked by palpating the inframammary fold and transferring this to the surface of the breast. The new areolar position is marked with a 6 cm cookie cutter. The midclavicular line to the areolar

M.A. Shiffman (ed.), *Mastopexy and Breast Reduction: Principles and Practice*,
© Springer-Verlag Berlin Heidelberg 2009

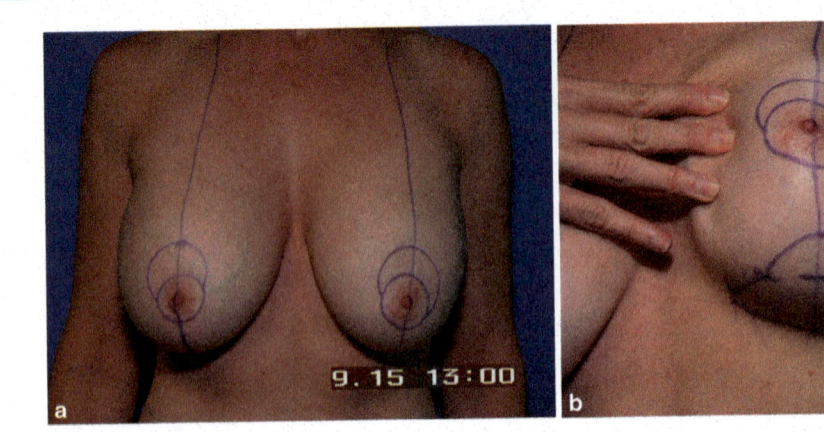

Fig. 29.1 (a,b) Marking the breast

superior pole is measured to be 19 cm, and if planning to place an implant, this measurement should be 20 cm. This precaution should be taken to make sure that the areolar does not sit too high and will show through the patient's bikini top or the bra. Be conservative because the areolar position can be raised higher at a later time, but once it is pulled too high it would be very difficult to lower the position. A 5 cm line is drawn from the inferior pole of the new areolar position.

The inframammary line is drawn such that the line cannot be seen when the breast is placed in a relaxed position. The medial and the lateral aspect of the inframammary breast line is marked and then marked 1 cm medially from each side. This will ensure that the incision will not be visible after the surgery. The breast is retracted laterally and a straight line is drawn from the end of the 5 cm line to the inframammary fold. The breast is then retracted medially and another line is drawn to the medial mark of the inframammary fold line. This will create a triangle that would be later cut to act as a support and shape the breast.

The 5 cm vertical line can sometimes be extended if planning to place a large implant depending on the shape of the patient chest and the size of the implant. Double checking is done again to make sure that the inframammary marking is not seen when the patient is standing. Sometimes if the breast is too ptotic and there is too much skin, the marking is modified to have a vertical scar only in the inferior aspect at 2 cm from the inframammary line. This is usually hidden by the bottom pole of the breast when the surgery is completed.

29.3.2
Technique

The patient is placed in a supine position and the breast prepped with Betadine. If breast reduction, lift, and augmentation are to be performed, the procedure is begun with the reduction. Tumescent fluid is injected into the breast until it is moderately firm and full. The tumescent fluid consists of 1 L of saline with 2 ml of 1:1,000 epinephrine and 500 mg of lidocaine. Approximately, 500 ml is injected into each breast.

Liposuction may be performed to reduce the breast using a 5 mm open spiral cannula and a 4 mm cannula to fine-tune the area. The superior pole of the breast is usually not liposuctioned so that there is good projection after surgery. If the breast is to be reduced by 500 g, then 500 ml is liposuctioned from each breast. This will require a lot of palpation to make sure that it feels the same in both breasts.

Incisions is made along the preoperative markings around the areola as well as along the new position of the areolar complex (Fig. 29.2). Deepithelialization of the skin is done, as well as 1 cm undermining.

The areolar is lifted and anchored to its new position using the 4-0 Monocryl. The four quadrants are evenly distributed and sutured to the areola using the 4-0 Monocryl. The skin is closed using the 5-0 nylon. There is going to be some pleating when the areolar is completely closed. This will usually resolve and the skin will become evenly retracted. If there are some pleating that persists after 6 weeks, be patient because essentially all patients resolve by 6 months. If for some reason it did not resolve after 6 month, revision can be performed to even out the pleating.

The inframammary incision is performed and the dissection taken down to the pectoralis fascia. A pocket is developed in the subglandular plane. In reduction mammoplasty, the implant is generally placed in a subglandular plane unless the skin in the medial superior region is thin or the patient requests submuscular placement. In either situation, a pocket is developed and the implant is placed in after proper hemostasis and antibiotic irrigation.

29.3 Surgical Procedure   239

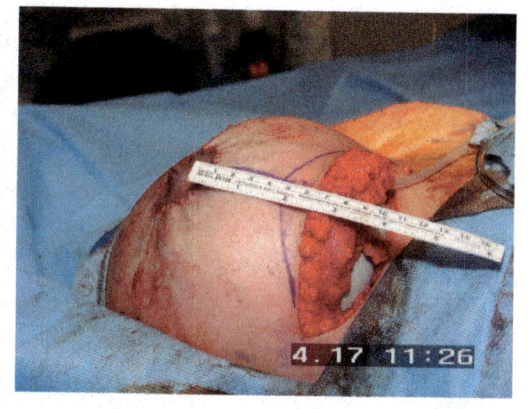

Fig. 29.3 The line from the lowest aspect of the areola to the superior point of the lower triangle should be 5 cm but can be adjusted to accommodate an implant

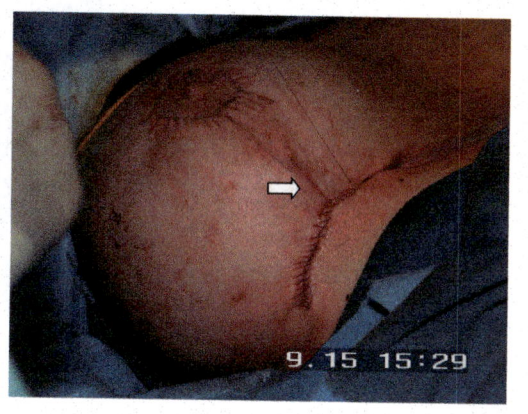

Fig. 29.4 Modify the markings to include an inferior vertical scar 2 cm long if skin is too loose

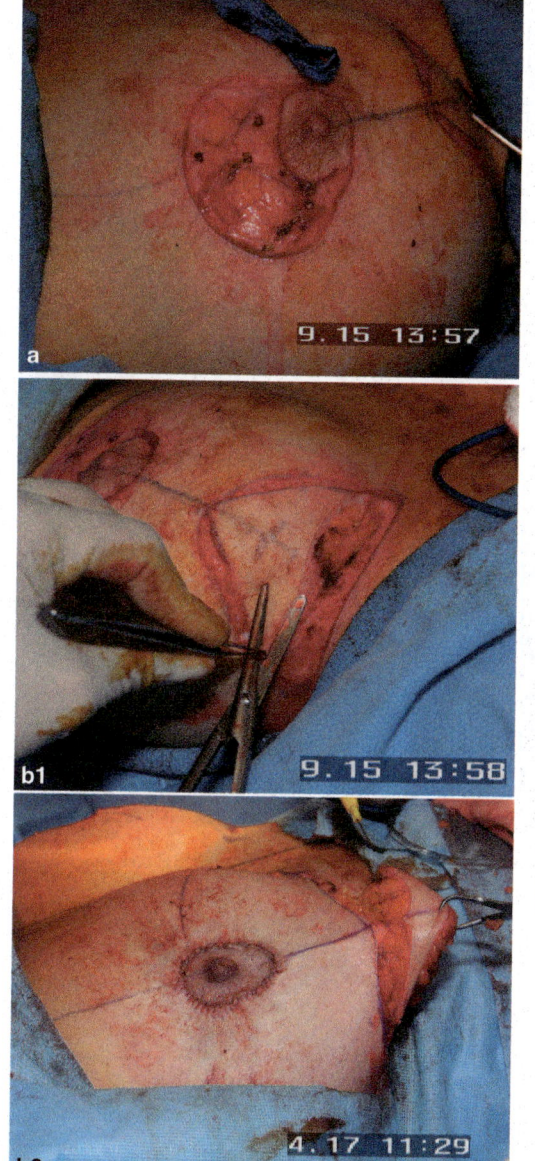

Fig. 29.2 (a) The areola is incised and the excess skin deepithelialized. (b1,2) The inferior triangle is incised and deepithelialized or can be resected if breast reduction is to be performed

The triangle that is preoperatively marked is resected with the breast tissue (Fig. 29.2). This is where the preoperative marking has to be modified depending on the size of the implant. The 5 cm line can be 6 cm or longer depending on the size of the implant (Fig. 29.3). The incisions may be modified to include an inferior vertical scar if the skin is too loose (Fig. 29.4). After taking out the triangle, the incision is closed using a 4-0 Monocryl subcutaneously and the skin is closed using a 5-0 nylon. A compression dressing is applied.

29.4 Postoperative Care

The patient should be seen on the first postoperative day. The dressing is changed and the compression dressing left off. In this technique of reduction mammoplasty or mastopexy, there is no real concern about nipple–areolar necrosis as there is no vertical incision. The patient is examined for proper implant position, hematoma, and incision healing. Patients are told to apply

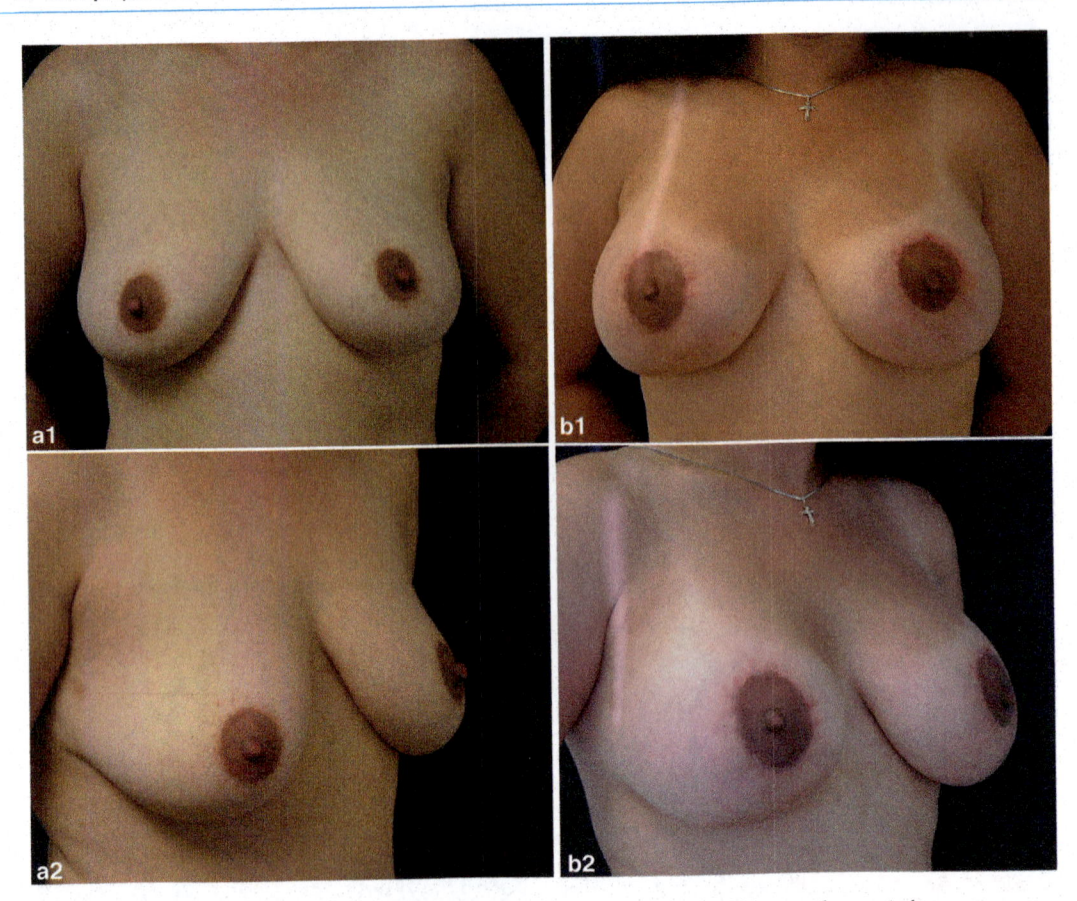

Fig. 29.5 (**a***1,2*) Preoperative patient. (**b***1,2*) Postoperative without visible inframammary fold scar and no vertical scar

antibiotic ointment to the incision and change the dressings daily. Patients are given simple arm exercises and can take showers starting 48 h after the surgery. Patients are told to continue taking Keflex 500 mg twice daily and 2,000–3,000 mg vitamin C daily.

29.5
Complications

Other than one patient having hypertrophic scarring around the areola, there has not been any other complication. Sometimes when the implant size is large, there is an indentation in the center that will stretch out in time. There is always some settling or some times bottoming out of the lift with time, but this is a problem that can happen with any lift or reduction procedure.

29.6
Conclusions

This is a lift that avoids the most unwanted and the most obvious scar associated with a breast lift or reduction procedure, the vertical scar (Fig. 29.5). There have been many different types of lift that have been introduced in text books or the literature, but they mostly involve the vertical scar that this technique avoids. Patient satisfaction is high and the complication rate is very low.

Breast Reduction and Mastopexy with Vaser in Male Breast Hypertrophy

Alberto Di Giuseppe

30.1 Introduction

In the early 1980, few articles were published on suction lipectomy as part of a combined surgical solution for gynecomastia, and it was suggested to utilize SAL (suction assisted lipoplasty) in conjunction with sharp surgical resection of the subareolar breast bud and wherever necessary the parenchymal tissue (Fig. 30.1).

Courtiss [1] suggested extensive removal of fat with suction lipectomy, and used knife or scissors to remove the subareolar breast cone (Fig. 30.2). It was a general thought that it was impossible to remove parenchymal tissue via SAL alone, due to the resistance fibrosis of the gland.

Rosenberg [2] showed to be competent in using SAL alone to remove successfully fat and parenchymal tissue, without complications (Fig. 30.3). Histology confirmed the accuracy of fat as well as breast tissue cleaning in gynecomastia treatment using SAL.

Nydick [3] showed that there was an incidence of gynecomastia in 65% of pubertal males, and resolution almost always occurs, but in another study by Nuttal [4] of 306 adult males, clinical gynecomastia was seen in 36%, with a greater incidence (57%) in men over 44 years.

Regarding the etiology, an increasing responsibility has been addressed to drugs and medications, such as steroids, Zantac, Tagamet, Nizoral, as well as Marijuana. Anabolics, of course, can increase male breast volume [5]. Obesity is a part of the problem, as a certain deposit of fat in male breast is always connected with an increase in body weight by man, with intensification with age and loss of breast tone and pectoralis muscle power. Surgical intervention is the only real radical treatment, which does not interfere with hormone balance.

Nearly 80% of American plastic and cosmetic surgeons seem to approach gynecomastia with open surgical breast tissue excision with or without SAL as a support for defining contouring of the thorax-breast [6]. The consistency of the fibrous male breast can be expressively addressed with the new vibration assisted sound et resonance (Vaser) ultrasound-assisted technique.

Vaser (S.S.T. Denver, Co US) uses solid probes introduced via small cutaneous incisions to emulsify fat as well as breast tissue and dissolve them, thus aspirating the emulsion through a suction cannula.

30.2 Selection

The author has used Vaser system technology as the sole treatment of male gynecomastia for the past 4 years, including the treatment for all types of gynecomastia (pure fatty, mixed, or fibrous bud) depending on the incidence of type of tissue in the clinical case presentation (Fig. 30.4). The volume of tissue removed typically varies from 150 ml in a small gland up to 700 ml per side in an obese patient, including the tumescent solution. The infranatant aspirate may vary from 200 ml in minor cases and up to 1,800 ml in large volumes.

Ptosis correction may vary from virtually 0 up to 4 cm and in the postoperative period that is noticeable already 1 week after surgery.

Preoperative assessment is done with the patient standing. The central cone of breast is marked and areas of undermining, which include breast fat tissue or residual fibrous tissue, are marked. Lines of surgical incisions (axillary – inframammary crease – periareolar, if necessary) are marked. All cases are performed under tumescent anaesthesia, sometimes modified, with intravenous sedation.

Modified tumescent anesthesia includes the following:
1. Ringer lactate 1,000 ml
2. Adrenaline 1 ml
3. Lidocaine 750–1,000 mg
4. Sodium bicarbonate 12.5 meq

In multiple areas, general anesthesia is preferred, such as when gynecomastia is treated with abdomen contouring

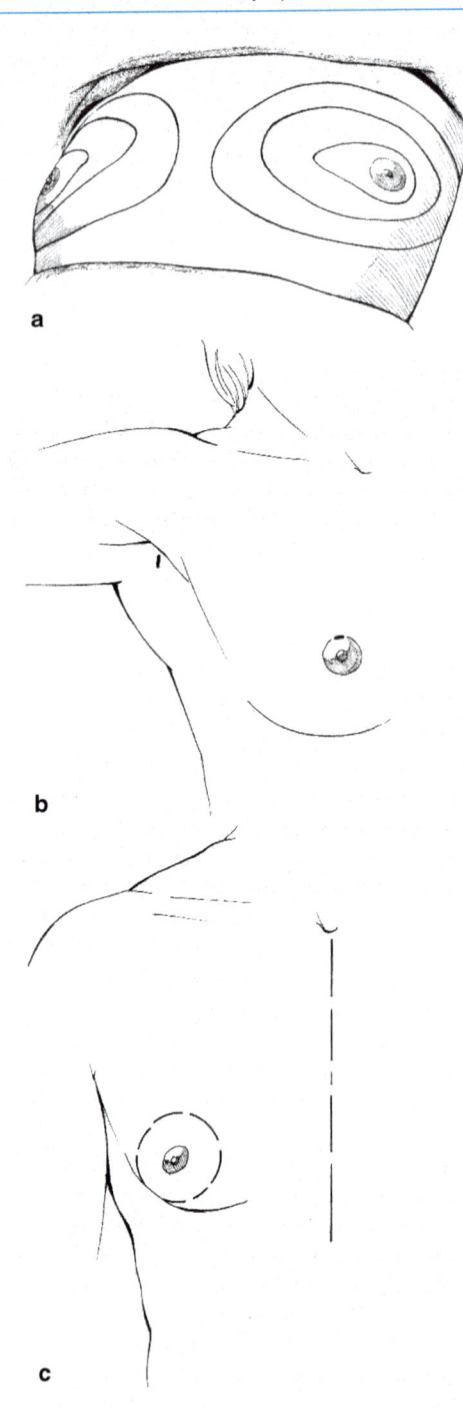

Fig. 30.1 (a) Planned fat removal. (b) Skin incisions: axilla-areola. (c) Subareolar adenectomy

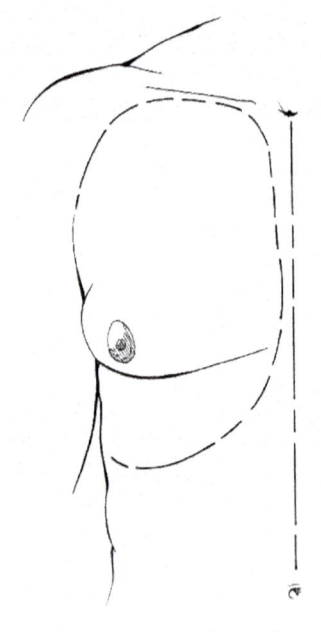

Fig. 30.2 Courtiss' original design of breast liposuction in large area of thorax

and or thighs contouring. When performed under general anaesthesia, lidocaine dose is reduced to some 100 mg l^{-1} only to provide postoperative analgesia, and bicarbonate is eliminated. Depending on the dimension of the breasts, total tumescent solution infused may vary from 500 ml to even 1,700 ml for each side. The infiltrated solution has approximately 2:1 ratio with the aspirate.

The Vaser system provides a set of solid probes with diameters of 2.9, 3.8, and 4.1 mm, and a recently introduced new probe, which has a sort of arrow tip expressively designed to target more aggressively the breast central bud (Fig. 30.5)

30.3
Technique

Via an inframammary incision, tumescent solution is infiltrated in the superficial as well as into the deep layers (Fig. 30.6). When completed, the infiltration should be uniform. A minimum of 15 min should be given for the adrenaline to have its effect. To prevent friction injuries at entrance site, a plastic skin protector should be used. To help its introduction, a special dilator and a skin protector are used (Fig. 30.7).

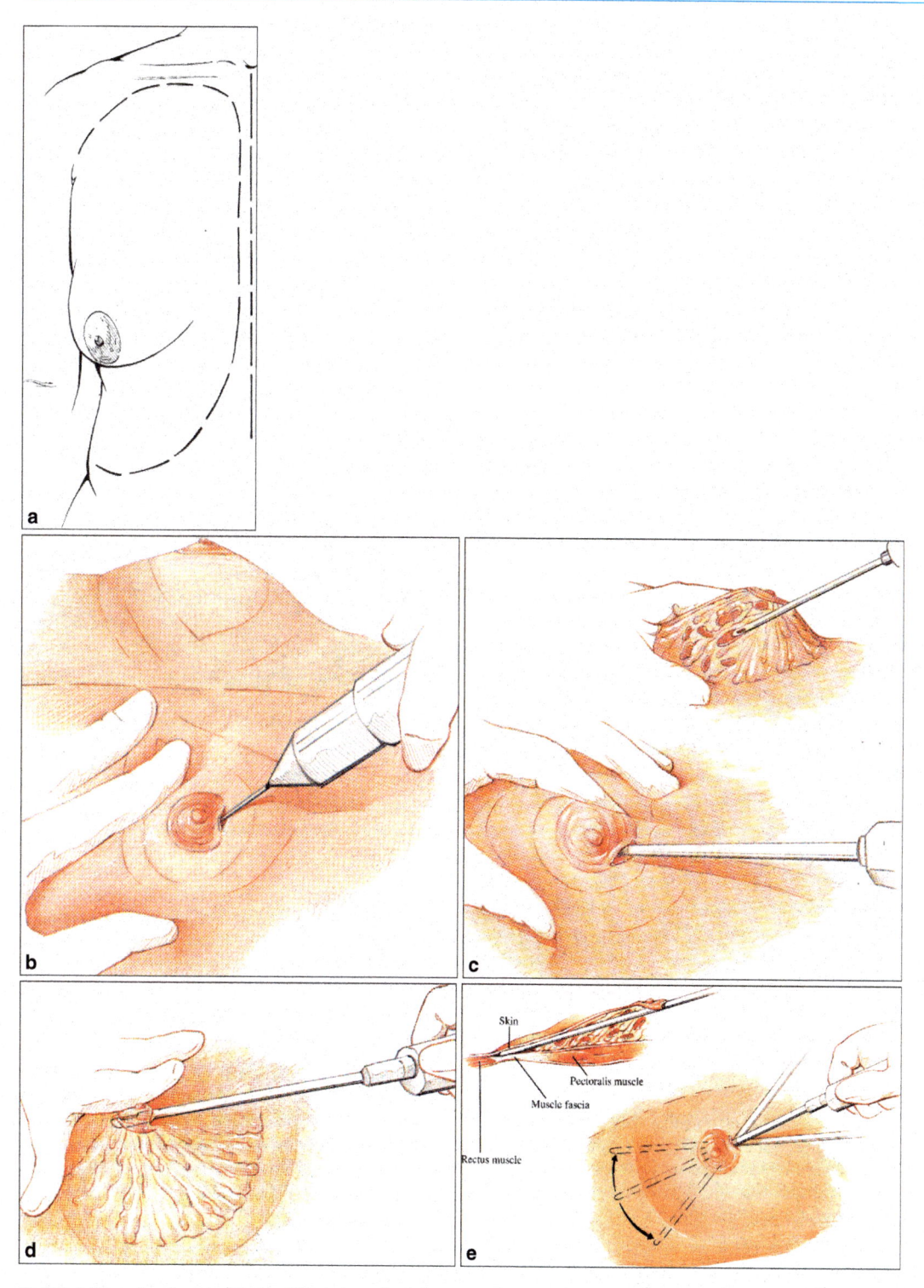

Fig. 30.3 (a) Rosenberg's original design. (b) Local anesthesia for periareolar approach. (c) Cannula for breast reduction. (d) Periareolar aggressive tissue removal. (e) Level of suction

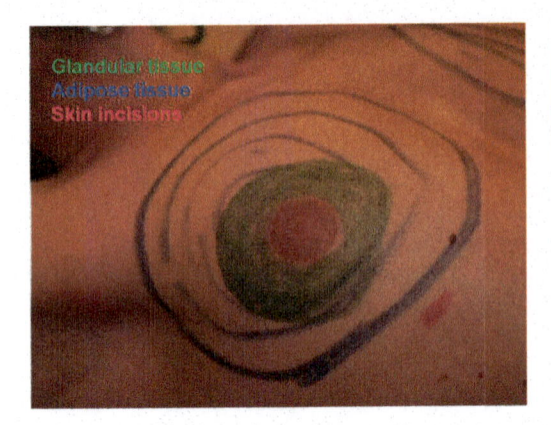

Fig. 30.4 Extent of liposuction marked

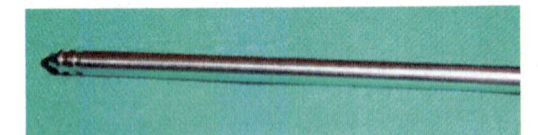

Fig. 30.5 New probe with arrow tip

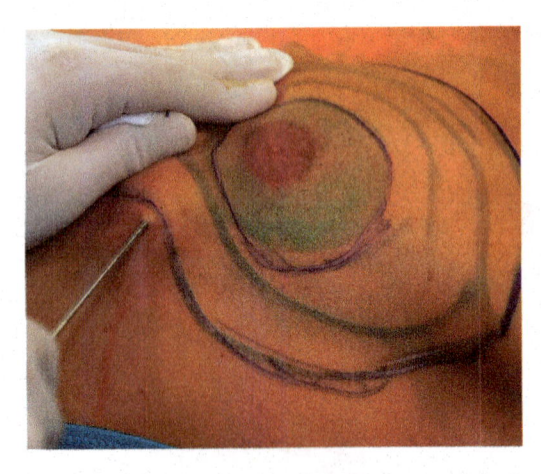

Fig. 30.6 With an inframammary incision, tumescent solution is infiltrated in superficial as well as deep layers

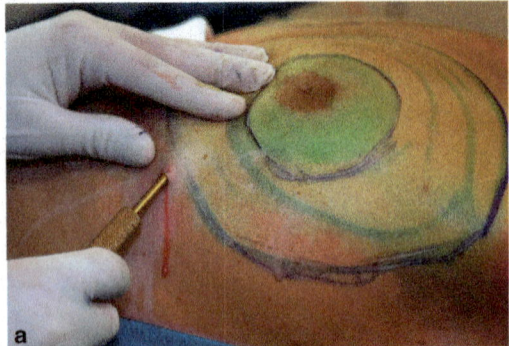

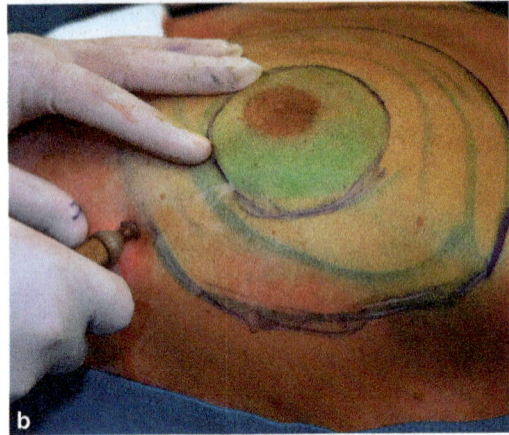

Fig. 30.7 (**a**) Skin dilator. (**b**) Skin protector in place

The initial phase, after setting the power of the Vaser at 80%–90% of its total, consists in undermining the skin of the thorax remaining in the subdermal plane (Fig. 30.8). This superficial undermining is performed using the 3.8 mm probe, with the Vaser system tuned to 70% of its total power. The continuous mode provides full administration of ultrasound energy on time.

The Vaser system provides what is called the Vaser mode, which means an interrupted administration of energy by time that diminishes the total energy given by half for fraction of time (thus increasing margin of safety of the instrument). The author believes that the continuous mode works well, as the probes are designed to emulsify the target tissue. The careful superficial undermining with the solid probe is essential to fully display the subcutaneous tissues at the subdermal layer from the deeper planes.

This extensive subdermal undermining is realized through the help of the solid titanium probe: with the proper tumescent infiltration. Vaser helps to find the correct cleavage plane preserving the supporting structures of the connective tissue, as vessels, nerves, collagen vertical fibres. In this way, Vaser realizes a selective emulsification of just the fat tissue, sparing

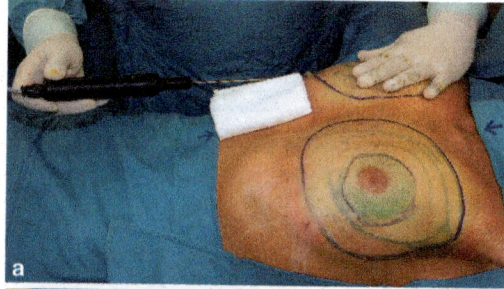

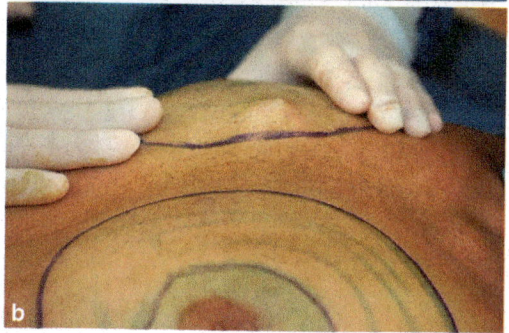

Fig. 30.8 (a) Superficial undermining with probe. (b) Note tip of probe at work

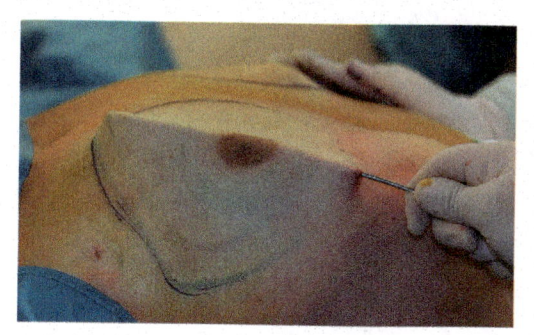

Fig. 30.9 Check flaps after removal of emulsified fat

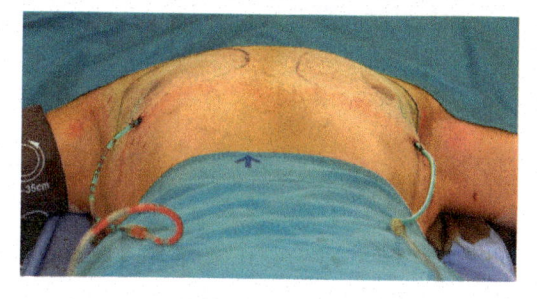

Fig. 30.10 Suction catheters in place and symmetry of result is verified with a double check

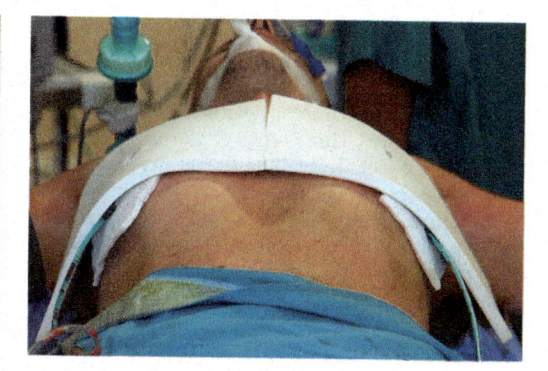

Fig. 30.11 Epifoam-Dressing

"noble" supporting structures of the dermis and the skin. Rudolph [7] stated that dermis plays a considerable role in skin retraction. As thin is the flap obtained with the probe undermining, as much skin retraction is achieved; this is best obtained raising subdermally a thin vascularized flap similar to what happens in subdermal liposuction.

The standard aspirate is not different from typically emulsified fat taken elsewhere in the body. This proves the high quality cavitation and efficacy of the designed probes, which have rings (one to three) at the tip to increase power and quantity of emulsified fat per unit time. The subdermal flap is checked to be correctly and uniformly raised (Fig. 30.9). Also the nipple areola area, where most of the fibrous parenchymal tissue is localized, is thinned carefully. Lack of zone of adherence is verified all the way around the undermined areas. Suction drainages are left in place for 24 h to prevent seroma collection. Symmetry of result is verified with a double check (surgeon and assistant) (Fig. 30.10).

A silicone-baked foam dressing (Epifoam) is positioned for 10–15 days to soften the underlying tissues (Fig. 30.11). An elastic compressive garment that helps obliterate dead space is left in place for 4 weeks.

With larger breasts or breast with ptosis and excess skin, cross-suctioning is used to improve the results. A 5 mm incision is made in the axilla, which is best to conceal the scar. Another incision, if necessary, is made at the areola to help defatting this area or better sculpturing and thinning the breast cone, which has to be flat (not overdone and depressed). Avoiding waviness and irregularity and destroying lumps and nodules of the breast parenchymal is essential to prevent postoperative sequelae and complications. In large gynecomastia and ptotic gynecomastia with excess skin, even the inframammary crease must be obliterated to allow proper redraping of the skin.

30.4 Complications

Vaser is a solid technology with high standard of quality and safety. Three types of alarms are present in the case of technical failure (never experienced in 4 years) or wrong use of probe or elevation of skin temperature. So burns, seroma, and skin slough that were a serious potential complication in previously used technologies are not really an issue with the present technology.

Two small hematomas that required aspiration and 10 cases of residual central bud that required secondary touch up revision under local anaesthesia occurred in a series of 200 patients.

30.5 Conclusions

With the new technology, Vaser UAL is safe and effective in all forms of gynecomastia (Figs. 30.12 and 30.13).

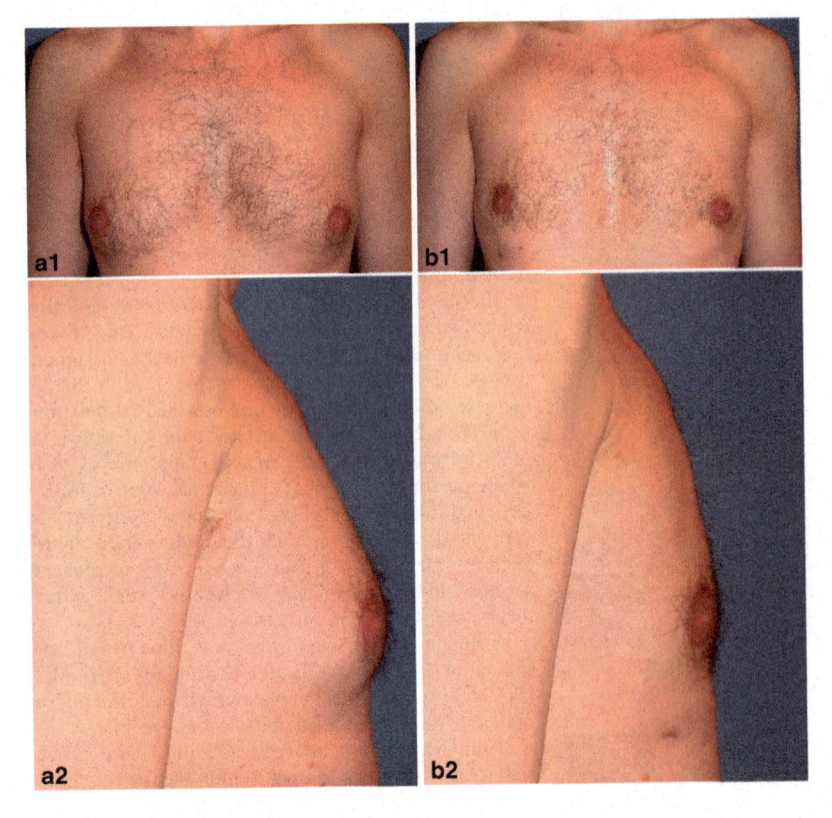

Fig. 30.12 (**a***1,2*) Preoperative patient with moderate pure gynecomastia with asymmetry. (**b***1,2*) Post-operative following 350 ml aspirate and Vaser 15 min each side

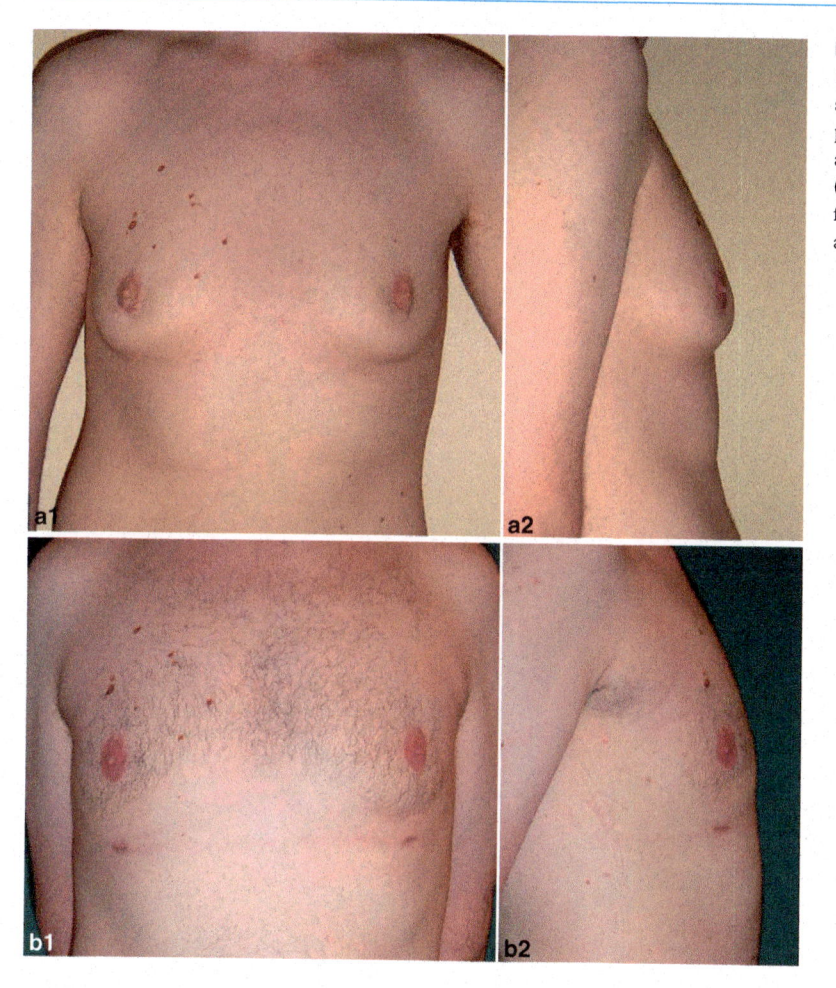

Fig. 30.13 (**a**1,2) Preoperative 19-year-old male with secondary gynecomastia, ptotic skin and gland, and abdominal laxity. (**b**1,2) Postoperative following Vaser and 1,100 ml aspirate from breasts

References

1. Courtiss EH: Mammoplasty with minimal scar. Annual meeting of the American Society of Plastic and Reconstructive Surgeons, Washington, D.C. 1992
2. Nydick M, Bustos J, Dale JH Jr, Rawson RW: Gynecomastia in adolescent boys. J Amer Med Assoc 1961;178: 449–454
3. Nuttal FQ: Gynecomastia as a physical finding in normal men. J Clin Endocrinal Metab 1979;48(2): 338–340
4. Rosenberg GJ: A new cannula for suction removal of parenchymal tissue of gynecomastia. Plast Reconstr Surg 1994;94(3):548–551
5. Letterman G, Schurter M: Gynecomastia. In: Courtiss EH (ed). Male Aesthetic Surgery. St Louis, CV Mosby 1976, pp 229–253
6. Mladick RA: Gynecomastia: liposuction and excision. Clin Plast Surg 1991;18:815
7. Spears SL: The Breast: Principles and Art. Philadelphia, Lippincott-Raven 1998
8. Rudolph R: The life cycle of the myofibroblast. Surg Gynecol Obstet 1977;145(3):389–394

Part V
Breast Reduction

History of Breast Reduction

Melvin A. Shiffman

31.1 Introduction

The history of breast reduction covers the innovative techniques of surgeons around the world. The ability of surgeons to report on a variety of techniques to accomplish a cosmetic reduction in breast tissue shows perseverance in finding better ways.

31.2 History

Durston (1670) [1] gave a description of gigantomastia occurring suddenly in a 23- or 24-year-old woman. This woman developed ulcerations of the breasts that were painful and became considerably larger [2]. In another publication the same year, Durston [3] described that she died and one breast weighed 64 pounds and the other about 40 pounds. No cancer was found.

Dieffenbach (1848) [4] reported on aesthetic breast surgery involving a "small" incision in the SMF.

Pousson (1897) [5] reported removing a crescent-shaped section from the upper anterior portion of the breasts to treat bilateral mammary hypertrophy. The skin and subcutaneous tissues were excised down to the pectoralis fascia and the breast was elevated and suspended by suturing to the pectoralis fascia.

Guinard (1903) [6] reported on a patient with macromastia using semicircular incisions in the submammary folds to remove a large amount of skin and breast tissue.

Morestin and Guinard (1908) [7] reported their experience with discontinuous resections of up to 1,400 g performed through an inframammary incision.

Thorek (1922) [8] reported on breast amputation and free nipple graft.

Kraske (1923) [9] described reduction of large breast.

Aubert (1923) [10] performed resection and transposition of the nipple.

Hollander (1924) [11] described an inferolateral excision of skin and breast tissue to eliminate the inframammary scar of the inverted T incision.

Biesenberger (1928) [12] noted the importance of leaving subcutaneous tissue attached to the skin. He performed extensive undermining and severing of the suspensory ligaments (Cooper's ligaments), and then wedge excisions of breast tissue in an inverted "S" shape involved the lateral aspect of the breast. This resulted in a high risk of skin and breast loss and the technique was largely abandoned.

Schwarzmann (1930) [13] fashioned a periareolar "cutis bridge" for maintenance of the blood supply to the nipple. This allowed a superiorly based dermoglandular pedicle to revascularize the nipple–areolar complex.

Schwarzmann (1937) [14] maneuver was developed that involved cleavage between skin and gland, preserving a periareolar zone stripped of the skin.

Maliniac (1938) [15] used strips of dermis graft for stabilization the breast.

Maliniac (1945) [16] presented a two-stage breast reduction to preserve the blood supply.

Bames (1948) [17] preserved the lateral and medial breast segments and resected the superior portion to preserve perforating vessels.

Aufricht (1949) [18] introduced an inferior pedicle technique and showed a geometric method to plan the reduction rather than using a free hand method and preserving perforating vessels by preserving the lateral and medial segments of breast and resecting the superior portion.

Reports on free nipple transplantation for reduction mammaplasty included Conway (1952) [19], Conway and Smith (1958) [20], Marino (1952) [21], and May (1956) [22].

Maliniac (1953) [23] did total gland excision, nipple areolar graft, and deepithelialized the inferior flap that was folded superiorly under the superior flap.

Wise (1956) [24] devised a pattern to predetermine the shape of skin flaps (Fig. 31.1) and a horizontal dermal parenchymal bridge for the preservation of the arteriovenous and cutaneous nervous system from above and below the dermal pedicle.

Arie (1957) [25] described a superior pedicle technique and Gillies and Marino (1958) [26] described the "periwinkle shell" (spiral rotation) technique for moderate ptosis.

M.A. Shiffman (ed.), *Mastopexy and Breast Reduction: Principles and Practice*,
© Springer-Verlag Berlin Heidelberg 2009

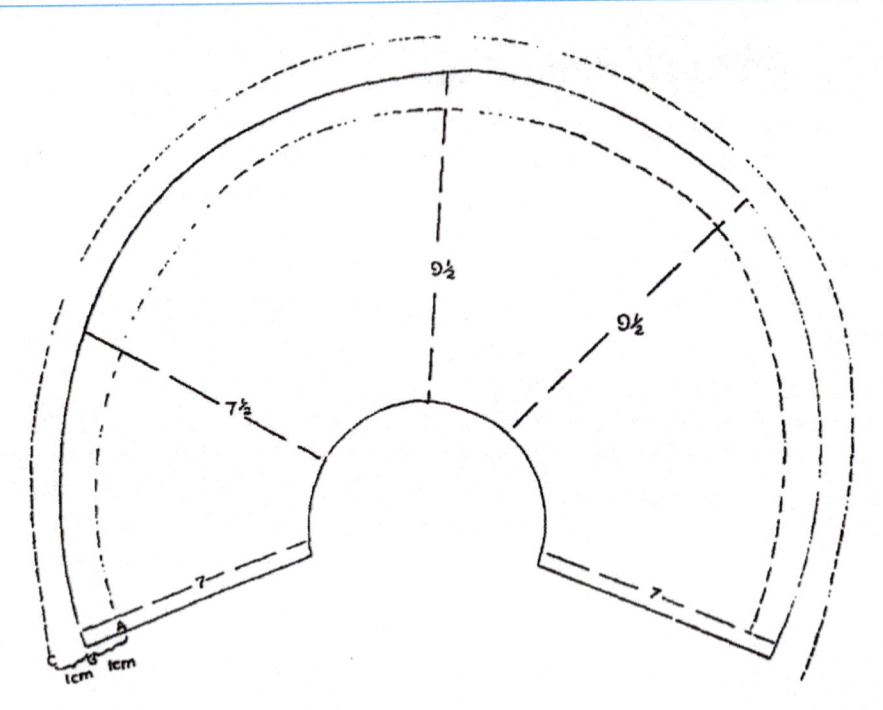

Fig. 31.1 Wise pattern. The solid line is Wise's technique compared to the dotted lines that are other authors' techniques

Strombeck (1960) [27] modified a keyhole pattern. He extended the concept of a dermal bridge technique described by Schwarzmann (1930) [14] to reintroduce the dermal pedicle for nipple transposition. He used a pattern similar to that described by Wise (1956) [24]. This was a horizontal dermal pedicle that consisted of the dermis of the two, lateral pedicles to transpose the nipple and create a fibrous "balcony" to prevent postoperative ptosis. The skin and gland above the areola were excised.

Pitanguy (1960) [28] performed a horizontal dermal bridge and "keel"-shaped resection of the gland from the inferior and central portions of the breast; it had excellent results when used for limited breast reductions (less than 300 g) and breast ptosis.

Dufourmental and Mouly (1961) [29] introduced the lateral wedge resection of skin, fat, and gland with a resultant inferior oblique lateral scar. Preoperative markings were made in the supine position.

Strombeck [30] reported the use of the horizontal bipedicle procedure for reduction mammaplasty.

Pitanguy (1961, 1962) [31, 32] described the superior dermal pedicle technique.

Wise et al. (1963) [33] used a modification of the breast amputation and nipple areola transfer.

Skoog (1963) [34] described a superior laterally based dermal flap separated from the gland at the subcutaneous level. He transposed the nipple on a unilateral skin flap, disconnecting nipple from gland. This was an intermediate procedure to free nipple transplantation.

Robertson (1967) [35] reported on the inferior flap mammaplasty in conjunction with free nipple grafting.

Hoopes and Jabalay (1969) [36] described amputation with nipple areola transplant and prosthesis.

Hoopes (1971) [37] performed amputation and mammoplasty for gigantomastia by using nipple areolar transplant and prosthesis.

Hinderer (1971) [38] described dermopexy with reduction, and reported attaching dermis strips to help fixate the breast to the chest wall to support the breast, in 1972 [39].

McKissock (1972) [40] described the bipedicle vertical pedicle for nipple transposition that had simplicity of design and safety.

Lalardrie (1972) [41] reported a dermopexy with reduction "Dermal Vault" technique.

Weiner et al. (1973) [42] described a modified superior dermal pedicle technique for nipple transposition. This technique cannot be used if the nipple site is to be more than 7.5 cm above its original position.

Pontes (1973) [43] described removal of the lower half of the breast starting 2 cm below the inferior edge of the areola after deepithelialization of the periareolar area and superior pedicle. The nipple–areolar complex is placed into position after closure of the breast.

Regnault (1974) [44] reported on a reduction mammaplasty using the B technique that resulted in a lateral oblique scar without a medial extension.

Lalarde (1974) [45] performed reduction with transposition of the nipple.

Gsell (1974) [46] described a superior-based dermal flap similar to the McKissock pedicle but transected at the inframammary end. This is risky as much of the blood supply to the parenchyma is transected. Nipple areola necrosis may occur.

Ribeiro (1975) [47] described an inferior pedicle technique. A vertical scar was avoided by bringing the nipple–areola complex under and through the superior skin flap and into position while tubing the inferior dermal pedicle.

Orlando and Guthrie (1975) [48] described a superior medial dermal pedicle.

de Castro (1976) [49] described a modified Pitanguy technique using curved incisions to define the medial and lateral breast flap borders and resection of the breast tissue on a horizontal plane. He believed that this modification produced breasts that were less tense and more desirable in shape.

Cramer and Chong (1976) [50] reported on a unipedicle cutaneous flap with areolar–nipple transposition or an end-bearing, superiorly based flap.

Weiner (1976) [51] described the modified superior pedicle technique.

Wise (1976) [52] discussed nipple transposition vs. nipple transplantation.

Courtiss and Goldwyn (1977) [53] described an inferior dermal pedicle technique as an alternative to free nipple–areola grafting in severe macromastia or ptosis. The inferior dermal pedicle extends transversely across the full length of the inframammary fold incision. A keyhole pattern, described by McKissock, was used.

Robbins (1977) [54] described the inferior dermal pedicle technique.

Georgiade et al. (1979) [55] performed reduction mammaplasty using an inferior pedicle nipple–areola flap.

Marchac and de Olarte (1982) [56] tried to prevent ptosis by fixing the gland to the pectoral fascia.

Ribeiro (1983) [57] reported on the inferior dermal pedicle technique.

Meyer and Kesselring (1983) [58] described closure with an L-shaped suture line.

Galvao (1983) [59] described a method of preserving the subdermal plexus of vessels with the nipple–areolar complex detached from the breast gland, leaving a completely free deepithelialized superior- and inferior-based dermal pedicle with only the subcutaneous fat that is folded and the breast closed after resection of the gland. The nipple–areola complex is brought out through the new position after complete closure.

Cardoso (1984) [60] used three dermal pedicles for nipple–areolar complex movement in the reduction of gigantomastia.

Hester et al. (1985) [61] performed breast reduction using the maximally vascularized central pedicle.

Renó (1985) [62] described the periareolar mastopexy.

Teimourian et al. (63) reported on reduction mammaplasty with liposuction.

Marshak (1988) [64] described a short horizontal scar mastopexy.

Benelli (1988) [65] reported on the periareolar mastopexy described as the "round block" technique.

Lejour et al. (1989) [66] introduced the vertical mammaplasty without an inframammary scar.

Georgiade (1989) [67] reported on the inferior pedicle technique.

Lejour and Abboud (1990) [68] described a vertical mastopexy without an inframammary scar combined with liposuction for breast reduction.

Sampaio-Goes (1991) [69] described periareolar mammaplasty with the double skin technique.

Menesi (1992) [70] reported on a distally based dermal flap for gland fixation.

Renó (1992) [71] reported on reduction mammaplasty with a circular folded pedicle technique.

Goes (1996) [72] performed the double skin technique with application of poyglactine or mixed mesh to fix the gland with allogenic mesh using a circular flap of dermis with a central pedicle.

31.3
Discussion

The progression of techniques and modifications of techniques speaks of the ingenuity of surgeons over the years. Cosmetic breast surgery of mastopexy and breast reduction is a continuously changing specialty and surgeons should maintain vigilance over the medical literature and attend meetings to keep up with these advances.

References

1. Durston W: Concerning a very sudden and excessive swelling of a woman's breasts. Phil Trans Vol IV for anno 1669, Royal Society, London 1670, pp 1047–1049
2. Durston W: Observations about the unusual swelling of the breasts. Phil Trans Vol IV for anno 1669, Royal Society, London 1670, pp 1049–1050
3. Durston W: Concerning the death of the big-breasted woman. Phil Trans Vol IV for anno 1669, Royal Society, London 1670, pp 1068–1069
4. Dieffenbach JF: Die extirpation der bruestdruese. In: Dieffenbach JF (ed). Die Operative Chirurgie, Brockhaus, Leipzig 1848, pp 359–373
5. Pousson: Bulletin et Memoire de la Societe de Chirurgie de Paris 1897

6. Guinard: Societe de Chirurgie de Paris 1903
7. Morestin H, Guinard A: Hypertrophie mammaire traitee par la reduction discoide. Bull Soc Chir (Paris) 1908;33:649
8. Thorek M: Possibilities in the reconstruction of the human form. N Y Med J 1922;116:572
9. Kraske II: Die operation der atropischen und hypertrophischen hangebrust. Munch Med Wschr 1923;60:672–673
10. Aubert V: Hypertrophie mammaire de la puberte. Resection partielle restauratrice. Arch Franco-Belg Chir 1923;3:284–289
11. Hollander E: Die operation de mammahypertrophie und der hangebrust, Deutsch Mede Wschr 1924;50:1400
12. Biesenberger H: Eine neue methode der mammaplastik. Zbl Chir 1928;38:2382–2387
13. Schwartzmann E: Die technik der mammaplastik. Chirurgica 1930;2:932–943
14. Schwartzmann E: Beitrag zur vermeidung von mamillennekrose bei einzeitiger mammaplastik schwerer falle. Rev Chir Struct 1937;7:206–209
15. Maliniac JW: Breast deformities. Anatomical and physiological considerations in plastic repair. Am J Surg 1938;39:54
16. Maliniac JW: Two-stage mammaplasty in relation to blood supply. Am J Surg 1945;68:55
17. Bames H: Reduction of the massive breast hypertrophy. Plast Reconstr Surg 1948;3:560
18. Aufricht GL: Mammaplasty for pendulous breasts: empiric and geometric planning. Plast Reconstr Surg 1949; 4:13–29
19. Conway H: Mammaplasty: analysis of 110 consecutive cases with end-results. Plast Reconstr Surg 1952;10(5):303–315
20. Conway H, Smith J: Breast plastic surgery: reduction mammaplasty, mastopexy, and mammary construction; analysis of two hundred forty-five cases. Plast Reconstr Surg 1958;21(1):8–19
21. Marino H: Glandular mastectomy: immediate reconstruction. Plast Reconstr Surg 1952;10(3):204–208
22. May H: Breast plasty in the female. Plast Reconstr Surg 1956;17(5):351–357
23. Maliniac JW: Use of pedicle dermo-fat flap in mammaplasty. Plast Reconstr Surg 1953;12:110–115
24. Wise RJ: Preliminary report on method of planning the mammaplasty. Plast Reconstr Surg 1956;17:367–375
25. Arie G: Una nueva tecnica de mastoplastia. Rev Lat Amer Cirug Plast 957;3:23–38
26. Gillies H, Marino H: L'opération en colimaçon ou rotation spirale dans les ptoses mammaires modérées. Ann Chir Plast 1958;3:90
27. Strombeck JO: Mammaplasty: report of a new technique based on the two pedicle procedure. Br J Plast Surg 1960;13:79–90
28. Pitanguy I: Breast hypertrophy. In: Wallace AB (ed). Transactions of the International Society of Plastic Surgeons, 2 edn. Edinburgh, UK, E&S Livingstone 1960, pp 509–522
29. Dufourmentel C, Mouly R: Plastie mammaire par la methode oblique. Ann Chir Plast 1961;6:45–58
30. Strombeck JO: Mammaplasty: report of a new technique based on the two pedicle procedure. Br J Plast Surg 1961; 13:79–90
31. Pitanguy I: Mammaplastias estudo de 245 casos consecutivos e apresentacao de tecnica pessoal. Rev Bras Cirurg 1961;42:201–220
32. Pitanguy I: Une nouvelle technique de plastie mammaire. Etude de 245 cas consecutifs et presentation d'une technique personelle. Ann Chir Plast 1962;7:199–208
33. Wise RJ, Gannon JP, Hill JR: Further experience with reduction mammaplasty. Plast Reconstr Surg 1963;32:12–20
34. Skoog T: A technique of breast reduction. Acta Chir Scand 1963;126:453–465
35. Robertson DC: The technique of inferior flap mammaplasty. Plast Reconstr Surg 1967;40(4):372–377
36. Hoopes JE, Jabaley ME: Reduction mammaplasty: amputation and augmentation. Plast Reconstr Surg 1969;44(5):441–446
37. Hoopes JE, Jabaley ME: Amputation and mammoplasty for gigantomastia. Mod Med 1971:137–138
38. Hinderer UT: Plastia mamaria modelante de dermopexia superficial y retromamaria. Rec Esp Cir Plast 1971;5(1):65
39. Hinderer UT: Remodelling mammaplasty with superficial and retromammary dermopexy. In: Transacta der III Tatung der Vereinigung der Deutschen Plastischen Chirurgen, Koln 1972,p 93
40. McKissock PK: Reduction mammaplasty with a vertical dermal flap. Plast Reconstr Surg 1972;49(3):245–252
41. Lalardrie JP: The "dermal vault" technique. Reduction mammaplasty for hypertrophy with ptosis. In: Transacta der III Tatung der Vereinigung der Deutschen Plastischen Chirurgen, Koln 1972, pp 105–108
42. Weiner DL, Aiache AE, Silver L, Tittiranonda T: A single dermal pedicle for nipple transposition in subcutaneous mastectomy, reduction mammaplasty, or mastopexy. Plast Reconstr Surg 1973;51(2)115–120
43. Pontes R: A technique for reduction mammaplasty. Br J Plast Surg 1973;26:365–370
44. Regnault P: Reduction mammaplasty by the "B" technique. Plast Reconstr Surg 1974;53(1):19–24
45. Lalardrie JP, Jouglard JP: Chirurgie plastique du sien. Paris, Masson et Cie 1974
46. Gsell F: Reduction mammaplasty for extremely large breasts. Plast Reconstr Surg 1974;53(6):643–646
47. Ribeiro L: A new technique for reduction mammaplasty. Plast Reconstr Surg 1975;55(3):330–334
48. Orlando J, Guthrie R: The superomedial dermal pedicle for nipple transposition. Br J Plast Surg 1975;28(1): 42–45
49. de Castro CC: Mammaplasty with curved incisions. Plast Reconstr Surg 1976;57(5):595–600
50. Cramer L, Chong J: Unipedicle cutaneous flap: Areolanipple transposition or an end-bearing, superiorly based flap. In: Georgiade NG (ed). Reconstructive Breast Surgery, St. Louis, C.V. Mosby Company 1976, p 143
51. Weiner DL: Reduction mammaplasty with a single superior dermal pedicle. In: Goldwyn RM (ed). Plastic and

Reconstructive Surgery of the Breast, Boston, Little-Brown & Co. 1976
52. Wise RJ: Treatment of breast hypertrophy. Clin Plast Surg 1976;3(2):2879–300
53. Courtiss EH, Goldwyn RM: Reduction mammaplasty by the inferior pedicle technique: an alternative to free nipple and areola grafting for severe macromastia or extreme ptosis. Plast Reconstr Surg 1977;59(1):500–507
54. Robbins TH: A reduction mammaplasty with the areola-nipple based on an inferior dermal pedicle. Plast Reconstr Surg 1977;59(1):64–67
55. Georgiade NG, Serafin D, Morris R, Georgiade G: Reduction mammaplasty utilizing an inferior pedicle nipple-areola flap. Ann Plast Surg 1979;3(3):211–218
56. Marchac D, De Olarte G: Reduction mammaplasty and correction of ptosis with a short inframammary scar. Plast Reconstr Surg 1982;69(1):45–55
57. Ribeiro L, Backer E: Inferior based pedicles in mammoplasties. In: Georgiade NG (ed). Aesthetic Breast Surgery. Baltimore, Williams & Wilkins Company 1983, p 260
58. Meyer R, Kesselring U: Reduction mammoplasty (twelve years' experience with the L-shaped suture line). In: Georgiade NG (ed). Aesthetic Breast Surgery. Baltimore, Williams & Wilkins Company 1983, p 219
59. Galvao MSL: Reduction mammaplasty with preservation of the superior, medial, lateral and inferior pedicles. In: Georgiade NG (ed). Aesthetic Breast Surgery. Baltimore, Williams & Wilkins Company 1983, p 175
60. Cardoso AD, Cardoso AD, Pessanha MC, Peralta JM: Three dermal pedicles for nipple-areolar complex movement in reduction of gigantomastia. Ann Plast Surg 1984;12(5):419–427
61. Hester TR Jr, Bostwick J III, Miller L, Cunningham SJ: Breast reduction utilizing the maximally vascularized central pedicle. Plast Reconstr Surg 1985;76(6);890–900
62. Renó WT: Mamaplastia periareolar em cone. Presented at 2nd Congresso Brasileiro de Cirurgia Plástica, Sessão Pinga-Fogo, Gramado, Brazil 1985
63. Teimourian B, Massac E Jr, Wiegering CE: Reduction suction mammaplasty and suction lipectomy as an adjunct to breast surgery. Aesthetic Plast Surg 1985;9(2): 97–100
64. Marchac D, Sagher U: Mammaplasty with a short horizontal scar. Evaluation and results after 9 years. Clin Plast Surg 1988;15(4):627–639
65. Benelli L: Technique de plastie mammaire: le "round block." Rev Fr Chir Esthet 1988;50:7
66. Lejour M, Abboud M, Declety A, Kertesz P: Reduction des cicatrices de plastie mammaire: De l'ancre courte a la verticale. Ann Chir Plast Esth 1989;35:369
67. Georgiade G, Riefkohl R, Georgiade NG: Inferior dermal-pyramidal type breast reduction: long-term evaluation. Ann Plast Surg 1989;23(3):203–211
68. Lejour M, Abboud M: Vertical mammoplasty without inframammary scar and with liposuction. Perspect Plast Surg 1990:4:67
69. Sampaio-Goes JC: Periareolar mammaplasty double skin technique. Breast Dis 1991;4:111
70. Menesi L: Mammaplasty with dermal flap. Transactions of the Xth Congress of the IPRS. Elsevier Science: Madrid, Vol III, 1992:122
71. Renó WT: Reduction mammaplasty with a circular folded pedicle technique. Plast Reconstr Surg 1992;90:65
72. Goes JC: Periareolar mammaplasty: double skin technique with application of polyglactine or mixed mesh. Plast Reconstr Surg 1996;97(5):959–968

CHAPTER 32

Principles of Breast Reduction Surgery

32

Melvin A. Shiffman

32.1
Introduction

Each form of reduction mammoplasty, depending on the vascular pedicle, has its own possible problems. Over the years some principles have evolved that may help keep the surgeon out of trouble.
Principles
1. Obtain all records of earlier breast surgeries and review the surgical reports prior to performing breast reduction.
   a. Beware of prior breast augmentation that has utilized an inframammary incision. An inferior-based pedicle probably cannot be used in this situation.
   b. In secondary breast reductions, do not cut across the prior pedicle, except if the earlier procedure was bipedicle then one pedicle can been transected.
2. Obtain a preoperative mammogram on all patients preferably, but at least those over 35–40 years of age.
   a. This may prevent the accidental incision into a cancer.
3. Obtain preoperative photographs on all patients.
   a. This will substantiate preoperative asymmetry or other deformities.
4. Always mark the breast for skin incisions and possibly glandular excisions before surgery.
   a. Mark in the sitting or standing position.
   b. Freehand artistry with a scalpel may be used with certain techniques, but is not for the novice.
      i. Freehand artistry is more prone to asymmetry, as it requires a large amount of experience to resect the correct amount of tissue.
   c. Freehand artistry requires training before attempting the technique.
5. Record the following measurements:
   a. Sternal notch and/or mid clavicle to nipples
   b. Nipples to midline
   c. Extent of ptosis: the degree of ptosis and/or measurement from nipple to inframammary fold and inframammary fold to lowest point of breast
   d. Inframammary fold to superior point of the planned areola
6. Remove only that amount of breast tissue to relieve the symptoms of enlarged breasts and to satisfy the patient as to cup size.
   a. Most patients do not wish to have an A cup following breast reduction from a D or larger cup size.
7. When estimating the position of the new nipple in very large breasts, lower the site of the new nipple between 1 and 2 cm from the level of the inframammary fold depending on the size of the breast.
   a. If the new nipple site is not lowered, the nipple–areolar complex may be too high and will show in a brassiere or bathing suit.
8. If the nipples are rotated laterally, use the distance from the midline (10–12 cm) to establish the new nipple position rather than the line from the mid clavicle or sternal notch to the nipple.
9. Pedicles
   a. Do not thin pedicle excessively.
   b. Long pedicles should be at least 6 cm in width.
   c. A superior pedicle over 12 cm in length may not survive [1].
   d. Observe for twisting of the long pedicle at the time of closure.
   e. Check the nipple–areolar complex at the completion of closure for early evidence of vascular congestion or cyanosis.
10. Breast skin flaps should be undermined minimally or not at all.
11. Consider nipple areola transplant in very large breasts.
    a. When the excision will be over 1 kg in weight [2] or when the distance from the inframammary

M.A. Shiffman (ed.), *Mastopexy and Breast Reduction: Principles and Practice*,
© Springer-Verlag Berlin Heidelberg 2009

fold to the upper rim of the keyhole pattern exceeds 35 cm [2].
   b. Place graft on a flat, deepithelialized bed, not on subcutaneous fat.
   c. See the patient on the first postoperative day to make sure there is no hematoma and that the nipple–areolar complex is not cyanotic.
   d. Venous refill of the nipple–areola complex should always be less than 6 s. If more than 6 s, the surgeon should seriously consider nipple areola transplant to prevent nipple areola necrosis.
12. Smoking should be stopped at least 2 weeks before and 2 weeks after surgery to prevent postoperative necrosis.

32.2 Conclusions

Surgeons should learn from the experience of other surgeons and avoid their mistakes. Be aware of those principles that will help reduce possible complications and possibly avoid litigation.

References

1. McKissock PK: Color Atlas of Mammaplasty. New York, Thieme 1991, p 45
2. McKissock PK: Color Atlas of Mammaplasty. New York, Thieme 1991, p 47

The Use of Epinephrine in Breast Surgery

Michael S.G. Bell

33.1 Introduction

Preoperative infiltration of dilute epinephrine 1:1,000,000 combined with 1/3% xylocaine is gaining acceptance as a standard technique in breast surgery. The principle of injecting large volumes of xylocaine epinephrine solutions into the breast applies to breast reduction, mastopexy, and breast augmentation. Blood losses are cut to half in breast reductions done using this technique, and opioid consumption postoperatively is also one-half [1, 2]. This solution allows mastopexy and breast augmentation to be done as an office procedure when combined with intravenous sedation techniques [3, 4].

33.2 History

The desire to reduce the sizeable amount of blood loss in breast reduction prompted initial studies in using epinephrine xylocaine mixtures, beginning with Bretteville-Jensen in 1974 [1] and Brantner and Peterson in 1984 [5]. All reported satisfactory significant reduction in blood loss. Klein [6] coined the term "tumescent technique" of using large volumes of dilute local anesthetic solutions with epinephrine. He reported the safety of using xylocaine 1% and epinephrine 1:1,000,000 solution up to doses of 35 mg kg^{-1}. Infiltration of local anesthetics has also been found to reduce discomfort and requirement of opioid after surgery [2, 3, 6–8].

33.3 Technique

The author has been using a solution of 0.35% xylocaine in 1:1,000,000 adrenaline over the past 15 years for breast reduction, mastopexy, and breast augmentation surgery. The solution is prepared preoperatively in the pharmacy using 3½ bottles of 2% cardiac xylocaine, each containing 50 ml of the solution. This is added to 825 ml of normal saline, giving a solution of 0.35% xylocaine. The solution can be stored in a refrigerator for up to 1 month. One milliliter of epinephrine 1:1,000 is added to this at the time of surgery.

All breast incisions are premarked with a surgical marking pen, and after general or intravenous anesthesia is administered, infiltration is done using a 12 gauge blunt tipped Wells Johnson cannula [No. 20–0008LL]. Up to 10 ml kg^{-1} of solution is injected dividing between the breasts (Fig. 33.1). A blunt cannula is necessary, as a sharp needle overly penetrates dense breast tissue, making injection difficult. The blunt cannula also follows planes more readily.

For breast reduction and mastopexies, the solution is injected subcutaneously along the skin incision lines and at the level of the pectoralis fascia. Injecting at the area of the planned pedicle is avoided, although there has never been any observed problem with nipple ischemia attributable to this solution. Care is also taken to inject back to the mid-axillary line, ensuring that the most efficacious block is achieved.

For breast augmentation, injections are done along the proposed incision line and also beneath the pectoralis major muscle running laterally along the ribs to the mid-axillary line. A smaller volume of the solution is usually used with breast augmentations and mastopexies than with breast reduction patients, as they are usually thinner and smaller. Usually 150–200 ml per breast would be average. For these patients where volume differences are so critical, we usually use a 20 ml syringe with three-way stopcock to precisely inject the solution. In breast reductions, where less precision is needed, we routinely use a pressurized intravenous (IV) bag and a three-way stopcock for efficiency and ease of injection of these larger volumes. There has been no problem observed with postoperative asymmetry because of confusion involving different volumes of solution.

M.A. Shiffman (ed.), *Mastopexy and Breast Reduction: Principles and Practice*,
© Springer-Verlag Berlin Heidelberg 2009

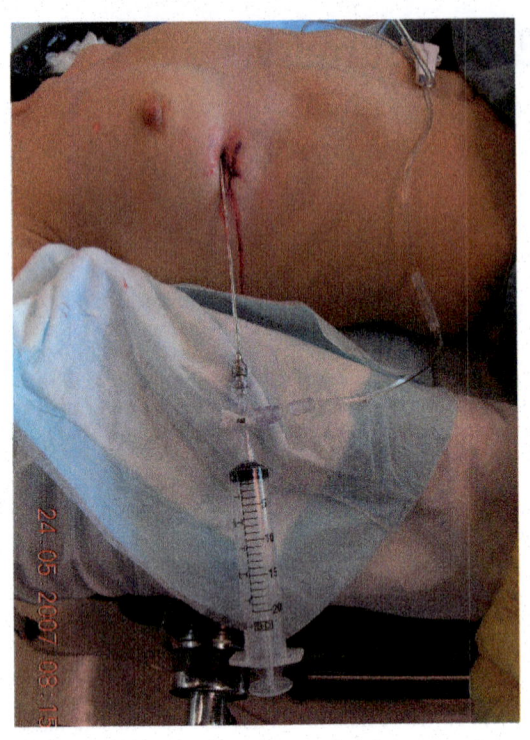

Fig. 33.1 Infiltration of tumescent solution in breast augmentation

33.4
Complications

There have been no problems with wound healing attributable to dilute xylocaine epinephrine injection in the breast. The effects of the anesthetic wear off by 6–7 h judging by visual analogue scale (VAS) pain testing. In the past 2,500 breast reductions, only two patients have been returned to the operating room with bleeding. This was felt to be due to relatively large veins that had not been cauterized. One could not logically blame this upon the adrenalin effect of masking a vessel from the potential to bleed.

33.5
Discussion

Healthy women undergoing elective surgery should not be placed at the risk of requiring homologous blood transfusions that are expensive and inconvenient. It has been a standard practice of many surgeons performing reduction mammoplasty in the past years to give blood because of the accepted large blood loss during these procedures. In contrast, the tumescent technique of infiltrating breast tissue along the lines of resection with large volumes of dilute local anesthetic and epinephrine is safe, cheap, and remarkably effective (Fig. 33.2). It reduces blood loss to half. It also eliminates the risk of

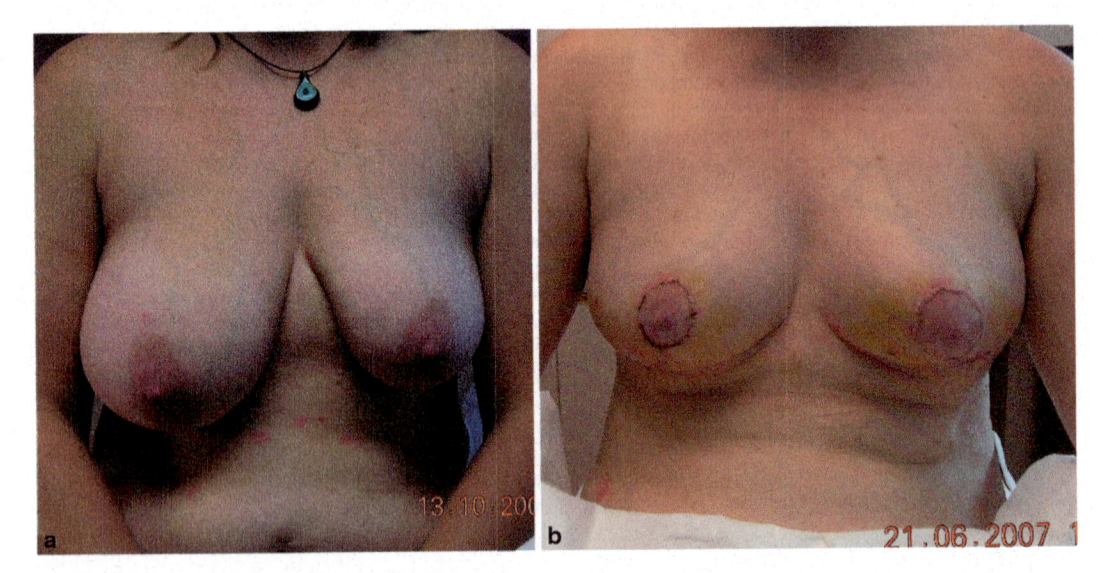

Fig. 33.2 (a) Preoperative patient with right mammary hypertrophy and left breast ptosis. (b) One week postoperative right breast reduction and left mastopexy using tumescent solution

blood mismatch and cost of autologous blood donation. It also avoids the morbidity of postoperative anemia and the lethargy and inability to resume usual activities seen so frequently in the past.

The second significant benefit pre-infiltration of the breast with local anesthesia is the reduction in postoperative pain noted immediately upon waking in the recovery room [2]. The total opioid consumption is reduced by 45%. Tumescent solution with 35–55 mg kg^{-1} of 0.1% xylocaine for liposuction procedures results in peak plasma levels 4–8 h after completion of the surgical procedure [6, 9]. Peak plasma xylocaine levels were well below toxic levels in all patients in these two reported studies.

The postoperative pain relief results from a prolonged residual nerve block likely caused by the slow release from tissue stores. This is presumably associated with the addition of epinephrine, which slows vascular absorption of the xylocaine. Decreased central sensitization as a result of the preoperative neural block may in part reduce the parenteral opioid consumption.

This technique is quite beneficial in that it allows the patient to have breast reduction surgery done reliably on an outpatient basis. Over night stay after breast reduction surgery remains the standard in most large centers. In the case of breast augmentations and mastopexy, there is a very low incidence of nausea and vomiting. Unfortunately, in breast reduction patients, the incidence of nausea and vomiting was 87%, which is the same as patients who did not have xylocaine epinephrine infiltration. In the case of breast reductions, the improved pain relief in the early postoperative period was not reflected in a shorter time for achieving fitness for discharge [2].

33.6
Conclusions

The use of large volume dilute xylocaine epinephrine solution is well established to significantly reduce blood loss in breast reduction and mastopexy procedures. It also reduces early postoperative pain in breast reduction, mastopexies, and breast augmentations, reducing the opioid consumption to about one-half. There have been no complications associated with the use of this solution either in wound healing or systemically. Unfortunately, this technique has not improved the 87% incidence of nausea and vomiting in breast reductions, so that same day early discharge seen in patients with breast augmentation and mastopexy was not achieved. Breast augmentation and mastopexy procedures can be done safely and with complete comfort in the office setting using this technique when combined with intravenous sedation [10].

References

1. Bretteville-Jensen G: Mammaplasty with reduced blood loss: effect of noradrenaline. Br J Plast Surg 1974;27(1): 31–34
2. Rosaeg O, Bell M, Cicutti N, Dennehy K, Lui A, Krepski B: Pre-incision infiltration with lidocaine reduces pain and opioid consumption after reduction mammoplasty. Reg Anesth Pain Med 1998;23(6):575–579
3. Quttainah A, Carlsen L, Voice S, Taylor J: Ketamine-diazepam protocol for intravenous sedation: the Cosmetic Surgery Hospital experience. Can J Plast Surg 2004; 12(3):141–143
4. Bell M: The use of epinephrine in breast reduction. Plast Reconstr Surg 2003;112(2):693–694
5. Brantner JN, Peterson HD: The role of vasoconstrictors in control of blood loss in reduction mammaplasty. Plast Reconstr Surg 1985;75(3):339–341
6. Klein JA: Tumescent technique for regional anesthesia permits lidocaine doses of 35 mg/kg for liposuction. J Dermatol Surg Oncol 1990;16(3):248–263
7. Mottura AA: Epinephrine in breast reduction. Plast Reconstr Surg 2002;110(2):705–706
8. Brown, MH: Epinephrine in breast reduction. Plast Reconstr Surg 2002;110(2):706
9. Ostad A, Kageyama N, Moy RL: Tumescent anesthesia with a lidocaine dose of 55 mg/kg is safe for liposuction. Dermatol Surg 1996;22(11):921–927
10. Bell M: Office anesthesia for breast augmentation made easy. Can J Plast Surg 2007;15(3):178

Choosing a Technique in Breast Reduction

Donald A. Hudson

34.1
Introduction

The perfect procedure to reduce the breast has been sought for centuries. Kraske [1], modifying the technique of Lexer [2], suggested an inverted T pattern consisting of an inferior vertical wedge glandular excision and a vertical and transverse ellipse of skin. However, lack of understanding of the blood supply to the nipple–areola complex (NAC) led to erratic results, and there was a time when a two-stage procedure was advocated.

Schwarzmann, in 1930 [3], advanced the concept of a dermal pedicle using a superior and medial dermal cutaneous pedicle bridge to the NAC. This improved the safety of the procedure. The search for a reproducible design led Wise [4] to modify the pattern of Nedhoff, which led to the keyhole markings. Wise used a full thickness graft for the NAC.

The inferior pedicle with the keyhole or inverted T pattern was popularized by Courtiss and Goldwyn [5], Robbins [6], and others, and is reported to be the most commonly performed technique used in the USA. In 1970, Lassus [7] described a short scar vertical mammoplasty, but it was Lejour [8] who popularized the technique. Hall-Findlay [9] subsequently simplified this technique.

Most techniques of breast reduction now employ a pedicle. This improves the results with respect to nipple sensation and increases the likelihood of breast feeding after reduction mammoplasty. Additionally, the irregular pigmentation after free nipple grafting is avoided.

The blood supply to the NAC arises from four major sources. The medial pedicle arises mainly from the perforators from internal mammary vessels. The inferior pedicle is supplied by the lateral row of intercostal perforators. There is also supply from the thoraco-acromial axis superiorly and laterally from the lateral thoracic vessels.

Theoretically, there are two factors to consider when reducing the breast: first, where is the tissue excess and how is reduction to be achieved? Concomitantly, the aesthetics of the breast needs to be addressed. In any real degree of macromastia, the excess tissue exists is in the inferior pole of the breast in both horizontal and vertical planes, and thus resection of the tissue in both these planes is required.

Another important factor to consider is breast aesthetics, especially the position of the nipple with respect to the rest of the breast and its relationship to the inframammary fold. While a number of articles have examined the "perfect breast," these criteria usually apply to young women with an ideal chest shape and good skin elasticity. In macromastia, the aim is to create a slightly pendulous breast rather than the breast of a nulliparous teenager. The aesthetic proportion is also age dependant and the new nipple position should be marked lower in the post partum patient, for example.

A reasonable ratio of suprasternal notch to the nipple distance vs. nipple to inframammary fold distance is 3:1 or even 4:1 The keyhole/inverted T has usually (rigidly) marked the vertical limb at 5 cm, irrespective of the new nipple position! This distance is often too short – it stretches out with time anyway and pseudoptosis is not an uncommon sequel. In contrast, in the vertical mammoplasty no horizontal skin excision is undertaken, and the distance from nipple to inframammary fold maybe disproportionately long.

Consider some commonly used techniques:

1. *Keyhole/Inverted T, Inferior Pedicle*: This technique was popularized in the 1970s and is based on clinical studies of its efficacy. The technique can be considered as an excision of two ellipses at 90 degrees to each other. This tissue excess is excised from the vertical and horizontal planes. This explains the versatility of the technique and explains why it is particularly useful in large reductions. The blood supply to the NAC is retained on a wide pedicle, which is reported to be safe at a length of 20–25 cm.

   While the inferior pedicle is reliable, it suffers from a number of "mechanical" disadvantages. First, the inferior pedicle is inferior and thus the excess tissue that is inferiorly situated cannot all be excised. More importantly, as the inferior pedicle lies under the point of maximum tension of the adjacent skin flaps, breakdown at the T is not uncommon. In fact, the more bulk in the pedicle, the more tension is

M.A. Shiffman (ed.), *Mastopexy and Breast Reduction: Principles and Practice*,
© Springer-Verlag Berlin Heidelberg 2009

applied to the T junction, with subsequent skin (and fat) necrosis. However, this is a versatile, safe technique, which explains its popularity.

2. *Inverted T/Keyhole with Superior-Medial Pedicle*: The superior medial pedicle has a number of advantages. It permits the excess tissue situated inferiorily to be excised without impedance. Additionally, the pedicle is rotated from an inferior position to a superior position, and theoretically at least, tissue is redistributed into a more appropriate location. However, whether these theoretical benefits translate into a better long-term result remain unproven.

   Perhaps a lesser known fact about the superior medial pedicle is the robustness of its blood supply. Anatomical studies by Palmer and Taylor [10] demonstrated that the dominant blood supply to the NAC is medial, and a recent study attests to its reliability in gigantomastia.

3. *Vertical Mammaplasty (VM)*: The technique (or its variations) has gained in popularity in recent years. While similar techniques were described in the 1950s, Lejour [8] championed its resurgence. The original technique described by Lejour was associated with an unacceptable complication rate. Hall-Findlay modified and simplified the technique and also improved its safety. The VM has a number of fundamental differences to the keyhole pattern:
   - A more limited skin incision – only a vertical ellipse of skin is excised, although parenchymal tissue is excised in both a vertical and inferior horizontal plane.
   - Parenchyma sutures are inserted. The two breast pillars that are created are sutured together, the so-called "parenchymal moulding." This is said to "cone" the breast and increase projection.
   - A superior or superior-medial pedicle is used.
   - Commonly (but not always) the original inframammary fold is destroyed, and a new fold is created superior to the original fold. The vertical scar should preferably not extend below the new inframammary fold, so the fold cannot be raised very much.

4. *Periareolar Reduction mammaplasty*: This technique, except perhaps in South America, has not gained widespread popularity. It has a limited skin resection and this technique is only really applicable to lesser degrees of breast hypertrophy. Additionally, the technique truncates the apex of the breast cone, resulting in a flat, poorly projecting breast. Furthermore, as the periareolar incision is cinched and reduced to the size of the new areola, a wrinkling of the skin occurs and a star burst appearance is not uncommon.

   No parenchymal remodeling occurs, which led Goes [11] to insert a mesh as an internal brassiere. This brings in a new component to the procedure in addition to expense.

5. *Liposuction*: Liposuction relies on skin retraction to achieve its improvement in shape, which is an obvious limitation in the breast. Liposuction cannot really remove (much) breast tissue, but only successfully removes fat, but Lejour noted that it is very difficult to determine preoperatively how much of the breast is actually fat. It has obvious advantage of limited scarring. Liposuction is useful as an adjunctive maneuver in breast reduction.

34.2
Conclusions

The problem with the inverted T/keyhole pattern technique is that it relies on the skin envelope to achieve and maintain its shape. Additionally there is a tendency to over-resect tissue, leading to a flat, poorly projecting breast. As tissue descends into the inferior pole with time, pseudoptosis is not an infrequent sequel. These latter problems can be overcome by not resecting too much tissue. Additionally, mark the new nipple position just below the inframammary fold. Finally, ensure that the vertical limb of the inverted T or keyhole pattern is marked proportionately. For example, if the new nipple position is marked at 24 cm, the vertical limb (excluding the areola) should be 6 cm to retain the aesthetics of 4:1.

In contrast, the VM tends to under-resect breast tissue. No skin resection is undertaken in the horizontal plane and there is a reliance on skin retraction, which is an obvious limitation in large reductions. This technique is also reported to require more frequent revisions. However, it does improve breast projection, and the scar hypertrophy medially and laterally with the inverted T technique is avoided.

Liposuction is a useful adjunctive procedure, particularly in the axilla and lateral breast. Choosing a technique requires an assessment of the patient, risk factors as well as the severity of macromastia and degree of ptosis. The vertical mammoplasty gives a predictable and satisfactory result in reductions of less than 500 g per breast. Achieving aesthetic results with larger reductions is more difficult. In contrast, the Keyhole/inverted T is a versatile technique for larger reductions. The choice of pedicle often depends on teaching and familiarity. The superor-medial pedicle has a robust blood supply and less tension is applied at the T junction.

References

1. Kraske II: Die operation der atropischen und hypertrophischen hangebrust. Munch Med Wschr 1923;60:672–673
2. Lexer E: Hypertrophie bei der mammae. Munchen Med Wochenschr 1912;59:2702
3. Schwartzmann E: Die technik der mammaplastik. Chirurgica 1930;2:932–943
4. Wise RJ: Preliminary report on method of planning the mammaplasty. Plast Reconstr Surg 1956;17:367–375
5. Courtiss EH, Goldwyn RM: Reduction mammaplasty by the inferior pedicle technique: an alternative to free nipple and areola grafting for severe macromastia or extreme ptosis. Plast Reconstr Surg 1977;59(1):500–507
6. Robbins TH: A reduction mammaplasty with the areola-nipple based on an inferior dermal pedicle. Plast Reconstr Surg 1977;59(1):64–67
7. Lassus C: A technique for breast reduction. Int Surg 1970;53:69
8. Lejour M: Vertical mammaplasty and liposuction of the breast. Plast Reconstr Surg 1994;94(1):100–114
9. Hall-Findlay EJ: A simplified vertical reduction mammoplasty: Shortening the learning curve. Plast Reconstr Surg 1999:104(3):748–759
10. Palmer JH, Taylor GI: The vascular territories of the anterior chest wall. Br J Plast Surg 1986;39(3):287–299
11. Goes JC: Periareolar mammaplasty with mixed mesh support. The double skin technique. Oper Tech Plast Surg 1996:3:199–205

Breast Reduction Techniques and Outcomes

Courtney Crombie, Irfan Ibrahim Galaria, Colette Stern, W. Bradford Rockwell

35.1 Liposuction-Assisted Reduction

Liposuction was first introduced as the sole technique for reduction mammaplasty in 1991 by Matarasso and Courtiss [1]. Surgeons who administer liposuction breast reduction feel that some of the complications associated with traditional breast reductions, such as infection, wound dehiscence, skin loss, numbness, and aesthetically unpleasing scars, may be avoided. This technique is most appropriately employed when the patient has minimal breast ptosis or if the ptosis is of secondary importance. If ptosis correction is a major concern to the patient, liposuction alone may not be the optimal technique. The elastic recoil of the skin following liposuction will improve ptosis to some degree, though the amount is unpredictable.

Breast reduction with ultrasound-assisted lipoplasty [2] is a technique that has been reported to be safe and effective in reducing the fatty volume and providing lift of the breast. Goes [3], Zocchi [4], and Di Giuseppe [2] review this technique and advocate the efficacy of ultrasound as an adjunct to liposuction breast reduction.

Patients with predominantly fatty, rather than glandular, breasts are the optimal candidates for liposuction breast reduction [5]. This ratio is difficult to determine by physical examination alone, though the ratio of fat to glandular tissue tends to increase with age. The amount of adipose deposits elsewhere on the body may also be helpful in predicting the amount of fatty tissue in the breasts.

35.1.1 Markings

The areas of increased fullness are marked preoperatively. The lateral breast and fold extending to the back is frequently an area of concern. If not addressed, this region may become more noticeable and concerning to the patient after reduction of the breast size. Breast asymmetry should also be noted preoperatively, brought to the patient's attention, and incorporated into the plan.

The additional percentage to be removed from the larger breast should be approximated in advance. The region between the clavicle and the upper pole of the breasts is marked and avoided, as the perforators in this region increase the chance of hematoma formation. If there is concern that an insufficient volume of breast parenchyma will be removed by liposuction only, the breasts may be marked for a resection technique as a standby option.

35.1.2 Technique

The procedure is performed with the patient in the supine position and arms secured on arm boards. Incisions about 5 mm are placed on the medial and lateral aspects of the breast, approximately 1–2 cm above the inframammary fold. The tumescent solution, usually consisting of 1 l of lactated Ringer's and 30 ml of 1% lidocaine and one ampule of epinephrine, is infiltrated bilaterally. Straight cannulas of 4 and 3 mm are used in a criss-cross fashion to obtain an adequate and symmetric reduction.

35.1.3 Outcomes

Gray reported his experiences with liposuction breast reduction in over 200 women [6, 7]. His average volume suctioned was 850 ml from each breast, with an average reduction in the nipple-to-sternal notch distance of 6 cm. All patients reported resolution of preoperative symptoms. There were no reported infections, loss of nipple sensation, skin loss, or inability to breastfeed. One hematoma and one seroma occurred, and one post-liposuction bilateral mastopexy and three breast cancer-associated unilateral mastopexies were performed.

Moskovitz et al. [8] performed an outcome study in liposuction breast reduction. Of the 78 patients who responded to their survey, 93% reported resolution of shoulder pain, 96% reported elimination or improvement of intertrigo, 88% reported elimination or improvement in their shoulder ruts, and 72% reported improvement in their posture. Seventy percent of the patients reported a decrease in ptosis, while 24% stated that ptosis was unchanged and 6% felt it had worsened. Overall patient satisfaction was high, with 92% stating that they would recommend this technique to a friend and 87% claiming that they would choose this method again.

In the appropriately chosen patient population, liposuction breast reduction is a reasonable alternative to traditional breast reductions. While postoperative nipple position and degree of ptosis correction is unpredictable, this technique provides the advantages of significantly smaller scars, high patient satisfaction, and an overall lower complication rate.

35.2
Inferior Pedicle Mammaplasty

Reduction mammaplasty with the nipple–areola complex based on an inferior dermal flap was first described by Ribeiro [9] in 1975. Since then, variations on this technique have been described by Robbins, Courtiss, and Goldwyn [10, 11].

35.2.1
Markings

The markings are performed with the patient in the standing position. Each vertical chest wall meridian is marked, with extension from the mid-clavicle to the inframammary fold. This line may not intersect the nipple. The new nipple position is determined by one of three ways, depending on the size of the breasts: at the level of the inframammary fold, 21–23 cm from the suprasternal notch, or at the level of the mid-humerus. According to Hall-Findlay [12], the inframammary fold is the most reliable position. In larger breasts, however, the nipple position may need to be lower. An inverted-V marking is drawn with the apex at the new nipple position. Each limb of the V is measured at approximately 7 cm, though this distance should be modified according to breast size. The distal extent of the limbs is extended medially and laterally to the inframammary fold. A pinch test is performed between the limbs to ensure that the planned skin resection is not overly aggressive. Symmetry of the markings should be checked by measuring the suprasternal notch-to-new nipple distance, as well as the inframammary fold-to-nipple distance, bilaterally.

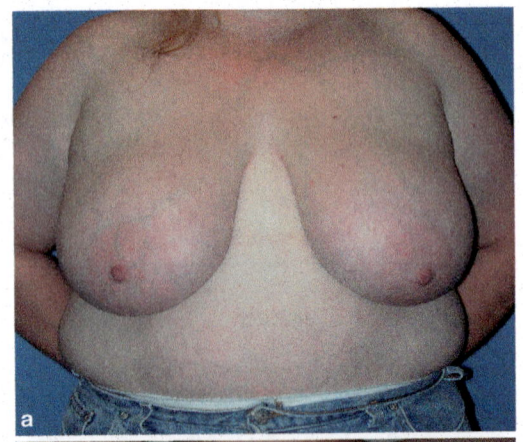

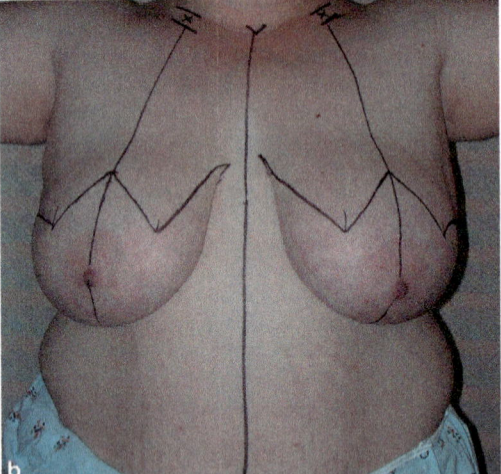

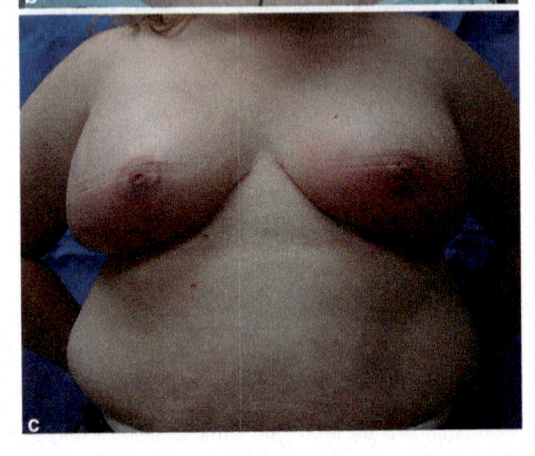

Fig. 35.1 (a) Preoperative patient undergoing inferior pedicle reduction. (b) Preoperative markings. (c) Postoperative

35.2.2
Technique

With the patient in the supine position, the patient is widely prepped and draped. A 38–42 mm areola marker is used to mark the new areola circumference. An inverted-U is marked around the new areola, extending inferiorly to the inframammary fold and delineating the inferior pedicle. The skin of the pedicle is infiltrated using local anesthetic with epinephrine and subsequently deepithelialized. The medial, lateral, and superior borders of the pedicle are incised down to the pectoral fascia, using caution to avoid undermining the pedicle. The inframammary fold is incised medially and laterally from the base of the pedicle. The adipocutaneous flap is then elevated off the chest wall superiorly to the level of the clavicles, medially to the sternum, and laterally to the border of the latissimus dorsi muscle. A layer of adipose tissue is maintained on the pectoral fascia in an attempt to preserve nerve supply. The remaining specimen within the inverted-V skin markings is excised. If further resection is need, the adipocutaneous flap and pedicle can be thinned.

Closure is initiated by placing a triangular stitch in the corners of the flaps to the midpoint of the pedicle base. Drains are placed, exiting in the mid-axillary line bilaterally. Interrupted, buried deep dermal sutures are placed along the inframammary incision. Similarly, the vertical limb is closed over the pedicle. The new nipple position is marked at the apex of the new breast mound using 38–42 mm nipple markers. The skin within the circumference is infiltrated using local anesthetic with epinephrine and deepithelialized. The dermis is scored at the 12, 3, 6, and 9-o'clock positions to allow for tension-free inset of the nipple–areola complex. If the viability of the nipple is in question, a free-nipple graft should be performed. If well-vascularized, the nipple–areola complex is tacked in place using interrupted, buried dermal sutures. A running subcuticular stitch is placed along the entire incision. All sutures used are absorbable, with the exception of the drain stitch. Steri-strips are placed, and the wounds are dressed.

35.2.3
Outcomes

The most common cause of patient dissatisfaction in breast reduction surgery is scarring [13–15]. Celebrier et al. [16] performed a retrospective review assessing patients' and surgeons' perspectives on the scar components after reduction mammaplasty using the inferior pedicle technique. They determined that patients were most satisfied with the periareolar scar and least satisfied with the inframammary scar.

Another potential aesthetic complication of the inferior pedicle technique is a "dog ear" at the medial or lateral edge of the inframammary incision. Dog ears should be prevented by noting and addressing them intraoperatively. Additional adipose tissue may be excised in these regions with beveling of the fat away from the incision.

Skin necrosis and wound breakdown are most likely to occur at the intersection of the vertical and transverse incisions, which is the region of maximum tension. Careful tissue handling, maintenance of flap thickness at the corners, and a low-tension closure may help to prevent devascularization from occurring. If wound breakdown does occur, local wound care is usually the adequate treatment.

35.3
Short Scar Techniques

35.3.1
Vertical Mammaplasty

Several short-scar reduction mammaplasty techniques have been introduced and applied in recent years; however, the vertical mammaplasty is the most widely used. Vertical mammaplasty was described as early as 1925 by Dartigues, but was popularized by Arie and Lassus [17–21]. The Lejour vertical reduction, first presented in 1989 [22], is a modification of Lassus' mammaplasty and is currently the most popular technique. Numerous adaptations of the Lejour technique have been proposed; however, it remains popular due to its shorter scar and more stable and pleasing results, as compared to other reduction mammaplasty approaches. The Lejour vertical reduction mammaplasty technique is described here.

35.3.1.1
Markings

With the patient in standing position, the midline of the chest is marked from the suprasternal notch to the abdomen. The inframammary crease is traced from the midline to the anterior axillary line. The meridian begins from a point 8 cm from the sternal notch – over the clavicle – and extends toward the nipple. The vertical axis of the breast is then marked on the upper abdomen at the level of the inframammary crease; this line usually measures 8–14 cm from the midline but will vary with chest width.

The initial mark for nipple/areola position varies depending upon personal preference. Typically, the inframammary crease is projected onto the anterior breast; the intersection of this line and the meridian delineates the new nipple position. Others have used either set measurements (19–22 cm) from the sternal notch to the meridian or have used the midpoint of the humerus to help define the nipple–areola position. The final position on either side can be adjusted to achieve symmetry.

The lateral resection margin is identified by gently rotating the breast medially and slightly superiorly; while maintaining this breast position, the vertical axis is extended from the upper abdomen onto the breast. After displacing the breast gently laterally, the vertical axis is again extended onto the breast to define the medial skin resection margin. The farther the breasts are displaced, the greater the volume of resection will be due to the increased distance between the lateral and medial borders.

A soft concave curve is used to join the medial and lateral marks inferiorly. This curve represents the inferior most aspect of skin resection and should be at least 2–4 cm superior to the inframammary crease. It is important to maintain an inferior margin above the starting of inframammary fold to prevent the vertical scar from extending distal to the final inframammary crease. In general, the larger the final desired breast volume, the higher this mark should be placed.

The superior edge of the areola will reach about 2 cm above the new nipple. An elliptical or dome is drawn around the superior half of the new nipple position to outline the areola. The inferior edges of this mark should connect with the medial and lateral breast markings. When the inferior edges of this semi-circle are pinched together to create a circle centered on the nipple, the total diameter should measure roughly 14–15 cm.

The new areola size, 38–42 cm, is marked while the nipple–areola is unstretched. A line roughly 3–4 cm below the inferior aspect of this newly measured areola is created to mark the superior margin of tissue resection.

35.3.1.2 Technique

Under general anesthesia, the patient is positioned supine on the operating room table with the arms abducted and secured at 70–90°. The patient should be placed in a sitting position prior to the final surgical preparation to confirm symmetric, desired positioning. Because it is difficult to determine preoperatively if a breast has glandular and fatty tissue that can be suctioned adequately, suction-assisted lipectomy is tried at the beginning of the case. The pillars should be aspirated

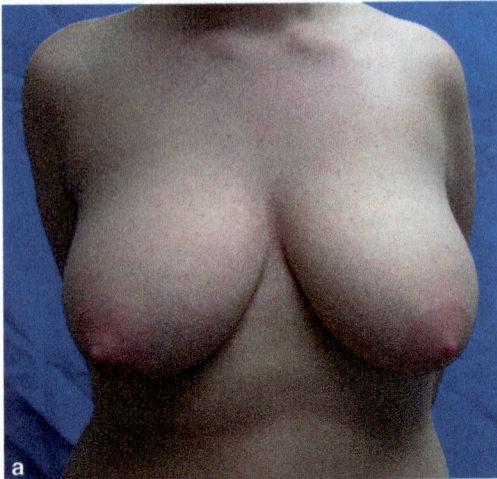

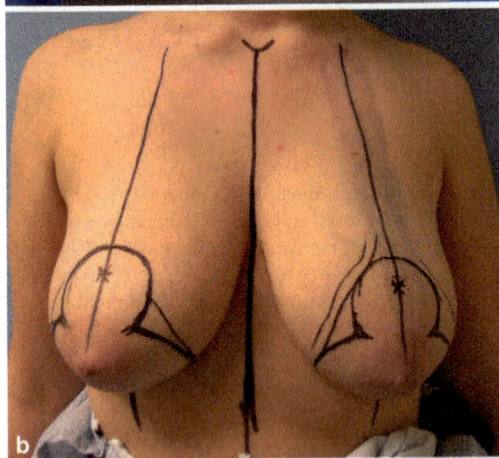

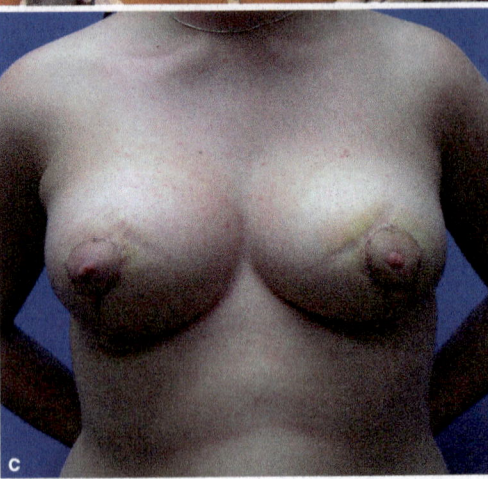

Fig. 35.2 (a) Preoperative patient undergoing vertical reduction. (b) Preoperative markings. (c) Postoperative

cautiously to avoid rendering them too soft and, subsequently, too difficult to suture.

Lidocaine (0.5%) with 1:100,000 epinephrine should be introduced in the area of resection, sparing the nipple areola region. The base of the breast should be constricted by tightly tying a penrose drain or lap sponge. The area around the areola within the marking should be deepithelialized to a point roughly 3–4 cm below the inferior most aspect of the areola.

The medial, lateral, and inferior markings are then incised. An inferior skin flap, roughly 1.5 cm in thickness, is raised extending down to the inframammary crease. The breast is then shifted laterally so that the medial breast markings are in line with the vertical axis of the breast as marked at the inframammary fold. The dissection is carried straight down to the pectoralis fascia. For the lateral breast dissection, the technique is repeated once the breast is shifted medially, so that the lateral breast marking is in line with the vertical axis. The central breast tissue between the medial and lateral pillars is elevated from the pectoralis fascia beginning at its inferior edge. This dissection is carried out until the level of the new nipple. Finally, the superior margin of resection is defined; an incision is made along the lower border of the deepithelialized tissue and extended down to the pectoralis fascia obliquely to create a superiorly based flap involving the new nipple–areola.

A heavy stitch is used to anchor the breast pedicle from its deep surface at the level of the new areola to the underlying fascia at the upper level of the retromammary dissection. The nipple–areola is next inset into its desired position. A drain may be placed not only to aspirate post-operative fluid and blood but also to help decrease dead-space. Medial and lateral pillars are approximated with sutures placed on the anterior surface of the gland as opposed to the cut edges of the pillars to promote breast projection. The dermis is approximated with a few interrupted sutures; the final subcuticular 3-0 Monocryl suture begins inferiorly and is used to gather the skin as it extends superiorly; a decrease in roughly a third of the wound length can be expected with this technique. The patient is placed in a surgical bra for 2–3 weeks. The drain is removed early post-operatively, usually within 24 h.

35.4 Technique Modifications

Hall-Findlay has adopted some modifications on the Lejour vertical reduction mammaplasty technique which, she argues, affords a more reliable and easier technique. These modifications include a different dermoglandular pedicle, the absence of pectoralis fascia sutures, limited liposuction, and lack of undermining the skin [23, 24]. Relying solely on the superior pedicle provided several unnecessary challenges. The pedicle was sometimes difficult to inset, it was difficult to apply to larger breast reductions greater than 800 g, and in these cases the pedicle was occasionally too long to ensure adequate blood supply to the nipple–areola complex. A superior pedicle required extensive undermining which would, on occasion, contribute to wound-healing problems. Because of these potential problems, the superior pedicle technique was a bit more difficult to master. Therefore, she uses a superior pedicle for only small breast reductions. The majority of her vertical reductions rely on a medial pedicle, even for small volume reductions. An inferior pedicle is used only when revision of a previous inferior based pedicle reduction is being performed. The lateral pedicle was reserved for mastopexies. Although the lateral pedicle provides safe support and good sensation, sometimes too much residual fullness remained when adopted for mammaplasty reductions.

There are a few important differences when marking the patient. Because this technique results in a greater amount of projection, the new nipple position should be marked 1–2 cm below that for a standard Wise pattern and slightly lower than that what would be used for a standard vertical mammaplasty reduction. A conservative area of skin should be resected, because the extra projection achieved by "coning" will require a larger skin envelope than what would be required with a more traditional technique.

The recommended base of the pedicle arbitrarily ranges from 6 to 12 cm depending upon the size of reduction from small to over 1,200 g, respectively. A greater effort is made to retain superiorly based breast tissue to maintain upper pole fullness, while resecting inferior and lateral tissue to avoid pseudoptosis and lateral fullness, accordingly. The dissection of the pedicle extends down vertically along the markings with no undermining and is carried down to just above but does not expose pectoralis fascia. This technique is believed to improve circulation to the tissue flaps and sensation to the pedicle.

During the closure, an attempt is made to "cone" the skin flaps to provide additional projection; the lower margins of the remaining breast tissue are brought together with interrupted 3-0 PDS first. "The sutures should start at an inferior and deep level and progress more superficially as they are placed more superiorly." This maneuver centralizes the lateral and medial fullness and shapes the final breast. Liposuction is reserved for contouring after closure.

35.5
Short Scar Periareolar Inferior Pedicle Reduction

The short scar periareolar inferior pedicle reduction (SPAIR) mammaplasty was popularized by Hammond with the aim of resolving some of the problems and frustrations with more traditional inferior-based pedicle and new vertical reduction techniques [25] (Figs. 35.1 and 35.2). The use of the more familiar inferior pedicle provides a pedicle that most surgeons are already comfortable with and provides greater control over the final breast shape. The inferior pedicle is believed to be easier to inset than a superior pedicle and the final on-table breast shape is more predictable of the final breast shape, as opposed to the often exaggerated final breast shape than can be encountered with other vertical breast reduction techniques. There are also two critical steps that further contribute to the final breast shape which help distinguish the SPAIR technique from others. First, internal sutures are sometimes placed, and second, Scarpa's fascia's attachment to the inferior mammary fold is left intact. The SPAIR mammaplasty is best reserved for reductions up to 1,000 g. Although possible in larger reductions, shaping the skin envelope becomes more challenging in these patients.

35.5.1
Markings

The breast meridian is marked from the clavicle down through the breast and across the inframammary fold. The inframammary crease is traced. A pedicle base of 8 cm in length is marked along the inframammary crease and is centered on the breast meridian. The breast is gently elevated superiorly and a distance of 8–10 cm is measured from the medial and lateral edge of the base of the pedicle onto the breast. This determines the amount of skin that will remain after the extra breast tissue is removed. The superior aspects of these two lines are then connected with a soft concave mark. The superior portion of the nipple–areola complex is marked by transposing the inframammary crease onto the anterior surface of the breast. The intersection of this imaginary line and the meridian is a good starting point and can be adjusted as necessary.

The medial and lateral margins of the skin resection are made by gently lifting the breast up and out and up and in, respectively. During these maneuvers, the breast meridian is connected to the meridian at the inframammary crease. Rotating the breast superiorly is designed to approximate the final breast size and shape. The superior, inferior, medial, and lateral edges are all connected; this final design resembles an elongated oval. At the level of the nipple, the medial skin resection margin should be at least 12 cm away from the midline to avoid too much tension on the closure. The new areola is marked 50 mm in diameter. The final shape of the inferior pedicle is drawn to incorporate the new areola.

35.5.2
Technique

The inferior pedicle with a 0.5 cm margin around the new areola is deepithelialized. Medial and superior flaps are raised; these flaps begin below the dermis and become roughly 4–6 cm thick as the pectoralis fascia is approached. The lateral flap maintains a thickness of roughly 2 cm throughout its length. The inferior pedicle is then dissected and the attachments of Scarpa's fascia at the inferior aspect of the breast are not disturbed. Once the extra breast tissue is removed, internal support sutures are sometimes required to help better shape the breast. Both the superior and medial breast flaps are undermined for almost 2–3 cm. The leading deep edge of the undermined superior flap is advanced superiorly, 4–6 cm, under itself and fixed to the pectoralis fascia. This advancement improves upper pole fullness. The medial edge is sutured to itself with interrupted suture. These sutures are separated by 2–3 cm. This rounds the breast contour medially. If the inferior pedicle is exceptionally floppy or loose, interrupted placation sutures can be placed into the pedicle itself to provide temporary stability until scar develops. However, patients who have no upper pole concavity, a thick texture to the subcutaneous fat, or a short breast do not require these internal fixation sutures.

The inferior skin envelope is designed by first placing the patient in a sitting position, 45°–60°, to allow gravity to pull down on the breast. The inferior pedicle is carefully drawn upward, which creates a fold in the inferior skin envelope both medially and laterally to the pedicle. The most dependent portion of each fold is pulled together and held in place with a temporary staple. Next, the medial and lateral flaps are pulled upward and are stapled together while imbricating the redundant tissue. The staples are adjusted as necessary to create a pleasing breast. The staples are removed and the redundant tissue is resected. The skin over the inferior pedicle portion of the lower skin envelope is deepithelialized. The medial and lower skin edges are sutured to each other.

The periareolar skin envelope is shaped by first placing a purse-string suture using CV-3 Gore-Tex to create a pocket that finally measures 4.5 cm in diameter. This newly defined border should be approximately circular in shape; small areas of skin at the border of this pocket can be de-epithelialized to create a more circular shape. The areola is inset and secured with absorbable suture.

35.5.3 Outcomes

Short scar techniques have gained in popularity because they have eliminated the horizontal scar, improved breast projection, and maintained the final breast shape for a greater period as compared to more traditional techniques. Although the learning curve is steeper, outcomes for vertical reduction mammaplasty techniques have been excellent. Despite initial concerns, large volume reductions (>1,000 g) have also been successfully performed, although with a slightly higher rate of complications in some studies. Massive volume reductions (>2,000 g) have also been successfully performed [26].

There are no good prospective, randomized trials evaluating and comparing various short scar techniques with other short-scar or more traditional approaches. Nonetheless, there are several large studies that have examined outcomes using various variations of the Lejour and Hall-Findlay techniques; these studies all reach similar conclusions; patient satisfaction and final breast form and function are excellent, while complications, in general, are low and acceptable. In one large study, the complication rate was 5.6%, with 2.2% superficial wound dehiscence and 1.2% hematoma as the two most common complications [27]. While, Lejour's relatively recent review of personal cases reports a complication rate of roughly 12%, with 5% seroma and 5.4% delayed wound healing as the two most common complications [28]. The rate of retained or improved nipple sensation was consistent with or slightly better (85%) than the rates seen with an inferior pedicle technique [24, 29–31]. Although poorly evaluated, the percentage of women who could breast feed following a vertical reduction appears to be not different than the percentage of women who could breast feed with an inferior pedicle-wise pattern technique; in a small study, 8/10 women who wanted to breast feed following vertical reduction mammaplasty were able to do so completely [32]. Rates of nipple loss were universally reported at <1%.

One of the most consistent criticisms of some of the short-scar techniques is the inability to visualize the final breast shape immediately postoperatively. A majority of the vertical techniques create an exaggerated breast contour, which ultimately requires some time for the breast to "settle" into its final shape. As a result two complications may sometimes develop: (1) the nipple-areola is often position too high, and (2) asymmetry between the breasts can be noted more frequently. To avoid these outcomes, it is important to create adequate lower pole support by tightly securing the medial and lateral poles to help prevent significant "bottoming-out." Some surgeons will also mark the nipple roughly 1–1.5 cm lower than the typical preoperative mark.

References

1. Matarasso A, Courtiss EH: Suction mammaplasty: The use of suction lipectomy to reduce large breasts. Plast Reconstr Surg 1991;87(4):709–717
2. Di Giuseppe A: Breast reduction with ultrasound-assisted lipoplasty. Plast Reconstr Surg 2003;112(1):71–82
3. Goes JC: Periareolar mammaplasty: double skin technique with application of polyglactin or mixed mesh. Plast Reconstr Surg 1996;97(5):959–968
4. Zocchi M: The ultrasonic assisted lipectomy (U.A.L.): physiologic principles and clinical application. Lipoplasty 1994;11:14
5. Moskovitz M: Breast reduction by liposuction alone. In: Spear S (ed). Surgery of the Breast. Philadelphia, Lippincott Williams & Wilkins 2006
6. Gray L: Update on experience with liposuction breast reduction. Plast Reconstr Surg 2000;108:1006–1010
7. Gray L: Liposuction breast reduction. Aesthetic Plast Surg 1998;22(3):159–162
8. Moskovitz R, Muskin E, Baxt S: Outcome study in liposuction breast reduction. Plast Reconstr Surg 2004;114(1):55–60
9. Ribeiro L: A new technique for reduction mammaplasty. Plast Reconstr Surg 1975;55(3):330–334
10. Robbins TH: A reduction mammaplasty with the areola-nipple based on an inferior dermal pedicle. Plast Reconstr Surg 1977;59(1):64–67
11. Courtiss EH, Goldwyn RH: Reduction mammaplasty by the inferior pedicle technique. Plast Reconstr Surg 1977;59(4):500–507
12. Hall-Findlay EJ: Reduction Mammaplasty. In: Nahai F (ed). The Art of Aesthetic Surgery: Principles and Techniques. St. Louis, Quality Medical Publishing 2005
13. Godwin Y, Wood SH, O'Neil TJ: A comparison of the patient and surgeon opinion on the long term aesthetic outcome of reduction mammaplasty. Br J Plast Surg 1998;51(6):444–449
14. Mizgala CL, MacKenzie KM: Breast reduction outcome study. Ann Plast Surg 2000;44(2):125–133
15. Brown AP, Hill C, Khan K: Outcome of reduction mammaplasty – a patients' perspective. Br J Plast Surg 2000;53 (7):584–587
16. Celebiler O, Sonmez A, Erdim M, Yaman M, Numanoglu A: Patients' and surgeons' perspectives on the scar components after inferior pedicle breast reduction surgery. Plast Reconstr Surg 2005;116(2):459–464
17. Dartigues L: Traitement chirurgical du prolapsus mammaire. Arch Franco Belg Chir 1925;28:13
18. Arie G: Una nueva tecnica de mastoplastia. Rev Latinoam Cir Plast 1957;3:23
19. Lassus C: A technique for breast reduction. Int Surg 1970;53(1):69–72
20. Lassus C: Breast reduction: evolution of a technique – A single vertical scar. Aesthetic Plast Surg 1987;11(2): 107–112

21. Lassus C: A 30-year experience with vertical mammaplasty. Plast Reconstr Surg 1996;97(2):373–380
22. Lejour M: Vertical mammaplasty: update and appraisal of late results. Plast Reconstr Surg 1999;104(3):771–781
23. Hall-Findlay E: A simplified vertical reduction mammaplasty: shortening the learning curve. Plast Reconstr Surg 1999;104(3):748–759
24. Hall-Findlay E: Pedicles in vertical breast reduction and mastopexy. Clin Plast Surg 2002;29(3):379–391
25. Hammond D: Short scar periareolar inferior pedicle reduction (SPAIR) mammaplasty. Plast Reconstr Surg 1999;103(3):890–901
26. Nahai F: Discussion on update on vertical mammaplasty. Plast Reconstr Surg 1999;104(7):2299
27. Lista F, Ahmad J: Vertical scar reduction mammaplasty: A 15-year experience including a review of 250 consecutive cases. Plast Reconstr Surg 2006;117(7): 2152–2165
28. Lejour M: Vertical mammaplasty: early complications after 250 personal consecutive cases. Plast Reconstr Surg 1999;104(3):764–770
29. Hamdi M, Greuse M, DeMey A, Webster MH: A prospective quantitative comparison of breast sensation after superior and inferior pedicle mammaplasty. Br J Plast Surg 2001;54(1):39–42
30. Mofid M, Dellon Al, Elias J, Nahabedian M: Quantitation of breast sensibility following reduction mammaplasty: a comparison of inferior and medial pedicle techniques. Plast Reconstr Surg 2002;109(7):2283–2288
31. Cruz-Korchin N, Korchin L: Vertical versus Wise pattern breast reduction: patient satisfaction, revision rates and complications. Plast Reconstr Surg 2003;112(6):1573–1578
32. Cherchel A, Azzam C, De Mey A: Breastfeeding after vertical reduction mammaplasty using a superior pedicle. J Plast Reconstr Aesthet Surg 2007;60(5):465–470

Breast Reduction Algorithm Using TTM Chart

Toma T. Mugea

36.1 Introduction

Breast surgery is one of the most difficult fields of aesthetic surgery, because of the complexity of surgical procedures and the relative guidelines defining the aesthetically perfect breast. The authors [1–7] present different dimensions as representative for the aesthetically perfect breast, which means something ideal, which needs no further improvement!

The perfect breast is aesthetically entirely appreciated on a perfect trunk and on a perfect body. It is also important to correlate the aesthetically perfect breast with the idea of beauty in different cultures. Many of the famous nude statues' breasts that in Ancient Greece were perceived as aesthetic would nowadays be slightly criticized as too small and therefore proposed for augmentation surgery, whereas the breasts of the nude models painted by Rubens in the Renaissance period would undoubtedly require reduction, according to the contemporary view.

At the same time, it is impossible to impose a single standard of breast beauty to women who are so entirely different from the point of view of their height, weight, and constitutional type.

The essential goals of breast reduction or mastopexy are to get a predictable result, retain nipple sensitivity, the possibility of lactation, and obtain an excellent aesthetic appearance.

36.2 Preoperative Assessment Using TTM Chart

A study was performed by the author using random cases, collecting different dimensions, and correlating the findings into (1) nonaesthetic breasts, (2) aesthetic breasts, (3) aesthetically perfect breasts, and (4) abnormal breasts.

A breast was considered normal if that was identified in the majority of females of the same age group and physiological status. A normal breast was reckoned to have a volume somewhere between 300 and 500 ml, depending on the physical build of the woman, to be located sagitally between the second and seventh rib and transversally between the sternal edge and the anterior axillary line. The "tail" of the breast should extend toward the axilla, and the nipple should project at the height of the fourth intercostal gap [8].

A breast was considered aesthetic if it had a pleasant appearance with a normal size and fullness, minimal ptosis, a conical to teardrop shape, and the nipple in the most anterior position, coming from a normal proportion, position, and projection.

The aesthetically perfect breast was one for which no common aesthetic procedures are needed. It perfectly fits with a perfect body and is in perfect harmony with regard to proportion, position, and projection [9]. This is "the top model" situation (Fig. 36.1).

Standards for the measurement technique were established and all measurements were made with the subject standing, with shoulders back and the head straight ahead (Fig. 36.2, Table 36.1). Each patient who was considered to have an aesthetic breast received a thorough physical examination and photographic examination, even from the back, to detect asymmetries.

36.3 Definition of the Points and Measurements Used in the TTM Chart

36.3.1 Points

Mn = Manubrium, the suprasternal notch
Pb = Pubis, the suvperior edge of the pubic bone
Ac = Acromion, the lateral edge of the acromion bone
Sp = Spine, the antero-superior spine of iliac bone
Ni = Nipple
PP = Ptotic point, the lowest point of the ptotic breast in the standing position. On the chart the distance in (cm) between this point and the nipple are noted.
BUP = Breast upper pole, anatomical landmark of the upper pole of the breast, corresponding to the second rib space

---

M.A. Shiffman (ed.), *Mastopexy and Breast Reduction: Principles and Practice*,
© Springer-Verlag Berlin Heidelberg 2009

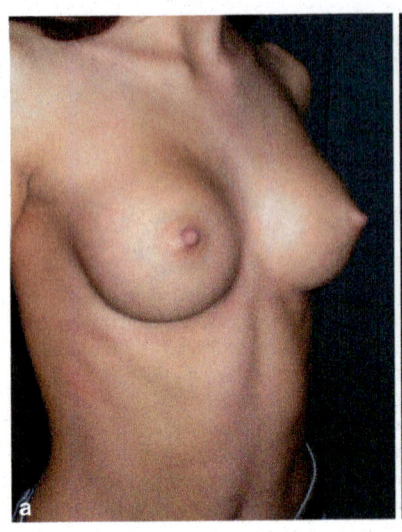

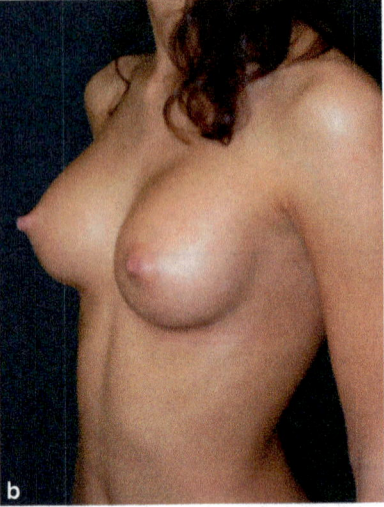

Fig. 36.1 (a,b) An example of the aesthetically perfect breast (no common aesthetic procedures are needed)

36.3.2 Distances

- Mn–Pb = The distance between manubrium notch and superior edge of the pubis, measured over the trunk and abdomen (in a skinny female patient, this distance is a straight line, but in an obese one, it is a large curve line, and even the abdomen apron is measured)
- Ac–Ac = The distance between the Acromion points
- Sp–Sp = The distance between the spine points (in a thin female patient, this distance is a straight line, and in an obese one, it is a large curve line)
- Mn–RNi = The distance between manubrium notch and the right nipple
- Mn–LNi = The distance between manubrium notch and the left nipple
- Ni–Ni = The distance between the nipples
- BVM = Breast vertical meridian represents the distance between and the inframammary fold and the anatomical landmark BUP, over the nipple
- PL = Perimeter length of the breast represents the distance between the inframammary fold and the upper edge of the breast mould, over the nipple (Fig. 36.3)
- BSM = Breast superior meridian represents the virtual line between the upper edge of the breast mould and the nipple
- BIM = Breast inferior meridian represents the virtual line between the lower edge of the breast mould and the nipple (this correspond to Ni-Infra distance)
- BHM = Breast horizontal meridian represents the longer distance between the axillary end of the inframammary fold and the sternal end of the inframammary fold, following the shape of the breast over the nipple
- BMM = Breast medial meridian represent the virtual line between the medial breast mould edge and the nipple (this correspond to St–Ni distance)
- BLM = Breast lateral meridian represents the virtual line between the lateral breast mould edge and the nipple (this correspond to Ax–Ni distance)
- BC = Breast circumference represents the longer distance between the axillary end of the inframammary fold and the sternal end of the inframammary fold following the shape of the breast over the nipple. In the aesthetic breast, breast circumference is identical with the breast horizontal meridian)
- Ni–PP = The distance between the nipple to the ptotic point
- BVD = Breast vertical diameter represent the distance between the breast anatomical landmarks in the sagital plane measured with a caliper
- BHD = Breast horizontal diameter represent the distance between the breast anatomical landmarks in the horizontal plane corresponding to the

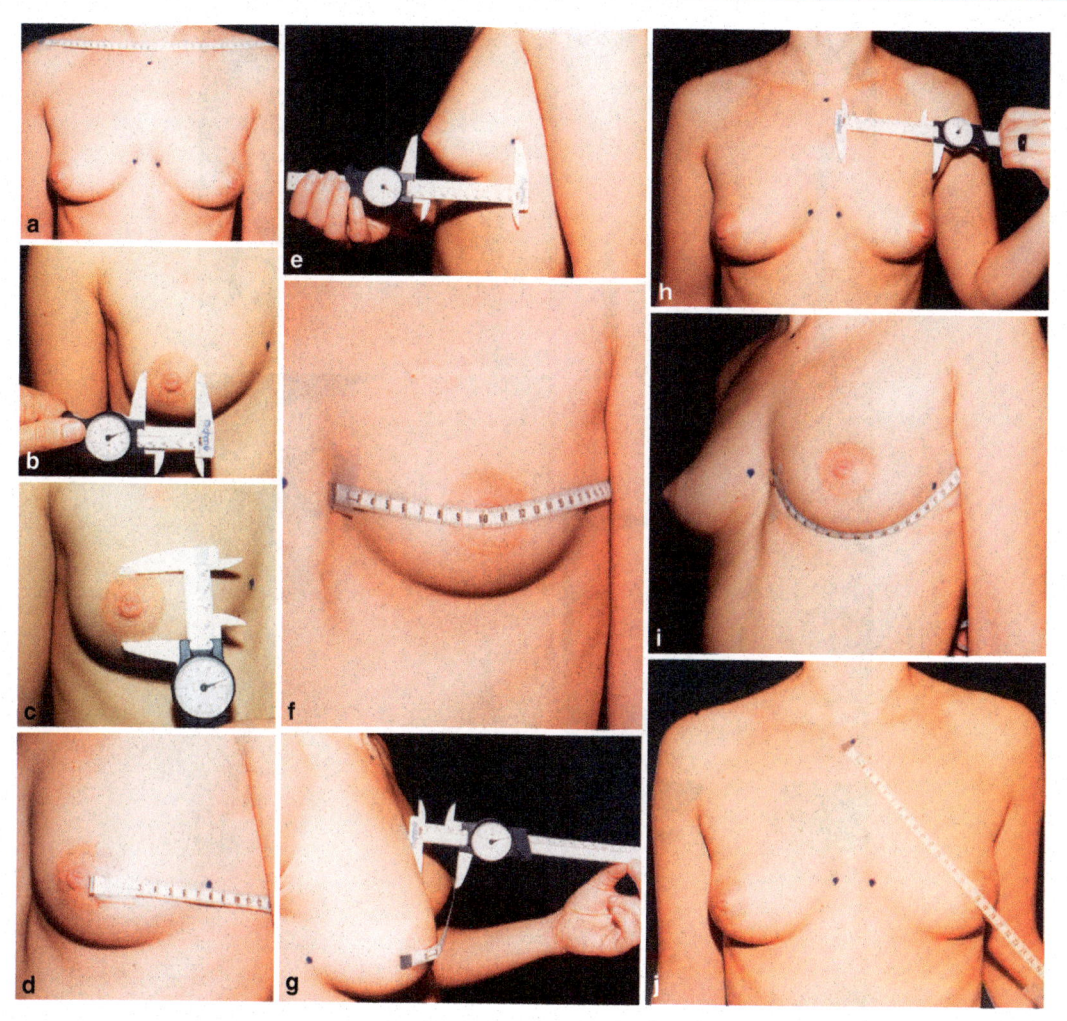

Fig. 36.2 Breast and trunk measurements in a young female from the "aesthetic breast" group. (**a**) Ac–Ac, (**b**) areola horizontal diameter, (**c**) areola vertical diameter, (**d**) Ax-Ni, (**e**) breast projection, (**f**) circumference, (**g**) cocktail view, (**h**) horizontal diameter, (**i**) infra length, (**j**) Mn–LNi, (**k**) Mn–Pb,

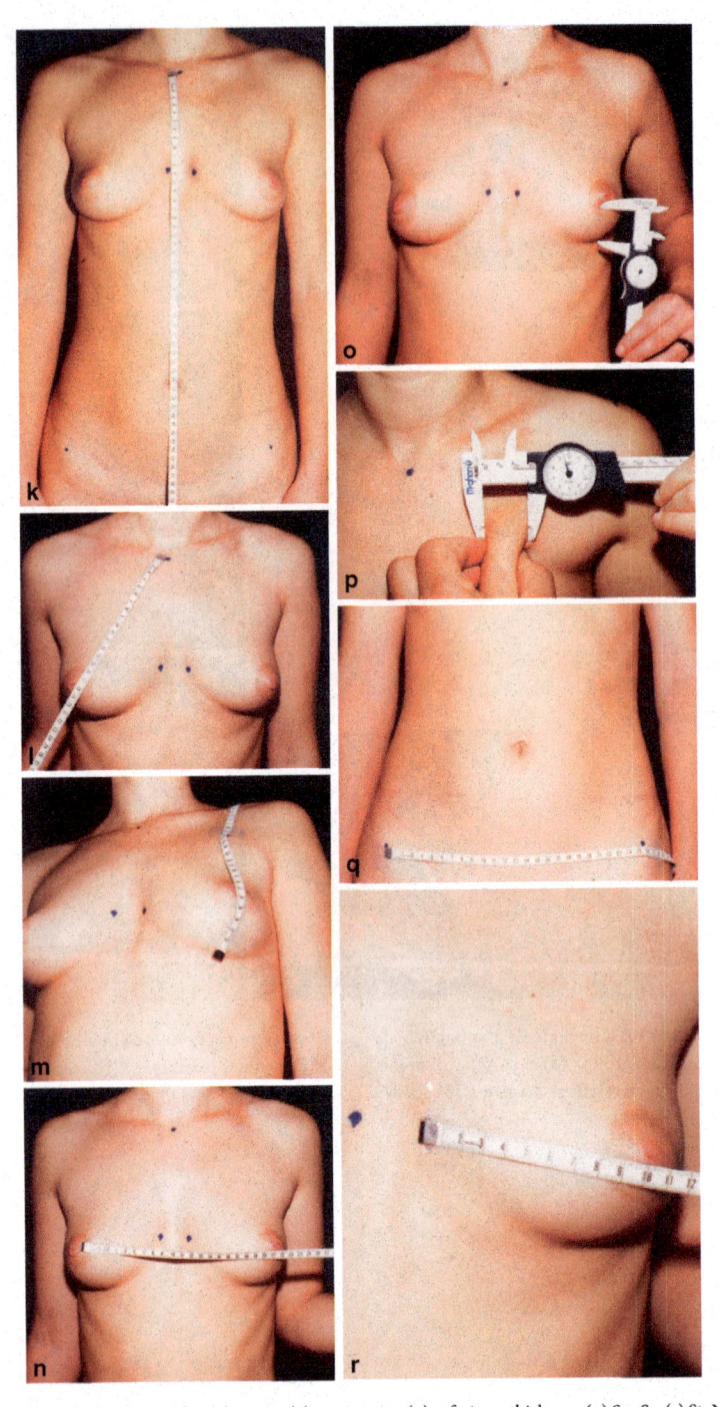

Fig. 36.2 *(continued)* (**l**) Mn–RNi, (**m**) Ni-Infra, (**n**) Ni–Ni, (**o**) ptotic point, (**p**) soft tissue thickness, (**q**) Sp–Sp, (**r**) St–Ni

Table 36.1 TTM chart with breast and trunk measurements of the patient from Fig. 36.2

TTM® Chart

CODE:

Name: XX   Date: YY

Height: 1,64   Weight: 50 kg   Pregnancies: 0   Weight Loss: 0

Pinch Test: P= 2   R= 4

Chest problems: NO

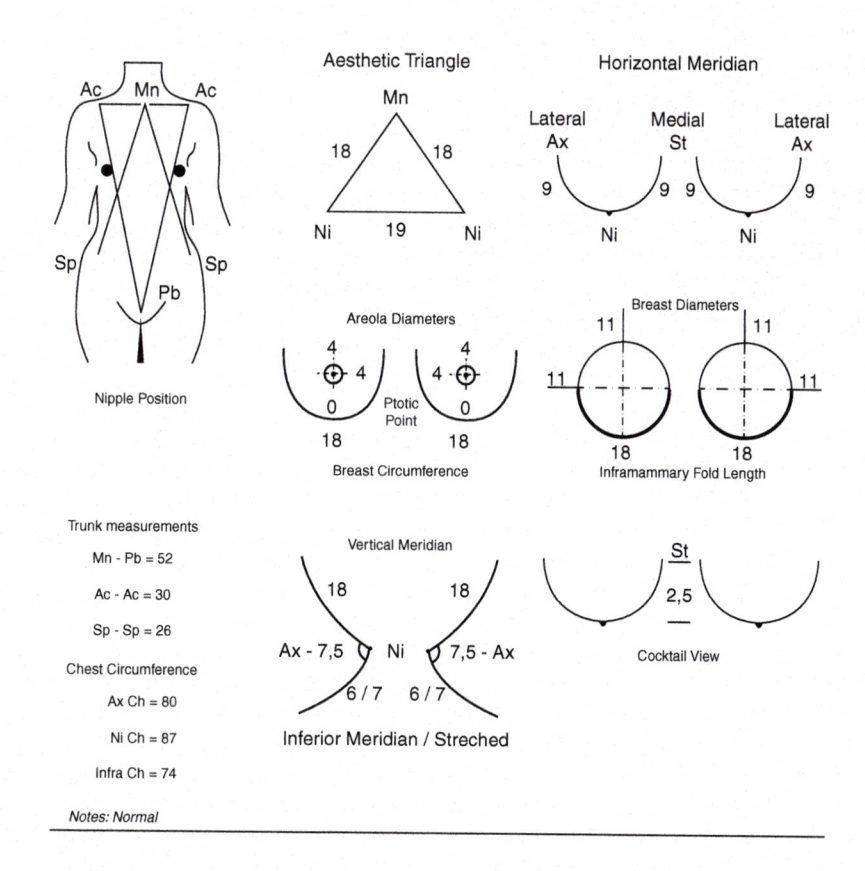

Aesthetic Triangle: Mn, 18, 18, Ni 19 Ni

Horizontal Meridian: Lateral Ax 9, Medial St 9 9, Lateral Ax 9, Ni, Ni

Nipple Position (Ac, Mn, Ac, Sp, Sp, Pb)

Areola Diameters: 4, 4, 4, 4, 0, Ptotic Point, 0
Breast Circumference: 18, 18

Breast Diameters: 11, 11, 11, 11
Inframammary Fold Length: 18, 18

Trunk measurements
Mn - Pb = 52
Ac - Ac = 30
Sp - Sp = 26

Chest Circumference
Ax Ch = 80
Ni Ch = 87
Infra Ch = 74

Vertical Meridian: 18, 18, Ax - 7,5, Ni, 7,5 - Ax, 6/7, 6/7
Inferior Meridian / Streched

Cocktail View: St, 2,5

Notes: Normal

---

medial and lateral edges of the inframammary fold, measured with a caliper

AvD = Areola vertical diameter (from margin to margin)

AhD = Areola horizontal diameter (from margin to margin)

Infra Length = The inframammary fold length, measured from the axillary end to the sternal end of the fold.

BP = Breast projection (the distance between the nipple and the anterior axillary line in standing position, measured as a straight line using a caliper)

CW = Cocktail view represent the distance between sternum and the horizontal line connecting the most anterior points of the breasts in standing position, measured as a straight line using a caliper)

Ax-Ch = Axillary chest circumference (the chest circumference measured at the axillary level)

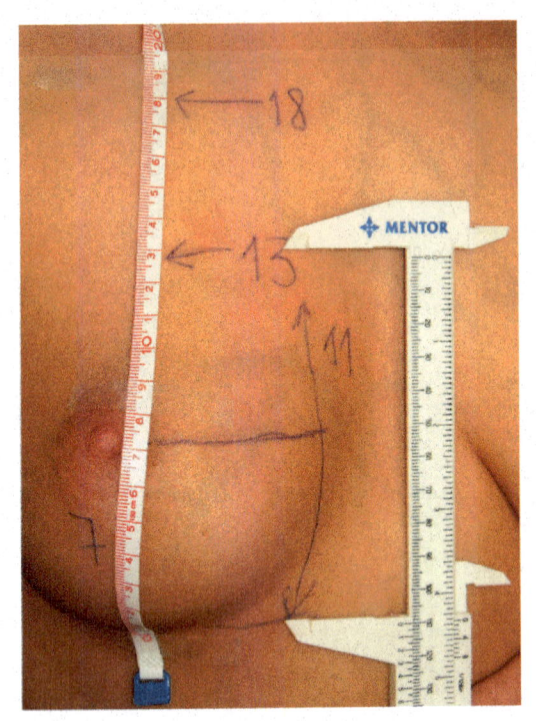

Fig. 36.3 Right breast vertical diameter is 11 cm, perimeter length of the breast mould is 13 cm, and the breast vertical meridian is 18 cm measured from the inframammary fold to the superior anatomical landmark, over the nipple

Ni-Ch = Nipple chest circumference (the chest circumference measured over the most projected points of the breasts, which may correspond to the nipple in a normal aesthetic breast or may not correspond to a ptotic breast)

Infra-Ch = Infra chest circumference (the chest circumference measured at the level of the inframammary fold)

In breast asymmetries, in some cases, an aesthetic situation and a ptotic breast can be found at the same time (Fig. 36.4).

Using the information collected from the TTM Chart of 50 aesthetic cases, the data was processed, and the correlations between the breast and the trunk measurements were found. Based on this information, a special computer program was created, able to list automatically the ideal breast dimension for a specific case, based on body weight, height, and trunk measurements. In the last 10 years, this program has been verified in our practice and demonstrates its accuracy.

After collecting the data in the TTM chart, the boxes nominated in the TTM computer program (Table 36.2) are filled in and organized in the following sections:

1. Patient identification data
2. Body weight, height (in cm), weight loss (in kg), and the number of pregnancies
3. Soft tissue thickness (in cm without coma), superficial pinch test (if can be done or not), and deep pinch test (in pinched and relaxed situation, measured in cm, without coma)
4. Chest problems associated to the case
5. Trunk measurements
6. Chest circumference (at axillary level, nipple level, and inframammary fold level)
7. Breast actual parameters including the following:
    a. Manubrium to nipple and nipple to nipple distances
    b. Areola vertical and horizontal diameters
    c. Ptotic point
    d. Breast circumference (similar to the horizontal meridian in the aesthetic breast)
    e. Inframammary fold length
    f. Cocktail view
    g. Lateral and medial breast meridians (Ax-Ni and St–Ni) for each breast
    h. Breast vertical and horizontal diameters
    i. Breast vertical meridian
    j. Breast projection (Ax-Ni)
    k. Breast inferior meridian (Ni-Infra) in stretched and relaxed situation

After filling in this data, the "calculate icon" situated in the right upper corner of the table is pressed and automatically the computer will list, in red color, the ideal breast dimensions if the patient has a normal body weight. If the patient is overweight, the computer will list, in red color, also the ideal overweight dimensions for each parameter.

The red colored ideal dimensions are listed just below each group of actual parameters of the breast, allowing the reader to see and compare this immediately.

If it is a case for breast augmentation, the reader will fill the icons situated in the right part of the table, colored in red on a grey background. After filling this, the calculate icon situated in the right upper corner of the table is pressed and automatically the computer will list, in blue colored icons, the selected implant from CPG Mentor catalogue.

The "K" number (the Key of the aesthetic breast or the "Breast Golden Number") is the result of the calculations

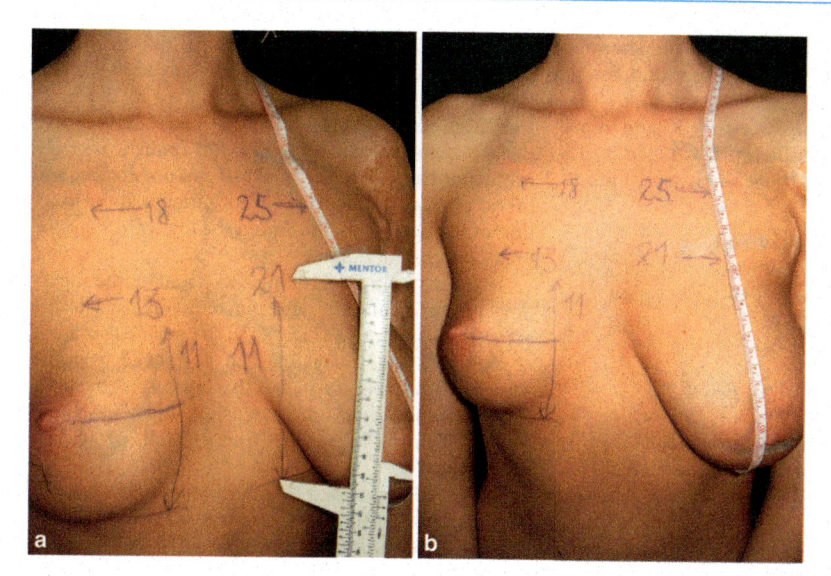

Fig. 36.4 (a) The ptotic breast on the left side shows the same breast vertical diameter as in Fig. 36.3 (11 cm), but 21 cm in the perimeter length. (b) The breast vertical meridian in the ptotic breast is 25 cm, compared with 18 cm in the right normal breast

Table 36.2 TTM computer program with actual dimensions of breast (*in black*) and the ideal parameters (*in red*) suggested by the computer for the patient shown in Fig. 36.2

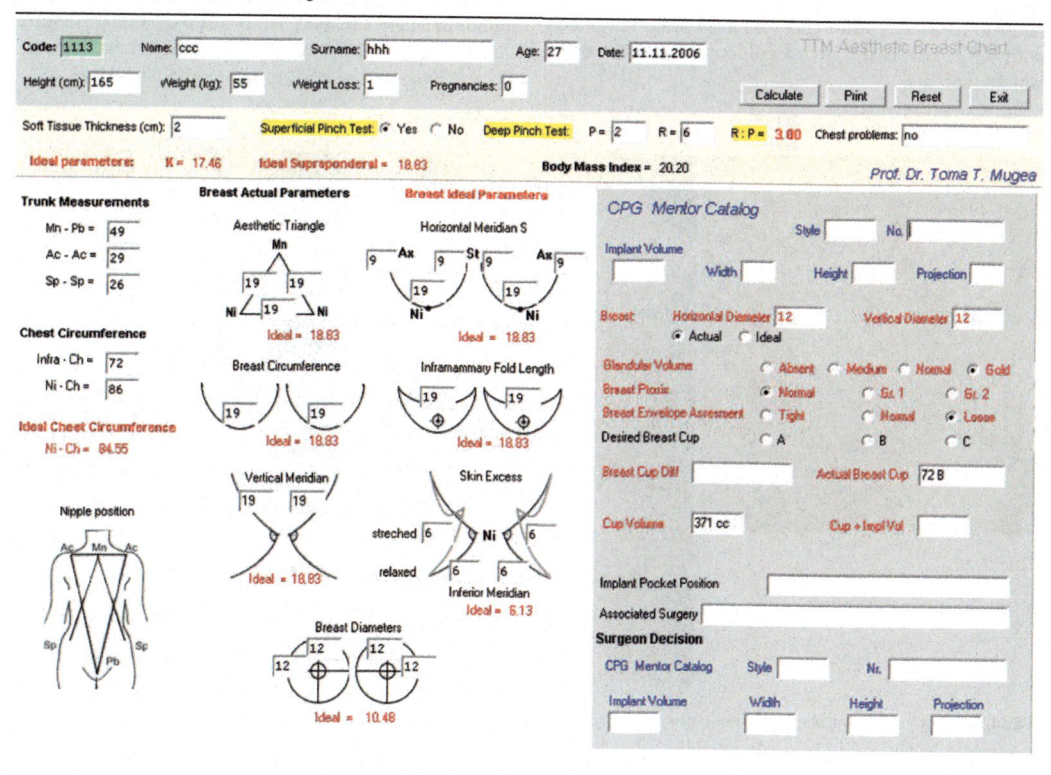

using a special program, designed to find and show the relationship between the breast and trunk dimensions in the case of an aesthetic breast.

The following connections between K and other distances were founded in aesthetic breasts (Fig. 36.5):

K = Ideal aesthetic triangle (between manubrium and nipples)
K = Inframammary fold length
K = Breast horizontal meridian
K = Breast circumference in the aesthetic breast
K = Breast vertical meridian
K: 2 = Breast medial meridian
K: 2 = Breast lateral meridian
K: 3 = Breast inferior meridian

The ideal breast measurements suggested by the computer program, based on trunk measurements, are suitable for thin or normal weight patients. In the cases of overweight ones, a correction factor was introduced, related to the body mass index (BMI). Because in overweight patients we have to deal mainly with breast reduction or mastopexy, and this new key is called Key for Breast Reduction (KBR).

For overweight patients, also the ideal aesthetic triangle, inframammary fold length, breast vertical meridian, and breast circumference all have the same value as with KBR. This is the breast golden number for overweight patients.

In Fig. 36.6 and Table 36.3, the trunk and breast dimensions of an overweight young lady are recorded. In her case, the dimensions correspond to the body weight, as can be seen on the TTM Chart. In this case, the breast golden number is 19 (ideal aesthetic triangle, inframammary fold length, breast circumference, and breast vertical meridian). Nipple location is at the junction of the upper two-thirds and the lower third on the breast vertical meridian.

To estimate skin tightening and elasticity, the superficial pinch test and the deep pinch test are used. In the superficial pinch test (Fig. 36.7), the smallest amount of skin and soft tissue that can be moved over the superficial fascia is grasped. If this test cannot be done, the skin is too tight, under tension, and breast augmentation cannot benefit from a full projection implant.

In the deep pinch test (Fig. 36.8), the largest amount of skin and soft tissues, without pectoralis musculofascial elements, that can be still moved over the deeper structures (pectoralis fascia) is grasped. If we mark the end of the stretched line with two dots and do measurements using the caliper arms, we can compare the two distances, in relaxed (R) and pinched (P) situation.

If the deep pinch test shows the ratio R:P < 2, this corresponds to a tight situation. The breast reduction procedure can benefit from the strong sustaining ligaments, and predictable long-term shape preservation can be done.

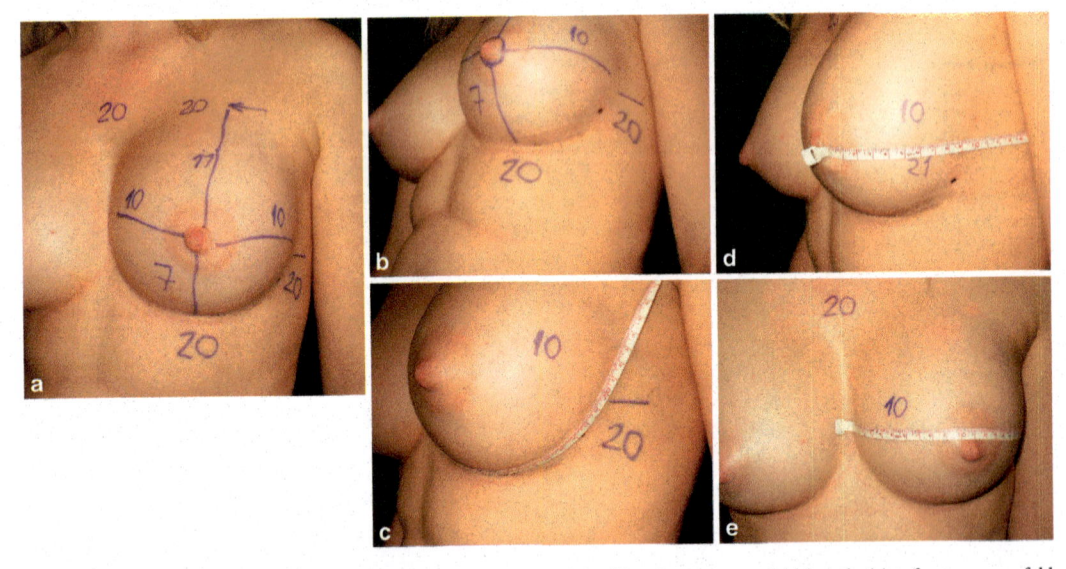

Fig. 36.5 Breast golden number and meridians. (**a**) horizontal meridian, (**b**) inframammary fold length, (**c**) inframammary fold length, (**d**) lateral meridian, (**e**) medial meridian

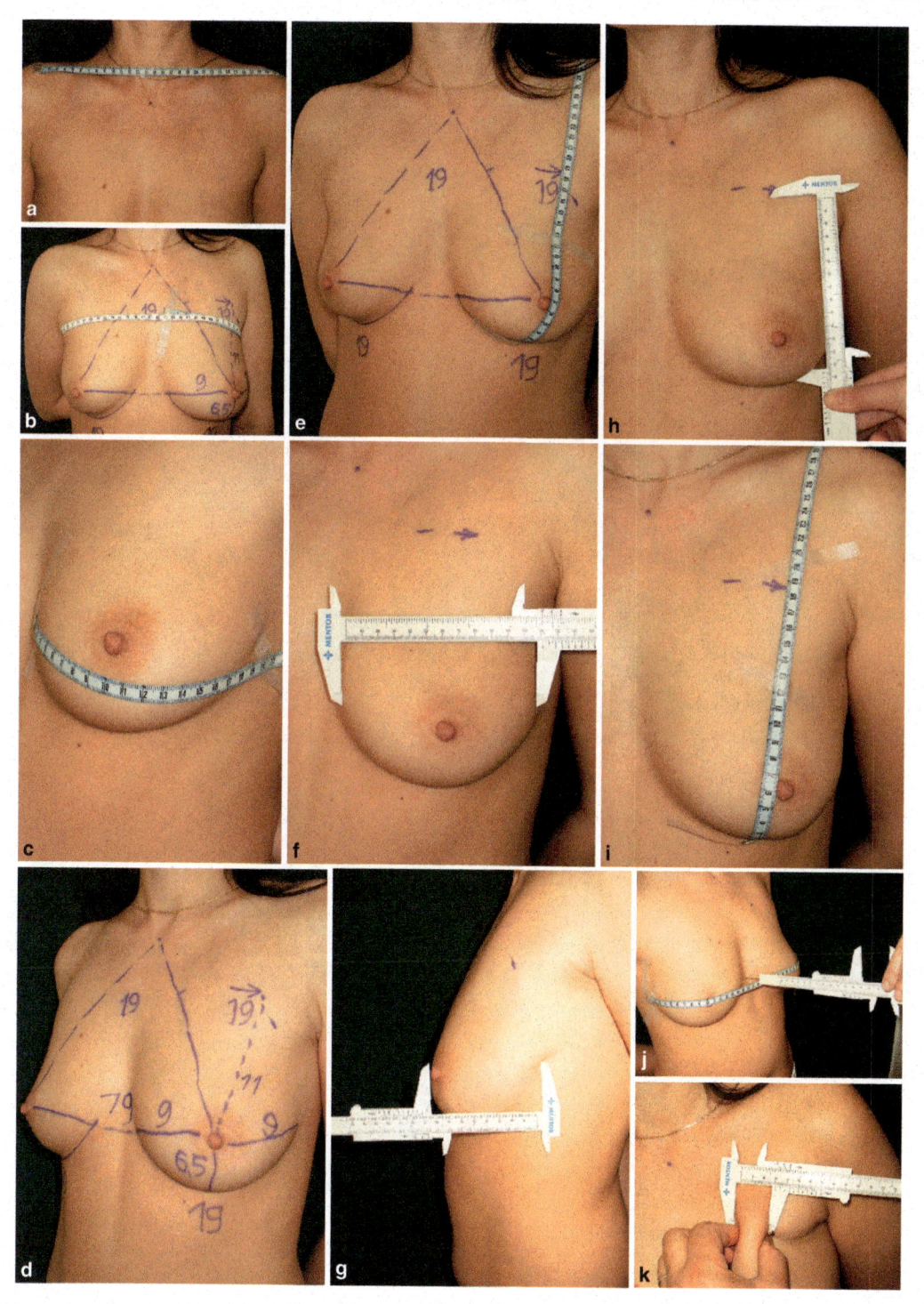

Fig. 36.6 Breast and trunk dimensions for an overweight patient. (**a**) Ac–Ac, (**b**) Ax-chest circumference, (**c**) breast circumference, (**d**) breast golden number, (**e**) breast golden number, (**f**) breast horizontal diameter, (**g**) breast projection, (**h**) breast vertical diameter, (**i**) breast vertical meri-dian, (**j**) cocktail view distance, (**k**) deep pinch test,

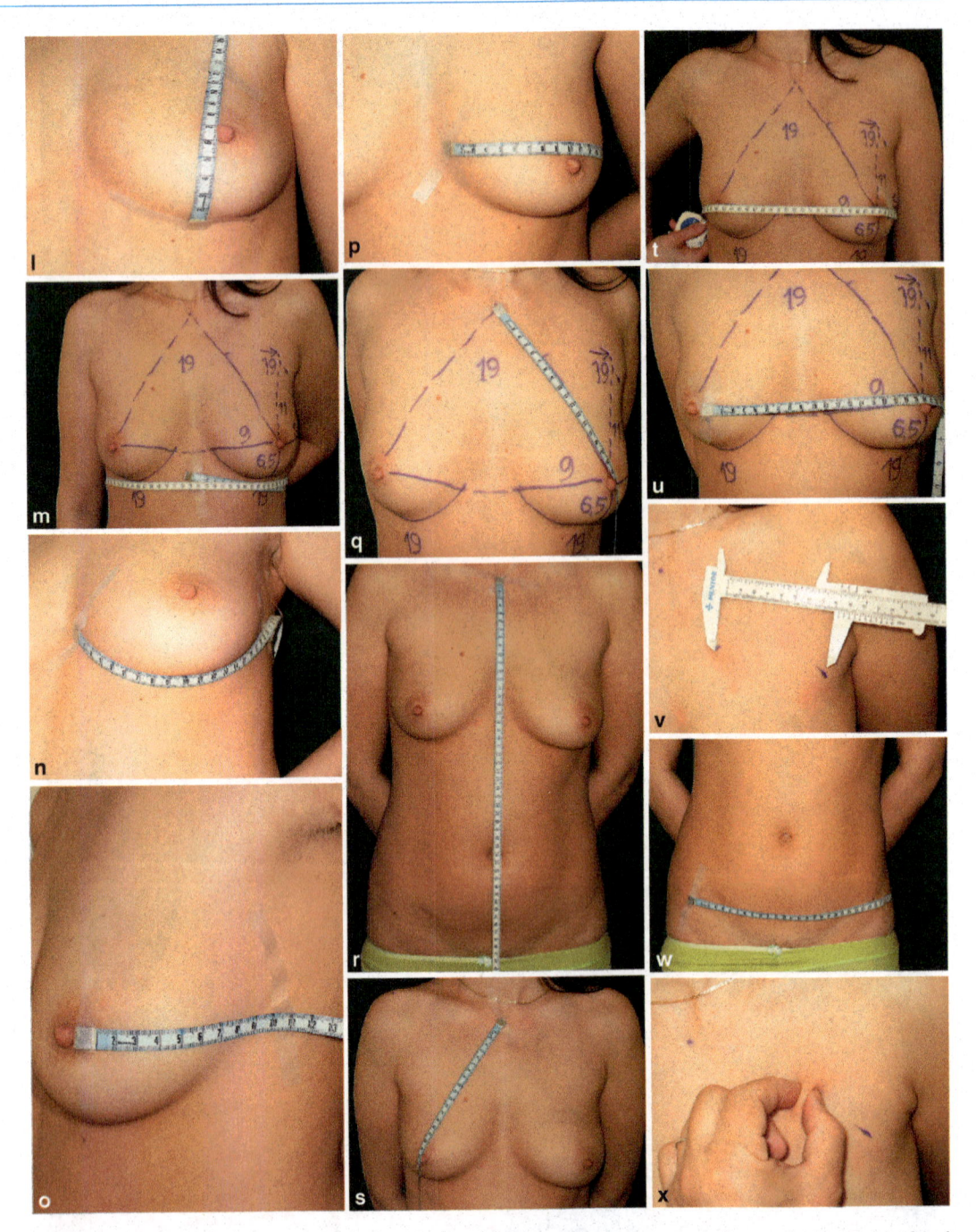

Fig. 36.6 *(continued)* (**l**) inferior meridian, (**m**) infra-chest circumference, (**n**) inframammary fold length, (**o**) lateral meridian, (**p**) medial meridian, (**q**) Mn–LNi, (**r**) Mn–Pb, (**s**) MnR–Ni, (**t**) chest circumference, (**u**) Ni–Ni, (**v**) relaxed soft tissue, (**w**) Sp–Sp, (**x**) superficial pinch test

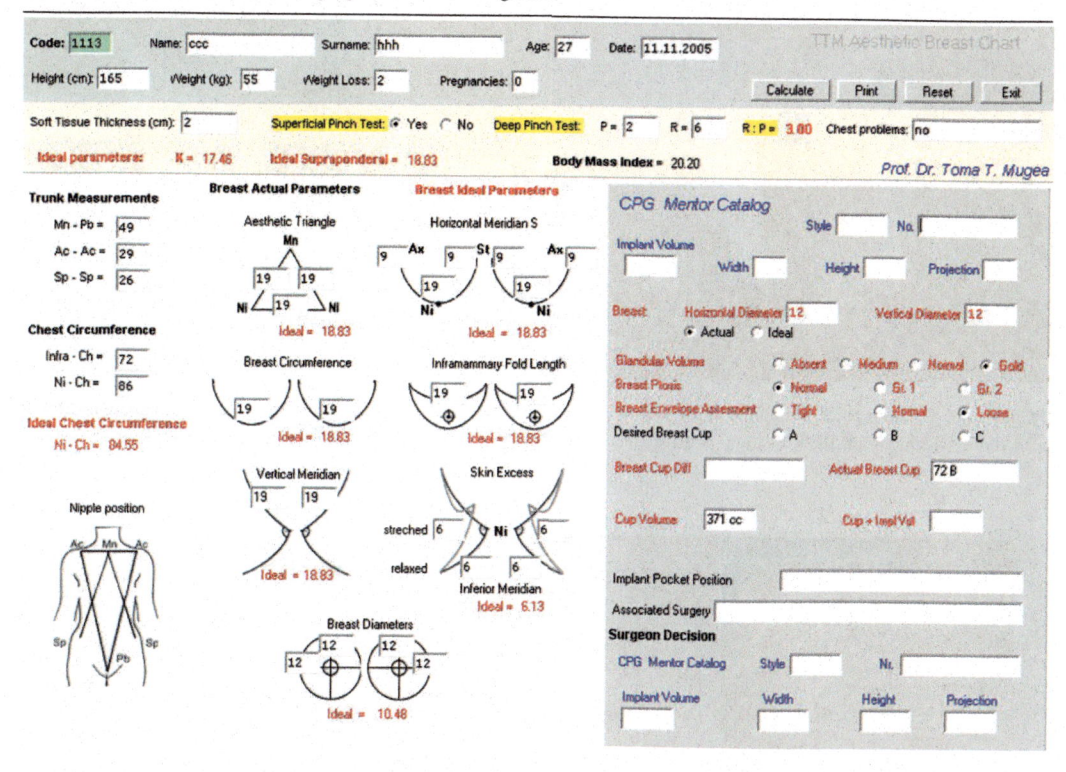

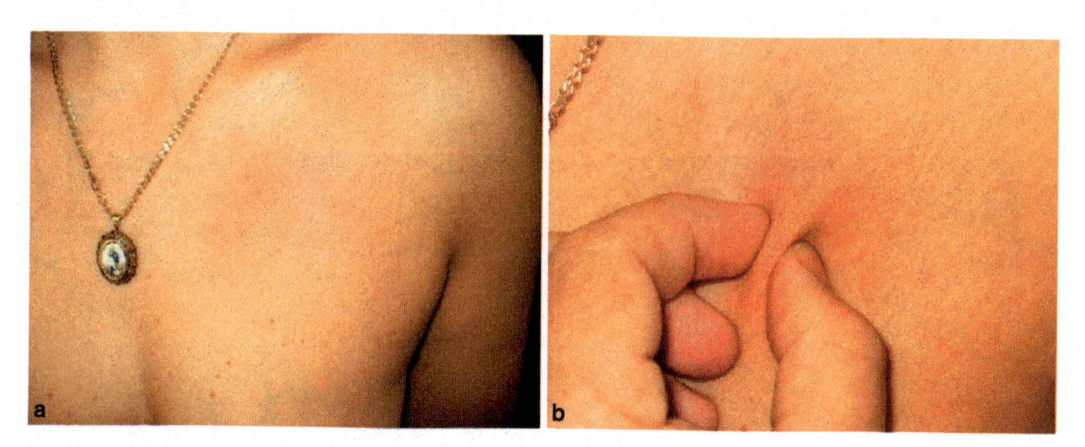

36.3 Definition of the Points and Measurements Used in the TTM Chart

Table 36.3 TTM chart for the overweight patient shown in Fig. 36.6

Fig. 36.7 (a,b) The superficial pinch test on the upper pole of the breast, showing normal tension in the superficial subcutaneous layer

If the deep pinch test shows the ratio R:P between 2 and 3, this corresponds to a normal soft tissue elasticity situation. Breast augmentation can be done according to the chart suggestions, with medium size projection.

If the deep pinch test shows the ratio R:P > 3, this correspond to a loose soft tissue or excess skin situation, as in a ptotic breast. The implant selected must have the largest projection for those specific breast diameters (Fig. 36.9), or an associated mastopexy procedure may be necessary.

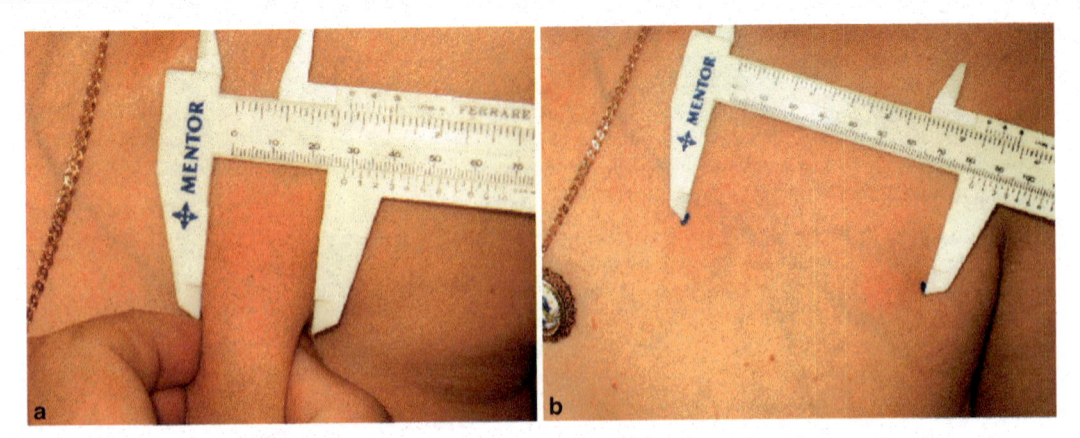

Fig. 36.8 (**a,b**) The deep pinch test on the upper pole of the breast, showing that the pinched distance is 2.5 cm compared with the relaxed one, which is 8 cm. The R:P ratio is larger than 3. This patient lost weight and the tissues cannot retract any more

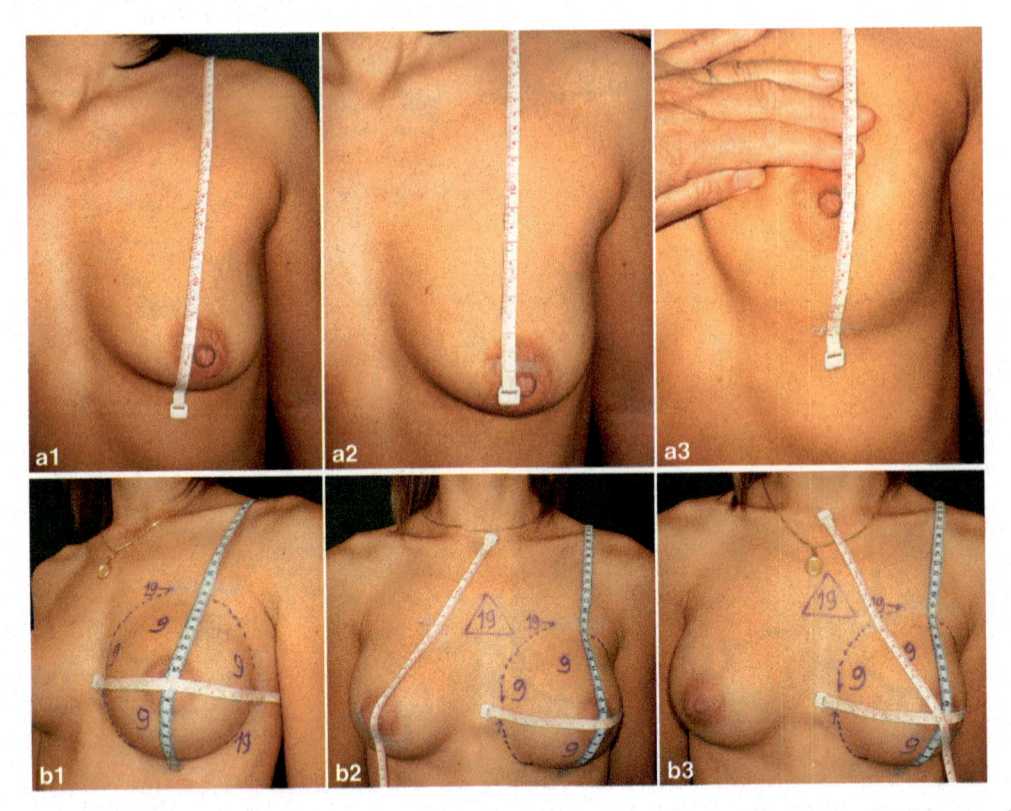

Fig. 36.9 (**a***1-3*) Patient vertical meridian is 16 cm, before the operation, with the relaxed inferior meridian. If we add the length of the superior meridian to the stretched inferior meridian, the vertical meridian will be 19 cm. This will correspond to the breast golden number, if the breast mould will be at the adequate volume. (**b**) Postoperative breast meridians and the breast golden number (19 cm), after the breast augmentation

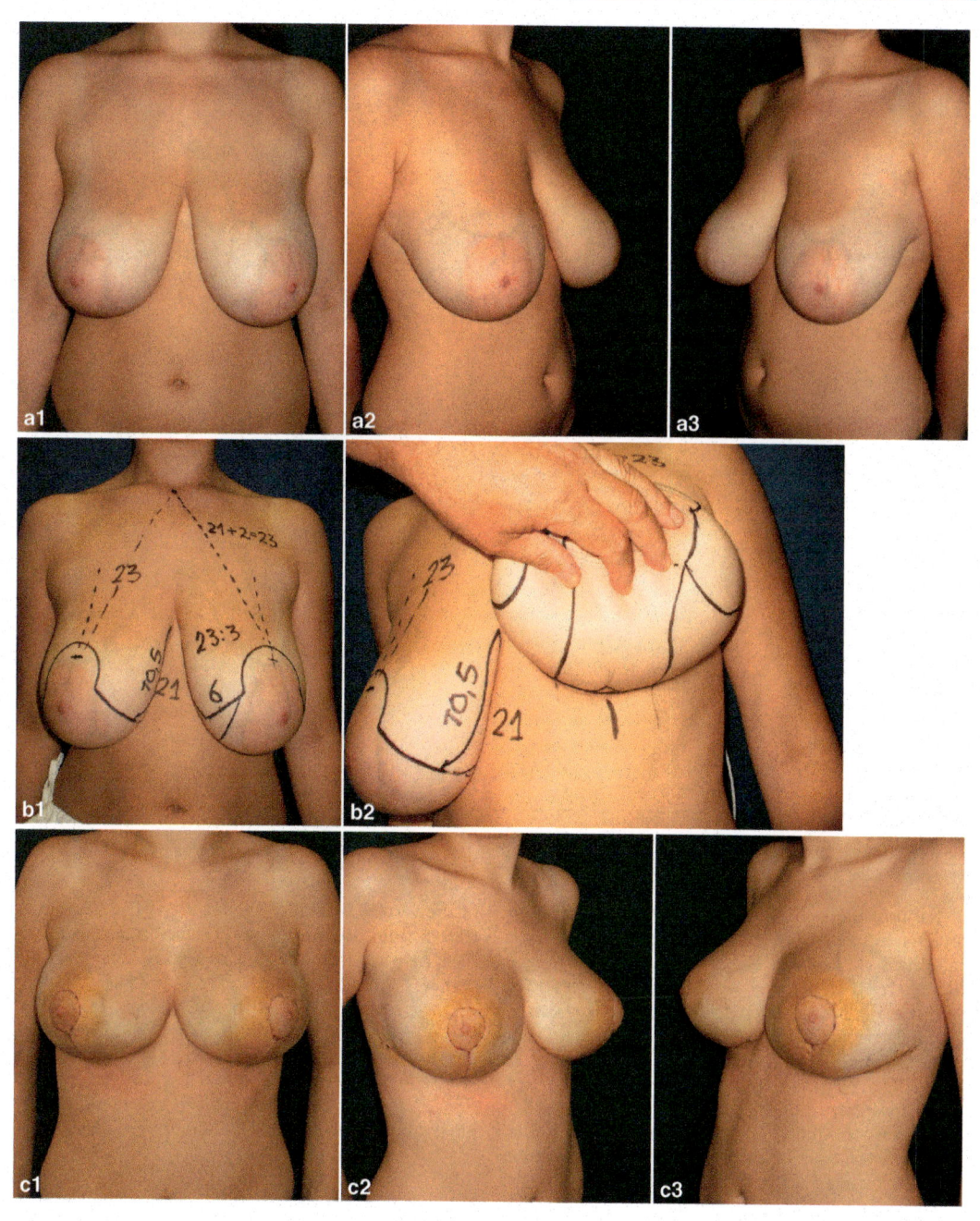

Fig. 36.10 (*a1-3*) Preoperative view of a case with breast hypertrophy and ptosis. (*b1-2*) Preoperative marking according to the suggested breast dimensions, based on 21 cm as the breast golden number. (*c1-3*) Seven days postoperative after breast reduction with inferior pedicle and inverted T scar

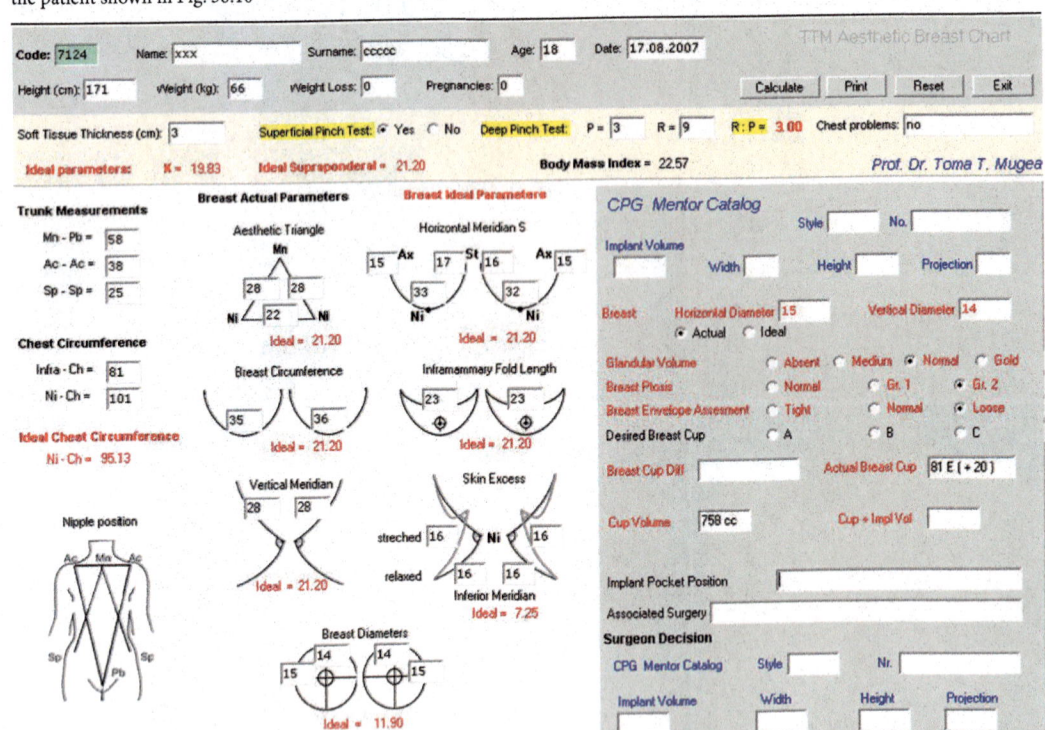

Table 36.4 TTM computer program with actual dimensions of breast and the ideal parameters suggested (*in red*) by the computer for the patient shown in Fig. 36.10

For breast reduction cases (Fig. 36.10), patient's body and actual parameters of breast have been introduced into the TTM program (Table 36.4), and the computer listed in red color the ideal parameters of her breast to be aesthetic. Her breast golden number should be 21 cm.

The inframammary fold length in her case is 21 cm, corresponding with the breast golden number. To calculate the distance from manubrium to the new nipple location, we mark 21 cm + 10% of this length as a correction according to the "pendulum rule." So, the distance between manubrium and the new nipple location should be marked at 23 cm (Fig. 36.10).

The inframammary fold length being 21 cm, half of this is 10.5 cm. The medial and the lateral cutaneous flap should have the same length on the drawing mark, in order to match the "arms" of horizontal part of inverted "T." The Ni–Infra distance at the end of the operation should be 1/3 from breast golden number with 10% correction, it means 23:3 = 7.6 cm. To calculate the length of the vertical branch of the inverted "T," 2 cm is subtracted from 7.6 cm, representing the distance between the nipple and the new areola margin. The length of the vertical "T" branch will be 6 cm.

The postoperative view of the patient (Fig. 36.10) shows an aesthetic appearance of the breast, with a natural shape and the nipple in the most anterior position on the breast mould. The inverted T scar is well positioned, without aesthetic major impairment on the breast and only the vertical branch being visible.

References

1. Penn J: Breast reduction. Br J Plast Surg 1955;7:357–371
2. Smith DJ, Palin WE, Katch VL, Bennet JE: Breast volume and anthropomorphic measurements: normal values. Plast Reconstr Surg 1986;78(3):331–335

3. Stark N, Olivari N: Breast asymmetry: an objective analysis of post-operative results. Eur J Plast Surg 1991;14:173
4. Brown RW, Cheng YC, Kurtay M: A formula for surgical modifications of the breast. Plast Reconstr Surg 2000;106(6): 1342–1345
5. Sommer NZ, Zook LG, Verhulst SJ: The prediction of breast reduction weight. Plast Reconstr Surg 2002;109(2): 506–511
6. Westreich M: Anthropomorphic breast measurements protocol and results in 50 women with aesthetically perfect breasts and clinical application. Plast Reconstr Surg 1997;100(2):468–479
7. Mugea TT: A new system for breast assessment using TTM chart – The 17th International Congress of the French Society of Aesthetic Surgery, Paris, 19–21 May, 2001
8. Georgiade NG, Georgiade GS: Reduction mammoplasty utilizing the inferior pyramidal dermal pedicle. In: Georgiade NG (ed). Aesthetic Breast Surgery. Baltimore, Williams & Wilkins 1983
9. Mugea TT: Aesthetic breast assessment – TTM chart, The 3rd International Congress of Cosmetic Medicine and Surgery, South American Academy of Cosmetic Surgery, Oct 19–21, 2001

CHAPTER 37

Template-Goniometer for Marking the Wise Keyhole Pattern of Reduction Mammaplasty

37

Dirk Lazarus

37.1
Introduction

Despite an increase in short scar mammaplasties, the Wise keyhole pattern still remains the most common skin incision used in reduction mammaplasty. It allows for flexibility in the method of nipple/areola transposition and gives a predictable result.

Wise and colleagues [1, 2] originally described special latex patterns of three separate sizes for accurate design of skin flaps. Wise stated that the patterns greatly simplified the procedure, allowing the surgeon to design the skin flaps rapidly and to attain a measured breast reduction with confidence. Predictable size, contour, and nipple placement and symmetry would be achieved. Strombeck [3] and Skoog [4] also used fixed patterns for preoperative marking.

Because the angle between the vertical limbs of the keyhole, in part, determines the volume of resection, a flexible, stainless steel wire pattern has been devised and successfully used to mark breasts preoperatively [5, 6]. This marker allows one to be able to vary the angle of the keyhole to accommodate the patient's individual requirements. But it is also important to be able to transfer the same angle from one breast to the other with accuracy to ensure symmetry of marking, or to be able to control the degree of adjustment in asymmetrical cases.

The Wise, Skoog, and Strombeck templates allow reproducibility, but only limited flexibility in design, whereas with the stainless steel wire method, reproducibility is difficult to achieve. A template-goniometer was thus designed to allow flexibility and reproducibility of design for the keyhole pattern for reduction mammaplasty.

37.2
Template-Goniometer

The template-goniometer [7] measures about 10 cm in height, and is easily portable in the pocket. It is simple to use and curtails the time required for preoperative marking. It consists of two P-shaped pieces of firm plastic or similar transparent material joined together by a rivet in the centre of the upper, round part of the P.

The rivet allows the two arms of the device to open and close, thus allowing the angle of the keyhole to be set and consistently carried across to the other breast. (Fig. 37.1). This upper part is marked in degrees as a goniometer for measuring the angle between the vertical limbs of the keyhole. The combined upper parts of the P form a circle of 4.5 cm in diameter. This part is used to mark the upper part of the keyhole, which will receive the areola. The vertical limbs of the P are marked in millimeters or centimeters for measurement of the length of the vertical limbs of the keyhole – the new nipple–inframammary crease distance.

Once the new nipple position has been determined, the volume of reduction desired and the amount of tissue laxity present are estimated. These measurements determine the angle at which the goniometer is set. Rough markings can be made freehand and then the template-goniometer is used to obtain smooth, regular lines. The template-goniometer is applied to the breast,

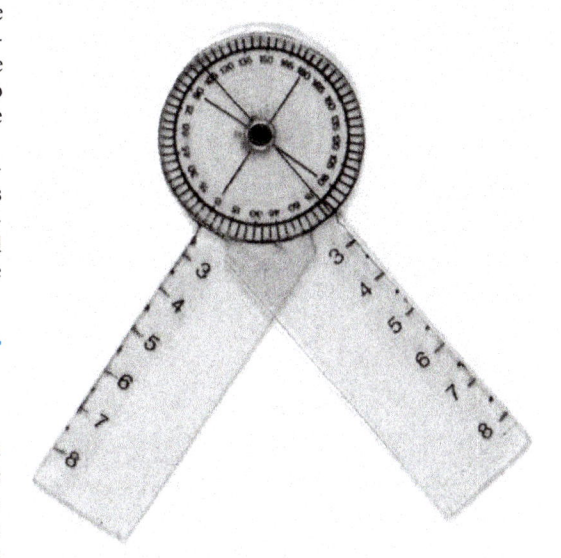

Fig. 37.1 Template-goniometer

M.A. Shiffman (ed.), *Mastopexy and Breast Reduction: Principles and Practice,*
© Springer-Verlag Berlin Heidelberg 2009

possible. The rest of the marking is done, and the procedure is repeated on the contralateral breast.

Since its creation, the template-goniometer has been used for all Wise keyhole pattern breast reductions performed by the author. Its use has resulted in a saving in marking time and has allowed marking to be reproduced between breasts and between patients. It also allowed a flexibility of design, especially with regard to the length of the vertical limbs of the keyhole and the angle between them. Once the upper circular part of the keyhole is marked at 4.5 cm, it is easy to make minor free-hand adjustments in size and shape, if these are required. Similarly, the vertical limbs of the keyhole are easily modified if necessary. The template-goniometer allows the keyhole pattern to be orientated vertically or canted medially or laterally. The device is useful as it allows not only recording of nipple height and the length of the vertical limbs in the patient's clinical notes, but also the angle of the keyhole can be documented.

Ultimately, the markings for reduction mammaplasty are based on the patient's morphology and the surgeon's artistry and experience. The template-goniometer has been found to facilitate preoperative markings for reduction mammaplasty and to allow not only reproducibility, but also flexibility of design.

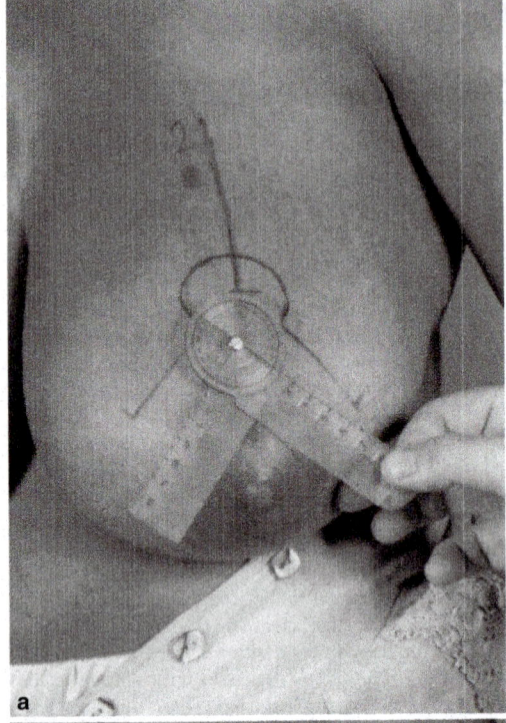

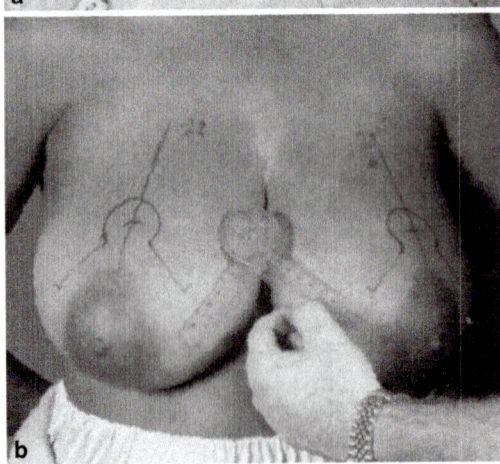

Fig. 37.2 (a,b) Method of using template-goniometer

with the riveted pivot point over the new nipple site and its outline traced onto the breast with a marking pen (Fig. 37.2). The marks are checked by moving and pinching the breast tissue to confirm that closure will be

References

1. Wise RJ, Gannon JP, Hill JR: Further experience with reduction mammaplasty. Plast Reconstr Surg 1963;12:32
2. Wise RJ: A preliminary report on method of planning the mammaplasty. Plast Reconstr Surg 1956;17:367–375
3. Strombeck JO: Mammaplasty: report of a new technique based on the two pedicle procedure. Br J Plast Surg 1960;13:79–90
4. Skoog T: A technique of breast reduction. Acta Chir Scand 1963;126:453–465
5. Georgiade NG: Breast Reconstruction Following Mastectomy. St. Louis, Mosby 1979, p 101
6. Georgiade GS, Riefkohl RE, Georgiade NG: Inferior pyramidal technique in reduction mammaplasty. In: Goldwyn RM (ed). Reduction Mammaplasty. Boston, Little, Brown and Co. 1990, pp 268–269
7. Lazarus D: A new template-goniometer for marking the Wise keyhole pattern of reduction mammaplasty. Plast Reconstr Surg 1998;101(1):171–173

Chapter 38

Individualized Wise Keyhole Pattern: An Aid in Reduction Mammaplasty of the Asymmetric Breasts

Aycan Kayikçioğlu, Yücel Erk

38.1 Introduction

Despite various modifications, the Wise keyhole pattern is the golden standard in planning the amount of reduction to be performed on the hypertrophic breasts [1–4]. Asymmetry of the breast remains a troublesome deformity, and achieving symmetry in volume and shape may be challenging. Because of the variations in the clinical presentation of asymmetric breasts, different combinations of either reduction or augmentation surgery would be required.

The authors have devised a technique for individualized keyhole pattern in the treatment of asymmetric breasts, when the surgical solution is simply the reduction and reshaping of the larger breast to fit to the smaller one.

38.2 Technique

The technique is applicable to a selected group of patients in whom only reduction mammaplasty of the larger breast to fit the other would suffice (Fig. 38.1). The whole surface of the smaller breast is covered with adhesive plasters preferably of thick and inelastic nature (Fig. 38.2). The inframammary sulcus is strictly obeyed. The nipple–areola complex and midclavicular line are depicted on the plaster coverage. Afterwards, the plasters are carefully elevated and the circle for the nipple–areola complex is cut off. The hole is connected to the inframammary sulcus (lower border of the plaster coverage) through the previously marked infraclavicular line in order to create the vertical limb in Wise's keyhole pattern. The mould is stuck to a transparent film or an X-ray and an individualized keyhole pattern is obtained ready to use on the larger breast (Fig. 38.2). The pattern helps to reflect the surface area of the smaller breast to the opposite breast. After the symmetric side for areola nipple complex is determined,

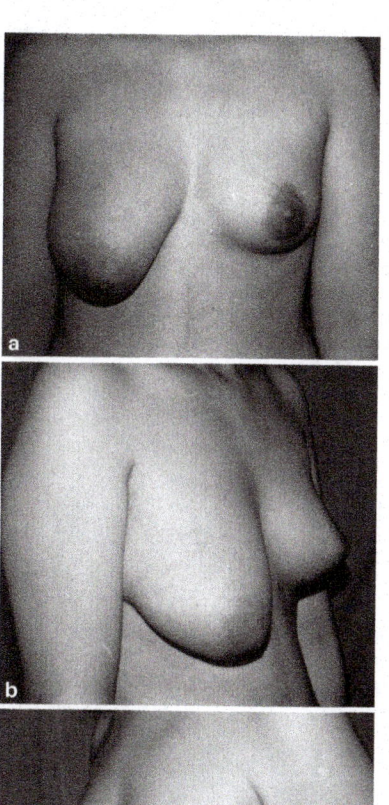

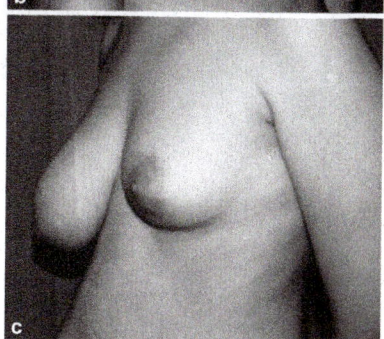

Fig. 38.1 (a–c) Preoperative 15-year-old girl who complained of marked asymmetry of her breasts. (a) anteroposterior view (b, c) oblique views

M.A. Shiffman (ed.), *Mastopexy and Breast Reduction: Principles and Practice*,
© Springer-Verlag Berlin Heidelberg 2009

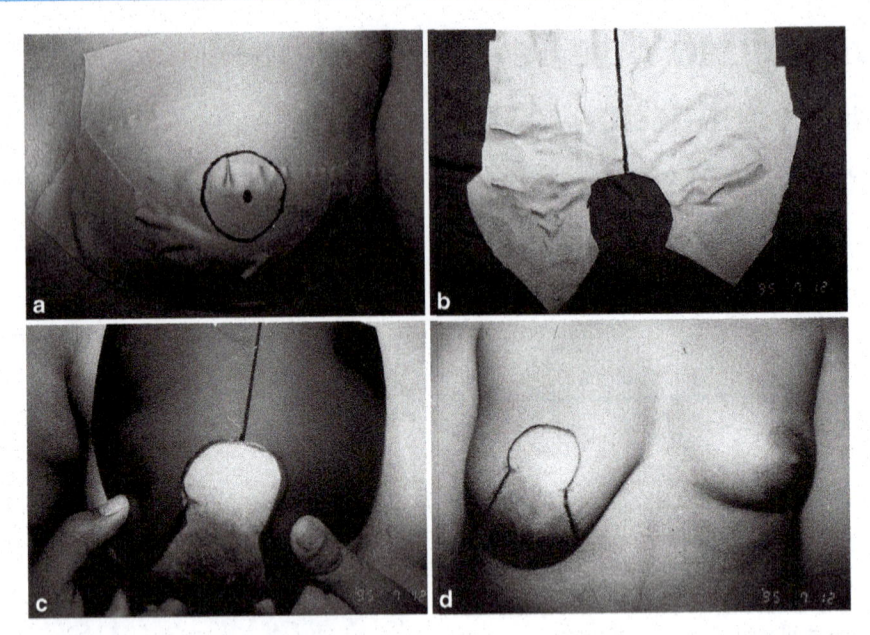

Fig. 38.2 (**a**) Covering of the left breast with adhesive plaster and marking of the nipple–areola complex. (**b**) After depicting the landmarks comprising the midclavicular line, areolar circle was excised, the hole was cut to the inframammary sulcus on the midclavicular line. A keyhole pattern was obtained. (**c**) The plaster mould was transferred on an X-ray film for better use on the breast. (**d**) After determining the new nipple position, the reduction was designed by using the mould

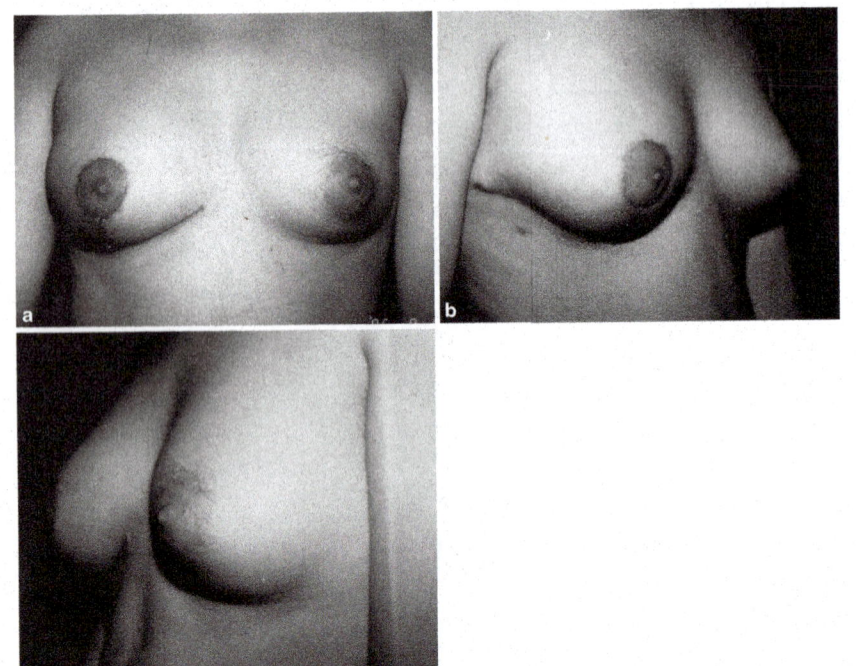

Fig. 38.3 (**a–c**) Postoperative after bipedicled vertical dermal flap technique of reduction mammaplasty of the right breast with 220 g excision. (**a**) anteroposterior view (**b, c**) oblique views

the reduction may be performed in regard to the depiction obtained (Fig. 38.3).

38.3 Discussion

The technique has been used for more than 15 years on a number of patients and we believe that it is an easy and fast technique for comparison of the breast sizes with each other. Since the asymmetric breasts may have great intrinsic variability of shape, volume, and contour not only between the breasts but also in different quadrants of the same breast, surgical experience remains the main factor to determine the success of the end result, but this simple method may contribute to the outcome.

References

1. Wise RJ: Preliminary report on a method of planning the mammaplasty. Plast Reconstr Surg 1956;17(5):367–375
2. Wise RJ, Gannon JP, Hill JR: Further experience with reduction mammaplasty. Plast Reconstr Surg 1963;32:12–20
3. Parsons RW: Versatile mammaplasty pattern of Wise. Plast Reconstr Surg 1975;55(1):1–4
4. Lazarus D: A new template-goniometer for marking the Wise keyhole pattern of reduction mammaplasty. Plast Reconstr Surg 1998;101(1):171–173

Double Dermal Keyhole Pattern

Elie Frederic Harouche

39.1 Introduction

The double dermal pattern was first described in 1995 [1] and is based on the traditional keyhole pattern with some modifications. Historically, the keyhole pattern has been a reliable, consistent technique with reproducible and predictable good results for breast reduction [2–5]. However, some drawbacks are well known and have been well documented. In particular, an area of weakness – the inverted T – has been troublesome and frustrating for many surgeons and patients [6]. Because of its placement, the weight of the breast, and various local wound factors, the inverted T has been the site of early postoperative dehiscences and later of widening of the scars [7]. Many attempts have been made to minimize the size of the incision with multiple reduction mammaplasty designs. Trials of periareolar incisions with or without a short vertical limb have been somewhat successful [8–11]. Nevertheless, the results are not always predictable and certainly not always reproducible, especially in large reduction mammaplasties. The best reduction mammaplasty closure, however, remains elusive.

39.2 Principles

The procedure is based on the principle that two dermal layers are superimposed on each other in the area of the inverted T. Two triangular flaps are incorporated, one on the lateral and the other on the medial flap of the keyhole pattern.

The technique is also based on the concept that these two superimposed dermal layers form a stronger support than one layer of dermis abutting another at the level of the inverted T.

39.3 Technique

This modified keyhole pattern is particularly suited for large or inferior pedicle-type reduction mammaplasty. It is, however, adaptable to any pedicle technique.

The keyhole pattern is drawn with each portion of the medial and lateral vertical limb measuring 5–6 cm from the areolar edge to the inframammary crease. A small triangle, ABC (Fig. 39.1), measuring approximately 3 cm is then drawn on the medial vertical limb of the keyhole pattern. The horizontal portion of this triangle is measured on the inframammary crease at a distance of 2 cm. A similar triangle, DEF, is drawn on the vertical limb of the keyhole pattern (Fig. 39.1).

Procedure for the reduction then proceeds as usual. The triangles are incorporated in the elevation of the medial and lateral flaps (Fig. 39.2). The lateral triangle is then deepithelialized (Fig. 39.3). It will then be noted that closure of the medial triangle, ABC, will be superimposed on the lateral triangle, DEF (Fig. 39.4). The closure is completed by suturing the skin edges of the triangles. Point A will meet point D, B will be sutured over point F, and E will be sutured under C (Fig. 39.5).

The end result of the closure is a gentle curved incision in the area of the T, with a double dermal layer at the level of the most stress (Fig. 39.6).

39.4 Discussion

Although this technique adds an additional 8–10 min to the procedure, it is well worth it. Once the lateral triangles are deepithelialized, care must be taken not to resect it with the specimen. When well executed, the double dermal keyhole pattern will reward the surgeon with headache free healing at the inverted T.

The double dermal closure provides strength and support where it is most needed. The cosmetic improvements obtained with this closure are evident, as the inverted T right-angle incisions have been eliminated and are not visible once they become curved as the wound heals. Although cut at various angles, the final result of this modified T incision is a soft, rounded, and less conspicuous closure (Fig. 39.6). There is less spread of the inframammary vertical incision, as the healing vector forces are both changed by this double dermal closure and incorporation of the triangular flap.

M.A. Shiffman (ed.), *Mastopexy and Breast Reduction: Principles and Practice*,
© Springer-Verlag Berlin Heidelberg 2009

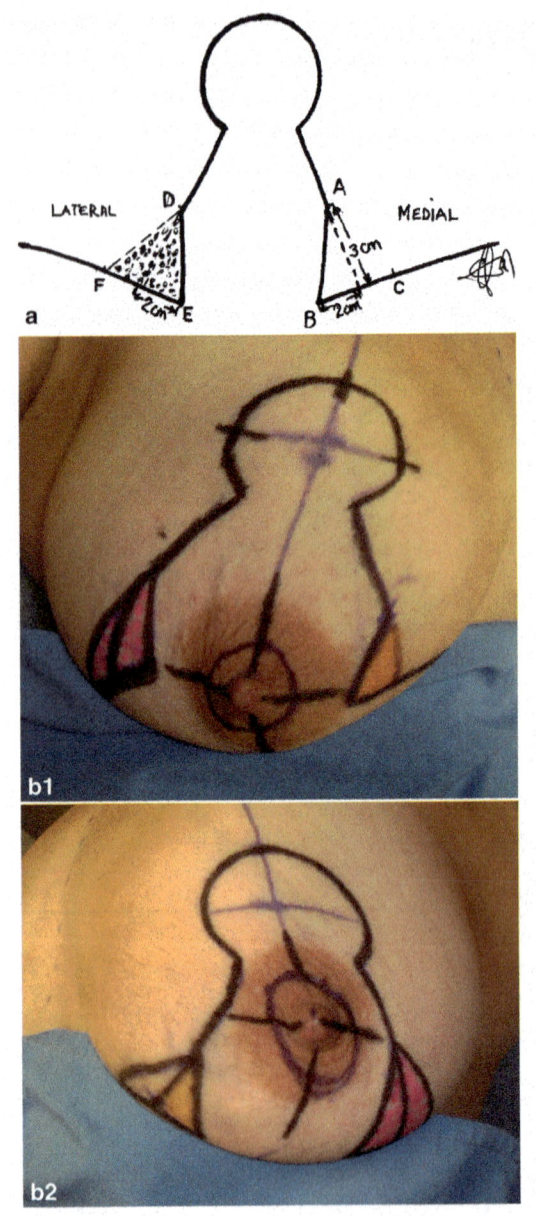

Fig. 39.1 (a) A small triangle, ABC, is drawn approximately 3 cm on the medial vertical limb of the keyhole pattern. The horizontal portion of this triangle is measured on the inframammary crease for a distance of 2 cm. A similar triangle, DEF, is drawn on the vertical limb of the keyhole pattern. (b1,2) The markings are completed

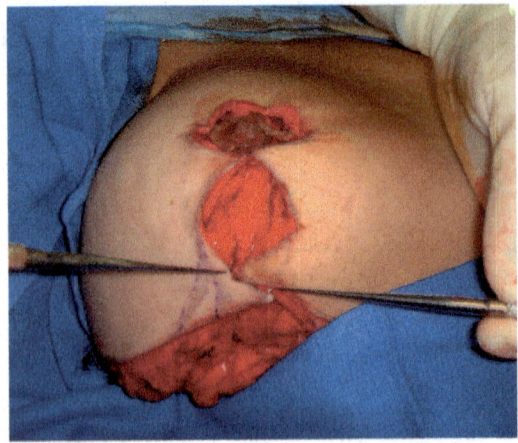

Fig. 39.2 The triangles are incorporated in the elevation of the medial and lateral flaps

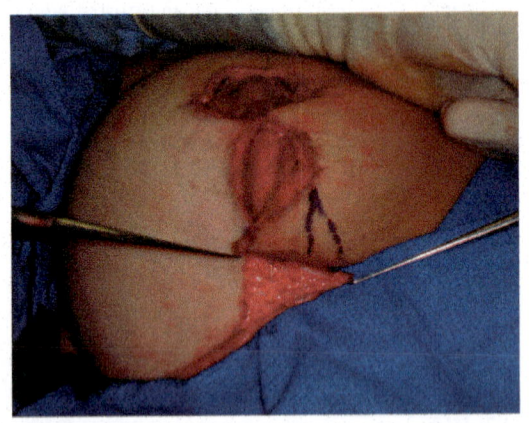

Fig. 39.3 The lateral triangle is deepithelialized

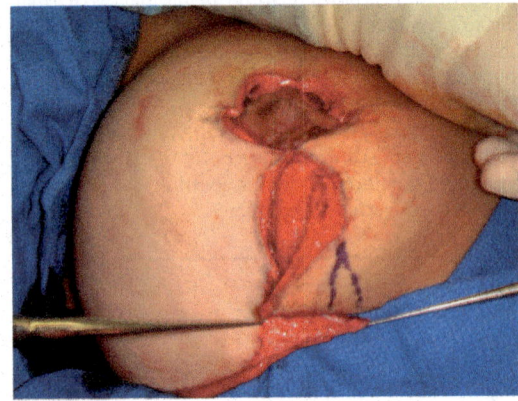

Fig. 39.4 The closure of the medial triangle, ABC, will be superimposed on the lateral triangle, DEF

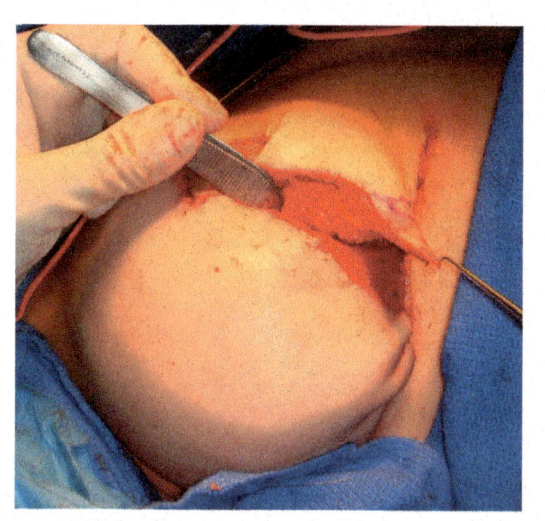

Fig. 39.5 The closure is completed by suturing the skin edges of the triangles. Point A will meet point D. B will be sutured over point F, and E will be sutured under C

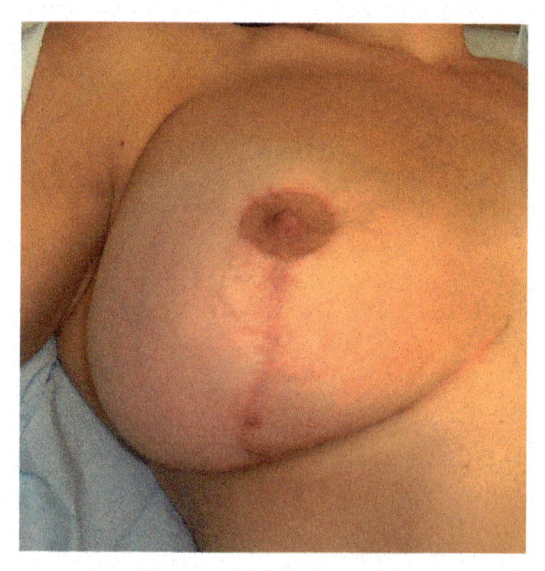

Fig. 39.6 The closure results in a gentle curved incision in the area of the T with a double dermal layer at the level of the most stress

39.5 Conclusions

The dermal modified keyhole closure is a simple, versatile, and adaptable method of closure regardless of the pedicle technique used for reduction mammaplasty. A triangular flap (skin and dermis) is incorporated on the medial keyhole flap. A deepithelialized dermal flap is created on the lateral keyhole flap. In the final closure of the wound, the medial triangular flap is sutured over the lateral deepithelialized dermal flap. A double dermal closure at the inverted T region is thereby created. The frequency of occurrence of wound spread and early postoperative wound dehiscence are decreased by this closure, which provides cosmetic improvement and wound support where it is most needed.

References

1. Harouche EF: The double dermal keyhole pattern for breast reduction. Plast Reconstr Surg 1995;96(6):1451–1453
2. Wise RJ: A preliminary report on a method of planning the mammaplasty. Plast Reconstr Surg 1956;17(5):367–375
3. Wise RJ, Gannon JP, Hill RJ: Further experience with reduction mammaplasty. Plast Reconstr Surg 1963;32:12–20
4. Strombeck JO: Mammaplasty: Report of a new techniques based on the two-pedicle procedure. Br J Plast Surg 1961;13:79–90
5. Bames HO: Resection of the massive breast hypertrophy. Plast Reconstr Surg 1948;3:560
6. Conway H, Smith J: Breast plastic surgery: reduction mammaplasty, mastopexy, augmentation mammaplasty and mammary construction; analysis of two hundred and fortyfive cases. Plast Reconstr Surg 1958;21(1):8–19
7. Rees TD, Flagg SV: Reduction mammaplasty. In: Goldwyn RM (ed). The Unfavorable Results in Plastic Surgery, Boston, Little, Brown 1972, pp 371–385
8. Chiari A Jr: The L short-scar mammaplasty. A new approach. Plast Reconstr Surg 1992;90(2):233–246
9. Lejour M, Abboud M: Vertical mammaplasty without inframammary scar and breast liposuction. Plast Reconstr Surg 1990;86:67–75
10. Lassus C: Breast reduction: evolution of a technique – a single vertical scar. Aesthetic Plast Surg 1987;11(2): 107–112
11. Benelli L: Technique de plastie mammaire, le "Round Bloc." Rev Fr Chir Esthet 1988;50:7

CHAPTER 40

Deepithelialization in Breast Reduction: A Simple Technique

40

Pierre F. Fournier

40.1 Introduction

In all cases of breast reduction, deepithelializing has to be done more or less around the areola. The deepithelialized areola, according to the technique, may or may not stay connected to the neighboring skin by one or two dermal glandular pedicles. Usually, this deepithelialization is performed using a knife.

With a knife, this deepithelialization may be excellent but sometimes may be irregular, too superficial, or too deep, particularly in the hands of a beginner. An identical layer thickness of the dermis has to be saved when the knife technique is used and this is difficult for beginners to learn because a cleavage plane does not exist in this procedure.

Consequently, being too superficial, in the immediate postoperative period or later, may result in a scar of poor quality. Months postoperatively, sebaceous cysts may appear or the scar is uneven. Localized infections may be present and frequently many sebaceous glands may have been included in the scar. Such unpleasant events should be avoided even if they are not serious. When performed too deep, the blood supply of the areola as well as the venous drainage may be hindered and necrosis of the areola may happen, either partially or totally.

For many years, the author has used a technique of deepithelialization that does not seem to be very well known [1, 2]. This technique has the advantage of being easy, quick, and extremely safe. An artificial cleavage plane into the dermis is created at the desired level.

40.2 Technique

The main thing is to apply a "Tourniquet" around the base of the breast. This nylon tourniquet has to be rather thick and should be very tight (Fig. 40.1). The tightness is maintained by a strong or several strong towel forceps passing through the tourniquet.

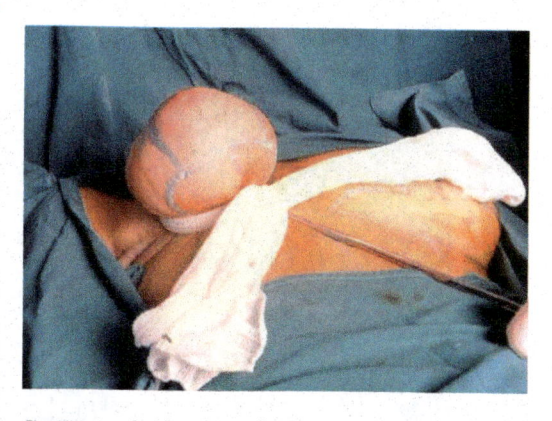

Fig. 40.1 A nylon "Tourniquet" is placed very tightly at the base of the breast

The larger the breast, the easier and more efficient is this maneuver. The breast strangulated is a firm mass, homogeneous, and tight, and this degree of tightness may be increased by using the hands of the assistant surgeon or the surgeon's hand.

Extreme tightness is indispensable to accomplish in this technique of deepithelialization. The surgeon has to incise the skin to the desired depth of the future cleavage plan. Strips of dermal-epidermis of 7–9 mm width are created, either concentric to the areola or horiz-ontal or vertical according to the place that has to be deepithelialized.

Each of such strips is dissected at one of its extremities for about 1 cm at the cleavage plane desired. This part of the strip is grasped firmly with an arterial forceps or needle holder (Fig. 40.2).

The grip has to be firm to avoid any slipping of the forceps. Moderate traction on the arterial forceps will give a dermal-epidermal strip neatly free from the depth, as if it was in a natural cleavage plane. This strip is regular and identical to itself in its whole length without any incursion into the deep aspect of the dermis (Fig. 40.2). Each strip is removed in the same manner in a few seconds (Fig. 40.2), and when the deepithelialization is finished, the tourniquet is removed and the rest of the operation is performed (Fig. 40.2).

M.A. Shiffman (ed.), *Mastopexy and Breast Reduction: Principles and Practice*,
© Springer-Verlag Berlin Heidelberg 2009

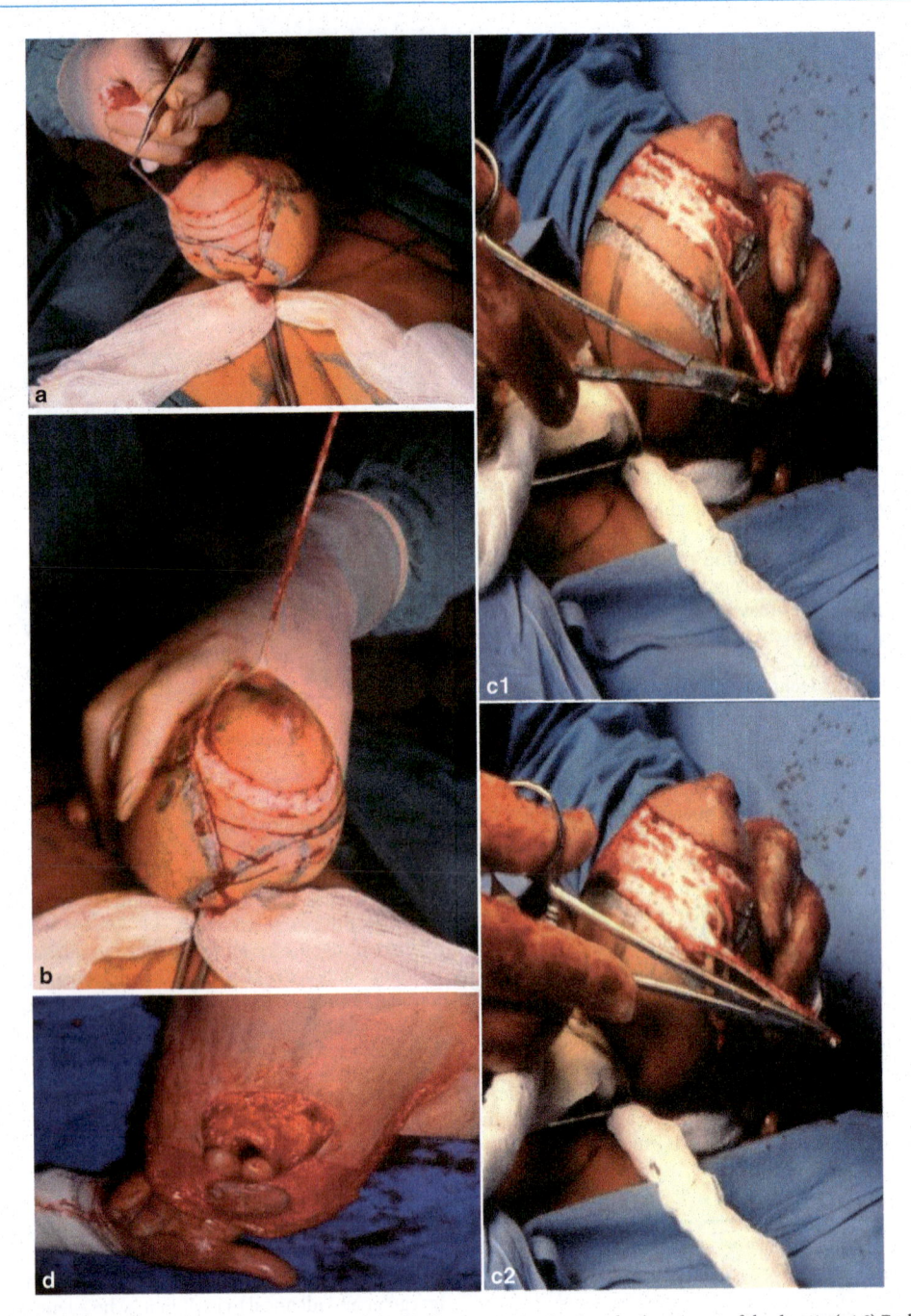

Fig. 40.2 Strips marked on the skin are incised and removed with arterial forceps. (**a**) The strip is dissected at one end for about 1 cm in the cleavage plane desired. This part of the strip is grasped firmly with an artery forceps or needle holder. (**b**) The strip is regular and identical to itself in its whole length without any incursion into the deep aspect of the dermis. (**c1,2**) Each strip is removed in the same manner in a few seconds. (**d**) When the deepithelialization is finished, the "Tourniquet" is removed and the rest of the operation is performed

This procedure is possible only above the tourniquet. If more skin has to be deepithelialized below the tourniquet as is done in dermal mastopexy, this technique cannot be applied. Deepithelialization has to be done with knife, scissors, or electrical cautery. Deepithelialization done this way is excellent. There is no damage to cutaneous or subcutaneous vessels and no sebaceous cysts or their complications are part of this procedure.

References

1. Fournier PF: Un procedemiento de desepidermisacion. Secundo Congresso Argentino de Cirurgia Estetica, Buenos Aires, Marzo 1974
2. Fournier PF: Un procédé pour désépithélialiser dans les réductions mammaires. In: Faivre J (ed). Rhinoplasties, Ptoses et Hypertrophies Mammaires Modérées, Maloine S.A. 1984, pp 263–268

A Specially Designed Ruler and a Triangular Suture to Simplify Reduction Mammaplasty

Gottfried Wechselberger, Petra Pülzl

41.1 Introduction

Although reduction mammaplasty using a superiorly [1] or inferiorly [2] based dermal pedicle is a well-established technique suitable for many cases, inaccurate preoperative marking frequently causes visible, displaced scarring, which mars the results. To prevent this common pitfall, we recommend herein a simple method for marking exact resection lines preoperatively by using a specially designed ruler [3]. The ruler is made of transparent plastic and has a triangular shape (Fig. 41.1). Two straight sides have centimeter scales and at a right angle. The ruler has a red midline and also four black lines marking a five-degree distance to the next line. The corner of the scaled borders is the top of the ruler. However, unless the resection lines are marked exactly prior to the en bloc resection of the inferior portion of the breast preoperatively, the results may be flawed by "dog-eared" scaring outside the original submammary fold.

To ensure exact marking, we place a strong temporary suture [4] at three marked points which will later be sutured to form the junction point of the inverted T-line. All the excess tissue volume, which will be resected later, now protrudes medially and laterally as a big dog-ear. Once this dog-ear is submerged, the correct resection lines become visible.

41.2 Technique

The initial measurements for the eventual size of the breast and nipple location are carried out in an upright position. The upper sternal notch and the midclavicular lines are marked. Point A, the new position of the nipple–areola, is marked on the midclavicular line at a level slightly lower than the projection of the inframammary crease. Then, the top of the pattern is placed on point A with the midline of the ruler corresponding to the midclavicular line (Fig. 41.2). Lateral borders of the ruler are then marked using an angle of 90° for normal skin or 100° if the skin is flaccid. In the second case, the ruler must be turned to the next black line, which is at 5° from the midline. The points for resection are designated B and C. The length of the lateral borders (distances AB and AC) varies from 8 to 9 cm depending on the size and shape of the breast to be achieved. A greater angle will result in a smaller breast. At last, the submammary fold is marked together with the horizontal incision lines. The lateral incision should not enter the anterior axillary line. The distance from the midsternum to each areola should be the same and will vary between 8 and 10 cm, depending on the patient's size. The point of intersection between midclavicular line and inframammary crease is point D (Fig. 41.3).

The operation is performed under general anesthesia with the patient in a 30° upright position. A temporary triangular suture is placed to approximate points B, C and D to mark the medial and lateral extension of the excision (Fig. 41.4). The placement of the triangular suture causes a projection of redundant tissue medially and laterally (Fig. 41.5). Using a forceps, the redundant tissue is pushed inward (Fig. 41.6). This procedure enables the surgeon to control and, if necessary, correct the estimated lines of the medial and lateral resection.

The reduction mammaplasty is performed using a superiorly (Höhler-Pitanguy [1]) or inferiorly (Robbin [2]) pedicle technique. After the resection, the breast is reshaped by bringing the medial and lateral skin flaps together starting with suturing both of the lower corners (point B and C) to the appropriate place in the submammary fold (point D). The upper 4–4.5 cm of these flaps is temporarily closed (Fig. 41.7). The vertical suture line and the inframammary suture line are closed in the usual manner. At last, the patient is brought into a semiupright position. The final detailed placement of the nipple–areola is always carried out by comparing one side with the other by fixing two circular patterns (Fig. 41.8). The range of the final location is up to 2 cm. The marked area is denuded and the temporary suture is removed. Now, the nipple is placed in this area (Fig. 41.9).

M.A. Shiffman (ed.), *Mastopexy and Breast Reduction: Principles and Practice*,
© Springer-Verlag Berlin Heidelberg 2009

Fig. 41.1 Mammaplasty-Ruler

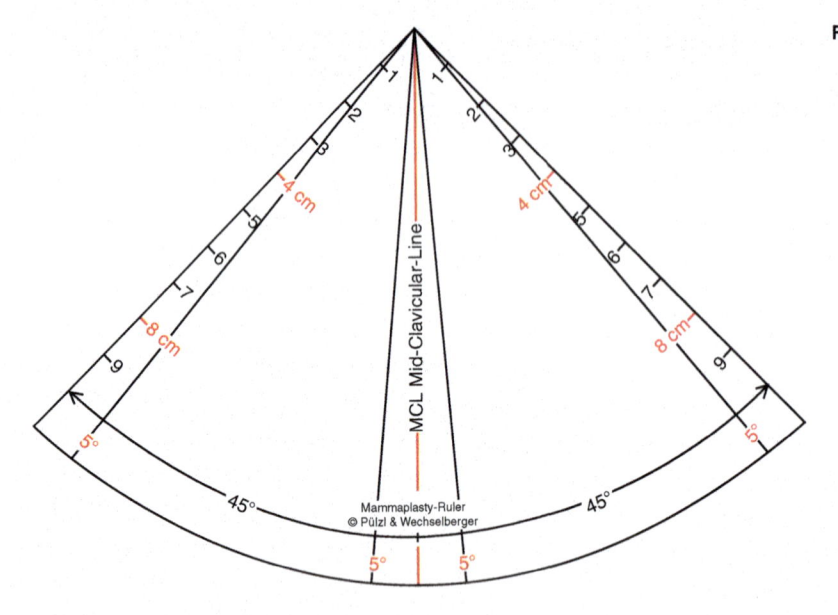

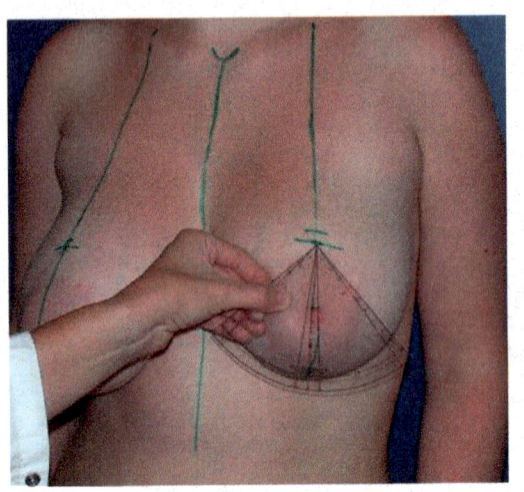

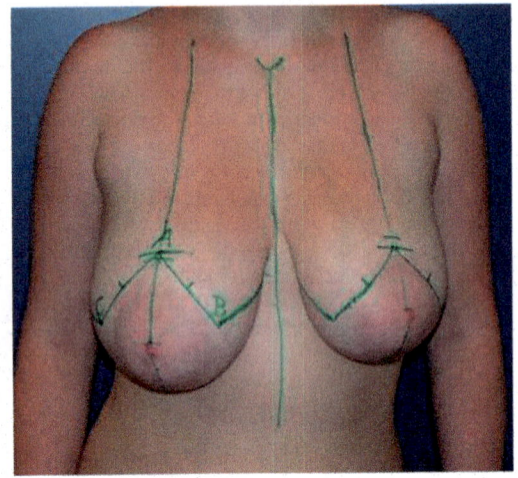

Fig. 41.2 The *top* of the pattern is placed on point A, the new position of the nipple–areola. The *midline* of the ruler must correspond to the midclavicular line

Fig. 41.3 Preoperative marking

41.3 Discussion

Imprecisely marking preoperative lines for the resection will result in a dog-ear at the medial and/or lateral end of the scar in the submammary fold. Should the drawing deviate from the ideal line, the whole scar line will be displaced from the submammary fold. The triangular suture is an easy method for controlling preoperative marking. This procedure helps to carry out an accurate resection of breast tissue, particularly on the medial and lateral sections. In addition to the cosmetic improvement, this technique further benefits the patient by the avoidance of intraoperative corrections or adjustments.

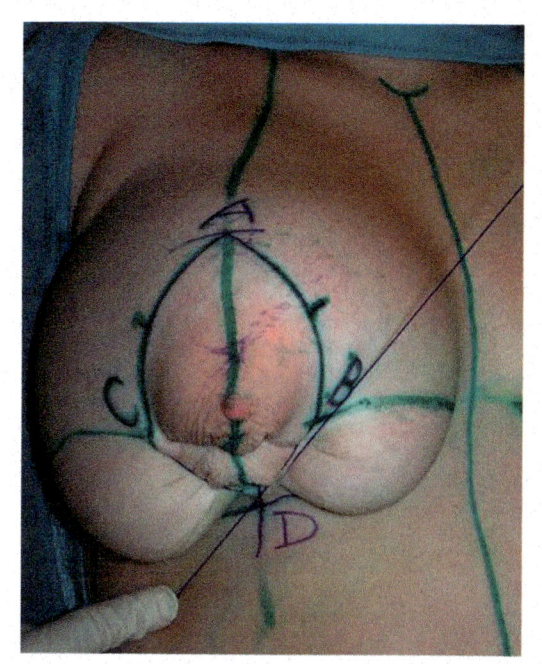

Fig. 41.4 The temporary triangular suture is set in place. It is approximated and the central areola complex is submerged with a hook

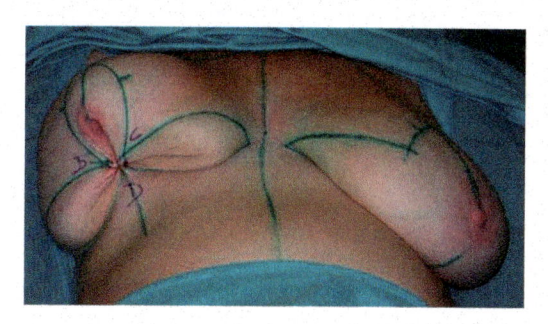

Fig. 41.5 The triangular suture is tightened and the redundant tissue becomes visible as a medial and lateral dog-ear

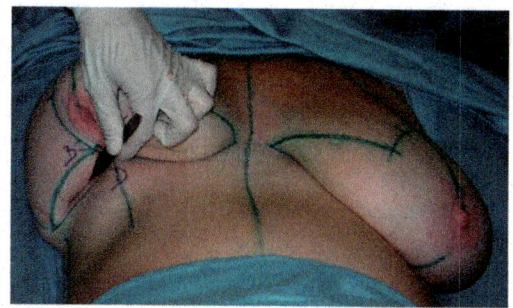

Fig. 41.6 The dog-ear is submerged and the shortest resection line without further dog-ears becomes visible

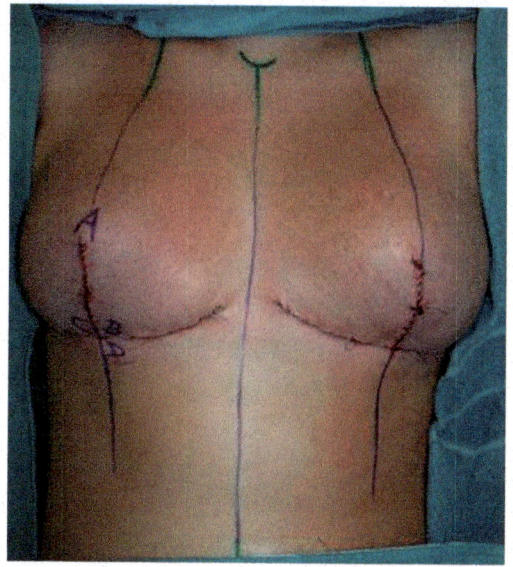

Fig. 41.7 The upper 4–4.5 cm of these flaps is temporarily closed

The authors' modification of the Robbins technique [2] is the final detailed placement of the nipple–areola. After suturing the flaps, one side is compared with the other by fixing two circular patterns (Fig. 41.9). Now, it is possible to vary the position of the areola–nipple complex. The range of the final location is up to 2 cm. After denuding the marked area, the nipple is delivered and sutured in this final position. In the superiorly based dermal pedicle technique as described by Pitanguy in 1962 [1], the nipple is never marked beforehand, because they found that its position is governed by the newly formed breast and its position being the logical consequence of a well-oriented glandular resection. Comp-aring one side with the other and after the initial sutures, its final detailed placement is carried out.

To avoid visible scars, it is very important that the lateral incision should not enter the anterior axillary line. If there is any mismatch between the length of the horizontal incision lines and the inframammary incision lines, we start suturing laterally reaping the longer distance of the incision lines. This causes ripples in the early postoperative period, which will disappear within

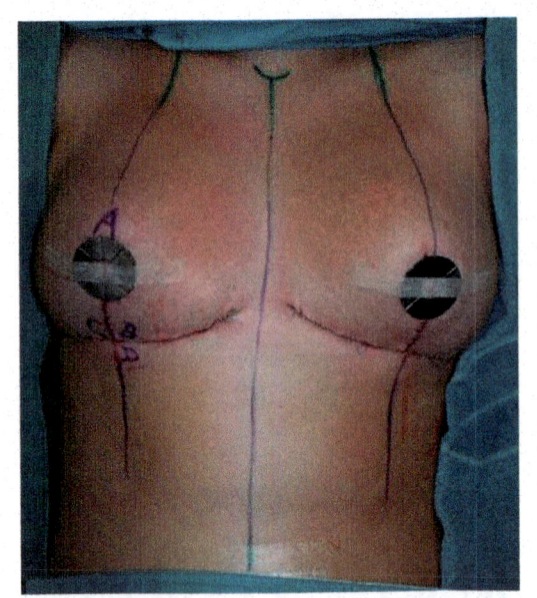

Fig. 41.8 The final detailed placement of the nipple–areola is always carried out by comparing one side with the other by fixing two circular patterns

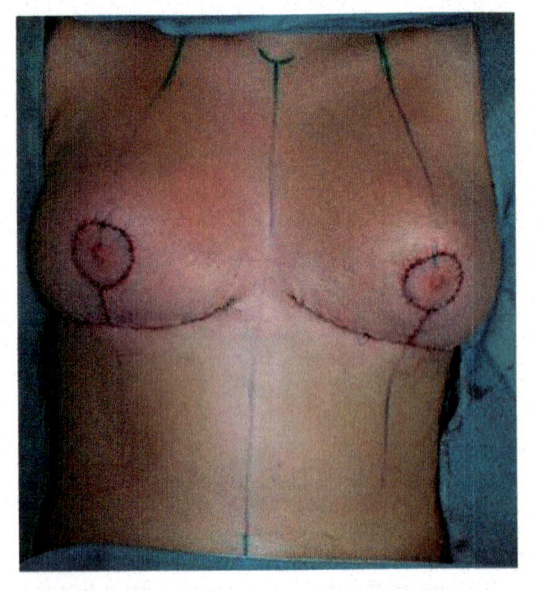

Fig. 41.9 The nipple is placed in the marked denuded area

1 or 2 weeks. Medially, we also avoid elongating our incision in case of length mismatch by using the same technique as lateral.

The distance from the inferior border of the nipple to the inframammary fold should not exceed 4–4.5 cm. Within 6 months, because of the weight of the breast this scar would be enlarged and a natural form with a slight ptosis will result. If the distance is more than the suggested length, the nipple will be located high and the volume of the breast will sag. The projection of the breast can be built by the length of the lateral borders and the angle between the two borders. If the skin is very flaccid, we use not more than 4 cm in length and an angle of 100°.

The authors use a plastic ruler to have more flexibility, which allows flexion over the breast. The transparency of plastic offers better visualization of the midclavicular line, which must correspond to the midline of the ruler.

41.4
Conclusions

This technique is to facilitate the correct preoperative marking for resection in inferiorly and superiorly based mammaplasty by using a specially designed ruler. The triangular suture is an easy method for controlling preoperative marking. This procedure helps to carry out an accurate resection of breast tissue, particularly on the medial and lateral sections.

References

1. Pitanguy I: Surgical treatment of breast hypertrophy. Br J Plast Surg 1960;20:78
2. Robbins TH: A reduction mammaplasty with the areola-nipple based on an inferior dermal pedicle. Plast Reconstr Surg 1977;59:64
3. Pülzl P, Schoeller T, Wechselberger G: Simplification of reduction mammaplasty using a specially designed ruler. Aesthetic Plast Surg 2006;30:622
4. Wechselberger G, Schoeller T, Papp C: A triangular suture to simplify reduction mammaplasty. Aesthetic Plast Surg 1998;22:451

Endoscopic Mastopexy and Breast Reduction

Marco Aurelio Faria-Correa

42.1 Introduction

New concepts regarding skin elasticity were introduced in the field of plastic surgery by way of innovative techniques of liposuction and circum-mammary breast reduction [1–3]. These new concepts, which concern the capacity of the skin to retract, allowed the author to investigate the feasibility of applying endoscopic methods to subcutaneous tissue to avoid skin resection. The author began by modifying the mini-abdominoplasty technique as well as the techniques for breast reduction and mastopexy – endoscopy was also used as an aid for the flap harvesting and placement of tissue expanders – and developed promising research regarding axillary and inguinal lymph node dissections [4].

Video endoscopic methods have been used in different surgical fields such as gynecology, orthopedics, and general surgery where many advantages have been shown. There are less tissue trauma, lower rates of infection, and minimal scars [5].

Laparoscopic procedures use pressurized CO_2 gas to create a space between the laparoscope and the tissue to allow visualization. In the subcutaneous tissue, however, pressured gases are not recommended because of the risk of embolism. To circumvent this risk, the author developed the "subcutaneous tomoscope" which is an instrument that transfers into a transparent capsule the needed space for illumination and visualization. The optical cavity functions much the same way as a scuba diving mask does while serving as a blunt dissector because of its wedge-shaped capsule [4]. Specially designed retractors were developed to increase the necessary working space as well as other instruments such as special needle holders and needles (Fig. 42.1). All of these instruments were designed to work through minimal incisions.

With video endoscopy, delicate processes can be performed through minimal incisions that can be made at strategically placed and remote sites avoiding visible scars. This is an important goal in the field of aesthetic surgery where scars are undesirable and may sometimes compromise the final aesthetic result.

42.2 Endoscopy for Mastopexy and Breast Reduction

Endoscopic versions for mastopexy and breast reduction were first performed in November 1992. Since then, the endoscopic technique has been used to treat 182 patients. The patients ranged in age from 14 to 58 years. They presented with first- or second-degree ptosis with or without hypertrophy. Patients were selected on the basis of having good skin elasticity without significant excessive skin. Breastfeeding and striae were not considered contraindications as long as the patient maintained good skin elasticity. Premature moderate ptosis recurrence was observed when the endoscopic technique was applied to patients presenting with skin flaccidity An important application for this technique is in patients with a small degree of breast asymmetry, particularly in young patients. The larger breast can be reduced with no visible scar or loss of sensation to match the smaller, unoperated breast.

42.3 Technique

The traditional video endoscopic system and the subcutaneous tomoscope, associated with endoscopic instruments, were used to create an optical space. Thus, monitor control could be used without CO_2 distension. Some instruments were modified and new ones were developed creating a set of instruments that facilitate this procedure. Regular laparoscopic for-ceps and scissors connected to the electrocautery were used.

42.4 Positioning of the Patient and the Team

Proper positioning of both the patient and the surgical team is important for facilitating this procedure. The monitor is placed over the patient's head and the anesthesiologist stays beside the patient's head. The surgeon works beside the patient. The surgical table must be

M.A. Shiffman (ed.), *Mastopexy and Breast Reduction: Principles and Practice*,
© Springer-Verlag Berlin Heidelberg 2009

310   42 Endoscopic Mastopexy and Breast Reduction

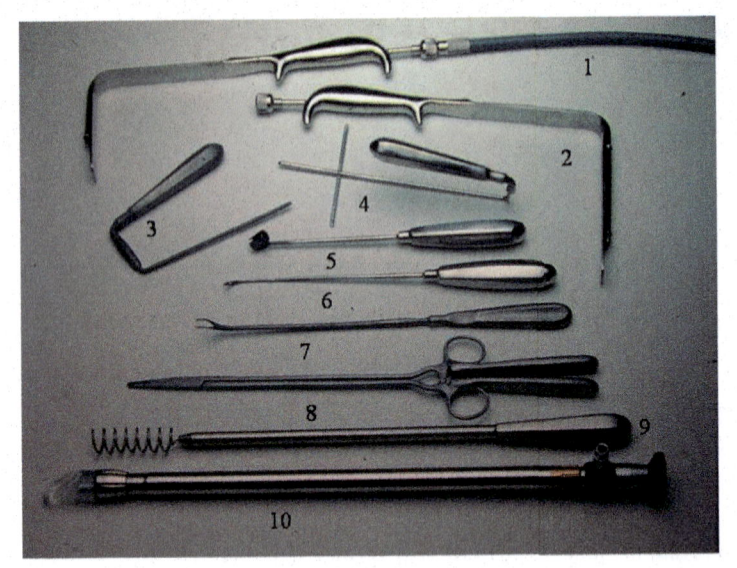

Fig. 42.1 Set of instruments developed by the author from superior to inferior: light source retractors; single and cross puncture elevators; transcutaneous suture set – guide, a modified riverdain needle, and a fondue fork; a modified needle holder; "screw-suture"; "subcutaneous-tomoscope"

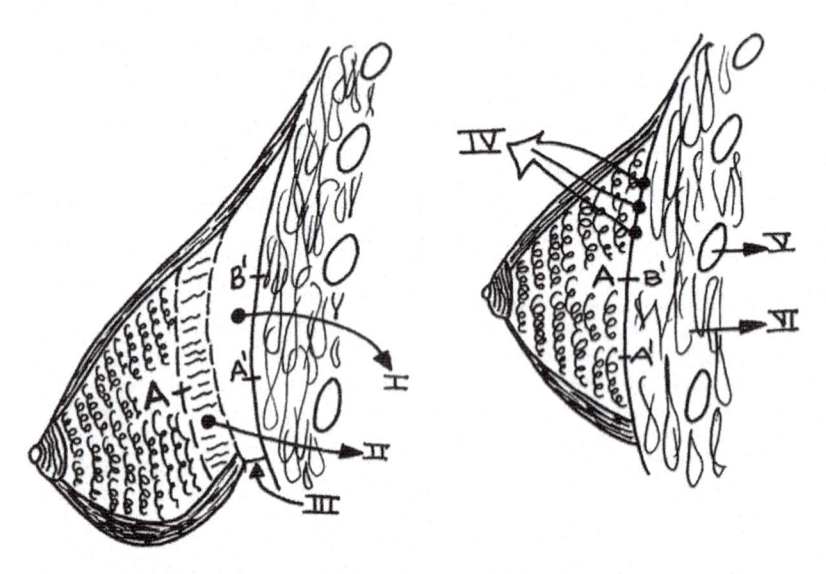

Fig. 42.2 Video-endoscopic breast reduction and mastopexy technique: A and A'- level point, B'- upper position, I–retro-mammary pocket, II–tissue resection area, III–submammary sulcus incision, IV–sutures to fix the gland in its new position at the pectoralis fascia, V–ribs, VI–muscle

adequate to allow change in the patient's positioning from supine to sitting.

42.5 Planning

In planning the mammoplasty, the breast must be observed as a three-dimensional structure (Fig. 42.2–42.4). Working endoscopically and considering the three-dimensional breast volume as a cone, looking upward the bottom of the cone can be seen (Fig. 42.5). Goal is to work on the base of the glandular cone. The first step is to plan the undermining of an enlarged area between the breast and the pectoralis fascia, thus, creating a retromammary pocket. Both gland advancement (mastopexy) and breast tissue reduction are planned to be proceeded from the bottom of the cone. If only mastopexy is needed, the incisions are demarcated at the inframammary fold. If breast reduction is intended, the incisions must be placed a little above the fold.

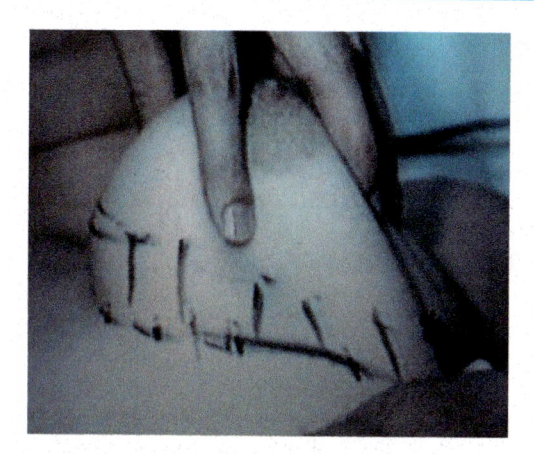

Fig. 42.3 *Marking* shows externally the breast tissue to be resected from the bases of the glandular cone

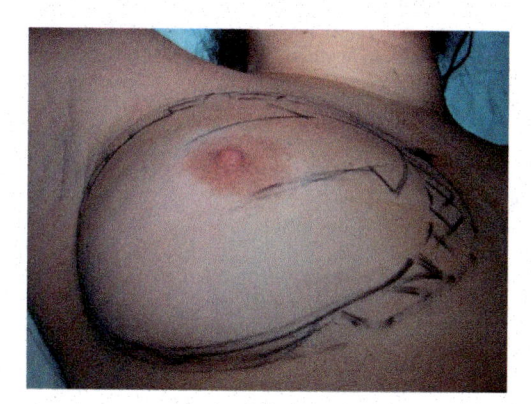

Fig. 42.4 *Arrow* shows the direction of the mastopexy towards upper-medial

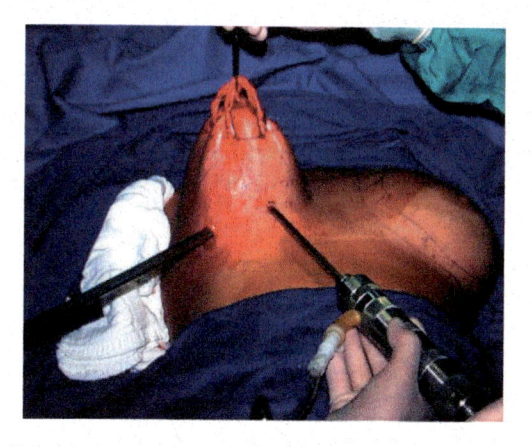

Fig. 42.5 Trans-operative view showing two small incisions (2 cm) at the submammary sulcus, through which the shaver and scope are introduced. Transcutaneous lifting sutures are used to maintain the optical cavity

42.6
Anesthesia and Infiltration

General, epidural or local anesthesia can be used. To reduce bleeding, the process is begun by the infiltration of epinephrine/saline solution (1:500,000). This is infiltrated at the base of the breast in the area to be undermined as well as inside the breast tissue.

42.7
Incisions

One or two incisions (1–2 cm) are made in the submammary sulcus. If necessary, a third incision can be made at the axilla to help tissue resection or suture placement.

In traditional open surgery, we carry out work in three dimensions; however, when working exclusively with monitor view, the third dimension is lost. This can be improved by simultaneously working through two different ports such that we "triangulate" to a focal point. This provides us with a depth-of-field feeling in the operative area. The best performance is achieved with a triangulation of approximately 30–45° (Fig. 42.5).

42.8
Dissection

A retromammary pocket is created between the breast and the pectoralis fascia (Fig. 42.2). This undermining must be wide enough to allow the advancement of the ptotic gland from the lower lateral to the upper medial position on the chest wall. This also provides an ample area of internal scar between the chest wall and the deep part of the breast tissue. This ample retromammary pocket is created with the aid of the tomoscope by blunt dissection under endoscopic control. The dissection area is similar to that where breast implants are placed. The bleeding is controlled endoscopically by the use of laparoscopic forceps connected to the electrocautery maneuvering them under monitor view. The dissection of the retromammary pocket is completed by using laparoscopic scissors connected to the electrocautery. The use of pressured gases to create and maintain the work space is avoided. The optical cavity can be provided with the aid of specially designed long and thin elevators and retractors that are introduced through the work ports. An external lift can be used by placing sutures placed through the anterior portion of the cone of the breast (Fig. 42.5).

42.9
Breast Tissue Resection

The tissue resection is performed at the base of the gland under endoscopic control, preserving the anterior cone and glandular ducts. A video arthroscopic shaver can be used to reduce the breast. The shaver works as a punching aspirator. There are two cannulas, one rolling inside of the other (Fig. 42.6); both are equipped with windows through which the breast tissue is aspirated and resected. Some breast glands may be too rigid, so its tissue cannot be resected by this punching aspirator. Thus, the procedure is performed by the use of a knife, scissors, electrocautery, or laser. This type of breast is the one that is seen on mammography presenting with a large amount of white fibrous tissue.

By resecting only the base of the breast cone, function and sensation are preserved. This is a physiologic mammoplasty. The axillary pole and bottom of the mammary cone are resected. There is no resection of even small amounts at the upper pole of the gland. Working endoscopically, the internal breast volume can be felt externally by hand palpation. By properly planning the tissue resection, the breast is modeled and sculptured into its new shape.

42.10
Breast Lifting Fixation

After obtaining adequate hemostasis, the next step is to lift and fix the gland into its new position (Fig. 42.7). Sutures are used to position the mammary gland and fix it to the pectoralis fascia. Suturing can be performed with laparoscopic needle holders. As many sutures as needed are placed to help in positioning the breast so that it will be held in place during the maturation of the internal cicatrix, which ultimately will fix the breast permanently in position. Patients with good skin quality are good candidates for this procedure and gain an aesthetic advantage with the repositioning of the gland, as this recreates an upper pole to the breast.

42.11
Dressings and Postoperative Care

Suction drains are used during the first 12 h and then removed. A Micropore tape dressing (Fig. 42.8) helps in repositioning the gland in its new site. This dressing is maintained for 20 days for long-term support. Continuous use of a supporting bra is recommended for at least 3 months thereafter and as long possible throughout the patient's life.

42.12
Complications

Among the 182 cases, five cases of hematoma have been observed in patients in whom no drains were used and early ptosis recurrence was observed in 12 patients because of poor skin elasticity.

42.13
Discussion

The endoscopic breast reduction and mastopexy techniques preserve the breast function and sensation with minimal scars [6–17] (Fig. 42.9 and 42.10). An important goal is to treat mammary asymmetry without using prostheses or adding long scars on breasts as opposed to the traditional procedures.

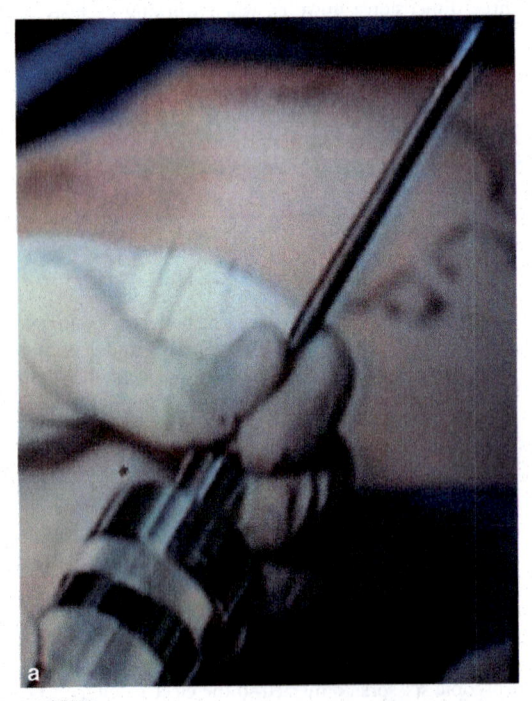

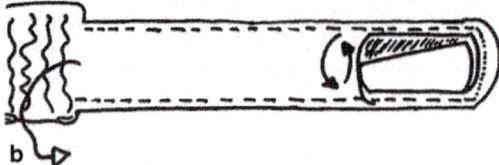

Fig. 42.6 (a) Shaver – a video arthroscopic instrument, originally employed to resect meniscus and debride fibrotic tissue inside the knee, used to carry out breast reduction. (b) Shaver instrument cannula. There are two cannulas, one rolling inside the other, a punching aspirator

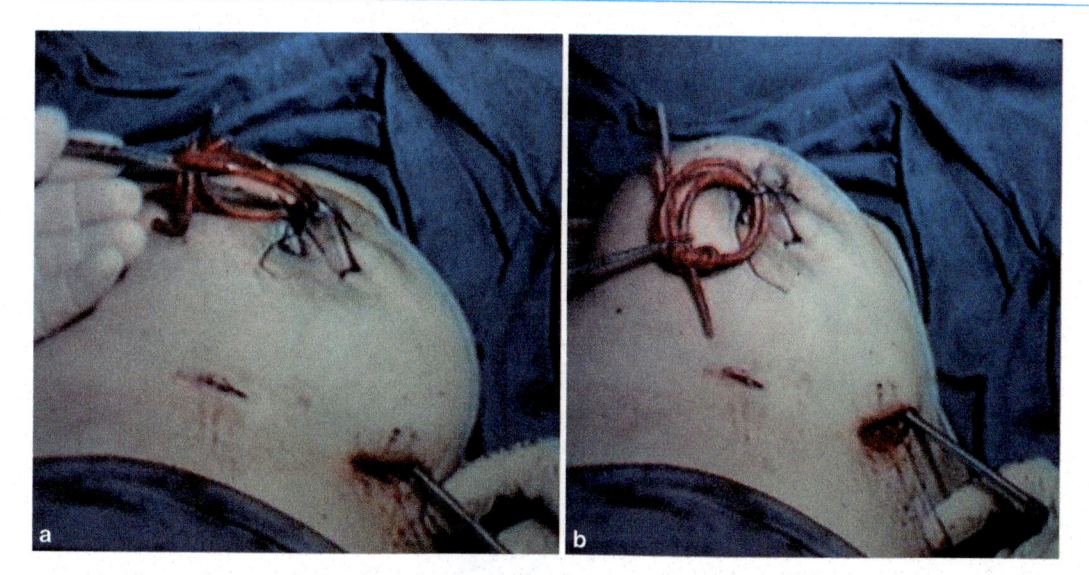

Fig. 42.7 (a,b) Grasping and testing the right position for placing the sutures

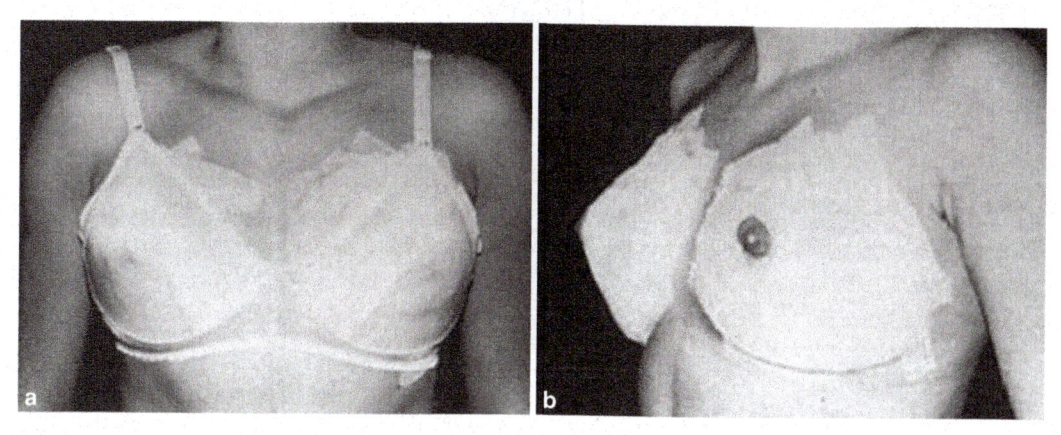

Fig. 42.8 (a,b) Micropore modulator dressing and drainage

Breast is an anatomic structure that grows perpendicularly from the chest. The effects of gravity will pull the breast down whether the patient is old or young, or operated or not. The maintenance of a long-term good result does not depend only on the technique used by the author. The maintenance of the mastopexy depends on the skin elasticity for retraction. Successful long-term follow-up relies on breast weight and precautions taken by the patient such as the use of a steadfast modulator bra especially during the practice of sports.

In patients whose skin does not have the capacity to retract, the results have been transitory as in usual mastopexies. Nevertheless, a characteristic of this minimally invasive technique that has been attracting patients' interest is the lack of visible scars as well as the maintenance of sensitivity and function.

42.14
Conclusions

The results of 15 years follow-up in 182 patients permit us to recommend its use in first-degree ptosis as well as for breast reductions in younger patients.

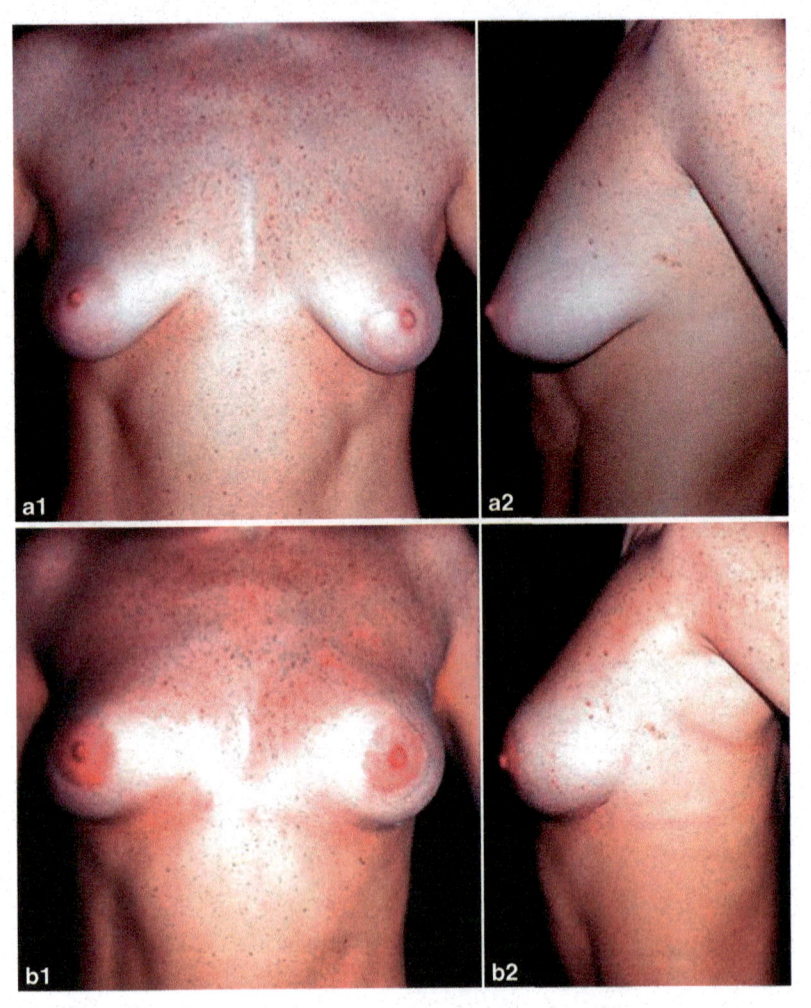

Fig. 42.9 (*a1,2*) Preoperative 32-year-old patient, breastfed two children, presenting with breast ptosis, moderate amount of striae, and moderate degree of flabbiness. (**b***1,2*) Eight months after endoscopic breast lift

The technical procedure presented shows its utmost effectiveness and best aesthetic results in young patients who present with a small amount of hypertrophy or asymmetry but with good skin elasticity and who do not have significant excess skin. The author believes that the use of these endoscopic techniques is a new trend in plastic surgery when properly applied.

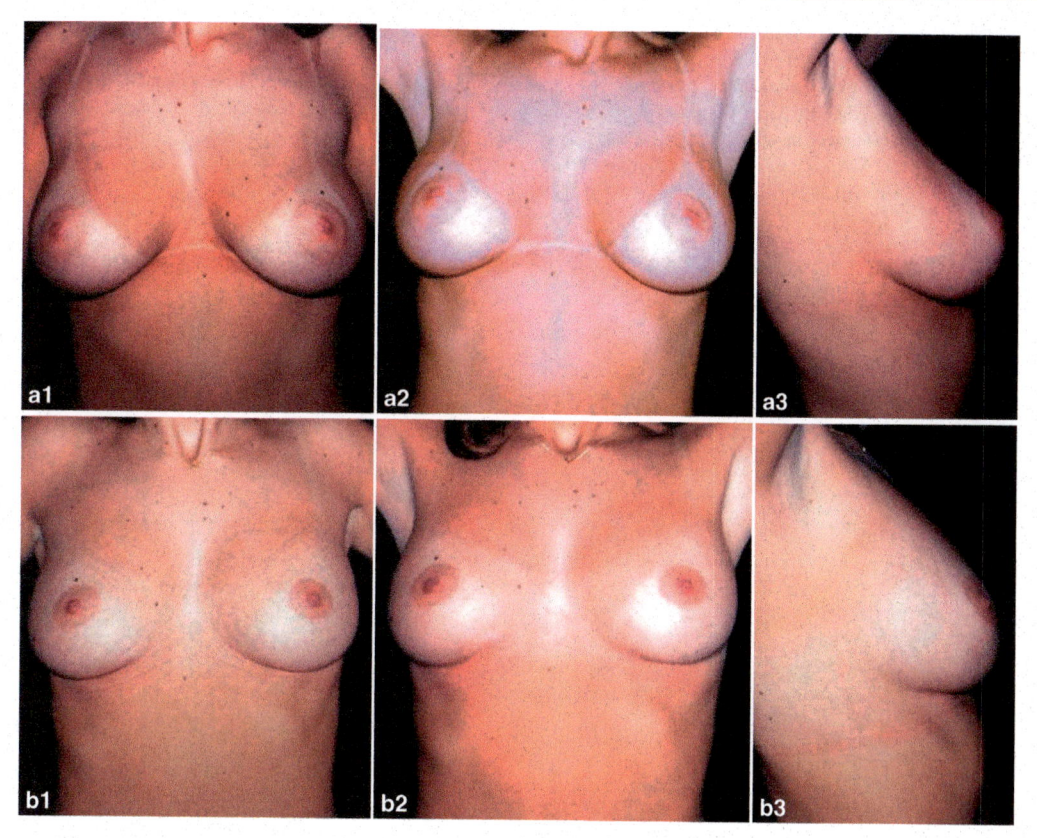

Fig. 42.10 (**a***1-3*) Preoperative 20-year-old patient with good skin elasticity, no striae, breast hypertrophy, and ptosis. (**b***1-3*) Two years after video-endoscopic breast reduction and lift (120 g each breast) showing a nice upper pole, good skin retraction, no function or sensation damage, and no visible scars

References

1. Avelar M, Juarez-Illouz YG: Lipoaspiração. Hipocrates 1986;3:320
2. Peixoto G: Reduction mammoplasty. A personal technique. Plast Reconst Surg 1980;65(2):217–226
3. Ribeiro L: Cirurgia Plástica da Mama. Rio de Janeiro, Medsi 1989
4. Faria-Corrêa MA: Videoendoscopy in plastic surgery: Brief communication – A videocirurgia na cirurgia plástica: Rev Soc Bras de Cir Plastica Est Reconstr 1992;7:80–81
5. Verbicaro E: Histórico. In: Cruz O (ed). Manual de Cirurgia Videoendoscópica. Rio de Janeiro, Revinter 1993
6. Faria-Corrêa MA: Endoscopic abdominoplasty, mastopexy and breast reduction. Clin Plast Surg 1995;22(4): 723–745
7. Faria-Corrêa MA: Breast lift and reduction. Endosc Plast Surg 1995:194–202
8. Faria-Corrêa MA: Endoscopic mammaplasty. World J Plast Surg 1995;1:118–119
9. Faria-Corrêa MA: Videoendocopic subcutaneous techniques for aesthetic and reconstructive plastic surgery. Plast Reconstr Surg 1995;96(2):446–453
10. Faria-Corrêa MA: Mamoplastia por endoscopia. Rev Cirurg Plast Ibero-Latino-Americana 1994;20:121–127
11. Faria-Corrêa MA: Mamoplastia videoendoscópica. Arquivos Catarinenses Med 1994;23:116–118
12. Faria-Corrêa MA: Mamoplastia videoendoscópica e abdominoplastia videoendoscópica (subcutaneoscopica). In Tournieux AAB (ed), Atualização em Cirurgia Plástica Estética. São Paulo, SP, Robe 1993:411–418
13. Faria-Corrêa MA: Mamoplastia por endoscopia. J Cirurg Plast Ibero-Latino-Americana 1994;20(2):121–127

14. Faria-Corrêa MA: Mamoplastia videoendoscópica. Rev Soc Bras Med Estét 1994;4:33–36
15. Faria-Corrêa MA: Endoscopic mammoplasty. In: Transactions of the 7th Asian Congress of Plastic and Reconstructive Surgery, Bangkok, Holistic 1994
16. Faria-Corrêa MA: Mamoplastia videoendoscópica. In: Tournieux AAB (ed), Atualização em Cirurgia Plástica Estética e Reconstrutiva. Sao Paulo, Robe, SP 1994
17. Faria-Corrêa MA: Redução e pexia mamária por videoendoscopia. In: Saltz R (ed), Cirugia da Mama – Estética e Reconstrutiva de Ricardo Ribeiro. Livraria e Editora Revinter 2000, pp 319–327

Reduction Mammoplasty: The Use of Contact Tip ND:YAG Laser

Jung I. Park

43.1 Introduction

The dizzying pace of scientific discoveries and their application in medical technology during the past 50 years has been beyond anybody's expectation. Since the introduction of ruby laser by Maiman in 1960, the laser application can be found in every walk of life and in every corner of the medical field.

Reduction mammoplasty requires extensive dissection in developing skin-fat flap and removing excess breast tissue. There are two issues associated with dissection; a significant blood loss and the need to preserve necessary core blood flow to the nipple–areolar complex. While the use of scalpel allows free flow of blood during dissection, the use of electric cautery creates extensive lateral thermal damage. The use of contact tip Nd:YAG laser compliments the use of either of the surgical instruments. It provides coagulation of blood vessels while dissecting with lesser degree of lateral thermal damage [1]. The CO_2 laser is also used widely in various surgical dissections. However, the ability of CO_2 laser to coagulate is very limited making it impractical for use in massive surgical dissection that involves larger blood vessels. CO_2 laser also lacks contact feedback. Contact tip Nd:YAG laser is unique among the medical laser equipments for its ability to use solid tip to deliver laser energy as opposed to free beam. This feature satisfies many surgeons' need for a contact feedback that is so crucial in order to maximize fine surgical tissue handling. There have been limited experiences with mastectomy and cosmetic breast surgery utilizing the contact tip laser [1–3].

43.2 Consultation

There is a wide range of perception of breast size in describing bra size. A patient may describe her breast size as double D cup size while another may consider the same size as merely C cup size. Despite the large size, some patients may simply wish to lift the breasts rather than reducing their size. Most patients, however, wish to reduce their sizes significantly smaller to the extent it may jeopardize survival of nipple–areola complex if her desire should be met. For those whose goals appear to be lifting the breasts and regain fullness of the upper breasts, the need for mastopexy and concurrent use of breast implants should be advised. The patient is informed of the possibility of early complications, i.e., bleeding, hematoma, seroma, wound dehiscence, infection, loss of nipple–areola complex, etc. and long-term complications, i.e., loss of nipple sensation, hypersensitivity, inability to lactate, unsightly scar, calcification, asymmetry of the breasts, disfigurement, etc.

43.3 Marking

The markings are made in the holding room with the patient in a standing position. The distances between the sternal notch and the nipples are measured and recorded. Next, the distances between the nipple and the mid inframammary line are measured. Information on symmetry of the breasts and decision on choice of surgical approach are made based on these data. Unless there is a significant discrepancy in the positions of the inframammary lines between the breasts, the markings are made following the inframammary creases from the medial breast at the sternum to the lateral chest wall. A mid inframammary point is marked. Similar point is marked on the opposite side at the same distance from the midline. These two points become reference "T" junctions during the breast mound construction. The index fingertip placed at the "T" is used as a guide to mark the surface representation of the "T" on the surface of upper breast. This point on the breast is designated as point "A." Two curvilinear lines in an inverted "V" shape is drawn around the nipple–areolar complex from point A down to the inframammary line. The distance between the lines is determined by pinch test on the breast skin for the evaluation of skin redundancy. Next, points are marked on the inverted V lines at 10–11 cm from the point A. These points are designated as points B1 and B2. The distances are determined by the anticipated final breast volume after breast tissue resection. The goal is to build the key hole to receive the new nipple–areolar complex (NAC) with the diameter of 5 cm and the length of vertical line between the inferior aspect of the key hole and the "T" junction to 4.5–5 cm. Redundancy in measurement is corrected at the time of breast mound construction by trimming any excess of the skin flap. Horizontal lines are then drawn between point B1 and lateral aspect of inframammary line, point "C," and between point B2 and medial end of the inframammary line, point "D." New and reduced nipple–areolar complexes are marked after the patient is fully prepped using a cookie cutter.

43.4 Procedure

Following sterile prepping and draping, diluted local anesthetic with epinephrine of 1:500,000 is injected under the planned incision lines and dissection planes prior to incision. The incisions are made through the skin with a No. 10 Bard-Parker blade. Although lateral thermal damage by the contact tip Nd:YAG laser is minimal compared to other modality, scalpel is superior in avoiding thermal damage to the skin. The area between the new nipple–areolar complex and the inverted "V" is deepithelialized using the knife.

The breast tissue in the lower pole is then removed in a shaving fashion using contact tip Nd:YAG laser following the vascular pedicle leading to the nipple–areolar complex. The dissection begins along the lines B1C and B2D, and along the curvilinear line 2–3 cm inferior to the lower margin of the nipple–areolar complex. The breast is tightly stretched away from the planned dissection plane with the use of skin hook or Allis forceps while the breast is held up away from the chest wall in order to align the feeding vessels in a straight line coming up from the chest wall toward the NAC. The 0.8-mm contact tip Nd:YAG laser with frosted side is used with the power of 16–18 W continuous mode controlled by a foot pedal or a button on the handpiece. One-millimeter tip with a higher power of 20 W is used for a rapid dissection and hemostasis. Pressing the tip into the breast tissue reduces the effectiveness in cutting. The tip has to be held lightly and the target tissue touched under tension without any pressure. Because of the stretch, the tissue separate rapidly as the laser tip touches the surface. Once the dermis is divided, the loose fatty tissues split with ease as soon as the fibrous septi are vaporized by the touch of the contact tip. Because of this unique dissection method, the blood vessels are exposed unharmed and visualized clearly. This is the reason why the operative field is exceptionally dry when Nd:YAG contact tip is used for dissection.

The dissection plane is followed simply by following the direction of the vascular channel down to the chest wall. The vessels are seen to increase their sizes as they are approaching to their larger caliber stems. When it is necessary to transect the vessels, it is carried out by touching with the frosted side of the contact tip if the vessel size is small or ligating and cutting in the usual fashion. Removal of the inferior pole breast is far more conservative in comparison to the cases of superior pedicle technique. The removal also follows the principle of central pedicle technique by preserving the central vascular pedicle in the lower pole area as described above. The skin in the lateral and medial aspect of the lower pole is included in the resected lower pole breast. As the dissection approaches the chest wall, it meets the inframammary line by remaining tangential to the surface in order to validate the concept of shave excision. The remaining upper breast skin and underlying subcutaneous tissue of the medial, upper, and lateral aspect are elevated as a flap with thickness of about 2–2.5 cm. The breast tissue of the medial, upper, and lateral aspect is removed from the periphery of the breast in a shaving fashion following the vascular pedicles similar to the lower-pole dissection. The breast mound is constructed by bringing the medial and the lateral skin flap to the central "T" point. The opposing lines of medial and lateral skin flaps are sutured together temporally. The inferior aspect of both medial and lateral flap that are B1C and B2D are also sutured temporarily to the inframammary line. The skin flaps at the lines of sutures are folded over, as needed in the process of shaping the breast mound. The redundant portions of the flaps will eventually be trimmed prior to the final closure.

The breast mounds are viewed from the front with the patient in a sitting position. Any necessary adjustment of breast mound is made. While the patient is still sitting, the positions of new NACs (keyholes) are determined and marked with a cookie cutter just inferior to the most prominent portion of the breast mound. The patient is placed back in the supine position and keyholes are made by cutting out the skin within the cookie cut. The nipple–areolar complex is brought out and sutured to the key hole. The redundant skin flaps of the vertical closure and along the inframammary line are trimmed. The flaps and key hole are sutured in layers using 3-0, 4-0, and 5-0 Monocryl sutures. Seven-mm Jackson-Pratt suction drains are inserted one on each side prior to the flap closure.

43.5 Discussion

Laser light energy, when in contact with tissue, behaves in four different ways: absorption, scattering, transmission, and reflection [4–6]. Absorption is when the light energy is taken up by the tissue and converted into heat. Scattering is when the light energy bounces back and forth inside the tissue until it finds the tissue that absorbs the energy and produce heat. Transmission is when the laser energy simply passes through the tissue. Reflection is when the light energy bounces back on the surface. The light energy that is absorbed by the tissue will generate intense heat. CO_2 laser is absorbed at the laser–tissue interface generating intense heat. It generates a rapid temperature elevation to above 100°C creating vacuolization of the cells and sharp cutting without lateral thermal damage. Nd:YAG laser, when it is used as a free beam, results in a larger area of coagulation because of wide scattering before it is absorbed. Owing to slow rise in temperature, the tissue coagulates before the temperature reaches vaporization point. As a result, free-beam Nd:YAG laser is not used as a cutting tool. The contact tip was designed to resolve this difficulty associated with scattering of laser energy. In the contact laser surgery, the technique exists to uncouple the temperature distribution from its dependency on the absorption characteristics of wavelength. Nd:YAG laser contact tip is an optical device attached to the fiber optic system. The tip works by total internal reflection in a fashion similar to the conveyance of light in the fiber optic itself (Fig. 43.1). The difference is that as the light reaches the tapered section of an optical material, heat is generated at the tip–tissue interface instead of normal scattering fashion. Unlike free beam Nd:YAG laser, the contact tip laser causes a rapid rise in temperature at the laser–tissue interface like CO_2 laser. The contact tip thus converts coagulating characteristics of free-beam Nd:YAG laser into cutting mode. During vaporization with a noncontact laser beam, more than 40% of the energy can be lost due to reflection and backscattering from the tissue. In addition, more than 10% of the incident energy will be lost in the escaping vapor (Fig. 43.2).

The main benefit of using Nd:YAG laser over CO_2 laser is the ability to use flexible fiber optic system to deliver the laser energy instead of heavy and rigid CO_2 laser equipment with multiple cumbersome joints. The materials used in contact laser surgery are synthetic sapphire and fused silica. Sapphire has a much higher melting point of 1,800°C compared to fused silica, which has a melting point of 900°C. The contact tip made of sapphire is superior optically and mechanically, and is resistant to degradation during the surgery [7, 8]. Wavelength conversion effect treated contact tip function by absorbing a predetermined amount of the laser energy at the tip–tissue interface (Figs. 43.3 and 43.4). This then raises the tissue temperature at a determined level. By passing the laser energy through a contact tip, the Nd:YAG laser can alter its temperature gradient from low-absorbing wave length to heat generation, which provides a steep temperature gradient at the incision site. The final determinant of the laser's therapeutic effect is the temperature gradient created in the tissue. With modification of the shape of the laser tip, the temperature gradient can be changed to a desired curve to effectively coagulate, or vaporize and coagulate as needed. Although the tissue effect occurs at the laser tip, the lateral surface of this contact tip can be roughened or frosted to allow some of the energy to disperse. The tip can then provide coagulation at the margin of the incision [8].

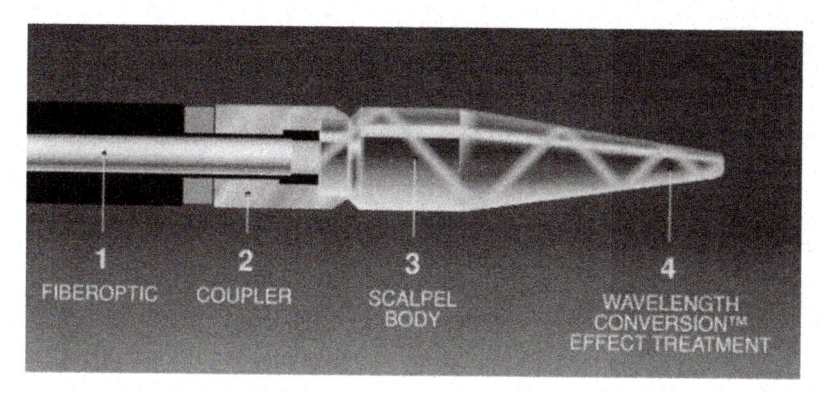

Fig. 43.1 Detachable Contact Laser™ tip and fiber optic

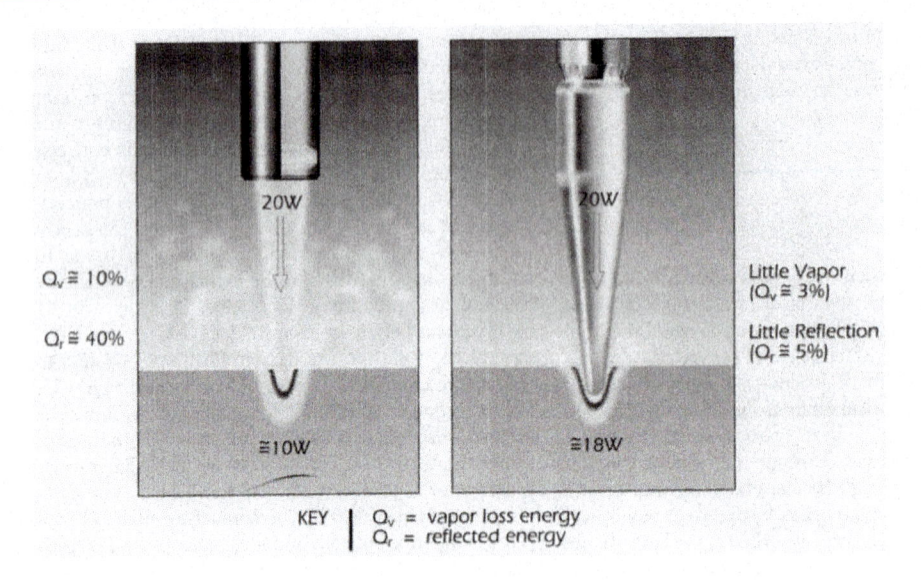

Fig. 43.2 Noncontact vs. Contact Laser™ surgery

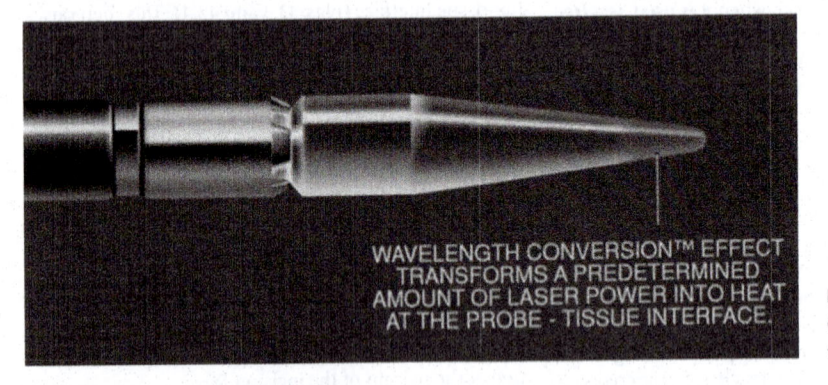

Fig. 43.3 Wavelength Conversion™ Effect surface treatments

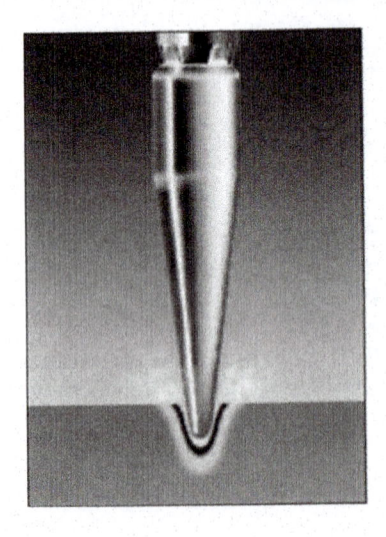

Wavelength Conversion™ Effect
- Create Many Temperature Profiles With One Laser

Easy To Use
- Tactile Feedback
- Omni Directional (Endoscopic)
- Uniform Performance in All Soft Tissue

Highly Efficient
- Little Reflection
- Little Smoke

Ability To Cut, Coagulate &/Or Ablate Tissue

Fig. 43.4 Contact Laser™ surgery features

CO_2 laser has only limited capability of coagulation because of its steep temperature gradient. It can cut through tissue with limited lateral thermal effect, entering medium-sized blood vessels in the deep plane before they can be identified and coagulated. As a result, blood extravasates, creating a field that is higher in water content. Since CO_2 laser has the highest absorption by water, all the laser energy will be immediately absorbed by the blood, preventing any further dissection. As the blood boils by the laser, char forms to further impede the effectiveness of CO_2 laser penetration. With the Nd:YAG contact tip laser, blood vessels, nerves, and other structures can be easily identified and skeletonized before they are transected or coagulated owing to its ability to dissect slow, but cleanly. There is a built-in safety feature in contact laser surgery. The laser beam, once it exits the end of contact tip, scatters very widely so that the harmful effect of the laser beyond the laser tip is negligible. The lateral thermal effect for coagulation is controlled in such a way that it does not produce extensive tissue damage seen with electrocautery.

In the histopathologic study, Miyazaki et al. [9] observed 20–50 $\propto$m of tissue coagulation when a ND-YAG contact laser technique was used. This is in contrast with incision done by electric scalpel which resulted in a width of coagulation over 100 $\propto$m. The features of the contact tip Nd:YAG laser are gaining freedom from the wavelength dependency, maintaining the precision of the laser, and hemostasis with excellent control of the depth of the tissue.

Blood loss during Nd:YAG laser surgery was studied by Kurono et al. [10]. In this study, mean blood loss during radical neck dissection with the contact Nd:YAG laser was 99 ml as compared to 730 ml with the conventional technique. Wyman and Rogers reported an average blood loss of 132 ml in their series during modified radical mastectomy using Nd:YAG contact-tip laser surgery. The blood loss in this type of surgery using conventional techniques, in their experience and that of others, was described as being on the order of 500 ml.

Proper traction and countertraction maneuvers are particularly important in laser dissection. Traction and countertraction allows the tissue to be quickly removed from the heat source. This maneuver brings a new tissue plane quickly into contact with laser energy for rapid dissection. The contact tip laser assures precision, control, and versatility in cutting and coagulation while eliminating the chance of inadvertent tissue damage as seen in free-beam laser surgery, i.e., CO_2 laser. Tactile feedback of the contact mode provides security to the surgeon and enhances visual control.

Nd:YAG contact laser dissection allows much easier identification of blood vessels, since the operative field is dry and the anatomy is clear. When the blood vessel is identified, one uses the frosted side of the laser tip to coagulate the vessel before it is transected. The diameter of the laser tip varies between 0.2 and 1.2 mm. A tip with a smaller diameter produces a sharper incision. The finest tip has a depth of penetration of 0.3 mm, which is equivalent to that of a CO_2 laser in terms of lateral thermal damage. However, the skin incision is always made with a knife, since the knife is the only device that causes no lateral thermal damage. The tip with a larger diameter provides a higher intensity laser. For most fine flap development, 0.6 mm tip is used.

For gross dissection, 0.8 and 1.0 mm tip are used. Each tip has a maximum allowed power delivery to avoid excessive heat, which causes tip deformation. The laser energy recommended for longevity of the tip is between 10 and 20 W. It is important not to activate the laser tip while the laser is not in contact with the tissue, since the focused laser can burn the laser tip itself. The laser tips are designed not to adhere to the tissue. When sticking occurs, the surgeon should pull the laser after reactivating the laser to release the tip from the adherent tissue. Burning the tissue that is adherent to the laser tip causes tip deformation because of extreme temperature rise. The tissue should be gently wiped with hydrogen peroxide or saline-soaked gauze. On rare occasions, when the tip is separated from the fiber delivery system, the fiber should be clamped quickly to prevent accidental discharge of free laser energy and the machine should be turned off at the same time. The laser tip has to be handled as an optical device rather than as a mechanical instrument. For example, while dissection is being carried out, the surgeon should not press the laser tip against the tissue hoping for a quicker dissection. Unlike the scalpel, forcing does not facilitate dissection, but causes deterioration at the junction between the tip and the fiber. The laser can be activated by pushing a button on the hand piece or by using a foot switch. The surgical dissection is carried out using a continuous mode.

43.6
Conclusions

With the Nd:YAG contact tip laser, blood vessels, nerves, and other structures can be easily identified and skeletonized before they are transected or coagulated owing to its ability to dissect slowly but cleanly. Because of the fiber optic system, it is more mobile in physical handling than the CO_2 laser. The laser can be activated by pushing a button on the handpiece or by using a foot switch (Figs. 43.5 and 43.6).

322   43 Reduction Mammoplasty

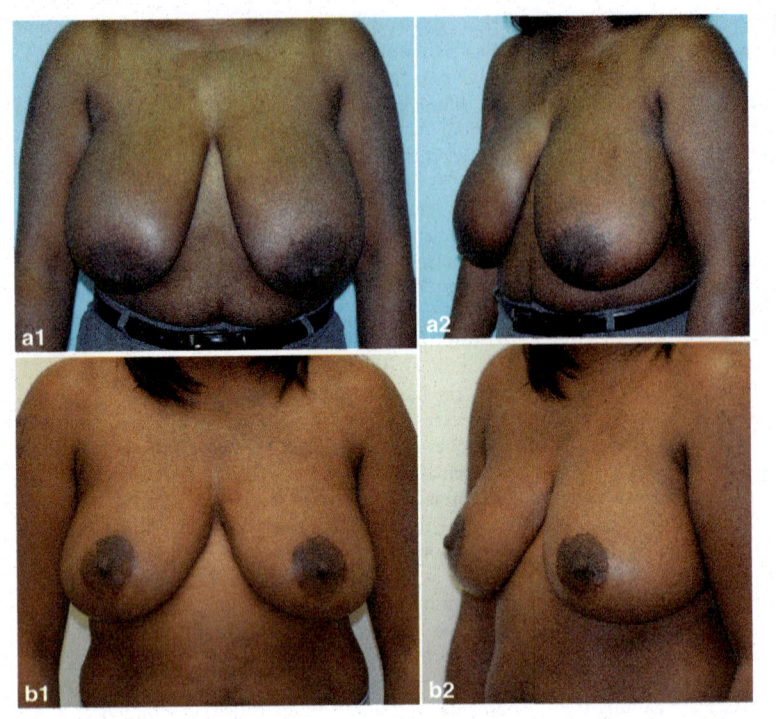

Fig. 43.5 (**a***1,2*) Preoperative. (**b***1,2*) Postoperative

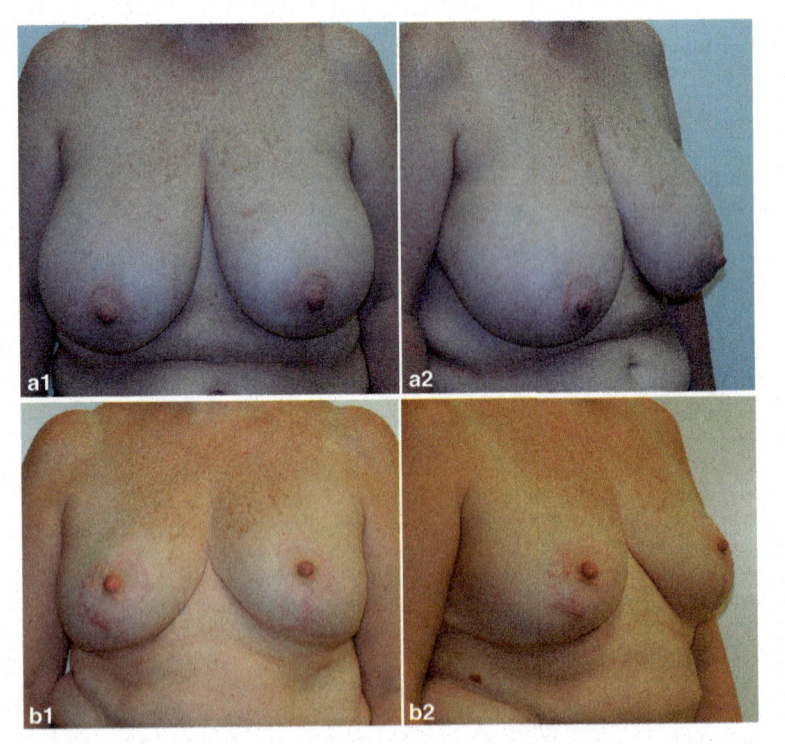

Fig. 43.6 (**a***1,2*) Preoperative. (**b***1,2*) Postoperative

References

1. Wyman A, Rogers K: Radical breast surgery with a contact Nd:YAG laser scalpel. Eur J Surg Oncol 1992;18: 322–326
2. Maker VJ: Technique of modified radical mastectomy with contact Neodymium YAG laser. Contemp Surg 1991;38(2):11–15
3. Park JI: Reduction mammoplasty using Nd:YAG contact tip laser. Am J Cosm Surg 1993;10:201–206
4. Laudenslager JB: Ion-molecule processes in lasers. In Ausloos P (ed), Kinetics of Ion-molecule Reactions. New York, Plenum 1978
5. Brau CA: Rare gas halogen excimers. In Rhodes CK (ed), Excimers Lasers. New York, Springer 1979
6. Beck OJ, Wilske J, Schoenberger JL, Gorisch W: Tissue changes following applications of lasers to the rabbit brain: results with CO2 and neodymium:YAG laser. Neurosurg Rev 1979;1:31–36
7. Daikuzono N, Joffe SN: Artificial sapphire probe for contact photocoagulation and tissue vaporization with the Nd:YAG laser. Med Instrum 1985;19(4):173–178
8. Fuller TA: The thermal surgical lasers, a technical monograph. Oaks, PA 1993, p 50
9. Miyazaki Y: Comparison of the tongue response to injury by contact Nd:YAG laser and carbon dioxide laser. Presented at the International YAG Laser Symposium, Tokyo 1986
10. Kurono Y, Mogi G, Ichimiya I: Nd:YAG laser in head and neck surgery. Presented at the International Nd:YAG laser symposium, Tokyo 1986

Axillary Reduction Mammaplasty

Yhelda Felicio

44.1 Introduction

The first description of reduction mammaplasty in the literature was in the seventh century when Durstin [1], in 1669, described breast reduction surgery. Beisenberg [2] treated gynecomastia, but it was only at the beginning of the past century that the major contributions related to the issue began to be cited in the literature such as studies by Arié [3], Mouly and Dufourmentel [4], Strombeck [5], Pitanguy [6], Andrews [7], and Peixoto [8]. These authors brought new contributions to the development of breast reduction techniques. According to many authors, the surgical techniques for treating breast hypertrophy and ptosis should be the ones the surgeon is best at. The negative aspects pointed out for classical reduction mammaplasty are the size of the scars, a fact with which most patients agree.

The results of an interactive survey on mastoplasty carried out at the XXI Sao Paulo Plastic Surgery Day in Campos do Jordao, Sao Paulo, June 2001 showed that patients' major complaints referred to inappropriate scars (59.4%), late postoperative ptosis (16.5%), inadequate shape (11.4%), and breast asymmetry (7.6%); 5.1% did not have any one of the given complaints.

In January 1984, the author began using a less-aggressive reduction mammaplasty with an areolar access technique that preserves a larger number of central mammary lobules and presents only an areolar scar. The experience with this technique by the author has been described elsewhere in literature [9–14]. Over a period of 9 years, the technique was performed on five hundred patients (one thousand breasts). After this, the conclusion was that the breast could be submitted to a mammaplasty utilizing the axillary route without any visible scar. The experience with the technique was initially described in 1993 [15] and then in other articles [16–20].

The problem most common to all mammary reductions is the patient dissatisfaction due to breast scarring or lateralization of the breast. Despite whether the resected tissue is in the upper, lateral, or inferior pole, many operated breasts in a late postoperative phase started showing excessive tissue with ptosis in the extreme lateral quadrant of the breast.

Axillary access to breast reduction surgery was described in the literature as early as 1924 by Dártigues [21]. Many other reports have described it, although the technique has not become popular to date.

A high satisfaction rate was obtained in one research study with two hundred breasts operated on by the axillary route reduction technique (Tables 44.1–44.5).

44.2 Technique

The surgery is performed with the patient in the supine position with extended arms under local or epidural anesthesia and sedation.. The incision should be around the entire axilla and fusiform in character (Fig. 44.1). The detachment has to be very careful and the axillary region anatomy must be carefully studied (Fig. 44.2). After the axillary fat resection, the level of tissue should be very well identified before beginning the excision of the breast tissue which should be done little by little (Fig. 44.3). Through this access, the breast tissue can be resected in all the quadrants. Radiowave surgery (high frequency) is used, which avoids major bleedings (Fig. 44.4). Skin retraction takes place and the settlement of the breast tissue into its new form will occur after the axillary and breast lift is done (Fig. 44.5). The procedure requires four sutures (Vicryl 3-0 s and Monocryl nylon 3-0, 4-0, and 5-0), for both axillas. Suction drainage in the breast and compression bandage must be applied below the axilla for 24 h postoperatively (Fig. 44.6). Twenty four hours after the surgery, it is removed with the drain and the patient can take baths and take off the bandage. Cold thermal packs (criocurativos or equivalent) should be used on the breasts and axillas for 15 min, 5 times daily for the next 10 days. The ecchymoses will disappear within approximately 10 days. A brassiere should be worn for 3 months after the surgery. Antibiotic therapy should be given for 7 days, pre-and postoperatively.

M.A. Shiffman (ed.), *Mastopexy and Breast Reduction: Principles and Practice*,
© Springer-Verlag Berlin Heidelberg 2009

Table 44.1 Axillary reduction mammaplasty: diagnosis (March 1993–March 1997)

Diagnosis	Number	Percent
Hypertrophy	132	66.0
Ptosis	36	18.0
Asymmetry	21	10.5
Silicone Prosthesis Associated	7	3.5
Tumor	4	2.0
Total	200	100.0

Table 44.2 Types of breast pathology (March 1993–March 1997)

Pathology	Number	Percent
Normal breast with hypertrophy	104	52.0
Fibrocystic disease	51	25.5
Lymphadenitis	40	20.0
Fibroadenoma	2	1.0
Blue dome cyst	1	0.5
Mastitis	1	0.5
Lipoma	1	0.5
Total	200	100.0

Table 44.3 Age of Patients (March 1993–March 1997)

Age group	Number	Percent
16–25	46	23.5
26–35	46	23.5
36–45+	108	53.0
Total	200	100.0

Table 44.4 Amount of breast tissue ressected (March 1993–March 1997)

Grams of breast tissue	Number	Percent
50–100	6	3.0
101–200	26	13.0
201–300	46	23.0
301–400	46	23.0
401–500	26	13.0
501–2,000	50	25.0
Total	200	100.0

Table 44.5 Complications (March 1993–March 1997)

Complications	Number
Keloid	5
Hypertrophic scar with seroma	5
Hematoma with short dehiscence	3
Hypersensitivity of the arm	2
Total	15

44.3 Conclusions

This technique was based on the philosophy of the cicatricial retraction of skin as described by Fournier [22] on liposculpture by syringe. Nevertheless, scarring is still a major problem in the Brazilian environment (Fig. 44.7). Brazilian people's (especially northeastern) skin is pigmented and easily susceptible to hypertrophic and keloidal scars. Moreover, in a breast with severe ptosis a lateral quadrant ptosis correction is a difficult task with any surgical procedure.

The author considers the concept to be a very good one (Figs. 44.8 and 44.9). This technique has the following advantages:

1. It is less aggressive when compared to classical techniques and any breast quadrant may be approached by the axillary route. Moreover, resection is mainly approached by lateral quadrants, as they are responsible

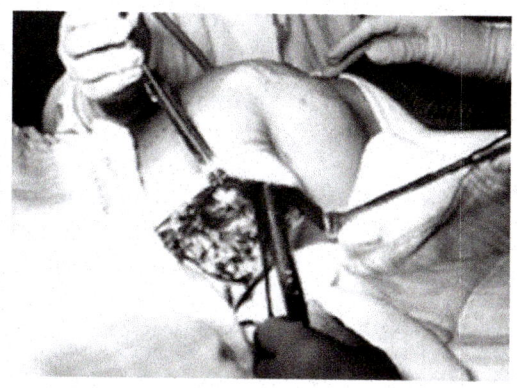

Fig. 44.2 Detachment in order to achieve a good cleavage plan

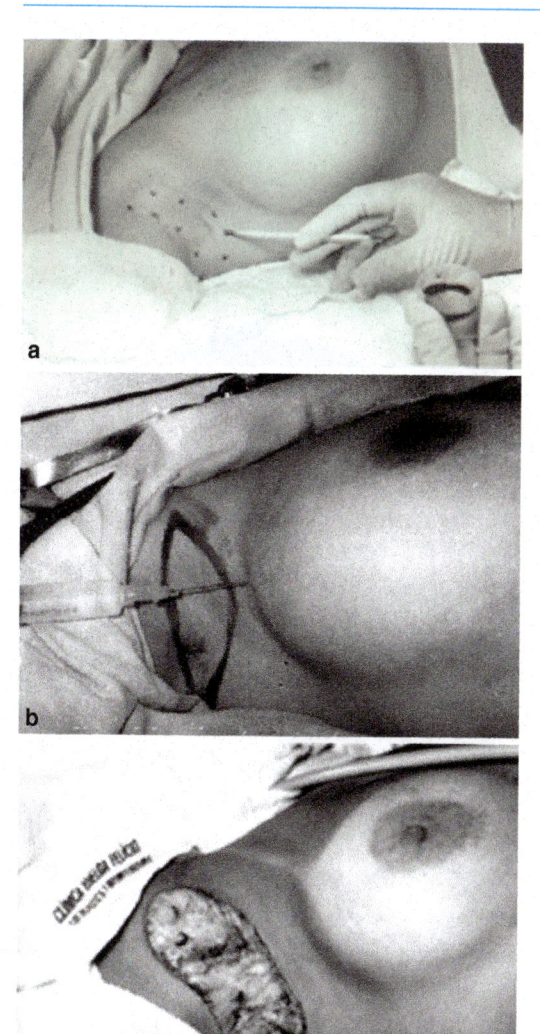

Fig. 44.1 (a) Fusiform demarcation in axilla. (b) Local anesthesia of the axilla and the external lateral quadrant of the breast. (c) Incision at intraaxillary fossa

for the inelegant aspect of most patients in the late postoperative period.
2. It can be performed under either local or epidural anesthesia.
3. It is more economical, since it only requires four sutures for both axillas.
4. Its major advantage is that it avoids any scar in the breast because the axillary scar is hidden by natural folds.
5. Less trauma is believed to occur in the axillary route technique if compared to the inverted T technique, mainly because of immediate patient recovery (maximum of less than 40 days) and the absence of breast scars, yielding a single axillary scar of approximately a third of the size of inverted T surgery scars; but neither one technique invalidates the other. Conversely, in the inverted T technique, there is complete scar retraction at 6 months postoperatively and breast swaying and tilt only occurring a year after surgery. Both are believed to differ in the follow-up because the axillary technique is a closed technique while the inverted T is open. Breasts operated on by the axillary route, at 6 months postoperative, present little scarring retraction and a similar memory to the aspect of the initial breast. Only after 1 year, complete scarring retraction and a very different aspect from the original breast, approximately 50% smaller than the initial volume, are observed.

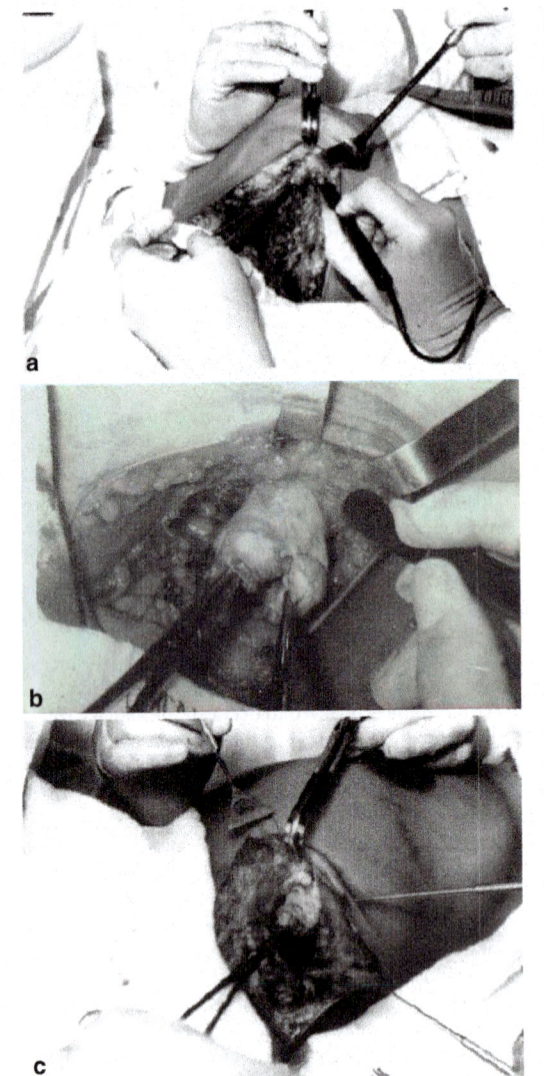

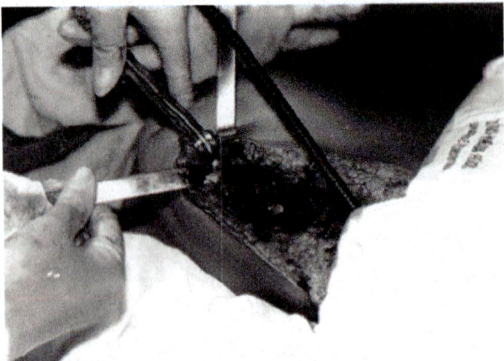

Fig. 44.4 The mammary tissue of all the quadrants can be resected by high-frequency electrocoagulation surgery which results in minimal bleeding. The mammary resection should be stopped when there is no leftover tissue over the pectoral muscles

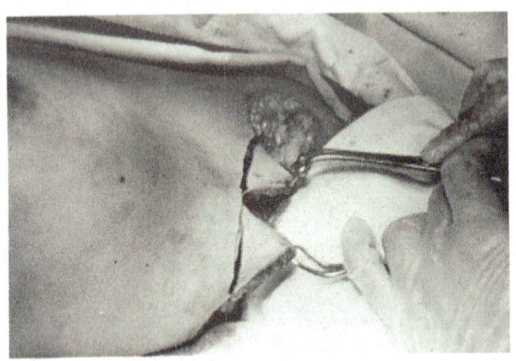

Fig. 44.5 Axillary and breast lifting

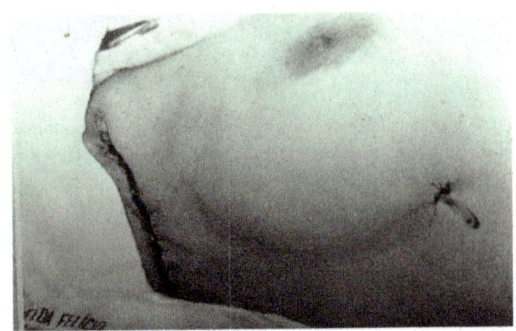

Fig. 44.3 (a-c) Resection of the mammary tissue by high-frequency electrocoagulation surgery, little by little

Fig. 44.6 Final suture with Vicryl 3-0 and nylon 3-0, 4-0, 5-0. Four sutures for both axillas. Drain in breast

44.3 Conclusions 329

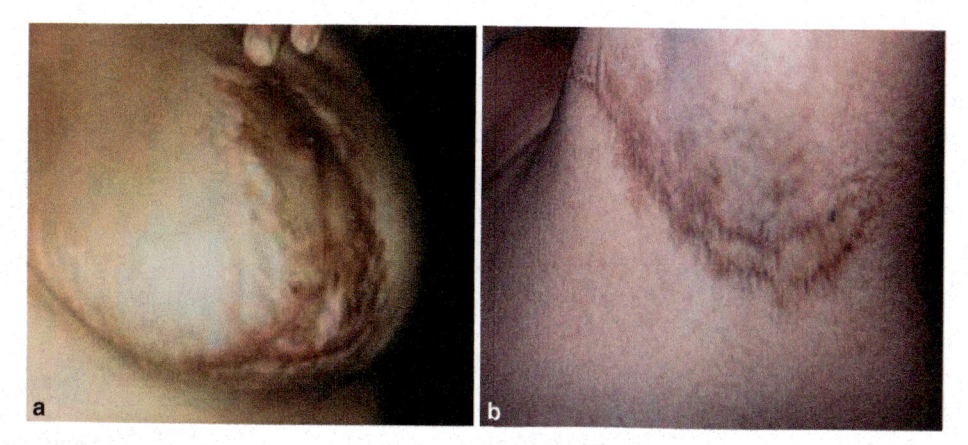

Fig. 44.7 Complications in different techniques. (**a**) Inverted T keloid. (**b**) Axillary keloid

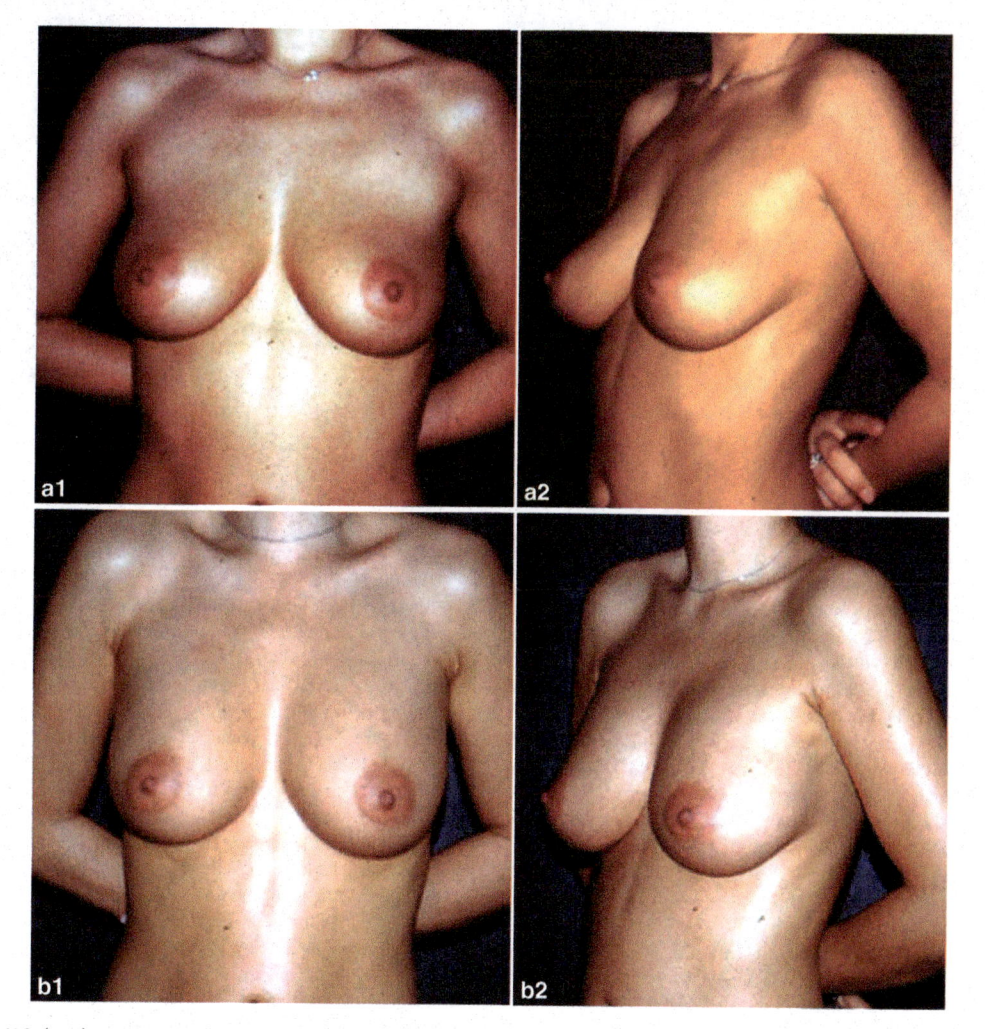

Fig. 44.8 (**a***1,2*) Preoperative. (**b***1,2*) Six months postoperative after mastopexy (resected 150 g for each breast) associated with breast implant, silicone gel, 200 ml in each breast

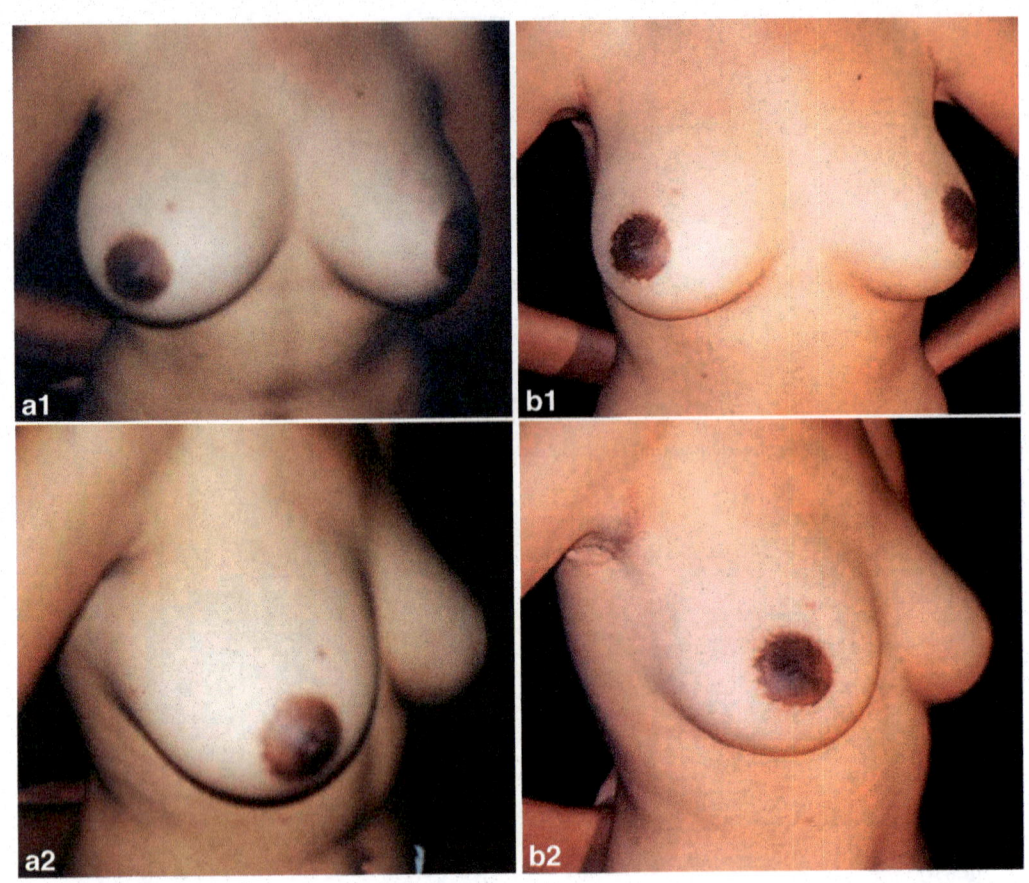

Fig. 44.9 (*a1,2*) Preoperative. (*b1,2*) Postoperative five years late

References

1. Durston W: Concerning a very sudden and excessive swelling of a woman's breasts. Phil Trans Vol IV for anno 1669:1047–1049, Royal Society, London 1670
2. Biesenberger H: Deformitaten und Kosmetishe Operationen der Wieblichen Brust. Wien, Maudrich 1931
3. Arie G: Una nueva técnica de mamaplastia. Rev Lat Amer Cir Plást 1957;3:23–28
4. Mouly RY, Dufourmentel C: Plasties mammaires par la méthode oblique. Ann Chir Plast 1961;6:45
5. Strombeck JO: Breast reconstruction. I. Reduction mammaplasty. Mod Trends Plast Surg 1964;16:237–255
6. Pitanguy I: Surgical treatment of breast hypertrophy. Br J Plast Surg 1967;20(1):78–85
7. Andrews JM, Yshizuki MM, Martins DM, Ramos RR: An areolar approach to the reduction mammaplasty. Br J Plast Surg 1975;28(3):166–170
8. Peixoto G: Reduction mammaplasty. Plast Reconstr Surg 1984;8:231–236
9. Felicio Y: Mamaplastia redutora com incisão periareolar. Presented at Sul Bras Cirurg Plást, in Florianopolis, Santa Catarina 1984, pp 307–311
10. Felicio Y: Periareolar reduction mammaplasty. Plast Reconstr Surg 1991;88(5):789–798
11. Felicio Y: Réduction mammaire peri-aréolaire. La Rev Chirurg Esthét Langue Franç 1991;16(64):19–26
12. Felicio Y: Periareolar reduction mammoplasty by Yhelda Felicio. In: Mole B (ed), Actualités de Chirurgie Esthétique. Paris, Masson 1992, pp 91–106
13. Felicio Y: Periareolar reduction mammaplasty. Plast Reconstr Aesthet Surg 1993;74:287–291
14. Felicio Y: Truthfullness and Untruthfullness of the periareolar mammoplasty by Yhelda Felicio. In: Mole B (ed), Actualités de Chirurgie Esthétique, 2° série. Paris Masson 1993, pp 161–175

15. Felicio Y: Plastie mammaire de réduction sans cicatrice mammaire, avec radio-chirurgie. La Rev Chir Esthét Langue Franç 1993;18(73):53–58
16. Felicio Y: Mamaplastia redutora via trans-axilar com proximate. In: Tournieux AAB (ed), Atualização em Cirurgia Plástica Estética. Sao Paulo Robe, 1994, pp 371–375
17. Felicio Y: Mastoplastia de reducción por la técnica de Yhelda Felicio. Rev Iberolatinoamericana Cir Plast 1994; 20(2):141–146
18. Felicio Y: Axillary reduction mammaplasty. Ann Plast Surg 2000;45(5):570–571
19. Felicio Y: Axillary reduction mammaplasty – Yhelda Felicio's technique. Aesthetic Plast Surg 1997;21(4):268–275
20. Felicio Y: Comparison of the inflammatory response to trauma in the inverted T technique and axillary access technique for breast reduction surgery. Rev Soc Bras Cir Plást 2002;17(2):57–68
21. Dartigues L: Chirurgie réparatrice. In Lépine R (ed), Plastique et Esthétique de la Poitrine et de l'Abdomen, Paris 1924, pp 44–47
22. Fournier P: Liposculpture: The Syringe Technique. Paris, Arnette 1991

Periareolar Mammaplasty with Transposition of Flaps

Pedro Djacir Escobar Martins, Pedro Alexandre da Motta Martins, David Ponciano de Sena, Marcelo Marafon Maino

45.1 Introduction

Reduction mammaplasty techniques can achieve good results: shapes and sizes in harmony with each patient's biotype and meet the patient's expectations. The operation may leave an inverted "T" scar, or a periareolar scar around the entire circumference of the areola or only around its lower half. A good knowledge of the anatomic structures of the breast, particularly its vascularization and innervations, ensures complete mastery in handling mammary parenchyma.

Tissue resections and flap mobilizations may be safely performed regardless of the preoperative size and shape of the breast, and fully satisfactory results may be achieved.

However, technical and philosophical approaches should adapt to the skin of each breast. Its proportion with mammary content should be taken into consideration because scars will be shorter if less skin is redundant. Some factors may positively affect the reduction of scars, such as the conditions of skin elasticity, the patient's age and ethnic characteristics. Other factors affect it negatively or are contraindication for surgery, such as smoking, drinking and use of drugs.

Peixoto [1], in 1984, discussed skin retraction which occurs on all cutaneous areas of the body surface at different rates according to some well-known factors. Skin retraction varies according to anatomic region, but the integrity of skin elastic fibers and their texture, identified mainly by the absence of striae, plays an important role. An aged skin becomes less elastic and its retraction is impaired.

In mammaplasty, shape should never be compromised when reduced scars are sought. Techniques used to achieve reduced scars will have better results when carefully indicated, particularly for young patients with a skin without striae and mammary parenchyma with little or no fat infiltration.

45.2 Indications

Short scars left by reduction mammaplasty are obtained with the use of periareolar techniques. Their indications are limited and according to the author's experience represent not more than 10% of the patients. The periareolar approach is indicated for patients who meet the following conditions:

1. Size and shape: Small and moderate hypertrophies. Resection weight should not be greater than 300 g per breast, in general. It is an excellent indication for tuberous breasts.
2. Parenchyma: Gland tissue should have little or no fat infiltration.
3. Skin: Healthy, with good elasticity and without striae.
4. Age: Preferably young patients; younger than 40 years.

45.3 Contraindications

1. Size and shape: Large hypertrophies, resections greater than 500 g per breast.
2. Severe ptosis.
3. Skin with poor elasticity or striae.
4. Patients older than 50 years.
5. Habits including smoking, drinking, or use of drugs.

45.4 History

In the last 20 years, several authors [2–7], particularly some Brazilians, described mammaplasty techniques using a periareolar approach. Some [3, 5, 8] elevate all the breast skin; the breast remains connected to the thorax and has its vascular supply and sensation preserved by perforating branches of the intercostal vessels and nerves.

M.A. Shiffman (ed.), *Mastopexy and Breast Reduction: Principles and Practice*,
© Springer-Verlag Berlin Heidelberg 2009

Some surgeons [3, 5, 8] use meshes of alloplastic materials or nylon threads to provide suspension and avoid later breast ptosis. Others [2, 6, 7], like this author, detach skin only from the lower half of the breast, and the upper half keeps its intact skin cover, except around the nipple–areola complex.

The author's technique adopts some basic concepts of the Pitanguy's [9] technique for breast reduction: the inferior pedicle flap [10] and skin retraction [1].

45.5
Preoperative Marking

Marking may be made with the patient awake, sitting, and slightly leaning backwards, or already under anesthesia on the operating table in supine position, with the upper extremities in abduction and the head of the bed elevated at 30°. Initially, as for most techniques, the midclavicular lines are drawn passing over the nipples and crossing the inframammary folds at a distance of about 8–10 cm from the midsternal line which is also drawn.

The cardinal points, A, A', B, C, D and E, are marked on the areola and on the skin around the circumference that marks the area to be deepithelialized. These points should facilitate the distribution of skin. Point A, described by Pitanguy, corresponds to the future position of the nipple. Point A' is located on the midclavicular line 2 cm above Pitanguy's point A (Fig. 45.1). It corresponds to the upper limit of the border of the new areola which will have a 4 cm diameter. Point B is located

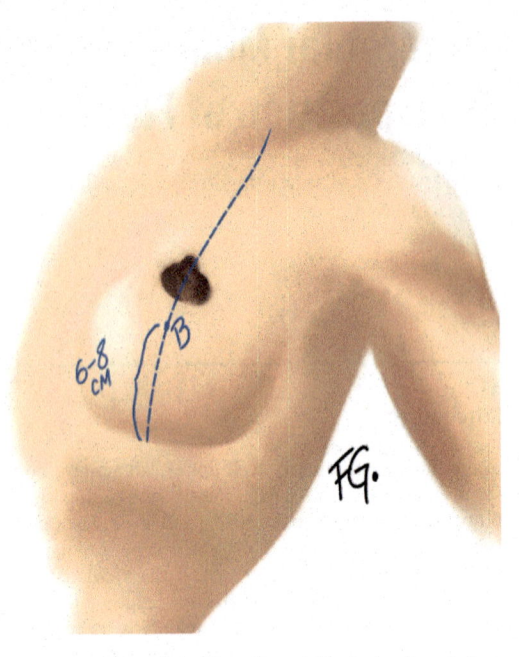

Fig. 45.2 Point B is located on the midclavicular line, 6–8 cm from the inframammary fold, and corresponds to the lower margin of the new position of the areola

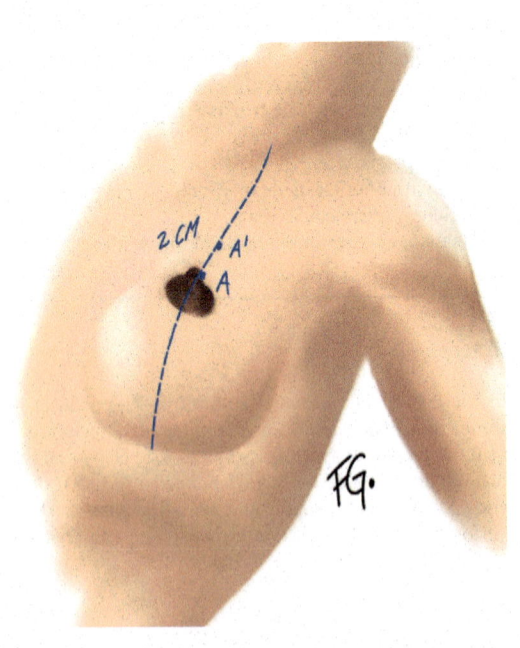

Fig. 45.1 Point A' is located 2 cm above Pitanguy's Point A

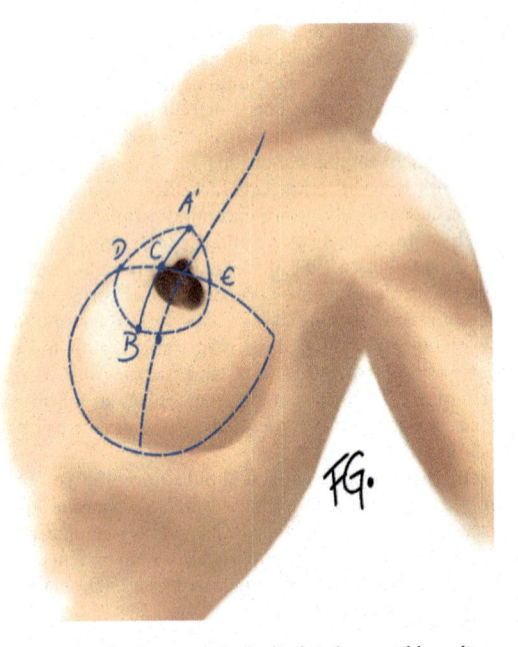

Fig. 45.3 The A'–B line is medially displaced to avoid lateralization of NAC. The greater circumference A'–D–B–E drawn with a *dotted line* around the areola theoretically corresponds to the maximum area of skin that may be deepithelialized

on the midclavicular line, 6–8 cm from the inframammary fold and corresponds to the lower margin of the new position of the areola (Fig. 45.2).

To avoid nipple–areola lateralization, a parallel line at 0.5–1 cm to the midclavicular line is drawn in the medial direction between points A' and B. This line will centralize the circumference drawn around the areola, an area that will be deepithelialized (Fig. 45.3). Therefore, the nipple–areola complex will move medially to the correct position. Keeping points A' and B in place, the periareolar circumference can be reduced medially and laterally, and will then have an elliptical shape with the greatest diameter in the longitudinal direction (Fig. 45.3).

Point C is located in the midpoint between points A' and B, and corresponds to the longest radius of the circumference of skin that will be deepithelialized around the areola (Fig. 45.3). Point D is located medially and point E is located laterally. They are the transversal limits of the circumference of skin that will be deepithelialized around the areola (Fig. 45.3).

After the first breast is marked, point A' is transferred to the opposite side so that the upper border of the areola is at the same height. Point B will be marked at the same distance, 6–8 cm from the inframammary fold on both sides. The medial margins of the skin circumference should be equidistant to the midsternal line so that the nipple–areola complexes are symmetrically positioned.

45.6 Technique

1. Deepithelialization of the marked area around the areola (Fig. 45.4).
2. Incision that runs 2 mm from the lower border of the areola to divide the breast in two halves (Fig. 45.4): upper half of the breast that will contain the nipple–areola complex and not undergo any skin detachment; and lower half of the breast that will be fully detached from the skin and which will be used to prepare a glandular tissue pad which will provide shape and support to the reduced breast. The breast is elevated by the assistant to facilitate the incision that will divide it into two halves. Initially, this incision is directed perpendicularly to the nipple–areola complex at a depth of about 2 cm. After that, the scalpel blade is tilted perpendicularly to the fascia of the pectoralis major muscle and slightly moved cephalad to ensure a good vascular supply from perforating branches for the lower half of the breast. The upper half of the breast is then detached from the fascia of the pectoralis major muscle at the plane where a retromammary prosthesis is usually placed, so that later the glandular tissue pad is positioned there (Figs. 45.5 and 45.6).
3. A linear incision on the deepithelialized surface at 2 mm from the margin of the skin in the upper half of

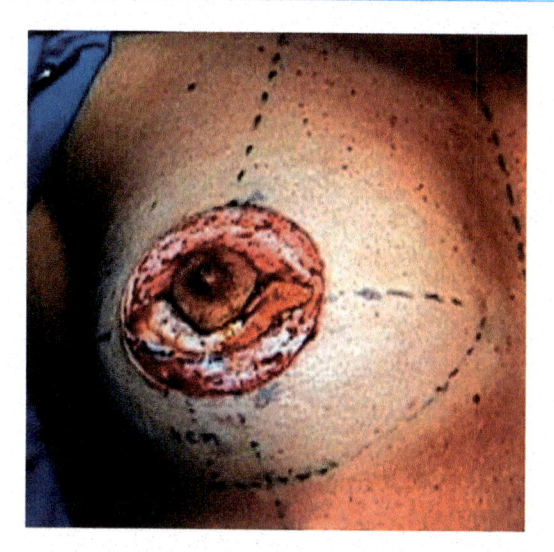

Fig. 45.4 Deepithelialization of the marked area around the areola; Incision at 2 mm from the lower border of the areola to divide the breast in two halves

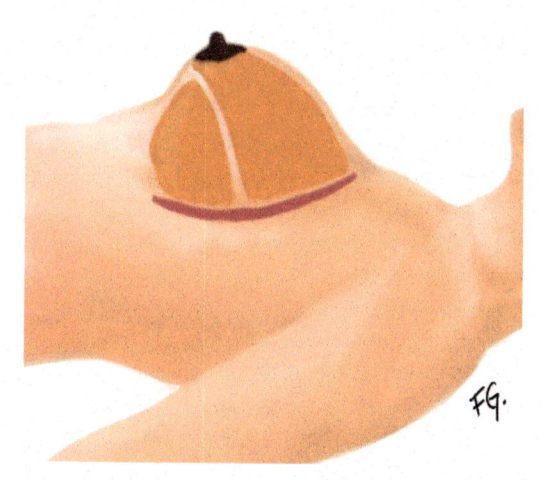

Fig. 45.5 Division of the breast into two halves

the breast is the initial procedure to release this part of the mammary gland (Fig. 45.7). Skin is distended by assistants to facilitate its detachment, which is superficial, at the level of subcutaneous tissue and extends to the inframammary fold. Lower half of the breast will be totally released from the skin and rest of the mammary gland (Fig. 45.8). Its vascular supply will be ensured by perforating branches mainly from the fourth and fifth intercostal spaces. Therefore, two flaps will be raised: a glandular inferior pedicle flap that will be used to shape the breast and a skin flap that will cover it.

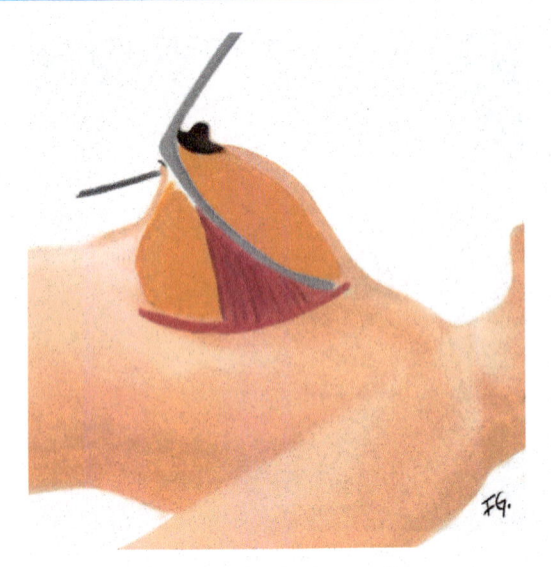

Fig. 45.6 The upper half of the breast is detached at the plane where a retromammary prosthesis is usually placed

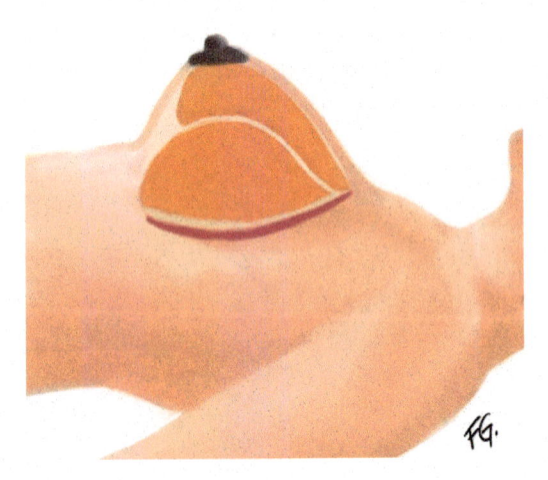

Fig. 45.7 New position of the glandular tissue pad

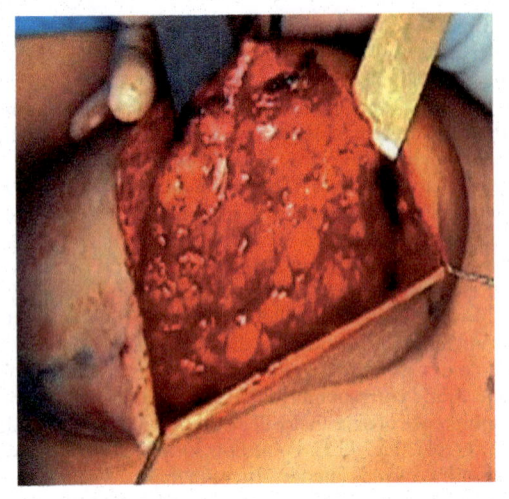

Fig. 45.8 Linear incision 2 mm from skin margin to detach all skin from lower half of the breast

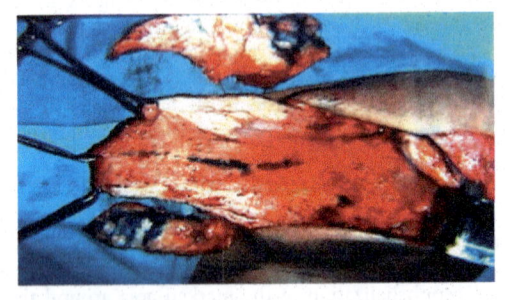

Fig. 45.9 Medial and lateral resections in lower half of the breast

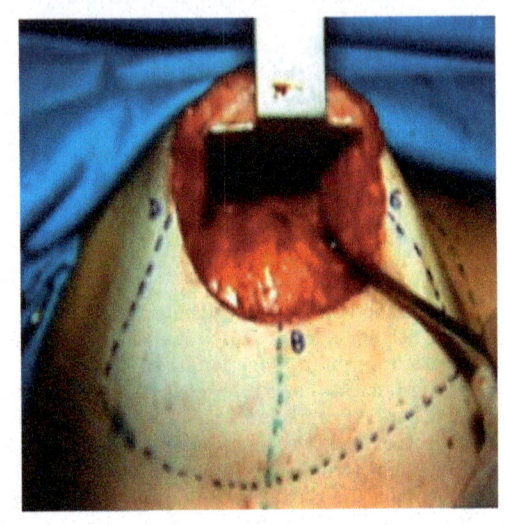

Fig. 45.10 A glandular tissue pad made up with tissue from lower half of the breast in the shape of a mammary prosthesis

4. Mammary reduction is achieved by medial and lateral gland resections in the lower half of the breast (Fig. 45.9). In the upper half of the breast, a wedge is removed as prescribed by Pitanguy, or glandular tissue is resected from the base of the breast as prescribed by Peixoto [9].

With the remaining tissue of the lower half of the breast, a glandular tissue pad is prepared in the shape of a mammary prosthesis. This pad is fixed with 3-0 monofilament nylon suture to the fascia of the pectoralis major muscle. Its distal end is sutured at the level of the second intercostal space (Fig. 45.10).

5. The upper half of the breast is reconstructed following a technique similar to Pitanguy's, surrounding the glandular pad so that no dead space is left. The nipple–areola complex should be positioned at the apex of the new breast.
6. Aspiration drainage should be performed through the small incision in the axillary region.
7. To distribute skin better, U-shaped sutures are performed to unite the four cardinal points of the areola and of the skin which were previously marked. After that, a continuous subdermal purse-string suture, called the round block, is applied to make the circumference of the breast skin meet the areola skin.
8. Micropore tape is used all around the breast to ensure the correct coaptation of tissues which were manipulated.

45.7
Postoperative

1. Continuous drain is maintained for at least 24–48 h or until the volume drained daily is negligible.
2. Micropore bandaging is kept for 2 weeks, and may be changed if necessary.
3. Periareolar sutures are exposed to facilitate their handling and the access to cleaning with saline or antiseptic solution and dressing. Stitches are removed between the seventh and tenth postoperative day.
4. Because extensive areas of skin and tissue were detached and manipulated, prophylactic antibiotics should be prescribed. It is important to warn patients that the result will improve with time, when the skin retracts and tissues accommodate.
5. Some folds around the areola may be seen, but will disappear in at the most 3 months. At 6 months, the breasts will have a normal and pleasing appearance. The periareolar scars may improve even further with time and become practically imperceptible.
6. The mammary gland functions should be preserved as much as possible during surgery.

45.8
Discussion

Reduction mammaplasties with minimum scarring, particularly those performed with a periareolar approach, depend on the skin capacity of retraction. The skin should adequately shape itself when it covers the new breast. The indications for this type of surgery are, therefore, limited because there should not be a great difference between the amount of skin and the mammary content.

The circumference of skin to be deepithelialized should not be much greater than that of the areola. The smaller the difference in size of these circles, the better the result of periareolar scars. When disproportion is large, the areola will become larger in the late postoperative period because of the centrifugal action of the skin. To avoid this, the area to be deepithelialized around the areola should be limited.

When the mammary parenchyma has substantial fat infiltration, a bipedicled suspension flap from the pectoralis major muscle may be used [11, 12] which will be fixed to the basis of the glandular tissue pad of the lower pedicle.

Early ptosis may be prevented by using fixation with two crossed superior pedicled flaps, one medial and one lateral, that will be fixed around the glandular tissue pad. This procedure favors long-term results (Fig. 45.11 and 45.12).

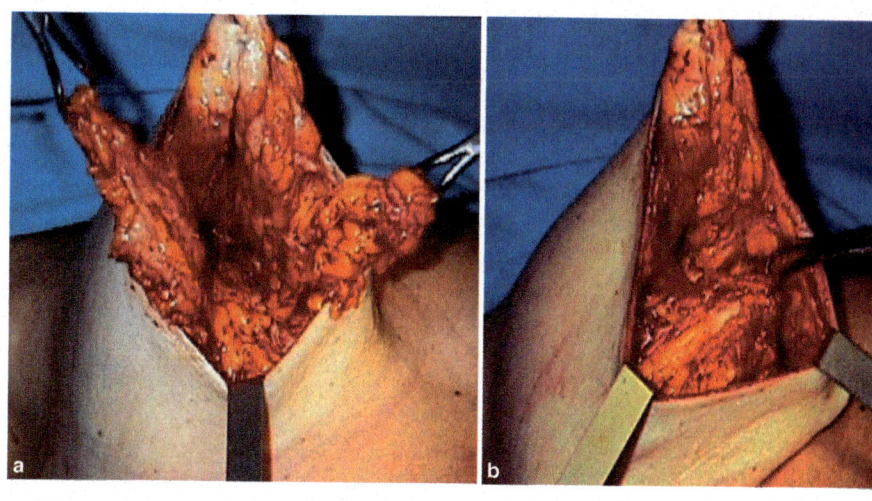

Fig. 45.11 (a,b) Crossed pedicled flaps

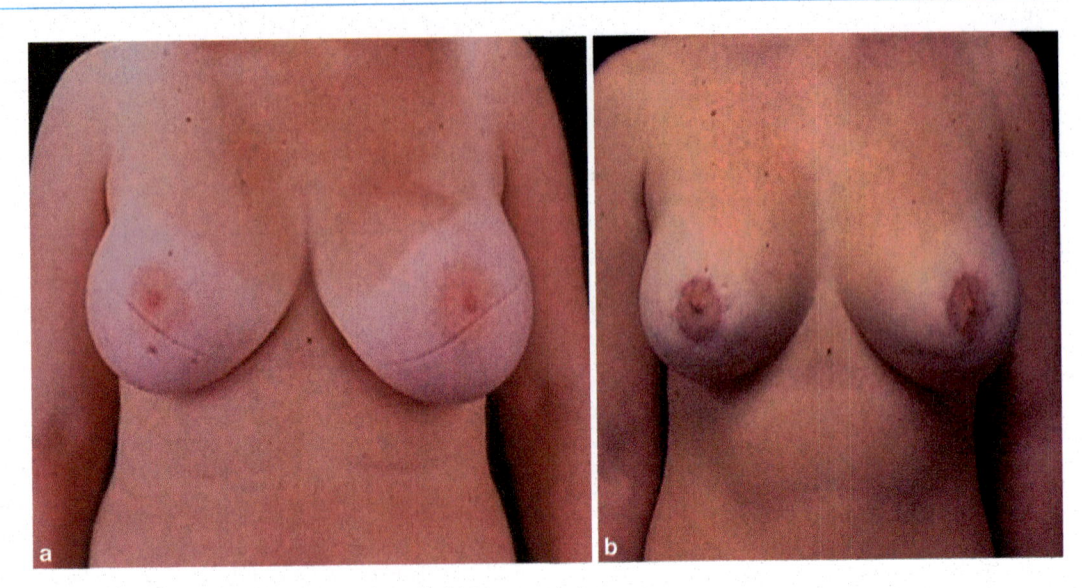

Fig. 45.12 Crossed pedicled flaps. (**a**) Preoperatively. (**b**) Postoperatively

When the nipple–areola complex is correctly positioned and the skin is healthy, it is not necessary to resect it. This technique can be performed through minimal incision in the lower border of the areola (Fig. 45.13).

In some cases, when the skin circumference is much greater than that of the areola, it is recommended to remove a triangular piece of detached skin from the lower half of the breast. This resection is centered on the midclavicular line and will result in a vertical scar which should not run beyond the inframammary fold.

In severe hypertrophies, when the percentage of reduction is very large and it is necessary to resect a large amount of skin, a large scar is inevitable.

In most cases of severe ptosis in which the skin has striae and poor elasticity, it is useless to shape the mammary content if the supporting effect of the skin is compromised. The resection of a large amount of skin is necessary to have an adequate skin container for the shaped breast.

45.9 Conclusions

In reduction mammaplasty, the most important factor to determine the extension of scar is the container-to-content ratio. The greater the disproportion of this ratio, the longer is the scar. This disproportion is a limiting factor for scar reduction.

Although there has been great progress in the approaches to dealing with mammary tissue, not much has been found about how to deal with the skin; an important field of study that poses a challenge for the future.

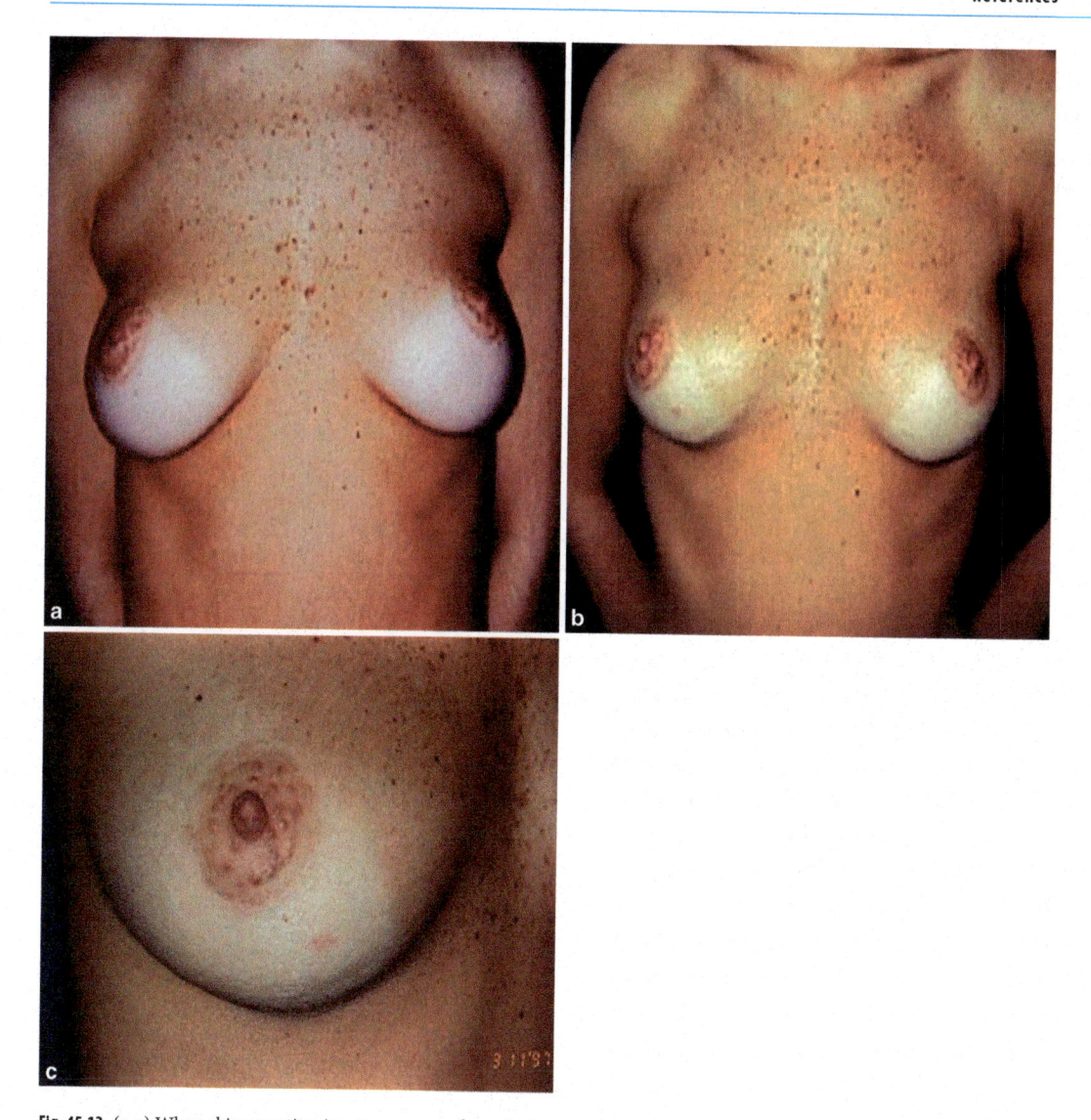

Fig. 45.13 (a-c) When skin resection is not necessary, the technique can be performed with only one Webster-type incision at the lower half of the areola. Observe the decrease in diameter of the operated breast and the imperceptible scar in late postoperative

References

1. Peixoto G: Reduction mammaplasty, a personal technique. Plast Reconstr Surg 1980;65(2):217–226
2. Benelli L: Technique de plastie mamaire: le round block. Rev Chir Esthét 1988;50:12
3. Bustos RA, Loureiro LEK, Tame CE: Mamoplastia redutora com retalho glandular trilobulado de pedículo inferior por incisão periareolar. In: Hochberg J ed. Anais XXIV Congr Bras Cir Plast Porto Alegre, 1985:484–489
4. Felicio Y: Mamoplastia redutora com incisão periareolar. Anais da 1°, Jorn. Sul Bras Cir Plast 1984;307
5. Goes JC: Mamoplastica periareolar, técnica da dupla pele. Rev Bras Cir Plast 1989;(23):55
7. Pitanguy I, Sangado F, Radwansky: Tratamento das deformidades benignas da mama. In: Dias EM, Caleffi M, Silva

HMS, Figueira ASS (eds), Mastologia Atual. Rio de Janeiro, Revinter 1994, pp 363–378
8. Ribeiro L, Muzzi S, Accorsi Jr A: Mamoplastia reductiva – Técnica circunferencial. Cir Plast Ibero-Lat-Am 1992; 17(3):249
9. Valle Pereira JF, Cirillo P: Mastoplastia riductiva e mastopessi con incisione periareolare. Riv Ital Chir Plast 1992;24:373
10. Pitanguy I: Mamoplastias: estudo de 245 casos consecutivos em apresentação de técnica pessoal. Rev Bras Cir Plast 1961;42:201
11. Ribeiro L: Cirurgia Plástica da Mama. Rio de Janeiro, MEDSI 1989:185–266
12. Daniel MJ: Mamoplastia com retalho de músculo peitoral. Uma abordagem dinâmica e definitiva para ptose mamária. Arquivos Catarinenses de Medicina 1994: 23–37
13. Martins PDE: Mamoplastia periareolar com suporte musculoaponeurótico. Arquivos Catarinenses de Medicina 1994;23(Suppl. 1):57

Inverted Keel Resection Breast Reduction

Ivo Pitanguy, Henrique N. Radwanski

46.1 Introduction

Patients presenting with breast hypertrophy invariably complain of physical discomfort, especially of the skeletal system. Psychological evaluation many times reveals a state of unhappiness and self-consciousness, and may result in difficult social adaptation. In warm climates, as in Brazil, where participation in outdoor activities and sports is stimulated year-round, and where the media promote the use of lighter and more revealing attire, aesthetic complaints because of large, cumbersome breasts become more relevant. In our country, breast hypertrophy is among the most common contour deformities that present for surgical correction.

A personal modification of Arié's technique was initially presented in 1959, and published in the following year [1]. With the description of point A, which is the projection of the submammary sulcus along the midclavicular line, the vertical incision was extended above the nipple–areolar complex, with more satisfactory and longer-lasting results. Soon after, with the same principles, the Pitanguy technique [2], with the inverted keel resection, was developed for the treatment of large breast hypertrophy. These two procedures have served the purpose of approaching most aesthetic deformities of the breast, such as hypertrophy with or without ptosis, and represent the technical basis of many subsequent procedures.

The senior author will focus on his techniques for breast reduction and mastopexy that involve the inverted keel approach to resection, covering a personal experience of over five decades. The following principles are emphasized: all resection is limited to the lower pole of the breast; no dissection of parenchyma is done, thus eliminating dead space and maintaining the intimate relationship between skin and parenchyma; the great feasibility of these procedures, allowing easy understanding and replication of the technique.

46.2 Historical Considerations

The personal techniques for breast reduction developed from comprehension of, and respect for, breast embryology. Breast buds develop from vertical thickening of the ectoderm, thus establishing an intimate relationship between skin and gland. The continuity between breast parenchyma and skin should be preserved in all breast reduction operations. This principle may be stated as such: the "continent" should not be separated from the "content."

In a historical context, previous techniques, principally the Biesenberger [3] approach, included extensive skin undermining, resulting in poor upper pole definition and ptosis in the postoperative follow-up, along with a high rate of complications. Other techniques, such as Lexer's [4] and Arié's [5], were quite popular, but they did not address the projection of the upper pole, and the results were generally lacking in producing a pleasing breast cone. This aspect has currently become more important with the popularization of breast augmentation, where patients seek specifically a fuller upper pole.

The authors' modification of Arié's technique [1] described point A as the initial landmark, from which the other points are developed. With this concept, the lower pole undergoes a rotation to the upper pole, filling up the breast and assuring a long-term aesthetic result. Later, when the limitations of the single vertical scar were perceived in larger breasts, an improvement was presented using the inverted keel resection, then called the Pitanguy technique, where a greater amount of skin and parenchyma can safely be removed, assuring the ascension of the nipple to a new position, where point A is located, and finishing with very acceptable scars. The technical points of interest in the teaching of my techniques are the following:
1. Maintain function and sensibility
2. Achieve satisfactory volume and lasting form
3. Reduce scars
4. Allow a greater feasibility in teaching the techniques

46.3 Personal Technique

46.3.1 For Large Hypertrophy

General anesthesia is almost always used. The patient is intubated and then placed in a semisitting position, flexed at 45° and with the arms out-stretched.

M.A. Shiffman (ed.), *Mastopexy and Breast Reduction: Principles and Practice*,
© Springer-Verlag Berlin Heidelberg 2009

Two long sutures are placed along the midline, one at the sternal notch and the second at the xyphoid. These will help the surgeon check for symmetry during demarcation and at the end of the procedure. The midclavicular line is drawn passing through the nipple–areola complex (NAC) all the way to the sulcus. Point A is determined along this line, at or slightly lower than the breast sulcus. This point determines the future position of the NAC. Points B and C are determined by pinching excess skin. They form a triangle with point A. The surgeon should, at this moment, feel how much tissue will be sufficient to allow for a pleasant final conical shape. Two strong hooks, on either side, help determine the amount of resection. The last two points, D and E, define the medial and lateral extension of the horizontal incision. Care should be taken not to extend beyond the midline and the anterior axillary line. The lines uniting these points are either straight or curved when excess skin is present.

The periareolar incision is done along the new diameter of the areola, previously determined with an appropriately sized demarcator. The area between points ABC is deepithelialized (Schwartzmann's maneuver). This assures the maintenance of the dermal capsule of the superior pole, which is considered the third neurovascular pedicle of the NAC.

Glandular resection is always restricted to the inferior pole and is straight when the breast is composed mainly of fatty tissue or in an inverted ship's keel fashion if the parenchyma is more glandular.

The inverted keel resection allows for the creation of two pillars, medial and lateral, that will be brought together after removal of adequate parenchyma. If a wedge-like space is not created in breasts that are very dense, bringing the remaining tissues together will cause excess tension and will also make it very difficult to ascend the nipple–areola complex. The inverted keel addresses this by allowing the upper-pedicled NAC to slide upwards as the pillars are approximated. On the other hand, the straight resection in fatty breasts permits the ascension of the NAC because the two pillars will be defined once the assistant raises the remaining tissues using a long hemostatic forceps.

After resection and hemostasis have been done, the operated breast is wrapped in moist towels and the same procedure is done on the opposite breast. The two are then lifted by the assistant, and inspected from a distance to compare remaining parenchyma, one side with the other.

Tissues are now brought together with one main suture, bringing points A–B–C to the midline. Sutures are done from deep to superficial planes. The new position of the NAC is determined. The breast mound should be seen as a cone, with the NAC resting on its top. The NAC on both sides is demarcated and symmetry is checked once again, using the two long sutures. This is one of the main advantages of this technique: the surgeon feels that he is free to demarcate the new position of the NAC, and is not bound to fixed measures as in other techniques.

When all excess skin has been trimmed and fine sutures placed, a useful procedure has been adopted in our service, which consists of a mold made of plaster, placed over the dressing, which guarantees the immobilization of the breast. It has been noted that this firm pressure has resulted in a very low rate of serosanguinous collection over the years. This plaster shield is removed in 24 h, when the breast is inspected. Placement of drains is not routinely used, as all dead space has been closed (Figs. 46.1–46.3).

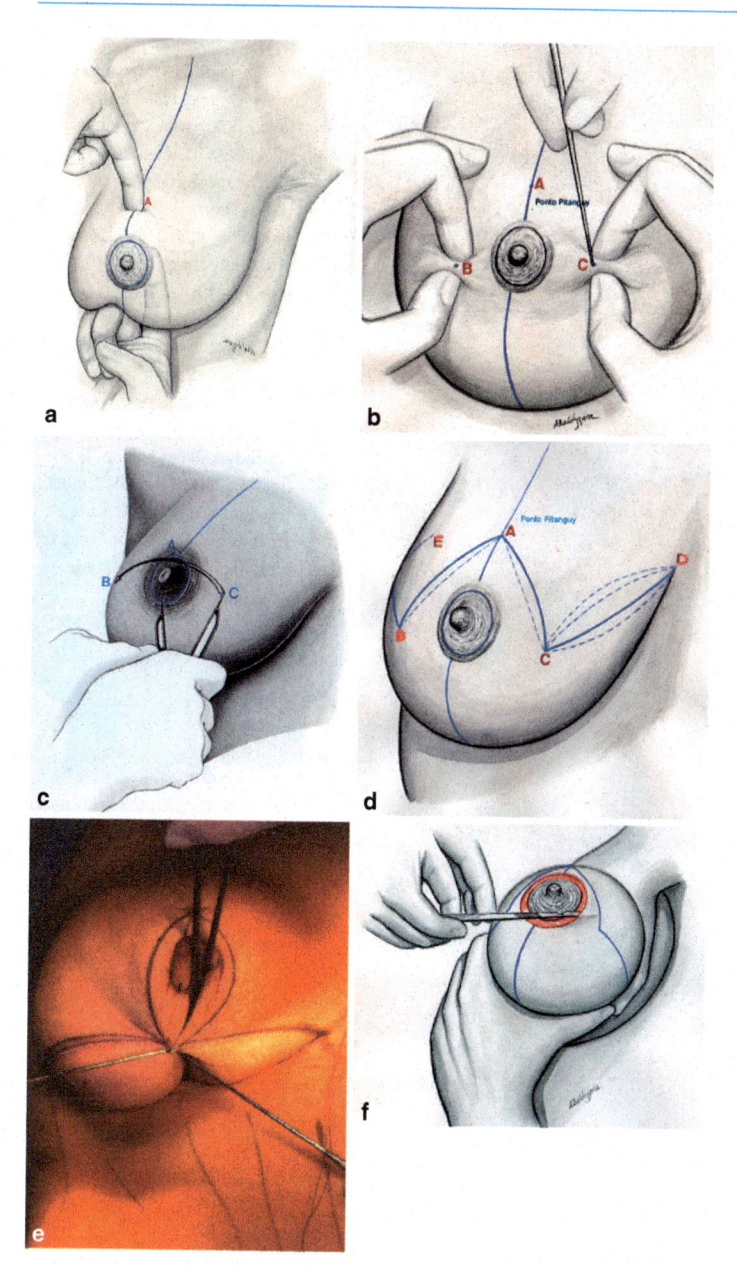

Fig. 46.1 (**a**) Point A (also called Pitanguy's Point) is found at the level of the submammary sulcus, along the mid-clavicular line. (**b**) A pinching maneuver allows the surgeon to estimate how much parenchyma should be removed. (**c**) Final demarcation is checked with long sutures and a compass. (**d**) Lines of resection are curved to permit removal of excess skin. (**e**) Finally, two strong hooks are pulled together to ascertain that demarcation is correct. (**f**) Deepithelialization around the nipple-areolar complex (Schwartzmann's maneuver) guarantees the vascular integrity of this important structure.

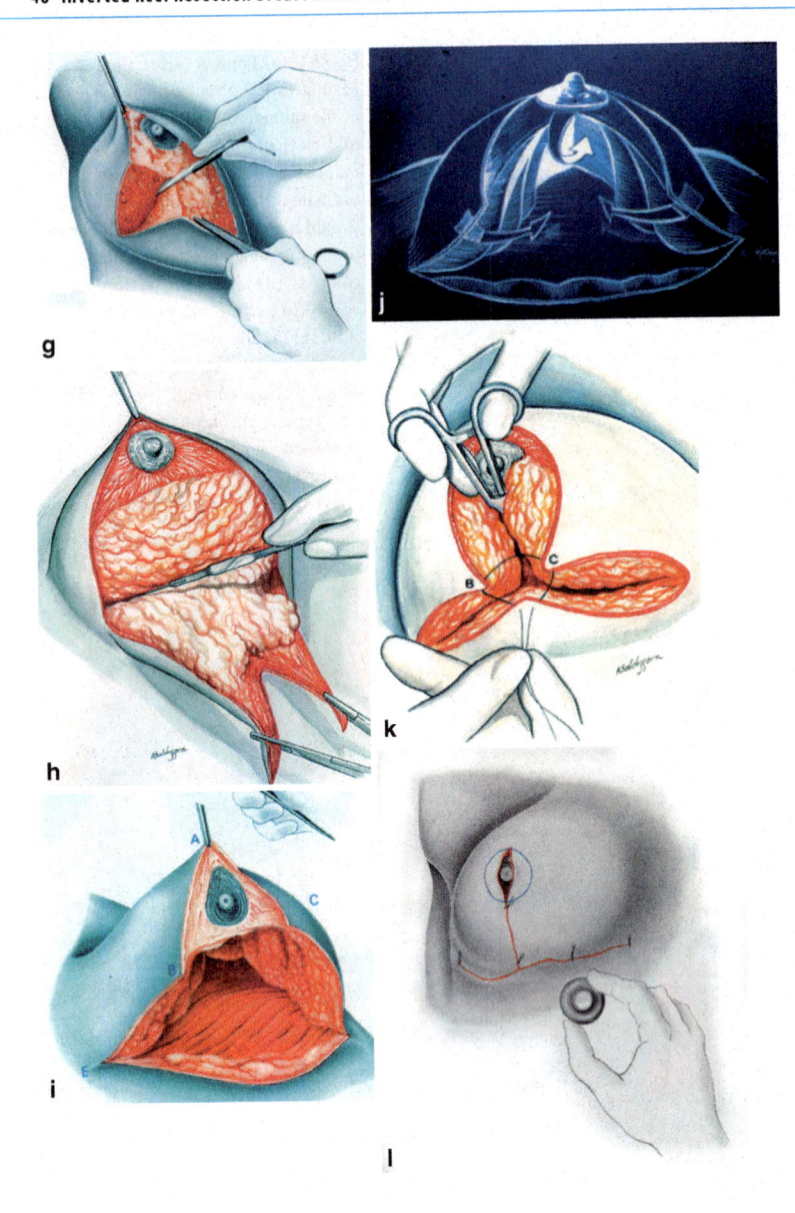

Fig. 46.1 *(continued)* (**g**) Resection of breast tissue is always restricted to the lower pole. (**h**) A straight resection is indicated in breasts that are mostly fatty in nature. (**i**) The inverted keel resection should be applied to breasts that are mainly composed of glandular tissue. (**j**) With the inverted keel resection, the surgeon creates two pillars; this also allows the NAC to rise to its new position. (**k**) Closing of the pillars eliminates all dead space. (**l**) The final position of the NAC, which will lie around Point A, is not a fixed measurement, but depends on the aesthetic feeling of the surgeon

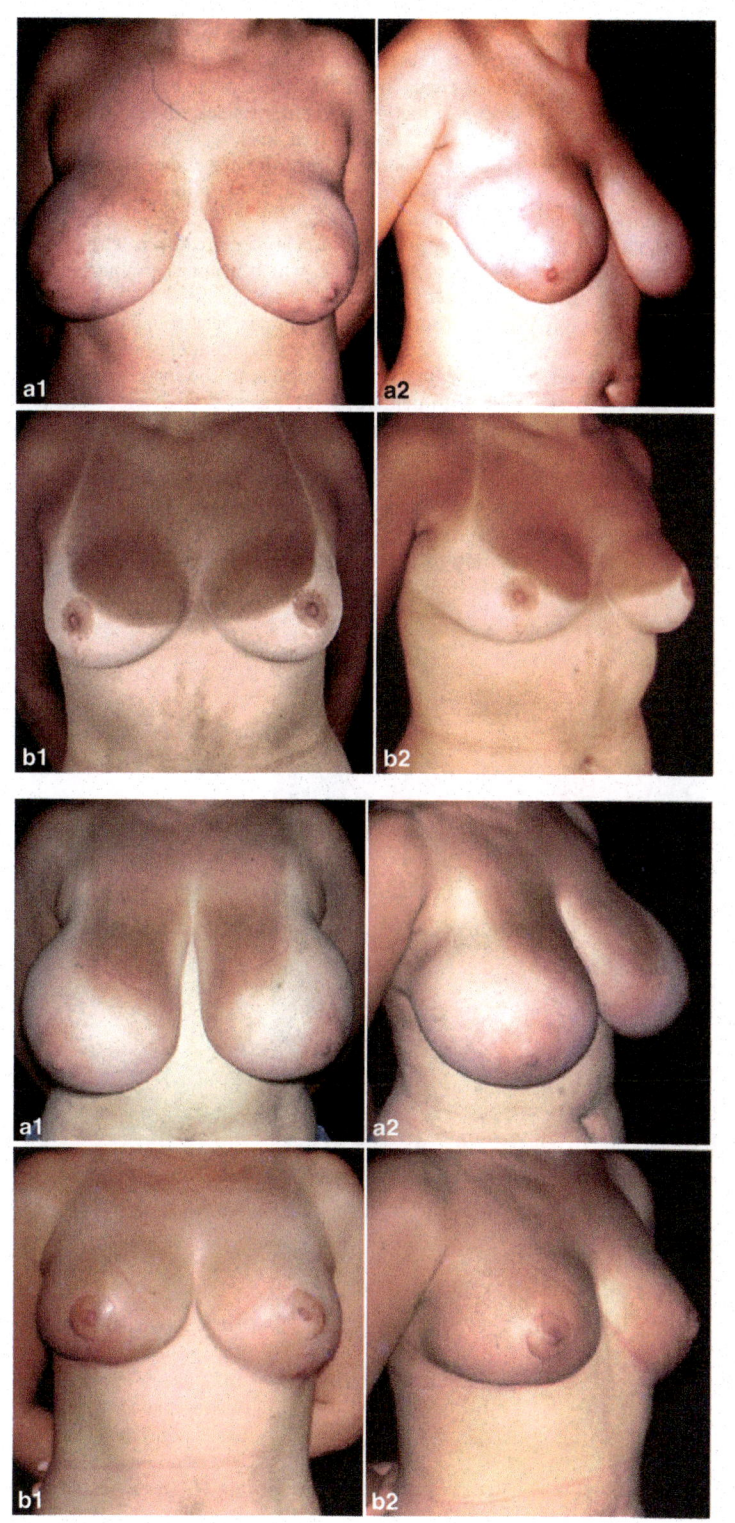

Fig. 46.2 (**a**1,2) Preoperative 41-year-old female. (**b**1,2) Postoperative after reducing very large breasts with the classic Pitanguy approach (inverted keel)

Fig. 46.3 (**a**) Preoperative 25-year-old female with breast asymmetry. (**b**) Postoperative following inverted keel approach

46.4 The Rhomboid Technique

46.4.1 For Moderate Hypertrophy, With or Without Ptosis

This technique, also called the Arié–Pitanguy procedure, has an initial rhomboid demarcation and finishes with a single vertical scar. It has these indications: mild-to-moderate hypertrophy, breast ptosis, and ptosis with hypoplasia (augmentation procedure) (Figs. 46.4–46.6).

Initially, point A is determined as previously described, along the midclavicular line at the level of the submammary sulcus. By pinching the medial and lateral skin on either side of the nipple, the surgeon "feels" how much skin must be removed, and points B and C are determined. Point D, which should not be lower than the sulcus, will complete the elliptical demarcation. The final incision is a vertical scar, ending at (or slightly below) the submammary sulcus.

Resection can be restricted to skin when simple ptosis is present, or can include a variable amount of breast tissue from the lower pole, when the patient desires reduction in volume. As described in the classic technique, the inverted keel resection creates two pillars or columns. Once these are approximated, the superior pole is defined and the nipple will rise to the new position.

The appropriate areola demarcator is chosen for placement of the NAC, which, again, is around the area of point A.

The rhomboid technique is very suitable for resection of excess skin and for placement of a breast implant, resulting in a single vertical scar. The surgeon should be careful to demarcate the excess skin envelope but not too much, as the implant will tend to fill up the breast cone.

When necessary, the final vertical incision can be complemented with a small horizontal component, converting the single scar into an "L" or inverted "T" so as not to extend the scar beyond the sulcus (Fig. 46.4–46.6).

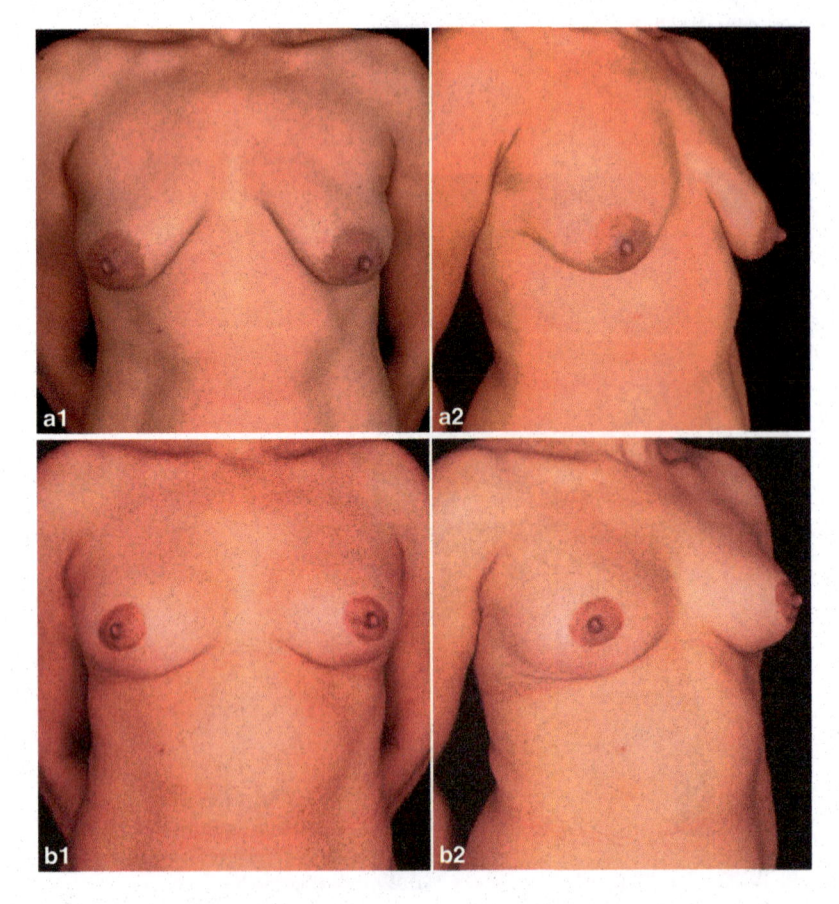

Fig. 46.4 (**a1,2**) Preoperative 26-year-old female. (**b1,2**) Postoperative after mastopexy done through the Pitanguy rhomboid procedure. Breast tissue was used to fill the upper pole

46.4 The Rhomboid Technique 347

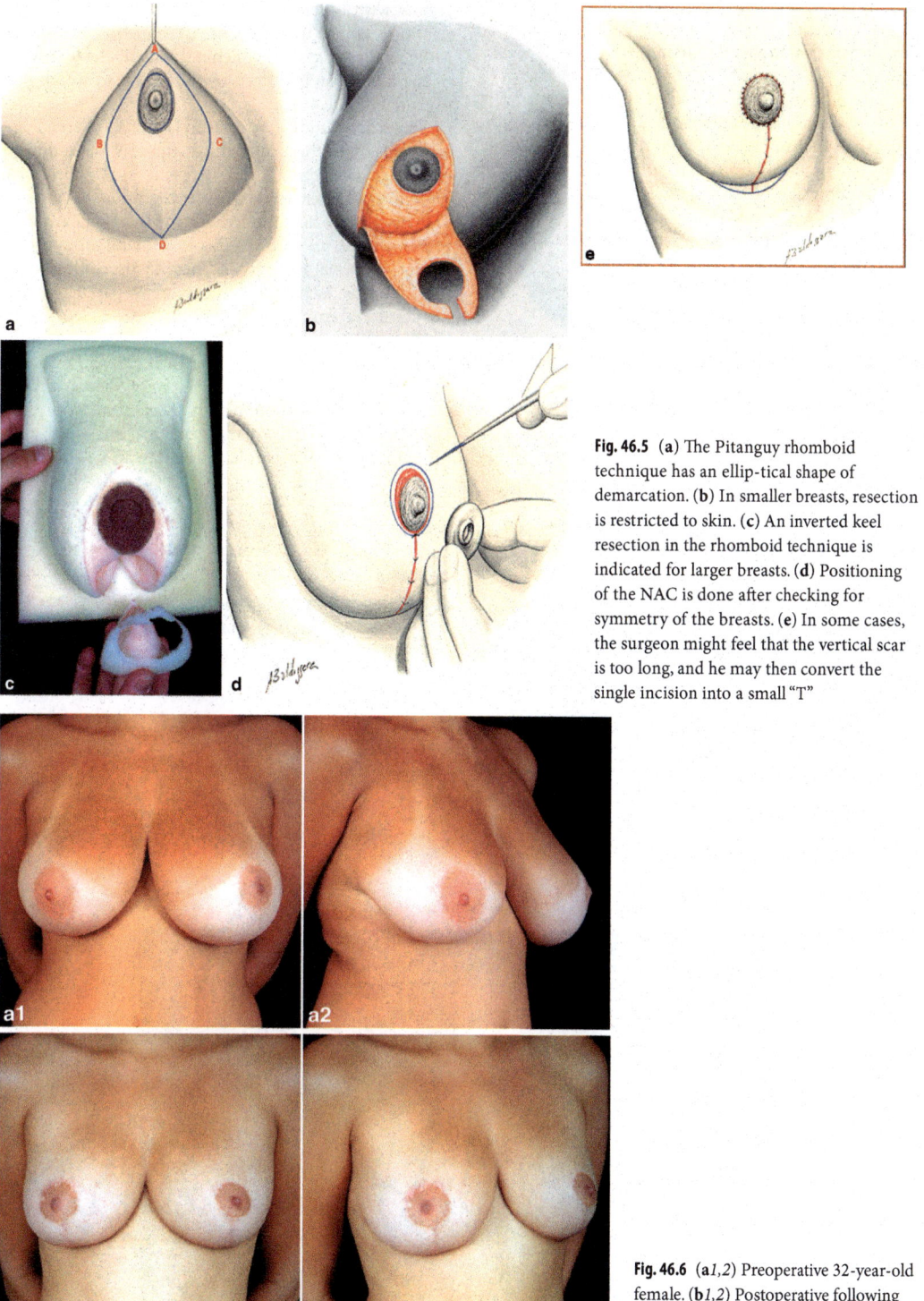

Fig. 46.5 (**a**) The Pitanguy rhomboid technique has an ellip-tical shape of demarcation. (**b**) In smaller breasts, resection is restricted to skin. (**c**) An inverted keel resection in the rhomboid technique is indicated for larger breasts. (**d**) Positioning of the NAC is done after checking for symmetry of the breasts. (**e**) In some cases, the surgeon might feel that the vertical scar is too long, and he may then convert the single incision into a small "T"

Fig. 46.6 (**a***1,2*) Preoperative 32-year-old female. (**b***1,2*) Postoperative following Pitanguy rhomboid technique applied to large breasts

46.5 Complications of Breast Reductions

The rate of complications for both techniques is very small, because all dead spaces are closed with the approximation of the two columns of breast tissue. Flap ischemia is also avoided, since no undermining is done between skin and parenchyma. A certain degree of hypesthesia of the NAC can occur, which usually resolves in the first 2 months postoperative (Table 46.1).

46.6 Discussion

These procedures have been adopted and systematized by the author, producing satisfactory and predictable results with a very low rate of complications [6–14]. An important aspect of the breast reduction techniques is the relative ease with which it is taught. The feasibility of the technique is proven by the ease with which it is executed (Table 46.2).

Sound anatomical principles and respect for physiology are the basis for these procedures. In breast reduction, as emphasized by the author since his first publications, resection of breast tissue is restricted to the lower pole. The vascularity and innervation of the NAC are thus preserved, and all dead space is closed with the approximation of remaining tissue. There is also little risk of flap or nipple ischemia, because breast parenchyma is not separated from overlying skin.

Depending on the degree of breast hypertrophy, the surgeon may choose to perform either the rhomboid technique or the classic Pitanguy breast reduction technique. Although it is possible to apply the rhomboid approach to larger breasts, this is not recommended, as the single vertical scar will become

Table 46.1 Breast Hypertrophy: 1957–2006. Complications
Ivo Pitanguy Clinic (IPC) – 3,476 cases
38th Ward of the Santa Casa (SC) – 6,403 cases
Total cases: 9,879

Complications			IPC	SC
Dehiscence of incision		Lesser	1.3	6.0
		Larger	0	1.2
Dehiscence of areola		Lesser	0.1	2.0
		Larger	0.3	0.4
Heamatoma			0.2	0.4
Hypertrophic scars			0.6	7.0

Table 46.2 Breast Hypertrophy: 1957–2006. Ages of Patients
Total cases: 9,879
Ivo Pitanguy Clinic – 3,476 cases
38th Ward of the Santa Casa – 6,403 cases

Idade	IPC	SC
10–19 years	4.0	11.0
20–29 years	26.0	33.0
30–39 years	32.0	29.0
40–49 years	21.0	17.0
50–59 years	14.0	7.0
≥60 years	3.0	3.0

Table 46.3 Breast Hypertrophy: 1957–2006. Techniques Used

	Cases
The Ivo Pitanguy clinic	3,476
38th Ward of the Santa Casa	6,403
Total	9,879

PITANGUY TECHNIQUE 58.9 %
PERIAREOLAR TECHNIQUE 2.9 %
PITANGUY ROMBOIDE TECHNIQUE 38.2 %

quite long. It is therefore more appropriate to utilize the classic technique. In either case, the inverted keel resection has allowed for safe removal of excess parenchyma of the lower pole, facilitating closure of remaining tissues, leaving no dead space and assuring the rising of the nipple to its new position. The periareolar approach has been mostly abandoned, as the final results have not been consistently favorable (Table 46.3).

Plastic surgeons have noted that patients are requesting a fuller upper pole and this may be due to what the media has emphasized as the result of a breast augmentation. The two techniques allow for a projection of the superior aspect of the breast following rotation of the lower to the upper pole.

References

1. Pitanguy I: Breast hypertrophy. In: Wallace AB (ed). Transactions of the International Society of Plastic Surgeons. Second Congress, Edinburgh, Livingstone 1960, p 509
2. Pitanguy I: Une nouvelle technique de plastique mammaire: Estude de 245 cas consecutifs et presentation d'une technique personelle. Ann Chir Plastique 1962;7(3):199–208
3. Biesenberger H: Eine neue methode der mammaplastik. Zentrabl Chir 1928;38:2382–2387
4. Lexer E: Zur operation der mammahypertrophie und der hängebrust. Dtsch Med Wochenschr 1925;51:26
5. Arié G: Una nueva técnica de mastoplastia. Rev Latinoamericana Cir Plast 1957;3:23
6. Pitanguy I: Contribuição a técnica do enxerto livre para a correção das grandes hipertrofias mamárias. (Personal contribution to the free-grafting technique in very large breasts). Rev Lat Americana Cir Plástica 1963;7(2):75
7. Pitanguy I: Surgical treatment of breast hypertrophy. Br J Plast Surg 1967;20(1):78–85
8. Pitanguy I: The breast. In: Pitanguy I (ed). Aesthetic Plastic Surgery of Head and Body. Berlin, Springer 1981
9. Pitanguy I: Reduction mammaplasty by the personal technique. In: Chang WHJ (ed), The Breast: An Atlas of Reconstruction. Baltimore, Williams and Wilkins 1984, pp 75–160
10. Pitanguy I: Personal preferences for reduction mammaplasty. In: Georgiade ND (ed). Aesthetic Surgery of the Breast. Philadelphia, Saunders 1990, p 167
11. Pitanguy I: Principles of reduction mammaplasty. In: Georgiade ND (ed), Aesthetic Surgery of the Breast. Philadelphia, Saunders 1990, p 191
12. Pitanguy I: Reduction mammaplasty: A personal odyssey. In: Goldwyn RM (ed.). Reduction Mammaplasty, Boston, Little, Brown 1990, p 95
13. Pitanguy I, Radwanski HN: Philosophy and principles in the correction of breast hypertrophy. In: Mang WL, Bull HG (eds). Ästhetische Chirurgie. Germany, Einhorn-Presse 1996, pp 216–232
14. Pitanguy I: Evaluation of body contouring surgery today: A 30-year perspective. Plast Reconstr Surg 2000;105(4): 1499–1514

General References

Goin MK: Psychological aspects of aesthetic surgery of the breast. In: Georgiade, N.D. (ed.). Aesthetic Surgery of the Breast. Philadelphia, Saunders 1990, p 19

Gifford S: Emotional attitudes toward cosmetic breast surgery: Loss and restitution of the "ideal self." In: Goldwyn RM (ed). Plastic and Reconstructive Surgery of the Breast. Boston, Little, Brown 1976, p 103

Rees TD: Concepts of beauty. In: Rees TD (ed). Aesthetic Plastic Surgery. Philadelphia, Saunders 1980, p 1

Baroudi R: Preoperative evaluation for breast surgery. In: Georgiade ND (ed). Aesthetic Surgery of the Breast. Philadelphia, Saunders 1990, p 19

McCarty KS Jr, Glaubitz L, Thienemann M, Riefkohl R: The breast: Embryology, anatomy and physiology. In: Georgiade ND (ed.), Aesthetic Surgery of the Breast, Philadelphia, Saunders 1990, p 3

Superior Vertical Dermal Pedicle for the Nipple–Areola

Antonio Carlos Abramo

47.1 Introduction

The goal in reduction mammaplasty and mastopexy is to achieve a pleasing balance among size, shape, and projection of the breast with optimal sensation and appropriate blood supply for the nipple–areola and breast, accompanied by breastfeeding after the surgery. Anthropomorphic measurements of the female breast and thorax are useful as guidelines in planning reduction mammaplasty [1].

Size, shape, and projection of the breast and its landmarks are distorted in massive breast hypertrophy and severe breast ptosis. Measurements are employed in an attempt to achieve symmetry between the breasts and its correlation with the torso shape, also to establish its position on the thorax. The traditional treatment for massive breast hypertrophy or severe breast ptosis is amputation of the inferior portion of the breast with free grafting of the nipple–areola [2]. The usual complications of free nipple–areola graft technique include temporary or permanent loss of sensation, necrosis, hypopigmentation, and flatness of the nipple–areola.

The relatively high number of complications and the disadvantage of the free nipple–areola graft led to the development of numerous pedicle techniques to avoid nipple–areola deformities. Age, smoke, body mass index, and amount of mammary tissue resected must be taken into account to choose the appropriate pedicle technique for the nipple–areola in reduction mammaplasty. However, the main criteria in deciding the suitable pedicle technique for nipple–areola are the surgical parameters. The length and the thickness of the pedicle rather than the amount of mammary tissue resected are the most important limiting factors for the transposition of the nipple–areola [3].

Several pedicle techniques were proposed to avoid vascular compromise and loss of sensation of the nipple–areola in reduction mammaplasty for massive breast hypertrophy and severe ptosis. Inferior pedicle techniques are usually reported as the main support pedicle for nipple–areola in heavy hypertrophy and ptosis of the breast [4]. Superior pedicle techniques have also provided a safety transposition of the nipple–areola in reduction mammaplasty for moderate and large breast hypertrophy and ptosis [5]. A variation of the superior pedicle techniques is the vertical orientation of the pedicle. It addresses a straight transposition for the nipple–areola avoiding a winding course of the pedicle to lead the nipple–areola to the new location without distortion [6]. Although the medial pedicle technique originates from the superomedial pedicle technique it was developed for all breast hypertrophy, especially management of severe mammary hypertrophy [7]. Another alternative for transposition of the nipple–areola is a dermoglandular latero-central pedicle that was proposed to reduction mammaplasty for moderate breast hypertrophy [8].

No matter what pedicle technique is used, the excessive length and thickness of pedicle can cause torsion, twisting, and compression over the pedicle during the transposition of the nipple–areola with damage of the vascularity and sensibility of the nipple–areola. To appraise nipple–areola viability after transposition, an intraoperative evaluation of the blood supply can be carried out independent of the pedicle technique used for the nipple–areola. It is performed by applying an intravenous injection of fluorescein sodium 10% and watching the coloring of the nipple–areola exposed to ultraviolet light in a darkish operating room [9]. Otherwise, temporary loss of sensation of the nipple–areola is a common occurrence in reduction mammaplasty with extensive resection of the breast tissue or excessive raise of the nipple–areola. Recovery of sensation of the nipple and areola can result from the regeneration of the cutaneous branches of the intercostal nerves or from the remaining cutaneous innervation of the breast rather than the preserved adjacent cutaneous branches [10]. Quantitative tests using Semmes-Weinstein monofilaments or computer-assisted neurosensory testing are employed to quantify the sensibility of the breast and nipple–areola after reduction mammaplasty [11, 12]. Subjective tests as crude touch with cotton and light pressure with needle are also employed

M.A. Shiffman (ed.), *Mastopexy and Breast Reduction: Principles and Practice*,
© Springer-Verlag Berlin Heidelberg 2009

to identify, not quantify, sensation on the breast skin and nipple–areola after reduction mammaplasty [13]. Prospective studies have demonstrated that nipple–areola sensation at month 6 was statistically similar compared to reduction mammaplasty with superior and inferior pedicle techniques for the nipple–areola [14]. No statistically significant difference was found on breast and nipple–areola sensation regarding the amount of breast tissue removed [15]. No difference was found in the aesthetic outcome and complications between superior and inferior pedicle techniques in reduction mammaplasty [16].

47.2
Dermal Pedicles Review

Reduction mammaplasty with dermal pedicle for the nipple–areola derives from the study of Schwarzmann [17] that reported the nipple–areola as integrant part of the skin of the anterior chest wall. He emphasized the blood nourishment of the breast skin developing a dermal bed for the nipple–areola. To support this concept numerous dermal pedicles were created for nourishment of the nipple–areola.

Arie [18] developed a vertical mammaplasty with the nipple–areola superiorly, medially, and laterally supported in a dermal bed to ensure a safety transposition for the nipple–areola.

Strombeck [19] proposed a horizontal double pedicle for the nipple–areola maintaining the dermal portion joined to the subjacent mammary tissue.

Skoog [20] described a lateral dermal pedicle supported by a thin layer of mammary tissue without attachments to the fascia pectoralis to ensure a wide arc of rotation for the pedicle.

McKissock [21] reported a long vertical dermal flap with double pedicle for the nipple–areola. The amount of mammary tissue attached to the inferior portion of the vertical dermal flap is thicker than the superior one and its base is supported on the inframammary skin and pectoralis muscle. The superior portion of the vertical dermal flap is not thick to allow its overlap to accommodate the nipple–areola in the new location.

Weiner et al. [22] also reported a vertical dermal flap for the nipple–areola with pedicle supported superiorly. The mammary tissue located underneath the dermal bed is released from the pectoralis muscle to allow a transposition of the nipple–areola without retraction.

Courtiss and Goldwyn [23] developed an inferior dermal pedicle for the nipple–areola based along the inframammary fold to make use of the intercostal arteries as blood supply for the nipple–areola.

Abramo [13] advocated a vertical dermal pedicle based superiorly without mammary tissue attached to the pedicle creating only a dermal bed to support the nipple–areola. It is performed to attempt a long distance transposition of the nipple–areola without twist or distortion of the pedicle. Modifications regarding the thickness, length, and location of the dermal pedicles are extended so far to ensure the viability of the nipple–areola after its transposition in reduction mammaplasty.

47.3
Anatomical Review

Usually the breast and nipple–areola derive arterial blood supply from the internal mammary, lateral thoracic, and intercostals arteries. O'Dey et al. [24], performing microdissections of the anterior chest wall, found four arterial sources for the blood supply of the nipple–areola. The main supply is established through the branches of the lateral thoracic artery, followed by the internal mammary artery, the anterior branches of the intercostal arteries and branches from the highest thoracic artery. According to Serafin [25] the anterior perforating branches of the internal mammary artery arise mainly from the 2nd and 3rd intercostal spaces, becoming intradermal at the level of the nipple–areola. The lateral thoracic artery has two branches running parallel to the lateral contour of the breast; the medial branch turns medially and superficially toward the nipple–areola, to form anastomosis with branches of the internal mammary artery at the upper pole of the breast. The intercostal arteries end in an anastomotic plexus with the lateral thoracic and internal mammary arteries, in the lower quadrant of the breast. The breast parenchyma is reached by the posterior perforating branches of the internal mammary, lateral branches of the lateral thoracic and intercostals arteries.

As the course and distribution of the nerves supplying the nipple–areola and breast skin change between individuals, different information can be found in the literature. Lockhart et al. [26] reported the supraclavicular nerve as responsible for the innervation of the skin and gland of the upper pole of the breast, and the 6th intercostal nerve supplying the lower pole of the breast. The lateral and anterior cutaneous branches of the 3rd, 4th, 5th, and 6th intercostal nerves were reported as supplying nerves to the nipple–areola. Schelenzs et al. [27] described the lateral and anterior cutaneous branches of the 3rd, 4th, and 5th intercostal nerves as supplying nerves to the nipple–areola, and the lateral and anterior cutaneous branches of the 2nd and 6th intercostals nerves as supplying nerves to the breast skin.

A classification to distribute adequately the enlargement and ptosis of the breast was proposed considering the diameter of the breast circumference and the measured distance of the nipple–areola located below the inframammary fold [13]. Massive breast hyper-trophy was settled by enlargement of the breast circumference over 20 cm transcending the anterior axillary line. Severe breast ptosis was determined by the distance from the inframammary fold to the nipple–areola more than 10 cm.

47.4 Marking

Breast measurements are obtained with the patient standing. A clavicle–nipple line is drawn from a point marked on the clavicle, 7 cm from the suprasternal notch. Point A is defined by the projection of the inframammary fold on the clavicle–nipple line. From point A, a keyhole pattern composed by an internal circle with 7 cm diameter and 5 cm straight limbs arising from the internal circle with opening angle of 125° between them is placed over the breast so that its midline coincides with the clavicle–nipple line (Fig. 47.1). The keyhole pattern is outlined on the breast skin. The ends of the vertical straight limbs are connected with the inframammary fold medially, remaining 5 cm distant from the mid sternal line and laterally, to the anterior axillary line (Fig. 47.2).

47.5 Operative Technique

The outline of the keyhole pattern and its extension to the inframammary fold are superficially incised. A vertical flap is marked from the new site of the nipple–areola, determined by the internal circle of the pattern, to 1 cm below the areola diameter (Fig. 47.3). The pedicle of the vertical flap is supported in the upper pole of the breast. The width of the vertical flap is the areolar diameter aiding 1–1.5 cm of margin around the areola diameter, in accordance with the degree of the breast hypertrophy and ptosis. The length of the vertical pedicle also changes according to the breast hypertrophy and ptosis. It can be more than 15 cm in massive breast hypertrophy and severe ptosis. The vertical flap is deepithelialized providing a dermal bed for the

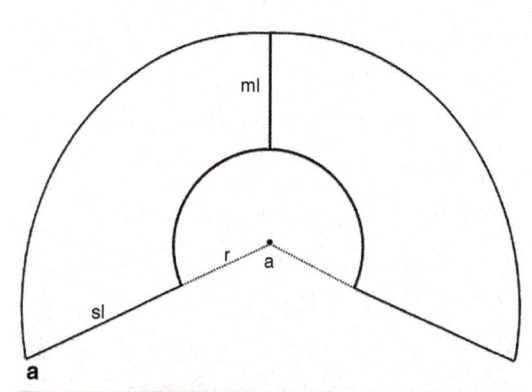

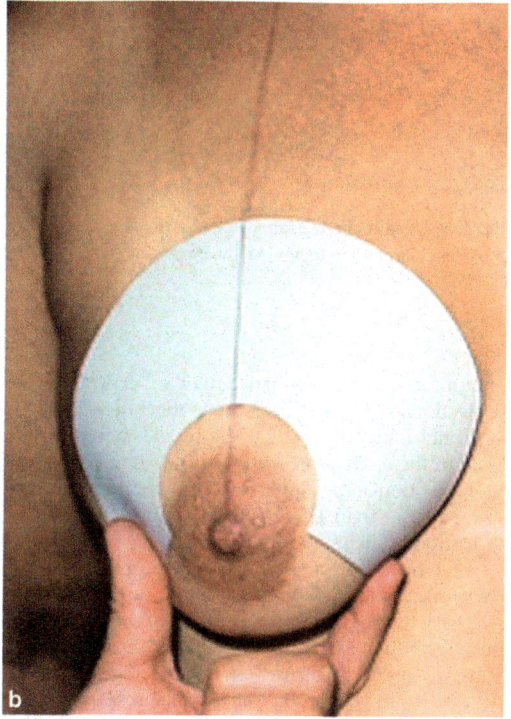

Fig. 47.1 (a) The keyhole pattern comprises an internal circle 3.5 cm radius (r), two divergent 5 cm long straight limbs (sl) originating from the center of the internal circle with 125° opening angle (a) and an external circle arising from the end of the straight limbs to define the middle line of the pattern. (b) The middle line of the pattern coincides with the clavicle–nipple line to provide a nipple–areola transposition without distortion

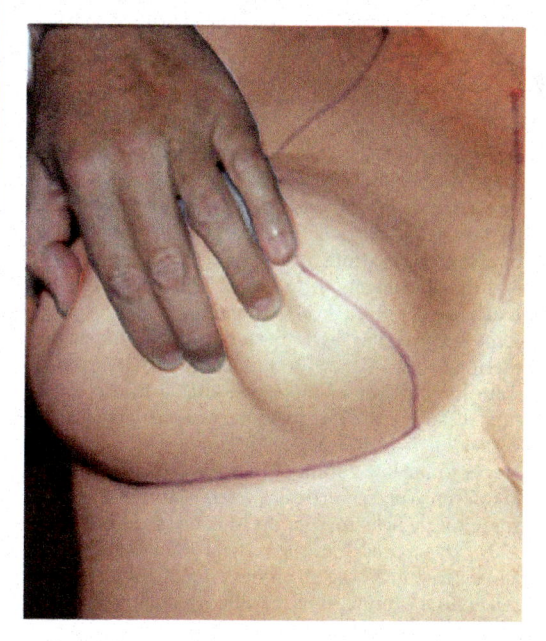

Fig. 47.2 Junction of the end of the straight limb with the inframammary line is done 5 cm away from the thorax midline

Fig. 47.3 A vertical flap to support the nipple–areola is outlined from the proximal end of the straight limbs to the lower border of the areola, 1.5 cm farther than the areolar diameter

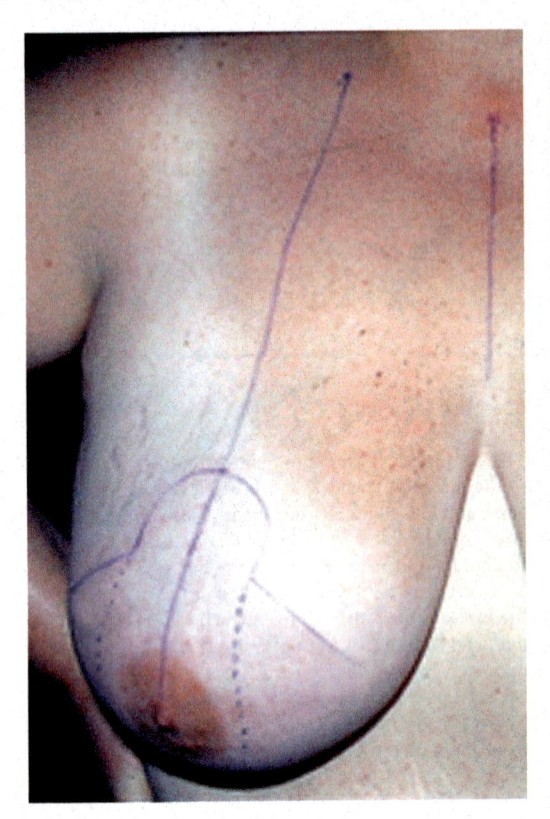

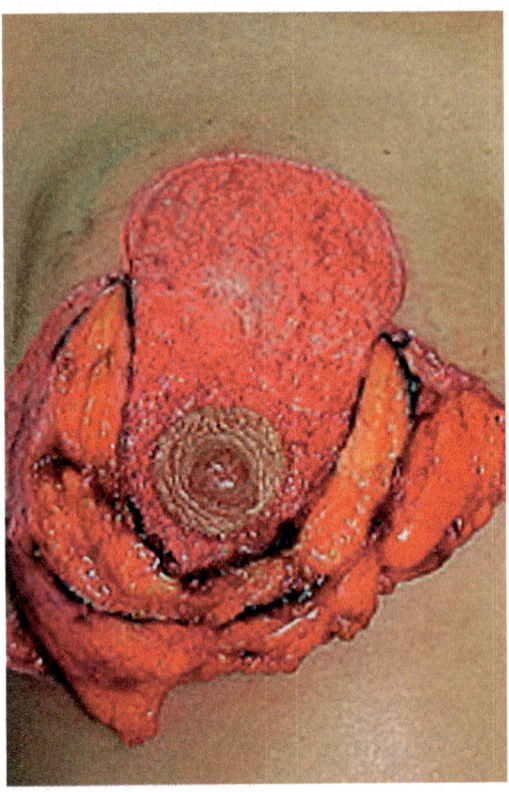

Fig. 47.4 Deepithelialization of the outlined vertical flap provides a dermal bed to nourish the nipple–areola

nipple–areola (Fig. 47.4). The mammary tissue of the lower pole of the breast inside the boundaries of the pattern is removed, creating two vertical pillars for the breast. The length of the vertical pillars is the length of the straight limbs of the pattern. The upper pole and its attachments to the chest wall are maintained intact except by a keel of mammary tissue deeply removed over the fascia pectoralis at the upper pole meridian (Fig. 47.5). The tunnel created is extended from the new site of the nipple–areola to the second intercostal space. The mammary tissue beneath the vertical flap is thoroughly removed from its distal aspect to the lower limit of the new site of the nipple–areola creating a vertical, merely dermal, flap with superior pedicle to support the nipple–areola (Fig. 47.6). The approach of the vertical pillars provides the advancement of the mammary tissue of the upper pole into the tunnel at its meridian, reducing the breast circumference with enhancement of central breast projection (Fig. 47.7). Then the vertical dermal flap is vertically folded up so that the nipple–areola can be fixed in the circle representing its new site (Fig. 47.8). Transposition of the nipple–areola can be safety accomplished more than 15 cm without flatness, traction, or distortion of the nipple–areola.

After the nipple areolar flap is held in position, the color, and capillary refill of the nipple–areola is evaluated to detect torsion or compression of the flap around its longitudinal axis. The test with fluorescein sodium is not regularly performed. It is only employed when the nipple–areola presents signals of vascular compromise after the transposition. In that case, an intravenous injection with 10 cc of fluorescein sodium 10% is applied. The operating room is darkened and the color of the nipple-areola is evaluated with ultraviolet light. In the absence of vascular compromise the nipple–areola acquire an yellow-green color 1 min after the intravenous injection of fluorescein sodium increasing the color until the minute six (Fig. 47.9). Return to the natural color occurs until 8 min since the intravenous injection of fluorescein sodium. When vascular suffering is established nipple–areola acquires a dark blue color that remains after 8 min of the intravenous injection of fluorescein sodium. If impending nipple–areola necrosis is observed at the end of the operation the nipple–areola dermal flap is converted to a free nipple–areola graft.

47.6
Appraisal and Complications

Reduction of breast circumference with enhancement of central breast projection is achieved in reduction mammaplasty with a superior vertical dermal pedicle for the nipple–areola to massive breast hypertrophy and severe ptosis (Fig. 47.10). Deformities of the nipple–areola as flatness, distortion, and traction are not encountered. By no means is breast feeding possible with a superior vertical dermal pedicle for the nipple–areola.

Loss of sensation and vascular compromise can occur. To better evaluation of the sensibility and vascular viability the nipple is analyzed separately from the areola that is divided into four quadrants. Subjective cutaneous contact tests employing crude touch with cotton and needle pressure are used to evaluate nipple–areola sensation (Fig. 47.11). It is expressed by contraction after crude touch with cotton and pain after needle pressure. No permanent loss of sensation of the nipple–areola occurred after reduction mammaplasty with a superior vertical dermal pedicle for the nipple–areola. The level of nipple–areola sensory perception can decrease by using a dermal pedicle for the nipple–areola but it is not frequently. Response of the nipple–areola sensation to crude touch and needle pressure take place at the same time. Return of the nipple sensation occurs until month

Fig. 47.5 The *arrow* shows the tunnel created by the keel of mammary tissue removed at the meridian of the upper pole of the breast

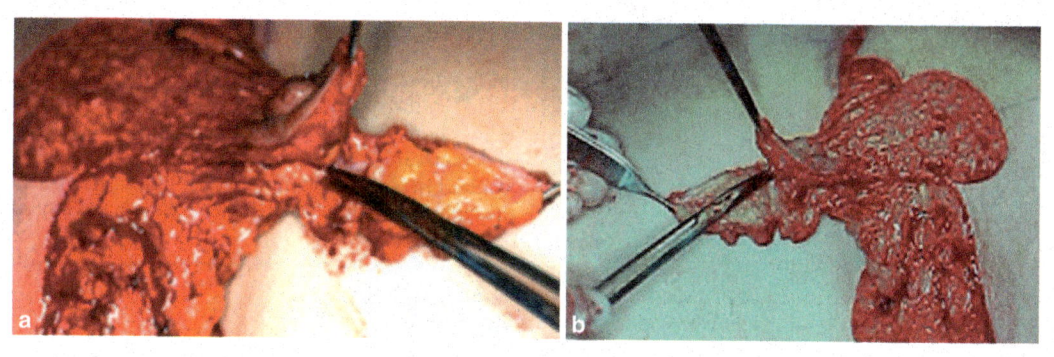

Fig. 47.6 (a) The mammary tissue is removed from the vertical flap. (b) A dermal flap supported on the upper pole of the breast supplies the nipple–areola

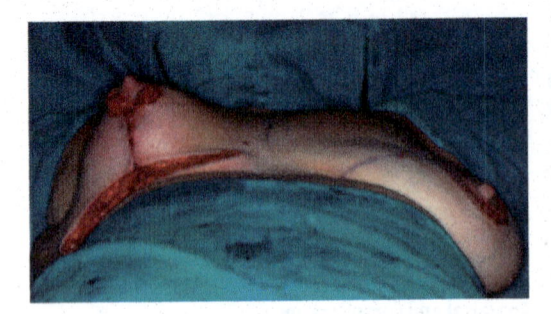

Fig. 47.7 Increase of the breast projection with a reduction of its diameter occurs after the approach of vertical pillars. They become evident compared to the right breast with the left one

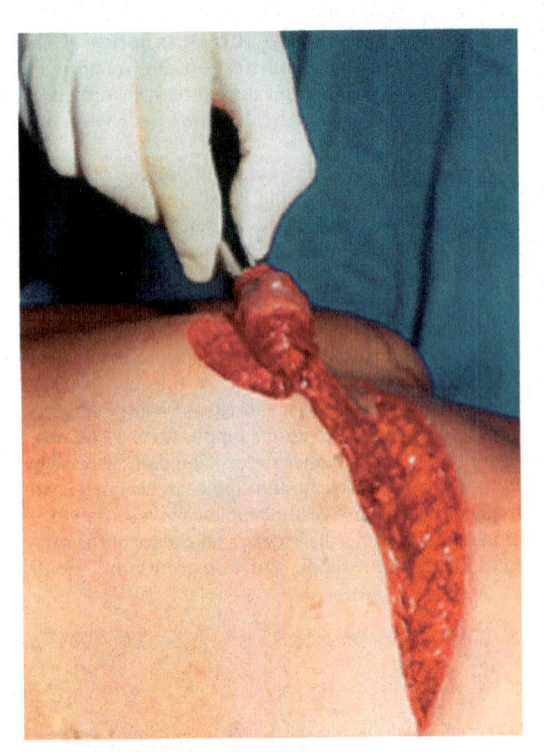

Fig. 47.8 Transposition of the nipple–areola is safety accomplished without distortion

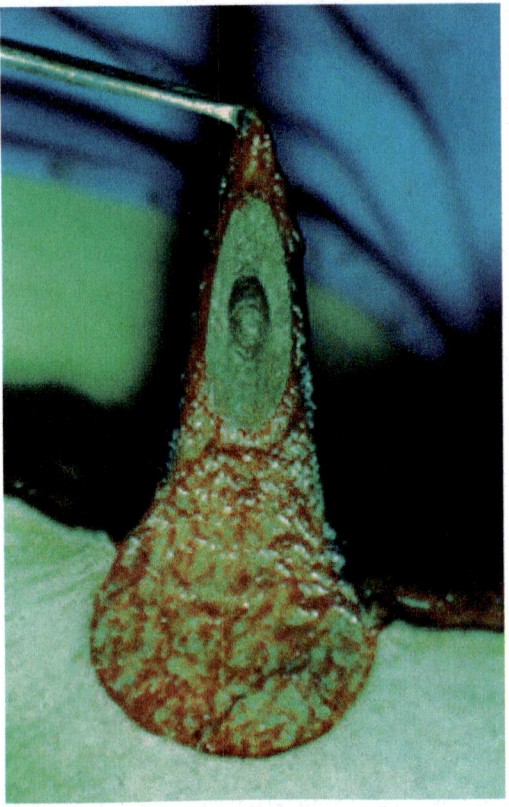

Fig. 47.9 A *dark yellow-green color* is observed in the nipple–areola after 6 min of intravenous injection of fluorescein sodium 10%

1 after the surgery. Recovery of the areola sensation begins firstly on the superior medial quadrant followed by the superior lateral quadrant, inferior medial quadrant, and the inferior lateral quadrant. It is recovered in all quadrants at month 6 postoperatively. A significant difference in the return of sensation between the superior and inferior quadrants of the nipple–areola occurs until the third month after the surgery. Return of the nipple-areola sensation is more delayed, the more nipple-areola is elevated and the more breast tissue is removed. The dark blue color observed during the test with fluorescein sodium always shows clearly the vascular compromise of the nipple-areola. However, yellow-green color ordinarily ensures the viability of the nipple–areola. Necrosis of the nipple-areola supported by the superior vertical dermal pedicle compromises more the lower quadrants than the superior quadrants. The superior medial quadrant of the nipple-areola presents less compromise (Fig. 47.12). Necrosis of the nipple and entire areola is not a common situation.

47.7
Discussion

Measurements in reduction mammaplasty are helpful to address an appropriate correction of the breast deformities that are acquired with pregnancy, age, and excessive amount of weight loss. Westreich [28] established the

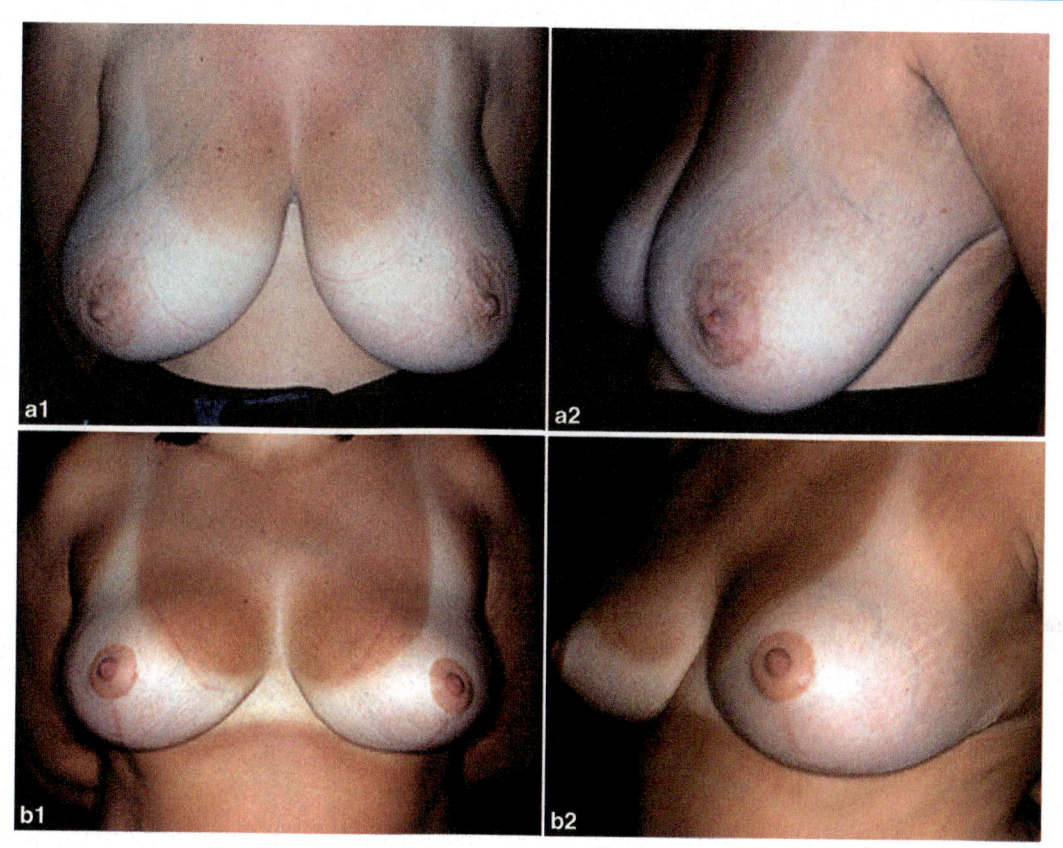

Fig. 47.10 (*a1,2*) Preoperative view of massive breast hypertrophy with severe breast ptosis causing mild asymmetry with the left breast more hypertrophic than the right one. (*b1,2*) At month 10 postoperatively, the length of the superior vertical dermal pedicle was 14 cm long. The amount of mammary tissue removed on the right breast was 1.345 g and on the left breast 1.670 g

nipple–clavicle line from a clavicular point placed 5 cm laterally to the manubrial–clavicular joint, as guideline for displacement of the nipple–areola. Translate the nipple–clavicle line to a point 7 cm distant from the suprasternal notch, and allow to counteract the lateral deviation of the breast and nipple–areola that occurs in massive breast hypertrophy. It also avoids medial distortion of the vertical dermal flap during nipple–areola transposition. The distance from the areola to the inframammary fold is settled in 5 cm, since it represents a close approximation to the median values founded in a normal female population [29]. Also, the short distance between the nipple–areola and the inframammary fold restrains the down advancement of the breast.

Breastfeeding after reduction mammaplasty with a superior vertical dermal pedicle for the nipple–areola is not possible because of the absence of mammary tissue in the pedicle.

The skin and the superficial mammary tissue of the upper pole have a rich intradermal blood supply next to the nipple–areola created by the superficiality of the anterior perforating branches of the internal mammary artery [25]. Likewise, the skin of the upper pole has a rich dermal innervation provided by the supraclavicular nerves [30]. The subcutaneous course of the anterior cutaneous branches of the 3rd, 4th, and 5th intercostal nerves becomes more superficial as they approach the areola also creating a dermal innervation for the nipple–areola [31].

The deep resection of mammary tissue at the meridian of the upper pole does not compromise its superficial vascularity and innervation at the level of the nipple–areola. Despite its thinness, the superior vertical dermal pedicle preserves the blood supply and sensation of the nipple–areola through its dermal connection, because it is based on the skin and superficial mammary tissue of the untouched upper pole of the breast.

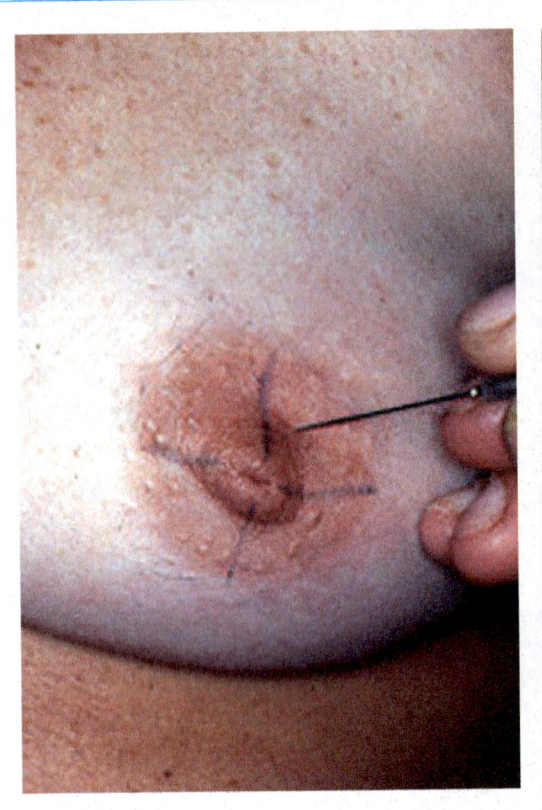

Fig. 47.11 Qualitative evaluation of the nipple–areola sensation with crude touch using needle pressure. Nipple–areola was divided into four quadrants for better evaluation

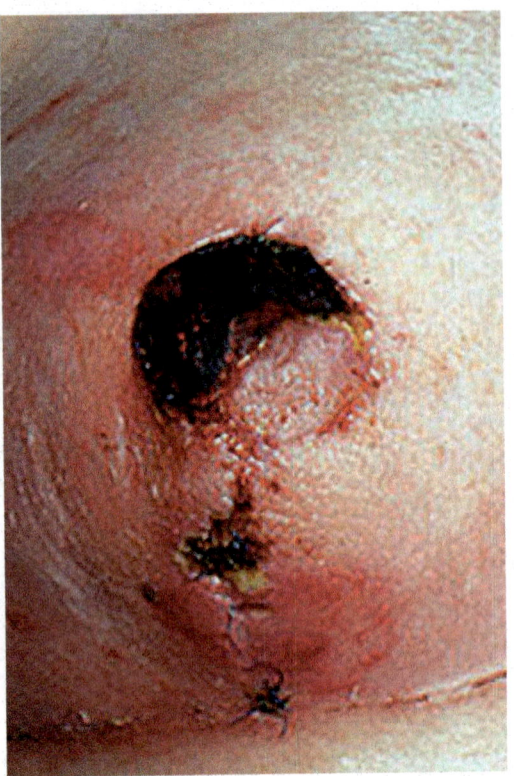

Fig. 47.12 Vascular compromise involving superior quadrants and the lateral inferior quadrant of the nipple–areola

An excessive long and thick flap folded over itself can compromise its blood supply and sensibility. The excess inelastic glandular tissue beneath the folded flap can squeeze and twist either the flap or the pedicle causing ischemia of the nipple–areola. Unlikely, the minimal thickness of the vertical dermal flap with superior pedicle does not cause pressure over itself or against its pedicle allowing a safe nipple–areola transposition without distortion. The lack of breast tissue under the top of the mammary cone, provided by the deep resection of mammary tissue at the upper pole meridian, avoids pressure over the pedicle of the folded dermal flap preserving the blood supply and sensation of the nipple–areola [31].

The test to evaluate the viability of the nipple–areola with fluorescein sodium 10% has partial relevance. It is effective to identify the compromise of the blood supply when the nipple–areola exhibits dark blue color, but it does not exclude the possibility of later suffering of the nipple–areola when yellow-green color is exhibited [32]. However, when impeding nipple–areola necrosis develops after transposition the dermal flap of the nipple–areola is converted to a free graft. It is performed at the end of the operation, to enhance the possibility of a devascularized nipple–areola viable as a free graft and to avoid patient return to the operating room a few hours later, as proposed by Wray and Luce [33].

47.8
Conclusions

The vertical dermal flap with superior pedicle for the nipple–areola is an alternative to free graft of the nipple–areola in reduction mammaplasty for massive breast hypertrophy and severe ptosis of the breast.

References

1. Vandeput JJ, Nelissen M: Considerations on anthropometric measurements of the female breast. Aesth Plast Surg 2002;26:348
2. Romano JJ, Francel TJ, Hoopes JE: Free nipple graft reduction mammaplasty Ann Plast Surg 1992;28:271
3. Jackson IT, Bayramicli M, Grupta M, Yavuzer R: Importance of the pedicle length measurement in reduction mammaplasty. Plast Reconstr Surg 1999;104:398
4. Robbins TH: Reduction mammoplasty by the Robbins technique. Plast Reconstr Surg 1987;79:308
5. Hugo NE, McClellan RN: Reduction mammaplasty with a single superior-based pedicle. Plast Reconstr Surg 1979;63:230
6. Abramo AC: Pattern for reduction mammoplasty that uses a superior vertical dermal pedicle. Aesthetic Plast Surg 1991;15:265
7. Nahabedian MY, McGibbon BM, Manson PN: Medial pedicle reduction mammaplasty for severe mammary hypertrophy. Plast Reconstr Surg 2000;105:896
8. Blondeel PN, Handi M, Van de Sijpe KA, Van Landeryt KH, Thiessen FE, Monstrey SJ: The latero-central glandular pedicle technique for breast reduction. Br J Plast Surg 2003;56:348
9. Reynolds JEF, Trasad AB: Fluorescein sodium. In: Martindale, The Extra Pharmacopea, 28 edn. Great Britain, Farmaceutical Society, The Farmaceutical Press 1982
10. Hamdi M, Greuse M, Nemec F, Deprez C, De Mey A: Breast sensation after superior pedicle versus inferior pedicle mammaplasty: anatomical and histological evaluation. Br J Plast Surg 2001;54:43
11. Schlenz I, Rigel S, Schemper M, Kusbari R: Alteration of nipple and areola sensitivity by reduction mammaplasty: a prospective comparison of five techniques. Plast Reconstr Surg 2005;115:743
12. Santanelli F, Paolini G, Bitarelli D, Nofroni I: Computer-assisted evaluation of nipple-areola complex sensibility in macromastia and following superolateral pedicle reduction mammaplasty. Plast Reconstr Surg 2007;119:1679
13. Abramo AC: Reduction mammaplasty with superior vertical dermal pedicle. Dissertation presented at Paulista Medicine School, Federal University of São Paulo to obtain Master Degree in Plastic Reconstructive Surgery. São Paulo 1988
14. Hamdi M, Greuse M, De Mey A, Webster MH: A prospective quantitative comparison of breast sensation after superior and inferior pedicle mammaplasty. Br J Plast Surg 2001;54:39
15. Wechselberger G, Stob S, Schoeller T, Oehlbauer M, Peza-Katzer H: An analysis of breast sensation following inferior pedicle mammaplasty and the effect of the volume of resected tissue. Aesth Plast Surg 2001;25:443
16. Kreithen J, Caffee H, Rosenberg J, Chin G, Clayman M, Lawson M, Seagle MB: A comparison of the Lejour and Wise pattern methods of breast reduction. Ann Plast Surg 2005;54:236
17. Schwarzmann E: Die technic der mamoplastik. Chirurgentagung 1930;2:932
18. Arie G: Una nueva técnica de Mastoplastia. Rev Latinoam Cir Plast 1957;3:23
19. Strombeck JO: Mammaplasty: Report of a new technique based on the two-pedicle procedure. Br J Plast Surg 1960;13:79
20. Skoog T: A technique of the breast reduction. Acta Chir Scand 1963;126:453
21. McKissock PK: Reduction mammaplasty with a vertical dermal flap. Plast Reconstr Surg 1972;49:245
22. Weiner DL, Aiache AE, Silver L, Tittiranonda T: A single dermal pedicle for nipple transposition in subcutaneous mastectomy, or mastopexy. Plast Reconstr Surg 1973;51:115
23. Courtiss EH, Goldwyn RM: Breast sensation before and after plastic surgery. Plast Reconstr Surg 1976;58:1
24. O'Dey D, Prescher A, Pallua N: Vascular reliability of nipple-areola complex-bearing pedicles: An anatomical microdissection study. Plast Reconstr Surg 2007;119:1167
25. Serafin D: Surgical anatomy of the breast. In: Georgiade NG (ed). Breast Reconstruction Following Mastectomy. C.V. Mosby, St. Louis, Toronto, London 1979, pp 35–53
26. Lockhart RD, Hamilton GF, Fyfe FW: Anatomy of the Human Body, 2 edn. London, Faber and Faber 1959
27. Schlenz I, Kasbari R, Gruber H, Holle J: The sensitivity of the nipple-areola complex: An anatomic study. Plast Reconstr Surg 2000;105:905
28. Weistreich M: Anthropomorphic breast measurement: Protocol and Results in 50 Women with aesthetically perfect breasts and clinical application. Plast Reconstr Surg 1997;100:468
29. Smith DJ, Palin WE Jr, Katch VL, Bennett JE: Breast volume and anthropomorphic measurements: normal values. Plast Reconstr Surg 1986;78:331
30. Farina MA, Newby BG, Alani HM: Innervation of the nipple-areola complex. Plast Reconstr Surg 1980;66:497
31. Schlenz I, Rigel S, Schemper M, Kusbari R: Alteration of nipple and areola sensitivity by reduction mammaplasty: a prospective comparison of five techniques. Plast Reconstr Surg 2005;115:743
32. Abramo AC, Oliveira LMF, Milan RC, Mateus S: Evaluation of nipple-areola complex sensibility after reduction mammaplasty by superior vertical dermal pedicle. Rev Soc Bras Cir Plast 1999;14:7
33. Wray RC, Luce EA: Treatment of impending nipple necrosis following reduction mammaplasty. Plast Reconstr Surg 1981;68:242

Liposuction and Superior Pedicle

Felix Giebler, Eva Giebler

48.1 Introduction

Most of the vascularization of the breast comes from superiorly the lateral thoracic artery, from the perforators of the internal mammary, and from the intercostal perforators three to six [1, 2]. The nipple–areolar complex (NAC) is perfused by superficial dermal vessels [3] that are important for cosmetic procedures and deepithelialization. The lymphatic drainage of the breast is established by the axillary lymph nodes and the parasternal (interthoracic) primary lymph nodes.

The vascularization and the innervation (from the superior portion of the supra clavicle nerves and from the third to fifth branches of the clavicle plexus) are highly important for the formation and the function of a flap or pedicle [4]. A cosmetic procedure on the breast should not interfere with the sensitivity or the vascularization of the NAC, in order to not hamper its function and its erotic function, too. Whichever technique is used, it is important to preserve the nipple sensation [5].

48.2 History

The reduction techniques in breast surgery started at the beginning of the last century and were subsequently improved on in order to get better aesthetic result with less scarring and sufficient functioning. The first reduction plasty was the transposition of the NAC that was established by Lexer in 1912 [6] and was republished in 1923 by Kraske [7]. The superior pedicle techniques are the modern ones that started with Pitanguy in 1957 [8]. Afterwards, there were a lot of techniques described that are named partly after the closure technique of the skin such as the vertical "T" technique from Strömbeck [9] that was reduced to a vertical or "L" technique by Lassus [10] and Lejour [11]. The superior pedicle technique allows the free resection of the inferior tissue, leaving the superior vascular base intact. Parenchymal resection may be performed medial and lateral to the pedicle but not superior to the NAC. Combination of the reduction techniques with liposuction opened new horizons [12, 13]. "Preoperative" liposuction reduces the volume of the breast before the resection and makes it possible, even in cases of a larger breast, to have a well vascularized NAC flap instead of the necessity of a free nipple graft. The disadvantages are delayed healing by more bruising and the calcifications, which may interfere with mammography (Table 48.1).

48.3 Technique

The superior pedicle technique is best applied to moderate breast reductions of 500 g [14]. In cases of larger breast volumes, combination with the liposuction procedure is advisable [15] (Fig. 48.1). Accessory liposuction after deepithelialization helps to reduce the breast size before the coned form or keel resection so that the removal of 750 g on each side is still safe, with the required length of the superior pedicle of 10–12 cm. The thickness of the pedicle should be at least 1.5 cm and the width not less than 6 cm. Liposuction is implemented after infiltration with Klein solution [16] with blunt three-hole cannulas 1–4 mm in diameter. It is wise not to form the pedicle with liposuction in order to not interfere with the vascularization.

After transposition, the NAC should be fixed on to a deepithelialized area that contains the small vessels, which give contact to the dermis of the pedicle and check the vascularization of the NAC. Swelling or dark blue coloring are signs of a hampered vascularization.

One sequela of the vertical reduction technique is sometimes lateral fullness of the breast. This lateral fullness can be the result of insufficient rotation of the lateral pillars to the midline or leaving too much tissue laterally. Especially in this case, liposuction of the breast can remove the fullness prior to the suturing of the pillars. There is still the possibility of contouring the lateral breast after the pleating of the pillars (Figs. 48.2, 48.3).

The superior pedicle technique may be applied with the inverted "T" technique and the vertical skin technique. We personally combine the superior pedicle technique with the free positioning of the NAC after deepithelialization,

Table 48.1 Advantages of Liposuction in the Breast

Breast is more supple and pliable
Sculpturing of the lateral and subaxillar fat
Shaping of the lower breast to prevent dog ears
Correction of asymmetry at the end of the operation
A more stable result?
Reducing the volume of the breast before the resection in order to get a shorter vertical scar

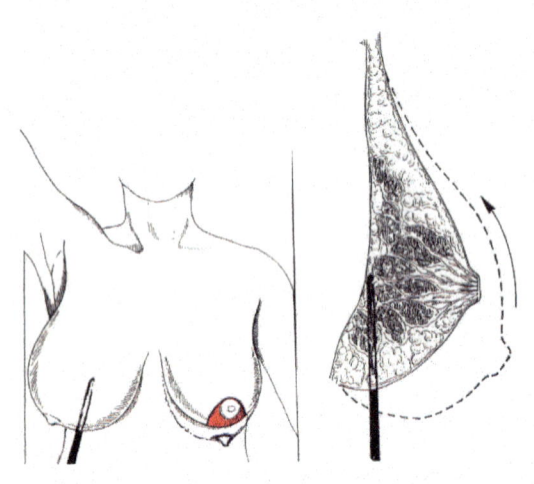

Fig. 48.1 Scheme of liposuction of the breast before tissue excision. Notice the reduction of volume and the associated rising of the NAC

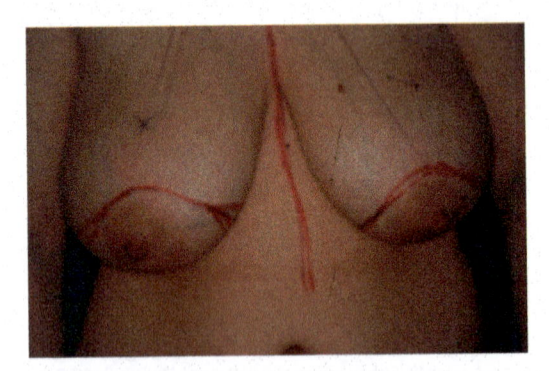

Fig. 48.2 Marking the midline preoperatively shows the preoperative asymmetry. In only 12% symmetry is to be found

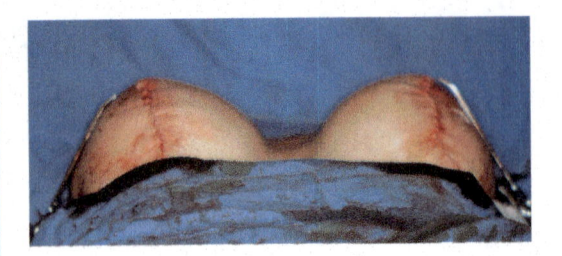

Fig. 48.3 Checking for symmetry from the foot of the bed. The base of the left breast is wider. The next step is free nipple positioning with sizer and deepithelialization

after first doing a specified glanduloplasty, combined with the coned form resection of the gland with a superficial zigzag plasty of the lower breast and ends up with a vertical scar [18]. The combined liposuction of the breast is bound to a good quality and elasticity of the skin (Fig. 48.4).

48.4 Complications

Complications after mammoplasty with a superior pedicle and liposuction result usually from errors in judgement, planning, and technique. Exceeding the length of the pedicle by more than 15 cm and elevating the nipple by more than 10 cm may cause trouble. The possible slough of the nipple with deformation of the NAC and changes in the sensibility, especially the possible loss of erotic sensibility, may change the quality of life and has to be explained to the patient [19, 20].

48.5 Discussion

The vertical technique combined with a superior pedicle and a free nipple transposition gives the mammoplasty the possibility of a more freehand approach. This technique allows more flexibility of the nipple positioning than the preformed keyhole pattern technique. In particular, when combined with the liposuction technique established directly after the first deepithelialization or established to correct the lateral aspect of the breast at the end of the glanduloplasty gives the possibility of a more creative and individualized operative result. Especially, in the case of macromastia, liposuction gives the possibility of ending the operation with a smaller vertical scar [21].

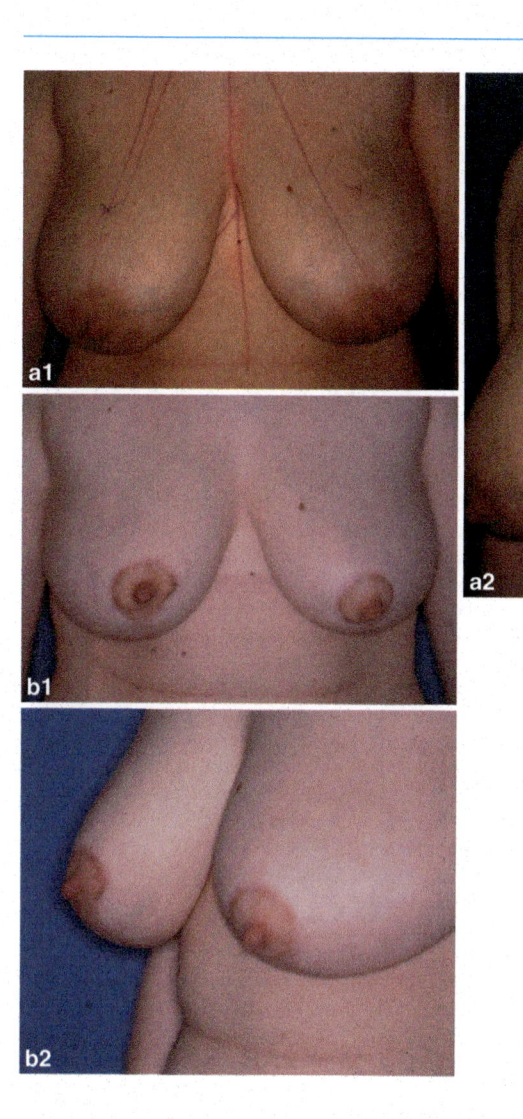

Fig. 48.4 (**a***1,2*) Preoperative 30-year-old patient. (**b***1,2*) Six months postoperative after resection of 270 g from each side and liposuction 100 g from each side (supranatant fat). Notice the rising of the NAC of about 2 cm. It is important to place the nipple at the end operation too low in order to prevent a sky-scraping deformation

48.6 Conclusions

The aim of the cosmetic breast surgery is to form an aesthetic breast with sufficient projection, central NAC position, and functional preservation. The preservation of the feeding function of the breast is seen in most of the cases, although patients are informed of a positive result of only 50% [22]. Beyond statistical summations, it is of importance to inform your patients about all possible complications (this requested by law). The doctor is legally obliged to fully disclose all information to his patient that is necessary to enable the patient to choose intelligently whether or not to accept an operation. Each point should be countersigned by the patient in the written consent (Table 48.2).

The first step towards this goal is the exact forming of the breast hillock. The refinements at the end of the operation, possible "dog ears," for example, may be corrected by liposuction after free contouring of the new breast and free positioning of the NAC with the superior pedicle that enables a good result.

Table 48.2 What to tell the patient? Total information requested by law

Asymmetry of the breasts	10%
Scarring	15%
Haematoma	6–10%
Necrosis of the NAC	0.5–7%
Deformation of the NAC immediately p.o.	10%
Deformation of the NAC permanent	1%
Nipple retraction	1–4%
NAC asymmetry	10%
NAC unequal in height	10%
Loss of sensibility	8%
Loss of erotic sensibility	1%
Hyper-sensibility of the NAC	4%
Loss of breastfeeding function	50%
Interference with mammogram	100%

A long learning curve shows you the way from the pattern linked reduction techniques to the more free hand techniques, which are better suited for this important symmetrical dual pedicle organ [23]. The individualized technique is supported by the superior vertical pedicle technique, liposuction, and vertical resection [24].

References

1. Edwards E: Surgical anatomy of the breast. In: Goldwyn RM (ed). Plastic and Reconstructive Surgery of the Breast. Boston, Little Brown 1976
2. Rohen JW: Topographische Anatomie. Stuttgart, Schattauer 1971, pp 95–99
3. Mitz V, Lassau JP: Etude des rapports entre les vascularisations arterielles glandulaires et cutanees du sein. Arch Anat Path 1973;21(4):365–374
4. Maliniac JW: Arterial blood supply of the breast: revised anatomic data relating to reconstructive surgery. Arch Surg 1043;47:329
5. Wuringer E, Mader N, Posch E, Holle J: Nerve and vessel supplying ligamentous suspension of the mammary gland. Plast Reconstr Surg 1988;101(6):1486–1493
6. Lexer E: Hypertrophie beider mammae. Munch Med Wochenschr 1912;59:2702
7. Kraske H: Die operation der atrohischen und hypertrophischen hangbrust. Munch Med Wochenschr 1923;60: 672–673
8. Pitanguy I: Une nouvelle technique mammaire. Etude de 245 cas consecutifs et presentation d'une technique personelle. Ann Chir Plast 1962;7:199–208
9. Strombeck JO: Mammaplasty: report of a new technique based on the two pedicle procedure. Br J Plast Surg 1960; 13:79–90
10. Lassus C: Breast reduction: evaluation of a technique – a single vertical scar. Plast Reconstr Surg 1995;3:189–198
11. Lejour M: Vertical mammaplasty for breast hypertrophy and ptosis. Operative technique. Plast Reconstr Surg 1996;3:189–198
12. Hohler H: Die reduktionsplastik der weiblichen brust. Zeitschrift Plast Chir 1978;2:68–91
13. Lejour M: Vertical mammaplasty and liposuction of the breast. Plast Reconstr Surg 1994;94(1):100–114
14. Teimourian B, Massac E, Wiegering CE: Reduction suction mammoplasty and suction lipectomy as an adjunct to breast surgery. Reduction suction mammoplasty and suction lipectomy as an adjunct to breast surgery. Aesthetic Plast Surg 1985;9(2):97–100
15. Zocchi M: Ultrasonic liposculpturing. Aesthetic Plast Surg 1992;16(4):287–298
16. Klein JA: The tumescent technique for liposuction surgery. Am J Cosm Surg 1987;4:2163–267
17. Skoog T: A technique of breast reduction – transposition of the nipple on a cutaneous vascular pedicle. Acta Chir Scand 1963;126:453–465
18. Giebler FRG: Vertikale reduktionsplatik. Aesth Trib, Wiesbaden 2006;7:15
19. Hamdi M, Greuse M, Nemec E, Deprez C, DeMay A: Breast sensation after superior pedicle versus inferior pedicle mammaplasty: anatomical and histological evaluation. Br J Plast Surg 2001;54(1):43–46
20. Craig RD, Sykes PA: Nipple sensitivity following reduction mammaplasty. Br J Plast Surg 1970;23(2):167–172
21. Toledo LS, Matsudo PKR: Mammaplasty using liposuction and the periareolar incision. Aesthetic Plast Surg 1989; 13(1):9–13
22. Schlenz I, Kuzbari R, Gruber H, Holle J: The sensitivity of the nipple-areola complex: an anatomic study. Plast Reconstr Surg 2000;105(3):905–909
23. Hinderer UT: Mammaplasty techniques in the treatment if the ptotic breast with hypertrophy, of average size, or with hypoplasia. In Zaoli G (ed). Advances in Aesthetic Plastic Surgery. Padova, Piccin Nuova Libraria 2001, pp 409–450
24. Lewis JR Jr: Reduction mammaplasty. Borrowing the good points of many techniques. Aesthetic Plast Surg 1976;1: 43–55

Superior Medial Pedicle Breast Reduction and Auto Augmentation

Mike Huntly, Ronald Finger

49.1 Introduction

For most plastic surgeons emerging from residency programs in the 1980s, the central pedicle or inferior pedicle breast reduction technique was the method of choice. This technique, incorporating the Wise pattern, was reliable and produced good results often maintaining the ability to breast feed. Disadvantages were extensive dissection of breast tissue, long operating times, and a tendency to "bottom out" over time. Nipple movement more than 15 cm vertically could become unreliable and if nipple loss occurred, reconstruction could be difficult because skin and underlying breast tissue could be lost. For larger breast reductions, the authors, like many, adopted a breast amputation technique with free nipple graft. This technique had advantages including simplicity, easy reproducibility, and shorter operating times. This involved removal of the lower segment of the breast as a horizontal ellipse and removal of a vertical wedge of central breast tissue, which when closed created the projection and desired shape. The nipple–areola complex was reapplied as a full thickness skin graft. The upper segments of the breast were left relatively undisturbed including blood supply from medial and lateral perforators and the innervation from intercostal nerve branches (Fig. 49.1). This method yielded excellent shape which could easily be reproduced on the second side. Surprisingly good preservation of nipple sensation was achievable. Disadvantages of this technique were that some loss of nipple projection and changes in texture of the skin of the areola and occasionally loss of pigmentation in patients of color could result. Over time, in my experience, shape held up very well with less tendency for "bottoming out."

Dr. Ronald Finger's superior medial pedicle technique was essentially identical to the breast amputation technique with free nipple–areola graft with the exception that the nipple–areola was transferred on a superior medial pedicle. The breast tissue resection and restoration of breast shape were otherwise identical. The superior medial pedicle proved to be a simple reliable method of moving the nipple–areola complex and preserving normal areola skin texture and nipple appe-arance. Furthermore, this method reduced operating time by approximately 15 min per breast to an average of 45–60 min for an average size breast reduction per side with one surgeon suturing. In the occasional situation where there was concern about nipple–areola circulation, conversion to a nipple graft technique was an easy second option before the end of the procedure. Results have been gratifying for both patient and surgeon in more than 350 cases or 700 plus breasts over the last 10 years.

49.2 Technique

Breasts are marked for reduction in the upright position using the standard Wise pattern centered on the premarked meridian of the breast. The new nipple position is planned in the range 22–27 cm from the sternal notch depending on the patient's stature and desired final breast size. The most common nipple position that corresponds roughly to the position of the inframammary fold or half way between shoulder and elbow with the patient upright is 25 cm.

After prepping the patient, the inframammary fold and lower breast parenchyma is injected with 0.25% Marcaine with epinephrine and 1% lidocaine with epinephrine to reduce intraoperative bleeding and help with postoperative anesthesia. The upper breast segments and in particular the pedicle should not be injected. The breast skin is stretched, and the areola is marked with a cookie cutter using 38–42 mm size range depending on the final size of the reduced breast.

The superior medial pedicle is then deepithelialized. The deepithelialized bed should resemble the appearance of a split thickness skin graft donor site with pinpoint dermal bleeding. The pedicle is incised along line GCEFB, extending into the breast parenchyma (Fig. 49.2). Two double pronged skin hooks are applied

M.A. Shiffman (ed.), *Mastopexy and Breast Reduction: Principles and Practice*,
© Springer-Verlag Berlin Heidelberg 2009

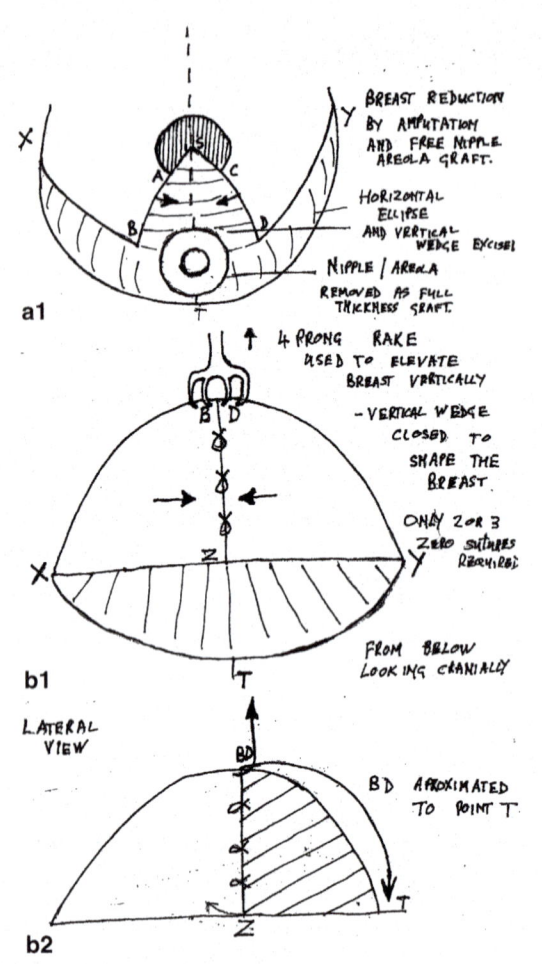

Fig. 49.1 Breast reduction by amputation and free nipple–areolar graft. (*a1*) Nipple–areola complex. removed as a full thickness graft. (*b1,2*) Vertical wedge closed to shape the breast

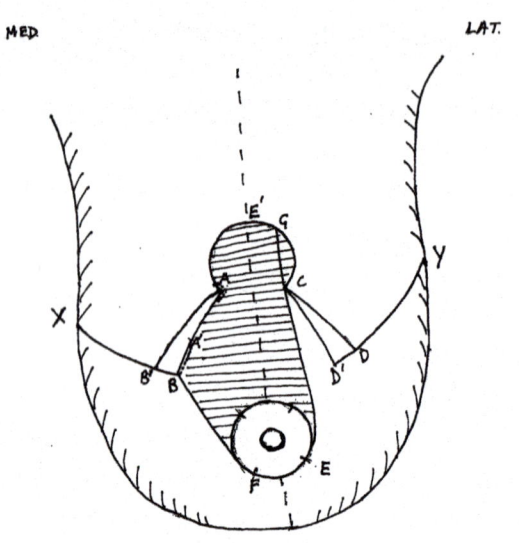

Fig. 49.2 The pedicle is incised along line GCEFB, extending into the breast parenchyma

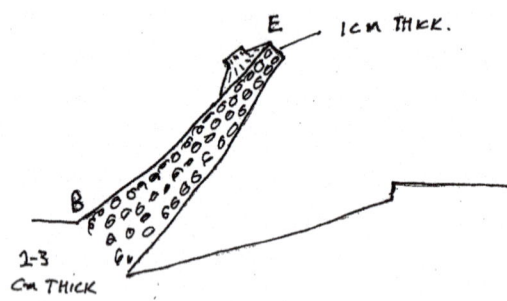

Fig. 49.3 The nipple–areola complex and a thin layer of parenchyma are elevated off the breast

at points E and F and the pedicle is incised on the under surface with a size 10 blade applying gentle vertical traction on the skin hooks. The nipple–areola complex and a thin layer of parenchyma are elevated off the breast (Fig. 49.3). The pedicle is tapered in thickness from 1 cm at the areola to approximately 2–3 cm at the base, with the pedicle slightly stretched. Thinning is done carefully with a #10 blade trying to preserve axial vessels where possible. Pinpoint cautery is used to control bleeders. The undermining should not proceed any further than line A–B. The nipple–areola complex is then rotated upwards approximating points E to E' with a single absorbable monofilament 3-0 or 4-0 buried deep dermal suture. An imaginary line B–E is the radius of the circle of rotation and point E is chosen to maximize length B–E. In situations where B–E is shorter than ideal, A–B can be adjusted to line A–B'. Deepithelializing this additional area will lengthen B–E to B'–E. A corresponding medial shift of C–D to C–D' may be required. The angle between the limbs of the Wise pattern, i.e., between the line A–B and line C–D, is adjusted during preoperative marking to achieve approximate equality in the lengths of lines X–B + D–Y and X–T + T–Y. Occasionally in smaller breasts where the vertical distance the nipple must be transposed is shorter, the pedicle will also be shorter. In these situations, a backcut along B to A' through the dermis and into the breast tissue, can help lengthen the pedicle.

With the nipple/areola relocated at the 12 o'clock areola position, resection of the breast tissue can proceed. When resecting breast tissue the back of the bed should be flat to ensure the parenchyma incision line XBDY is perpendicular to the chest wall. An upright bed back position can result in over resection of breast tissue. Line XBDY is made. A 4-prong facelift rake retractor approximates B and D and another 4-prong rake is placed on the opposite side of the incision. The breast is elevated with vertical traction on both rakes. The breast is split horizontally down to the pectoral fascia and the lower segment of the breast is removed in the form of a horizontal ellipse of skin and breast tissue. Care should be taken to avoid over resection with this initial cut, leaving more tissue on the upper segments of the breast. This is assured by avoiding inclination of the back of the bed and also avoiding downward (caudal) traction on the lower retractor during the initial incision through the breast tissue. The vertical wedge of breast tissue is then excised removing wedge HSCDZ (Fig. 49.4). Staying deep into the pedicle, a 4-prong rake is used to approximate B and D lifting the breast tissue vertically. Additional trimming and shaping of the medial and lateral segments of the remaining breast tissue can be performed. Hemostasis is achieved and the vertical wedge is closed with two or three 0 absorbable sutures. A suction drain is placed and line X–B is approximated to X–T and D–Y to T–Y using staples, advancing the medial and lateral flaps toward the meridian of the breast. This narrows the breast and optimizes shape and projection. The staples can be easily adjusted until shape is optimized. Once satisfied with the breast contour, the staples are replaced with buried deep dermal sutures of absorbable 4-0 or 3-0 monofilament. Generally, it is best to inset the areola prior to closing the vertical incision in case a back cut adjustment is necessary to minimize tension. A small 90° incision through the dermis at point A in the area shown is made. This promotes approximation of points A and C over the pedicle without tension. Generally the smaller breast is operated on first to ensure that weight reduction requirements are met. On the first breast, note is taken of the distance from the midline to point T and attempts are made to reproduce this distance on the second breast, which helps with symmetry.

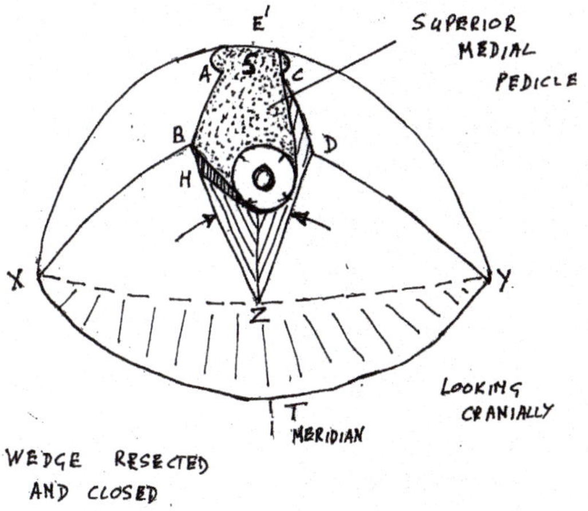

Occasionally the patient preoperatively will have medially displaced nipples, secondary to overgrowth of the lateral segments of the breast. In these patients, a superior lateral pedicle can be used to get the required pedicle length, which would not be available with the superior medial pedicle technique. This is designed exactly the same way only basing the pedicle superior and lateral.

At the end of the procedure, if there is any concern about the viability of the nipple areola complex, it is simple to convert to a full thickness nipple areola graft technique. The nipple–areola is simply harvested and thinned appropriately and the recipient bed is repaired with absorbable sutures, prior to application of the nipple–areola graft. This is secured with a bolster dressing with perforations in the graft, to allow fluid drainage.

All wounds are reinforced with longitudinally applied one inch wide paper strips, followed by a soft dressing of fluff rolls in figure of eight fashion secured with foam or micropore tape.

A soft bra is used. Drains are usually removed on postoperative day 2. The patient can then shower. Paper strips are changed weekly for 4 weeks to support the healing wounds. Ambulation is encouraged starting with the day of surgery. Aerobic activity is allowed in moderation after 3 weeks with a good support bra. Patients are usually kept overnight for observation and pain control. Fitted compression stockings are used perioperatively until the patient is ambulating. Lovenox 40 mg subcutaneously is given to patients at high risk of DVT.

49.3 Results

Patient satisfaction with this technique has been excellent. Breast shape has been well retained with less long term "bottoming out" of the lower pole (Figs. 49.5, 49.6). Nipple sensation has been retained at least as well as with inferocentral pedicle reductions. This has not been a topic of concern for the patients. Often patients with breast hypertrophy have diminished sensation preoperatively, probably as a result of skin stretching which increases the distance between nerve endings. Pedicles as long as 30 cm have been successfully used with this technique. The possibility of conversion to graft technique is discussed with all patients before surgery. Problems with nipple circulation can be minimized by avoiding smoking preoperatively and we insist on a minimum of 3 weeks smoke free before surgery. Tight closure should also be avoided. It is better to resect a little more tissue than close with too much tension on the pedicle. Placing the Wise pattern a little lower on the

Fig. 49.4 The vertical wedge of breast tissue is then excised removing wedge HSCDZ

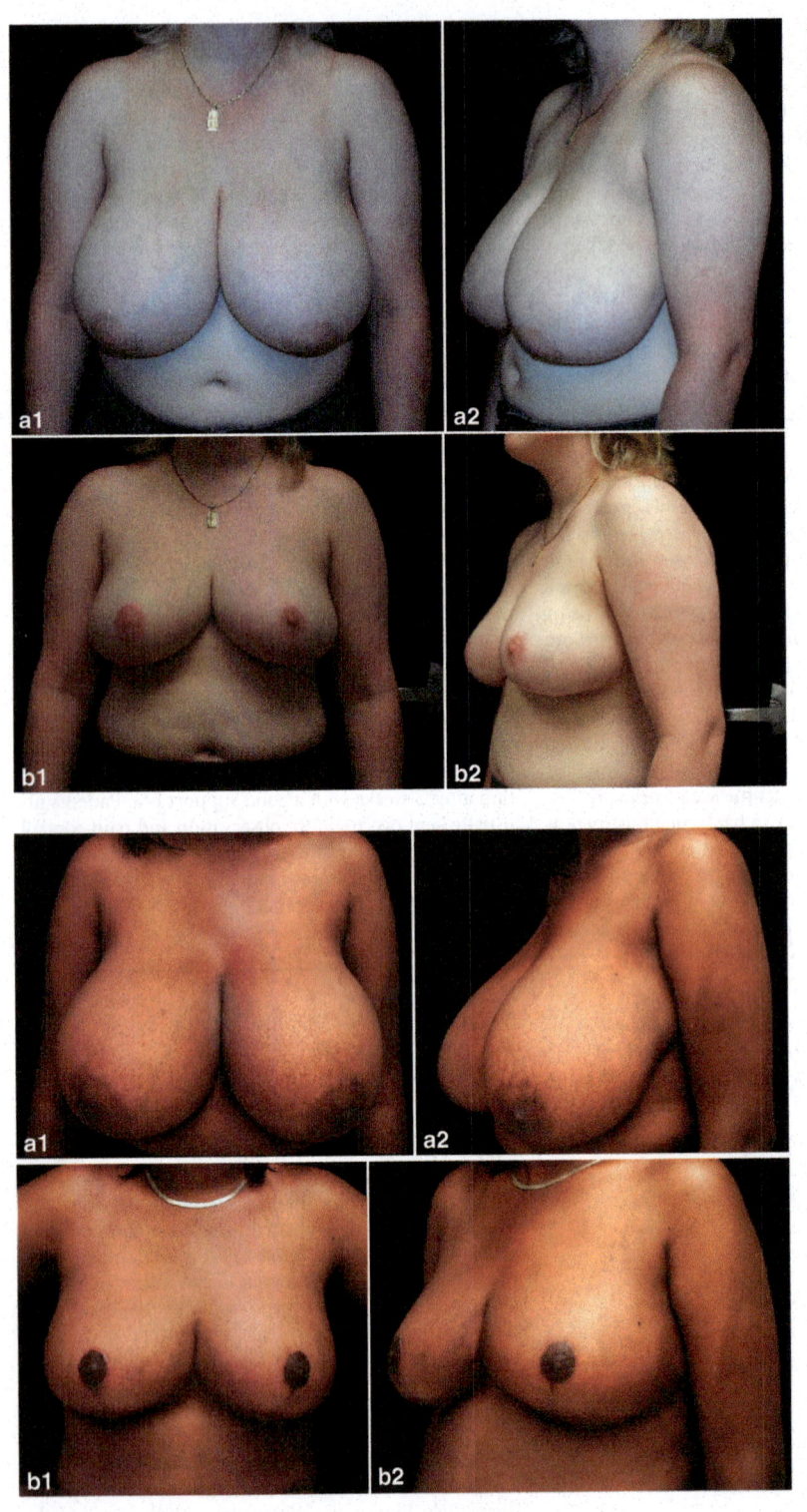

Fig. 49.5 (**a***1,2*) Preoperative 36DD cup size. (**b***1,2*) Post-operative with reduction of 500 g each side. Now is 36C cup size

Fig. 49.6 (**a***1,2*) Preoperative. (**b***1,2*) Postoperative after excision of 1,900 g from each side

breast preserves more skin and for a given breast size will reduce tightness. Avoidance of local anesthetic with epinephrine in proximity to the pedicle is again emphasized. The incidence of conversion to nipple–areola graft has been very low, certainly less than one in fifty breasts.

49.4
Auto Augmentation

Use of the superior medial pedicle or superior lateral pedicle technique frees up the central or inferior pedicle of the breast for auto augmentation. Patients with ptosis and at least a C cup, who do not want to significantly reduce their breast size, can benefit from this concept. The patient is marked for breast reduction placing the pattern a little lower than usual, to preserve skin to avoid a tight closure. This is important because there is more tissue to cover with skin since the lower pole breast tissue is being retained rather than discarded as in breast reduction. The superior medial pedicle is developed as described and transposed. The inferior breast tissue instead of being resected is deepithelialized, trimmed, and shaped into a living breast implant (Fig. 49.7). A central prepectoral pocket is dissected avoiding getting too superficial laterally and medially, which could interfere with innervation and circulation. The implant of living breast tissue is placed in the pocket and secure to the pectoralis fascia with sutures (Fig. 49.7). This restores upper pole fullness and helps secure a sagging or mobile inframammary fold in a more youthful elevated position.

This is a useful alternative for ptosis patients who have intrinsically poor quality skin which is likely to stretch after a standard mastopexy with relapse of breast shape. With this auto augmentation technique the breast tissue heals to the chest wall at a higher level which gives better long term support to maintain breast shape and position (Fig. 49.8).

49.5
Gynecomastia

Severe gynecomastia can also be treated with the superior medial or superior lateral pedicle thinning out the medial and lateral upper pole breast segments to

Fig. 49.7 Auto augmentation. (**a**) Central pedicle is deepithelialized, trimmed, shaped, and buried in the prepectoral space. (**b**) The central/inferior pedicle is buried and secured to the fascia

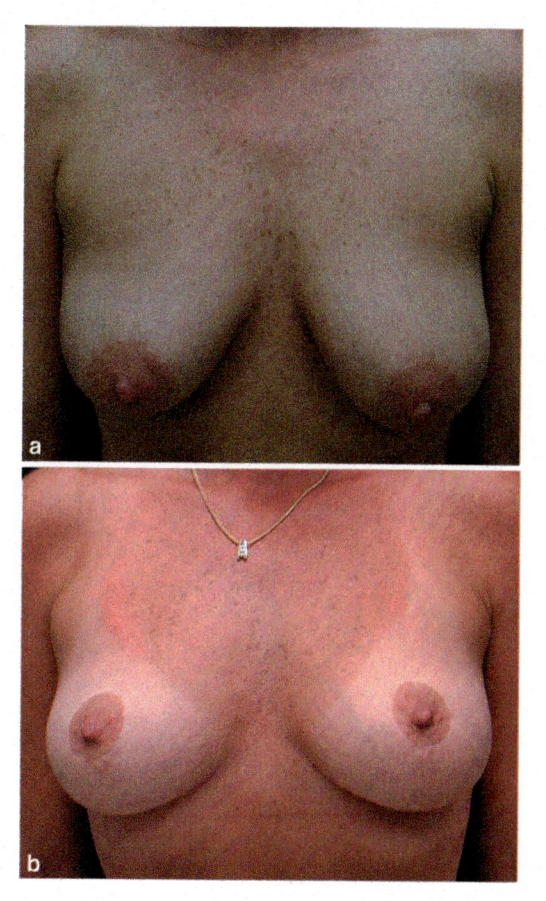

Fig. 49.8 Auto augmentation. (**a**) Preoperative. (**b**) Eighteen months after reduction and auto augmentation

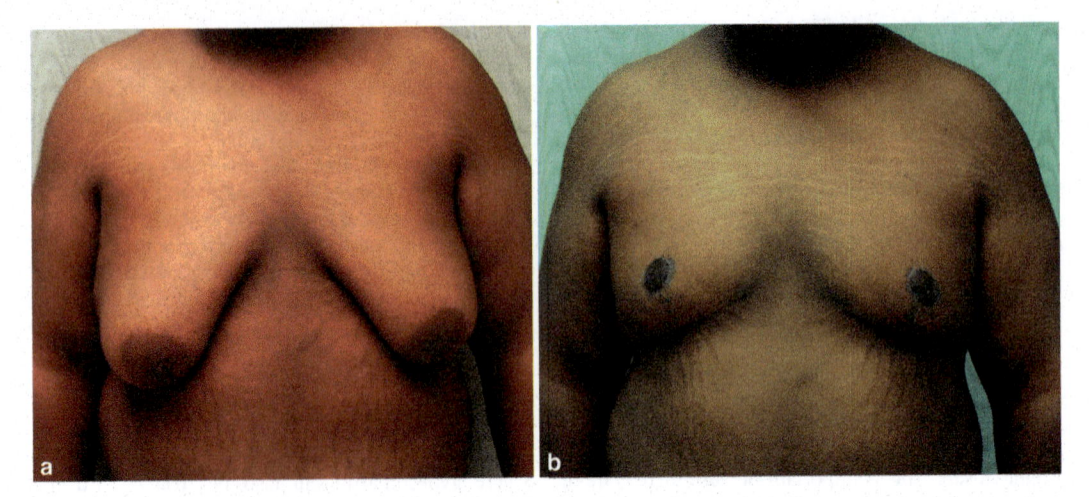

Fig. 49.9 (a) Preoperative male with gynecomastia. (b) Postoperative

achieve desired shape. A central or inferior pedicle may be too thick and bulky to achieve a satisfactory contour (Fig. 49.9).

49.6 Conclusions

This is a simple technique, which can easily minimize dissection of breast tissue and operative time. It involves three basic steps that are pedicle elevation, lower pole resection, and central wedge resection. A little trimming laterally and medially can optimize shape. Nipple–areola graft is an easy secondary option in the rare event of a compromised nipple. Auto augmentation and severe gynecomastia are useful applications of this technique. Initially this method should be utilized on moderate reductions where nipple movement in the range 8–15 cm is required until experience is gained.

Reduction Mammoplasty with the Supero-Lateral Dermoglandular Pedicle Technique

Lázaro Cárdenas-Camarena

50.1
Importance of the Mammary Gland

The female mammary gland is an organ with numerous and varied functions. Although lactation is the function for which it exists, it is not the only one nor the principal one. Lactation is a function that, in addition to providing the best source of food for a newborn, helps establish a close correlation between mother and child. With the passage of time, however, the mammary gland has become the organ of greatest importance in a woman's sensuality. For this reason, it is not currently considered exclusively as an organ with the single function of breastfeeding. The breast, as an isolated structure, has become the sensual part par excellence in all existing cultures and ethnic groups. The differences that the mammary gland can present as an innate part of the idiosyncrasy of each culture in no way limit the beauty that each race or ethnic group confers on it. Therefore, women, based on very particular concepts and ideals, search day to day for the ways and means of having a more pleasing and beautiful breast that will provide them with the desired size and shape.

One of the main problems that the woman faces in the constant search for this ideal is a large breast size. Notwithstanding the fact that often the size she has is only a little larger than the existing aesthetic canons, at other times the size is such that is produces true disabilities and functional alterations. Low self-esteem, personal insecurity, and changes in posture are only a few of the effects that large breasts can cause, and they are often not considered as causal to indicating breast surgery. Although larger sizes may lead to more severe functional and medical problems, such as dermatitis, lumbago, and physical disability, the problems that a large breast generates in the personality of the woman who suffers from it are sometimes more important and significant than the real functional problems it originates.

Mammary hypertrophy therefore constitutes one of the pathologies most often requested to be treated by a plastic surgeon. Taking into account the functions that the mammary gland performs it is undeniable that in its treatment providing the best possible result must be foremost at all times. Its function, aesthetics, and sensual symbolism are only some of the factors that should always be kept in mind when deciding to perform reduction mammoplasty. Assessment of the patient, empathy with her problem, and complete integration of all the factors that affect the environment of her pathology are of primary importance. So much so that one must remember that a patient entrusts us with much more than a mammary gland when it is decided to treat mammary hypertrophy. She trusts that we will return her self-esteem and her sensuality, which she has often never had.

50.2
Factors to be Considered

The techniques of reduction mammoplasty are numerous and varied [1]. New surgical alternatives for the functional aesthetic handling of a hypertrophic breast are constantly being designed and published. The passage of time and the experience acquired have substantially improved the scope and benefits that surgical techniques offer patients. The existence of so many surgical techniques is true testimony that there is no single ideal surgical technique, nor that a single one can solve all the problems that exist with the hypertrophic breast. Undoubtedly, when choosing a particular technique, we should consider and assess all the advantages and disadvantages that the technique itself can provide us. Weighing all these factors is what gives greater value to the choice of a technique that fully meets the need, which we seek for our patients and for ourselves as aesthetic surgeons.

Whatever technique is used in reduction mammoplasty, there are basic concepts that we should always bear in mind. From the anatomical physical point of view, we should conceptualize the breast as a structure that should have a round base and a conical shape [1–3]. This cone may have variations in projection, but the geometric concept must not be lost. Therefore, when

M.A. Shiffman (ed.), *Mastopexy and Breast Reduction: Principles and Practice*,
© Springer-Verlag Berlin Heidelberg 2009

doing a reduction, we should consider achieving a breast with a round base and a conical shape as an ideal that is an aesthetically beautiful breast. Obviously the shape is not everything nor the most important thing sought when doing reduction mammoplasty. There are elements and factors that will finally determine which technique we decide to add to our surgical options. The three physiological anatomical elements are of vital importance when designing or choosing a reduction mammoplasty technique are the vascularity of the nipple–areola complex (NAC), the sensitivity of the NAC, and integrity of the galactophorous ducts. Undoubtedly, if from the aesthetic point of view we want a conical breast with a round base, we also want a breast with a viable NAC, good vascularity, with adequate sensitivity, and with the ability to exercise its lactation function. Preserving an aesthetically beautiful breast meets the requirement of pleasing the eye. Adequate sensitivity allows preserving its sexual–erotic function, and integrity of the galactophorous ducts provides its functionality, which is what the mammary gland exists for. Obviously, these ideal results are not easy to obtain, but in the search for the ideal lies the achievement of perfection.

Like any anatomical structure, a hypertrophic mammary gland presents increased volume in its two basic structures, the container that is the skin, and the contained that is the breast tissue. When it is decided to do reduction mammoplasty, how to treat both structures must be considered, because it is definitely mandatory to do so. The great diversity of existing surgical techniques is due precisely to the fact that management of the skin and mammary parenchyma is numerous and varied. Likewise, the characteristics themselves of the skin and breast tissue are going to determine in large part the result obtained in surgery, even if the technique is the same. Breast tissue with a predominance of fat is a soft and amorphous tissue and, therefore, difficult to mold. It is the opposite with a breast tissue that is predominantly glandular where the firm tissue allows appropriate molding and handling and which provides more lasting and more aesthetically appropriate results. Because the excess of the breast is in the base and lower portion of the cone of the breast, resection of the tissue is performed primarily in this area [1, 2].

Skin quality is a determining factor of the surgical result as well as the choice of how to treat and remove excess skin. Firm, high-quality skin will have a better result than loose, low-quality skin. The former will favor proper retraction and a better postsurgical readjustment than the latter. Firm skin will provide better cutaneous support for more permanent results. Whatever the case, resection of the skin is always necessary. Since there is always an excess in the vertical portion of the breast, the large majority of surgical techniques employ elliptical resection of the skin in the shape of a vertical spindle [2]. As there is also an excess in the horizontal portion, skin resection in this portion is handled in different ways. Most techniques eliminate the excess with a horizontal spindle at the base of the breast, producing the classic "inverted T" scar [3–8]. However, there are many techniques that attempt to compensate for this excess in different ways. Some with a single vertical incision, distributing all the excess skin in this incision, leaving it to readjust over time [9–12] or with a unilateral resection outwardly, leaving a scar in the shape of an "L" or "J" [13–18]. Still others handle the skin with only a periareolar incision allowing readjustment of the skin to be slow [19, 20]. Clearly, these latter techniques are more successful when the skin quality is good [2, 21].

50.3
Surgical Techniques

Considering the basic premises of preserving a mammary gland with a round base and conical shape, preserving the vascularity and NAC sensitivity to the fullest, as well as the integrity of the galactophorous ducts, the techniques are numerous and varied. Their classifications can be made taking as a base a great variety of concepts. If we take into account the way the nipple–areola complex is preserved, they may be classified as superior [22, 23], inferior [5–7], medial [24], lateral [3], central [19, 20], and bipedicle, either horizontal [25] or vertical [8]. If the classification is based on the thickness of the pedicle, they can be dermal [3] or dermoglandular [5–7, 19, 20]. If the factor by which they are classified is handling of the skin and the resultant scar, they can be periareolar [19, 20], with a vertical scar [9–12], with an "L" or "J" scar [13–18], and with an inverted T scar [3–8]. Clearly, there are combinations of these classifications.

According to a 2002 survey of plastic surgeons in the U.S. [21], the most frequently used incision is the inverted T in 75% of cases and the most used pedicle is the inferior pedicle in 44% of patients, with limited incisions such as the periareolar or the vertical in only 15% of patients, superior pedicle or Wise pattern in 20% of cases, and McKissock in 5%, and the lateral pedicle being used in less than 1% of patients. The techniques of wide inferior pedicle incisions are the most used [21]. The reasons are due to the fact that for patients the wide incision techniques provide greater satisfaction than the limited incision techniques [21] since the number and percentage of complications are fewer and the aesthetic results are better with wide incision techniques [21]. Inferior pedicle techniques [5–7] are much used because they assure NAC vascularity in addition to being easy to perform and to learn in spite of the fact that they have disadvantages in the width of the scarring and the long-term secondary ptosis produced by a lack of support of the mammary parenchyma [21].

Limited incision techniques, initially described by Lassus in 1964 [9], have the great advantage of providing the patient with a smaller scar than the traditional

inverted Lassus' original technique has been modified by numerous authors [10–13] and to these limited incision techniques have been added those of the periareolar approach [19, 20]. However, they are not very satisfactory for surgeons because they are considered difficult to perform, with a long learning curve, and satisfactory results are not easily reproducible [21]. Also, patients are not very satisfied with the shape of the breast and because revisions are more frequent than with the wide incision techniques [21].

50.4 Why the Supero-Lateral Dermoglandular Technique

In the 1970s, Skoog [3] described a surgical technique for reduction mammoplasty in which the fundamental premise is preservation of NAC vascularity by a lateral pedicle. In his original design, a thin dermal flap was used that he later modified making it thicker at the base to avoid venous congestion. The concept of his technique was based on the excellent vascularity that this pedicle presented in the lateral vessels of the breast. This vascularity is referred to from anatomical studies done by Cooper in 1840 [26], where it was found that the breast is vascularized in its lateral portion by branches of the external and acromiothoracic arteries, both deriving from the axillary artery, while in the medial portion, vascularity came from direct branches of the internal mammary artery. Cooper explains that the trajectory of these vessels is quite variable since many branches are superficial while others enter the breast from below, coming from the intercostal arteries. Marcus, in 1934 [27], confirmed Cooper's findings and demonstrated a great vascularity of the NAC thanks to a periareolar system of superficial anastomosis, which alone is enough to preserve the vascularity of the NAC. Skoog's original design of a lateral dermal pedicle in his technique for reduction mammoplasty was born based on the descriptions of Cooper and Marcus. Skoog prefers to use a dermal flap instead of a dermoglandular flap to protect the vascularity of the breast tissue to the fullest, since he states that if there are problems with the dermal pedicle, the only thing lost is the areola, while with dermoglandular flaps necrosis occurs in a broad sector of the gland including the areola. Likewise, he states that handling the areola and the mammary parenchyma separately provides a more stable long-term result. He also mentions that, although there are alterations of sensitivity in most patients in whom this technique is used, it is recovered significantly a year after surgery. Unfortunately, the use of a dermal flap sections the galactophorous ducts, and it is not possible to achieve the lactation function when using this surgical technique [3].

Observing favorable concepts and advantages and disadvantages of the original technique described by Skoog, the author set about the task of designing a technique to take advantage of its attributes to the fullest but trying to eliminate or improve upon its disadvantages. It was thus that over 15 years ago, the author [28] designed a superolateral pedicle technique, but with a dermoglandular component, instead of only the dermal one described by Skoog.

Vascular safety is one of the most interesting factors of the superolateral dermoglandular pedicle. In a recent study by O'Dea et al. [29] it was determined that the best pedicle for performing reduction mammoplasty is the superolateral pedicle. In a study of 7 cadavers, O'Dea found six sources for NAC vascularity. The lateral thoracic artery was found in 100% of the cadavers studied, and the internal mammary artery vascularized the NAC in 86% of cases, these two arteries therefore being the principal ones providing vascularity to the NAC. These data also relate to Nakajima's findings [30]. He determined that the thickness of the pedicle is as important as its placement, since thin pedicles do not carry the same vascularity as dermoglandular flaps. Therefore, according to this study, the choice of the superolateral dermoglandular pedicle to preserve NAC vascularity is the surest, since it bears dominant branches originating from the lateral thoracic artery, branches that are consistent and thick, in addition to having minor supplementary arteries coming from the anterior and posterior branches of the intercostal arteries, from upper thoracic artery, superficial thoracic artery, and thoracoacromial artery [29] (Fig. 50.1).

NAC sensitivity is provided by the cutaneous branches of the 3rd, 4th, and 5th intercostal nerves [31] (Fig. 50.1). It has been found in numerous studies that the 4th intercostal nerve is the most important in NAC sensitivity [32–38]. Schlenz et al. [31] found, in an anatomical study of 28 cadavers, that the lateral cutaneous branch of the 4th intercostal nerve is the most consistent of all, being present in 93% of cases, while the anterior cutaneous nerve of the 3rd and 4th intercostal nerves was found in 57% of cases. The most interesting data show that the anterior cutaneous branches have a subcutaneous trajectory and terminate in the superomedial portion of the areola, while lateral cutaneous branches are deep in 93% of cases and superficial in only 7% of cases [31]. These superficial and deep trajectories have been described previously [32–34, 38]. These deep nerves come out of the pectoral fascia, cross the entire gland, and reach the NAC, and the thickness of the nerves that come from the lateral branches is five times greater than that of the medial branches [31]. So to avoid damaging the lateral cutaneous nerves, deep resections of the glandular parenchyma must be limited, and if preservation of the superficial innervations of the anterior intercostal nerves is desired, superficial cutting in the superomedial portion of the areola must be avoided [31]. Therefore, alteration of sensitivity in reduction mammoplasty does not depend on the amount of tissue resected but rather on the surgical technique used and the way the cuts

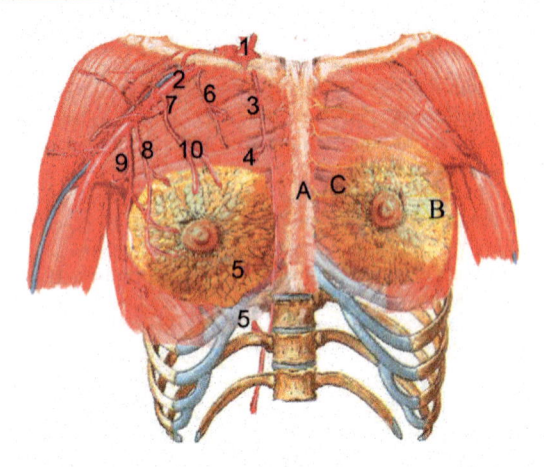

Fig. 50.1 Vascular supply and sensitivity of the mammary gland. The mammary gland has two main sources of vascular supply; one is deriving from the descendent aorta, and the other one from the subclavian artery. The subclavian artery (1) creates the axillary artery (2) and the internal mammary artery (3), also called the internal thoracic artery. When the internal mammary artery descends produces several perforators to supply the areola and nipple on the medial area (4), and also the anterior branches of the intercostals arteries (5). These branches join the posterior intercostals arteries deriving from the descendent aorta. After crossing the first rib, the subclavian artery is called axillary artery (2), and during its course delivers several branches that irrigates the breast: The highest thoracic artery (6), the thoracoacromial artery (7), the superficial thoracic artery [8], and the lateral thoracic artery (9) also called external mammary artery. The thoracoacromial artery creates the pectoral branch that goes to the mammary gland (10). The nipple and areola are innervated by the anterior (**a**) and lateral (**b**) cutaneous branches of the 3rd, 4th, and 5th intercostal nerves. The anterior cutaneous branches emerge at the parasternal line and goes to the breast through the medial branch (**c**). This branch innervates the medial part of the areola and nipple, and runs almost subcutaneous. The lateral cutaneous branches emerge at the lateral border of the breast and innervate the lateral border of the areola and nipple, but have superficial and deep branches that cross the breast gland

are made [31, 39]. Surgical techniques in which the base of the breast is resected, like those of the superior or dermal pedicles, affect sensitivity more [39], while the inferior pedicle techniques preserve greater sensitivity [31, 40]. Undoubtedly, the superolateral dermoglandular pedicle contributes greatly to preserving NAC sensitivity, since it avoids damaging the principal, most consistent branches that provide sensitivity, which are precisely the lateral cutaneous branches of the intercostal nerves [31].

Numerous studies have shown that lactation function following reduction mammoplasty does not depend on the location of the pedicle, rather on how it is composed. Pedicles that include the mammary gland, whether they are superior, medial, inferior, or horizontal bipedicled, have no significant differences among them in lactation capacity [41, 42], nor compared to nonsurgery patients [42]. Therefore, any pedicle that maintains the integrity and connection of the galactophorous ducts to the NAC will be able to preserve the lactation capacity. In these cases, the principal limitation on lactation is the amount of glandular tissue the woman has to be able to do it. But this is a limitation present not only after surgery. Consequently, the supero-lateral dermoglandular pedicle while preserving breast tissue and integrity of the galactophorous ducts is also a pedicle capable of sustaining the lactation function.

All of this supports the preference of a dermoglandular flap over a thin one, as Skoog originally described it. Including the mammary parenchyma in the pedicle definitively allows us to have integral vascularity throughout the tissue, provides us with greater sensitivity, and preserves the lactation function, at the same time achieving the proper aesthetic results, with satisfaction for the patient as well as for the surgeon.

50.5
How it Should be Done

The author has performed this surgical technique for more than 15 years, in more than 300 patients, and has learned more about it while achieving better results. It is a surgical technique that has been employed for moderate hypertrophies to gigantomastias, with breast resections from 300 up to 1,380 g, and with NAC migrations from 5 to 16 cm. This technique is not recommended in NAC displacements of less than 5 cm because rotation of the pedicle is at a very closed angle and that causes compression of the pedicle. Unlike what Skoog describes, the author's pedicle is dermoglandular instead of only dermis and subcutaneous cellular tissue. Unlike Skoog's design, the birth of the pedicle does not present a fixed constant taking into account the lateral branch but is based on the position of the NAC.

All marking is done preoperatively with the patient seated, with the surgeon facing her, and with her arms at her sides. Five key references are marked, to paint the technique design later: suprasternal notch, mid-sternal line, submammary groove, anterior axillary line, and the central meridian of the breast (Fig. 50.2). The central meridian of the breast corresponds to the midclavicular line and will determine the direction of upward migration of the NAC. If there is significant medial or lateral displacement of the nipple-areola complex preoperatively, the midpoint of the clavicle can be placed at a lesser or

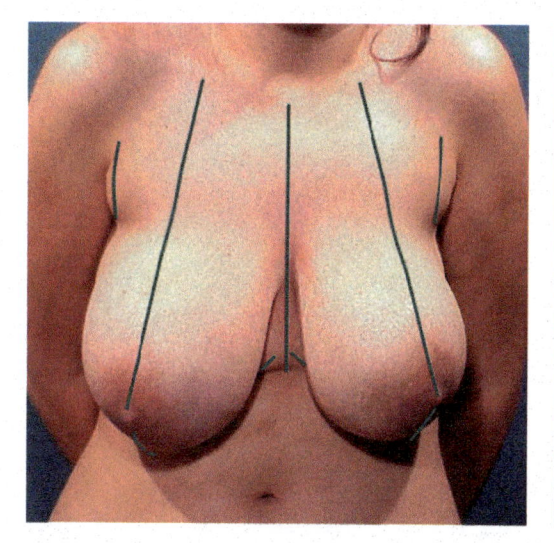

Fig. 50.2 For the design of the technique it is necessary to draw 5 lines or marks on the breast: Suprasternal notch, midclavicular lane, breast middle line, submammary crease, anterior axillary line and middle sternal line

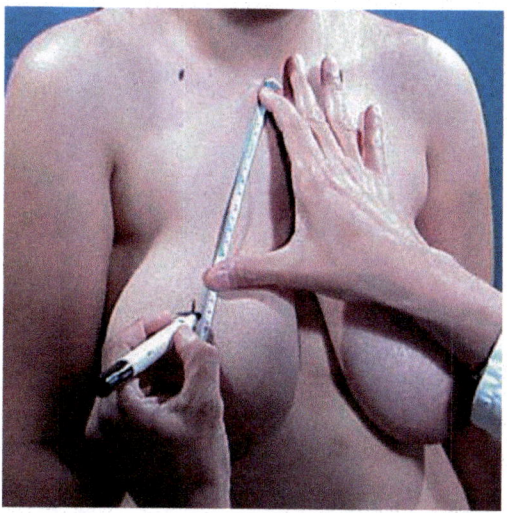

Fig. 50.3 The new position of the CAP is usually marked at approximately 21 cm. from the suprasternal notch. This distance can vary depending on the patient's height

greater distance from the suprasternal notch, as the case may be. This is to displace the breast meridian according to the preoperative breast characteristics and thus compensate for the upward displacement at the time of moving the nipple–areola complex.

With these points indicated, the new position that the midpoint of the nipple–areola complex will have is located. There are several ways to identify the new location point of the nipple–areola complex [43]. The author prefers to use as a reference the normal distance that should exist between the suprasternal notch and the NAC, depending on the patient's height and the new volume of the breast, confirming this position by projecting the position of the submammary groove over the breast meridian The author usually takes as a base a distance of 21 cm ± 1 cm from the suprasternal notch over the central meridian of the breast (Figs. 50.3, 50.4).

With the new location point of the NAC marked, a pattern is used made of a flexible, semirigid material to design the superior cuts in the surgery (Fig. 50.5). This pattern was designed expressly for that purpose and basically consists of an oval 6 cm wide by 4 cm high that would correspond to the new NAC. It has two lateral branches, with a 120° opening and a length of each branch of 9 cm, starting from the center of the NAC (Fig. 50.6). The pattern has markings for the width of its opening and the length of the branches, to facilitate decreasing or increasing those values according to the needs of the design. Larger widths in the degrees of the

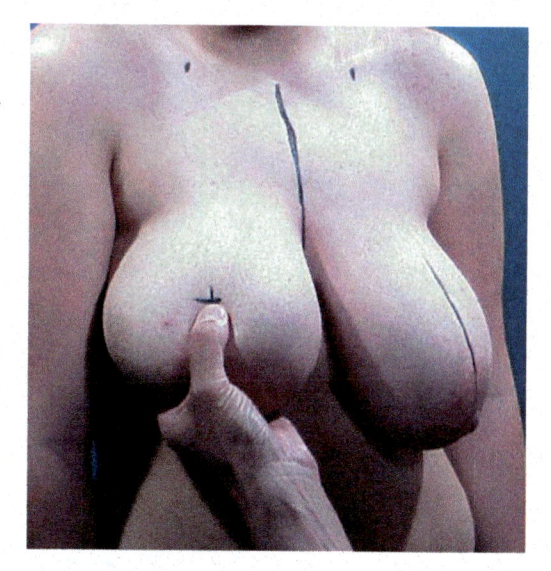

Fig. 50.4 The new position of the CAP is confirmed by placing four fingers on the submammary crease, and opposing the thumb to the middle finger

resection opening will clearly leave a smaller breast, which would also require a vertical incision of no more than 5 cm while a smaller width of the branches will mean leaving a larger breast whose vertical scar could

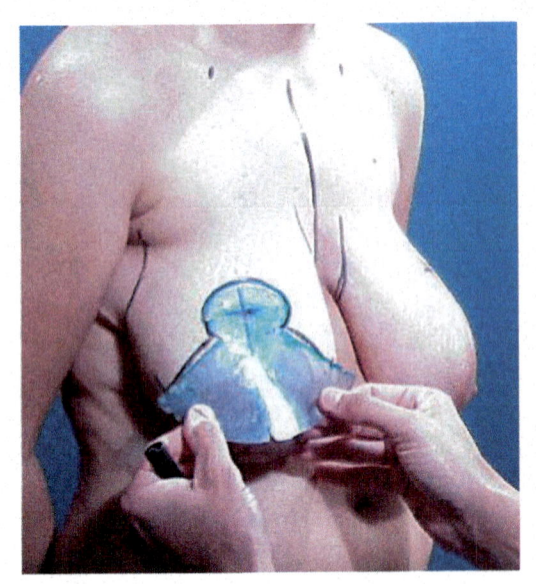

Fig. 50.5 With the new position of the CAP confirmed, a special pattern is used to make the superior drawing of the design

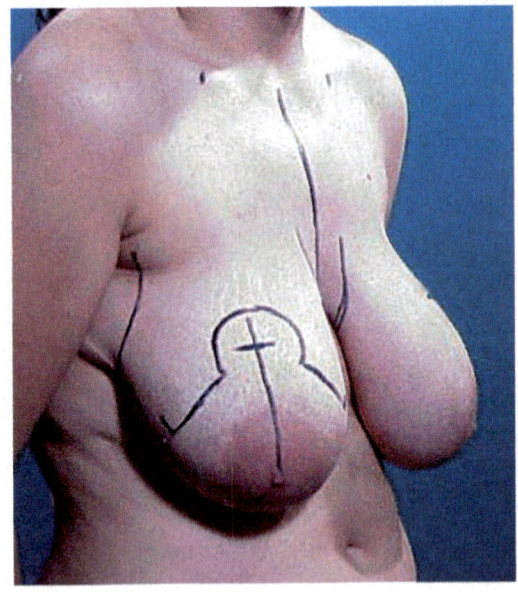

Fig. 50.7 Superior design of the technique where the pattern was used. The new CAP and the lateral lines of the pattern have been marked

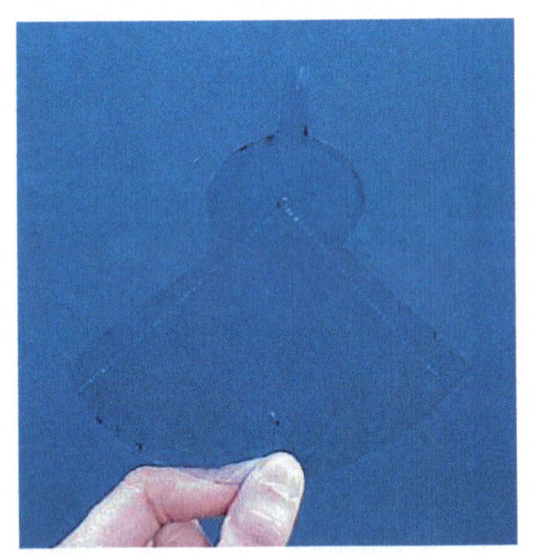

Fig. 50.6 The pattern is made using a flexible material and has several marks to allow the possibility to make variations during the design

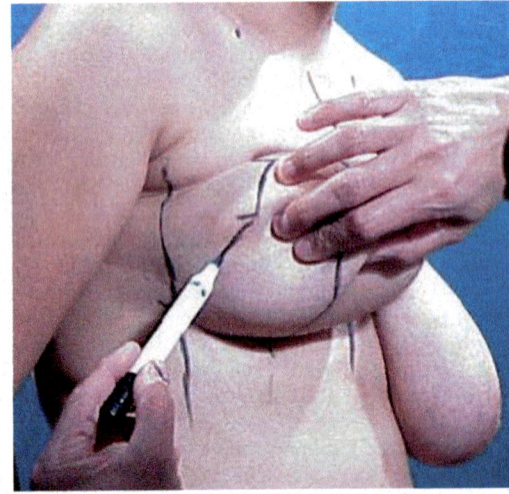

Fig. 50.8 The lines of the superior design are connected to the submammary crease. The lateral line must be inside the anterior axillary line to avoid lateral displacement and a noticeable scar

be from 6 to 7 cm (Fig. 50.7). With the two lateral branches marked, prolongation toward the new submammary groove is performed, which is traced 1 cm above the original groove. The anterior axillary and midsternal lines are used as references so that the union between the submammary groove and the lateral and medial branches is more symmetrical. The lateral branch should not go beyond the anterior axillary line, to keep the horizontal scar from moving outside this line and becoming obvious (Fig. 50.8). The medial branch must

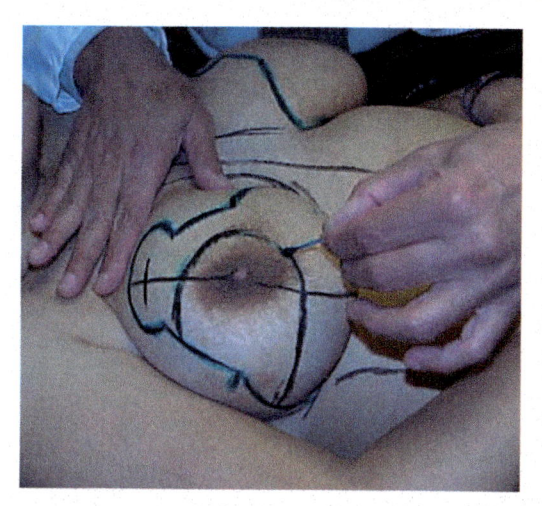

Fig. 50.9 Lateral design of the pedicle with the patient in supine position. The design is totally lateral, but when the patient stands up, the position is superolateral

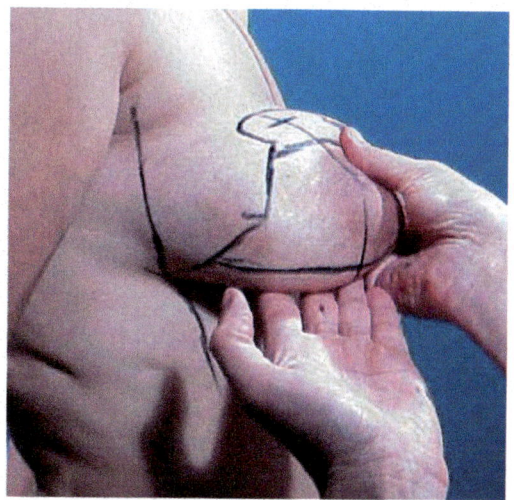

Fig. 50.11 If the breast is lifted, the pedicle is lateral again. That is why this pedicle has both components, superior and lateral

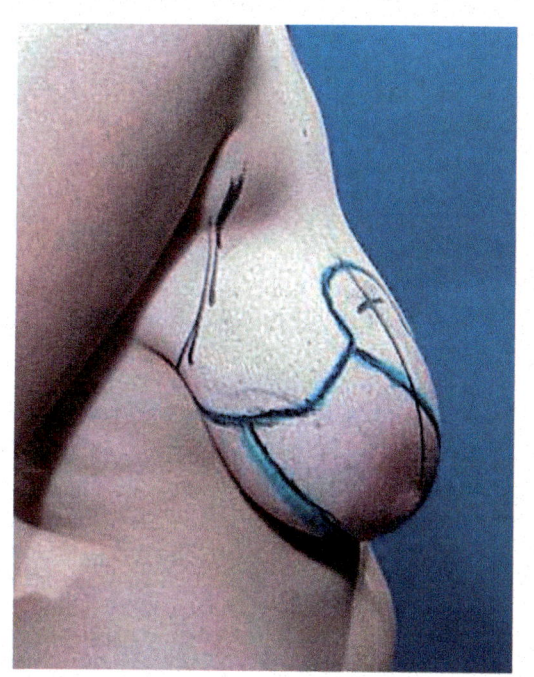

Fig. 50.10 The pedicle that was designed is lateral with the patient lying down and is converted into superolateral when the patient stands up

be left, at most, 2 cm from the midsternal line to avoid its being seen in the medial portion.

Having delineated the design of the surgical resection, the vascular pedicle of the nipple–areola complex is marked. This pedicle will have a lateral base of approximately 7–8 cm, depending on the new volume that is to be given to the mammary gland, and it will surround the new NAC size as usual, at approximately 2–4 cm from it. The tissue that is left distal on the pedicle is very important for giving shape and volume to the upper part of the breast when the pedicle enters that position. The location of the pedicle is predominantly lateral, but with a superior component. This means that it should be marked with the patient lying down and be placed fully horizontal above the NAC, toward the lateral portion of the mammary gland (Fig. 50.9). Situated this way and with the patient standing up, the position and direction of the pedicle becomes completely superolateral (Figs. 50.10, 50.11). It is important to consider this point, since in our first cases, the pedicle was situated taking as a reference Skoog's original marking. On Skoog's design the pedicle began exactly at the beginning of the lateral branch, starting from the NAC. This design with a dermal pedicle does not affect the rotation of the pedicle much. But in the case of a dermoglandular pedicle, its rotation is more problematic because of the volume of tissue the pedicle carries, with which the risk of vascular compromise from compression and torsion of the pedicle is feasible. Because of that, after experiencing this problem, the author

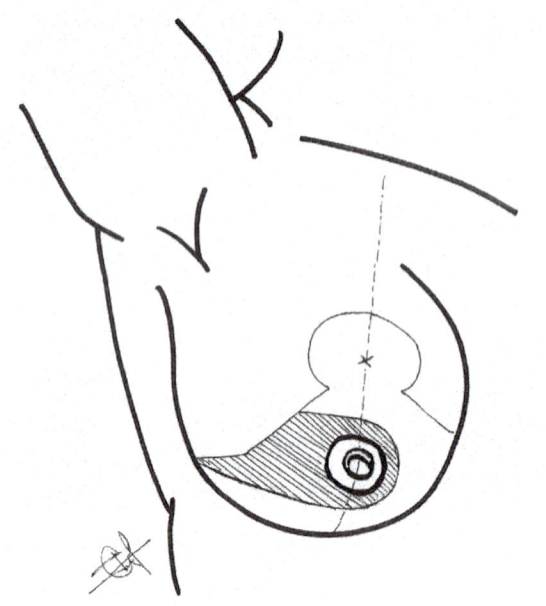

Fig. 50.12 Technique totally designed. The new CAP's position is marked at the breast meridian, and the pedicle is delimitated on the correct place

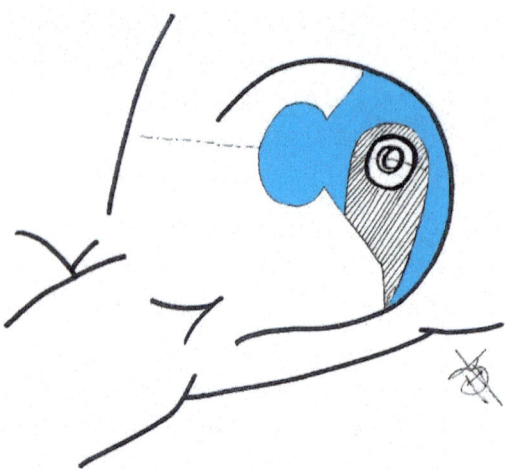

Fig. 50.14 In blue is the breast tissue that has to be eliminated totally and adjacent to it the pedicle that has to be deepithelialized

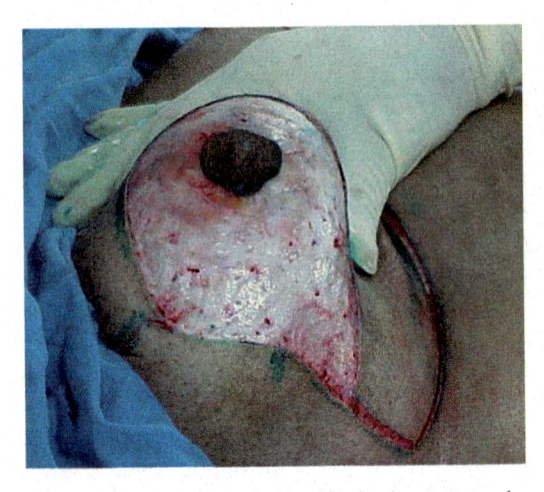

Fig. 50.13 The pedicle is totally deepithelialized maintaining the CAP and the dermis

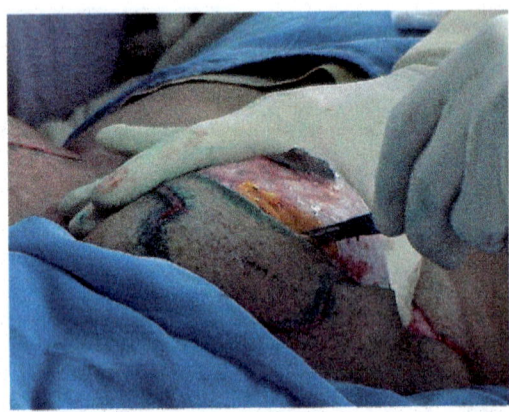

Fig. 50.15 All the tissue resection has to be made with perpendicular cuts to the ribs. This allows pedicle's vascularity, and avoids flaps' undermining

decided to modify the position of the pedicle and make it less superior and more lateral. Therefore, with small migrations of 6–8 cm, the pedicle can begin at 3–4 cm from the center of the new nipple-areola complex. With greater migrations of 8 cm, the pedicle must be situated in a lower position to avoid a very marked rotation with torsion of the pedicle and vascular compromise. In these cases, the beginning of the pedicle can be located more than 5 or 6 cm from the center of the new nipple–areola complex, and go beyond what will be the lateral branch of the new breast with no problem (Fig. 50.12).

This surgical procedure can be performed under an epidural block or general anesthesia. Depending on the breast's size we prepare 300 ml of isotonic saline 0.9% solution + 1 ml of epinephrine or 600 ml of isotonic saline 0.9% + 2 ml of epinephrine. In this manner we have a dilution of 1:300,000. The surgical area is infiltrated with amounts of up to 0.5 l per mammary gland to achieve adequate vasoconstriction. The cutting areas are superficially marked with a scalpel to avoid losing the design during surgery. The first step consists of deepithelialization of the vascular pedicle, maintaining the deep dermis and respecting the new size of the nipple–areola complex, which is 4 cm in diameter (Fig. 50.13). All of the demarcated area outside the vascular pedicle and inside the presurgical design is completely extirpated (Fig. 50.14). This area to be resected comprises the lower portion, a medial portion, and an upper portion of the breast. Within this upper portion is found the oval where the pedicle is going to enter the NAC and, therefore, the tissue within this oval must also be resected up to the costal grid to allow entry of the pedicle. One of the most important points and a primary characteristic of this technique that is always observed is that resection of the tissue and the vascular pedicle cuts must be completely perpendicular to the costal grid (Figs. 50.15, 50.16), so that the pedicle of the complex will be dermoglandular, maintaining completely the integrity of the nipple–areola complex toward the mammary gland and toward the costal grid (Fig. 50.17). The size of the new gland will depend on how wide the dermoglandular pedicle is left, as well as its length. Once the breast tissue to be extirpated is resected, the complex rotates toward its new position (Figs. 50.18–50.20). A final important detail in the development of the technique is that the pedicle must be fixed to the costal grid with nonabsorbable sutures (Prolene 2-0) to give it greater support (Fig. 50.21). The inferior part of the pedicle can even be plicated over itself to achieve greater conification of the breast (Figs. 50.22, 50.23).

Complete closure of the breast by planes is performed using absorbable sutures (Monocryl 2-0 and 3-0), to avoid their removal postsurgically (Fig. 50.24). Negative pressure drains are left for 24–48 h, discharging the patient 24 h after surgery. Following withdrawal of the drains, a breast support is used for a time span of approximately 3–4 weeks.

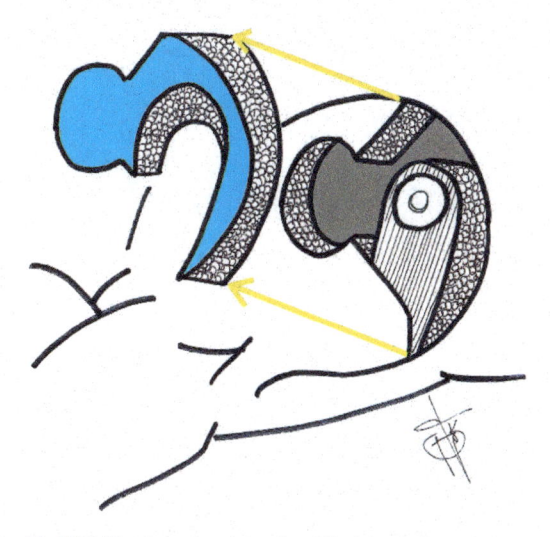

Fig. 50.16 The tissue is removed en-block, and the pedicle is maintained in the same manner

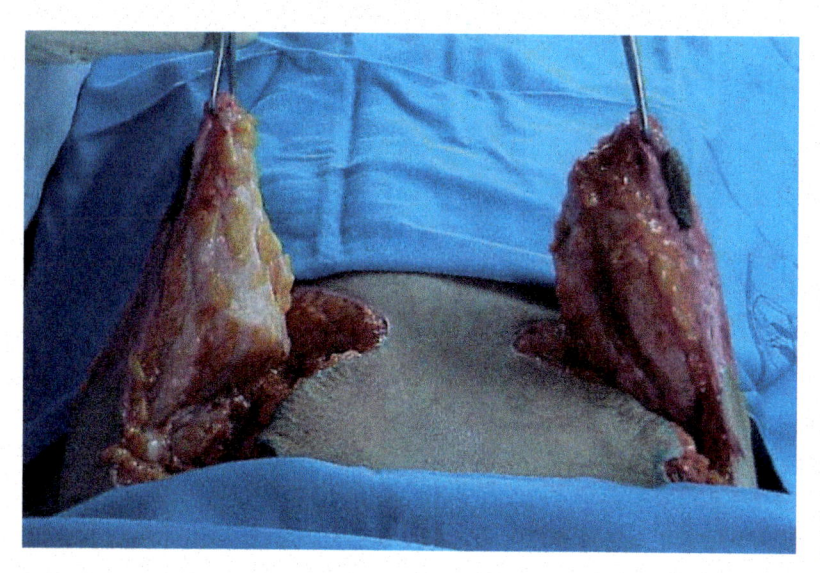

Fig. 50.17 The pedicles are attached and connected to the pectoral fascia. This permits nerves, vessels and galactic ducts integrity

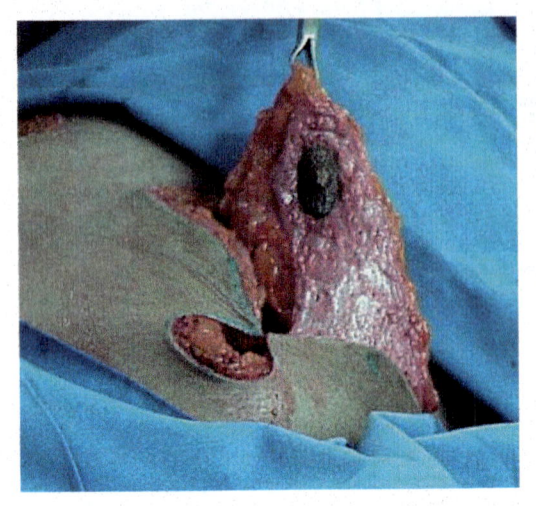

Fig. 50.18 The superolateral pedicle is ready to be rotated. Note the thickness and the dermoglandular component

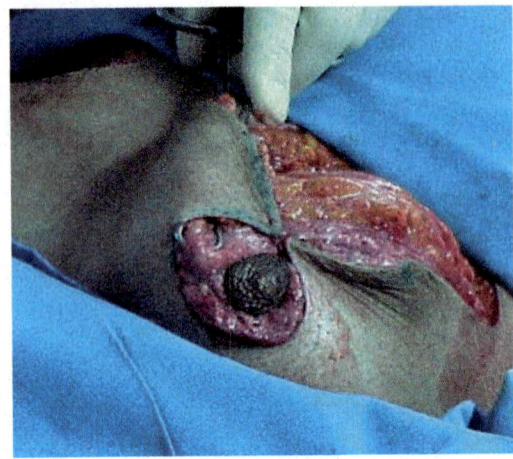

Fig. 50.20 The pedicle has been rotated to the new CAP's position. There is no tension, and there are no problems to reach the place

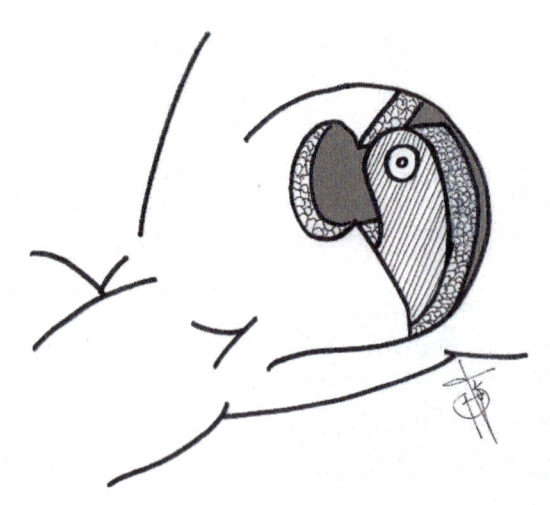

Fig. 50.19 With the breast tissue totally eliminated on the marked area the pedicle's rotation is very easy

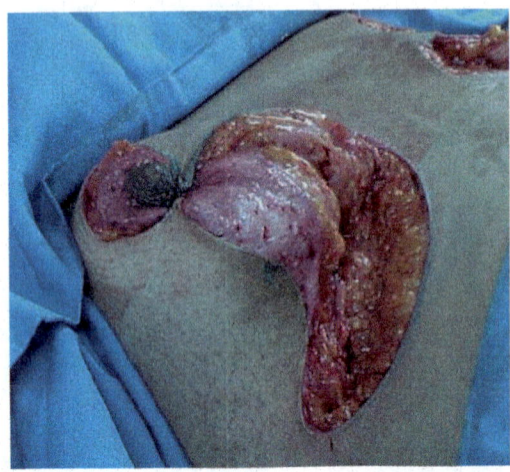

Fig. 50.21 The pedicle is fixed to the thoracic wall with non-absorbable sutures. This is done to obtain the breast conic shape and diminish skin tension

50.6
Care of Complications

As with any reduction mammoplasty technique, the superolateral dermoglandular pedicle is not exempt from complications. In a multicenter study conducted by Cunningham et al. [44], wherein multiple surgical techniques performed by different surgeons were analyzed, it was found that the most important factor in the appearance of complications is the amount of tissue to be removed. The importance of the tissue to be removed and the incidence of complications were reported by Strombeck [25] more than 40 years ago. The more breast tissue that is resected, the greater the risk and the higher

50.6 Care of Complications

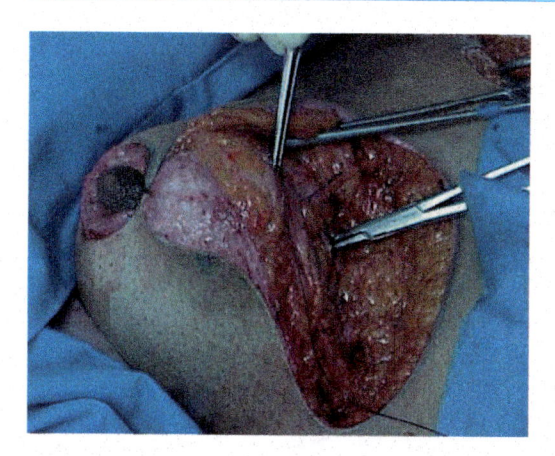

Fig. 50.22 The breast tissue is totally configured in its conic shape and its maintaining that position without needing the skin to give the contour

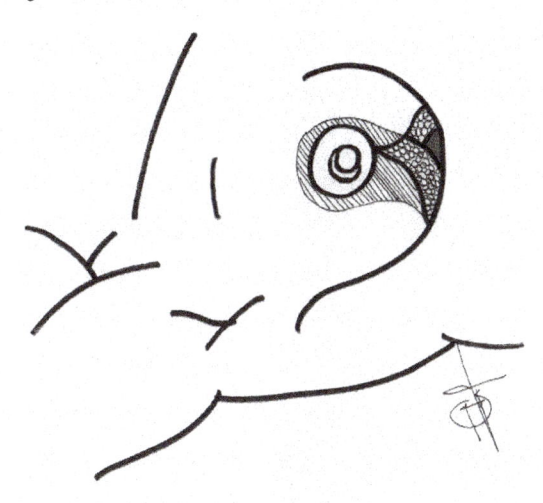

Fig. 50.23 The pedicle is in position and the skin is ready to be closed

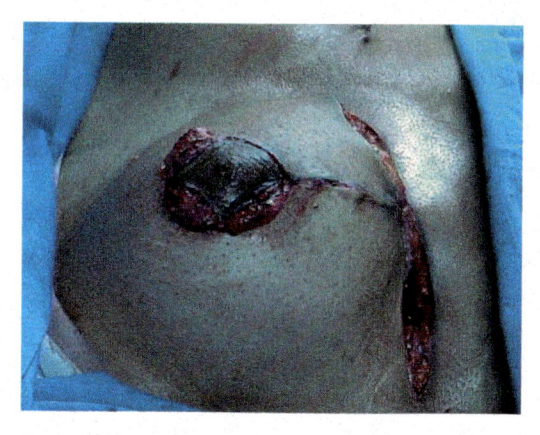

Fig. 50.24 The skin is closed without tension

percentage of complications there are. The younger and the less surgical time employed, the more the number of complications decreases. The breast size and smoking have a significant bearing on the onset of complications.

The most severe complication that the author has had is two patients with total unilateral necrosis of the NAC. One of them, a smoker of more than 20 cigarettes a day for several years, presented with partial necrosis of the other NAC, while the other patient, over 50 years of age, started the problem 5 days after being free from any alteration, apparently from some secondary vascular problem in the pedicle. In the latter case, the other complex had no alteration at all. In both patients, the resected breast tissue was over 1,000 g per breast, and both were overweight, although not obese. Overweight has also been mentioned as an important factor in the presence of complications [45–51].

The complication most commonly reported by almost all authors is delayed healing that also occurs in the author's technique. However, this problem has improved substantially by maintaining the shape and position of the breast with sutures and giving more support to the breast tissue. With this, the weight of the breast is maintained, avoiding the tension on the suture line, above all at the level of the union of the two incisions in the submammary groove. Reaction to the suture material that is a frequently reported complication [21] has been substantially improved by eliminating in the surgical procedure use of absorbable sutures braided with polyfilament and exchanging them for Monocryl monofilament, absorbable sutures. Polyfilament braided sutures have the disadvantage of leaving necrotic tissue between its filaments that makes its removal difficult and encourages reaction. It is common to observe fat necrosis in breasts with a significant predominance of fatty tissue and, therefore it is necessary to take this consideration into account when handling glands with these characteristics. A measure that the author consistently takes and which has decreased this complication is not tensing the suture too much when plicating the pedicle to avoid vascular compromising of the fat. The fat remains more vascularized from the characteristics of this technique where no undermining of breast tissue is done, since cuts are always perpendicular to the costal grid and flaps are not undermined. This same technical detail has allowed the author to avoid cutaneous necrosis in the flaps, which has never occurred. There have not been problems or dissatisfaction secondary to significant alterations of sensitivity or lactation capacity.

As with any inverted T technique, scars constitute the main problem and are where the greatest dissatisfaction can be caused for the patient in the postsurgical result. However, and although it seems paradoxical, inverted-T techniques provide greater satisfaction to patients and surgeons [21]. The aesthetic results in the shape and position of the breast are greater with wide-scar techniques than with limited scarring [21], the number of complications is much lower with wide-scar techniques [21, 44], and the likelihood of achieving satisfactory results with wide-scar techniques is much greater than with limited incision techniques. For that reason, the need for retouching in these latter cases is high [21]. Fortunately, with the new techniques and implements that exist for improving the scarring process this has ceased being a main problem. So much so that despite the breadth of the scar, the degree of satisfaction and conformity in the author's patients with this surgical technique surpasses 93% of cases.

50.7
Conclusions

Obviously, every surgical technique that exists for performing reduction mammoplasty has its advantages and disadvantages. The results with many of them are excellent. The technique of superolateral dermoglandular pedicle has many advantages, but three fundamental premises must be kept in mind to achieve success and avoid complications to the fullest. First, the pedicle must

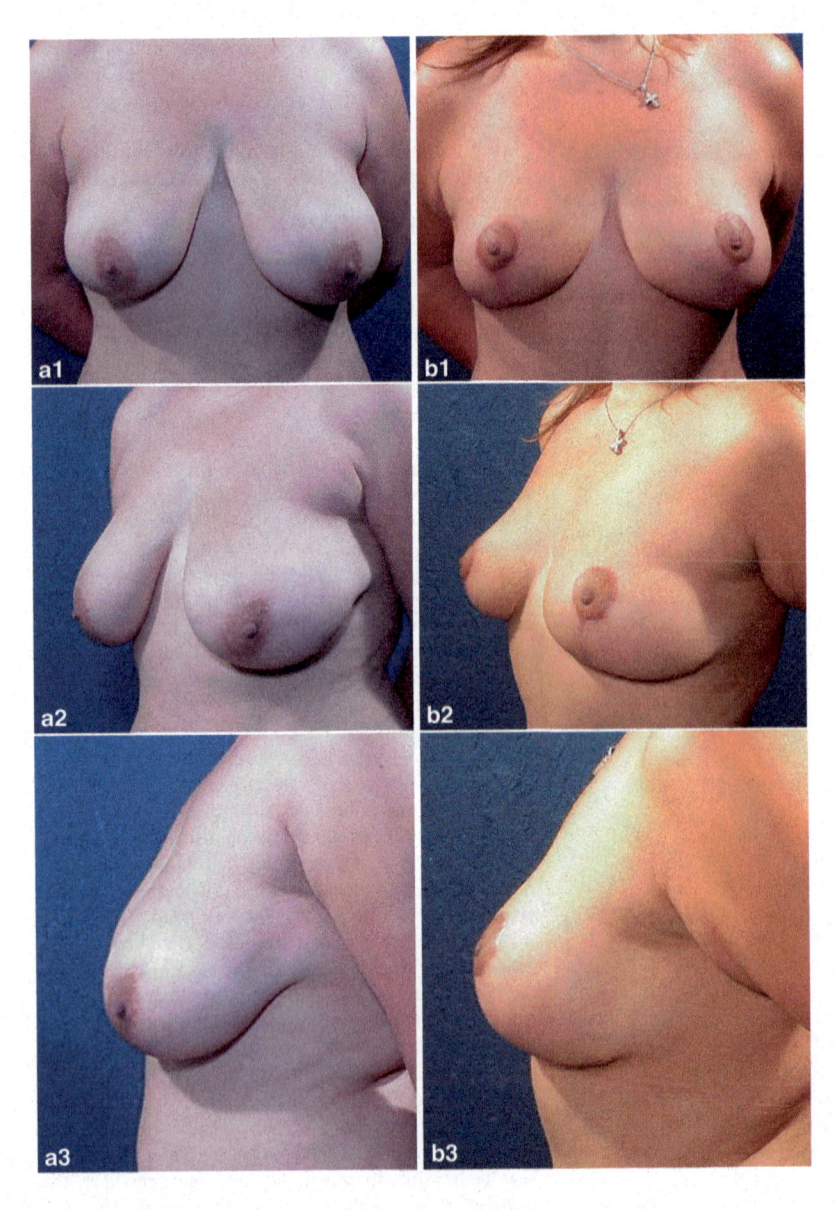

Fig. 50.25 (**a***1-3*) Preoperative. (**b***1-3*) Eight months postoperative after 425 g were removed from each side and CAP was elevated 7 cm. Skin quality and conical shape are good

always be situated in a more lateral direction than a superior one and must be used on breasts where the NAC needs to migrate more than 5 cm. This is for the purpose of avoiding torsion and vascular compromise of the pedicle. Second, all cuts should be made perpendicular to the costal grid, for the purpose of avoiding thinning the pedicle more than is appropriate, as well as the cutaneous flaps and the breast pillars. And third, the gland must be molded by affixing the pedicle to the costal grid or by plication over itself. This is for the purpose of achieving a better aesthetic result by giving a conical shape to the breast, as well as avoiding excessive pressure on the suture line and allowing cutaneous closure without tension.

The reduction mammoplasty technique with a superolateral dermoglandular pedicle is considered an excellent surgical option (Figs. 50.25, 50.26). It is a very

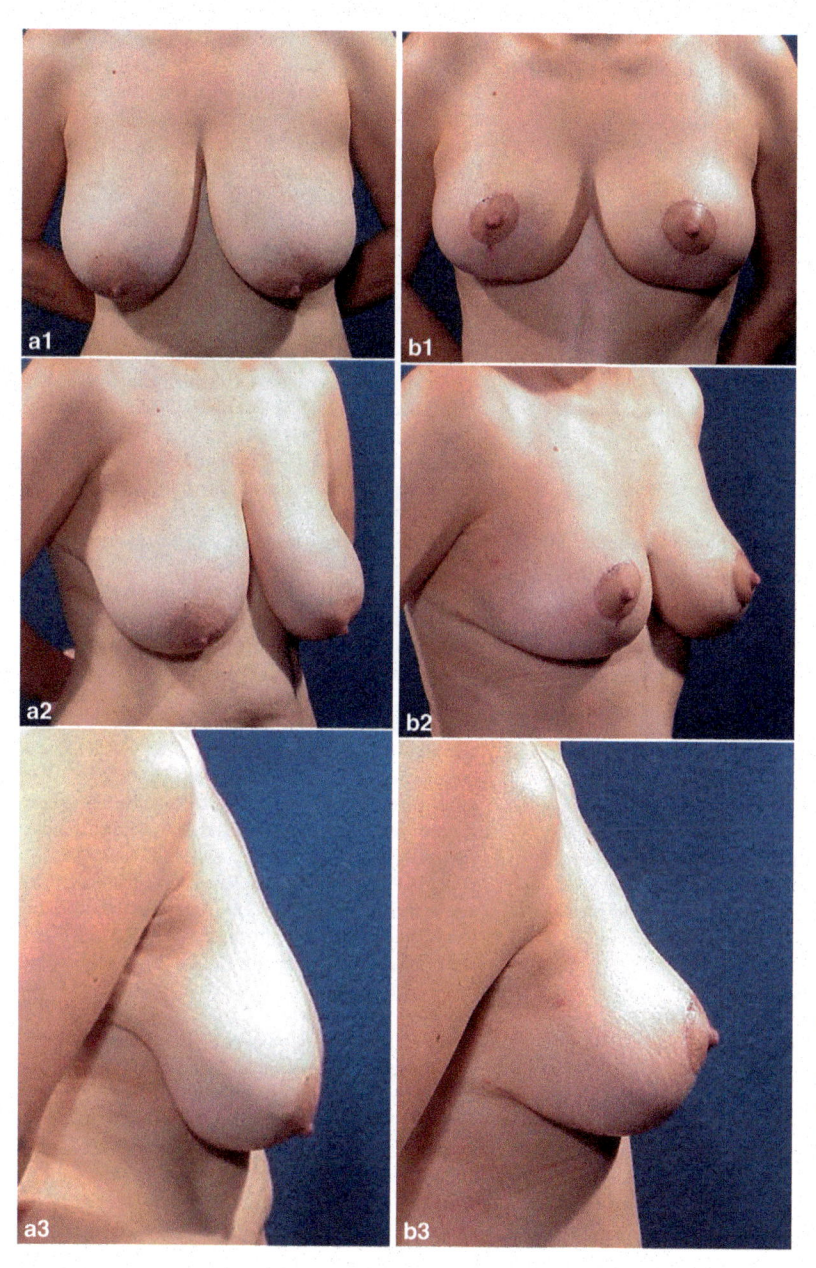

Fig. 50.26 (a1-3) Preoperative 32-year-old female. (b1-3) Three months following removal of 525 g from one side, 500 g from the other side, and CAP elevation of 9 cm. The breast base has good dimensions and skin quality is good

simple technique to design and perform and, therefore, its learning curve is fast and the results are reproducible. The security of the pedicle is unbeatable, since the vessels it contains are numerous and consistent. The sensitivity it provides is ideal, since the nerves remain contained within the pedicle, and they are most important in NAC sensitivity. The galactophorous ducts remain intact and joined to the mammary parenchyma, so the functionality of the gland is preserved. Therefore, the external dermoglandular pedicle preserves to the utmost three characteristics sought in reduction mammoplasty: vascularity, sensitivity, and functionality. The aesthetic results are excellent. That is why this is a preferred technique in the treatment of mammary hypertrophy and gigantomastia.

Acknowledgments

The author would like to thank Gisela Gonzalez and Joel Encinas MD, who helped on the design and preparation of the photographic material

References

1. Goldwyn RM: Reduction Mammaplasty. Boston, Little Brown 1990
2. Hudson DA: Some thoughts on choosing a technique in breast reduction. Plast Reconstr Surg 1998;102:554–557
3. Skoog T: Plastic Surgery. New Methods and Refinements. Stockholm, Almqvist and Wiksell 1974
4. Pereira JJ: Aesthetic breast surgery with inverted-T scar placed above the inframammary sulcus. Aesthetic Plast Surg 1997;21(1):16–22
5. Courtiss E, Goldwyn RM: Reduction mammaplasty by the inferior pedicle technique: An alternative to free nipple and areola grafting for severe macromastia or extreme ptosis. Plast Reconstr Surg 1977;59(1):500–507
6. Georgiade NG, Serafin D, Morris R, Georgiade G: Reduction mammaplasty utilizing an inferior pedicle nipple-areolar flap. Ann Plast Surg 1979;3(3):211–218
7. Robbins TH: A reduction mammaplasty with the areola-nipple based on an inferior pedicle. Plast Reconstr Surg 1977;59(1):64–67
8. McKissock PK: Reduction mammaplasty with a vertical dermal flap. Plast Reconstr Surg 1972;49(3):245–252
9. Lassus C: A technique for breast reduction. Int Surg 1970;53(1):69–72
10. Lejour M, Abboud M, Declety A, Kertesz P: Reduction des cicatrices de plastie mammaire de l'ancrecourte à la verticale. Ann Chir Plast Esthet 1990;35(5):369–379
11. Hall-Findlay EJ: A simplified vertical reduction mammaplasty: Shortening the learning curve. Plast Reconstr Surg 1999;104(3):748–759
12. Leone MS, Franchelli S, Berrino P, Santi PL: Vertical mammaplasty: A personal approach. Aesthetic Plast Surg 1997;21(5):356–361
13. Renault P: Reduction mammaplasty by the "B" technique. Plast Reconstr Surg 1974;53(1):19–24
14. Bozola AR: Breast reduction with short L scar. Plast Reconstr Surg 1990;85(5):728–738
15. Chiari A Jr: The L short-scar mammaplasty: A new approach. Plast Reconstr Surg 1992;90(2):233–246
16. Born G: The "L" reduction mammaplasty. Ann Plast Surg 1994;32(4):383–387
17. Chiari A Jr: The L short-scar mammaplasty: 12 years later. Plast Reconstr Surg 2001;108(2):489–495
18. Meyer R: "L" technique compared with others in mammaplasty reduction. Aesthetic Plast Surg 1995;19(6):541–548
19. Benelli L: A new periareolar mammaplasty: The "round block" technique. Aesthetic Plast Surg 1990;14(2):93–100
20. Sampaio-Goes JC: Periareolar mammaplasty double skin technique. Breast Dis 1991;4:111
21. Rohrich RJ, Gosman AA, Brown SA, Tonadapu P, Foster B: Current preferences for breast reduction techniques: a survey of board-certified plastic surgeons 2002. Plast Reconstr Surg 2004;114(7):1724–1733
22. Pitanguy I: Mammaplasty. Study of 245 consecutive cases and presentation of a personal technique Rev Bras Cir 1961;42:201–220
23. Pontes R: Reduction mammaplasty–variations I and II. Ann Plast Surg 1981;6(6):437–447
24. Schwarzmann E: Die technik der mammaplastik. Chirurg 1930;2:932–943
25. Strömbeck JO: Report of a new technique based on the two pedicle procedure. Br J Plast Surg 1960;13:79–90
26. Cooper AP: On the Anatomy of the Breast. London, Longman 1840
27. Marcus GH: Untersuchungen über die arterielle blutversorgung der mamilla. Arc Klin Chir 1934;179:361
28. Cárdenas-Camarena L, Vergara R: Reduction mammaplasty with superior-lateral dermoglandular pedicle: Another alternative. Plast Reconstr Surg 2001;107(3):693–699
29. O'Dey D, Prescher A, Pallua N: Vascular reliability of nipple-areola complex–bearing pedicles: An anatomical microdissection study. Plast Reconstr Surg 2007;119(4):1167–1177
30. Nakajima H, Imanishi N, Aiso, S: Arterial anatomy of the nipple-areola complex. Plast Reconstr Surg 1995;96(4):843–845
31. Schlenz I, Kuzbari R, Gruber H, Holle J: The sensitivity of the nipple-areola complex: An anatomical study. Plast Reconstr Surg 2000;105(3):905–909
32. Craig RD, Sykes PA: Nipple sensitivity following reduction mammaplasty. Br J Plast Surg 1970;23(2):165–172

33. Gonzalez F, Brown FE, Gold WE, Walton RL, Shafer B Preoperative and postoperative nipple-areola sensibility in patients undergoing reduction mammaplasty. Plast Reconstr Surg 1993;92(5):809–814
34. Slezak S, Dellon AL: Quantitation of sensibility in gigantomastia and alteration following reduction mammaplasty. Plast Reconstr Surg 1993;91(7):1265–1269
35. Courtiss EH, Goldwyn RM: Breast sensation before and after plastic surgery. Plast Reconstr Surg 1976;58(1):1–13
36. Serletti JM, Reading G, Caldwell E, Wray RC: Long-term patient satisfaction following reduction mammaplasty. Ann Plast Surg 1992;28(4):363–365
37. Mofid MM, Dellon AL, Elias JJ, Nahabedian MY: Quantitation of breast sensibility following reduction mammaplasty: A comparison of inferior and medial pedicle techniques. Plast Reconstr Surg 2002;109(7):2283–2288
38. Wechselberger G, Stoss S, Schoeller T, Oehlbauer M, Piza-Katzer H: An analysis of breast sensation following inferior pedicle mammaplasty and the effect of the volume of the resected tissue. Aesthetic Plast Surg 2001;25(6):443–446
39. Schlenz I, Rigel S, Schemper M, Kuzbari R: Alteration of nipple and areola sensitivity by reduction mammaplasty: a prospective comparison of five techniques. Plast Reconstr Surg 2005;115(3):743–751
40. Mitrofanoff M, Dallassera M, Bourkis T, Baruch J: Clinical study of breast sensitivity before and after reduction mammaplasty. Report of 44 cases. Ann Chir Plast Esthet 1997;42(4):314–323
41. Kakagia D, Tripsiannis G, Tsoutsos D: Breastfeeding after reduction mammaplasty: a comparison of 3 techniques. Ann Plast Surg 2005;55(4):343–345
42. Cruz N, Korchin L: Lactational performance after breast reduction with different pedicles. Plast Reconstr Surg 2007;120(1):35–40
43. Gulyás G: Marking the position of the nipple-areola complex for mastopexy and breast reduction surgery. Plast Reconstr Surg 2004;113(7):2085–2090
44. Cunningham BL, Gear AJ, Kerrigan CL, Collins ED: Analysis of breast reduction complications derived from the BRAVO study. Plast Reconstr Surg 2005;115(6):1597–1604
45. Strombeck JO: Reduction mammaplasty. Surg Clin N Am 1971;51(2):453–469
46. Dabbah A, Lehman JA Jr, Parker MG, Tantri D, Wagner DS: Reduction mammaplasty: An outcome analysis. Ann Plast Surg 1995;35(4):337341
47. Menke H, Eisenmann-Klein M, Olbrisch RR, Exner K: Continuous quality management of breast hypertrophy by the German Association of Plastic Surgeons: A preliminary report. Ann Plast Surg 2001;46(6):594–598
48. Zubowski R, Zins J E, Foray-Kaplon A, Yetman RJ, Lucas AR, Papay FA, Heil D, Hutton D: Relationship of obesity and specimen weight to complications in reduction mammaplasty. Plast Reconstr Surg 2000;106(5):998–1003
49. Economides NG, Sifakis F: Reduction mammaplasty: A study of sequelae. Breast J 1997;3:69
50. Lejour M: Vertical mammaplasty: Early complication after 250 personal consecutive cases. Plast Reconstr Surg 1999;104(3):764–770
51. Mandrekas A D, Zambacos GJ, Anastasopoulos A, Hapsas DA: Reduction mammaplasty with the inferior pedicle technique: Early and late complications in 371 patients. Br J Plast Surg 1996;49(7):442–446

Superior-Medial Pedicle Technique for Large Breast Reduction

Jorge I. de la Torre, James N. Long, Luis O. Vásconez

51.1 Introduction

The surgical techniques of reduction mammoplasty combine both the reconstructive and aesthetic aspects of plastic surgery [1]. While the primary goal of reduction mammoplasty is to decrease the weight and size of the breast, aesthetic improvement is a high priority. Current refinements in breast reduction techniques strive to provide relief of physical discomfort while preserving breast function and maximizing aesthetic results.

Reduction mammoplasty has been described for more than 100 years; early techniques involved mastectomy or simple amputation of the breast. The procedure has evolved significantly from the lower pole amputation and free nipple graft described by Thorek in 1931 [2]. Schwarzmann [3] proposed preserving the subdermal arterial and venous supply of the nipple/areola complex. This approach increased nipple survival and led to the practice of deepithelializing the pedicles of the breast flaps, which is still practiced today. In 1956, Wise expanded this concept, resulting in the inverted T scar still commonly used [4]. To increase nipple viability, various approaches were developed to maintain the nipple areolar complex on a pedicle of both dermis and subcutaneous tissue. Breast resection was performed above and below the level of the nipple areolar complex (NAC). Variation in parenchymal resection included Strömbeck's horizontal bipedicle, Skoog's lateral pedicle, McKissock's vertically oriented, bipedicle flap, Ribeiro's inferiorly based dermoglandular flap, Weiner's superiorly based pedicle and the central-mound technique described by Balch [5–10]. Each of these techniques attempted to preserve vascularity, innervation and lactation of the nipple areolar complex.

While the inferior pedicle remains the most popular technique in the United States today, the superomedial based techniques are becoming increasingly popular. Lejour's and Lassus' utilization of the vertical scar mammoplasty emphasized resection of breast tissue rather than skin and advocated the use of suction assisted lipectomy to shape the breast [11–14]. These techniques preserve the dermoparenchymal microvasculature which in turn minimizes the risk of skin and fat necrosis. The superiorly based pedicle techniques include less skin undermining and simplified resections resulting in reduced operative time. Shaping the breast mound, which can be difficult with techniques that disrupt the dermoparenchymal relationship, becomes more easily achievable with intraparenchymal pillar suturing which are part of these techniques.

Subsequent variations of the vertical reduction mammoplasty include utilization of the superomedial pedicle and durability of the superomedial variant has been demonstrated by advocates such as Hall-Findlay [15, 16]. Her results show this approach provides an elegant synthesis of the superomedial pedicle and vertical closure, maintaining the dermoparenchymal unit yielding excellent long term results. The experiences of the author have also demonstrated the superomedial reduction to be a simple method of vertical reduction mammoplasty with excellent long term aesthetic results having low complication rates and safety even in larger volume reductions. The safety profile is maintained in larger volume reductions up to 2,750 g and in patients otherwise considered to be high risk.

51.2 Surgical Anatomy

There are three critical principles that affect the shape of the breast: the inframammary fold, projection and ptosis. The inframammary fold is a distinct histologic structure which consists of fibrous connections between the dermis and chest wall. It confines the lower pole of the normal breast and it can move superiorly with a significant reduction of the breast. Projection is defined as the transverse diameter over the surface of the breast from the midsternal line to the anterior axillary line. It is important to recognize preoperative projection deficits in order to maximize the three-dimensional fullness of the breast. To provide projection of the breast,

M.A. Shiffman (ed.), *Mastopexy and Breast Reduction: Principles and Practice*,
© Springer-Verlag Berlin Heidelberg 2009

the base diameter is decreased and the remaining breast tissue is coned. Ptosis is the vertical dimension, which extends from midclavicle, through the nipple, to inframammary fold. Regnault described a grading scale to quantify the degree to which glandular tissue is inferior to the inframammary fold [17]. To address ptosis, the breast parenchyma must be tightened, the excess skin must be removed and the nipple areolar complex transposed superiorly. Breast symmetry requires consideration of the changes in projection, the degree of ptosis and the location of the inframammary fold.

Innervation of the nipple is primarily via the lateral cutaneous branch of the fourth intercostal nerve. Preservation of nipple sensation occurs by avoiding injury to the lateral cutaneous branch of the fourth intercostal nerve during elevation of the vascular pedicle. Because the nerve courses deep to the pectoralis fascia as it traverses the chest wall from lateral to medial, keeping the dissection superficial to the fascia will usually avoid compromise of the nerve. Additional sensory innervation to the breast includes the supraclavicular nerves of the cervical plexus, which supply the superior aspect of the breast and the anterior cutaneous divisions of the second through seventh intercostals, which supply the breast medially.

The breast has three main arterial axes. The medial portion which is supplied by medial perforators of the internal mammary artery, accounts for 60% of the perfusion to the breast. The lateral portion of the breast supplied via the lateral thoracic artery provides an additional 30%. The remaining blood supply, approximately 10%, is provided by the variable anterior and lateral branches of the intercostals arteries. The significant collateral supply between these vascular networks allows for a variety of pedicles to safely maintain perfusion of the nipple areolar complex. The venous drainage of the breast consists of two systems. The internal mammary veins and the superficial veins of the neck drain the superficial aspect of the breast, while the deep venous system drains primarily into the internal mammary vein with additional drainage to the axillary vein.

51.3
Preoperative

Accurate preoperative marking of patients undergoing the medial pedicle mammary reduction is essential for obtaining consistent results. The markings include the chest midline, each breast meridian, the inframammary fold, the new NAC position nipple and the skin resection. The most important element is properly marking the new level of the transposed nipple areolar complex. Traditionally, this has been at the level of the inframammary crease, however in the vertical/short-scar medial pedicle reduction this level should be lowered approximately 1–1.5 cm to accommodate the increased projection of the breast mound. This will leave the nipple at the prominence of the breast and just at or slightly above the inframammary crease pointing anteriorly. It is important to avoid placing the nipple too high since this is a difficult problem to correct.

Proper nipple location can be determined by transposing the level of inframammary fold to the anterior aspect of the breast with the patient in the standing position and providing gentle support to the breast. This mark, usually between 20 and 23 cm from the sternal notch, should be used to indicate the most cephalad aspect of the NAC transposition rather than the location of the nipple proper. The shape of the areola inset is designed to be wider than its height to accommodate the vertical tension that will occur as the breast settles in the postoperative period. Either an ellipse or mosque-shaped areolar window is suitable; however the total length of the incision should be approximately equal to or slightly larger than the total circumference of the nipple-marker used (approximately 15 cm for a 45 mm nipple marker).

Once the appropriate nipple location is decided, the remaining skin incisions are marked accordingly. As in the vertical resection reduction mammoplasty, the breast parenchyma is mobilized medially and the lateral resection is marked from the nipple–areola complex (NAC) to the inframammary fold with the medial incision marked in a similar fashion. No markings are required for the inframammary resection; rather the minimal resection is performed to remove any resultant tissue redundancies.

General anesthesia is routinely required. The arms are wrapped and the patient is placed in reverse Trendelenburg position. This reduces or eliminates the need to sit the patient upright but it permits some appreciation of the effects of gravity. The breasts are liberally infiltrated with lidocaine with epinephrine and in the cases of larger breasts, a tumescent infusion pump is used with a 22-gauge spinal needle to expedite infiltration. The local anesthesia not only permits the use of laryngeal mask anesthesia rather than endotracheal intubation but it also facilitates sharp resection rather than extensive use of electrocautery. The authors find sharp resection to be more expedient and precise than dissection electrocautery.

The specific technique selected for reduction mammoplasty is modified based on the degree of ptosis. Patients with limited ptosis are candidates for a superior pedicle and vertical reduction. Moderate to severe ptosis usually requires a superior-medial pedicle and either a vertical incision or a short inframammary resection (inverted T). The superior-medial approach can be employed even in very large reductions (i.e., exceeding 1,500 g). Only cases of very severe ptosis require the use of an inferior pedicle, particularly if the inframammary fold to nipple distance is relatively short and the medial pedicle length exceeds 25 cm.

51.4 Technique

The medial pedicle, vertical incision technique described by Hall-Findlay is one of the most versatile and effective methods for breast reduction. It allows reduction of a large breast, maintains nipple function and viability, and yields an excellent aesthetic result (Figs. 51.1 and 51.2).

The superior-medial pedicle is based on perforators from the internal mammary vascular axis as well as direct perforators from the pectoralis nusor. The skin is deepithelialized within the entire pedicle pattern exclud-

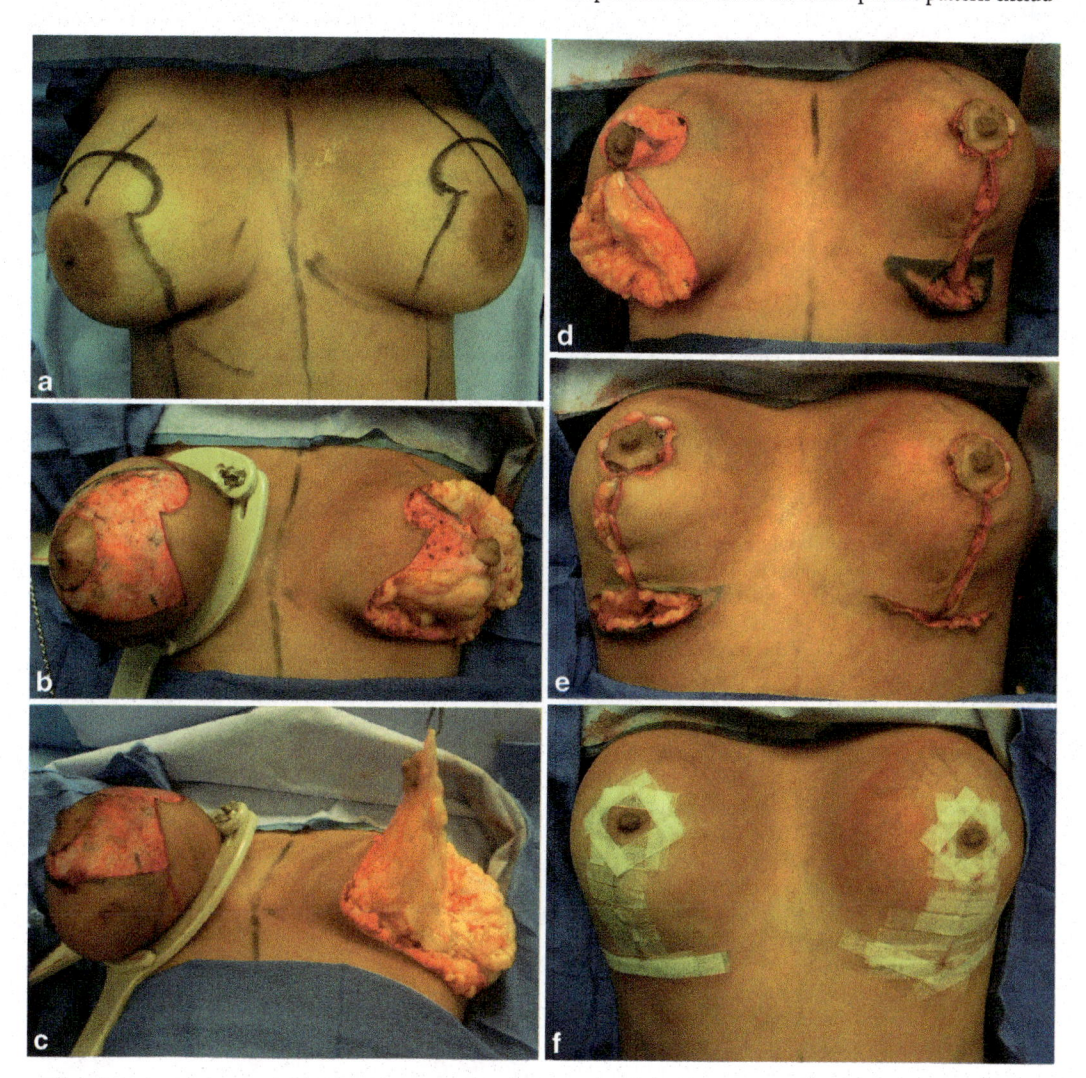

Fig. 51.1 (a) Preoperative marking with the patient supine on the operating table. Note that the circumference of the nipple window (keyhole) is 15 cm. The widest portion of the resection, just below the original NAC is approximately 15 cm. (b) The right breast has had the superior medial pedicle deepithelialized. Note that the Mammostat is in place to facilitate the deepithelialization and initial resection of the breast. The left breast has had the initial resection complete from the superior, lateral and inferior breast. (c) The deep perforators to the pedicle are preserved as noted by elevation of the left pedicle. Note how the use of epinephrine reduces bleeding even when the scalpel is used to resect. (d) The initial transposition of the right breast. The left NAC is completely inset and the vertical incision is closed except for the skin. The short inframammary resection is marked. (e) The right breast NAC and vertical incision are closed and the inframammary resection is being approximated. The closure of the right breast is complete. (f) Both breasts are completely closed with tape closure in place

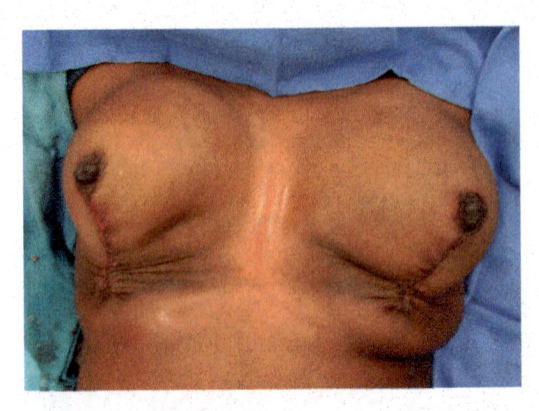

Fig. 51.2 Intraoperative patient with a 1,200 g reduction and closure of both sides using a medical pedicle, vertical reduction mammoplasty. Suction lipectomy has been performed on the left to reduce the inframammary fullness. The vertical incisions have been pleated to reduce the length of the vertical incision; however, the incision extends below the level of the inframmary fold

ing the sized nipple–areola complex. Resection is performed around the superior-lateral margins of the keyhole pattern perpendicular to the plane of the skin. In addition, the breast parenchyma inferior and lateral to the nipple is removed without undermining the pedicle. The lateral excision extends to the anterior axillary line but leaves a thick lateral pillar. The pedicle is further resected as needed to provide the desired volume reduction, making sure that the base of pedicle is at least 6 cm wide. The pedicle is rotated and inset from the apex of the pedicle to the 12 o' clock inset position. The medial and lateral parenchymal pillars are approximated which cones the breast, decreasing the base diameter and increasing projection. The deep dermal layer is approximated with interrupted sutures. The inferior skin excess of the breast and adipose tissues are then removed (similar to the limbs of the Wise pattern skin resection). Sharp resection, suction lipectomy, or both are used to thin out the area under the skin, decreasing dog-ear formation and reducing the length of the inframammary skin resection. Typically the vertical incision is kept less than 7 cm and the inframammary skin can be resected if this distance is too long. Additional suction lipectomy can be performed at this point to further reduce the breast or improve symmetry without taking down the closure. The vertical incision, and when needed the inframammary incision, are closed with a running subcuticular absorbable suture.

51.5
Postoperative Care

Following skin closure, tape, a light dressing, and a surgical support bra are placed and left intact for 24 h. Patients can then shower and begin using a soft support bra of their preference. Drains are not needed but if used, removal occurs by postoperative day 3–4 if the drainage is less than 30 ml per day [18]. Skin tape is left in place for 10–14 days to minimize discomfort at the time of removal. Exercise and strenuous labor can be resumed 10–21 days postoperatively as tolerated. Swelling and settling of the breast can take as long as 3 months to become final. Postoperative photographs should be obtained after this point. At 6 months a postoperative baseline mammogram can be performed and the patient can then resume routine cancer surveillance measures.

51.6
Complications

The author's review of 692 consecutive patients who underwent reduction mammoplasty with the previously described approach has revealed an acceptable complication rate. As with many plastic surgical procedures, postoperative dissatisfaction typically arises out of aesthetic concerns. Although improvement in physical symptoms following reduction mammoplasty is consistently reported in the literature, one of the most common complaints patients express is that their desired breast size and appearance were not met [19]. Breast asymmetry is extremely common, but in the majority of cases it is minimal and usually an improvement with respect to the preoperative asymmetry. Significant asymmetry which the patient notices or which requires further surgical revision occurs less than 10% of the time. Complications such as partial nipple slough are uncommon (less than 1%) and of minimal risk to the patient but can be disfiguring and can require revisional procedures. Thickened or poor quality scars can be seen in approximately 5% of patients; however the use of the short inframammary scar actually improves the quality of the inferior aspect of the vertical incision. Fat necrosis was noted in 4% of patients and decreased subjective sensibility in 2% of patients. The medial pedicle does not appear to affect the capacity to lactate or successfully breast-feed, but

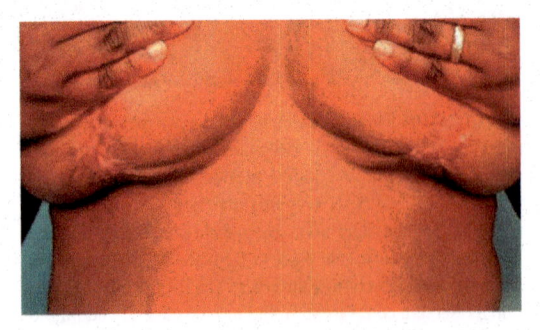

Fig. 51.3 Postoperative poor scar healing following a vertical only reduction mammoplasty

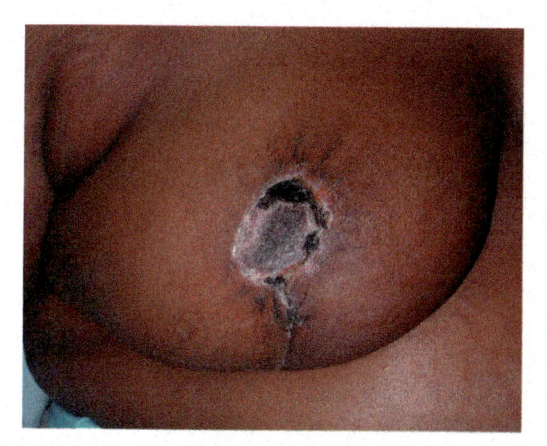

Fig. 51.4 Partial nipple areolar complex necrosis following an 1,800 g reduction in a diabetic patient

patients should be made aware of the potential risks. Obesity in patients with a body mass index (BMI) that exceeds 40 should be given extra consideration as candidates for reduction mammoplasty, as their risk of complication is significantly elevated. Those that are candidates for surgery are often encouraged to start weight loss programs. Facilitated by their increased mobility, these pt's can be brought to quite succesful results. Additional risks are those complications that accompany any operation including infection, bleeding, seroma, and pulmonary emboli. Proper precaution for deep vein thrombosis (DVT) formation and appropriate use of antibiotics should be employed (Figs. 51.3 and 51.4).

51.7 Conclusions

The medial pedicle technique is a simple method of vertical reduction mammoplasty with excellent long term aest-hetic results (Fig. 51.5–51.7). It achieves fullness in the upper pole while excising tissue in the inferior and lateral breast, and limits the tendency for a bottomed out appearance. This results in a rounder, more conical breast mound, with better projection. Complication rates are similar to or better than other techniques, and there is no increase in the rate of complications with in

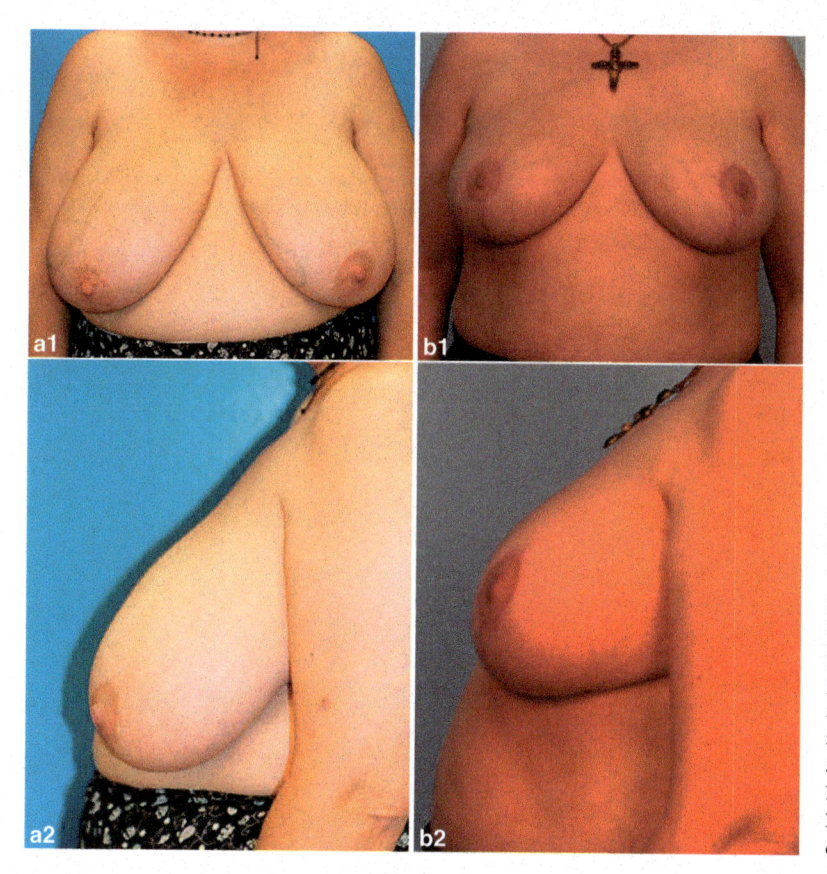

Fig. 51.5 (**a1,2**) Preoperative patient being seen for a large volume reduction mammoplasty. Note Nipple–Sternal notch distance is greater than 30 cm. (**b1,2**) Four months postoperative following medial pedicle reduction mammoplasty (1,750 g *left side* and 1,820 g *right side*). Note slight elevation of the NAC secondary to bottoming out of breast tissue

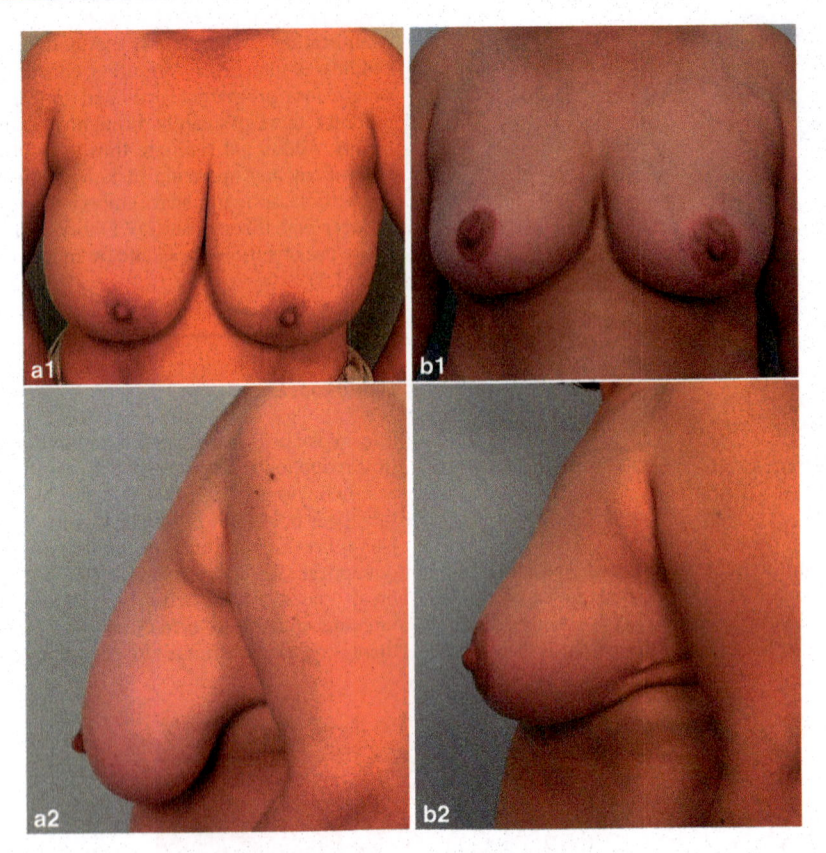

Fig. 51.6 (*a1,2*) Preoperative patient being seen for reduction mammoplasty with significant ptosis following bariatric weight loss. (*b1,2*) Postoperative following medial pedicle reduction with inframammary resection (750 g reduction per side). Note inframammary scar is relatively long to address the skin laxity and breast ptosis

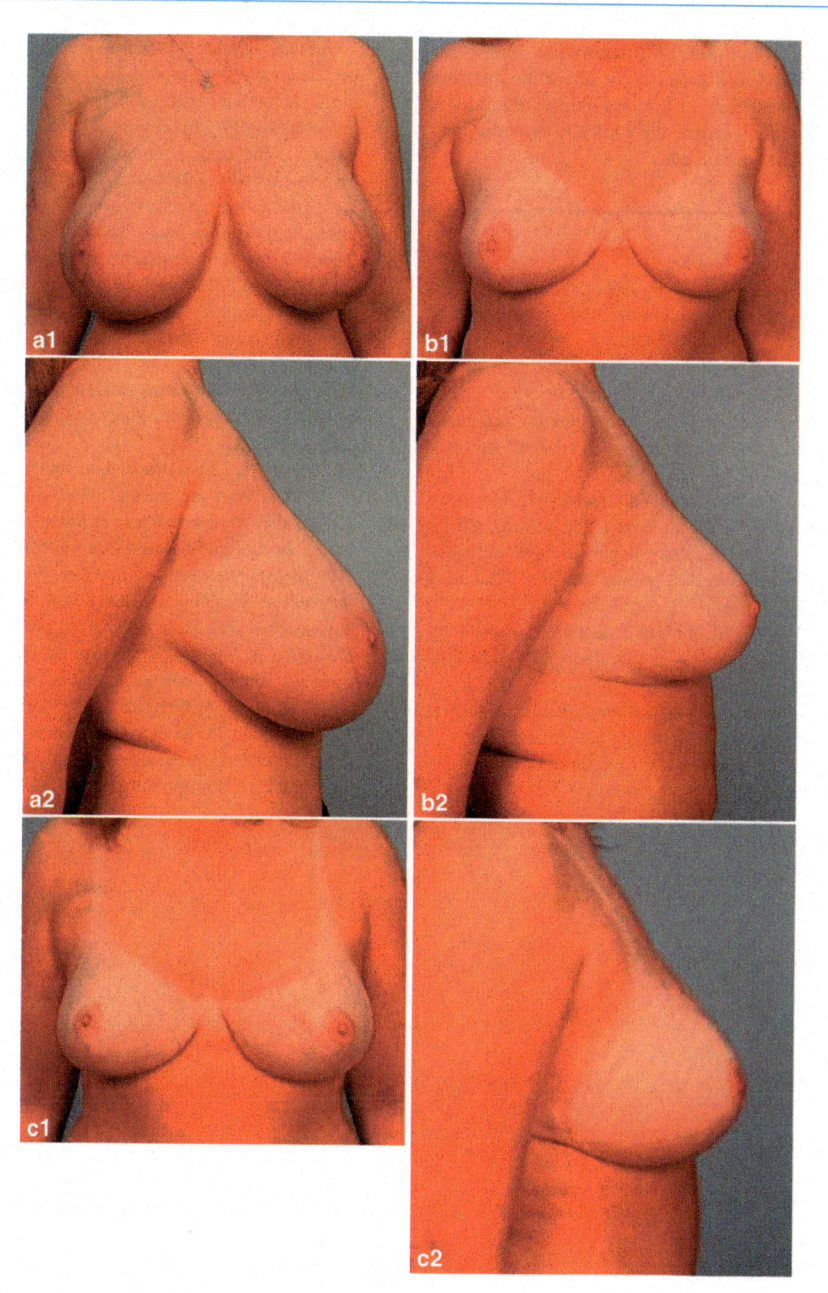

Fig. 51.7 (**a1,2**) Preoperative. (**b1,2**) Three months postoperative following medial pedicle short scar reduction mammoplasty (1,050 g on the right and 980 g on the left). (**c1,2**) Eighteen months postoperative demonstrating the long-lasting results possible with appropriate preoperative marking of the NAC and proper approximation of the medial and lateral pedicles

larger volume reductions. This technique for breast reduction is reliable and as safe as, or safer than, inferior pedicle techniques even in larger volume reductions. Addition, it is easily learned, and typically provides better long-term aesthetic results.

References

1. Schnur PL, Hoehn JG, Ilstrup DM, Cahoy MJ, Chu CP: Reduction mammaplasty: cosmetic or reconstructive procedure? Ann Plast Surg 1991;27(3):232–237
2. Thoreck M: Possibilities in the Reconstruction of the Human Form. NY Med J Rec 1922;116:572
3. Schwartzmann E.: Beitrag zur vermeidung von mamillennekrose bei einzeitiger mammaplastik schwerer falle. Rev Chir Struct 1937;7:206–209
4. Wise RJ: A preliminary report on a method of planning the mammaplasty. Plast Reconstr Surg 1956;17(5):367–375
5. Strömbeck JO: Mammaplasty: Report of a new technique based on the two pedicle procedure. Br J Plast Surg 1960;13:79–90
6. Skoog T: A technique of breast reduction. Transposit ion of the nipple on a cutaneous vascular pedicle. Acta Chir Scand 1963;126:453–465
7. McKissock PK: Reduction mammoplasty with a vertical dermal flap. Plast Reconstr Surg 1972;49(3):245–252
8. Ribeiro L: A new technique for reduction mammoplasty. Plast Reconstr Surg 1975;55(3):330–334
9. Weiner DL, Aiache AE, Tirriranonda T: A single dermal pedicle for nipple transposition in subcutaneous mastectomy, reduction mammaplasty, or mastopexy. Plast Reconstr Surg 1973;51(2):115–120
10. Balch C: The central mound technique for reduction mammoplasty. Plast Reconstr Surg 1981;67(3):305–311
11. Lassus C: A 30-year experience with vertical mammaplasty. Plast Reconstr Surg 1996;97(2):373–380
12. Lassus C: Update on vertical mammaplasty. Plast Reconstr Surg 1999;104(7):2289–2304
13. Lejour M: Vertical mammaplasty: early complications after 250 personal consecutive cases. Plast Reconstr Surg 1999;104(3):764–770
14. Lejour M: Vertical mammaplasty: update and appraisal of late results. Plast Reconstr Surg 1999;104(3):771–781; discussion 782–784
15. Hall-Findlay E: Vertical breast reduction: a critical analysis of 400 cases. Plast Surg Forum 1998;21:133
16. Hall-Findlay EJ: A simplified vertical reduction mammaplasty: shortening the learning curve. Plast Reconstr Surg 1999;104(3):748–759; discussion 760–763
17. Regnault P, Daniel R: Breast Ptosis. Aesthetic Plastic Surgery. New York, Little Brown 1984, p 539
18. Matarasso A, Wallach SG, Rankin M: Reevaluating the need for routine drainage in reduction mammaplasty. Plast Reconstr Surg 1998;102(6):1917–1921
19. Jones SA, Bain JR: Review of data describing outcomes that are used to assess quality of life after reduction mammoplasty. Plast Reconstr Surg 2001;108:62–67

The Central Mound Technique for Reduction Mammaplasty

Bret R. Baack

52.1 Introduction

The central mound technique (also known as the central pedicle technique) of breast reduction was first described by Hester et al in 1985 [1]. This technique is extremely versatile in that it involves separation of the breast skin from the gland, direct reduction of the glandular tissue, and custom tailoring of the skin to obtain projection while controlling the amount of tension on the closure. This method maintains the robust vascular supply to the gland which consists of branches of the lateral thoracic and thoracoacromial arteries superiorly and laterally. Additional vessels enter the gland posteriorly consisting of pectoralis major perforators supplied by the anterolateral and anteromedial intercostal perforators, and the internal mammary perforators. The primary sensory nerve to the nipple is the lateral cutaneous branch of the fourth intercostal nerve which is preserved with this technique. The majority of the lactiferous ducts and underlying glandular tissue are maintained, allowing breast-feeding postoperatively for most patients. Extensive clinical experiences attest to the safety and reliability of this technique even in patients requiring large reductions or with marked ptosis, therefore obviating the need for free nipple/areola grafting [2–5].

52.2 Technique

The preoperative markings are relatively straightforward compared to other breast reduction techniques, allowing the surgeon flexibility in shaping the breast as well as the final nipple–areola complex (NAC) position. The sternal notch and inframammary fold (IMF) are marked with the patient in a sitting position. The level of the fold is then projected anteriorly onto the meridian of the breast which will serve as the approximate final position of the nipple (Fig. 52.1). Symmetry is assured between these points in respect to the sternal notch and chest midline. Typically the sternal notch to nipple distance measures between 21 and 25 cm. The distance from the nipple to the midline is measured, and this distance from the midline marked on the inframammary fold to ensure that the vertical line of the closure will not be skewed medially or laterally. This measurement is usually 10–12 cm. A 5–6 cm wide pedicle is then centered about this point on the IMF and vertical lines drawn superiorly to just skirt around the existing areola to the new nipple location (Fig. 52.2). The pedicle can be made even narrower if there are concerns about the amount of skin laxity present to avoid a tight skin closure, as the inferior dermal pedicle does not contribute significantly to the blood supply of the areola.

If available, paravertebral blocks administered by the anesthesiology service prior to induction will provide significant pain reduction in the first 10–12 h postoperatively. The patient is positioned with the arms secured to arm boards at 90° and the knees flexed over a pillow and the heels padded. Sequential compression devices are placed prior to induction, and prophylactic intravenous antibiotics administered (cefazolin 1 g for weight <80 kg, 2 g for weight >80 kg, substituting clindamycin if the patient has an allergy to cefazolin). A test sit-up to 90° is performed prior to prepping and draping to assure that all equipment is secure and functioning.

The operation is begun by marking a new areola with a template of 38–43 mm. in diameter. The breast is infiltrated with approximately 60 cc of tumescent solution with an epinephrine concentration of 1:1,000,000 for hemostasis. The skin outside of the new areola marking within the pedicle is de-epithelialized. Although deskinning has been proposed to save time [6], the author prefers to leave the dermis intact. Intact dermis around the areola helps minimize shear forces on the nipple/areola complex. If there is breakdown along the vertical closure or most commonly at the T-juncture of the vertical and horizontal scars, the exposed dermis should hasten re-epithelialization of the wound. Skin flaps are elevated approximately 1.5–2.0 cm in thickness, first medially,

M.A. Shiffman (ed.), *Mastopexy and Breast Reduction: Principles and Practice*,
© Springer-Verlag Berlin Heidelberg 2009

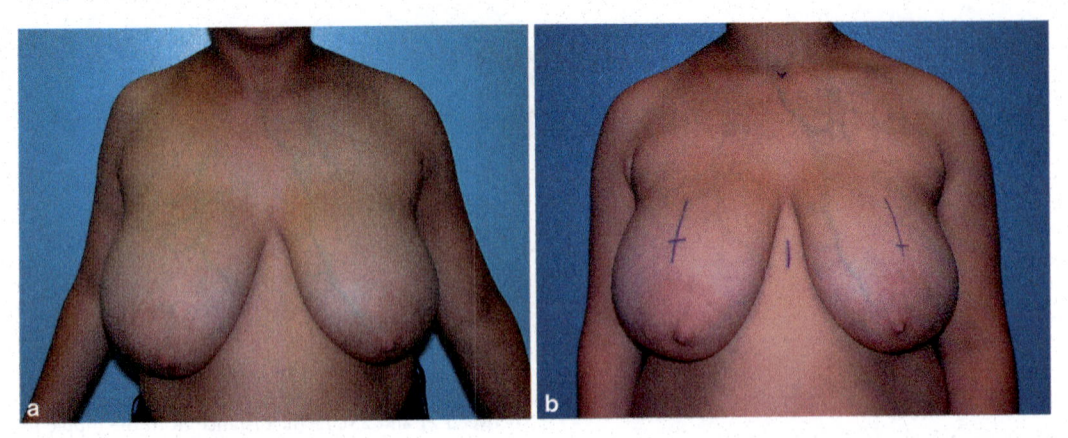

Fig. 52.1 (a) A 20-year-old patient with symptomatic macromastia. (b) The approximate position of the nipple is marked by transposing the inframammary fold (IMF) anteriorly onto the meridian of the breast. Symmetry is ensured with respect to the sternal notch and midline

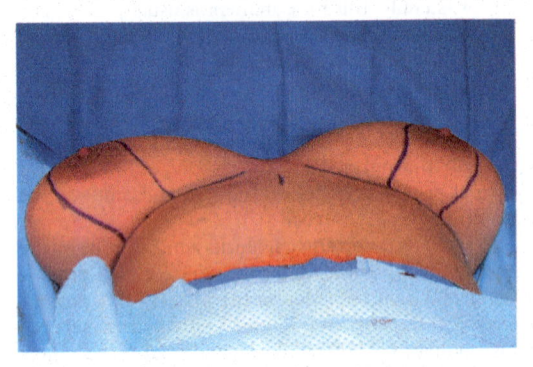

Fig. 52.2 A pedicle of 5–6 cm. in width is centered on the meridian of the IMF and drawn to just skirt around the existing areola up to the marked nipple point

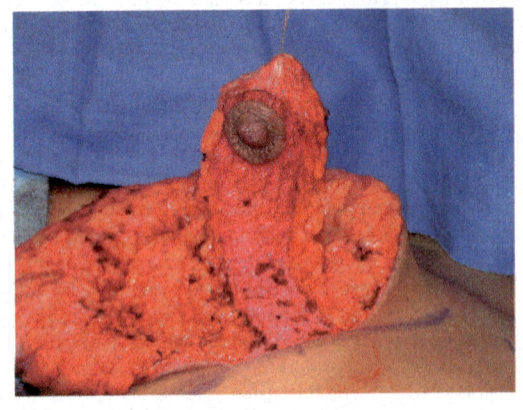

Fig. 52.4 Tangential excision of breast tissue is performed, leaving 2 cm of tissue overlying the pectoralis fascia

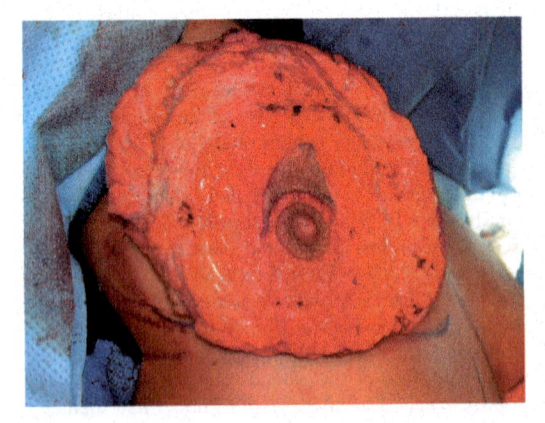

Fig. 52.3 The pedicle is deepithelialized, and the skin flap elevated

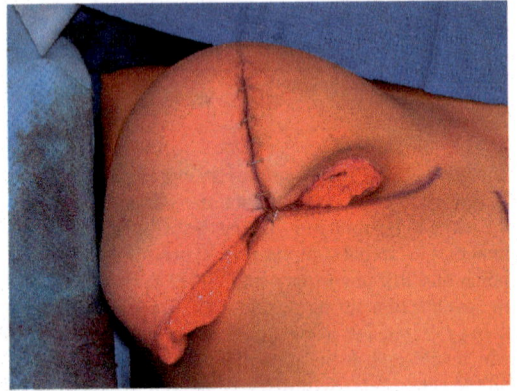

Fig. 52.5 The vertical limb is temporarily closed under mild tension, creating medial and lateral dog-ears which are marked and excised

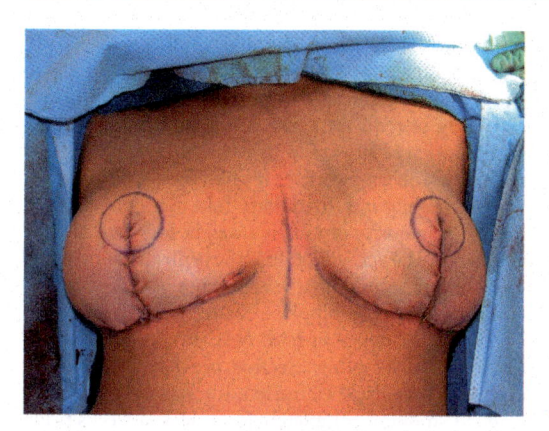

Fig. 52.6 The patient is placed in a sitting position on the operating table to assess size and symmetry. The desired position of the nipple is marked

then laterally, and finally superiorly. The dissection should leave approximately 2 cm. of tissue on the pectoralis fascia to preserve the neurovascular supply (Fig. 52.3).

The nipple/areola complex is retracted anteriorly, and glandular reduction performed in a tangential fashion, with the majority of the tissue excised from the superior and lateral aspects of the breast. This can usually be accomplished quickly with a scalpel with minimal blood loss if tumescent solution is used. Conservative resection is performed medially to prevent postoperative flattening of the breast in this area. Reduction is performed until the desired size is achieved or the pedicle is the circumference of the overlying areola (Fig. 52.4). This results in a freely mobile nipple–areola centered on a conical section of glandular tissue behind it, which gives shape and projection. All excised tissue is placed in separate containers for the right and left breast for weight evaluation during the procedure and eventual pathologic examination, as there is a small (approximately 1 in 500) but definite risk of finding occult breast cancer in the specimen [7].

Skin reduction is performed by pulling the skin flaps towards the center of the base of the pedicle. A temporary vertical closure is performed with staples. The skin flaps should be brought together with minimal tension while producing an aesthetic breast shape (Fig. 52.5). The vertical limb usually measures 8–10 cm. Excessive tension should be avoided, especially on the inferior aspect of the vertical limb at the inframammary fold, as this will commonly lead to breakdown in this area postoperatively. The resultant dog-ears medially and laterally are marked and excised, and the skin temporarily stapled into position.

The patient is placed in the sitting position to check for size, shape, and symmetry. After any adjustments are made, the desired nipple–areola positions are marked with a template, with measurements made from the sternal notch, inframammary fold, and midline to ensure symmetry (Fig. 52.6). The skin inside the markings is removed as is the excess skin along the vertical closure. A closed suction drain is placed within the breast prior to closure and brought out through the lateral aspect of the breast. The areola is inset and skin closure performed with interrupted buried absorbable suture for the dermis, followed by a running subcuticular closure with Monocryl (Ethicon). A mild compressive dressing is applied.

The dressings are removed the following day as are the drains. Patients are allowed to shower at that time and wear a snug sports bra day and night for the first 4 weeks. Normal activities are permitted in 2–3 weeks.

52.3 Complications

The author performed 238 cases in the 9-year period between July 1997 and June 2006. Of these, 228 had complete records available for review with at least 3 months of follow-up. The average age was 36, with a range of 16–69. The average amount of tissue excised was 639 g per breast, with a range of 100–1,903 g.

There was no loss of the nipple–areola complex, either total or partial, in any of the patients. Infection consisting of localized cellulitis developed in 1.5% of breasts, all of which responded to a course of oral cephalexin. Six patients reported diminished sensation in one breast at 3 months follow-up (1.3%). The most common complication was delayed healing due to tissue breakdown at the T-juncture in 4.4% of breasts. The average amount of tissue excised in these breasts was 966 g, as opposed to an average weight of

Table 52.1 Complications after Central Mound Reduction Mammaplasty in 228 patients (456 breasts)

Complication	Number of Breasts	Percentage
Total loss NAC	0	0.0
Partial loss NAC	0	0.0
Hematoma	0	0.0
Infection[a]	7	1.5
Loss of NAC sensation	6	1.3
Delayed healing	20	4.4
Fat necrosis	4	0.9
Revision required	6 patients	2.6
Deep vein thrombosis	0	0.0

[a]Cellulitis, all responded to oral antibiotics

626 g removed from breasts without healing complications. As noted by Lejour [8], breast weight is a major factor in the incidence of postoperative complications, especially delayed healing. Fat necrosis developed in 4 breasts (0.9%) and 6 patients required scar revisions (2.6%). There were no cases of hematoma, seroma, or deep venous thrombosis in this series (Table 52.1).

52.4
Discussion

It is important for plastic surgeons to be proficient at more than one technique of breast reduction, as one operation should not be applied to all breasts. Short-scar techniques are deservedly becoming more popular and are quite applicable to breasts requiring less than 600–800 g of reduction with minimal ptosis and good skin elasticity. However, the vertical mammaplasty techniques do not work well in women with inelastic skin and a long inframammary fold to nipple distance (as in the majority of massive weight loss patients), or who require larger reductions. The central mound technique allows for maximal preservation of the neurovascular supply to the nipple/areola complex, as attested by the 0% incidence of total NAC loss in the author's series. As in all other elective procedures in which extensive skin flaps are raised, the patient must have stopped smoking completely for at least 4 weeks prior

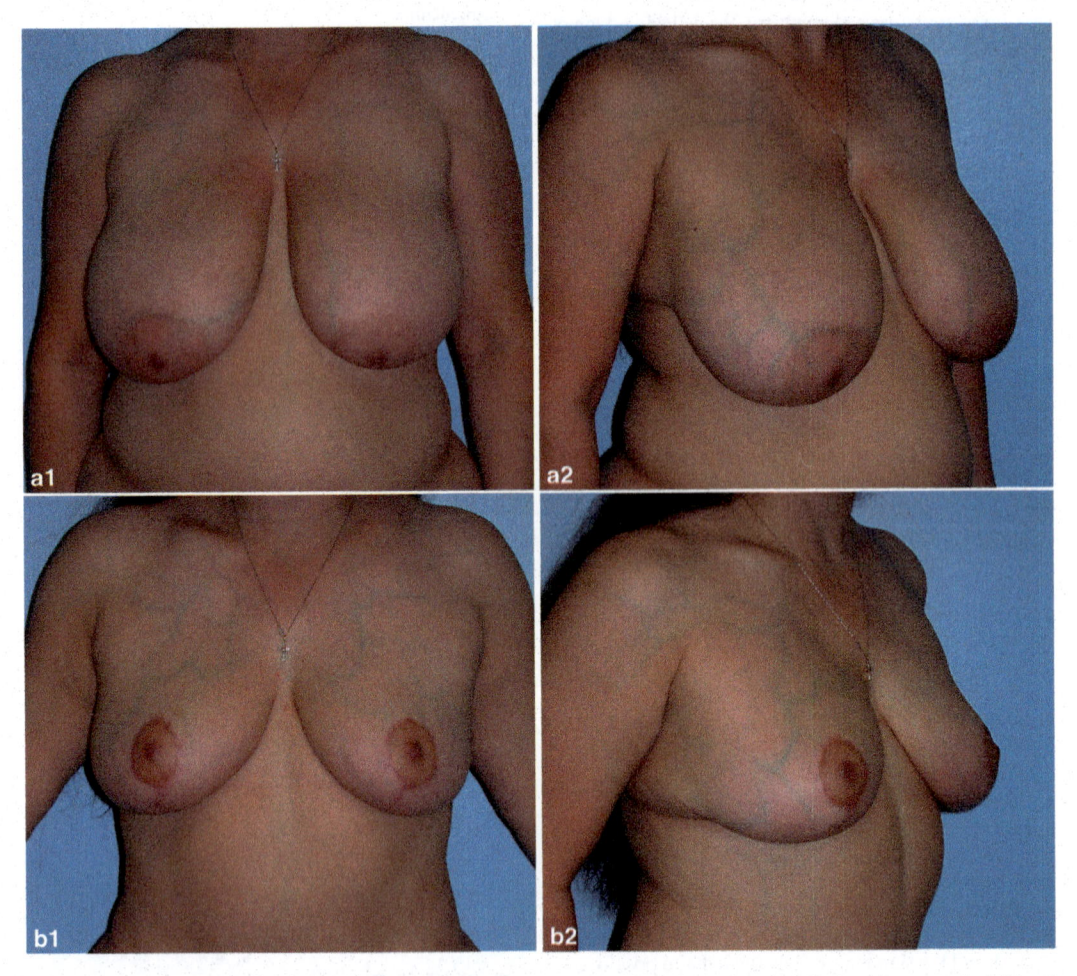

Fig. 52.7 (*a1,2*) Preoperative 32-year-old woman with grade 3 ptosis. (**b***1,2*) The result at 3 months following the removal of 600 g of tissue from the right breast and 540 g from the left breast

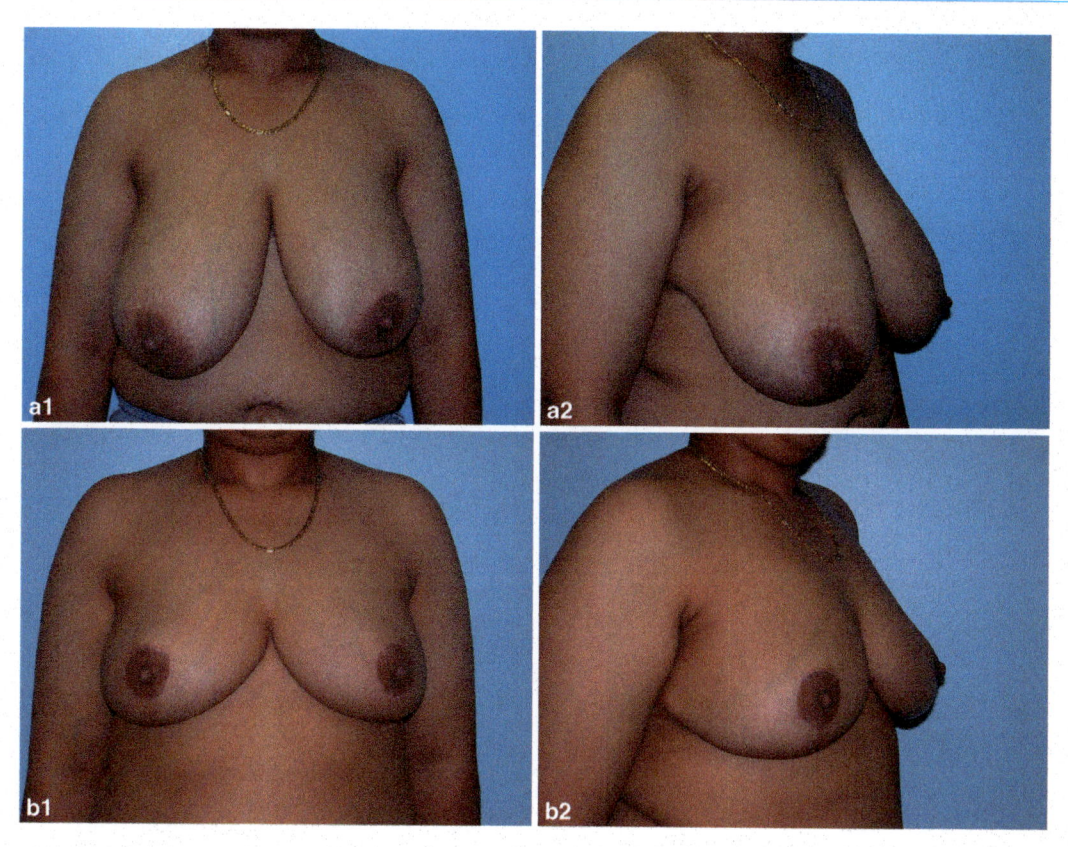

Fig. 52.8 (**a1,2**) Preoperative 30-year-old woman with marked asymmetry. (**b1,2**) The result at 6 months following the removal of 965 g of tissue from the right breast and 775 g from the left breast

to surgery (if there are any doubts, a cotinine level is obtained prior to surgery). The complication rate is low, but there is an increased incidence of delayed healing in larger reductions (greater than 1,000 g per side) and in patients with a history of smoking [4]. The position of the NAC is adjustable intraoperatively, and avoids positioning the nipple too high which can occur in other techniques where the nipple position is set in advance. This may account for the fact that the author has not seen a patient postoperatively with the complaint of "bottoming out."

The central mound technique allows for maximal freedom in breast shaping on the operating table while controlling the amount of tension on the skin closure, allowing for a pleasing aesthetic shape in the immediate postoperative period (Figs. 52.7 and 52.8). Long term follow-up shows excellent preservation of shape with a very high patient satisfaction rate.

References

1. Hester TR, Bostwick J 3rd, Miller L, Cunningham SJ: Breast reduction utilizing the maximally vascularized central breast pedicle. Plast Reconstr Surg 1985;76(6):890–900
2. Balch CR: The central mound technique for reduction mammaplasty. Plast Reconstr Surg 1981;67(3):305–311
3. Levet Y: The pure posterior pedicle procedure for breast reduction. Plast Reconstr Surg 1990;86:67–75
4. White DJ, Baack BR, et al: Clinical applications of the central pedicle technique of breast reduction. In: Operative Tech in Plast Reconstr Surg 1996;3(3):176–183
5. Grant JH, Rand RP: The maximally vascularized central pedicle breast reduction: evolution of a technique. Annals Plastic Surg 2001;46:584–589
6. Iwuagwu OC, Drew PJ: Deskinning versus deepithelialization for inferior pedicle reduction mammaplasy: a prospective comparative analysis. Aesthetic Plast Surg 2005;29(3):202–204
7. Colwell AS, Kukreja J, Breuing KH, Lester S, Orgill DP: Occult breast carcinoma in reduction mammaplasty specimens: 14-year experience. Plast Reconstr Surg 2004;113(7):1984–1988
8. Lejour M: Vertical Mammaplasty and Liposuction. St. Louis, MO, Quality Medical Publishing 1994

Central Mound Technique for Breast Reduction

Richard C. Hagerty, Andre Uflacker

53.1 Introduction

As Western women, particularly American women, have grown significantly over the last two decades, so have women's breast sizes and the symptoms that accompany them. This phenomenon has led to an increased number of women seeking breast reduction, as well as an increase in the amount of breast tissue to be reduced. Many excellent techniques for breast reduction have been described and are utilized today [1–6]. The larger amount of breast to be reduced commensurately reduces the surgical options. The greater the reduction size, the greater the risk of nipple necrosis and fat necrosis secondary to decreased blood supply because of an increased length of the pedicle. Unfortunately, weight loss and exercise discipline in these patients has not resulted in any meaningful reduction in the size of the breasts. Therefore, a surgical solution is usually necessary.

In general, if the nipple needs to be moved 10 cm or less superiorly and (if there are no underlying medical problems such as diabetes or environmental problems such as smoking that would interfere with the vascularity), the central mound technique is used [1, 4, 5]. This technique has the best chance of preserving sensation and viability of the nipple and reducing bottoming out of the breast inferiorly in the long term. The central mound technique also has the advantage of giving a good conical shape to the breasts. When the nipple needs to be moved superiorly more than 10 cm and the reduction is greater than fifteen hundred grams, the nipple graft technique is considered. The inferior pedicle technique, where no vertical component of the scar is necessary is also an excellent option. The authors decline to electively operate on any patient whom we know is actively smoking.

Large, heavy, pendulous breasts can be the source of significant difficulties, both mental and physical. In the young they can be a cause of considerable embarrassment, resulting in marked limitation of activities and social contacts. The breast can cause multiple functional problems through traction on the shoulders and spine, resulting in poor posture, neck strain, headaches, back pain and dermatitis. Without support, the weight of the breast pulls the shoulders forward and down, resulting in poor posture. With support from a brassiere, the weight of the breast is transferred to the shoulder straps, compressing the underlying soft tissue and the brachial plexus, which may result in paresthesias.

The patient is frequently overweight, compensating for the abnormal proportions of her breasts, and reducing the disparity of contour. Many patients with large breasts have a poor body image. Reduction mammoplasty can eliminate the symptoms and reduce the psychological distress. The goal in breast reduction surgery is to reduce the above symptoms and obtain breasts of appropriate size, symmetry, and sensation.

53.1.1 Anatomical Considerations

The breast receives its vascular supply mainly from the branches of the internal mammary artery medially, and from the lateral thoracic artery laterally (Fig. 53.1). Further vascular supply to the gland and nipple areolar complex comes from the thoracoacromial and intercostal perforating arteries. The majority of the blood comes from the base.

Innervation is supplied to the nipple and the areola by the branches of the anterior and lateral cutaneous nerves, which derive mainly from the fourth intercostal nerve. They pass through the subcutaneous tissue, through the base of the breast close to the underlying fascia and on to the center of the breast where they then progress to the nipple areolar complex, mostly from the upper medial pole. Consequently, with regard to the neurovascular supply to the nipple areolar complex, the medial upper pole of the breast tissue is preserved as much as possible.

M.A. Shiffman (ed.), *Mastopexy and Breast Reduction: Principles and Practice*,
© Springer-Verlag Berlin Heidelberg 2009

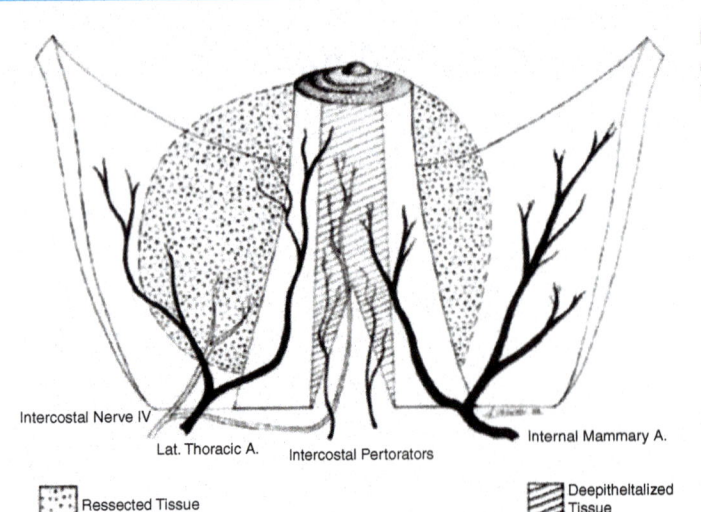

Fig. 53.1 Inferior view of the central mound showing preservation of the neurovascular bundle, and the larger lateral resection

53.2 Procedure

53.2.1 General Considerations

The patient is placed in the sitting or standing position. A vertical line is marked between the sternal notch and the umbilicus (Fig. 53.2). A second vertical line is made from the mid clavicle to the new nipple areolar complex, usually between 18 and 21 cm. The longer measurement is to allow for the stretching of the heavier breast. This mark loosely coincides with the level of the inframammary crease. A circle 5 cm in diameter is marked out which represents the new position of the nipple areolar complex. The circle is deepithelialized and the nipple–areola is advanced to the new position. A mark is made from the centerline along the inframammary crease of 10 cm bilaterally to mark the center of the breast.

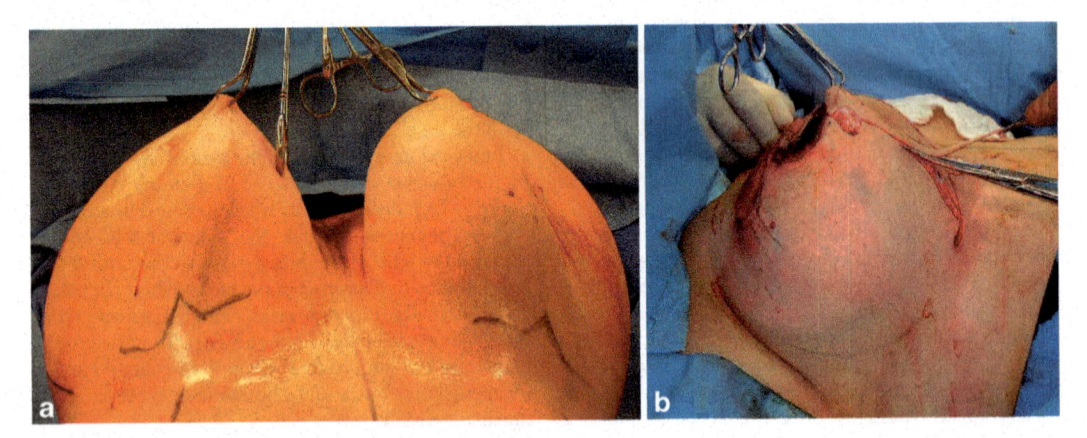

Fig. 53.2 (a) Novel technique for breast suspension, showing the breasts suspended by towel clips to a tenaculum attached to the ether screen bar. (b) Suspended breast and inferior deepithelialization

The new inframammary crease is marked about 1–2 cm above the actual inframammary crease and a triangle is marked as well, superior to the inframammary crease. Leaving this triangle reduces tension problems in this "T" area of healing. Any asymmetry is noted and the amount of breast reduction to be resected is marked. When present, the excess tissue in the axilla is circled.

The patient is taken to the operating room where she is placed in the supine position with arms extended and padded. The arms are wrapped for additional support. After general anesthesia, the back of the patient is brought up to thirty degrees. An ether screen is normally placed over the head of the patient. The nipple areolar complex is marked in Methylene Blue at 38 mm in diameter. Vertical incisions are made above the areola to the 5 cm circle that was previously drawn and then down to the triangle as well. This is usually about 3–4 cm in width.

Tumescent fluid is placed in each axilla when there is excess tissue and conservative liposuction is done (Fig. 53.3). Care is taken to make the liposuction area separate from the breast reduction area. Liposuction of the breast itself is avoided because of the possibility of compromising the blood supply to the nipple areolar complex. Once the axillary suctioning is completed, the inferior and superior pedicles are deepithelialized.

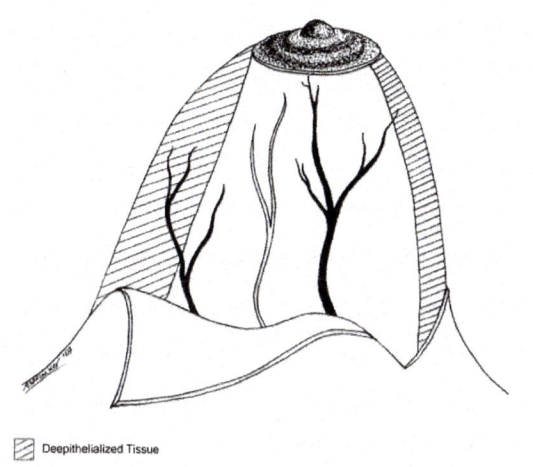

Fig. 53.3 Central mound showing preservation of the neurovascular bundle and deepithelialized tissue superiorly and inferiorly

53.2.2
Novel Technique for Breast Suspension

The authors normally suspend the breasts during the operative procedure. Suspension allows for static mobilization of the breasts for more accurate, efficient and elegant surgical manipulation. The first assistant is no longer required to manually suspend the breast, and is free to help the operating surgeon with both hands.

The suspension can be done with readily available instruments and equipment in the operating room. The technique is adaptable and easily learned. Equipment includes a tenaculum, towel clips, and an ether screen. After the patient is intubated, an ether screen is placed approximately 20 cm horizontally above the chin. The patient is draped and the breast is exposed. The head of the bed is elevated to the about thirty degrees. A tenaculum clamp is placed through the drape around the horizontal ether screen bar in the midline. Large towel clips are placed into the breast dermis at about the apex of the new areolar complex and adjusted appropriately. These clips are attached to the tenaculum with either large or small towel clips suspending the breast. After the liposuction and deepithelialization of the breast is completed, the clips are readjusted. The skin flaps are elevated medially and laterally and are left about 1 cm in thickness. The recipient area for the nipple areolar complex, the 5 cm diameter, is deepithelialized. Normally there is no incision beyond the deepithelialization from the 9 to 3 O'clock position to help preserve blood supply through the superior pedicle.

Classically, in the original description of the central mound technique, this bridge is divided; however, by preserving the deepithelialized bridge, there is greater blood supply to preserve to the nipple. The greater the distance from the sternal notch to the nipple, the greater we make the length from the clavicle to the new nipple areolar complex, because the weight of the breast is pulling this tissue down and distorting the measurement. The skin flaps are elevated and the breast resection is done with more towel clips suspending the breast parenchyma and the flaps. The suspension towel clips are adjusted to allow for the desired three-dimensional shape of the breast. Using the larger towel clips, the skin to be reduced from the flaps is marked out and appropriate resections are completed.

The towel clip suspension technique allows for excellent intraoperative three-dimensional visualization of the breast. The suspension technique can initially look quite alarming, but is greatly appreciated by the operating room staff. Manual suspension of the breasts, particularly large ones, can result in back and neck strain on the assistant. Suspending the breast as described eliminates much of the strain on the assistant. The use of this technique can reduce operating room time by 30 min or more because of elimination of constant adjustment by the human suspender.

53.2.3
Remainder of the Procedure

Most of the reduction is done laterally with only moderate resection medially (Fig. 53.4). Minimal resection of the medial upper pole preserves the main neurovascular blood supply to the nipple. The central mound is normally left 3–5 cm in thickness, depending on the desired shape and size of the breast to be left. With the help of the towel clips the exact design of the skin takeouts are made. The normal length from the nipple areolar complex to the inframammary crease triangle can be anywhere from 7–10 cm. All clips are removed except the superior clip suspending the nipple areolar complex so that the surgeon can design the three dimensional breast. The excess skin is excised and the wounds are closed with 3-0 Monocryl. One or two deep Monocryl are placed under the lateral flap and the breast parenchyma to obliterate dead space laterally. There is no manipulation directly to the central mound to avoid torsion that would compromise blood supply to the nipple.

The inferior deepithelialized pedicle is advanced superiorly and incorporated into the vertical closure of the flaps. This technique decreases bottoming out. Draping of the medial and lateral flaps dictates projection and shape. The flap design can be modified intraoperatively. The towel clip technique allows for accurate intraoperative planning. The larger the flap is made from the areola to the inframammary crease, the shorter the medial and lateral scar. The nipple areolar complex is advanced to its recipient bed and closed with 4-0 Monocryl interrupted sutures and 5-0 Prolene running suture. The remaining incisions are similarly closed (Fig. 53.5). A suture of 3-0 Monocryl is placed from the 12 o'clock position of the nipple areolar complex to the 12 o'clock position of the recipient bed to line the breast up initially and is left in place throughout the procedure. Drains are not normally used. Twenty millilitre of 0.5% plain Marcaine is placed in the lateral pocket through the suture line using a syringe with the needle off. Sterile dressings are applied along with a front-opening surgical bra, which the patient has been previously asked to bring to the operating room. The bra is placed on the patient postoperatively by turning her from side to side; this eliminates the awkwardness of raising the patient's back off the table.

In the central mound technique, the majority of the reduction is lateral. Only a moderate amount is medial. There is no resection superiorly or medially to protect innervation and blood supply to the nipple areolar complex. The deepithelialized inferior pedicle is sutured to the vertical line, which reduces bottoming out. The medial and lateral skin flaps should be kept at least 1 cm in width and in the larger reductions the larger flap lift will be maintained to help minimize problems with poor vascularity and healing.

The new nipple areolar complex is 5 cm in diameter and then is deepithelialized. There is no incision beyond the deepithelialization from the 9 to 3 o'clock position to help preserve blood supply through the superior pedicle.

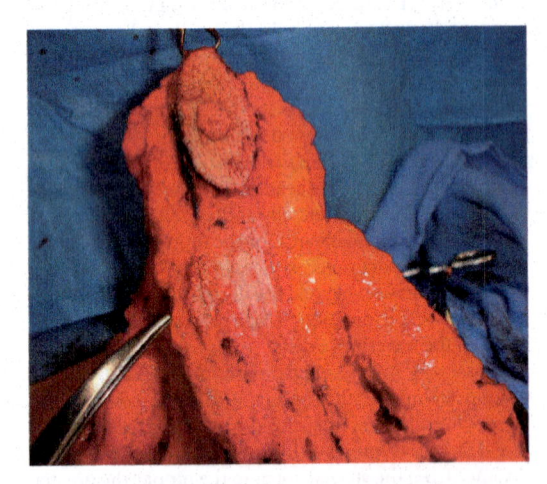

Fig. 53.4 Central mound before closure of the skin flaps

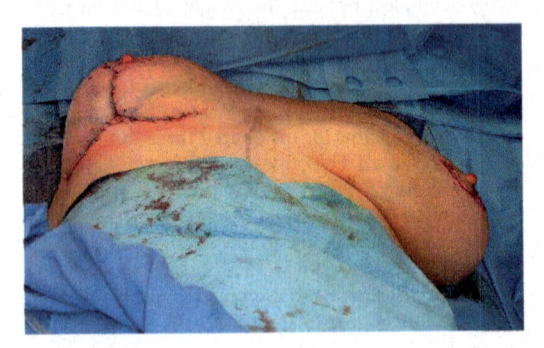

Fig. 53.5 Right breast after closure of the skin flaps around the central mound showing superb upright positioning of the reduced breast

53.3 Discussion

The authors use the central cone technique and its minor modifications for almost all of our cases of breast reduction (Figs. 53.6 and 53.7). Maintenance of the base of the cone in its central core provides the best possible blood and nerve supply to the breast and nipple areolar complex. Over the past 10 years we have performed over six hundred breast reductions using this technique. Skin flap necrosis occurred in twelve of these patients, and healed by secondary intervention. Complete nipple loss was observed in one patient who was in her seventies, as well as partial nipple loss in three patients that did not require grafting. One required a skin graft and she had a smoking history.

The weight removed from a single breast ranged from four hundred grams to nineteen hundred grams with an average of about eight hundred grams. There has not been any significant nipple retraction with this technique. There were several cases where lactation and breast feeding have been preserved after the procedure.

Patient satisfaction has been high. Symptoms of back pain and neck pain have been significantly reduced. Educating the patient preoperatively is essential. Once the patient understands the procedure and her responsibilities, complications are reduced. Normally, patients are told to walk at least 2 miles a day, 5 days a week, for at least 1 month prior to surgery.

In many cases the patient has to lose a certain amount of weight prior to surgery and the patient is not allowed to be scheduled until that weight loss goal is met. Obviously, the results of these regimens can be variable. However, the better shape the patient is in, the better the patient heals and more the compliant the patient is, as well as more responsible. Many people actually do quit smoking, exercise, and try to lose weight. If the patient is not compliant with weight loss and exercise prior to surgery, the patient is probably not going to be compliant postoperatively. There is high patient satisfaction with breast reductions in general and with the central mound technique in particular.

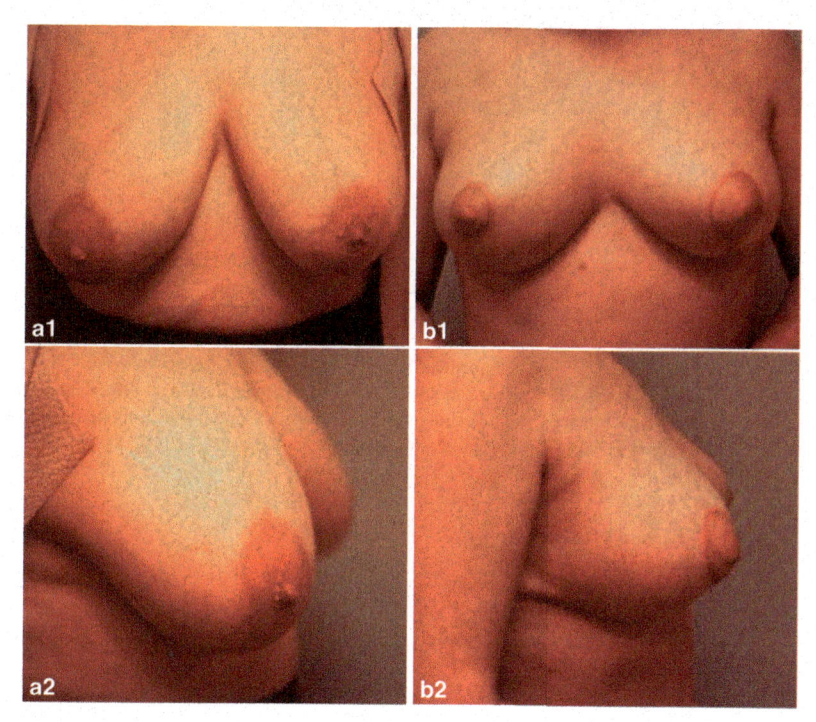

Fig. 53.6 (**a1,2**) Preoperative patient. (**b1,2**) Postoperative patient

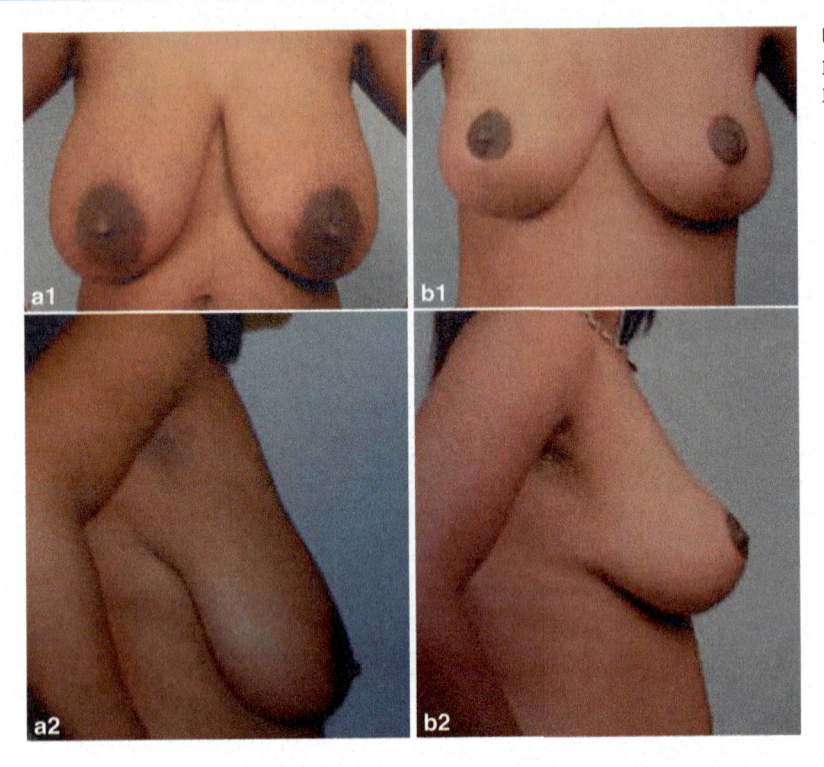

Fig. 53.7 (**a1,2**) Preoperative patient. (**b1,2**) Postoperative patient

References

1. Balch C: The central mound technique for reduction mammoplasty. Plast Reconstr Surg 1981;67(3):305–311
2. McKissock PK: Reduction mammoplasty with a vertical dermal flap. Plast Reconstr Surg 1972;49(3):245–252
3. Nahabedian MY, McGibbon BM, Manson PN: Medial pedicle reduction mammoplasty for severe mammary hypertrophy. Plast Reconstr Surg 2000;105(3):896–904
4. Hagerty RC, Hagerty RF: Reduction mammoplasty: Central cone technique for maximal preservation of vascular and nerve supply. South Med J 1989;82(2):183–185
5. Hester TR Jr, Bostwick J III, Miller L, et al: Breast reduction utilizing the maximally vascularized central breast pedicle. Plast Reconstr Surg 1985;76(6):898–900
6. Hagerty RC, Nowicky DJ: Integration of the central mound technique with the vertical skin takeout reduction mammoplasty. Plast Reconstr Surg 1998;102(4):1182–1187

The Robbins Inferior Pedicle Reduction Mammaplasty

Richard J. Restifo

54.1 Introduction

The inferior pedicle reduction mammaplasty is currently the most commonly performed reduction mammaplasty technique in the United States [1]. The method incorporates an inferior dermoglandular pedicle and an inverted-T closure. It produces consistently satisfactory results in a variety of situations [2], and is applicable for moderate to extremely large reductions [3, 4], with excellent nipple–areola survival and a low complication rate [5, 6]. Excellent aesthetic outcomes are readily obtained and nipple sensation is commonly preserved [7]. The technique is straightforward to master and is readily taught to resident staff. These manifold advantages likely underlie the popularity of the inferior pedicle reduction mammaplasty technique.

54.2 History

The inferior pedicle reduction mammaplasty was described in 1977 by both Robbins [8] and Courtiss and Goldwyn [9], each independently of the other. The descriptions of the technique were very similar and remain essentially unchanged today. A minor conceptual evolution in which the inferior flap was tailored with increasing parenchymal width towards the chest wall was described in 1979 as the "pyramidal" technique by Georgiade et al. [10]; this was not a substantially different technique but rather incorporated some modest modifications. As experience with these techniques accrued, their popularity increased, and recent publications [11, 12] offer only operative efficiency, outcome, and safety insights to a technique that was already excellent in its conception.

54.3 Technique

54.3.1 Preoperative Markings

With the patient standing upright a hand is placed in the inframammary fold and the opposite hand used to palpate the IMF level through the breast (Fig. 54.1). The intersection of this point and the central meridian of each breast is marked. This is the most critical point of the markings. An upright triangle of 7 cm to a side is then drawn downwards from this point. Alternatively, if the surgeon prefers to use one of the common wire areolar keyhole instruments, the top of the areolar keyhole is placed at this point. Also marked are the medial extent of the inframammary fold as well as the center point of the axillary roll as it intersects the anterior axillary line. These two points are then connected in a slightly curvilinear fashion to the lower corners of the previously drawn triangle. The dermal component of the pedicle is then designed, typically 8–10 cm in width at its base and centered on the central breast meridian, then tapering upwards and curving over the top of the areola with a margin of several centimeters. The dimensions described above are approximate and may be modified as appropriate; for example, the divergence of the triangle may be more or less depending on whether the laxity of the skin envelope and the width of the dermal pedicle may be greater, up to the entire inframammary fold in cases of severe macromastia. Ideally the sum of the lengths of the medial and lateral components of the upper markings, without the triangular divergence, will approximate the length of the inframammary fold marking (Fig. 54.3).

M.A. Shiffman (ed.), *Mastopexy and Breast Reduction: Principles and Practice*,
© Springer-Verlag Berlin Heidelberg 2009

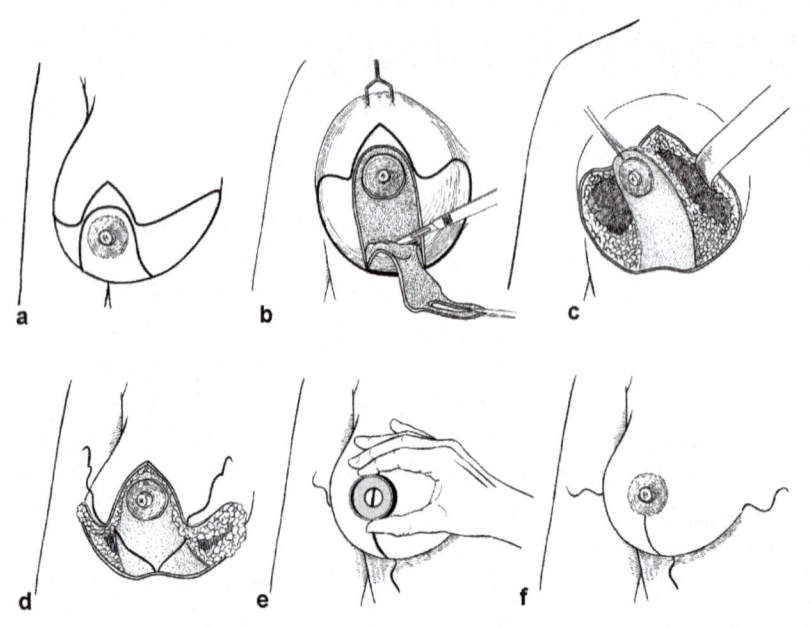

Fig. 54.1 (a) Preoperative skin markings. (b) Deepithelialization of dermal pedicle. (c) Pyramidal dermoglandular pedicle. (d) Inverted-T closure. (e) Designation of areolar circle. (f) Final inset and closure

54.3.2
Operative Procedure

The breast is held under moderate tension by an assistant and a 42 mm "cookie cutter" or similar circular template is used to inscribe the areola, with subsequent deepithelialization of the inferior pedicle (Fig. 54.2). The upper skin flap as marked is then elevated from the parenchyma, about 2 cm thick at the margin with gradually increasing thickness towards the chest wall. The divergent triangle is resected as the flap is elevated. The elevation of the upper skin flap affords exposure to the majority of the parenchyma. The parenchyma is then retracted upwards by traction on the top of the deepithelialized zone and simultaneous parenchymal pedicle development/parenchymal resection is commenced in a top to downwards direction. The parenchymal pedicle is approximately 3–5 cm thick at its apex beneath the areola, gradually increasing in width and thickness as the base is approached. The operator should consciously and affirmatively bevel away from the pedicle as the dissection progresses to assure an appropriately thick pedicle; this beveling is especially important at the lateral base of the pedicle where the distal continuation of the fourth anterolateral intercostal nerve emerges from the lateral border of the pectoralis muscle. In order to avoid injury to this nerve the pectoralis muscle or fascia should not be exposed but rather left covered by a layer of fat and breast tissue. Once the pedicle is defined, resection of medial, central, and lateral breast parenchyma is completed, joining the dissection plane of the previously elevated upper skin flaps. The pedicle should have a pyramidal configuration, roughly square at its base (Fig. 54.3). Further elevation of the upper skin flaps at the upper chest wall may be necessary to allow cephalad placement and elevation of the pedicle into the upper pole of the reconstituted breast.

Preliminary closure is now performed. The two lower triangle points are brought together at the midline inframammary fold and the incisions closed with a skin stapler. The bed is placed in the upright position and the breasts are assessed for size, shape, and symmetry. Once these are optimized by further glandular resection or skin tailoring, if necessary, the areolar cutout is determined by measuring 4.5 cm from the lower incision up the vertical limb, and a 38 mm cookie cutter this time is used to inscribe the areolar cutout (Fig. 54.2), which is resected full-thickness through the skin of the upper

54.3 Technique 409

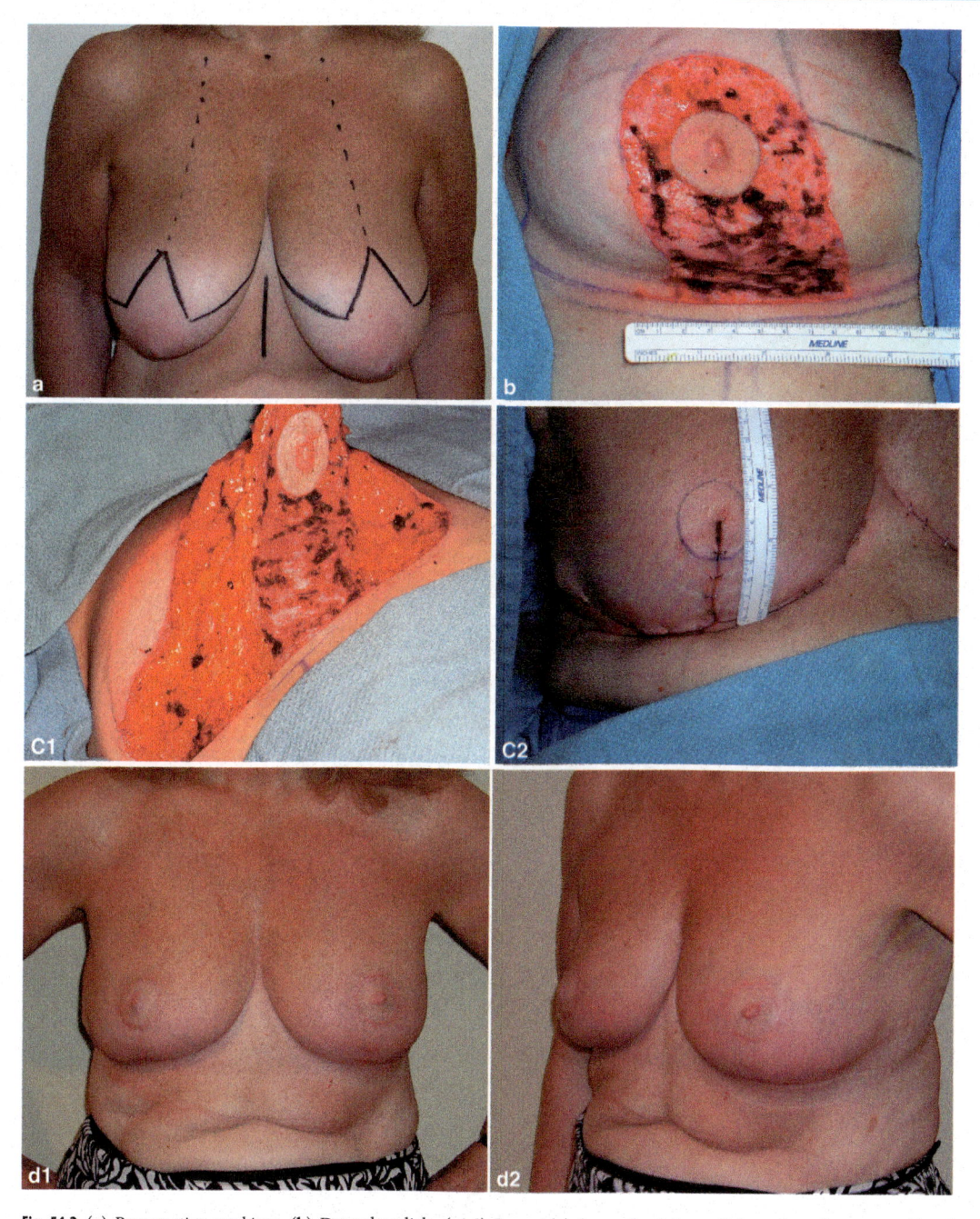

Fig. 54.2 (**a**) Preoperative markings. (**b**) Dermal pedicle. (**c1,2**) Pyramidal dermoglandular pedicle and areolar cutout. (**d1, 2**) Postoperative pedicle resection of 417 g from right and 553 g from left

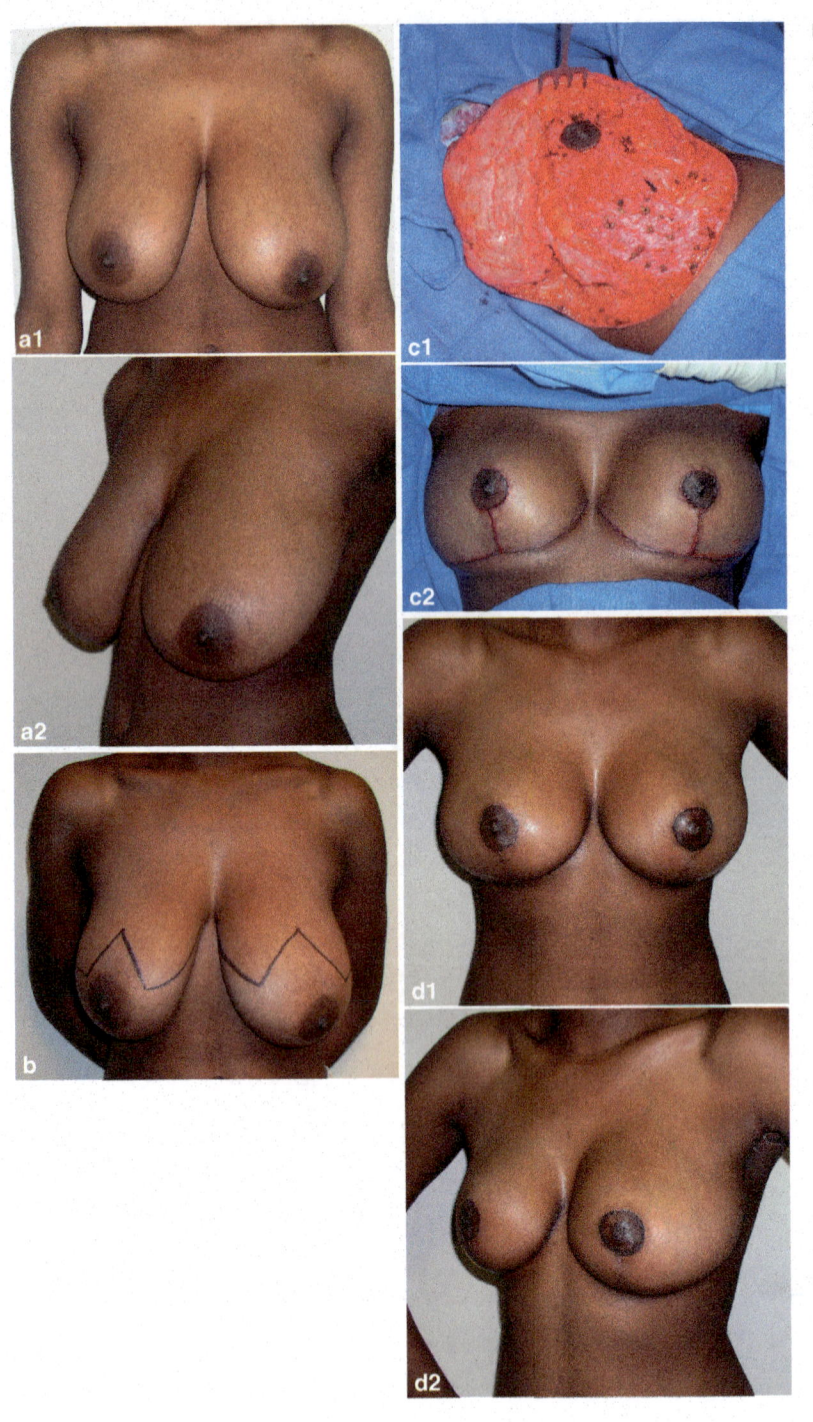

410 54 The Robbins Inferior Pedicle Reduction Mammaplasty

Fig. 54.3 (**a***1,2*) Preoperative. (**b**) Preoperative markings. (**c***1,2*) Dermoglandular pedicle and closure. (**d***1,2*) Post-operative after resection of 412 g from right and 630 g from left

flap. The incisions are now reopened for a final check for hemostasis and closed suction drain placement. The nipple–areola complex is inset into the areolar cutout pattern. The highly mobile inferior pedicle will usually allow this inset without tension or retraction, although with longer pedicles it may be necessary to fold the pedicle gently upon itself. Inset and incisional closure are achieved in layers and a dressing of choice and a modest compression wrap or brassiere is applied. Usually the drains are removed in 2–3 days and a patient wears a sports bra for a month (Figs. 54.4, 54.5).

54.3.3
Complications and Their Avoidance

Complications are relatively infrequent and are of the usual distribution. [5, 6] A hematoma will occur in approximately 4% of patients. Some authors feel that a tumescent technique with subcutaneous epinephrine injection will reduce blood loss, although meticulous surgical technique and hemostasis is probably the most effective way to minimize blood loss and prevent hematoma formation.

The rate of significant nipple necrosis is under one percent; this can be minimized by judicious deepithelialization of the inferior dermal pedicle and by respecting the width and thickness of the glandular component of the pedicle. Also important in minimizing the ischemic nipple is recognition that it is relatively easy to unintentionally undercut the pedicle during dissection. Appropriate patient selection is of obvious importance as well. For larger reductions or lengthier nipple–areola transpositions it is advisable to increase the width of the pedicle, up to the entire width of the inframammary fold in severe cases.

Minor wound dehiscence or delayed incisional healing occurs in 5–10% of patients, most commonly at the T junction. This complication can be minimized by appreciating the role of tension or ischemia in its etiology; a small triangular skin flap may be designed in the midline inframammary fold to reduce tension at the T junction. Excessive thinning or operative trauma to the lower aspects of the skin flaps, especially near the T-junction, should be avoided in order to minimize these wound healing problems.

Tension and ischemia also underlie hypertrophic scarring. Appropriately planned and well vascularized skin flaps and precise tension-free closure with fine sutures are probably the most effective ways to minimize scarring.

Significant wound infection is rare and the role of prophylactic antibiotics is unclear. However, prophylactic antibiotics should be considered as there is some evidence that they reduce wound dehiscence and hypertrophic scarring.

The rate of fat necrosis is about one percent and can be minimized by careful surgical technique and avoidance of partially detached fat, especially at the distal pedicle.

Although nipple sensory loss is somewhat subjective and varies with the method of measurement, sensory loss may be related to the amount of tissue removed and is probably less with the inferior pedicle reduction as compared to other techniques [7, 13]. Anatomically this is due to the potential for preservation of the fourth anterolateral intercostal nerve in the lateral aspect of the inferior pedicle. If the lateral pedicle dissection leaves the pectoralis fascia unexposed and covered by a layer of fat and parenchyma the nerve is less likely to sustain injury.

54.4
Optimization of Aesthetic Results

Some aesthetic issues can be addressed by simple operative considerations:

1. A round, as opposed to oblong or teardrop, areola can be promoted by designing and performing the areolar cutout after the vertical limb is closed.
2. A conspicuous medial scar should be avoided by limiting the extent of the incision to a point 2 cm from the midline sternum and by designing it to fall within the inframammary fold so that it is hidden by the ptosis of the breast.
3. A more conical shape is achieved by greater divergence of the triangle. A balance must be achieved so that excessive divergence does not lead to tightness at skin closure. This judgement is based upon the laxity of the skin envelope as determined by examination.
4. Bottoming [14] is the tendency of the inferior pedicle to prolapse downwards over time, leading to a long lower pole and an upwards-directed nipple–areola complex. This aesthetic liability is best counteracted by the initial design of the mammaplasty pattern; the vertical limb below the areolar cutout should be less than 5 cm in length and the position of the top of the nipple–areola complex should be at or preferably 1 or 2 cm below the original inframammary fold level.

54.5
Conclusions

The inferior pedicle reduction mammaplasty, essentially unmodified from its original description, is possibly the most useful reduction mammaplasty technique yet conceived. It is the "workhorse" method in the United States. It offers versatility, simplicity, safety, consistently good

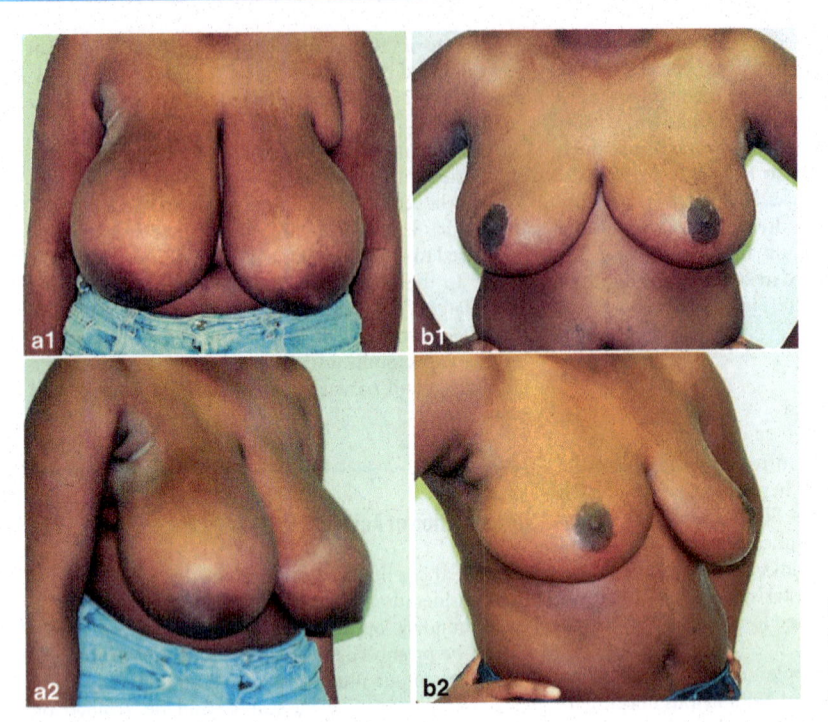

Fig. 54.4 (**a**1,2) Preoperative. (**b**1,2) Postoperative after resection of 2,275 g from right and 2,450 g from left

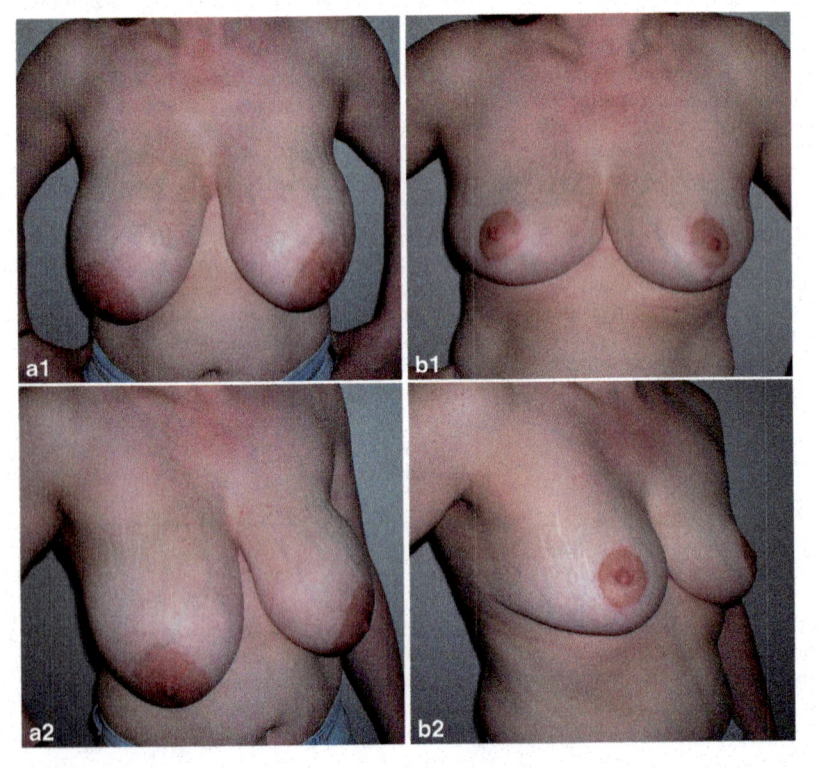

Fig. 54.5 (**a**1,2) Preoperative. (**b**1,2) Postoperative following resection of 716 g from right and 715 g from left

aesthetics, and maximal preservation of breastfeeding and nipple–areola sensitivity. The principle disadvantages of the inferior pedicle reduction mammaplasty as compared to other techniques are the long inframammary incision, a tendency towards "bottoming," and minor healing problems at the inverted T-junction. Overall the inferior pedicle reduction mammaplasty is an excellent technique that offers a high satisfaction rate among patients and plastic surgeons alike.

References

1. Rohrich RJ, Gosman AA, Brown SA, Tonadapu PT, Foster BF: Current preferences for breast reduction techniques: A survey of board-certified plastic surgeons 2002. Plast Reconstr Surg 2004;114(7):1734–1736
2. Georgiade NG, Serafin D, Riefkohl R, Georgiade GS: Is there a reduction mammaplasty for "all seasons?" Plast Reconstr Surg 1979;63(6):765–773
3. Lacerna M, Spears J, Mitra A, Medina C, McCampbell E, Kiran R, Mitra A: Avoiding free nipple graft during reduction mammaplasty in patients with gigantomastia. Ann Plast Surg 2005;55(1):21–24
4. Gerzenshtein J, Oswald T, McCluskey P, Caplan J, Angel MF: Avoiding free nipple grafting with the inferior pedicle technique. Ann Plast Surg 2005;55(3):245–249
5. Mandrekas AD, Zambacos GJ, Anastasopoulos A, Hapsas DA: Reduction mammaplasty with the inferior pedicle technique: early and late complications in 371 patients. Br J Plast Surg 1996;49(7):442–446
6. O'Grady KF, Thoma A, Dal Cin A: A comparison of complication rates in large and small inferior pedicle reduction mammaplasty. Plast Reconstr Surg 2005;115(3):736–742
7. Schlenz I, Rigel S, Schemper M, Kuzbari R: Alteration of nipple and areola sensitivity by reduction mammaplasty: A prospective comparison of five techniques. Plast Reconstr Surg 2005;115(3):743–751
8. Robbins TH: A reduction mammaplasty with the areola-nipple based on an inferior dermal pedicle. Plast Reconstr Surg 1977;59(1):64–67
9. Courtiss EH, Goldwyn RM: Reduction mammaplasty by the inferior pedicle technique. Plast Reconstr Surg 1977;59(4):500–507
10. Georgiade NG, Serafin D, Morris R, Georgiade GS: Reduction mammaplasty utilizing an inferior pedicle nipple areola flap. Ann Plast Surg 1979;3(3):211–218
11. Scott GR, Carson CL, Borah GL: Maximizing outcomes in breast reduction surgery: a review of 518 consecutive patients. Plast Reconstr Surg 2005;116(6):1640–1641
12. Wallace WH, Thompson WO, Smith RA, Barraza KR, Davidson SF, Thompson JT II: Reduction mammaplasty using the inferior pedicle technique. Ann Plast Surg 1998;40(3):235–240
13. Mofid MM, Dellon AL, Elias JJ, Nahabedian MY: Quantification of breast sensibility following reduction mammaplasty; A comparison of inferior and medial pedicle techniques. Plast Reconstr Surg 2002;109(7):2283–2288
14. Reus WF, Mathes SJ: Preservation of projection after reduction mammaplasty: Long term followup of the inferior pedicle technique. Plast Reconstr Surg 1988;82(4):644–652

CHAPTER 55

Modification of the Inferior Pedicle Technique

Sanjay Azad

55.1 Introduction

An ideal breast reduction technique should produce a breast of desired size and shape; preserving function and sensibility and avoiding all complications and scars. In practice, the results achieved by current techniques are far from ideal. Breast reduction surgery leaves visible scars and possibly soft tissue complications, to achieve a breast of desired volume and shape [1, 2].

The field of reduction mammaplasty has been a contentious area in which numerous techniques have been proposed [3]. The inferior pedicle inverted "T" scar technique is a popular technique, which was initially described simultaneously by various authors [4–6]. This technique results in a pedicle with a highly reliable vascularity. As a consequence, there is reduced incidence of necrosis of the nipple–areola complex, retention of nipple–areola sensation, retention of the ability to lactate, and a good aesthetic result. But this is offset by the extensive and prominent inverted T scar, bottoming out and the high incidence of T junction breakdown [7, 9].

Numerous modifications have been suggested for the inferior pedicle technique, over the passage of time. These basically relate to making the operation safe and give more reliable cosmetic results.

55.2 Historical Background and Technique Modifications

Operations describing procedures to reduce and shape the breast, but maintaining function have been described by Lexer [10], Beisenberger [11], Gillies and McIndoe [12] among many others. Schwarzmann in 1930 [13] proposed the concept of subdermal blood supply to the nipple. This theorem spawned the use of the deepithelialized dermal pedicle of the modern era.

Wise [14] described his method of planning the mammaplasty in 1956 using the keyhole pattern. This was followed by the use of horizontal bipedicled technique [15] and vertical bipedicle technique [16]. Robbins [17] is credited with the use of the inferior pedicle technique which was subsequently elaborated by Courtiss and Goldwyn [18] and Georgiade et al. [19].

The initial issues in inferior pedicle technique were of pedicle reliability and operation safety. However with better understanding of blood supply, the emphasis has shifted to cosmetic. With the upsurge of superior pedicle techniques and variants, there has been a search for better methods of using the inferior pedicle technique.

The modifications of the inferior pedicle technique are:
1. Type of inferior pedicle in relation to tissue (glandular, dermal, or both).
2. Position of the inferior pedicle (inferolateral, true central, inferomedial).
3. Width of pedicle.
4. Pedicle hitch and pedicle with mesentery.
5. Methods of mobilization of inferior pedicle.
6. Inferior pedicle vertical scar technique and its variants to limit chest wall scarring.

55.3 Type of Inferior Pedicle in Relation to Tissue

It was initially popular to use mainly dermal pedicle, but with better understanding of blood supply, the most common pedicle now in use is the dermoglandular pedicle. There is no particular thickness of pedicle which gives complete reliability, but figures between 2–4 cm thickness at the areola and between 4 and 10 cm at the base are described [6].

55.3.1 Width of the Pedicle

Pedicle width is typically kept between 6 and 8 cm wide. A heavier pedicle will result in more bottoming out and there is an argument for limiting pedicle width to minimize this well-known, long-term complication.

M.A. Shiffman (ed.), *Mastopexy and Breast Reduction: Principles and Practice*,
© Springer-Verlag Berlin Heidelberg 2009

55.3.2
Position of the Inferior Pedicle

The position is either inferocentral or more lateral. The advantages for the latter are the advantages of more ductal and nerve preservation. This would translate into better nipple sensation and a higher likelihood of lactation. However no studies relating to this are available.

55.3.3
Pedicle Hitch and Pedicle with Mesentery

The inferior pedicle can be hitched to the pectoral fascia in an effort to reduce bottoming out. However this can result in pedicle kinking and a broad lower pole which would affect results. This is not reported as a commonly used technique.

Preservation of mesentery of breast tissue on the pectoral fascia is an excellent way to preserve nipple nerve supply and also reduce ultimate "pedicle drop." This is a modification which is useful for anyone practising the inferior pedicle technique. It basically means not lifting the pedicle completely of the chest wall and leaving adequate adherence in situ.

55.3.4
Methods of Mobilization of Inferior Pedicle

This can be done using one of a number of methods. The author tends to use the bucket-handle approach [20]. Basically the assistant and the surgeon both firmly grasp the maximum possible breast mound between thumb and all four fingers. The position of grasp is on either side of one of the proposed vertical pedicle incisions. The effect of this manoeuvre is to change the shape of the breast into a prominent, compressed, vertically oriented, bucket-handle shape. Ensuring a firm grasp on the breast, the surgeon uses a no. 20 blade to dissect the pedicle. The incision is made at the junction of the pedicle with the breast and is carried progressively vertically down until the pectoral fascia is visualized. This is done on both sides. Finally, the two vertical incisions are joined together by incising the small remaining bridge of dermoglandular tissue above the nipple–areola complex.

55.3.5
Inferior Pedicle Vertical Scar Technique

The extensive chest wall scarring with a standard Wise pattern inferior pedicle technique has resulted in an effort to limit it. A recent randomized study has emphasized the cosmetic importance of this issue [21].

One such technique is the spair (short scar periareolar inferior pedicle reduction) mammaplasty described by Hammond in 1999 [22]. The technique essentially involves using an inferior pedicle and results in a vertical scar. The planning of the technique involves creation of two circles. The outer circle at 12 o'clock position measures 18–23 cm from the midclavicular point. The sternum to 3 o'clock position measure 10–12 cm and inframammary fold to 6 o'clock is 7–8 cm. The outer rim is deepithelialized along with the pedicle. The inferior pedicle is isolated and the resection is carried out in a superior, then lateral and medial aspect of the breast. The flaps are closed and the vertical segment of excess tissue is deepithelialized and closed. This is an excellent method, but with a rather complex surgical design.

The author now uses a combination technique which combines the inferior pedicle, and a single vertical scar [23]. The author terms this as the "inferior pedicle vertical scar technique." This technique has been used in 100 patients with a total of 196 breasts over the last 10 years. The technique gives a sensate, natural-shaped breast with limited scars. It has a short learning curve, is versatile and can be used for all breast sizes including mastopexy. The prospective study of this cohort of patients suggests that it is associated with a shorter hospital stay and a low complication rate. The technique is comparable in outcomes and complications to any of the standard methods described in the literature. This is a useful technique for large size breast reductions, in older patients with resection of over 500 g.

55.4
Operative Technique

55.4.1
Breast Marking

The markings are essentially very similar to that of the vertical scar superior pedicle [9], except for certain essential differences (Fig. 55.1). Markings are made with the patient in the sitting position. First the midline and the inframammary fold are marked. Then the vertical axis of the breast is drawn and is extended from inframammary fold. This is usually 10–12 cm from the midline and forms the landmark based on which the margins of skin excision are drawn.

Next the position of the new nipple is marked out. This is usually positioned at about 21–23 cm from the suprasternal notch on the mid-mammary line. This point usually corresponds to the inframammary fold projected on to the anterior surface of the breast. In this technique the nipple is marked slightly lower than with the standard inferior pedicle technique. Following this the margins of the skin excision are determined. Pushing the breast medially and rotating it upwards the lateral

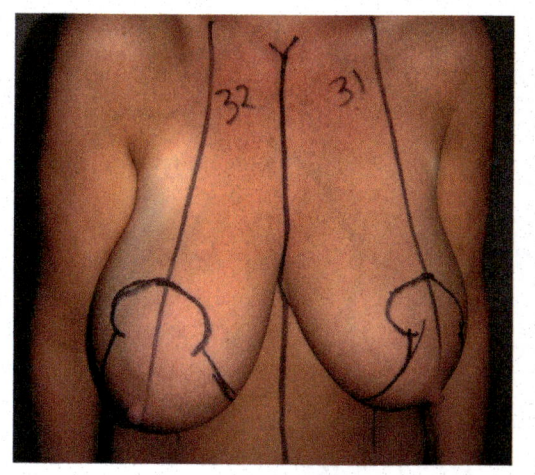

Fig. 55.1 Lejour markings for inferior pedicle vertical scar

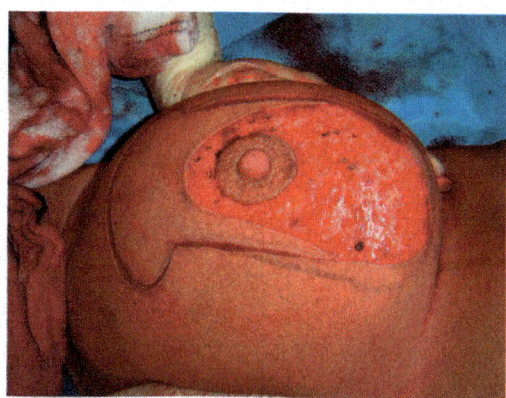

Fig. 55.2 Inferior pedicle deepithelialized before it is dissected free

margin of excision is drawn, in continuity with the midmammary line. Similarly the breast is pushed laterally with an upward rotation to mark the medial margin of excision. These two vertical lines are tapered to a point 3–4 cm above the inframammary fold.

Following this, the site of the future nipple–areola complex is marked out. The dome-shaped marking advocated by Lejour, each limb of the dome measures 7–8 cm. The lower end of the dome is joined to the medial and lateral margin of excision.

After this the areola is made taut and a circle with a radius of about 2.5 cm from the nipple is marked out on the areola so that a nipple–areola complex of about 5 cm diameter will be transposed to the new position.

Finally the inferior pedicle is marked out as in standard inferior pedicle technique. The pedicle is marked out no broader than 6 cm [6]. Broad pedicles leads to tight closure and contribute to nipple ischemia (as mentioned by the senior author of the paper). The only difference is that the pedicle is tapered in its inferior aspect to a point 3–4 cm above the inframammary fold so that the scar does not extend below this postoperatively.

55.5 Operative Procedure

The procedure is started by deepithelializing the inferior pedicle (Fig. 55.2). This is done in the standard way except that the pedicle is tapered to a point 3–4 cm above the inframammary fold. Incisions are then made on the medial and lateral margins of inferior pedicle and gradually deepened down to the pectoral fascia. These incisions are joined above the nipple areola complex to complete the elevation of inferior pedicle. Once the pedicle has been defined the breast is mobilized on a plane above the pectoral fascia (avascular plane). This mobilization is more extensive laterally to correct the axillary fullness that is often present.

The margins of the skin excision within the Lejour pattern are incised to facilitate glandular excision. The excision is started from the medial margins of skin excision and is done in a shelving manner on either side. The flap consisting of the skin and breast tissue is kept quite thin (1–1.5 in.) to start with and gradually with the shelving excision the flap gets progressively thicker depending on the size of the breast and the amount of tissue that needs to be excised. The glandular tissue is excised mainly from the medial, lateral, inferomedial, and inferolateral aspects of the breast. The excision at the superior aspect is kept to the minimum so that the breast achieves sufficient projection and superior fullness.

An incision is made through the dermis of the inferior margin of the pedicle. The lower margin of the pedicle is then gently mobilized. A few key sutures are then placed and the size of the breast is assessed and if deemed necessary, more breast tissue is excised to achieve the desired shape and projection.

Once the glandular excision is complete the nipple–areola complex is transposed to the new site and fixed with a few 3/0 monocryl subcutaneous sutures. Then the vertical scar is stitched up with some interrupted subcutaneous 4/0 monocryl stitches. The vertical scar is then stitched with subcuticular 4/0 monocryl, gathering the excess skin up with each stitch, so that finally it gives a pleated appearance. These result in a vertical scar about 6–7 cm long. At the end of the procedure, the breast appearance shows adequate projection with a bulge in the upper part (Fig. 55.3).

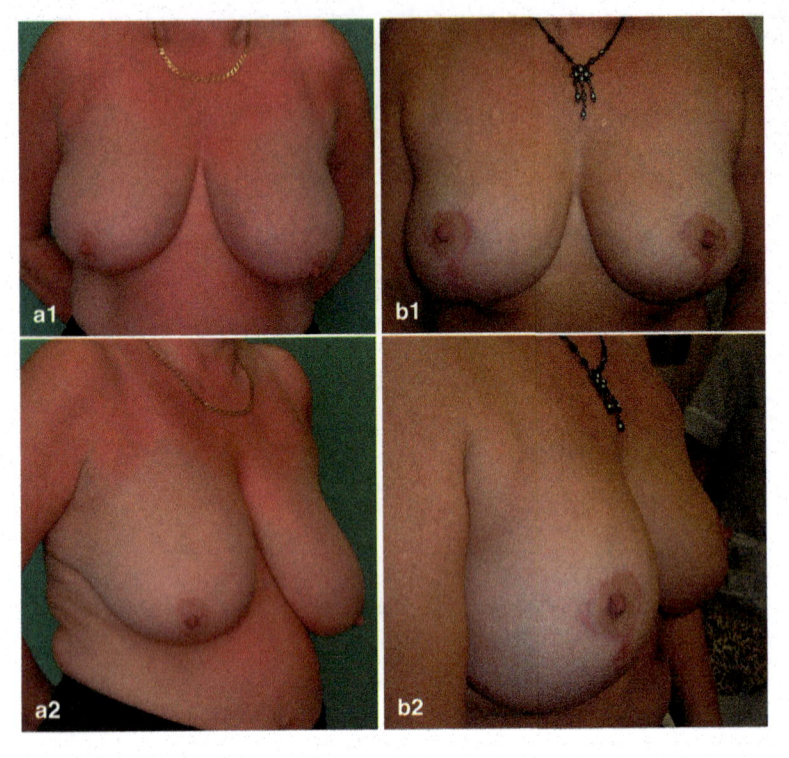

Fig. 55.3 (**a**1,2) Preoperative patient. (**b**1,2) Three months postoperative after inferior pedicle vertical scar technique, removing 325 g from right breast and 475 g from left breast

55.6 Conclusions

There are numerous modifications of the inferior pedicle technique which can help to make the procedure safer with a better cosmetic outcome. Limiting scars but using the safe inferior pedicle is an advance in the right direction in this common plastic surgical operation.

References

1. Godwin Y, Wood SH, O'Neill TJ: A comparison of the patient and surgeon opinion on the long-term aesthetic outcome of reduction mammaplasty. Br J Plast Surg 1998;51:444–449
2. Marchac D, De Olarte G: Reduction mammaplasty and correction of ptosis with a short inframammary scar. Plast Reconstr Surg 1982;69:45–55
3. Strombeck JO: Mammaplasty: Report of a new technique based on the two-pedicle procedure. Br J Plast Surg 1960;13:79–90
4. Robbins TH: A reduction mammaplasty with the areola-nipple based on an inferior dermal pedicle. Plast Reconstr Surg 1977;59:64–67
5. Courtiss EH, Goldwyn RM: Reduction mammaplasty by the inferior pedicle technique. Plast Reconstr Surg 1977;59:500–507
6. Georgiade NG, Serafin D, Morris R, Georgiade G: Reduction mammaplasty utilizing an inferior pedicle nipple-areolar flap. Ann Plast Surg 1979;3:211–218
7. Dabbah A, Lehman JA, Parker MG, Tantri D, Wagner DS: Reduction mammaplasty: An outcome mammaplasty. Ann Plast Surg 1995;35:337–341
8. Wise RJ: A preliminary report on a method of planning the mammaplasty. Plast Reconstr Surg 1956;17:367–375
9. Lejour M: Vertical mammoplasty and liposuction of the breast. Plast Reconstr Surg 1994; 94:100–114
10. Lexer E: Hypertrophie bie der mammae. Munch Med Wochenschr 1912;59:2702
11. Beisenberger H: Deformitaten and Kosmetische Operationen der Weiblichen Brust. Wien, W Maudrich 1931
12. Gilles H, McIndoe AH: The technique of mammaplasty in conditions of hypertrophy of the breast. Surg Gynecol Obstet 1939;68:658
13. Schwartzmann E: Die technik der mammaplastik. Chirurgica 1930;2:932
14. Wise RJ: Preliminary report on method of planning the mammaplasty. Plast Reconstr Surg 1956;17:367–375
15. Strombeck JO: Mammaplasty: report of a new technique based on the two pedicle procedure. Br J Plast Surg 1960;13:79–90
16. McKissock PK: Reduction mammaplasty with a vertical dermal flap. Plast Recontr Surg 1972;49(3):245–252

17. Robbins TH: A reduction mammaplasty with the areola-nipple based on an inferior dermal pedicle. Plast Reconstr Surg 1977;59(1):64–67
18. Courtiss EH, Goldwyn RM: Reduction mammaplasty by the inferior pedicle technique: An alternative to free nipple and areola grafting for severe macromastia or extreme ptosis. Plast Reconstr Surg 1977;59(1):500–507
19. Georgiade NG, Serafin D, Morris R, Georgiade G: Reduction mammaplasty utilizing an inferior pedicle nipple-areola flap. Ann Plast Surg 1979;3(3):211–218
20. Azad S, Bell D, Mohammed P, Erdmann MWH: Technical refinement in breast reduction using inferior pedicle technique. Plast Reconstr Surg 2002;109:2604–2605
21. Cruz-Korchin N, Korchin L: Vertical versus Wise pattern breast reduction: Patient satisfaction, revision rates, and complications. Plast Reconstr Surg 2003;112:1573–1578
22. Hammond DC: The SPAIR mammaplasty. Clin Plast Surg 2002;29:411–421
23. Kumar PV, Krishnakumar K, Azad S, Ramkumar: Breast reduction with inferior pedicle using single vertical scar: a new approach. J Plast Reconstr Aesth Surg

Short Scar Periareolar Inferior Pedicle Reduction Mammaplasty

Richard J. Restifo

56.1 Introduction

Although mammaplasties utilizing an inverted-T closure remain the most popular techniques in use today, in recent years there has been an increase in the use of "limited scar" techniques that limit the excursion of the scar into the inframammary fold [1]. The short scar mammaplasty with the highest utilization has been the vertical mammaplasty initially popularized by LeJour [2] in the early nineties. There have been several potential problem areas [3, 4] with this technique, especially early in an operator's experience. These include an excessive lower pole length, malpositioning or distortion of the nipple–areola complex, excess skin at the inframammary fold, and a poor immediate postoperative appearance with relative unpredictability concerning the final shape. These issues may lead to a high secondary revision rate. Furthermore, the vertical mammaplasty is based on a superior pedicle that is less familiar to many surgeons and may have less potential to preserve nipple sensitivity [5, 6] and breast feeding capacity. It is perhaps for these reasons that the vertical mammaplasty has not been universally adopted in the plastic surgery community, although experienced operators have reported excellent results with the technique [7, 8].

Another more recent option for limited scar mammaplasty is the short scar periareolar inferior pedicle reduction (SPAIR) [9–11] mammaplasty devised by Hammond. This technique carries the nipple–areola complex on the very familiar inferior pedicle. The SPAIR mammaplasty apportions the skin resection between the lower pole and central breast skin, with subsequent reconciliation at the vertical and periareolar closures, respectively (Fig. 56.1). An important component of the SPAIR mammaplasty is the periareolar pursestring ("round block" [12]) technique used to stabilize the periareolar closure. The potential advantages to this technique are the preservation of vascularity and sensitivity inherent in the inferior pedicle, the potential elimination of the inframammary scar, and a fairly stable immediate postoperative appearance that does not rely upon postoperative settling to achieve an acceptable shape.

56.2 Indications

As a general rule the SPAIR mammaplasty is indicated for modest to moderate reductions and mastopexies. Approximate limits are nipple–areola transpositions up to 10 cm and resections up to 600 g. Novices should attempt lesser resections and transpositions, but as experience is accrued the above "limits" may be exceeded.

56.3 Preoperative Markings

The SPAIR mammaplasty may require intraoperative modifications of the skin envelope by the process of "tailor-tacking," [11, 13, 14] with the patient upright on the operating table, as described below. Nonetheless, accurate preoperative markings will minimize the extent of these intraoperative maneuvers. The apex point is critical and represents the top of the areolar cutout pattern and is determined in much the same way as in other mammaplasties (i.e., the intersection of the central meridian of each breast with the level of the inframammary fold). As with other mammaplasty techniques it is far better to err on the side of placing this point "too low," and in general the distance from the suprasternal notch to the top of the areolar cutout is 21 cm or greater. Next, in the marking maneuver that is the most difficult to master, each breast is rotated in turn medially and laterally, each time dropping a vertical line straight down from the apex point (Fig. 56.2). These vertical lines will meet again at the inframammary fold, separated by the 6–8 cm width of the pedicle

Fig. 56.1 (a) SPAIR concept: skin resection and redistribution is allocated between central and lower pole skin (b) preoperative markings, (c) parenchymal resection

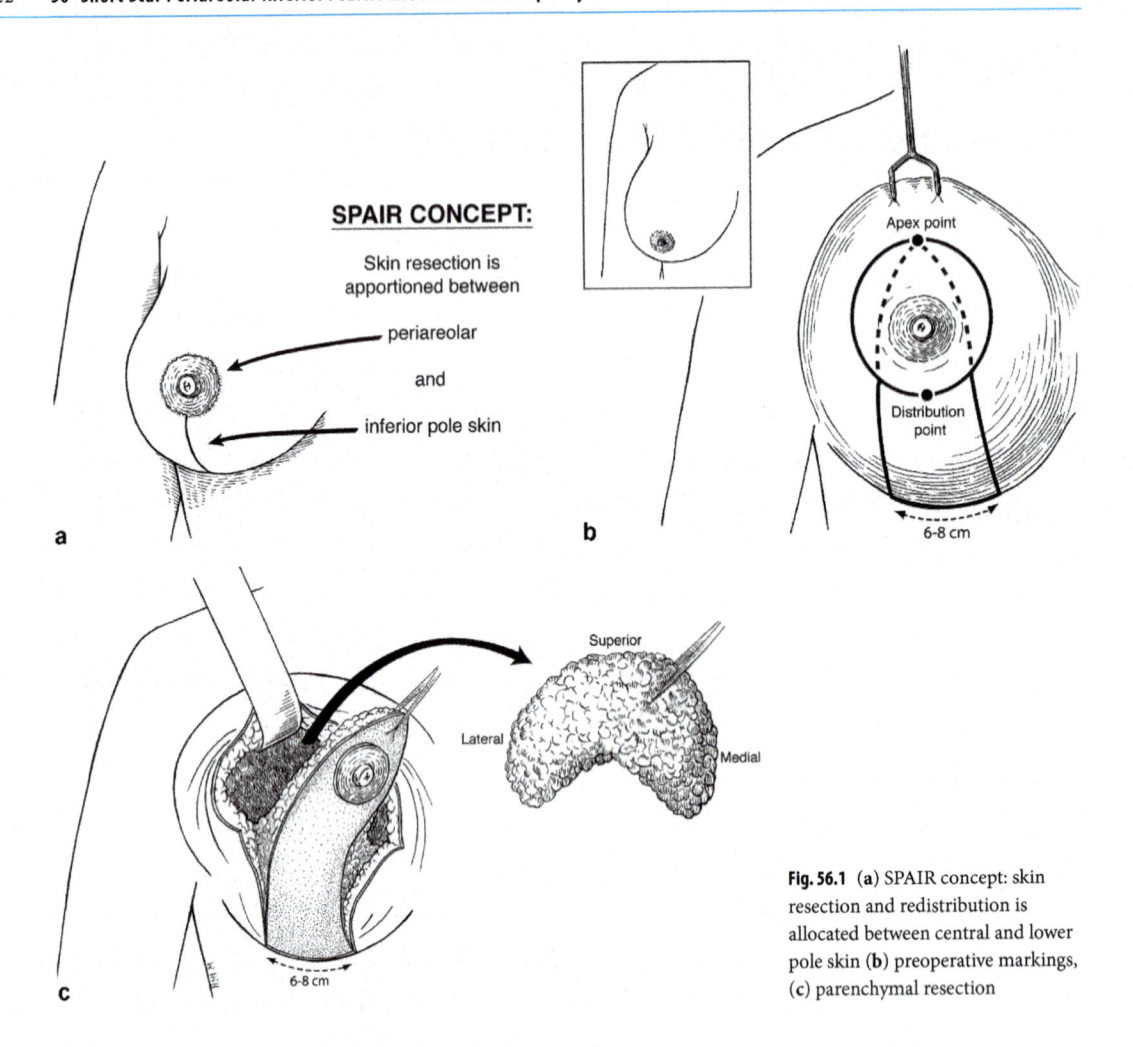

base. This is similar to the first steps of the marking procedure described by Lejour and results in a vertically oriented pattern that encompasses the nipple–areola complex and the inferior pedicle. The vertical dimension of this pattern is divided into "vertical" and "periareolar" segments based upon the relative contributions of resection of lower pole skin and central breast skin, respectively, to the total skin removal. This distribution varies, depending upon breast size and degree of nipple–areola transposition, and is estimated by pinching skin between thumb and forefinger until the desired shape is achieved. This junction of the vertical and periareolar patterns is the distribution point, which is typically around 8 cm up from the inframammary fold. The periareolar pattern is drawn by joining the apex and distribution points in an oval with a height-to-width ratio of approximately 1.3:1. A 6–8 cm wide inferior pedicle is then designed at the base of the vertical pattern at the inframammary fold (Fig. 56.2).

56.4
Operative Technique

A 42 mm cookie cutter is used to inscribe the areola with deepithelialization of the inferior pedicle. Starting at the upper margin of the areolar pattern the skin is incised and the upper skin/breast flap is elevated. This

56.4 Operative Technique

muscle for several centimeters in a cephalad direction; this mobilization of the thick upper flap contributes to upper pole fullness in the end result, as described below (Fig. 56.3).

Attention is now directed towards the development of the inferior pedicle. The dermal component of the pedicle is mobilized first by incising down to the parenchyma, leaving a dermal connection at the base. The glandular component of the pedicle is then developed in a pyramidal configuration with gradually increasing thickness towards the base. The neurovascular supply to the nipple–areola complex is protected by adequate pedicle thickness, with particular attention to the infero-lateral pedicle at the pectoralis level. These considerations are similar to those for any inferior pedicle reduction. The glandular resection is performed, removing parenchyma medially, laterally and cephalad to the pedicle, resulting in a tissue specimen that is roughly "horse-shoe" shaped. At this point there is the option of advancing the deep portion of the upper skin/breast flap cephalad and suturing it to the chest wall with nonabsorbable sutures; this is done to promote upper pole fullness and to assist in the shaping of the upper breast.

Reconstitution of the breast and skin closure is now commenced. The lower pole is closed first, starting at the distribution point and working downwards towards the inframammary fold. It may be necessary to perform further deepithelialization of the inferior dermal pedicle as the inframammary fold (IMF) is approached in order to obtain smooth closure as the lower part of the pedicle is imbricated into the vertical closure; likewise, a short extension of the deepithelialization in a lateral direction along the IMF may be required. This will result in a mild L-shaping of the final scar. The lower deepithelialized pedicle may be conservatively freed from its dermal connections to the lower pole skin at the base of the pedicle, but the length of the dermal attachment at the IMF should be preserved at as close as possible to the original 6–8 cm length to maximize the cutaneous contribution to pedicle circulation. It is important that the lower pole have an appropriate length and shape; if this is not satisfactory some intraoperative skin modifications may be required, such as further removal or deepithelialization of the skin at the vertical closure or lowering of the distribution point to place more of the skin redundancy into the periareolar opening.

The inferior pedicle should lie readily in the central periareolar opening that is outlined by the upper skin/breast flaps and the lower pole closure. The periareolar closure is now performed. This is perhaps the most difficult part of the operation, as the relatively large, roughly oval defect has to be reduced to a secure, round, four centimeter diameter opening, and the so-called "round block" of the periareolar pursestring. Several technical considerations are necessary to successfully achieve this. Firstly, the skin at the margin of the periareolar closure

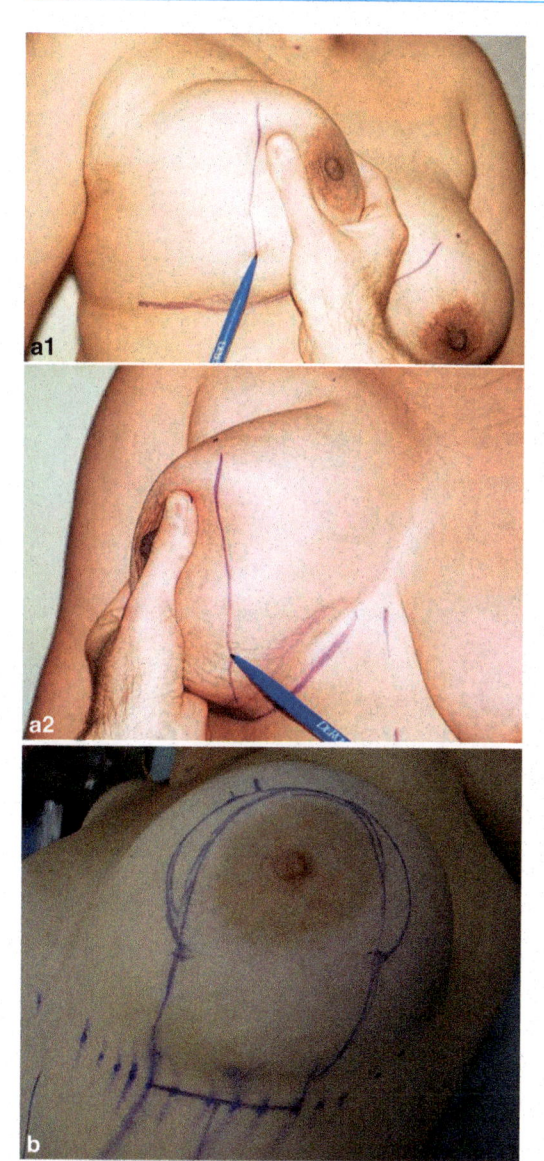

Fig. 56.2 (a) Preoperative markings: the breast is rotated in turn medially and laterally and a line parallel to the central breast meridian is drawn from the apex point to the inframammary fold. (b) Completed preoperative markings

flap is thin at the periareolar edge (to facilitate the subsequent purse-string periareolar closure) but becomes thicker as the dissection progresses upwards to the chest wall. At the chest wall the upper flap is approximately 3–4 cm thick and consists of skin and breast parenchyma. The upper flap is then elevated off of the

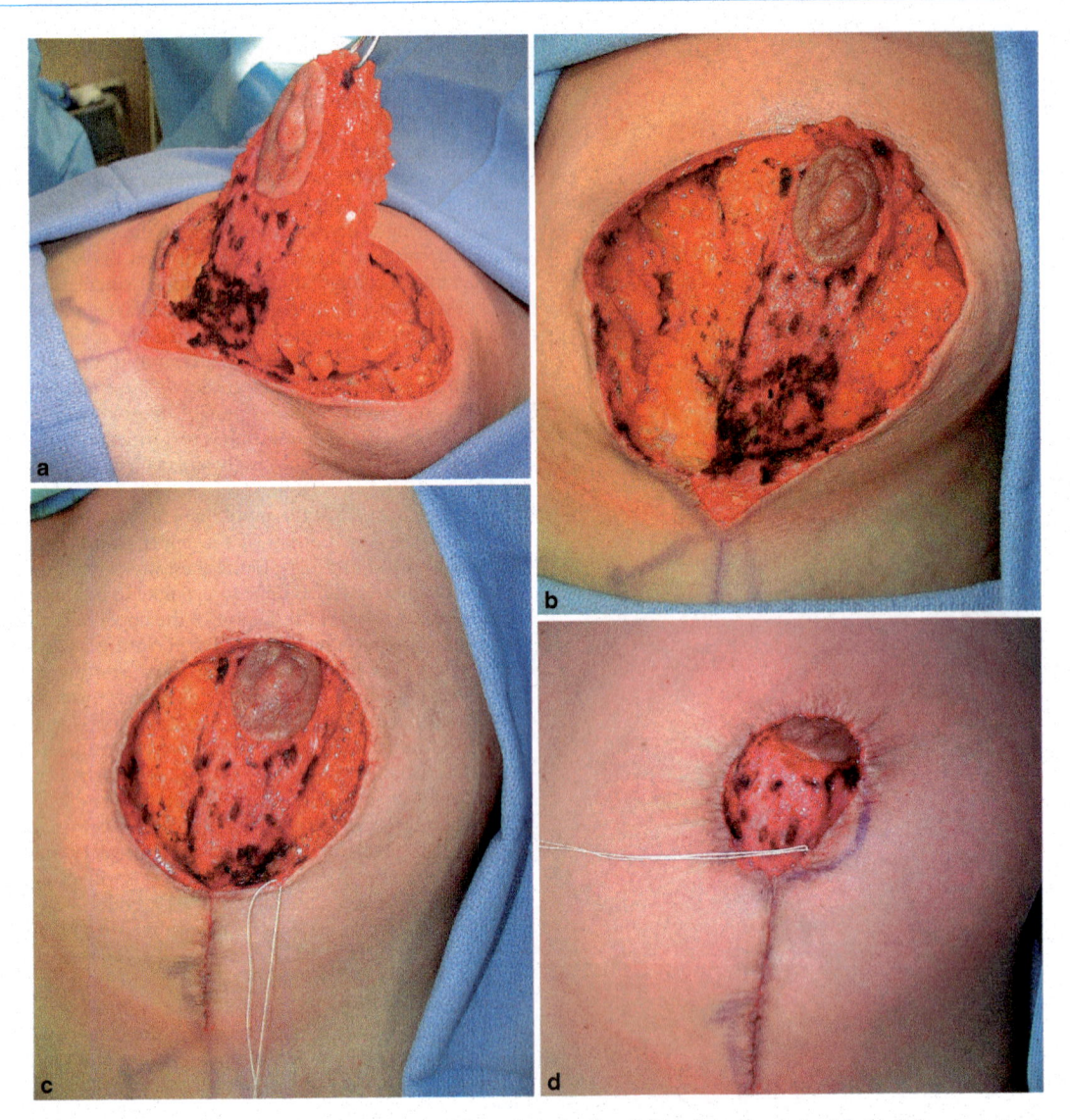

Fig. 56.3 Operative sequence. (**a**) Inferior dermoglandular pedicle developed. (**b**) Inferior dermoglandular pedicle prior to inset. (**c**) Lower pole closure. (**d**) Preliminary pursestring and correction of "roundblock"

should be sufficiently tapered and thinned so that the skin redundancy can be accommodated into the round block with a minimal amount of bunching, wrinkling and pleating. Another essential component is a Gore-Tex suture. This nearly frictionless suture material will allow the placement of many small tissue purchases around the perimeter of the areolar closure and still allow a smooth cinching down of the pursestring. It may be necessary, after observing the configuration of the areolar closure with the patient upright, to recut, trim or deepithelialize the skin margin in order to obtain a nearly perfect circle on final tightening of the Gore-Tex suture. An areolar "cookie-cutter" is very useful in this regard, both to ensure roundness of the skin opening and to determine the final diameter of the round block. It is of obvious importance to keep the Gore-Tex suture several millimeters deep to the skin surface and to adequately bury the single knot of the periareolar closure,

56.6 Complications and Their Avoidance   425

utilized to assist in determining the location and quantity of any further skin or parenchymal resection. In tailor-tacking preliminary sutures are placed until the breast is brought into an appropriate shape by the tightened skin envelope. Methylene blue or a marking pen records the temporary suture placement and after these temporary sutures are removed the skin to be resected or deepithelialized is evident. These intraoperative skin modifications typically involve four areas: increasing the tightness of the vertical closure, lowering the height of the distribution point, removing skin redundancy or "dog's ears" at the inframammary fold, and ensuring the symmetry and roundness of the "round block" after the Gore-Tex suture is tightened. As the operator becomes more experienced with preoperative markings the degree of these modifications will diminish. However, these modifications may be important as there is no significant evolution of the breast shape in the postoperative period as there may be in vertical mammaplasty. The important concept is that the breast should "look right" on the operating table.

56.6
Complications and Their Avoidance

As with any novel technique there are potential pitfalls that are most evident early on the "learning curve." The most frequently reported complications of the SPAIR mammaplasty are related to the periareolar pursestring closure, such as exposure of the Gore-Tex suture, asymmetry, periareolar scar widening and persistent wrinkling. Some concepts that will minimize difficulties are as follows.

56.6.1
Patient Selection

This is a technique that is primarily suited to small to moderate reductions or nipple–areola transpositions. As in all limited scar techniques, all skin envelope reduction must be reconciled through a shorter total incision length. Thus the technique is not appropriate if a massive amount of skin resection is required. In general the technique should be reserved for patients that are motivated by the aesthetic advantages of such a technique.

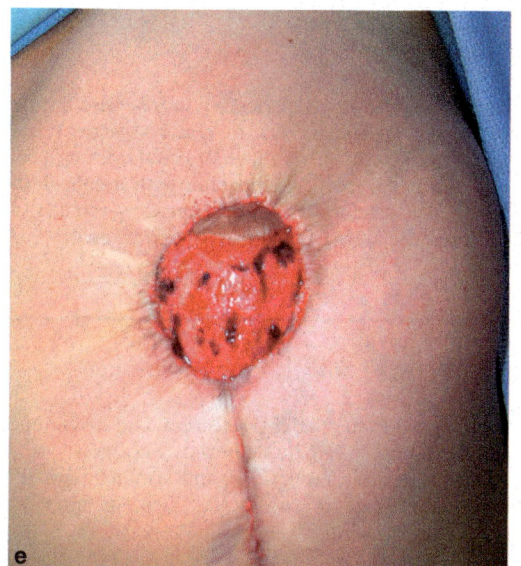

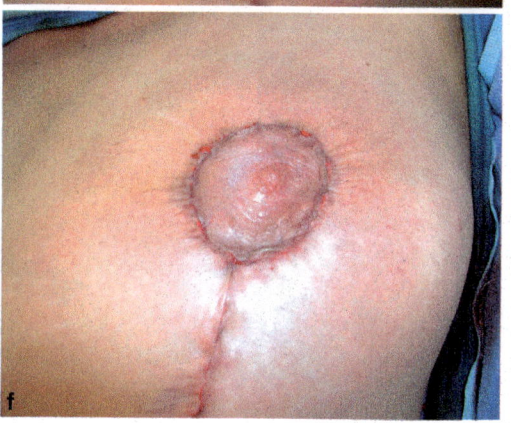

Fig. 56.3 *(continued)* **(e)** "Roundblock" finalized and secured, NAC ready for inset. **(f)** Final inset of NAC

as exposure of the Gore-Tex will usually necessitate its removal, leading to destabilization of the round block and widening of the areola postoperatively.

56.5
Intraoperative Modification of Preoperative Markings

It may be necessary to deviate from the preoperative markings based upon the appearance of the breast upon preliminary closure. This is especially true early in an operator's experience and argues for conservation of skin when placing the preoperative markings. After preliminary closure the result is judged with the bed in the upright position. The process of "tailor-tacking" may be

56.6.2
Periareolar Closure

The periareolar closure involves gathering a larger outer circumference skin opening down to the approximately 4 cm diameter of the areola. If this outer circumference exceeds approximately 8 cm there will be a high risk for periareolar scar problems such as excessive or persistent pleating, scar widening, and loss of areolar roundness. Likewise, excessive resection of skin from the central breast will lead to shape problems such as central flattening. Although the "round block" is a more advanced technique than the old "donut mastopexy" it is prudent to respect the classical limitations, such as limiting the outer to inner diameter ratio to less than 2:1 [15]. Conservatism in periareolar skin resection will avoid many complications.

56.6.3
Vertical Closure

When the vertical closure is excessively long, leading to an unsatisfactory shape of the lower pole, it is advisable to extend the closure into the inframammary fold in a limited fashion. Typically this is in a lateral direction. This does not represent "failure" of the technique but rather a proactive step to limit secondary revisions.

56.6.4
"Backup" Markings

Early in an operator's experience it may be wise, during the preoperative markings, to create separate Wise-pattern markings with a different color marking pen. This may be utilized if the operator finds it difficult to achieve a satisfactory result in the operating room. As a last resort the more familiar pattern may be used.

56.7
Results

With appropriate patient selection and technique excellent results can be achieved (Figs. 56.4, 56.5) with mastopexies, reductions, and symmetry procedures contralateral to TRAM flap or implant reconstructions.

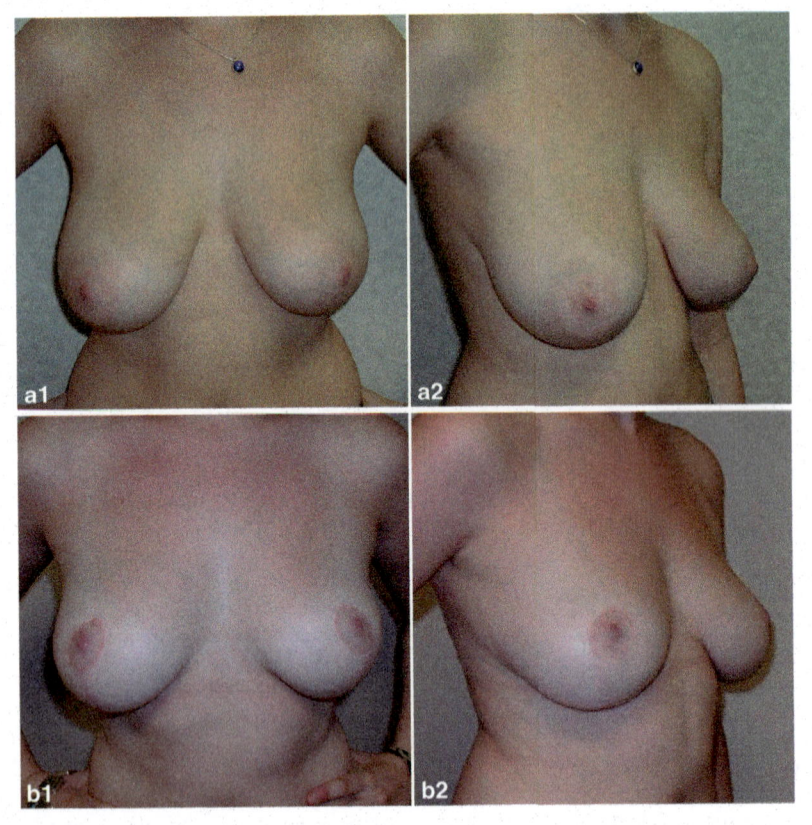

Fig. 56.4 (*a1,2*) Preoperative. (*b1,2*) Postoperative after SPAIR reduction; *right* 260 g, *left* 235 g

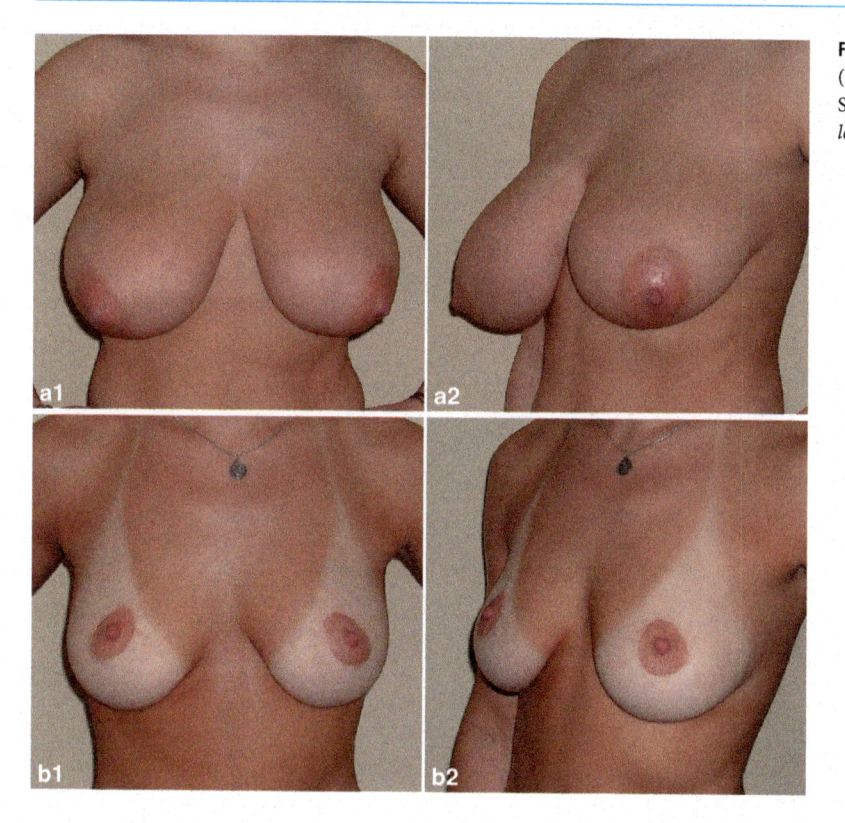

Fig. 56.5 (**a***1,2*) Preoperative. (**b***1,2*) Postoperative after SPAIR reduction; *right* 495 g, *left* 432 g

56.8 Conclusions

The SPAIR mammaplasty is a limited-scar technique with the advantages of an inferior pedicle. In contrast to the vertical mammaplasty, which places all of the skin redundancy into the vertical closure, the SPAIR distributes the excess skin between the vertical and periareolar areas. This leads to greater predictability in terms of the final shape of the lower pole. The SPAIR technique may require some "freehand" intraoperative skin envelope modifications and the periareolar closure may be challenging; these factors may be daunting for the inexperienced or infrequent breast reduction surgeon. However, if the technique is applied to moderate reductions or mastopexies, excellent results may be obtained. A high satisfaction rate among patients and surgeons has been reported for this technique [1]. The SPAIR mammaplasty is a useful alternative to vertical mammaplasty in situations where a limited-scar mammaplasty is indicated.

References

1. Rohrich RJ, Gosman AA, Brown SA, Tonadapu PT, Foster BF: Current preferences for breast reduction techniques: A survey of board-certified plastic surgeons 2002. Plast Reconstr Surg 2004;114(7):1724–1733
2. Lejour M: Vertical mammaplasty and liposuction of the breast. Plast Reconstr Surg 1994;94(1):100–114
3. Palumbo SK, Shifren J, Rhee C: Modifications of the Lejour vertical mammaplasty: Analysis of results in 100 consecutive patients. Ann Plast Surg 1998;40(4):354–359
4. Berthe J, Massaut J, Greuse M, Coessens B, De Mey A: The vertical mammaplasty: A reappraisal of the technique and its complications. Plast Reconstr Surg 2003;111(7):2192–2199
5. Schlenz I, Rigel S, Schemper M, Kuzbari R: Alteration of nipple and areola sensitivity by reduction mammaplasty: A prospective comparison of five techniques. Plast Reconstr Surg 2005;115(3):743–751
6. Mofid MM, Dello, AL, Elias JJ, Nahabedian MY: Quantification of breast sensibility following reduction mammaplasty; a comparison of inferior and medial pedicle techniques. Plast Reconstr Surg 2002;109(7):2283–2288

7. Hidalgo D: Vertical mammaplasty. Plast Reconstr Surg 2005;115(4):1179–1197
8. Hall-Findlay E: A simplified vertical reduction mammaplasty: Shortening the learning curve. Plast Reconstr Surg 1999;104(3):748–759
9. Hammond D: Short scar periareolar inferior pedicle reduction (SPAIR) mammaplasty. Plast Reconstr Surg 1999;103(3):890–901
10. Hammond D: Short scar periareolar inferior pedicle reduction (SPAIR) mammaplasty. Clin Plast Surg 2002;29(3): 411–421
11. Restifo R: Early experience with SPAIR mammaplasty: A useful alternative to vertical mammaplasty. Ann Plast Surg 1999;42(4):428–434
12. Benelli L: A new periareolar mammaplasty: The "round block" technique. Aesthetic Plast Surg 1990;14(2):93–100
13. Whidden P: The tailor-tack mastopexy. Plast Reconstr Surg 1978;62(3):347–354
14. Lassus C: A 30-year experience with vertical mammaplasty. Plast Reconstr Surg 1996;97(2):373–380
15. Spear S, Kassan M, Little J: Guidelines in concentric mastopexy. Plast Reconstr Surg 1990;87(6):961–966

Reduction Mammaplasty Using Inferior Pedicle Technique Combined with Dermal Suspension

Hülya Aydin, Burçak Tümerdem Uluğ

57.1 Introduction

Reduction mammaplasty is one of the most frequently performed aesthetic breast surgery. Among the different techniques that provide reliable results, inferior pedicle technique with inverted T-scar has been widely used for many years. It is a safe and simple technique especially for the patients with massive macromastia and severe ptosis [1]. The main disadvantage of this technique is loss of shape over time as a result of sagging of the remaining breast tissue behind the submammary fold and as a consequence, upward distortion of the plane of nipple–areola complex [2].

Many other reduction mammaplasty techniques also can produce good results, but few make it possible to prevent secondary ptosis as they rely on support of skin envelope that redrapes over the gland [3]. Additional measures to prevent ptosis are described in literature. These are fixation and suspension sutures of the remaining gland to the pectoral fascia [4, 5], glandular shaping and stabilization [4, 5] or allogenic mesh [4, 6, 7]. The use of strips of dermis graft for stabilization was indicated by Maliniac [8, 9], followed by Lewis [10], Da Silva [11], and Hinderer [12].

Menesi [13] presented his distally based dermal flap for glandular fixation and support. Goes [6] used a circular flap of dermis with a central pedicle in the areolar region. All these techniques aimed at achieving a permanent pleasant shape that would oppose gravitational forces that create continuous ptotic effect.

On the basis of the advantages of dermal suspension, we used inferior pedicle technique with inverted T-scar combined with suspension of two laterally extended triangular dermal flaps.

57.2 Surgical Technique

Markings are made on the patient, with the patient in upright position. The sternal notch and midclavicular points are marked. A point 7 cm lateral of the sternal notch is marked, and a straight line that connects this point with the center of the breast is drawn. The new nipple–areola position is determined using the inframammary fold as a landmark. The new inframammary fold is drawn 2 cm at the medial and 3–4 cm at the lateral side superior to the original fold. The width of keyhole limbs is estimated by pushing the breast medially and laterally to mark each limb in relation to the previously marked central axis of the breast. The height of vertical limb is 7 cm from the center of the keyhole presenting the nipple. The areola is marked peroperatively using a cookie cutter with a diameter of 4 cm. The medial line is drawn at the right angle and the lateral line is drawn in an S-shaped manner from the base of vertical keyhole limbs to intersect with the inframammary fold. The inferior dermaparenchymal pedicle is centered over the breast meridian with a width of 8–10 cm. The deepithelialization of the inferior pedicle is extended laterally to create two triangular dermal flaps (Fig. 57.1). Following dissection of dermal flaps, a classic Wise pattern resection is performed and nipple–areola complex is transposed to its new position by the inferior dermaparenchymal pedicle. After assessment of intact vascularity of triangular dermal flaps, they are transposed to the lateral aspects of the pedicle to cover and support the pedicle and are fixed to pectoralis fascia with 2-0 nonabsorbable sutures with adequate tension. This provides bra-like support for the breast tissue, giving a well-defined shape perioperatively (Fig. 57.2). Two suction drains are inserted on each side. The drains are taken out on the second postoperative day.

57.3 Complications

The author had one patient out of 20 with partial necrosis of the nipple–areola complex. Two patients had hypertrophic scar at the inframammary suture line. Two patients had minor superficial wound-healing problems at the corner of T-scar without clinical significance.

M.A. Shiffman (ed.), *Mastopexy and Breast Reduction: Principles and Practice*,
© Springer-Verlag Berlin Heidelberg 2009

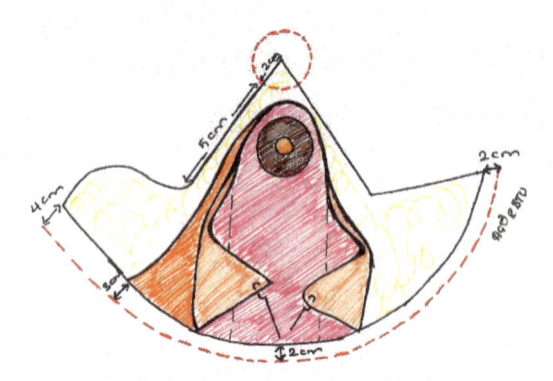

Fig. 57.1 Schematic drawing of new inframammary line and design of the inferior pedicle with laterally extended two triangular dermal flaps

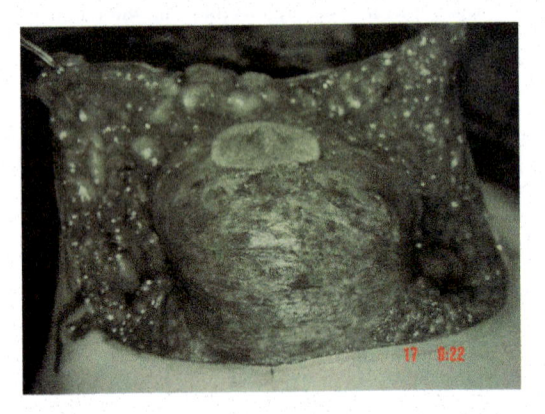

Fig. 57.2 Intraoperative basal view of the breast after fixation of dermal flaps to the pectoralis fascia, covering and suspending the inferior pedicle. Note that it provides bra-like support

All the patients were satisfied with the aesthetic outcome (Figs. 57.3, 57.4).

57.4 Discussion

Reduction mammaplasty is one of the most frequent procedures in plastic surgery. Many different techniques have been developed to improve the aesthetic outcome. However loss of breast projection and breast shape still represent challenges in aesthetic breast surgery. The inferior pyramidal pedicle technique is one of the most widely performed procedures among reduction mammaplasty techniques. Especially patients with massive macromastia and severe ptosis are ideal candidates for this procedure. The disadvantages of inferior pedicle technique include unpredictable settling of breast overtime with bottoming out the lower breast, extension of breast volume below the inframammary fold and hollowing out the upper breast [3]. The inferior pedicle weighs down the skin of inferior pole, which distends and increases the distance between areola and inframammary fold, lessening the volume of upper pole thereby making the areola and nipple appear upward [14].

Hammond [7] combined the concept of short periareolar and vertical scar with inferior pedicle reduction mammaplasty. He addressed the disadvantages of inferior pedicle technique by fixing the pedicle to the chest wall with nonabsorbable sutures.

Marchac and De Olarte [5] and Lejour used several sutures to shape the residual gland and to reposition it on the pectoralis fascia. On the other hand, it has been put forward that fixation and suspension sutures of the remaining gland may impair vascularization [3]. Additionally, they cannot prevent recurrence of ptosis [2]. Using dermis rather than breast parenchyma for fixation purposes spares the pedicle's circulation [15]. Dermafascial fixation incorporates two strongest structures, the dermis and the fascia to achieve more durable results [15]. For this reason, we have designed the inferior pedicle technique with the combination of dermal suspension to prevent sagging in the long term.

Hinderer [7] described a dermal suspension technique with a conventional inverted T-scar reduction mammaplasty. Goes [6] proposed repositioning all connective structures for the breast and treating the gland separately from cutaneous lining, which was duplicated by means of circular dermal flap with central pedicle in the areolar region. He used mixed mesh, which acted as an inner brassiere for this purpose. The disadvantages of the "double skin" technique by Goes [6] include a flattening of the breast, as in most periareolar reduction techniques and implantation of foreign material with the hazard of infection. Qiao et al [16] presented a new technique which is a combination of periareola/round block technique of Benelli [17], the mixed mesh support of technique of Goes [18], for shaping of the mound, laterally based scar including elements of the Regnault B technique and lateral wedge technique [19]. Menderes et al. [20] used a dermal suspension flap technique for the vertical bipedicled flap of McKissock's breast reduction and compared with the classical McKissock's technique. They found out that dermal suspension flaps for McKissock's vertical bipedicled flap technique provided additional advantages for prevention of secondary ptosis of reduced breasts in the long term. Frey [2] proposed a new technique that evolved from a combination of central pedicle, bra-like dermal suspension, and B-formed incision of skin.

Exner and Scheurler [3] described the incorporation of a superiorly pedicled dermal flap for better and long-lasting support in vertical scar reduction mammaplasty.

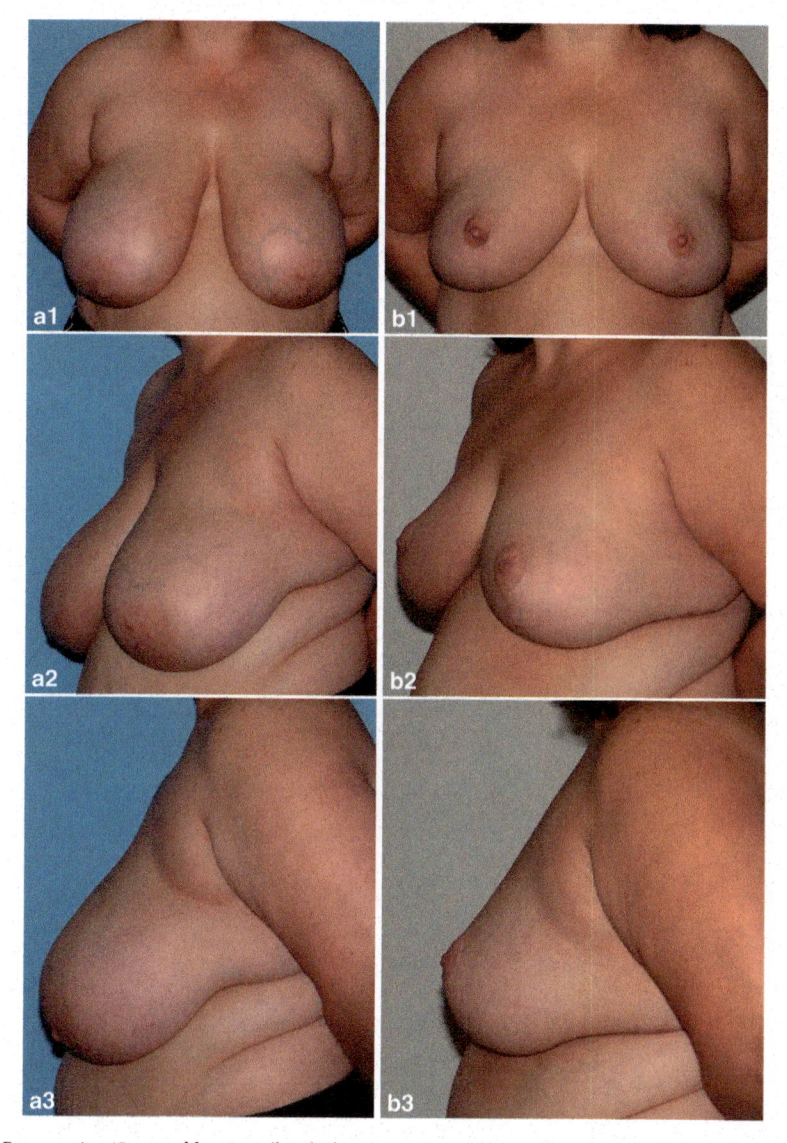

Fig. 57.3 (**a***1-3*) Preoperative 45-year-old patient. (**b***1-3*) Three years postoperative after inferior pedicle technique with dermal suspension breast reduction

De la plaza [14] used two horizontal crossed dermal flaps in Wise pattern reduction mammaplasty with a superomedial dernoglandular pedicle. He claimed that these flaps prevented the dehiscence with scar formation at the juncture of the vertical and horizontal suture lines and displacement of lower pole after a time.

Ceydeli et al. [15] modified short-scar technique by fixing an inferior dermal flap below the medial pedicle of pectoralis fascia in a superomedial direction.

On the basis of criticism for inferior pedicle technique and advantages of dermal suspension, the authors applied inferior pedicle technique with inverted T-scar combined with suspension of two laterally extended triangular dermal flaps. These laterally extended dermal flaps were fixed to the pectoralis fascia by covering and supporting the inferior pedicle. The flaps suspended the breast tissue in an internal brassiere form. This approach prevented lateral bulging of the breast and provided a good projection.

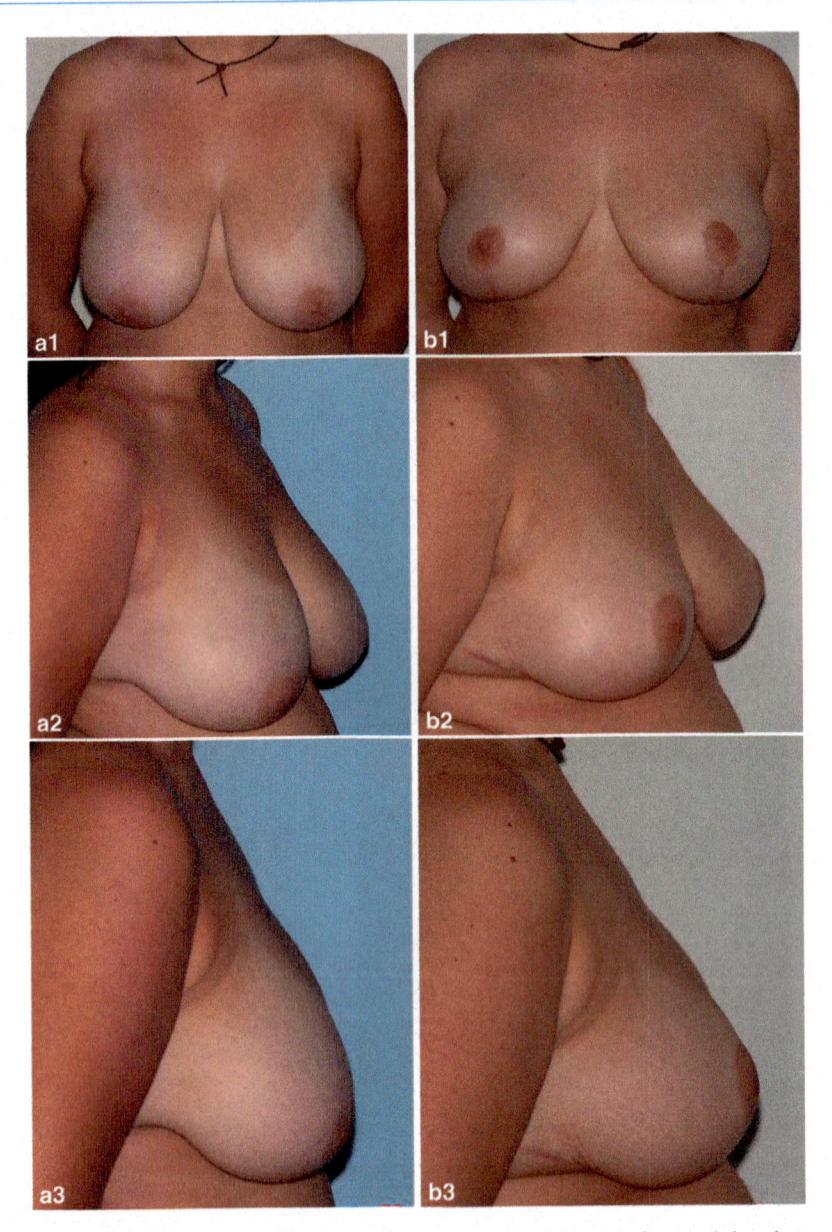

Fig. 57.4 (*a1-3*) Preoperative 18-year-old patient. (*b1-3*) One year postoperative following inferior pedicle technique with dermal suspension breast reduction

Besides preventing the ptosis of inferior pedicle, dermal suspension eliminated the tension in cutaneous suture due to tissue edema especially in early postoperative period. Therefore the likehood of healing problems at the corner of inverted T-suture line decreased and the quality of scars along vertical and horizontal suture lines improved.

Dermis suspension gives a well-defined shape preoperatively, which does not change significantly with time [3]. Therefore patient satisfaction is high, as the aesthetic result is an important aspect of the breast reduction in the long term. This is also suitable for mastopexies without reduction. The technique of dermis suspension provides a long lasting well-defined breast shape bringing a solution to the secondary ptosis.

57.5
Conclusions

Inferior pedicle technique with inverted T-scar is one of the most frequently performed procedures among reduction mammaplasty techniques. Despite its advantages, inferior pedicle technique may result in a flat breast with inadequate projection and the length of the vertical scar of the inverted T may increase due to ptosis of derma-glandular inferior pedicle in the long-term. To overcome these problems, the authors applied the inferior pedicle technique with inverted T-scar, combined with the suspension of two laterally extended triangular dermal flaps. This provided bra-like support for the breast tissue, giving a well-defined shape and projection peroperatively which does not change significantly with time.

References

1. Courtiss EH, Goldwyn RM: Reduction mammaplasty by the inferior pedicle technique. An alternative to free nipple and areola grafting for severe macromastia or extreme ptosis. Plast Reconstr Surg 1977;59(1):500–507
2. Frey M: A new technique of reduction mammaplasty: Dermis suspension and elimination of medial scars. Br J Plast Surg 1999;52(1):45–51
3. Exner K, Scheufler O: Dermal suspension flap in vertical-scar reduction mammaplasty. Plast Reconstr Surg 2002;109(7):2289–2298
4. Lejour M: Vertical mammaplasty and liposuction of the breast. Plast Reconstr Surg 1994;94(1):100–114
5. Marchac D, De Olarte G: Reduction mammaplasty and correction of ptosis with a short inframammary scar. Plast Reconstr Surg 1982;69(1):45–55
6. Goes JC: Periareolar mammaplasty: Double skin technique with application of polyglactine or mixed mesh. Plast Reconstr Surg 1996;97(5):959–968
7. Hinderer UT: Mammaplasty: the dermal brassiere technique. Aesthetic Plast Surg 1978;2:1
8. Maliniac JW: Breast deformities. Anatomical and physiological considerations in plastic repair. Am J Surg 1938;39:54
9. Gulyas G: Mammaplasty with a periareolar dermal cloak for glandular support. Aesth Plast Surg 1999;23(3):164–169
10. Lewis GK: A method of mastopexy with fascia lata transplants. J Int Coll Surg 1956;26(3):346–353
11. Da Silva G: Mastopexy with dermal ribbon for supporting the breast and keeping it in shape. Plast Reconstr Surg 1964;34:403
12. Hinderer UT: Plastia mamaria modelante de dermopexia superficial y retromammaria. Rev Esp Chir Plast 1972;5:521
13. Menesi L: Mammaplasty with dermal flap. Transactions of the Xth Congress of the IPRS. Madrid, Elsevier, Vol III, 1992, p 122
14. De la Plaza R, De la Cruz L, Moreno C, Soto L: The crossed dermal flaps technique for breast reduction. Aesthetic Plast Surg 2004;28(6):383–392
15. Ceydeli A, Gamboa M: Dermafascial fixation suture: A technique for a more durable projection with short-scar (vertical) reduction mammaplasty. Aesthetic Plast Surg 2006;30(5):592–594
16. Qiao Q, Sun J, Liu C, Liu Z, Zhao R: Reduction mammaplasty and correction of ptosis: dermal bra technique. Plast Reconstr Surg 2003;111(3):1122–1130
17. Benelli LA: A new periareolar mammaplasty: The "round block" technique. Aesth Plast Surg 1990;14(2):93–100
18. Grant JH III, Rand RP: The maximally vascularized central pedicle breast technique: Evolution of a technique. Ann Plast Surg 2001;46(6):584–589
19. Regnault P: Breast reduction: B technique. Plast Reconstr Surg 1980;65(6):840–845
20. Menderes A, Mola F, Vayvada H, Yilmaz C, Baytekin C: Dermal suspension flaps for McKissock's vertical bipedicle flap vs. classical McKissock's technique: comparison of aesthetic results and patient satisfaction. Br J Plast Surg 2005;58(2):209–215

Mckissock Bipedicle Breast Reduction

Melvin A. Shiffman

58.1 Introduction

The McKissock bipedicle breast reduction [1] preserves more of the vascular supply to nipple–areolar complex than single pedicle breast reduction. The breast arterial blood supply is from (1) the intercostal arteries, derived from the aorta, give off mammary branches from the 3rd, 4th, and 5th intercostal spaces, (2) the intercostal branches of the internal mammary artery supply to the breast, and (3) lateral thoracic artery, derived from axillary artery, through external mammary branch. Medial intercostal perforators are responsible for directly supplying inferomedial and central parenchyma inferior to the nipple. These perforators course upward through the breast tissue to supply the gland and are one source for nipple–areola complex perfusion. The nipple and areola blood supply arise medially and cranially from internal thoracic artery and laterally and inferiorly from lateral thoracic artery and intercostal arteries.

58.2 Technique

The patient is placed on oral antibiotics, Cipro 500 mg twice daily, 24 h before surgery or may receive intravenous antibiotic, Ancef 1 gm, 45–60 min prior to incision.

58.3 Marking

The patient is placed in a sitting or standing position for marking. The midline is marked. The midclavicle point is determined and a line drawn from the midclavicle to the nipple. The new nipple position is determined by placing a finger pointing outward at the inframammary fold and this is marked on the line from midclavicle to nipple. The mark is lowered by 1–2 cm depending on how heavy and pendulous the breast is. This will prevent the result of a high nipple since the skin stretches when the breast hangs in upright position (Fig. 58.1).

The Wise pattern is used to mark new areolar position and new inframammary fold that is 5 cm from the areola on each side. The Wise pattern results in a new areola of approximately 4 cm diameter. A line is drawn at inframammary fold, including a dart in the midline extending 1 cm superiorly onto the pedicle and 2 cm from the midline on each side. The dart will reduce the incidence of necrosis due to too much tension on the closure. The inframammary line is connected from a lateral point at the lateral axillary line to medial point at least 2 cm from the midline to the point 5 cm from the areola on the Wise pattern. Make sure that there is no pigmented areola from the original areola that remains. If pigmented areola skin is outside markings, the excess should be excised and the 5-cm-line position remarked on the new-excised area.

Mark the pedicle from the new marked areola to the inframammary fold. This should be at least 6–8 cm in width.

58.4 Surgery

The skin is incised in marked areas and pedicle deepithelialized.

Skin flaps are raised in subcutaneous tissues laterally and medially extending 2 cm from the skin incision starting at the inframammary fold and ending superiorly at a point on the areola that is one-third inferior to the top of new areola marking. The medial and lateral segments are incised (Fig. 58.2) by dividing the tissues down to the underlying pectoralis major muscle fascia and then excised from the fascia (Fig. 58.3). Care must be taken to maintain the width of the pedicle down to the underlying pectoralis fascia. This requires angling the incision laterally through the breast in the lateral excision and medially through the breast in the medial excision. The pedicle superior to the areola needs a deep portion to be excised starting at least 2 cm below the skin and extending to the underlying fascia (Fig. 58.4). This allows folding of superior portion of the pedicle for closure.

M.A. Shiffman (ed.), *Mastopexy and Breast Reduction: Principles and Practice*,
© Springer-Verlag Berlin Heidelberg 2009

436   58 Mckissock Bipedicle Breast Reduction

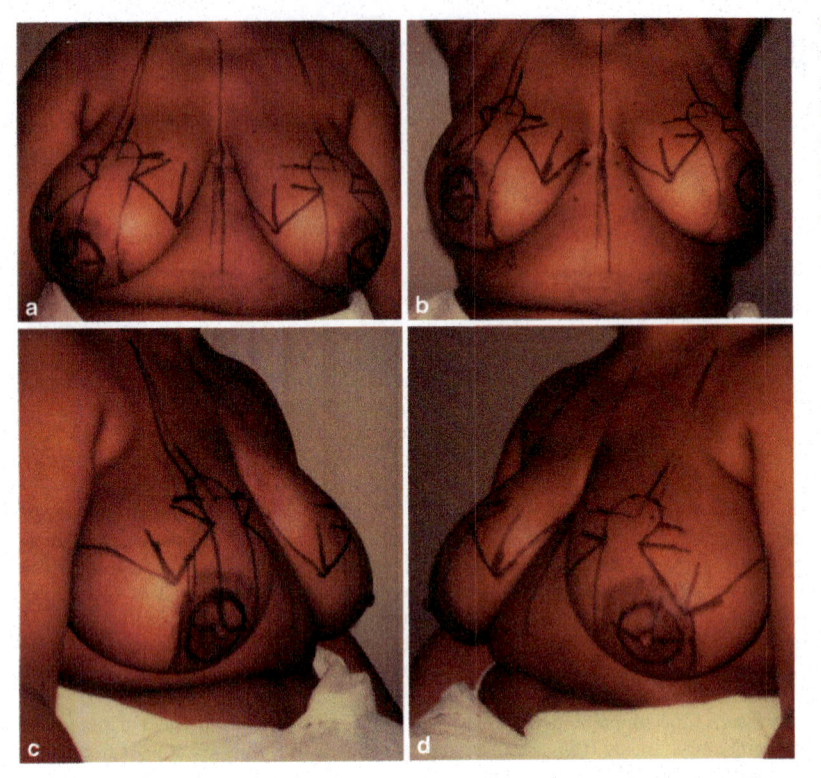

Fig. 58.1 Marking the breast using Wise pattern. The midclavicle line to nipple has been readjusted medially to new nipple point because of the extreme lateral position of the nipple when sitting

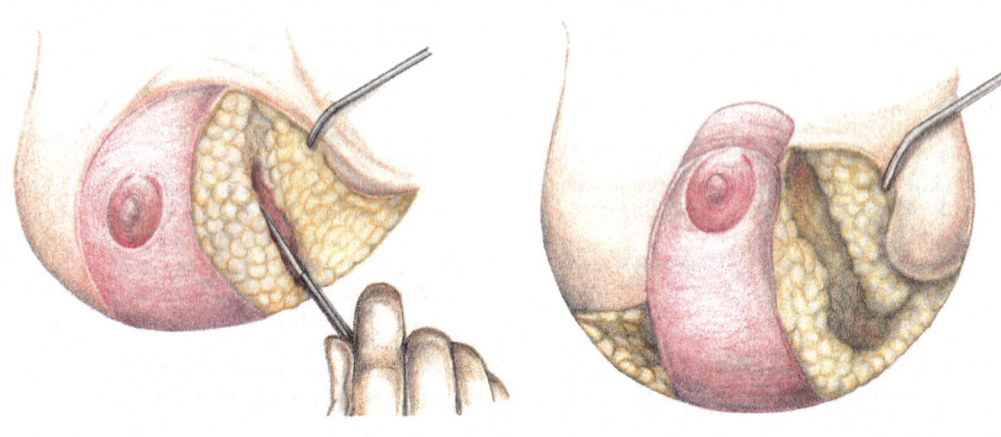

Fig. 58.2 After deepithelialization of the pedicle lateral and medial incisions are made along the pedicle down to the fascia

Fig. 58.3 The total lateral and medial segments are excised

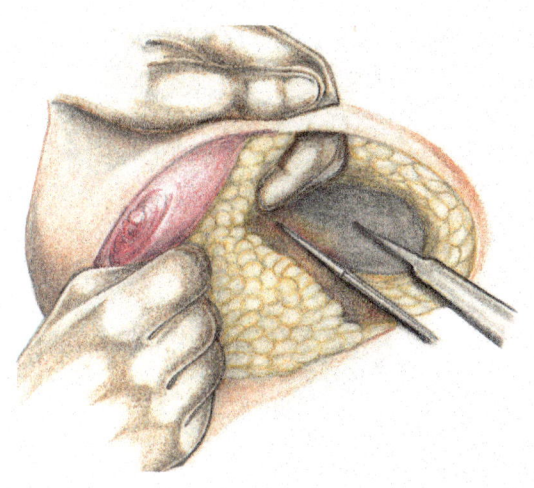

Fig. 58.4 Superior to the areola the breast is excised in a circular or oval fashion starting 2 cm below the skin and extending down to the fascia

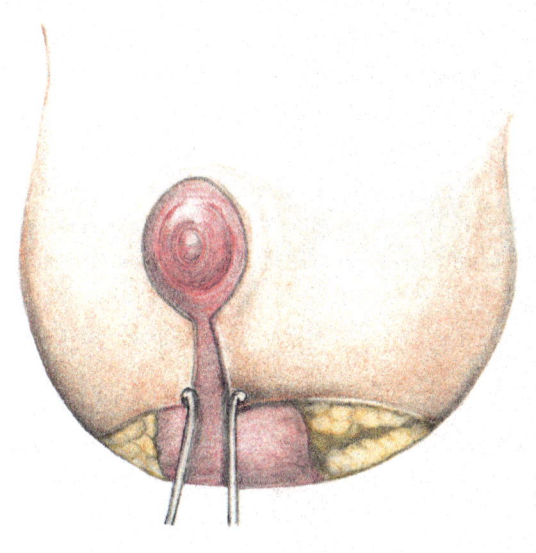

Fig. 58.5 The nipple–areola complex is brought superiorly into its new position and the incisions closed

After careful and complete control of bleeding with electrocoagulation, suction catheters are placed at the lateral edge of new inframammary fold and pulled through the opening in the superior portion of the pedicle into the medial aspect of the wound. The wound is closed with interrupted subcuticular 2-0 chromic sutures starting by folding the superior portion of the pedicle and suturing the areola to its new position (Fig. 58.5). The sutures are then used to close the inferior point of the areola to the vertical incision and then the vertical incision also closed and sutured to the new inframammary fold. During this portion of the procedure the pedicle should be checked to make sure it is not twisted. The inframammary incision is closed with the subcuticular sutures. The skin is closed with running or interrupted 5-0 nylon suture and sterile dressings applied. A bra is placed so that the inferior portion of the bra is at the inframammary fold.

58.5 Postoperative Care

The patient is placed on oral antibiotics, such as Cipro 500 mg twice daily, for 7 days if no intravenous antibiotic was given prior to surgery. An analgesic, such as Vicoden (1–2 tabs every 4 h as needed), can be prescribed.

Follow up is on the first postoperative day at which time the breast is checked for hematoma, asymmetry, and cyanotic changes of the nipple–areola complex (NAC). If cyanosis is present, the areola is checked for venous refill. If the refill time is less than 6 s, NAC can be observed on a daily basis until the cyanosis subsides or until the refill is over 6 s. If the refill is over 6 s, the incision should be opened around the inferior portion of areola and the whole vertical closure to inframammary fold. The breast can be checked at that time for torsion of the pedicle by careful external palpation under sterile conditions. If the cyanosis does not subside in 24 h after opening the wound, consideration should be given to a nipple–areolar complex transfer to the lower abdomen or upper thigh and transplanted to the breast when the tissues have healed or adequately granulated.

The next visit, if there are no problems, would be on the fourth postoperative day and the suction catheters removed if the drainage is less than 50 ml on each side.

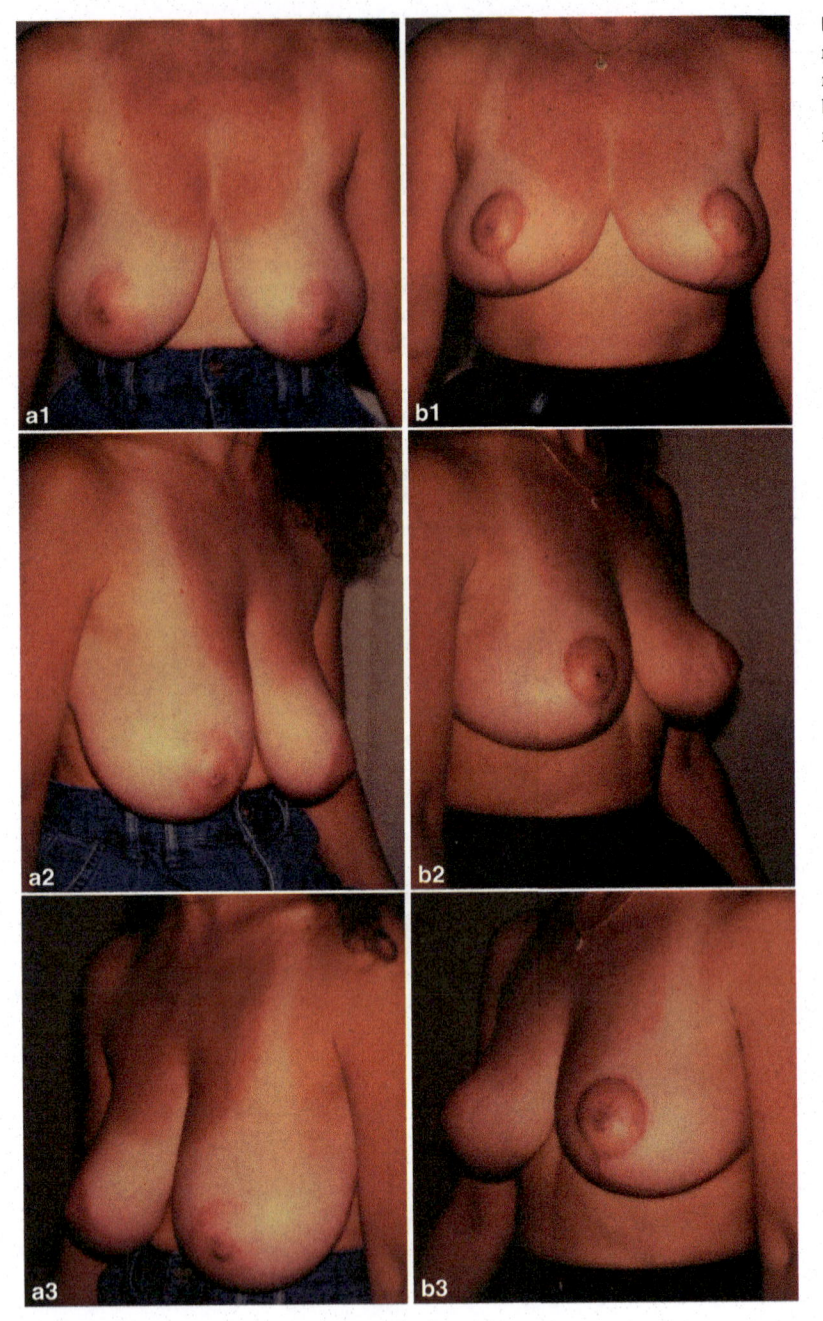

Fig. 58.6 (a1-3) Preoperative macromastia. (b1-3) Six months after McKissock bipedicle reduction mammoplasty

The patient is seen on the 7th postoperative day and the sutures removed and Steri-Strips applied. The patient is next seen in 30 days and in 6 months at which time postoperative photos are taken (Fig. 58.6).

58.6
Discussion

The procedure is simple to learn and the aesthetic results are usually excellent except for the scars. Scars may become hypertrophic or keloid.

Asymmetry, calcifications, infection, and bleeding may occur.

Vascular necrosis of the nipple–areola complex is a serious but rare complication after bipedicle dermal flap reduction.

58.7
Conclusions

The McKissock bipedicle breast reduction reduces the chance of nipple–areola necrosis (NAC) because of very adequate blood supply that is preserved to NAC. The procedure results in the maintenance of normal breast curves and leaves an adequate amount of breast tissue to fill the bra without having to add a breast augmentation.

Reference

1. McKissock P: Color Atlas of Mammaplasty. New York, Thieme 1991, pp 47–78

Strömbeck Technique

Pierre F. Fournier

59.1 Introduction

Choosing a technique of breast reduction today may be difficult for a young plastic surgeon. Will he choose a lateral technique or a technique with an inverted T? A bipedicle technique, horizontal or vertical? With one pedicle or two pedicles? Oblique, superior, or inferior? With skin undermining or no skin undermining? Which technique is the safest and gives the best results? Some techniques are praised and others are denigrated by experienced surgeons with a reliable opinion and being an authority in breast reduction. The choice of the young surgeon is in addition more difficult in the apparent difficulties of techniques that are described. But is it the technique which is bad or surgeon? The author believes anyhow the situation is simple.

Around 1960, this situation changed radically with the publication of Strömbeck [1] and his new concepts in breast reduction surgery. His concepts simplified so much the situation and were so successful that they have been copied, modified, adapted, faked up, disguised, republished, and his original technique is confused or mistaken and found with difficulty, in the middle of plagiarisms or modifications.

The author believes that in breast reduction surgery, we can distinguish:
Before Strömbeck
and
After Strömbeck.

We should credit those who make science and it is sometimes difficult to distinguish them. The author wishes to give to Strömbeck the place that he deserves in this difficult surgery that he has greatly simplified and made safer for the surgeon and for the patient.

59.2 Before Strömbeck

Breast reduction techniques were very numerous and large undermining that glandular remodeling was necessary. The consequence of such techniques was a lot of complications; bleeding hematomas, necrosis of different mammary tissues, or wound disruption. Evidently, it was impossible to have good results in many cases but an operation for breast reduction was often an adventure for the surgeon, even with an experienced one, as well as for the patient. The most common technique used at that time was Biesenberger [2] technique and lateral technique described by Marc [3].

59.3 After Strömbeck

The situation changed radically when Strömbeck described his two principles:
1. The dermal glandular resection has to be done as a block of tissue without any undermining, perpendicularly to the skin.
2. The areola and nipple are supplied by the skin and the flap on which the nipple may be carved (or cut?), in any direction, in the breast tissue.

In his technique, the flap is horizontal or curved with an upper concavity. The final result was a scar as an anchor with a superior resection of slight importance. This bipedicle flap, if necessary, could be severed. As time passed, sectioning this flap was done frequently and Strömbeck decided to increase the base of this flap with an additional deepithelialization to give more safety to this part of the operation.

The Strömbeck technique has been developed for big breast, with a long pedicle and in moderately hypertrophied breasts or mild hypertrophies with ptosis, the pedicle is short and needs to be sectioned to be placed in a higher position easily.

Origin of the Strömbeck technique: The amputation technique of Thorek [4] (Fig. 59.1).

In large hypertrophied breasts with ptosis the treatment of choice was the bloc amputation with areolar nipple graft. This operation was easy and quick, the only hazard was the "take" of the areolar nipple graft. Aesthetic results were good since Thorek, in 1922, added to the inferior resection, a superior wedge-shaped resection giving more conicity to the mammary gland.

M.A. Shiffman (ed.), *Mastopexy and Breast Reduction: Principles and Practice,*
© Springer-Verlag Berlin Heidelberg 2009

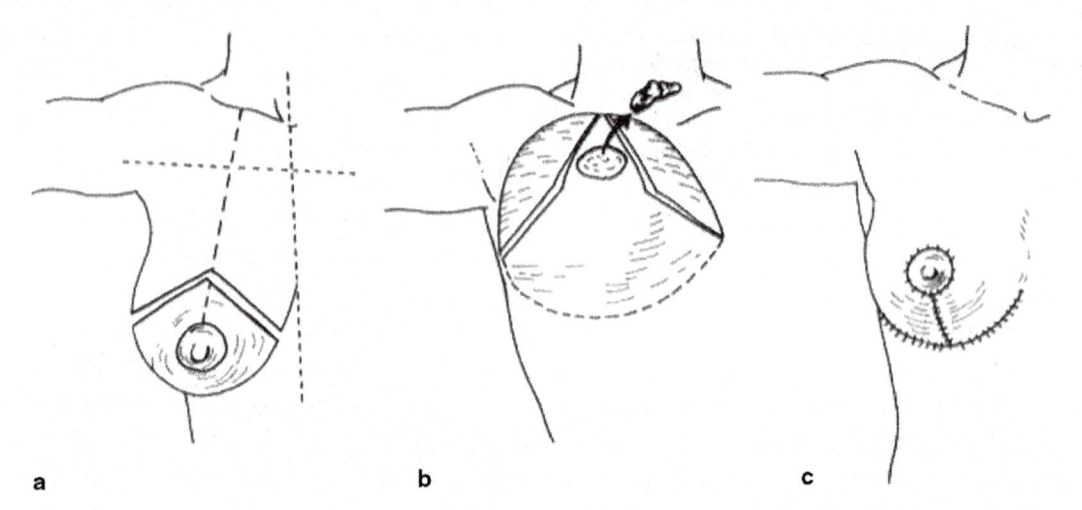

Fig. 59.1 Thorek amputation technique. (**a**) The lower side of the second rib is marked as well as the meridian line and submammary sulcus. (**b**) Submammary skin glandular tissue resection. (**c**) After nipple areolar graft

This Strömbeck technique is always good even today in large breast hypertrophy and gigantomastia. The majority of cases that the author has to treat, with or without ptosis, are average hypertrophies. If a patient may accept a possible risk of a nipple areolar necrosis for a gigantomastia, she will not accept this risk with an average hypertrophy and the surgeon will not accept the risk as well.

As a flap bearing the nipple areola is much safer than a free graft, Strömbeck decided to do (instead of a free graft as it is done in Thorek technique) a flap carrying the nipple areola complex. In the beginning, it was a bipedicle flap and later he decided to cut one side of this flap and to increase the deepithelialization of the base of this flap. Then it was possible to easily place the nipple areola complex in a higher position.

Block amputation of the mammary gland was a safe procedure with Thorek technique and has not been changed by Strömbeck. But with Strömbeck placing the nipple areola complex in a high position, this operation became easy and safe with the Strömbeck bipedicle technique or with one pedicle technique with increased deepithelialization of the base of the pedicle when it was necessary.

59.4
Sir Harold Gillies

"A graft is a piece of skin completely detached from the place where we took it, which is dead when you put it on and which comes back to life after.

A flap is a piece of skin which is incompletely detached from where you took it, which is alive when you put it on and who may die later."

If Strömbeck started from Thorek amputation technique for what is the dermal glandular resection, he has improved this technique transplanting the nipple areola complex with a bipedicle flap with upper concavity first and later when this flap was too short, he did not hesitate to section it, usually the lateral pedicle, to be able to rotate more easily without any tension this flap.

For more safety, when the surgeon has to section this pedicle, he should not hesitate, as Strömbeck did later to deepithelialize the base of this pedicle to increase the deepithelialized surface on one side. When the pedicle is long this deepithelialization has to be increased on both sides even when it is unnecessary to section one of them. The nipple areola complex will be transposed easily as both flaps are very long.

Since this last technical improvement, section of one pedicle after increasing the deepithelialized portion of its base, practically all cases of pure ptosis with average or important hypertrophy or even gigantomastia may be treated with this technique.

Montaigne, the French philosopher and writer of the 1800s:

"Whoever saw a physician using the recipe of one of his peers without adding or removing something."

A short time after Strömbeck publication one can see in the surgical literature minor modifications of the original technique of Strömbeck. They are named technique of Doctor… or of Professor… Such techniques are offered and praised as better than Strömbeck technique. We do not want to call such authors plagiarists but the humble modifications that they brought to Strömbeck technique even if the details that they offer are interesting and reliable, do not deserve to have their name given to this modification and to be proposed as "original techniques."

When looking at the diagrams of the newer "techniques" there are similarities to the Strombeck technique (Fig. 59.2). The dermal glandular technique is rigorously identical to the Strömbeck technique, that is to say to the Thorek technique. Only, the transposition of the nipple areola flap is different. The pedicle may be a bipedicle vertical instead of a horizontal one or a slightly upward concave one or aftersection of the medial implantation of a single pedicle with a lateral pedicle instead of a medial pedicle, an upper flap, a lower flap or a wide deepithelialization around the areola, creating a vital pedicle that will be buried after the inferior and intraglandular resection are performed.

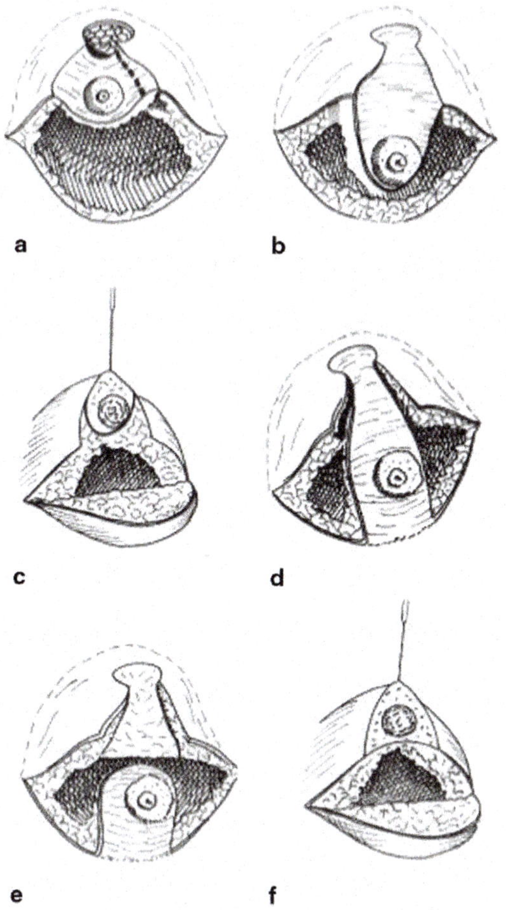

Such techniques are not new. They only consist in minor modification of the emplacement of the flaps bearing the nipple areola complex, associated with a dermal glandular resection identical to the Strömbeck technique only slightly modified. Such "techniques" have no other interest than to complicate the understanding of this operation for a surgeon beginning to learn breast reduction.

Strömbeck has modified completely the surgery of breast reduction and all the modification procedures of the flap bearing the complex nipple areola to a higher position do not change the concept of breast reduction given by Strömbeck even if they may be interesting. They do not deserve the name of a technique that only may be of "a different way to transpose the nipple areola complex."

Strömbeck is the only one to have made a giant step in the surgery of breast reduction bringing simplicity and safety. His principles are also adopted when doing a modern lateral technique.

Fig. 59.2 Inverted T techniques (*anchor shape* scar) drafted from Strömbeck technique. All of them are variations of the nipple areolar complex transposition. (**a**) External pedicle. (**b**) Long upper pedicle. (**c**) Sharp upper pedicle. (**d**) Vertical bipedicle. (**e**) Lower pedicle. (**f**) Extended periareolar deepithelialization without pedicle

59.5 Preoperative Marking

A good drawing will give a good result and all the steps of the operation will be easy. The immediate result and late result will be good. We could compare a breast reduction operation for pure ptosis, pure hypertrophy, or ptosis with hypertrophy to the readjustment of a garment too ample, after measuring, drawing, making pattern, cutting according to this pattern, and assembling and saving together the different parts of the pattern. During such steps, the most important will be done by the fashion designer, the surgeon. The sewing work, long, and tedious, whose future is dictated but who needs less experience, will be given to the assistants whose work has to be excellent and faultless. The final aesthetic result as well as its duration in time cannot be identical with all patients and it will be necessary to explain this to the patients before the operation and this may be sometimes difficult. A good result, aesthetically speaking as well as its duration in time, depends on one side the work of the surgeon and consequently the drawing and on another side the patient herself and tissues that she offers for the operation (Fig. 59.3).

Even if the marking is perfect, the breast obtained will not be identical in a woman of small stature, mature, multiparous with a thorax that may be too short or too wide, the implantation of the breast may be high or low

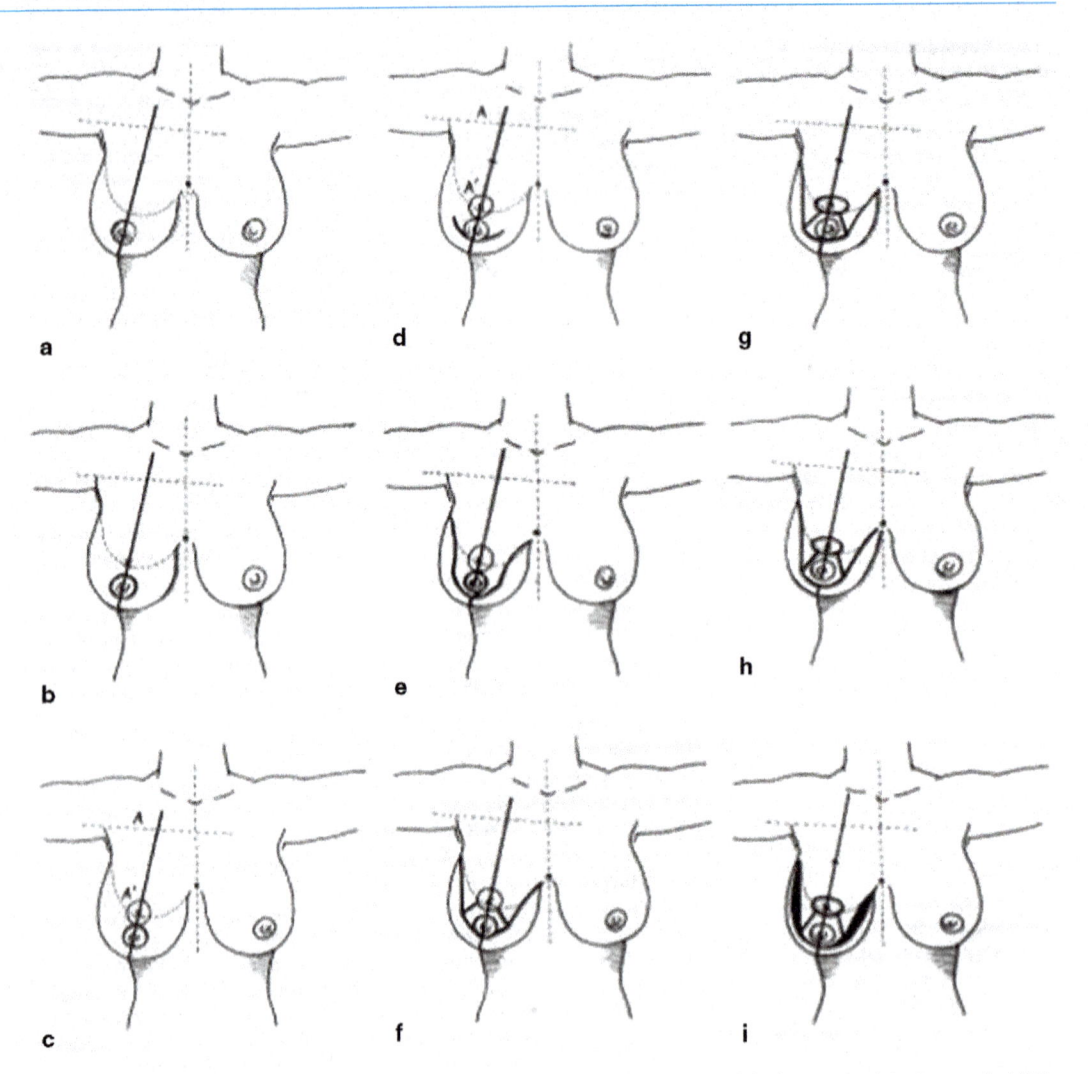

Fig. 59.3 (a) The lower side of the second rib, the meridian line, and the submammary sulcus are marked. (b) On the meridian line, the center of the future areolar is marked as well as on the present areola the circumference (*circle*) of future areola. (c) An identical circumference (*circle*) is marked around the center of the future areola. (d) The distance AA′ between the lower side of the second rib to the upper part of the new areola is measured (*marked*) and a curved line with an upper concavity is traced (*marked*) below the inferior side of new areola. This line is situated exactly at the middle of the AA′ distance. (e) It is on this curved line that we mark the two halves of the present submammary sulcus and they have the same length that the original half sulcus. (f) From the meeting point (or check point) a straight line will be drawn toward the new areola. (g) The angles of the new areola are joined by a curved line passing 1 cm above the areola that have to be transferred. The lower angles are joined by a curved line passing 2 cm below the limit of the areola that we have to transfer. (h) The circumference of the place of the new areola is increased with the distance between upper angles (generally 4 or 5 cm), in horizontal direction and reach the final drawing limiting the upper resection, the lower resection and the pedicles that we have to deepithelialize. (i) If the pedicles are long, widening of base has to be marked. In case of short pedicle, medial surface is broadened (increase) that has to be deepithelialized, and external pedicle is cut

or too wide, the skin may be thin with striae, and the inner tissues may be predominately fatty. Another patient may be younger, taller, nulliparous with a thorax, with nice proportions, and the implantation of the breast may be in a normal situation and of normal surface, neither too large, neither too narrow with a skin of good quality, thick and without striae and whose deep tissues are made essentially of glandular tissue.

We can say as the tailors say when making a garment:

"So is the material so will be the garment."

The surgeon may say also:

"So are the tissues so will be the result."

A great painter with a mediocre model will never paint the "Venus of Botticelli" and the great sculptor of the Antiquity could have wonderful statues with blocks of marble of great quality easy to be carved, polished and that could not be spoiled with time. All this has to be explained to the patient and also this has to be well understood by her. A patient believes sometimes that all is possible in aesthetic surgery, showing to the surgeon ladies' fashion magazines requesting the breast of such or such model. The preoperative discussions are very important to avoid any unjustified claims of the patients. As well as morphologic work, the surgeon has to do psychological work.

The marking gives at the end of the operation a scar as an anchor or an inverted T. The author has used the technique of Strömbeck for more than 40 years and this technique has not one single wrinkle. This marking can be also applied when using other techniques described by Skoog [5], Pitanguy [6], McKissock [7] or with an upper or lower pedicle, techniques which are only more modifications of Strömbeck technique.

The concept in modern breast reductions are:
1. Bloc resection of the skin and glandular tissue, only on the skin when we have a case of pure ptosis, on the skin and glandular tissue when we have cases of hypertrophy or ptosis with hypertrophy.
2. No skin undermining (or very little when necessary). Undermining severs Cooper's ligaments and may give haematomas or necrosis.

Marking the patient has to be done the night before the operation. The Wise pattern used by Strömbeck is unnecessary but may be useful at the beginning if it is adapted to the breast of the patient. It may be a source of errors and of bad results if it is used without being adapted to the breast.

"We have to do a tailor made work and not a ready made work."

All the markings used are wrong for 20% of patients that is more or less due to the deformations of the tissues. The idea is to do marking adapted to the breast that we have to operate on and this marking will be different according to the breast thorax of the patient. We have to use common point of reference. As well as in nose reduction, we have to respect the proportions between each other and the proportions of the nose on the face. In breast reduction, we have to respect the proper proportions of the breast in regard to the rest of the body. A centimeter tape, a marking pen, and metal rings of different diameters are necessary for the areola marking.

The patient will be standing and not seated but the surgeon will be seated. The first thing to check is whether the shoulders are horizontal. If they are oblique, this is a cause of pseudo mammary asymmetry. After establishing horizontal shoulders we have to check the implantation of the breasts on the thorax whether high or low and it is necessary to inform the patient about this. An eventual breast asymmetry may also exist preoperatively.

Further examination of the thorax and the breast will be done at this time checking the condition of the skin whether thin or thick, striae or no striae, the surface of the areola, condition of the nipple normal, invaginated, or overdeveloped, its color, and whether there is a scar from a previous operation.

The surgeon should also palpate the consistency of the breast, whether pure firm gland tissue, fat without any consistency, or intermediary condition. The patient will be informed of the result of this examination.

The midline of the body is traced first from the manubrium to the xyphoid process. Then, a horizontal line is traced again, on the second rib localized by palpation at the angle of Louis. The submammary sulcus is finally marked from the parasternal line to the anterior axillary line. This last marking has to be checked with the patient lying down as this sulcus is not always fixed but misplaced in a lower position in case of breast hypertrophy. The marking in the horizontal position will be adopted and this marking is usually 1 cm higher or more. This marking, with experience, has to be diminished as much as possible, on each side, mostly on the sternal side.

The second intercostal space and 6th intercostal space are the upper and lower limits of projection of a nonptotic breast that is located between these two limits.

The meridian of the breast has to be marked starting either 5 or 6 cm from the midline, on the collarbone or placing a centimeter tape behind the neck, on the nape of the neck, each end of this tape held by the patient. The tape is passed on a line to the areolas. This line has to be very well traced, the areola has to be exactly on it on the meridian of the breast. Its symmetry has to be checked measuring it in relation to the midline. This line is prolonged below the areola and divided into two parts at the submammary sulcus. The two parts have to be measured and marked on the skin. Too lateral or too medial jeopardizes the harmony and proportions of the future breast.

The placement of the center of the future areola has to be estimated finally. It will be on the breast meridian and to find the true placement one of the following maneuvers has to be done:

1. The forward projection on the meridian of the submammary sulcus; it is the most faithful maneuver.
2. By estimation (according to the thorax and degree of ptosis), this place is between 18 and 23 cm from the sternal notch, on a line starting from this place and crossing the meridian line. We have to remember that it is much better to place a new areola too low as it is always possible to correct it without scar sequelae. The reverse is not possible.
3. A horizontal line passing at the level of the mid portion of the arm or at the level of the xyphoid process after the ptosis has been corrected.
4. On a horizontal line passing at the level of the 6th rib: radiographic studies of the projection of the areola, on a nonptotic breast have shown that it was at the level of the 6th rib. This 6th rib is identified by palpation of angle of Louis.
5. Using the maneuver of Claoué: asking the patient to contract the pectoralis major muscle with the patient having her hands on her hips and in the supine position. The placement is given by crossing the line of cutaneous projection of inferior part of pectoralis major and meridian line. This is easily understood if we remember that the lowest palpable digitation of the pectoralis major is inserted on the 6th rib. With the arm in anatomic position, a horizontal line passing at the level of the nipple is marked on the midline. Then, the patient raises both arms vertically and a new horizontal line passing through the midline giving the new position of the areola. This maneuver is excellent but is good only for mild cases of breast ptosis. The difference between the two lines indicates the correction desired.

The placement of the future areola is then marked with a point. When the place of the center of the areola is made and marked with a point, on the meridian line, we have to choose the diameter of the new areola to be transposed and we have to mark it on the areola of the ptotic breast. If the areola is small or of normal size (4–5 cm), we shall keep it as it is. The most common diameter is 5 cm sometimes 4 but less often. It is better to do too large an areola instead of too small one.

We ask the advice of the patient but we have to guide her. The diameter of the future areola chosen by the surgeon and the patient is marked by an incision line with a metal ring of appropriate diameter. This ring has its center above the nipple and is applied firmly for a few seconds on the breast tissue. The line created on the skin by the pressure will be marked immediately after the ring has been removed. This maneuver is done when the patient is lying down, when the breast is a large one, and its weight could exaggerate the surface of the areola which at the end of the operation should be too small. Next marking is on the meridian line with this ring making an identical circle on the place chosen as center of the future areola. The length of this circle will be modified when the marking is finished.

Measure the distance between the upper line of the future areola that was just marked and the horizontal line passing at the level of the second rib. This distance is generally between 9 and 15 cm according to the thorax and ptosis. A slightly curved line is traced, parallel to the inferior marking of the new areola, at a distance which is half the upper measurement (that is to say 41/2 to 71/2 cm).

On a normal breast seen on profile, the areola submammary sulcus distance is half the distance from areola to second rib. A point has to be marked on this curved line, toward each of its extremities. Such points are parted from the extremity of each submammary sulcus by a distance equal to the distance parting the point of crossing of the meridian line, from the extremity of the corresponding submammary sulcus. Once marked, such points will be joined to the homologous extremity of the submammary sulcus by a curved line with an upper convexity or sometimes a lazy S. Two such lines are the upper edge of the future submammary sulcus divided into two, the lower edge being the inferior portion of the submammary primary sulcus marked before and divided into two by the meridian line. The two points are then joined at the center of the new areola with an oblique line above and medial. Such two points will be later joined together by a curved line. This line when at the level of the meridian line, will be 1 cm from the areolar marking to be excised. The points obtained by the crossing of the inferior side of the new areola by the oblique lines will be joined together by a curved line with an upper concavity that will be 2 cm from the upper side of the areola. Such four points and the lines joining (uniting) them are the limits of the cutaneous glandular bridge bearing the areola. All this surface is deepithelialized using conventional techniques or using the strip technique. The marking is finished except the final circumference of the placement of the future areola. The circumference delineating the areola will be increased by the distance between two superior points placed on the inferior side of the areola using a metal ring of appropriated circumference.

We have now:
1. An upper zone of resection.
2. A lower zone of resection.
3. A dermal glandular bridge bearing the nipple–areola complex with a medial and lateral pedicle.

In many cases, the length of this cutaneous glandular bridge is not long enough and it is not possible to raise the areola into its new position. It is necessary then to deepithelialize the medial pedicle (the lateral one may also be used). The lateral pedicle will be sectioned completely and the areola will ascend without any problem.

It is better to have only one pedicle with an excellent blood supply instead of two pedicles with a deficient blood supply. Such marking allows the surgeon to place the areola on an upper or a lower pedicle or to do a dermal mastopexy.

59.6 Surgical Technique

General anaesthesia with intubation. Often this operation is done in two steps one week apart to avoid blood transfusion and for a short anesthesia (Figs. 59.4, 59.5).

The patient is placed in a supine horizontal position on the table. The author starts on the right breast and from the same side of the patient, the left breast is operated on after the first one is finished.

Deepithelialization is performed on the pedicles and if it is scheduled, on the additional surface, on their base. The second step is the upper resection of skin and glandular tissue. It is necessary to leave some glandular tissue as Strömbeck advises. Resecting until the pectoralis major muscle may give an invaginated nipple. This resection is mostly useful to make room for the transplanted areola after the bearing flap has been sectioned. Hemostasis is done with electrical cautery during the whole operation.

The lower resection that is the true resection is done second. Either side can be started on, it does not matter! Under the base of the flap, the resection should be oblique. Only the dermis and a small amount of

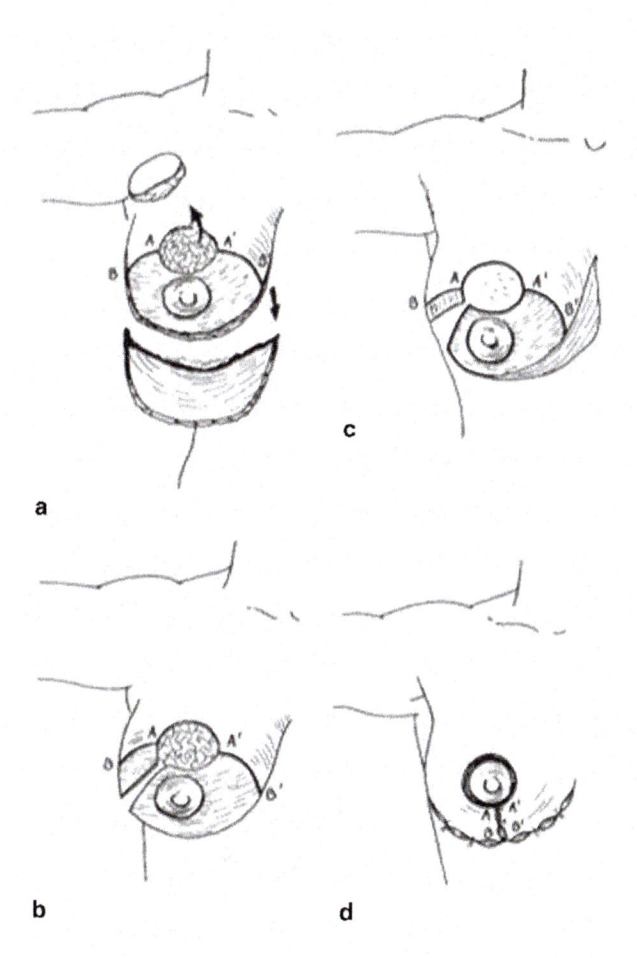

Fig. 59.4 (a) Upper resection, lower resection, and two deepithelialized pedicles. (b) The external pedicle is sectioned. (c) Widening of the base of the pedicle has to be done if we intend to cut the external pedicle and deepithelialization has to be done at this place. (d) Final result

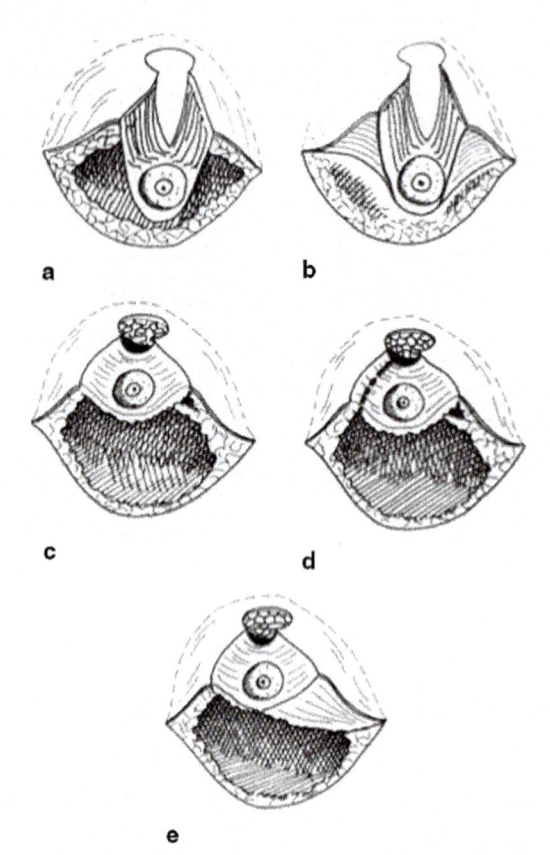

Fig. 59.5 Different possible pedicles when doing Strömbeck technique. (**a**) Long pedicles. (**b**) Long pedicles with widening of deepithelialized base. (**c**) Short pedicles. (**d**) Short pedicles. The external pedicle may be cut completely without widening the base. (**e**) Short pedicles with widening of bases

subcutaneous tissue have to be saved. After a careful hemostasis, the different elements are sutured together without any tension. A small conical piece of glan-dular tissue is resected between the upper and lower resection to allow the drainage of the upper resection.

If the marking has been correctly done there are no special difficulties and no modifications to do. Should the surgeon believe that there is too much tension he should resect some more glandular tissue even if it is necessary to go below the bearing flap.

Deep suture of Dexon® should give a firm breast with a low or very moderate tension.

The skin on the T line is sutured with a subcuticular nylon suture reinforced by a few interrupted sutures. An over and over continuous suture is done, on the areola. Suction drainage is a must. All the skin sutures are done when the two breasts are completed. The surgeon will suture one breast and his assistant the second one.

The breast tissue removed is weighed and placed in a sterile glass container filled with 500 ml normal saline. One container is used for each breast. This will allow an identical resection on both sides whatever the tissues resected, fat or gland. Fat and gland may be different in each breast and we are interested more in the volume resected than in the weight resected. The skin removed may be dissected and kept in a sterile container filled with normal saline and antibiotics and kept in the deep freeze. This skin may be used later (3 weeks) in case of wound dehiscence or infection. The periareolar sutures are removed after 1 week. The intradermal suture is removed after 3 weeks and interrupted sutures on the vertical part of the T, after 10 days.

59.7
Postoperative Care

The postoperative period is usually without problem. The drains are removed after 1 or 2 days. Antibiotics are given routinely. The patient may leave the hospital after 2 or 3 days. Blood is not given routinely. The breast tissue removed is sent for pathology study.

59.8
Complications

Necrosis of the areola or glandular tissue is not part of postoperative period as well as bleeding as it was seen with procedures involving large skin undermining and glandular tissue removal.

In case of large hypertrophy, the author may operate on the right breast first and 5 days later the second one. The marking on the second breast is kept visible until the second breast is done if we scratch the skin very slightly with the tip of a no. 11 blade. The reasons are to avoid too long general anaesthesia and a blood transfusion not desired by the patients.

59.9
Conclusions

The Strömbeck technique is a very safe one, giving excellent results, with minor complications [7–10] (Fig 59.6). The most important for the surgeon is to do very accurate markings preoperatively (Figs. 59.7, 59.8).

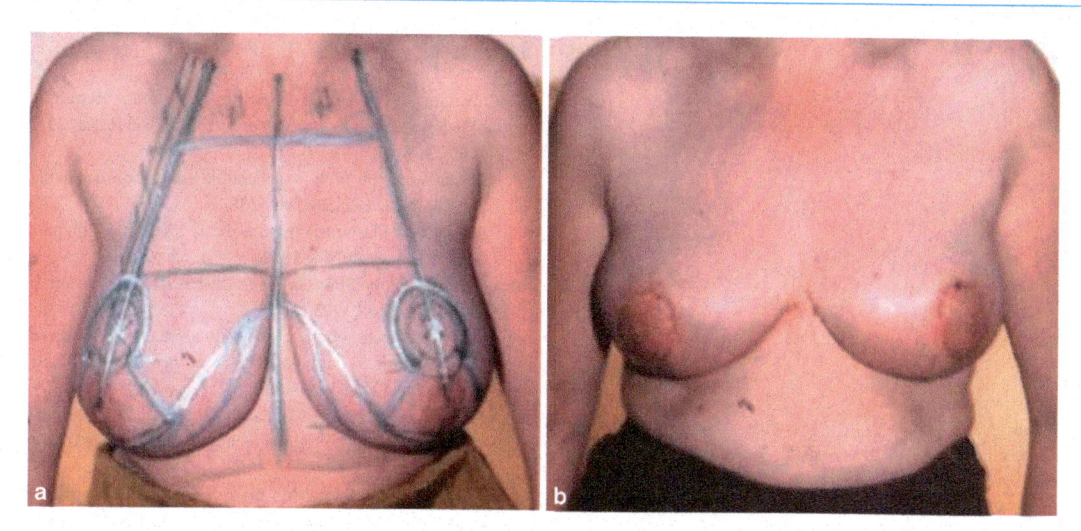

Fig. 59.6 (a) Preoperative. (b) Postoperative after Strombeck reduction

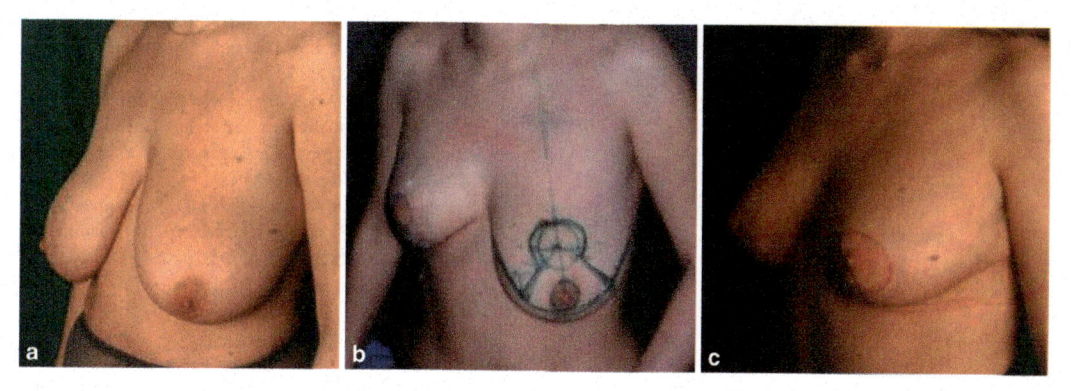

Fig. 59.7 (a) Preoperative. (b) One breast reduced to avoid blood transfusion and for a shorter anesthesia. (c) Left reduction done one week later

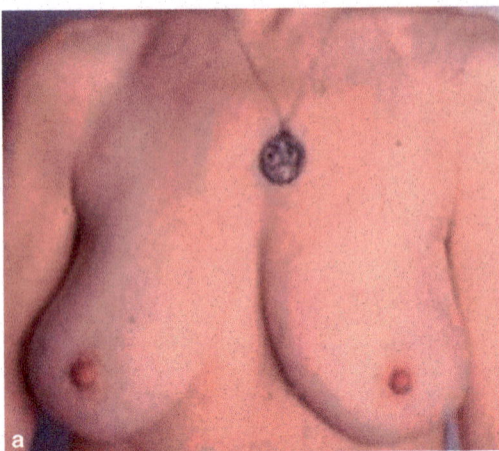

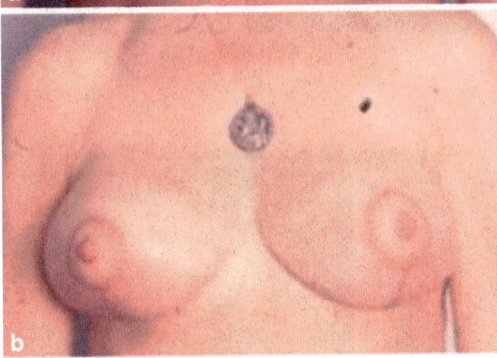

Fig. 59.8 (a) Preoperative. (b) Postoperative

References

1. Strombeck JO: Mammaplasty: Report of a new technique based on the two pedicle procedure. Br J Plast Surg 1960;13:79–90
2. Biesenberger H: Eine neue methode der mammaplastik. Zentrabl Chir 1928;38:2382–2387
3. Marc H: La Plastie Mammaire par la "Methode Oblique." Paris, G.Doing and Cie 1952
4. Thorek M: Possibilities in the reconstruction of the human form. N Y Med J 1922;116:572
5. Skoog T: A technique of breast reduction: transposition of the nipple on a cutaneous vascular pedicle. Acta Chir Scand 1963;126:453–465
6. Pitanguy I: Mammaplstias estudio de 245 casos consecutivos e apresentacao de tecnica pessoal. Rev Bras Cir 1961;42:201–220
6. McKissock PK: Reduction mammaplasty by the vertical pedicle flap technique: Rationale and results. Clin Plast Surg 1976;3(2):309–320
7. Fournier PF: Un procedemiento de desepidermisacion. Secundo Congresso Argentino de Cirurgia Estetica, Buenos Aires, Marzo 1974 -Cite in: Ulrich T. Hinderer (M.D.)
8. Fournier PF: The dermal brassiere mammaplasty. Clin Plast Surg 1976;3(2):355
9. Fournier PF: Un procédé pour désépithélialiser dans les réductions mammaires. In Faivre J (ed), Rhinoplasties, Ptoses et Hypertrophies mammaires modérées. Paris, Maloine S.A. 1984, pp 263–268
10. Fournier PF: La technique de Strömbeck. In Faivre J (ed), Rhinoplasties, Ptoses et Hypertrophies mammaires modérées. Paris, Maloine S.A. 1984, pp 201–216

Medial and Inferior Bipedicle Breast Reduction for Gigantomastia and Mammary Hypertrophy

Nicolae Antohi, Cristina Isac, Vitalie Stan, Tiberiu Bratu

60.1 Introduction

The excessive size of a woman's breasts causes her both physical and psychological impairment. Pendulous and heavy breasts cause back and shoulder pain, headaches, ulnar nerve paresthesias, grooves from the bra straps pressure. Breasts can even be painful by themselves. The skin in the inframammary fold skin can be chronically irritated and macerated (intertrigo) which can lead to recurrent fungal infections and mastitis; the spine can be deviated (scoliosis and kyphosis). The physical activity is limited. From the psychological point of view, very large breasts can be a troublesome focus of embarrassment for teenagers and even for the adult woman. Patients feel very limited in choosing clothes and in physical activities, like fitness, which leads to obesity. All these favor a very low self-esteem [1] and depression.

The goals of massively enlarged breast surgery are reducing the overall breast volume while maintaining nipple–areola viability and obtaining an aesthetically pleasing shape and a lasting comfort for the patient. There is no doubt that reduction mammaplasty gives a high degree of satisfaction to majority of patients and its efficacy has been well demonstrated throughout the years.

Many techniques have been described for breast reduction. They evolve and are being constantly refined. Classically, for severe breast hypertrophy and gigantomastia partial breast amputation with free nipple–areola grafting has been used. Disadvantages of this technique include loss of sensation, unnatural appearance of NAC, poor projection of the breast and inability to breast feed, which is extremely important for young women. Subsequently several different techniques have been developed successfully in order to avoid free-nipple grafting and to preserve sensibility and blood supply of the nipple–areola complex (NAC) through a dermoglandular pedicle. Among the most frequently used are inferior pedicle, vertical bipedicle, lateral pedicle, medial pedicle. These techniques are a testimony that no one technique is suited to all occasions and every method used has its own advantages and shortcomings.

The authors use a different technique of breast reduction based on medial and inferior pedicles. This technique can be successfully used in severe breast hypertrophy and gigantomastia with the possibility to preserve safely the vascularization of NAC through the pedicles.

60.2 History

One of the very early contributions came from Dieffenbach (1848) [2] who probably performed the first reduction mammaplasty. Before 1900 there was no concept of NAC transposition. Morestin [3] was the first to transposeNAC in 1909. Next, the importance of the subdermal blood supply to the skin and gland was recognized, so that attempts were made to preserve the skin over the underlying gland. At that time there was no theory of blood supply based on a pedicle, so that Thorek [4] proposed in 1922 breast amputation with free-nipple grafting probably to avoid compromise of NAC survival. In 1930 Schwartzmann [5] introduced the blood supply concept of the areola based on the subdermal plexus. He preserved a strip of deepithelialized tissue around the NAC which improved its blood supply and thus its viability. The whole range of pedicles concept followed, in which NAC was transposed on various deepithelialized dermoglandular pedicles. Various and excellent procedures have been described afterwards and all of them used the inverted T-scar.

Strombeck [6] described his horizontal bipedicle procedure in 1960 and later he used the medial pedicle in most cases of breast reduction. The superomedial pedicle was first described by Orlando and Guthrie [7], followed by Hauben [8] who found the technique suitable for breasts of moderate to larger size. The superior pedicle technique (introduced by Skoog [9] and Weiner [10], later modified by Pitanguy [11]) is reliable but cannot be used in large hypertrophies because of the

M.A. Shiffman (ed.), *Mastopexy and Breast Reduction: Principles and Practice*,
© Springer-Verlag Berlin Heidelberg 2009

difficulty in transposing NAC on long distances. McKissock [12] first described his vertical bipedicle technique for reduction mammaplasty in 1972. With this technique, the central breast is reduced to a vertical bipedicle flap in the form of a bucket which is folded on itself. This technique is preferred for the large breasts because of the reliability of NAC.

Described by Ribeiro (1975) [13, 14], Robbins (1977) [15], Courtiss and Goldwin [16], Ariyan [17] with variations regarding the width and thickness of the pedicle, the inferior pedicle is a safe and flexible technique, being one of the most frequently used nowadays.

In cases of severe breast hypertrophy and gigantomastia amputation of the lower pole of the breast with free nipple grafting, as first proposed by Thorek [4], has been advocated for a long time as a method of choice. Recently other techniques aforementioned have been adopted to avoid free-nipple grafting. These procedures entailed unipedicle (medial [18, 19], inferior [12–22], lateral [23]) or bipedicle (vertical bipedicle McKissock [12]) techniques. Encouraging results and few complications were published in the literature with these techniques which were applied safely in severe cases of breast hypertrophy and gigantomastia.

Central mound technique described by Hester [24] consists in wide undermining of the skin, the gland being tangentially reduced. The procedure is very safe and applicable to even large gigantomastia [25], it provides a better vascular and nerve supply to the nipple and does not damage the lactiferous ducts. Its drawback is the increased likelihood of bottoming out and recurrent ptosis, due probably to the separation of skin and gland.

Recently, emphasis has shifted towards technical refinements by means of shortening the postoperative scars. These include vertical techniques [26, 27] that are modifications of Lejour [28] technique, vertical reduction with a short horizontal scar, L-shaped scar techniques, periareolar technique, and inframammary scar technique). However, we consider that these procedures are not suitable for gigantomastia and not even for severe breast hypertrophy, although there are reports regarding the use of short vertical scar in gigantomastia [29] or even avoiding it [30].

60.3
Severe Breast Hypertrophy and Gigantomastia

Mammary hypertrophy is characterized by a breast volume at least 50% greater than normal [31]. Severe breast hypertrophy is in the breasts that weigh more than 1,500 g each and gigantomastia is reserved for those breasts that weigh more than 2,000 g each.

The aims of hypertrophic breast reduction surgery can be summarized as follows:

1. Reduction of the breast volume close to a theoretical one, relieving in this way symptoms, but achieving in the same time an aesthetically acceptable shape.
2. Stability of the breast.
3. Accurate placing of the nipple–areola complex without affecting its vascularization, innervation, and aspect.

There is evidence that women with larger breasts may have a statistically greater chance for developing breast cancer and that this risk is diminished by reduction mammaplasty [25].

60.4
Applied Anatomy: Blood Supply and Innervation

The main blood supply of the breast comes from three main sources: the internal mammary artery, notably through perforators from the second to fifth intercostal spaces [32] (which contributes up to 60% of total blood supply, mainly to medial part of the breast), lateral thoracic artery (from subclavian artery) which provides approximately 30% of blood flow and posterior intercostal arteries in the third to fifth intercostal spaces which supply the lower lateral part. There are also some perforating vessels from the thoracoacromial artery which add to blood supply in the superolateral part. The direction from which blood supply comes to the breast does not matter. Therefore, numerous techniques described in the literature are based on different types of blood supply. The areola receives its blood supply through a superficial and deep periareolar vascular plexus. The rationale for deepithelialization consists in keeping the dermis which protects the subdermal plexus.

The medial pedicle contains, therefore, perforating branches from internal mammary artery and the inferior pedicle contains the inferior perforators from internal mammary artery, musculocutaneous perforators from the thoracoacromial artery and terminal branches from the lateral thoracic artery.

The innervation of the breast comes from anterior rami of the third to sixth intercostal nerves laterally and medially from the second to sixth rami of the intercostal nerves [33]. The most important is the fourth intercostal nerve (from T4) which innervates the nipple–areola complex. The upper part of the breast is innervated by supraclavicular nerves from the cervical plexus (Fig. 60.1).

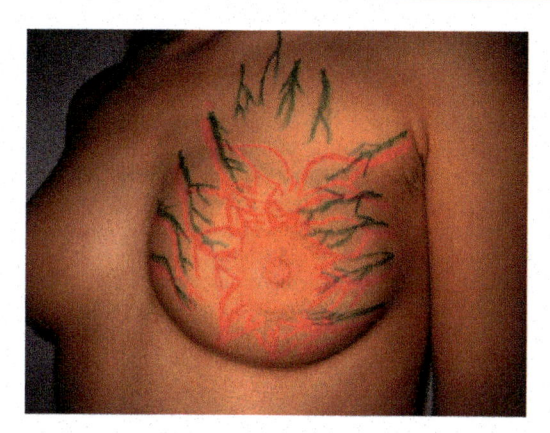

Fig. 60.1 Blood supply and innervation of the breast

60.5
Indications and Contraindications

The symptoms mentioned above represent criteria for surgical intervention (neck and shoulder pain, shoulder grooves, postural changes, intertrigo, limited daily activities). The criteria that the patients should meet are the usual ones for an elective surgery. Diabetes and hypertension should be controlled. The overweight patient is advised to lose weight preoperatively to a certain point where she thinks she may keep it in the future. Loosing excess weight is not desirable postoperatively, as it favors ptosis. Moreover, obese patients are prone to complications, such as wound dehiscence, infection, deep vein thrombosis.

Smokers should be warned that they are at increased risk of flap necrosis and they should stop smoking at least 30 days before surgery. They should be disallowed surgery in the event they cannot stop smoking. We add at the usual preoperative work-up a mammogram which should be obtained in all women over 35 and in those with a family history of breast cancer. There is no upper limit of age for surgery as long as the patient is in good health and the usual work-up lab results are within normal limits. The patient is advised to avoid medication that affects wound healing and blood coagulation for at least 2 weeks before the operation (aspirin and other prostaglandin inhibitors).

The authors consider contraindications for surgery to include extreme obesity, pulmonary, heart and renal failure, previous thromboembolism, blood clotting disorders.

60.6
Patient Selection

Selection of patients is one of the most important points that led to a successful operation with gratifying results for the surgeon and a pleased patient. The procedure is used in patients with bulky, ptotic breasts with additional risk factors and in whom nipple to inframammary fold distance exceeds 20 cm.

LaTrenta and Hoffman [34] recommend free-nipple grafting procedure beginning with 1,500 g tissue resected and in their opinion inferior pedicle technique works best for moderate macromastia which requires resection between 1,000 and 1,500 g per side. For less than 1,000 g breast tissue resected, techniques like McKissock, inferior pedicle, and central mound are advocated and for moderate resections of less than 500 g the Pitanguy (superior pedicle) seems most effective. Jones Glyn [35] uses breast amputation for resections more than 1,500–2,000 g per side and for resections between 500 and 1,500 g the authors recommend any of the procedures based on different types of pedicles.

Mathes [32] indicates larger limits: moderate reduction (less than 800 g), large reduction (800–2,500 g) and gigantomastia reduction (more than 2,500 g). He used the inferior pedicle technique for large reductions when the inferior pedicle has a length of up to 21 cm, preserving a width of 6–8 cm of the pedicle. In his opinion the procedure is not adequate for very large reductions, because the pedicle would be too long to assure the viability of the nipple, and, on the other hand, the bulkiness of pedicle would hamper achieving a pleasing shape and enough reduction of breast volume. In cases of gigantomastia (more than 2,500 g resected) he used nipple–areola grafted and inferior pedicle with the only goal to reestablish projection of the breast mound, as an auto augmentation.

60.7
Surgical Procedure

60.7.1
Preoperative Markings

The patient is marked in the standing position in the exam room. The midsternal line is drawn first, then breast meridian (the line which joins midclavicular point with the nipple and continues downward onto thoracic wall across inframammary crease). The inframammary fold and its midline are marked. The extremes of inframammary fold are kept as short as possible taking care not to encroach on the medial ends on the midline. This would result in a web scar. The lateral extent of inframammary fold is designed with a slight upward tilt that does not follow original inframammary fold. Then position of nipple is established by projecting inframammary fold on the anterior surface of the breast. The nipple will be positioned at this point or slightly lower depending on the amount of tissue which is supposed to be removed. The symmetry is checked by measuring the distance from nipple to midsternum. The areola is drawn with a diameter between 42 and 45 mm, depending on the breast size. The opening between medial and lateral limbs is established hand-freely by pinching the medial and lateral breast mounds and bringing them together or using a Wise pattern. The angle between medial and lateral limbs usually does not exceed 90°. Two points are marked at the desired opening and two diverging lines are drawn laterally and medially outlining the areola window; these lines measure usually about 7 cm and represent the lateral and medial limbs of the keyhole pattern. This distance represents the length of the future vertical scar and it can be modified according to the expected breast volume. We prefer to err with the length of this line on the longer side, as it is much easier to shorten it intraoperatively. The bottom corners of these lines are joined with the medial and lateral extremes of the inframammary fold. The medial pedicle is marked with a mean width of about 7 cm and can be extended up to 10–11 cm depending on the length of the pedicle. The longer the pedicle is, the wider we design its base. Its base corresponds exactly to the medial limb of the keyhole pattern with the possibility of being partially drawn inside the areola window if necessary.

The inferior pedicle is outlined with a width depending on its length. The authors use a width around 10 cm for large reductions and if the patient has a high risk for pedicle circulation impairment (smokers, obesity, collagen disease). For less reductions, a pedicle width of 6–8 cm is used. The drawing is observed for symmetry by checking upper borders of areolas and position of the nipples with a level. The patient is photographed before and after markings (Figs. 60.2, 60.3).

60.7.2
Operative Technique

Breast reduction is performed under general anesthesia. The patient is usually given one dose of antibiotic intravenously prophylactically. The patient is in the supine position with the arms abducted, well padded under the elbows and secured in order not to fall when she is going to be elevated. After prepping and draping, we mark the key points with sutures (upper pole of areola window, bottom points of the arms of the keyhole, extremes of the inframammary fold and its midline) (Fig. 60.4). The gland is infiltrated with a solution of saline with epinephrine 1:400,000, avoiding infiltration under the

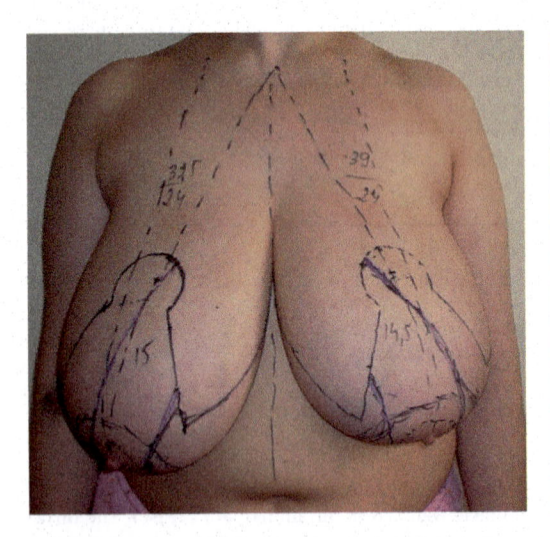

Fig. 60.2 Preoperative markings

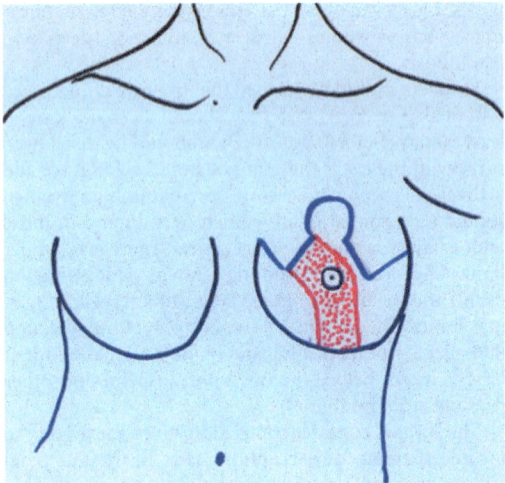

Fig. 60.3 The nipple–areola carrying medial and inferior bipedicle

nipple areolar complex (NAC) and the bases of the pedicles. The infiltration greatly reduces intraoperative blood loss. A 42 or 45 mm stainless steel "cookie cutter" is applied on the areola to outline the new areola circumference while the breast is held on moderate stretch. The new areola is incised to the dermis. With the breast kept under tension, the skin is deepithelialized according to preoperative marking using a no. 10 blade, taking care to leave the new nipple–areola intact and to preserve the underlying dermis (Fig. 60.5). The skin along the markings is incised through the dermis.

After the deepithelialization is completed the pedicles are outlined. The incisions are carried vertically down to the thoracic wall.

60.7.3
Creation of the Pedicles

The bipedicle is defined following the preoperative markings by incising the gland along the inferior edge of medial pedicle, curving downward along the inner part of the inferior pedicle (Fig. 60.6). The superior edge of the medial pedicle and the lateral one of the inferior pedicle is incised (Fig. 60.7). The incision is perpendicular to the chest wall and even slightly bevelling the incisions away from the base of the pedicles to ensure good viability of nipple–areola complex (Fig. 60.8). At this step both pedicles are left attached to the thoracic wall by a wide and thick base (Fig. 60.9). The gland is incised to create the pedicles by means of sharp scissors or scalpel. This is less traumatic for the pedicle vascularization than using the cautery. The medial pedicle is detached from the thoracic wall up to its base and two distal thirds of the inferior pedicle (Fig. 60.10). This step is undertaken in order to accommodate more easily the

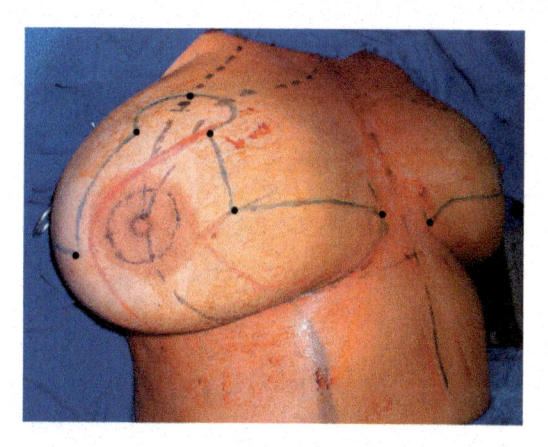

Fig. 60.4 Key-points markings before incisions

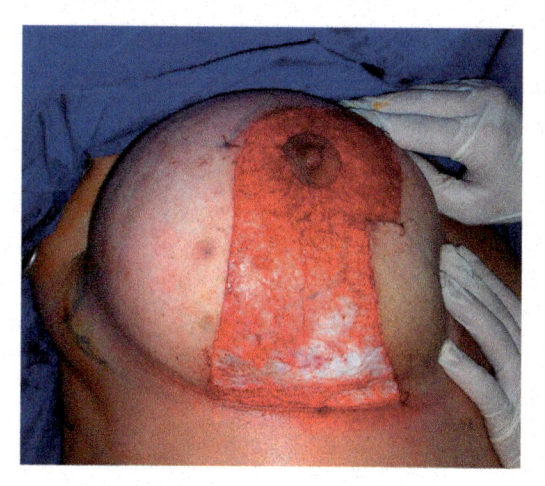

Fig. 60.5 Deepithelialization of the pedicles is completed

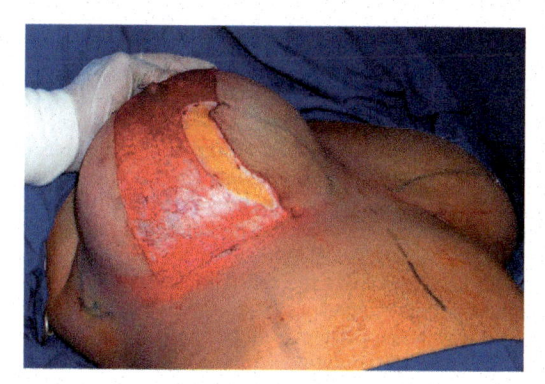

Fig. 60.6 Incision through the gland along the inferior edge of the medial pedicle curving downward along the inner part of the inferior pedicle

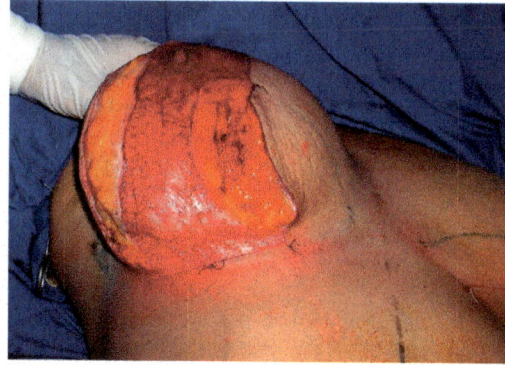

Fig. 60.7 Incising the superior edge of the medial pedicle and the lateral edge of the inferior pedicle

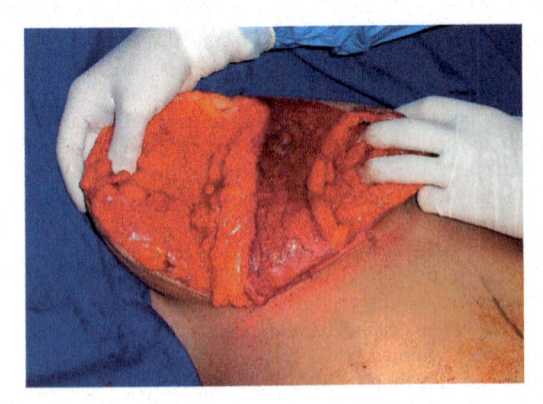

Fig. 60.8 The incisions along the pedicles are made perpendicular on the chest wall, even slightly beveled

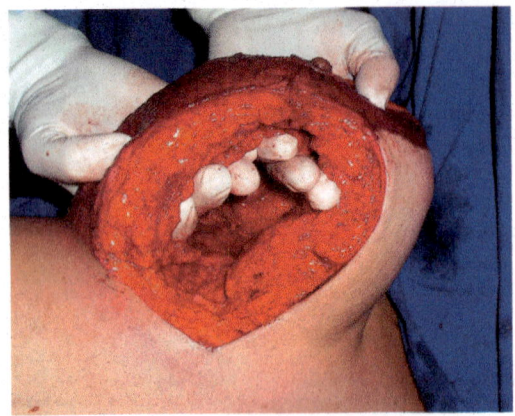

Fig. 60.10 The pedicles detached from the thoracic wall

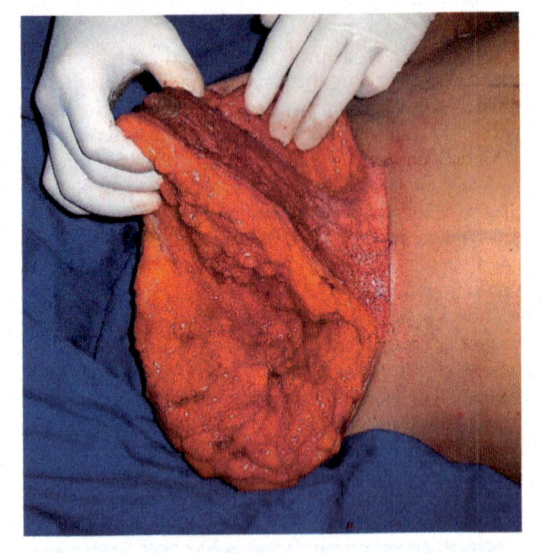

Fig. 60.9 Pedicles are left attached to the chest wall by a wide and thick base

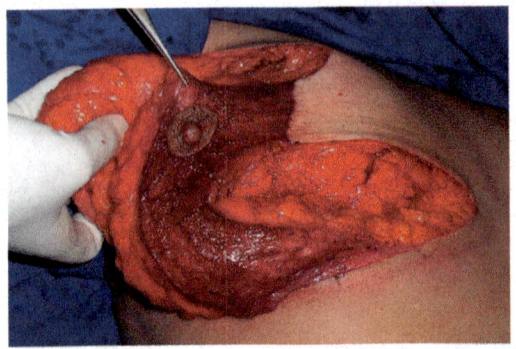

Fig. 60.11 Incision along the lateral limb of the keyhole and the incisions that delineate the lateral and medial skin flaps are performed

bipedicle bearing the nipple–areola complex in its new position.

60.7.4
Hemostasis is Carefully Controlled

Incisions are performed along the lateral limb of the keyhole, incisions that delineate the lateral and medial skin flaps. The inframammary crease incision is deepened to the fascia all along its way except the central part where the inferior pedicle is attached (Fig. 60.11). Rigorous hemostasis is very important through out the whole procedure.

60.8
Tissue Resection

The lateral wedge of breast tissue is dissected proceeding from inframammary crease superiorly. The resection is made by cutting along the inferior border of the lateral skin flap straight down through the full thickness of the gland, along the glandular pedicles till the pectoralis major fascia. The dissection is carried in such a way to avoid undermining the pedicle by drifting medially underneath it. Supporting the gland centralized on the chest wall by the assistant is of great help.

In this way, the dermoglandular triangular shaped lateral wedge is removed taking care to excise an adequate bulk of tissue. This is the largest amount of breast tissue removed. We thin the lateral skin flap. An incision

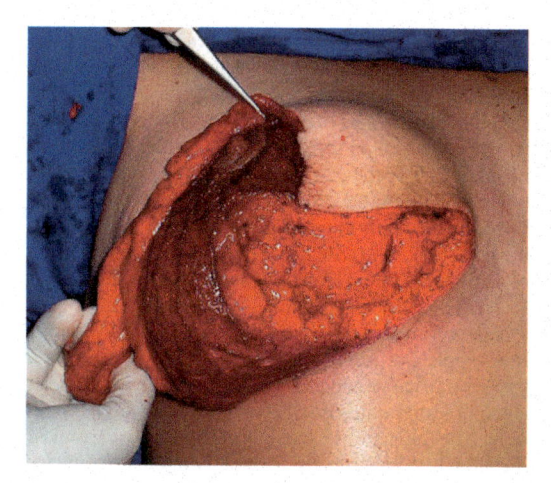

Fig. 60.12 Superior rotation of medial pedicle and advancement of inferior pedicle

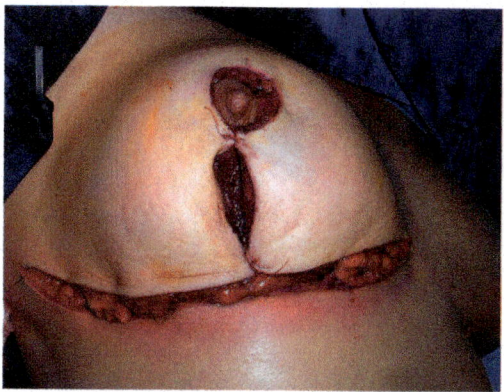

Fig. 60.13 The lateral and medial flaps approximated to each other and to midmammary fold

is made about 2.5–3 cm underneath the skin surface all along the lower edge of the flap. The excess tissue is resected from the undersurface of the flap all the way to its base.

The inferomedial wedge tissue is approached similarly.

Wedge excisions of dermoglandular tissue are thus performed laterally, superolaterally, inferomedially. Perforating branches to the breast tissue are coagulated.

The keyhole pattern is incised next. Enough breast tissue is incised above the superior margin of the medial pedicle, in the site of areola window, but at the same time not too much in order to prevent nipple areolar retraction. This allows superior rotation of the medial pedicle and insetting of NAC in place (Fig. 60.12).

60.9
Insetting the Pedicles and Shaping the Breast

The bipedicle is tucked in place without kinking or twisting. The two pedicles with full thickness are now ready for insetting. The pedicles are trimmed if necessary on the lateral aspects in order to accommodate the breast tissue and at the same time avoid compromise of the nipple areola blood supply by compression.

The lateral and medial flaps are approximated to the midline of inframammary fold and sutured to each other (Fig. 60.13). If after bringing together the flaps and shaping the breast any tension is present and there is difficulty in closing after approximating the flaps, more tissue is removed usually laterally and above the upper part of medial pedicle until no compression is observed. The excision of excess breast tissue is performed carefully protecting the base of the inferior pedicle (which contains perforating branches from the thoracoacromial artery and veins, lateral thoracic artery and anteromedial intercostal perforators) and of medial pedicle (which contains perforating branches from internal mammary artery). Usually the medial pedicle rotates easily 90° by itself. The superior part of the inferior pedicle to the pectoralis major fascia is advanced and attached using nonabsorbable sutures (one medial and one lateral) in order to align the pedicle in a central position and to achieve a more reliable long-term breast contour by preventing sagging of the breast tissue.

The areola apex is secured to the most superior point of areola window. Once the bipedicle is fixed in place, medial and lateral flaps are approximated and sutured above the inferior pedicle. Temporary sutures are used to close the breast.

The contralateral breast is approached similarly.

The two breasts are checked for shape and volume symmetry with the patient elevated. The amount of tissue resected in both breasts is weighed and compared. Areas of excess tissue may be assessed and removed until the amount resected appears adequate and the sizes of the breasts are compatible. Adjustments in the skin envelope can be made at this point. The patient is then lowered to the initial position and sutures are removed.

Suction drains are inserted bilaterally.

60.10
Skin Closure

The vertical limbs of the lateral and medial skin flaps are brought together and sutured to the center of the inframammary fold using a three-way suture. The flap

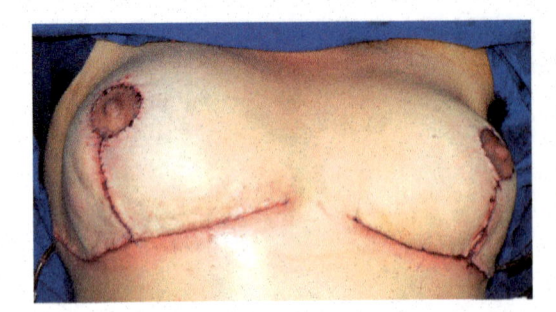

Fig. 60.14 Immediate postoperative view

tips should lie loosely together. Tension is avoided at the tips of the skin flaps (T junction) by suturing the skin from medial and lateral flaps respectively, towards the midline. The inframammary incision is closed in layers with deep buried dermal and subcuticular sutures. The areola is closed with deep buried interrupted 4-0 absorbable sutures and then a subcuticular or interrupted 5-0 nonabsorbable suture (Fig. 60.14).

Steri-strips are applied and usual dressings with Betadine cream covered with gauzes and adhesive tape are done.

Postoperatively, the drains are removed at 24 or 48 h depending on the amount of output recorded (we remove them when the output is less than 30 cc in 24 h). Analgesics are administered and antibiotics (we usually give antibiotics, a first generation cephalosporin for 5 days).

The patient is instructed to wear a bra the day following the operation. The authors usually keep the patients in hospital for 1 or 2 days. The sutures are removed at 14 days postoperatively.

Light physical activity is begun immediately, as well as walking. A mammogram is obtained 3 months following the operation in women over 30, as a baseline for cancer surveillance.

The patient returns to her everyday activities at about 10 days postoperatively avoiding strenuous efforts, lifting and fitness for 2 months. The bra is used for 2 months, day and night. Follow up is required at 1 month, 3 months, 6 months and 1 year. During the followup photos are taken and outcomes are recorded.

60.11 Discussion

Reduction mammaplasty is one of the most gratifying procedures for the patient, achieving improvement in lifestyle, social relationships, sense of self-esteem and body image.

The main goals of breast reduction procedure are weight and volume reduction, relief of neck, shoulder and back pain, as well as psychological and social improvement. There have been many debates about which technique is safer and more reliable and gives nicer and longer-term results. The outcome studies made until now have not reached consistent conclusions, so that many surgeons have different, even opposing opinions. As to which technique is superior in terms of achieving better results it is still a matter of debate.

Traditionally, severe breast hypertrophy and gigantomastia were addressed solely by free nipple grafting. Free nipple grafting is an effective technique used when there is particular concern about the viability of NAC. It is a simple and quick method used in substantial reductions. The indications for free nipple graft are various in the literature but mostly include women with gigantomastia presenting 2,500 g or more of breast tissue per side. Spear [36] recommends the technique to be used whenever the nipple–areola complex is to be elevated more than 15 cm.

The disadvantages of this technique are loss of nipple–areola sensation and erectile function, inability to breast-feed and hypopigmentation of NAC. Mathes [32] recommends breast amputation with immediate nipple reconstruction using the redundant breast skin at the apex of Wise pattern followed by areola tattooing. He states that tattooing the depigmented spots of the nipple and areola (which are inevitable, even with total apparent graft take) is useless because the dark brown color is never achieved. Another disadvantage is that NAC has a somehow unnatural appearance, lacking projection. Therefore, this technique should be preferably used in aged patients, rather than in the young or unmarried ones with gigantomastia. The free-nipple graft is used in severe breast hypertrophy, in which the pedicle would be too long to allow a safe transposition for NAC, in patients who have had previous breast surgery with the possibility to compromise pedicle vascularization,, in smokers, in aged patients and in those with systemic diseases where significant reduction in operating time is desired.

More recently, greater focus has been directed towards methods that preserve the viability of NAC, transposing it on various pedicles. Theoretically, we can regard the pedicle on which NAC is transposed as being an axial composite flap [37]. This means that we can design the pedicle with a length compared to its width according to Gillies' ratio of 3:1. Various authors reported on different procedures used in order to avoid breast amputation and its shortcomings.

The inferior pedicle technique is probably most frequently used worldwide nowadays. Many authors use it for even larger hypertrophies and gigantomastia [38]. Its popularity stems from its versatility, applicability, relative safety, preservation of neuro-vascular structures, low rate of complications, speed of execution, ease of teaching and fairly predictable results [25]. Another advantage is that it preserves nipple sensitivity, unlike free nipple grafting. Some surgeons use the inferior glandular, parenchymal technique, retaining more parenchyma on this inferior segment and overlying dermis. In this case, the length of pedicle can be augmented compared to width of base, making it possible to be safely used in larger hypertrophies and ptosis. Inferior pedicle may be difficult to be used in nipple to inframammary fold distance greater than 22 cm [35]. In Georgiade's opinion [32], the technique remains reliable even with pedicle length up to 28 cm. Some authors [39] advocate that the length of pedicle is the major determinant in nipple–areola necrosis rather than weight of breast removed. Jackson et al. [40] show that no matter how long the distance from sternal notch to nipple, the blood to nipple should always be satisfactory with inferior pedicle methods, especially when one uses Robbins method (inferior wedge technique). Their maximum length of inferior pedicle was 19 cm. They conclude that given security with inferior pedicle, free nipple grafting need never be considered. Inferior pedicle has been successfully used in a wide range of breast hypertrophies, including gigantomastia [22, 41]. Georgiade et al. [42] resected safely up to 2,500 g per breast with a mean nipple transposition of 18 cm and same author [43] reports a successful resection of 3,335 g on each side and a sternal notch to nipple distance of 52 cm using inferior pedicle. Chang et al. [21] reports on bilateral resections of 3,000–5,100 g with complications in 29.2% of cases. In 24 patients there was one nipple–areola necrosis.

Nahabedian et al. [19] use the medial pedicle for severe mammary hypertrophy. In their study the mean weight removed was 1,580 g on the right and 1,627 g on the left, the mean distance form the sternal notch to the nipple was 38.4 cm and the mean change in nipple position was 17.1 cm. The mean length of the pedicle was 14.8 cm (with the longest being 19 cm) and the mean base width of the medial pedicle was 9.4 cm.

Nahabedian [19] finds the medial pedicle technique safer than the inferior pedicle in severe breast hypertrophy. He states that medial pedicle is shorter than inferior one, which optimizes blood supply to NAC. Moreover the medial pedicle contains the main blood supply to the breast and nipple sensitivity is preserved in a higher percentage of cases compared to the inferior technique; breast shape and projection are improved comparing with the amputation and free- nipple graft and are equivalent to the results obtained by the inferior pedicle technique.

Abramson et al. [18] recommended the medial pedicle technique as a method of choice for resections ranging between 500 and 1,500 g per side. Both medial and inferior pedicle techniques retain nipple sensitivity and viability and achieve a reasonable shape. Studies showed [43] no difference in postoperative NAC sensitivity between inferior and medial pedicle techniques, although the medial one allowed for a greater mean weight reduction. Abramson et al. [18] finds that the medial pedicle technique is less prone to postoperative pseudoptosis or "bottoming-out" than the inferior pedicle.

Hefter [23] reports on using a wide lateral pedicle which has the same outcome and safety as the inferior pedicle even with large resections; widths of the pedicles ranged from 11 to 14 cm and the authors prefer the lateral pedicle as it is technically easier to dissect and transpose.

Another safe method still performed [44] in fairly large hypertrophies has been described by McKissock. In his technique, the deepithelialized vertical bipedicle flap carries nipple–areola and depends primarily on inferior parenchyma for blood supply. The method is easy, reliable and has a pleasing aesthetic result. Disadvantages of the vertical bipedicle are the "boxy" or square appearance of the breasts immediately postoperatively; they tend to be flat in the lower pole and have more fullness in the upper pole. The flatness of the lower pole resolves with time, however.

McKissock [45] stated regarding his technique: "if the length as determined by a measurement from the inframammary fold passed the nipple to the upper rim of the areolar window exceeds 35 cm, consider the breast outside acceptable limits of safety." McKissock's procedure seems to be reliable in patients with nipple to notch distance of up to 40 cm.

The authors' procedure is based on a vertical bipedicle medial and inferior. It is a safe procedure to be applied in extreme cases of breast hypertrophy regarding the viability of the nipple–areola complex.

The sine qua non for NAC to survive is its unaltered blood supply. Gillies [46] frequently lamented that "plastic surgery is a constant battle between blood supply and beauty." His words can be extended in the case of severe breast hypertrophy when the surgeon has to choose between two alternatives; to design the NAC on a pedicle undertaking the major risk of nipple–areola necrosis or to use a much simpler, easier, and safer technique – the free-nipple graft, with its disadvantages regarding sensibility, breast feeding and appearance. It is extremely important in our opinion for NAC to maintain its native blood supply in order to preserve both its viability and appearance. Even in extreme cases, in order to preserve the native nipple–areola blood supply the surgeon would be tempted to keep NAC on a pedicle, although free-nipple graft technique is much easier and quicker to perform. But obviously the appearance of NAC is improved when NAC is born on a pedicle. On the other hand, this pedicle would inherently be either too long or too thick on expense of the NAC's viability and of the shape of the breast. The longer the pedicle, the wider its base, and more difficult to accommodate. Thus, the problem in using a pedicle in cases of massive breasts consists in the difficulty of achieving an equilibrium between a small enough pedicle to sustain NAC and to reduce adequately the breasts. Therefore, a bulkier pedicle would preclude the achievement of an aesthetically pleasing shape (the bulky pedicle impedes on adequate amount of tissue excision) and would, at the same time, exert pressure on the vessels, compromising the nipple. The double pedicle in the technique we use can be safely either thinned or designed with a narrower base, having a safe back-up from the alternate pedicle. In this way, an improved breast shape can be achieved, decreasing the risk of nipple devascularization.

All the techniques described over the centuries struggled to achieve this goal, although, sometimes, even the safest technique used for a particular case cannot ensure the survival of such an important structure. We believe that an NAC based on its original blood supply fares much better in terms of survival and shape compared with a free-nipple graft; that is why we advocate pedicled procedures even in severe breast hypertrophies and gigantomastias.

The medial pedicle incorporates the main blood supply to the breast (perforators from internal mammary artery especially those from the second and third interspaces which are the largest [35]); the medial pedicle enhances the vascularity of NAC, thus its viability. At the same time, medial pedicle allows us to remove the bulkiness of lateral tissue. Patients with severe hypertrophy and gigantomastia usually have a high degree of ptosis which leads to an inherent lack of tissue in upper pole. The medial pedicle, besides contributing to a better blood supply of NAC, helps in giving upper pole fullness, mimicking the medial cleavage of the breasts.

In cases with severe ptosis we are particularly concerned about the viability of NAC transposed on a medial pedicle alone. That is why using the inferior pedicle beside the medial one adds to the safety of nipple–areola vascularity. The distal part of the medial pedicle coincides with that of inferior pedicle which corresponds precisely to the NAC site. Thus, vascularization of distal parts of both pedicles overlap, NAC receiving blood supply from two different sources which support each other. This dual blood supply enhances considerably its chances of survival. In the event that one distal part of one flap might suffer from a diminished blood supply, this area would be taken over by the alternate source (Fig. 60.15).

The thickness of the inferior pedicle varies according to its width. Its thickness can be reduced due to additional vascularity brought to NAC by the medial pedicle. Another role of the inferior pedicle consists in auto augmentation. It is used as an auto prosthesis of the breast after reduction, maximizing projection to the

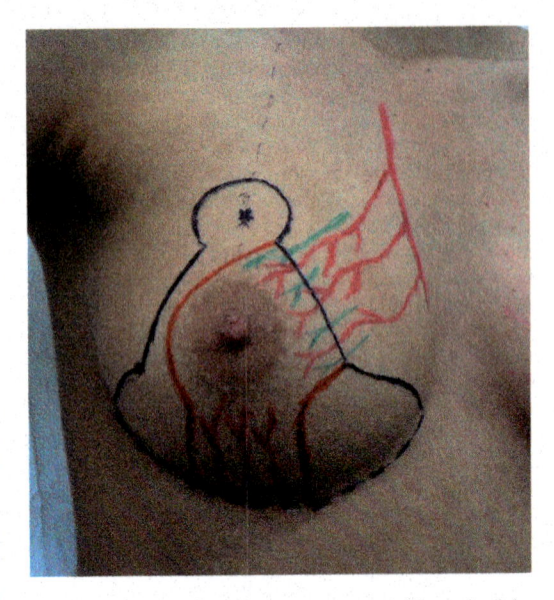

Fig. 60.15 Blood supply and innervation carried by each of the two pedicles

central breast and improving shape. It is also technically easy to inset the bipedicle. While the medial pedicle practically rotates by itself into the keyhole, the whole complex containing the nipple–areola slides upwards very easily, without any need to be tucked up. This avoids any kinking or twisting which would compromise the blood supply of the nipple.

Both the medial and inferior pedicles contain anterior branches from the intercostal nerves so that the nipple sensation is retained using this technique.

The improved shape of the breast is maintained long term due to suspension of the pedicle with nonabsorbable sutures to the pectoralis muscle fascia. Suspension sutures in mammaplasty have been variously described in the literature [47–49]. This procedure avoids "bottoming out."

The technique proposed combines the medial and vertical pedicles, making it obviously a safe method which enhances the chances of survival of NAC. Thus it can be used for gigantomastia and severe breast hypertrophy in which a single pedicle would be too long and unsafe. Moreover, combining the two pedicles, allows us to sum up the advantages of each technique applied separately and decrease their shortcomings (lack of upper pole projection and bottoming out encountered with the inferior pedicle only).

Always keep in mind that it is important what we leave behind and not how much tissue is taken out. On the other hand, it is not skin brassiere that gives final

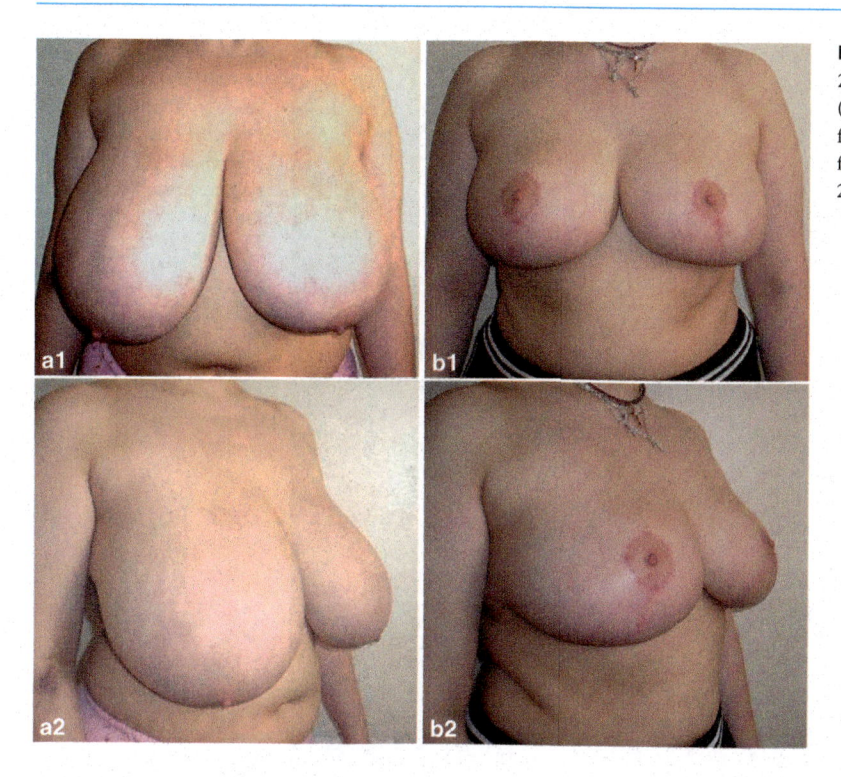

Fig. 60.16 (**a***1,2*) Preoperative 20-year-old woman. (**b***1,2*) Postoperative following removal of 2,650 g from the right breast and 2,480 g from the left breast

shape of breast, but the parenchyma beneath that is crucial to permanence and projection of reduced breast [35]. However, occasionally the bipedicle may be so bulky as not to allow us to excise an adequate amount of breast tissue. This may be considered one of the disadvantages of our technique. This procedure may also cause excessive fullness of lower pole and "boxy" appearance of the breast (Fig. 60.16)

With so many techniques published in literature as safe alternatives to free-nipple grafting, the authors would indicate breast amputation with free nipple graft only in selected cases in which the patient with severe hypertrophy or gigantomastia has additional poor risk factors (advanced age, heavy smokers, systemic diseases, severe obesity) and with resections of more than 2,000 g per side.

60.12
Complications

Early complications of the technique proposed, as in any other breast reduction surgery may include hematoma, seroma, partial nipple–areola necrosis, infection (due mostly to hematoma), fat necrosis (with resultant difficulty in mammographic screening), skin necrosis, and wound dehiscence. Late complications include hypertrophic scars (mostly in medial and lateral extremes of horizontal incision), asymmetries, dog-ears, NAC placed too high that leads to a glandular drop out (avoided by an accurate preoperative planning and measuring), insufficient reduction, change in sensation, inability to breast feed, recurrent hypertrophy.

60.13
Conclusions

It is unequivocal that reduction mammaplasty is extremely efficient in reducing both the physical and psychological symptoms, as many studies have proved. Drawing a conclusion is very difficult as results differ from surgeon to surgeon and even in the same surgeon because of differences in patients. Even the same technique in the hands of different surgeons does not give the same results. This type of surgery has a great degree of satisfaction for both the patient and the surgeon, however.

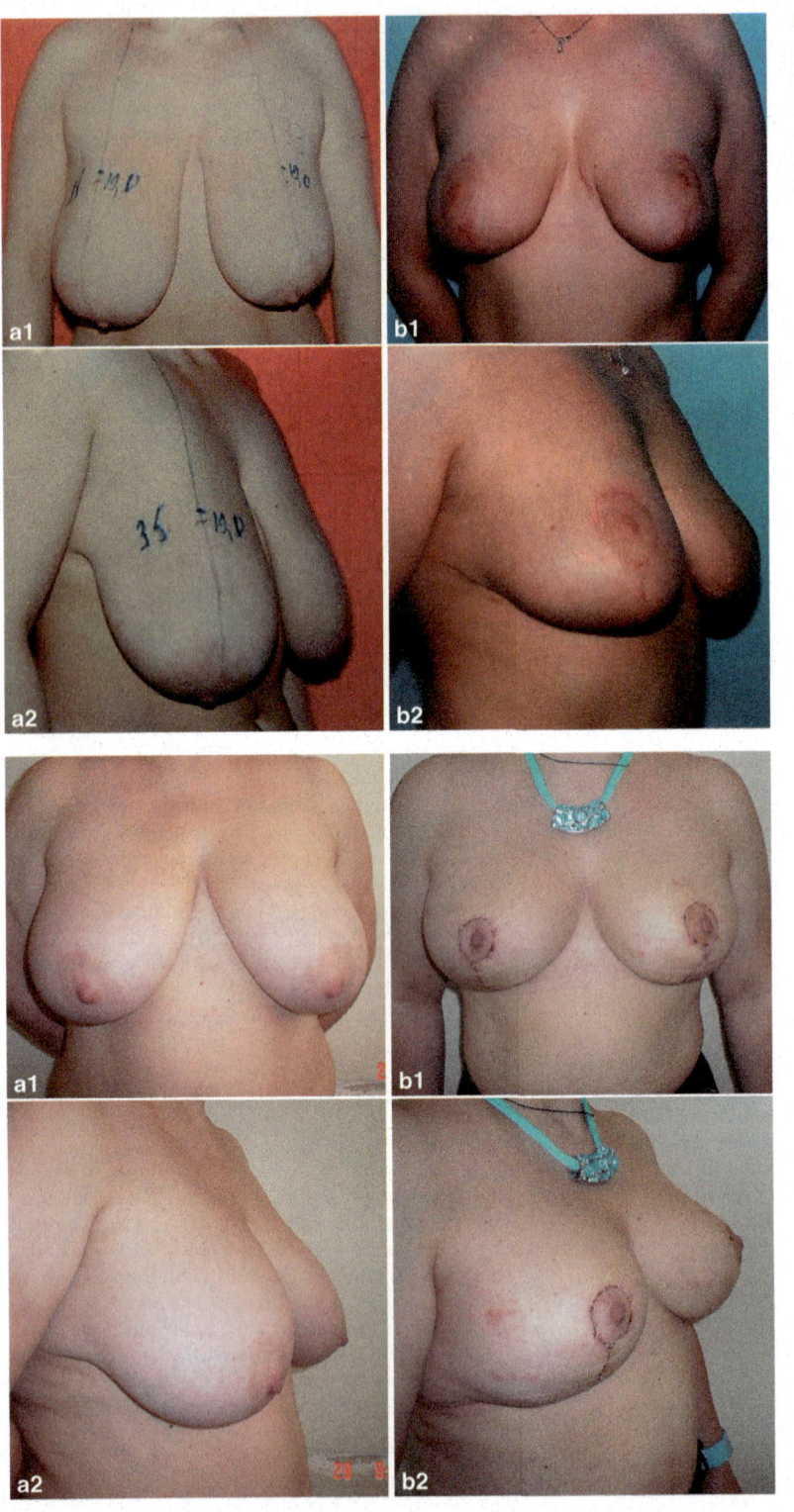

Fig. 60.17 (**a***1,2*) Preoperative 55-year-old woman with severe breast hypertrophy and ptosis. (**b***1,2*) Postoperative after removal of 1,150 g from right breast and 1,070 g from left breast

Fig. 60.18 (**a***1,2*) Preopoerative 35-year-old woman with moderate breast hypertrophy. (**b***1,2*) Postoperative following removal of 850 g from right breast and 780 g from left breast

There are numerous techniques used in breast reduction surgery but only few used for severe breast hypertrophy and gigantomastia. In most cases free nipple grafting and inferior pedicle are used for this kind of pathology.

Medial and inferior bipedicle breast reduction could be considered a good alternative to free-nipple graft and other techniques of breast reduction for severe breast hypertrophy and gigantomastia (Figs. 60.17, 60.18). The viability of NAC is enhanced by the dual blood supply from both medial and inferior pedicle. The procedure gives a good projection to the upper pole and central breast and minimizes shortcomings encountered with free-nipple graft (it preserves nipple sensibility and ability to lactate).

Being safe and reliable, the technique can be taken into consideration in most cases of severe breast hypertrophy and gigantomastia and also in those cases where additional risk factors exist. However, proper selection of patients is most important and minimizes the risk of complications.

References

1. Adams P. William: Reduction mammaplasty and mastopexy. Sel Readings Plast Surg 2002;9(29)
2. Dieffenbach JF: Die extirpation der bruestdruese. In: Dieffenbach JF (ed). Die Operative Chirurgie. Brockhaus, Leipzig 1848, pp 359–373
3. Morestin H: Hypertrophie mammaire. Bull Mem Soc Anat Paris 1905;80:682
4. Thorek M: Possibilities in the reconstruction of the human form. NY Med J 1922;116:572
5. Schwarzmann E: Die Technik der Mammplastik. Chirurg 1930;2:932–943
6. Strombeck JO: Reduction mammaplasty: A report on a new technique based on the two-pedicle procedure. Br J Plast Surg 1960;13:79–90
7. Orlando JC, Gutherie RH Jr: The superomedial dermal pedicle for nipple transposition. Br J Plast Surg 1975;28(1):42–45
8. Hauben DJ: Experience and refinements with the superomedial dermal pedicle for nipple-areola transposition in reduction mammaplasty. Aesthetic Plast Surg 1984;8(3):189–194
9. Skoog T: A technique of breast reduction; transposition of the nipple on a cutaneous vascular pedicle. Acta Chir Scand 1963;126:453–465
10. Weiner DL, Dolich BH, Miclat MI Jr: Reduction mammaplasty using superior pedicle technique. Aesthetic Plast Surg 1982;6(1):7–14
11. Pitanguy I: Personal preferences for reduction mammaplasty. In Goldwyn RM (ed). Plastic and Reconstructive Surgery of the Breast. Boston Little Brown 1976, p 167
12. McKissock PK: Reduction mammaplasty with a vertical dermal flap. Plast Reconstr Surg 1972;49(3):245–252
13. Ribeiro L: A new technique for reduction mammaplasty. Plast Reconstr Surg 1975;55(3):330–334
14. Ribeiro L, Accorsi A, Buss A, Marcal-Pessoa M: Creation and evolution of 30 years of the inferior pedicle in reduction mammaplasties. Plast Reconstr Surg 2002; 110(3):960–970
15. Robbins TH: A reduction mammaplasty with the areola-nipple based on an inferior dermal pedicle. Plast Reconstr Surg 1977;59(1):64–67
16. Courtiss EH, Goldwyn RM: Reduction mammaplasty by the inferior pedicle technique. Plast Reconstr Surg 1977;59(4):500–507
17. Ariyan S: Reduction mammaplasty with the nipple-areola carried on a single, narrow inferior pedicle. Ann Plast Surg 1980;5(3):167–177
18. Abramson D, Pap S, Shifteh S, Glasberg SB: Improving long-term breast shape with the medial pedicle Wise pattern breast reduction. Plast Reconstr Surg 2005;115(7):1937–1943
19. Nahabedian MY, McGibbon BM, Manson PN: Medial pedicle reduction mammaplasty for severe mammary hypertrophy. Plast Reconstr Surg 2000;105(3):896–904
20. Georgiade NG, Serafin D, Morris R, Georgiade G: Reduction mammaplasty utilising an inferior pedicle nipple-areola flap. Ann Plast Surg 1979;3(3):211–218
21. Chang P, Shaaban AF, Canady JW, Ricciardelli EJ, Cram AE: Reduction mammaplasty: the results of avoiding nipple-areolar amputation in cases of extreme hypertrophy. Ann Plast Surg 1996;37(6):585–591
22. Gerzenshtein J, Oswald T, McCluskey P, Caplan J, Angel MF: Avoiding free nipple grafting with the inferior pedicle technique. Ann Plast Surg 2005;55(3):245–249
23. Hefter W, Elvenes OP: Role of the size of the pedicle in reduction mammaplasty, Scand J Plast Reconstr Hand Surg 2006;40(1):13–18
24. Hester TR: Breast reduction utilising the maximally vascularised central breast pedicle. Plast Reconstr Surg 1985;76:890
25. White D, Maxwell P: Breast reduction. In: Achauer BM, Eriksson E, Guyuron B, Coleman JJ III, Russel RC, Vander Kolk CA (eds). Plastic Surgery: Indications, Operations, and Outcomes. St. Louis, Mosby 2002, pp 2705–2741
26. Graf R, Reis de Araujo LR, Rippel R: Reduction mammaplasty and mastopexy using the vertical scar and thoracic wall flap technique. Aesthetic Plast Surg 2003;27(1):6–12
27. Hall-Findlay Elisabeth: Vertical breast reduction with a medially-based pedicle. Aesthetic Surg J 2002;22(2):185–194
28. Lejour M, Abboud M, Declety A, Kertesz P: Reduction of mammaplasty scars: from a short inframammary scar to a vertical scar. Ann Chir Plast Esthet 1990;35(5):369–379
29. Heine N., Eisenmann-Klein M, Prantl L: Gigantomastia: treatment with a short vertical scar. Aesthetic Plast Surg 2007;32(1):41–47
30. Pribaz J: Eliminating the vertical scar in reduction mammaplasty. 14th European Course in Plastic Surgery, Abstract Book and Course Program 2005, p 171

31. Zdenko S: Breast reduction- Patient assessment and selection. 14th European Course in Plastic Surgery, Abstract Book 2005, p 165
32. Mathes S, Schooler W: Inferior pedicle reduction: techniques. In: Mathes S (ed). Plastic Surgery, 2nd edn. Philadelphia, W.B. Saunders 2006, pp 601–630
33. Fitzpatrick M: Vertical bipedicle reduction mammaplasty. In: Noone RB (ed). Plastic and Reconstructive Surgery of the Breast. St. Louis, Mosby 1991, p 207
34. LaTrenta GS, Hoffman LA: Breast reduction. In: Rees TD LaTrenta GS (eds). Aesthetic Plastic Surgery, 2nd edn. Philadelphia, WB Saunders 1992, pp 926–1003
35. Jones G: Breast reduction. In: Mathes S (ed). Plastic Surgery, 2nd edn. Philadelphia, W.B. Saunders 2006, pp 539–584
36. Spear L. Scott: Breast reduction: inverted technique. In: Thorne CH (ed). Grabb and Smith's Plastic Surgery, 6th edn. Philadelphia, Lippincott Raven 2007, p 614
37. Migliori M, Muldowney B: Breast reduction: the inferior pedicle as an axial flap. Aesthetic Surg J 1997;17(1):55–57
38. Lacerna M, Spears J, Mitra A, Medina C, McCampbell E, Kiran R, Mitra A: Avoiding free nipple grafts during reduction mammaplasty in patients with gigantomastia. Ann Plast Surg 2005;55(1):21–24
39. Erdogan B, Ayhan M, Deren O, Tuncel A: Importance of pedicle length in inferior pedicle technique and long-term outcome of areola-to-fold distance. Aesthetic Plast Surg 2002;26(6):436–443
40. Jackson IT, Bayramicli M, Gupta M: Importance of the pedicle length measurement in reduction mammaplasty. Plast Reconstr Surg 1999;104(2):398–400
41. Akpuaka FC, Jiburum BC: Reduction mammaplasty by the inferior pedicle technique: experience with moderate to severe breast enlargement. West Afr J Med 1998;17(3):199–201
42. Georgiade NG, Serafin D. Riefkohl R, Georgiade GS: Is there a reduction mammaplasty for "all seasons"? Plast Reconstr Surg 1979;63(6):765–773
43. Georgiade GS, Riefkohl RE, Georgiade NG: The inferior dermal-pyramidal type breast reduction: long-term evaluation. Ann Plast Surg 1989;23(3):203–211
44. Mofid M, Dellon A: Quantitation of breast sensibility following reduction mammaplasty: a comparison of inferior and medial pedicle techniques. Plast Reconstr Surg 2002;109(7):2283–2288
45. McKissock Paul: Color Atlas of Mammaplasty. Germany, Thieme 1991
46. Gillies H, Millard DR: The Principles and Art of Plastic Surgery. Boston, Little Brown 1957
47. Lockwood T: Reduction mammaplasty and mastopexy with superficial fascial system suspension. Plast Reconstr Surg 1999;103(5):1411–1420
48. Wuringer E: Refinement of the central pedicle breast reduction by application of the ligamentous suspension, Plast Reconstr Surg 2002;109(2):812–814
49. Pennington David: Improving the results of inferior pedicle breast reduction using pedicle suspension and plication. Aesth Plastic Surg 2006;30(4)

Modified Biesenberger Dual Pedicle Technique of Breast Reduction

Lloyd N. Carlsen

61.1 Introduction

The elusive goal of a surgical procedure is its successful application to a variety of clinical problems. In plastic surgery, a favorable result constitutes a further desideratum (something wanted or needed). Hence, the following account of a method of reduction mammoplasty. The author devised this method in 1966, presented it in 1974 [1], and published it in 1975 [2]. The procedure is more of a dual pedicle technique than a modification of the Biesenberger technique.

This method stems from the Biesenberger [3] approach, as modified by Gillies and McIndoe [4]. Following the advice of Pitanguy "to adapt the technique to the deformity rather than the deformity to the technique," the author has found this method to have a wide application permitting all grades of hypertrophy and/or ptosis to be corrected in one stage. Although the surgeon does not have the security of a preformed pattern, he does have the satisfaction of performing a procedure that has flexibility, permitting him the freedom to "cut as you go."

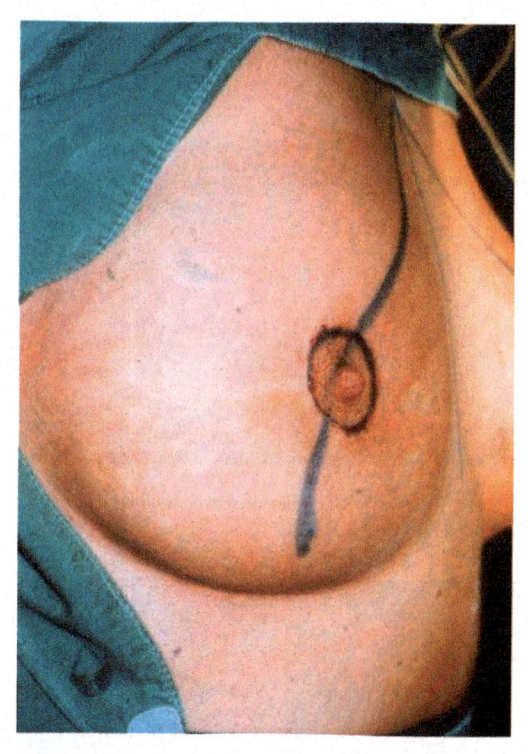

Fig. 61.1 A *black line* is drawn from the supersternal notch across the nipple/areola complex onto the breast. This acts a guideline for nipple placement

61.2 Technique

1. An oblique line is drawn from the sternal notch across the nipple areolar complex (NAC) onto the breast (Fig. 61.1). This acts as a guide for nipple placement. A vertical line is dropped mid sternum.
2. A circumareolar subepidermal incision is made for a distance of 3–4 cm (Fig. 61.2). At this level, the incision is made through the dermis, subcutaneous fat, and fascia.
3. Blunt dissection separates the skin envelope " with its intact blood supply" from the breast tissue. (Fig. 61.3).
4. The entire breast can now be delivered (Fig. 61.4).
5. An outline for the resection of a cone of tissue in the superior aspect of the breast and a wedge from below are outlined. The excess breast tissue is excised, a cone formed above the nipple areola, and a wedge below (cone and wedge vary in size as needed). The upper pillars of the breast are closed first. Suturing the cone allows the NAC to be projected outwards and downwards.

M.A. Shiffman (ed.), *Mastopexy and Breast Reduction: Principles and Practice*,
© Springer-Verlag Berlin Heidelberg 2009

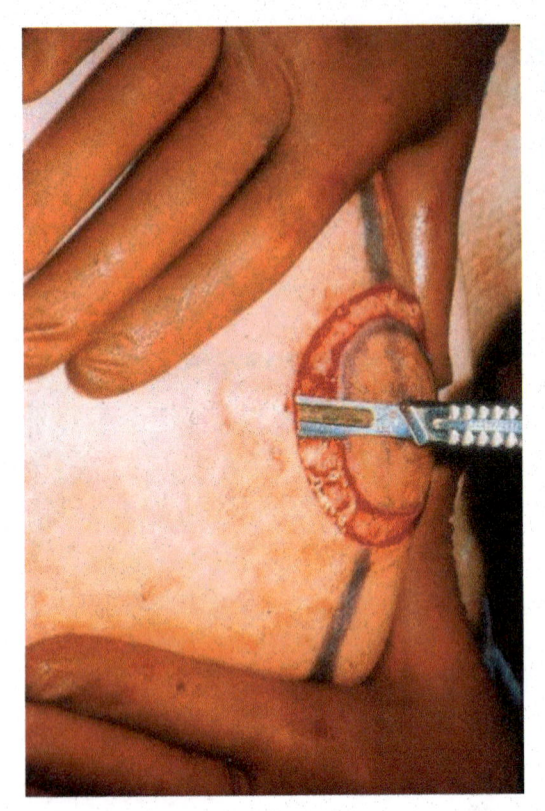

Fig. 61.2 A circumareolar subepidermal incision is made out for a distance of 4 cm. The dermis is then incised

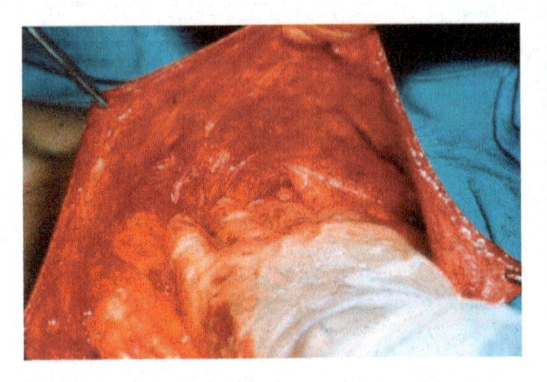

Fig. 61.3 The entire skin envelope is freed in the subfacial plane

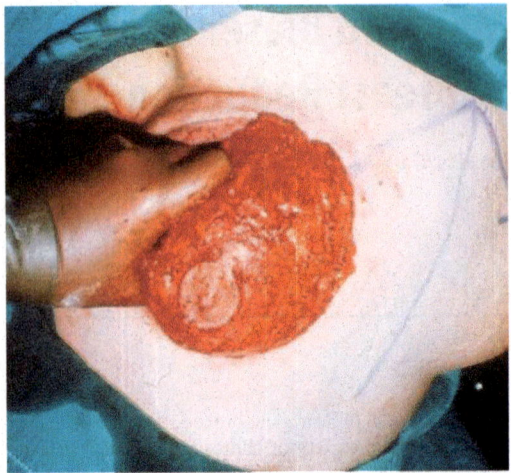

Fig. 61.4 The entire breast gland is delivered

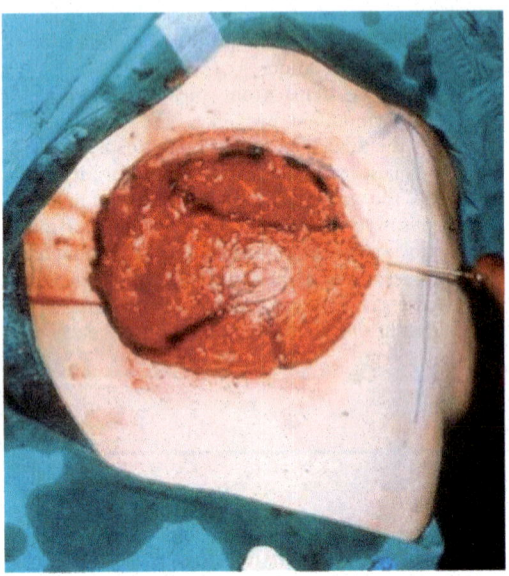

Fig. 61.5 An outline for the resection of a cone of tissue in the superior aspect of the breast and a wedge from below is drawn

6. This can be adjusted as required. The breast tissue is sculpted with O chromic absorbable sutures. The lower pillars from which a wedge of tissue has been removed are then closed (Fig. 61.5).
7. A cone of tissue in the superior aspect of the breast and a wedge from below are removed (Fig. 61.6).
8. The skin is held, pushing the lateral flap medially and bringing the medial flap laterally as one would close a double breasted coat (Fig. 61.7).
9. The tension of the lateral flap is judged by holding the dorsum of the hand against the skin and moving medially. A line is then drawn where one wants the scar to be in place (Fig. 61.8).

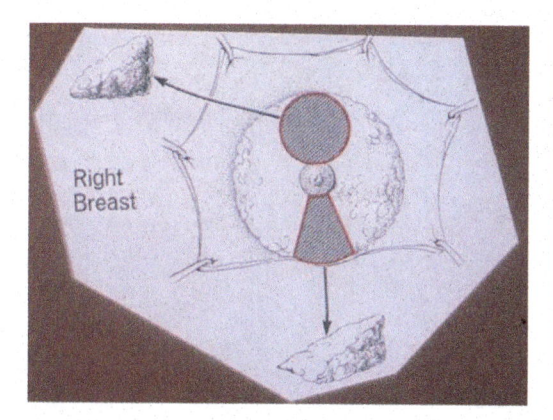

Fig. 61.6 A cone of tissue in the superior aspect of the breast and a wedge from below are removed

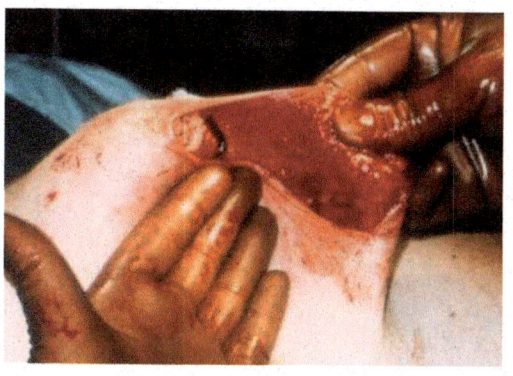

Fig. 61.8 The tension of the lateral flap is judged by holding the dorsum of the hand against the skin and moving it medially

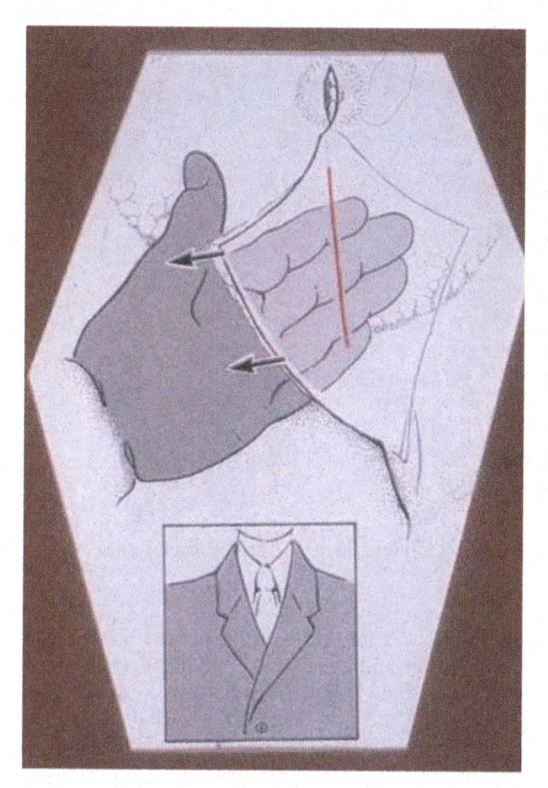

Fig. 61.7 The skin is then held, pushing the lateral flap medially, and bringing in the medial flap laterally, as one would close a double breasted coat

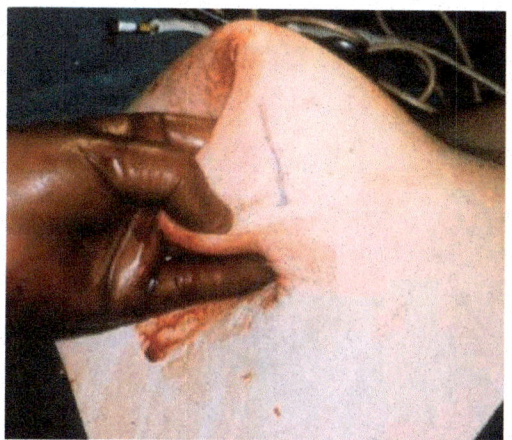

Fig. 61.9 Tension on the flaps required to secure the pyramid, is judged by the pressure of the dorsum of the hand against the lateral flap and the pull placed on the medial flap with the thumb and finger. A line is then drawn where one wants the scar to be placed

10. An incision is made through the medial flap. This creates a handle on the flap (Fig. 61.9).
11. The bucket handle of the medial flap is held with the thumb while the dorsum of that hand pushes the lateral flap medially. The desired pyramid with the appropriate tension on the two flaps is created. The fingers of the holding hand are slightly parted to allow marking on the lateral flap with an ink stick between the fingers (Fig. 61.10).
12. The lateral flap is incised and closure commenced with one had holding both of the bucket handles (Fig. 61.11). Two skin hooks are placed to hold the lateral flap in juxtaposition to the medial flap where suturing is commenced (Fig. 61.12).
13. The vertical component is closed (Fig. 61.13).

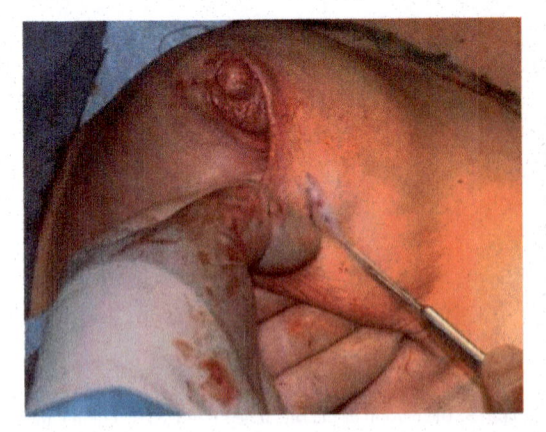

Fig. 61.10 The skin of the medial flap is then incised. This creates a handle on the medial skin flap

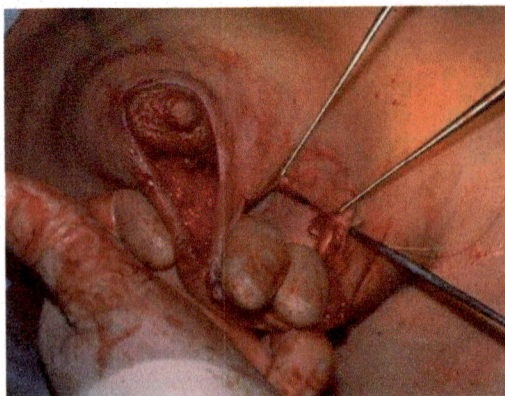

Fig. 61.12 The handle of the medial flap and lateral flaps are then held with the hand, while 2 skin hooks are placed to hold the lateral flap in juxtaposition to the medial flap, where suture is commenced

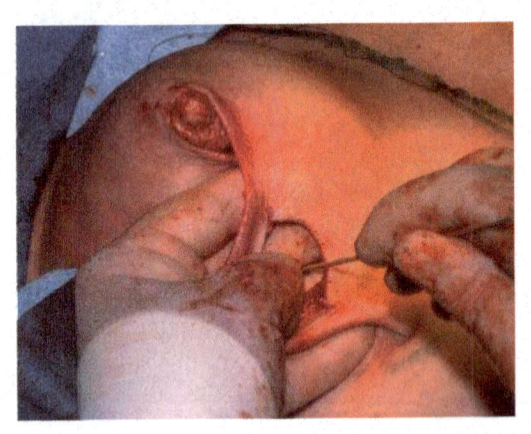

Fig. 61.11 With an ink stick, placed between the fingers of the holding hand, marks are made on the lateral flap for its incision. The lateral flap is then incised

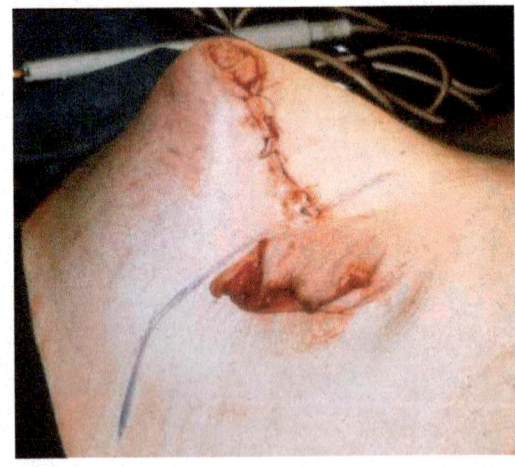

Fig. 61.13 Closure of the vertical component is carried out

14. The inferior redundant skin is excised to create the position of the breast on the chest wall that one desires (Fig. 61.14).
15. The NAC is brought out along the oblique line at a position of election (Fig. 61.15). The potential site of the nipple and areola should be decided last of all, bearing in mind the preoperative lines [5]. The areola is placed lower, rather than higher, to accommodate any secondary postoperative ptosis. The linear closure of the superior circular defect permits this formation. It can be adjusted to create or decrease fullness of the upper breast. A drain may be inserted infralaterally if necessary. Interrupted sutures are used.

The "cut as you go" nature of the method is evident in the selection and creation of the lateral and medial flaps. In the right breast, the lateral flap is grasped with the left hand and held beneath the medial flap, as one would hold a double-breasted coat before buttoning it. For the left breast, the lateral flap is grasped with the right hand. The vertical complement of the eventual inverted T-shaped scar is incised in turn. The excess skin is pulled laterally toward the tail of the breast allowing completion of the horizontal component of the inverted T. The skin brassiere is fashioned to fit the new form. It should be reasonably snug but not under tension.

A padded elastic dressing is important to help mould the shape and prevent hematomas. It is carefully applied and left undisturbed for 5–7 days. The drain can be removed by lifting up an edge of the dressing.

61.3 Discussion

This is a bipedicle technique that preserves the medial and lateral blood supply to the breast. It is a technique based on the original Biesenberger operation with concepts from other surgical techniques. Most breast reduction descriptions are combinations of multiple ideas that have been developed by various surgeons over the years.

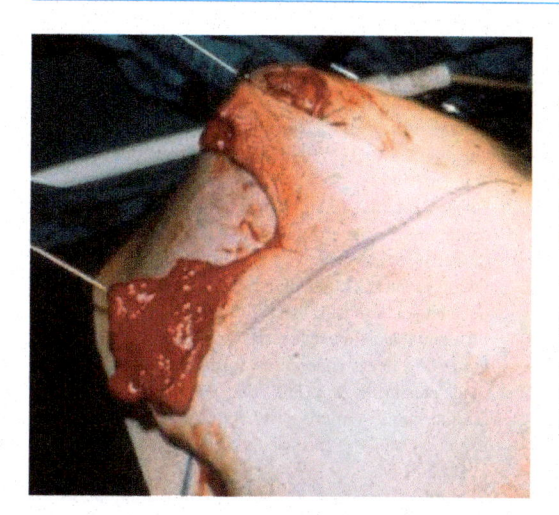

Fig. 61.14 The inferior, redundant skin is then excised to create the position of the breast on the chest wall that one desires

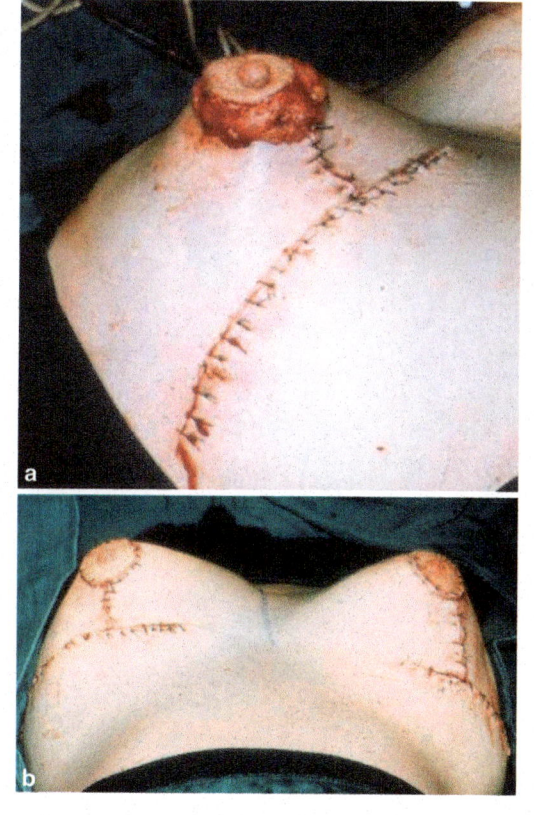

Fig. 61.15 (a,b) The nipple–areola complex is then brought out in position of election and sutured into position

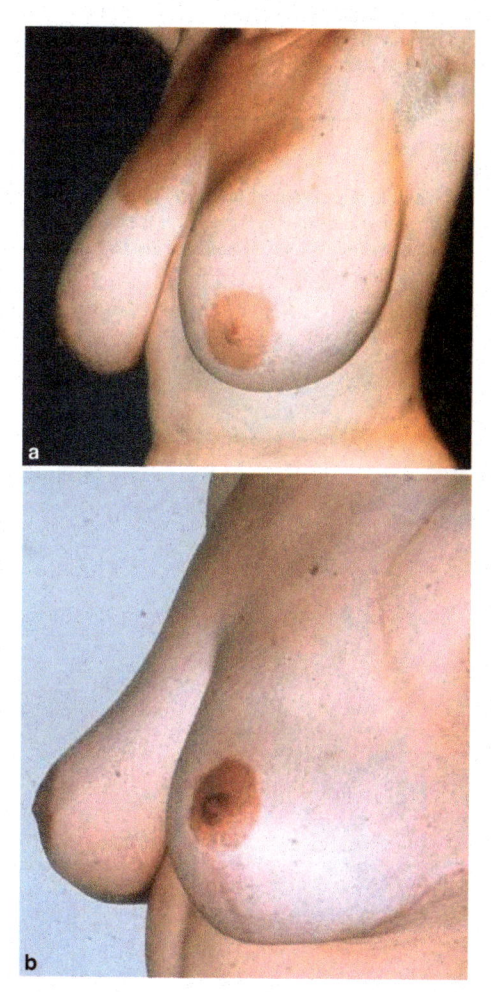

Fig. 61.16 (a) Preoperative. (b) Postoperative

From 1966 until 1980 the author did 224 reductions with this technique. During this period of time the Biesenberger [3], Pitanguy [6, 7], Strombeck [8], and Dufourmentel–Mouly [5] techniques were used by the author. The problems and complication rates with this technique were no different than with the other techniques. Now the author utilizes the vertical or inferior flap procedure and occasionally the dual flap procedure.

The one drawback with this technique is that one must be technically exact in separating the skin brassiere from the breast. It is important that the entire skin and subcutaneous fat is raised as one flap in order to preserve the plexus of blood supply to the skin. This is technically challenging.

The procedure is effective for mastopexy with thin skin. It produces a projecting conical shape and sculpts the breast without relying on the skin to produce or maintain shape (Fig. 61.16). The results are better breast contours and scars.

References

1. Carlsen L: A variation of the Biesenberger technique of reduction mammaplasty. Presented at the annual meeting of the American Society of Aesthetic Plastic Surgery, New Orleans, March 7, 1974
2. Carlsen L, Tershakowec MG: A variation of the Biesenberger technique of reduction mammaplasty. Plast Reconstr Surg 1975;55(6):653–656
3. Biesenberger H: Deformitaten und Kosmetische Operationen der Weiblichen Brust. Vienna, Wilhelm Mauderich 1921
4. Gillies H, McIndoe AH: The technique of mammoplasty in conditions of hypertrophy of the breast. Surg Gynecol Obstet 1939;68:659
5. Dufourmentel C, Mouly R: Plastie mammaire par la methode oblique. Ann Chir Plast 1961;6:45–58
6. Pitanguy I: Une nouvelle technique de plastie mammaire. Etude de 245 cas consecutifs et presentation d'une technique personelle. Ann Chir Plast 1962;7:199–208
7. Strombeck JO: Mammaplasty: Report of a new technique based on the two pedicle procedure. Br J Plast Surg 1960;13:79–90
8. Edholm P, Strombeck JO: Influence of mammoplasty on the arterial supply of the hypertrophic breast. Acta Chir Scand 1962;124:521
9. Goulian D Jr, Conway H: Correction of the moderately ptotic breast. A warning. Plast Reconstr Surg 1969;43(5):478–480
10. McIndoe A, Rees DT: Mammaplasty: Indications, technique, and complications. Br J Plast Surg 1958;10:307–320
11. McKissock PK: Reduction mammaplasty with a vertical pedicle dermal flap. Plast Reconstr Surg 1972;49(3):245–252

CHAPTER 62

Mammaplasty with a Circular Folded Pedicle Technique

62

Waldir Teixeira Renó

62.1 Introduction

Breast reduction surgery is one of the most challenging and difficult procedures that the surgeon faces in plastic surgery. Besides the frequent asymmetry, ptosis, and flaccidity, the patient's expectation is usually higher than what the surgeon can offer only because breasts are the most important prominence of the female silhouette. Even in an aged patient with overweight, large breasts and projected abdomen asking only for reduction without interest in cosmetic results, the image of sensual breasts is present and the surgeon must be prepared because she will demand it. On the other hand, we do not have conditions to define the perfect breast shape because there are no rigid criteria. Every epoch, every climate, and every culture has established a distinct concept of the ideal breast.

Recent concerns deal with obtaining long-term breast projection and minimized scarring. It is important not only to reduce, but also to redistribute, support, and stabilize the breast tissue. The author devised a central convergence of the breast tissues by a circumareolar dermo-glandular pedicle folded on itself. After cutaneous glandular excision in the inferior pole and glandular undermining under the perimeter of the pedicle, the pedicle is folded on itself to produce direct elevation of the nipple–areolar complex into its subsequent position, to act as a central support and to promote the global mobilization of the breast and surrounding thoracic skin. Only after completing the central pedicle will the extension and direction of the scars be determined in the inferior pole.

Since the first publication in 1992, this technique has evolved to become more selective and effective. One of the most important advances was the creation of a turned down flap based on the inframammary fold to fill and lower it in cases where the inframammary fold is too high and depressed. This flap was named the "Longacre Reverse Flap" [1, 2] and act as strut and a expander of the breast base in the inferior pole.

62.2 History

This technique was developed in the mid 1980s just as a periareolar technique and was named the "Conical Periareolar Mammaplasty" [3, 4]. Prior to that time the author used only a periareolar technique characterized by a pocket suture in the deepithelialized pedicle near the edge of the skin (Fig. 62.1). It was later named the "round block" by Benelli [5].

As a periareolar technique it is very selective and as at that time, the author wanted a technique for various breast deformities, an excision in the inferior pole was added with each case and the pocket suture was replaced with U shaped sutures to obtain better control over the distribution of the breast tissue and surrounding thoracic skin. [6] The technique was renamed the "Circular Folded Pedicle Technique" [7, 8].

62.3 Technique

Preoperaitve markings (Fig. 62.2) are performed in the office prior to hospital admission. With the patient standing, markings include the inframammary fold, point A (a point on the breast meridian at the level of the inframammary fold), the mid sternum line, and the anterior axillary line. Point A must be19 to 23 cm from the sternal notch depending on the size of the thoracic cage.

With the patient supine, the amount of skin and glandular excess in the central area is determined by digital maneuver. The amount of skin to be deepithelialized around the areola is estimated by the amount of skin that can be pinched between the thumb and middle finger while the index finger depresses the nipple. The point pressed medially is marked as point B and the point pressed laterally is marked as point C. This maneuver places the glandular tissue toward the superior pole by forcing it cranially so that the breast contour is projected

M.A. Shiffman (ed.), *Mastopexy and Breast Reduction: Principles and Practice*,
© Springer-Verlag Berlin Heidelberg 2009

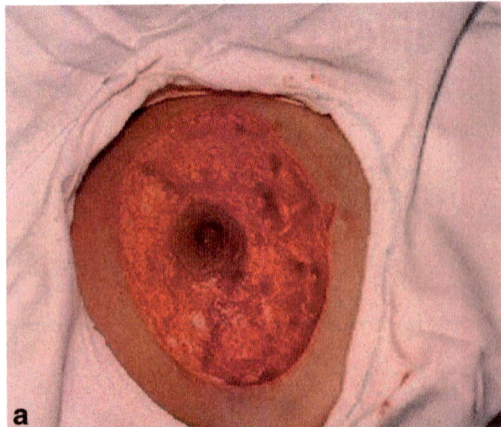

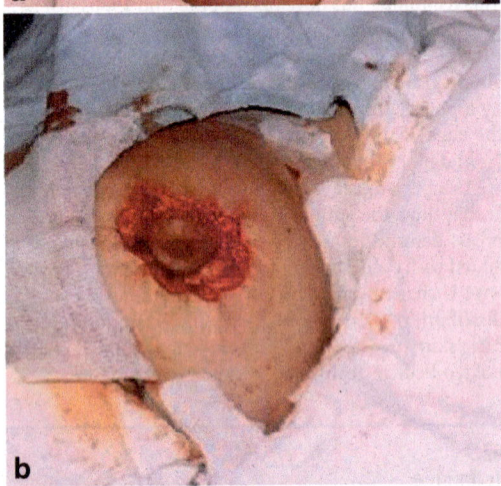

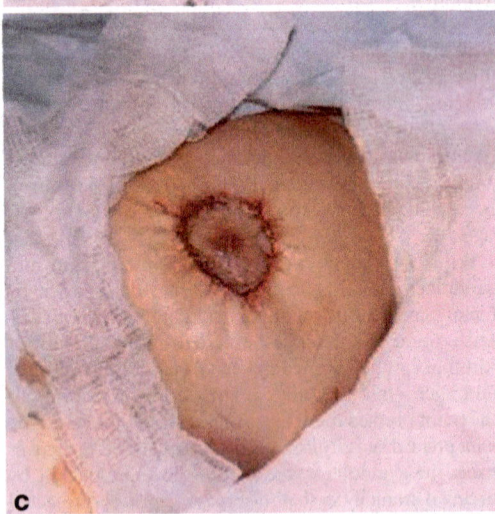

and easily marked. Point D is marked at one cm above the inframammary fold at the level of the anterior axillary line.

Point B must be medial to the areola and around 11 to 13 cm from the midsternal line. That will be the most medial point in the central area. Point C marked lateral to the areola must be 9–11 cm from the anterior axillary line and represents the most lateral point in the central area. A circular line is drawn touching points A, B, and C and the inferior limit in the central area. Its radius is around 4 cm.

Keeping the previous maneuver, the other hand grasps the inferior pole between the thumb and the other fingertips that projects a new shape to the inferior pole. The points where the fingertips grasp the skin should be marked. A line is drawn joining these points marked on each side along the inferior pole from the areola to point D. After that, four types of markings are possible in the inferior pole. Type I: when these points are coincident, the scar will only be periareolar. Type II: when these points form a fusiform drawing, only one scar will extend from the areola to the inferior pole varying between a vertical and oblique one (Fig. 62.3). Type III: after having concluded the fusiform drawing, a vertical breast excess in the inferior pole is observed and is marked transversely forming an inverted Y scar in the inferior pole (Fig. 62.4). Type IV: after concluding the markings, it is observed that there is insufficient mammary volume in the inferior pole, mainly at the inframammary fold, to support the breast mound. In this case a reverse flap is carried out at the inframammary fold (Fig. 62.5), and the final scar will be an inverted-T with a short medial branch (Fig. 62.6).

The anesthetist provides sedation or general anesthesia and infiltration with 0.25% lidocaine with 1:200,000 epinephrine injected under the planned incisions.

Deepithelialization is performed between the areola and the circular line previously marked. At least 1 cm of skin is deepithelialized along lines B–D and C–D (Fig. 62.7). When indicated, this is followed by the breast reduction starting from caudal to cranial and directed toward the pectoralis fascia (Fig. 62.8). As a result the walls of the inferior pole will be thin.

Fig. 62.1 (a-c) Conical Periareolar Technique (1985). Only a circumareolar pedicle is folded on itself by a pocket suture later named "round block". (a) A continuous suture is passed near the edge of the skin. (b) As the suture is stretched, the skin close around the areola. (c) Final aspect of the surgery with some short folds around the areola

62.3 Technique

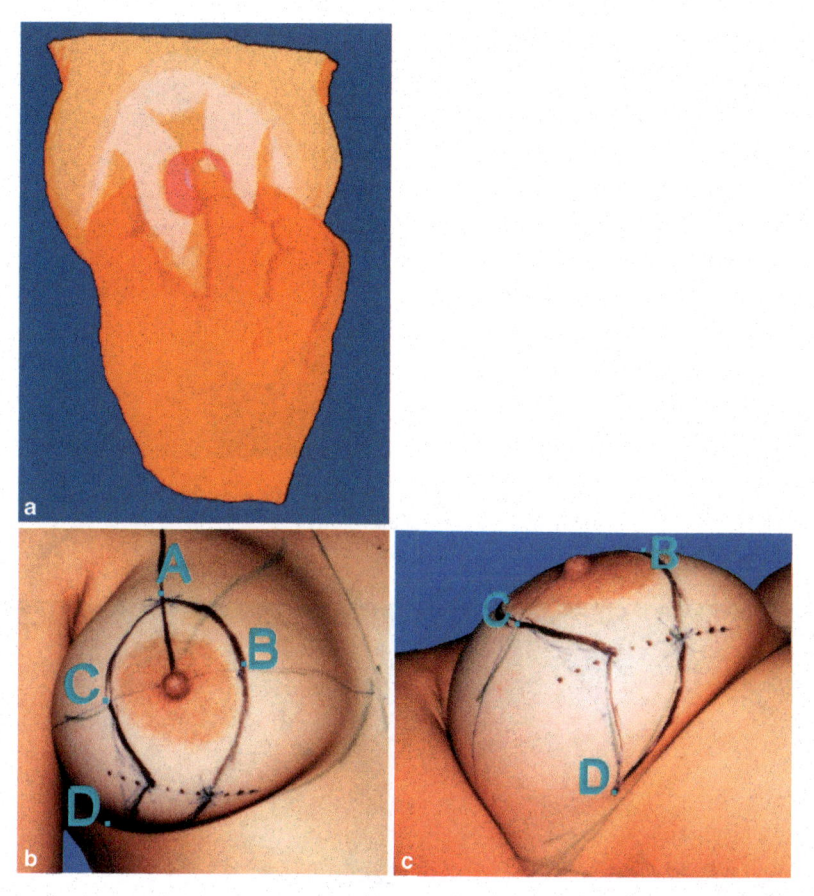

Fig. 62.2 Preoperative markings of the circular folded pedicle technique. (**a**) The amount of skin to be deepithelialized around the areola is estimated by the amount of skin that can be pinched together between the thumb and the middle finger while the index presses the areola around the nipple. (**b**) Usually point B is 11–13 cm from the midsternum line and point C is 9–13 cm from the axillary anterior line. Touching points A, B, C and the inferior limit of the areola, a *circular line* is drawn to delimitate the circular pedicle. Its radius is around 4 cm. (**c**) With the patient supine the inferior pole is grasped by digital maneuver to determine how this area will be treated. Most frequently, an oblique fusiform drawing is obtained, linking the central marking with point D

In the central area, the inferior border of the pedicle is held with two hooks. A special retractor is introduced under the deepithelialized circle that allows undermining in this area with a thickness of 1.5–2.0 cm. The deepithelialized circle surrounding the areola is folded on itself and fixed by cardinal U-shaped sutures placed between each side of the fold using nonabsorbable suture (nylon 4-0 and 5-0) (Fig. 62.9). The flaps in the inferior pole are approximated in the glandular, subcutaneous, and subdermal plane with buried nonabsorbable sutures (nylon 4-0 and 5-0). The skin is closed with continuous intradermal absorbable sutures (Poliglecaprone 25, 4-0) completed with a few simple sutures of nylon 6-0. Drains are used if needed.

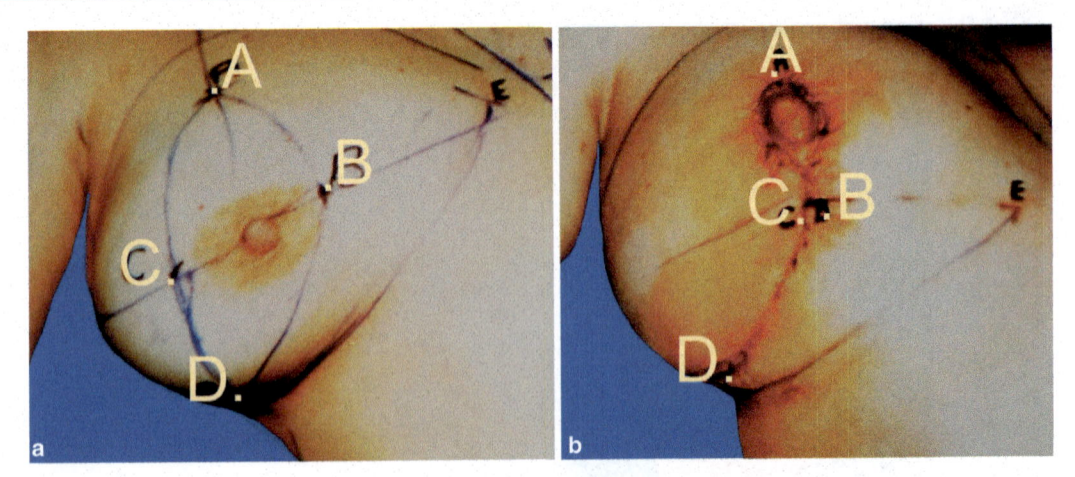

Fig. 62.3 Type II. (**a**) The points marked in the inferior pole result in a fusiform drawing. (**b**) Only one scar will extend from the areola to the inferior pole varying between a vertical to an oblique one

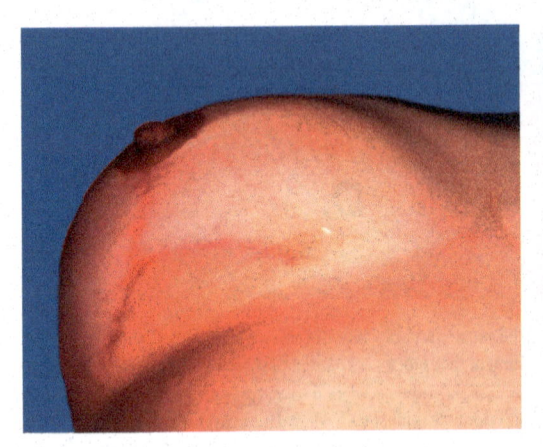

Fig. 62.4 Type III. An inverted Y scar is the result of a vertical breast excess in the inferior pole. Postoperative 3 months after the surgery

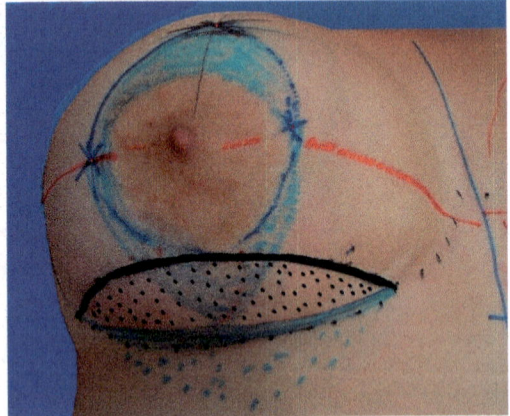

Fig. 62.5 Type IV. Reverse flap to improve a high and depressed inframammary fold. A transverse fusiform drawing based on the inframammary fold and filled with dotted black lines is marked in the inferior pole. The *blue dotted lines* below the inframammary fold are the superficial representation of the place where the reverse flap will be fixed

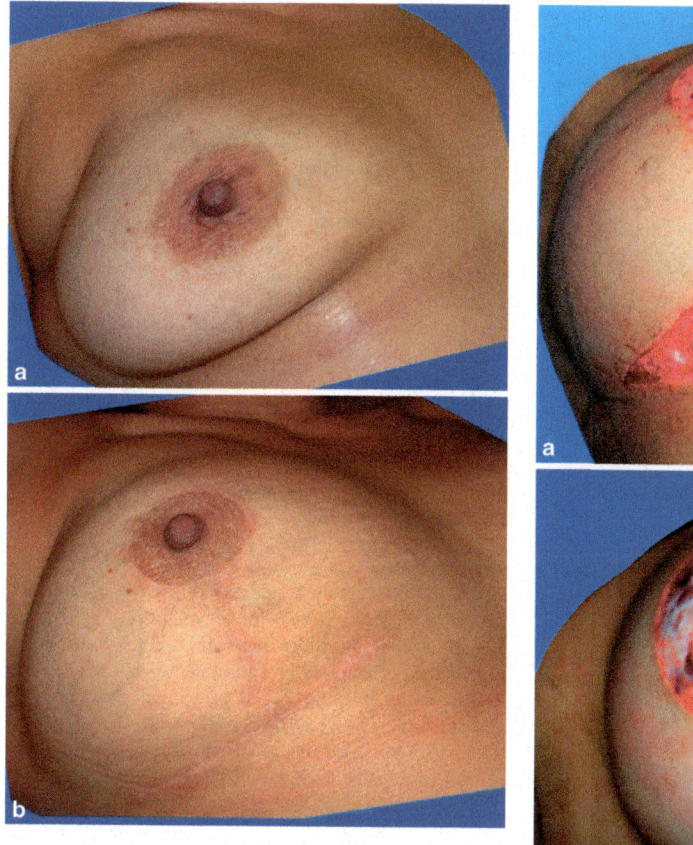

Fig. 62.6 (a) Preoperative revealing a depressed and atrophic inframammary fold. (b) Three months postoperative following mammaplasty with the circular folded pedicle technique associated with the reverse flap. The final scar is an inverted T with short medial branch

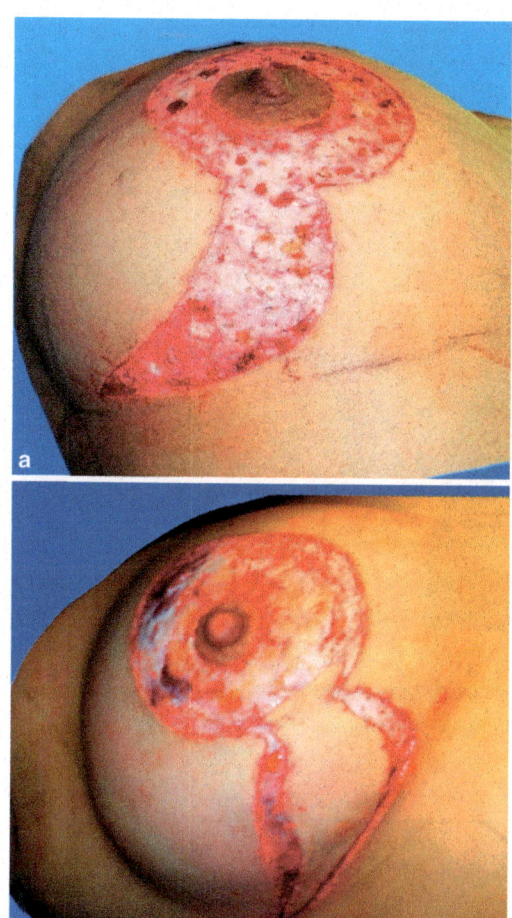

Fig. 62.7 (a) The pedicle and the area marked in the inferior pole are deepithelialized. (b) When the breasts present moderate to severe hypertrophy, at least 1 cm of skin must be deepithelialized in the inner border lines

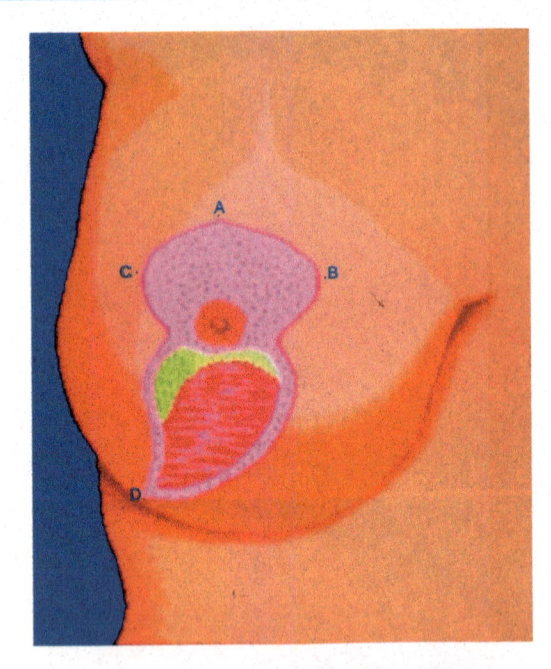

Fig. 62.8 Deepithelialization around the areola and in the inner border lines of B–D and C–D. The breast tissue is resected in the inferior pole by beveled incisions to the pectoralis fascia

62.4
Technology

The author has developed and implemented a special retractor for breast surgery (Patent No. U.S. 6,210,324B1, April 3, 2001). This retractor consists of a second-degree lever formed by two indented and parallel surfaces and a handle. After the initial incision to determine the thickness of the flap, the inferior indented surface of the retractor is introduced in the incision while the superior surface slides over the skin. Once the determined extension is obtained, the handle is turned up until the retractor is supported against the skin only by the superior surface extremity (Fig. 62.10). In this way there is a clear and ample view of the operative field making the sculpture of the breast easier, safer, and faster.

62.5
Complications

Results to date have been satisfactory to both patients and surgeon. The incidence of complications in 269 patients was 11.51%. Minor wound separation (1.5 cm or less) at the transition between the areola and latero-inferior scar was the most frequent complication occurring in 19 patients (7.06%). A transitory sensitivity decrease in the nipple–areola area was noted on only one side in three patients (1.11%). Four patients (1.49%) did not have adequate reduction. Three patients (1.11% developed hematomas that were drained without major sequelae. One patient (0.37%) had extensive steatonecrosis bilaterally and partial loss of the right areola. In all these patients the scars have been quite good.

62.6
Discussion

This technique was developed to obtain good projection with better quality and less extensive scars. In tropical areas the dress code is for very light clothes making it a difficult task to hide long scars that are unpleasant. The mixing of races can result in significant scars.

The ability to obtain good projection with minimal scarring and to prevent ptosis of the breast mound associated with superior displacement of the nipple areolar complex is clearly desirable in reduction mammaplasty. An understanding of the anatomic type and configuration and manipulation of the pedicle is clearly important in this regard. The trend over the last decade has been toward the transposition of dermal-glandular pedicles [9–12]. The changes in the relationship of the breast mound to its overlying skin will occur with time because of a lack of central support since the pedicle is stretched upward while the remaining breast is shaped downward.

A distinct advantage of this technique is that the pedicle is not stretched upward but rather is folded on itself carrying out a global movement of the breast directed around its central axis. Consequently, the breast tissue is enhanced centrally while stretched peripherally. Moreover, the pedicle folded on itself, provides a special support in the central area.

Up to now mammaplasties have been classified according to the configuration of the pedicle and a predetermined design of the scars. Dartigues [13] in

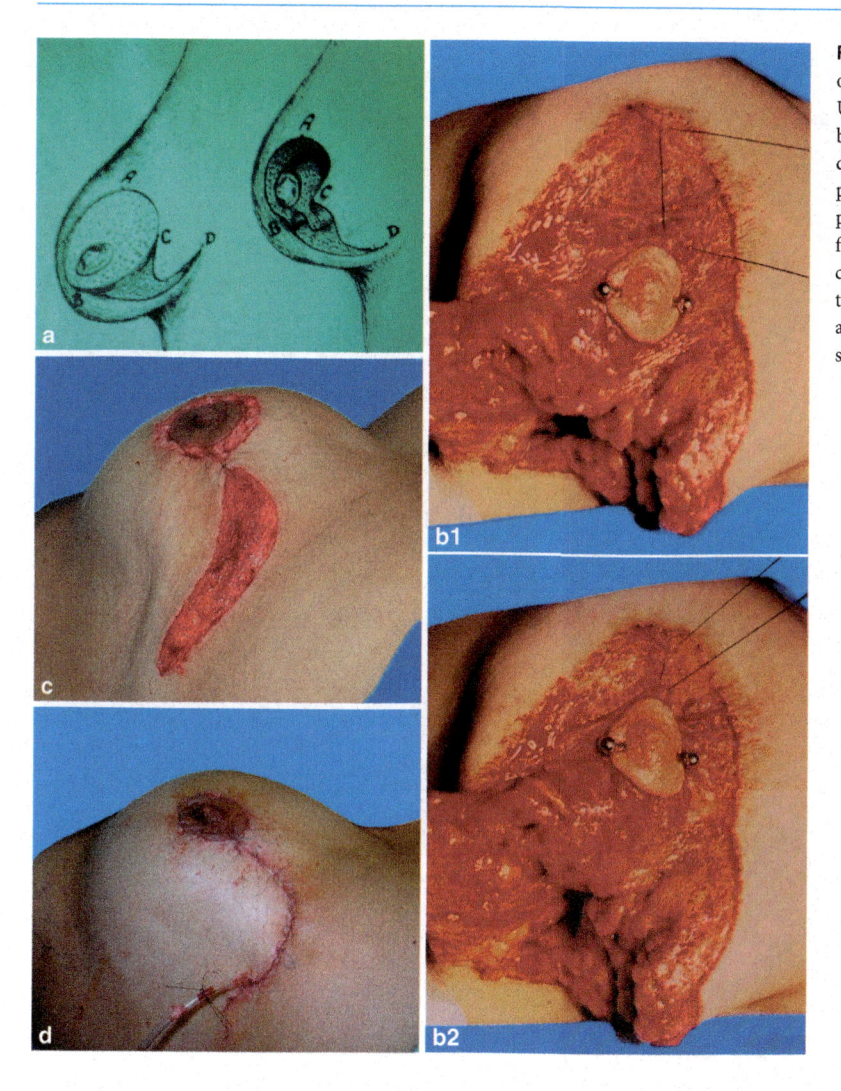

Fig. 62.9 (a) Pedicle folded on itself. (**b***1,2*) One of the U-shaped sutures placed between each side of the deepithelialized circular pedicle is tied to fold the pedicle on itself. (**c**) The folding maneuver is completed. (**d**) The flaps in the inferior pole are approximated and the skin is sutured

1925 was the first to describe the vertical technique followed by Arie (1957) [14], Lassus (1970) [15], and Lejour (1989) [16]. Dufourmental and Mouly (1961) [17] presented the oblique technique avoiding the inframammary fold. Biesenberger (1928) [18] and Pitanguy [19–21] popularized the inverted T technique. The author's technique has a folded pedicle that carries out the global mobilization of the breast and surrounding thoracic skin that will generate several possible configurations of scars. It means that the accommodation and shape planned for the new breast will define necessary access and the resultant scar.

In this technique, the extension of the scar is dependent on skin elasticity. Working on normal skin, it is

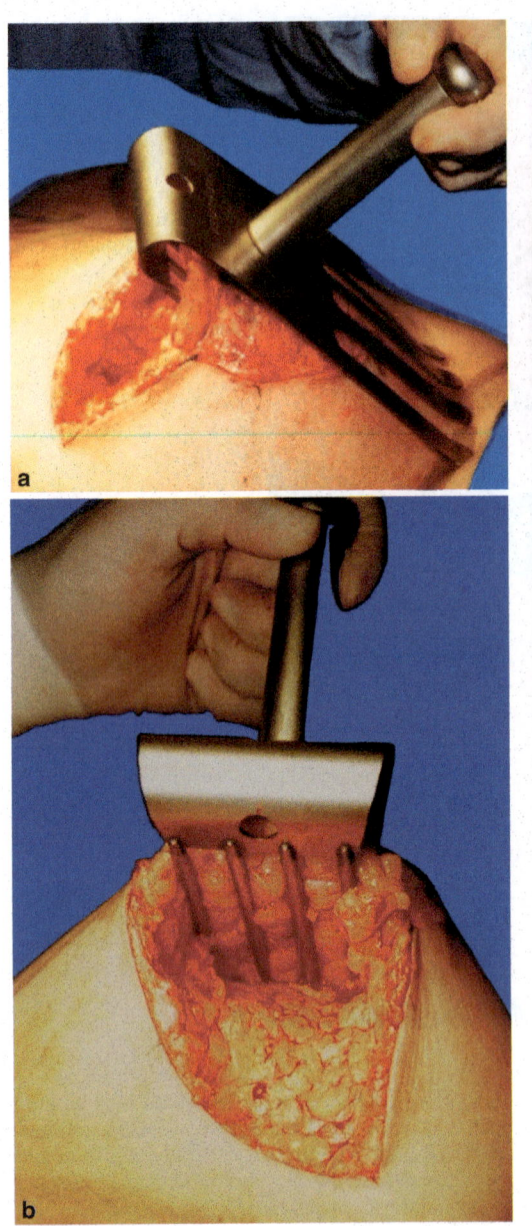

Fig. 62.10 (a) Handle of the retractor is turned up until the retractor is supported only by the superior extremity. (b) Clear and ample view of the surgical field is revealed

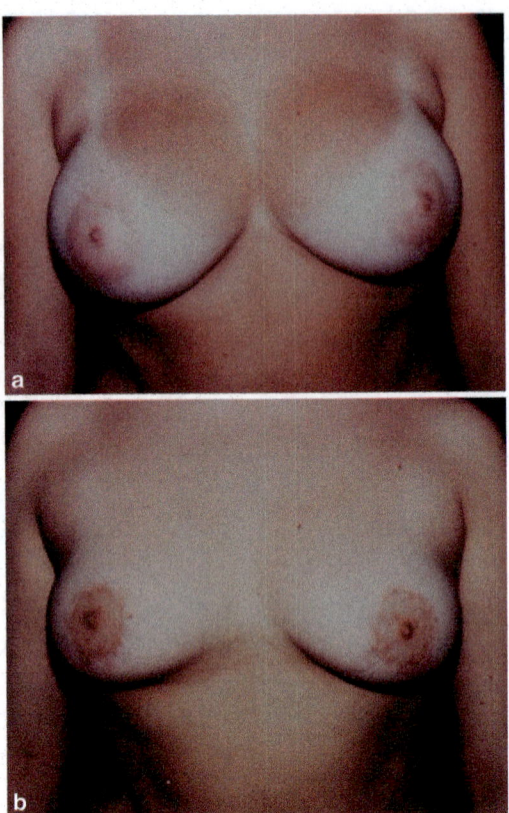

Fig. 62.11 Type I. (a) This 17-year-old patient presents with moderate hypertrophy and stressed skin. (b) One year postoperative after removal of 450 g from the right breast and 260 g from the left breast. Only a periareolar scar was seen

possible to minimize the scars but depending on the laxity of the skin, scars can be extended as well. In the same patient the configuration of the scars may be different in each breast. The patient must be informed of this fact.

Four types of scars are possible. Type I: in young breasts with stressed skin, glandular content, and small to moderate hypertrophy, the scar will be periareolar (Fig. 62.11). Type II: the most frequent, in breasts with moderate cutaneous flaccidity, glandular or lipoglandular content, with small to moderate hypertrophy, only one scar will extend from the areola to the inferior pole varying between a vertical and an oblique one in search of the ideal accommodation and shape for each breast (Fig. 62.12). Type III: in breasts with very flaccid skin, lipomatous content, and moderate to severe hypertrophy, the resulting scar is an inverted Y with a short medial branch that preserves the most medial part of the inferior pole (Fig. 62.13). Type IV: in breasts with high and depressed inframammary fold due to a deficient base in its vertical dimension, the resultant scar is similar to the inverted T (Fig. 62.14).

Either local anesthesia completes the sedation for minor breast procedures or general anesthesia is administered by the anesthetist. An average of 100 ml 0.25% lidocaine with 1:200,000 epinephrine is used in repeated doses for each breast. This decreases blood loss significantly, which in turn has essentially eliminated transfusion [22].

62.7 Conclusions

The circular fold pedicle technique provides central support that preserves long-term breast projection and stabilizes the nipple–areola to inframammary fold distance. It offers the versatility of dealing with various breast problems such as ptosis, hypertrophy, asymmetry, and breasts with a small base, while providing the possibility of minimal and excellent scarring, accuracy, and the option of surgical revision or even another surgery through the same approach without lengthening the original scar.

The development of a reverse flap to fill and lower the inframammary fold acts as an inferior support that strengthens the central support. The creation of a special retractor for breast surgery makes the surgery easier, faster, and less traumatic.

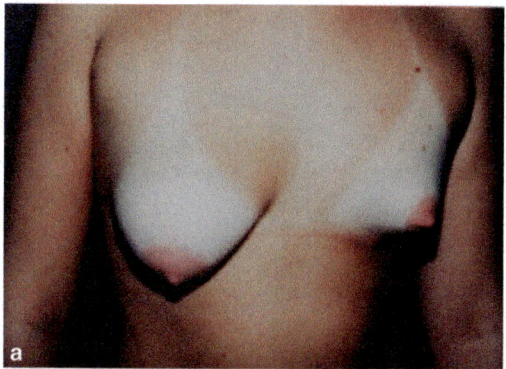

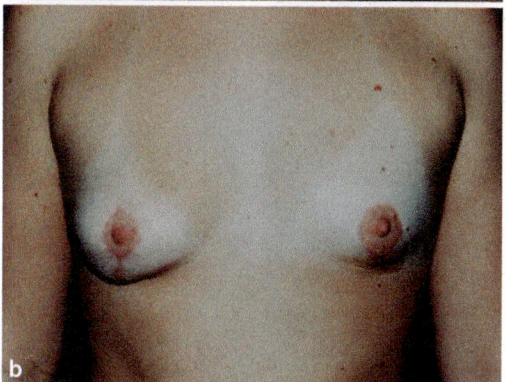

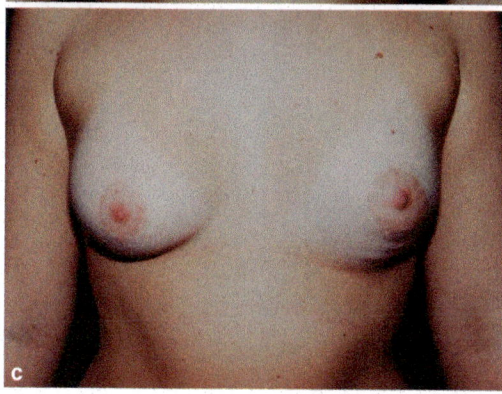

Fig. 62.12 Type II. (**a**) Preoperative 22-year-old patient with severe developmental breast asymmetry. (**b**) Six months postoperative after selective breast removal of 150 g from the right breast, and just before augmentation mammaplasty. (**c**) Two years postoperative after augmentation using round textured silicone gel-filled implants (right breast, 200 ml; left breast 220 ml)

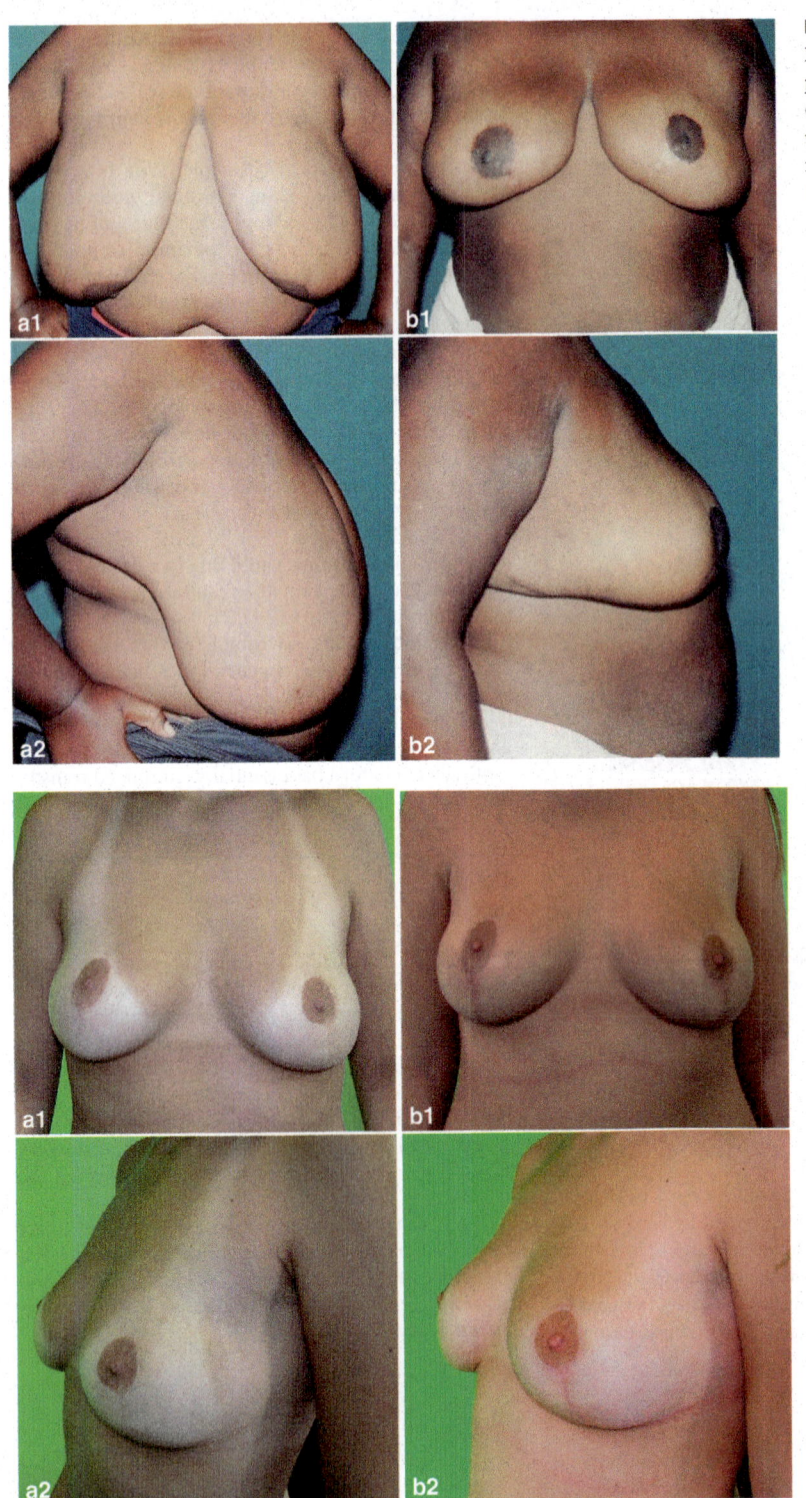

Fig. 62.13 Type III. (*a1,2*) Preoperative 26-year-old patient with gigantomastia. (*b1,2*) One year postoperative after removal of 1,600 g from the right breast and 1,800 g from the left breast

Fig. 62.14 Type IV. (*a1,2*) Preoperative 21-year-old patient with hypertrophy, ptosis, asymmetry, and high and depressed inframammary fold. (*b1,2*) Six months postoperative following mammaplasty with a circular folded pedicle technique associated with a reverse flap in the inferior pole

References

1. Longacre JJ: The use of local pedicle flaps for reconstruction of the breast after subtotal extirpation of the mammary gland and for correction of distortion and atrophy of the breast due to e excessive scar. Plast Reconstr Surg 1953;11(5):380–403
2. Longacre JJ: Correction of the hypoplastic breast with special reference to reconstruction of the "nipple type breast" with local dermofat pedicle flaps. Plast Reconstr Surg 1954;14(6):431–441
3. Renó WT: Mamaplastia periareolar em cone. Presented at 2nd Congresso Brasileiro de Cirurgia Plástica, Sessão Pinga-Fogo, Gramado, Brazil 1985
4. Renó WT: Mamaplastia periareolar em cone. Presented at 3rd Congresso Brasileiro de Cirurgia Plástica, Sessão Pinga-Fogo, Gramado, Brazil 1986
5. Benelli L: Technique de plastie mammaire: le "round block." Rev Fr Chir Esthet 1988;50:7
6. Renó WT: Central support in mammaplasty. Transactions of the Xth Congress of International Confederation for Plastic and Reconstructive Surgery, Madrid 1992
7. Renó WT: Reduction mammaplasty with a circular folded pedicle technique. Plast Reconstr Surg 1992;90(1):65–74
8. Renó WT: Cosmetic follow-up: Reduction mammaplasty with a circular folded pedicle technique. Plast Reconstr Surg 1999;104(6):1914–1919
9. Strombeck JO: Mammaplasty: report of a new technique based on the two pedicle procedure. Br J Plast Surg 1961;13:79–90
10. Skoog T: A technique of breast reduciton: transposition of the nipple on a cutaneous vascular pedicle. Acta Chir Scand 1963;126:453–465
11. McKissock PK: Reduction mammapolasty with a vertical dermal flap. Plast Reconstr Surg 1972;49(3):245–252
12. Ribeiro L: A new technique for reduction mammaplasty. Plast Reconstr Surg 1975;55(3):330–334
13. Dartigues L: Traitement chirurgical du prolapse mammaire. Arch Franco-Belg Chir 1925;28:313
14. Arie G: Una nueva technica de mastoplastia. Ver Latinoam Cir Plast 1957;3:23
15. Lassus C: A technique for breast reduction. Int J Surg 1970;53(1):69–72
16. Lejour M, Abboud M, Declety A, Kertesz P: Reduction des chicatrices de plastie mammaire: De l'ancre courte a la verticale. Ann Chir Plast Esthet 1989;35:369
17. Dufourmentel C, Mouly R: Plastie mammaire par la methode oblique. Ann Chir Plast 1961;6:45–58
18. Biesenberger H: Eine neue methode der mammaplastik. Zbl Chir 1928;38:2382–2387
19. Pitanguy I: Breast hypertrophy. Transactions of the Second International Congress of Plastic and Reconstructive Surgery, London 1959
20. Pitanguy I: Mamaplastias. Estudo de 245 casos consecutivos e apresentação de técnica pessoal. Rev Bras Cir 1961;42:201–220
21. Pitanguy I: Une nouvelle technique de plastie mammaire. Etude de 245 cas consecutifs et presentation d'une technique personelle. Ann Chir Plast 1962;7:199–208
22. Brantner JN, Peterson HD: The role of vasoconstrictors in control of blood loss in reduction mammaplasty. Plast Reconstr Surg 1985;75(3):339–341

The Modified Robertson Reduction Mammaplasty

Elvin G. Zook, Nicole Z. Sommer

63.1 Introduction

The Robertson technique of reduction mammaplasty was first reported in 1964 in an attempt to preserve the natural inferior breast contour for very large as well as small reductions [1–4]. The original technique used a bell-shaped incision and free-nipple grafting [1]. The procedure has since been "modified" to include inferior pedicled soft tissue encompassing the nipple–areola complex, retaining its sensation and viability [5, 6]. The bell-shaped curvilinear markings have the advantages of versatility, especially in larger reductions, inframammary crease preservation, easy intraoperative markings, good nipple projection, and reduction of "bottoming-out." Pseudoptosis or "bottoming-out" with this technique is minimized because the infraareolar dermal skin pedicle is not disrupted, maintaining stronger inferior support to the breast mass.

63.2 Surgical Technique

The markings for the modified Robertson reduction are performed after anesthesia is achieved (Fig. 63.1). The inframammary fold, vertical breast meridian, and body midline are marked. A slightly different variation of the skin markings compared with those previously described for the inferiorly based bell curve is used. Instead of making an 8–9 × 4 cm² rectangle square as traditionally described [2, 5], a 6–7 × 4 cm² rectangle is drawn and marked at the inframammary fold centered over the breast's meridian line. A gentle bell-shaped curve is then created from the rectangle and extended into the medial and lateral inferior poles of the breast. The medial extent of the incision is limited to no closer than 2 cm from the midline to avoid visible scarring in this area. A 38- to 44-mm washer is used to mark the size of the new nipple–areola complex. The inferiorly based dermal pedicle is marked as a cephalad extension of the bell curve to incorporate the nipple–areola complex.

The superior incisions are marked by gently retracting the breast inferiorly, drawing a horizontal line across the upper breast, and connecting the medial and lateral ends of the inferior markings. The more superior the upper incision is drawn, the greater the volume of breast tissue resected. This provides versatility for tailoring the breast to the desired volume of reduction. The superior incision is made only after the upper flap is drawn down to the bell shaped cut in order to ensure that it will reach. The authors compare the length of the upper and lower incision and attempt to closely match incision lengths between the two to facilitate closure without bunching of redundant tissue.

The dermal pedicle is deepithelialized after application of the breast tourniquet (Fig. 63.2). An inferiorly based parenchymal flap is created from the inframammary fold and midpoint of the bell curve superiorly to about 1–2 cm above the new nipple–areolar complex (Fig. 63.3). Excessive breast tissue is resected medially, laterally, and superiorly to the pedicle. The superior skin/breast tissue flap is undermined at the level of the pectoralis fascia, carefully tapering the tissue as needed to allow for adequate draping of the flap over the pedicle and nipple–areola suturing without tension. Irrigation, hemostasis, and evaluation for use of drains are completed. The superior flap is sutured to the inferior bell curve incision, advancing the lateral tissue toward the vertical breast meridian to provide breast projection (Fig. 63.4). The patient is seated upright for evaluation of nipple–areola location placement. The new nipple–areola complex site is marked with the appropriate sized washer, an oval parallel to the clavicle is marked in side to washer ring and excised full thickness (Fig. 63.5). I excised circular tension in the breast post surgery will elongate the areola into a vertical oval. The surgery is completed by delivering and insetting the nipple–areola complex into position with absorbable sutures. If the inferior pedicle is too long to provide adequate blood supply to the attached nipple–areola complex, the nipple–areola can be removed, the pedicle shortened so that the remainder (necessary to give bulk to the breast) is viable, and the nipple–areola is replaced at the appropriate site as a free graft.

M.A. Shiffman (ed.), *Mastopexy and Breast Reduction: Principles and Practice*,
© Springer-Verlag Berlin Heidelberg 2009

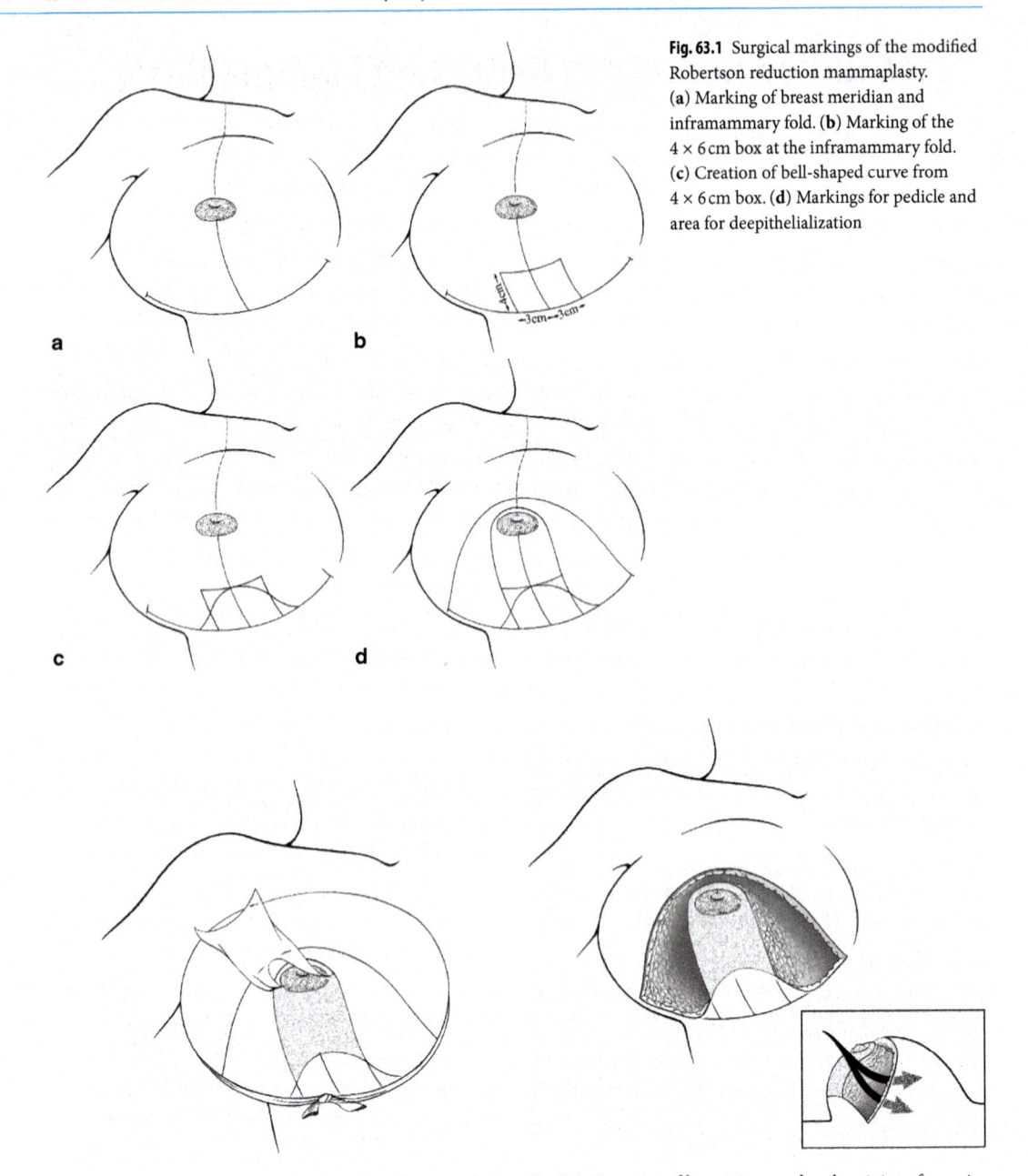

Fig. 63.1 Surgical markings of the modified Robertson reduction mammaplasty. (**a**) Marking of breast meridian and inframammary fold. (**b**) Marking of the 4 × 6 cm box at the inframammary fold. (**c**) Creation of bell-shaped curve from 4 × 6 cm box. (**d**) Markings for pedicle and area for deepithelialization

Fig. 63.2 Breast tourniquet applied and inferior pedicle deepithelialized

Fig. 63.3 Resection of breast tissue and undermining of superior flap

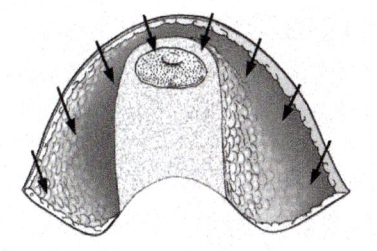

Fig. 63.4 Advancement of superior flap inferiorly for closure

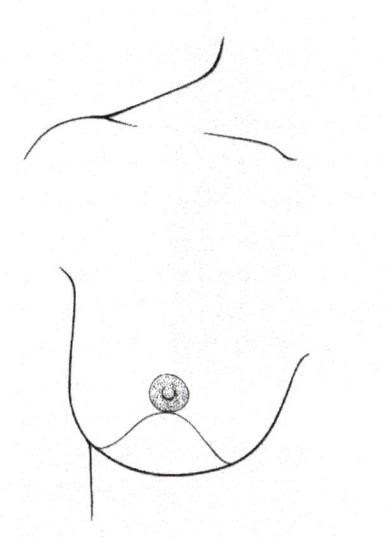

Fig. 63.5 Final scar location

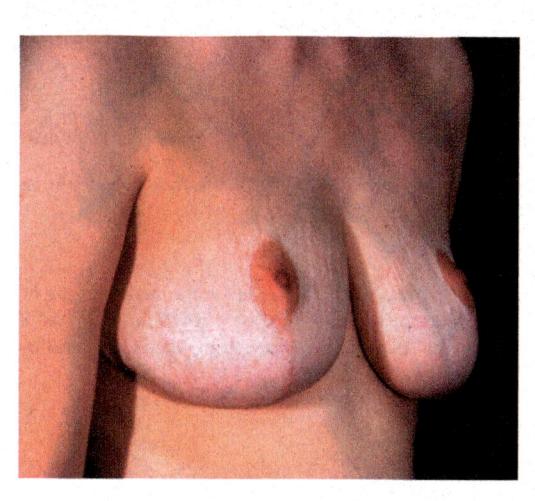

Fig. 63.6 Development of pseudoptosis after inverted T-incision

63.3 Complications

Of those patients who did not have free-nipple grafts, 88% reported normal nipple sensation before surgery and 65% post operation. Overall, 94% of patients were very satisfied with the results.

The relief of macromastia symptoms is comparable to other reduction techniques [8–14]. Eighty-one percent of the patients rated their scars as expected or better. Clearly, the fact that 19% found their scars worse than expected reiterates the need to discuss the procedure with patients to emphasize that this procedure is not primarily cosmetic in nature [7]. On average, patients' perception was that it took over 2 years for their scars to reach their final mature state, reflecting possibly a misunderstanding of the process of scar maturation described to them or that they are in fact truly noticing changes in the scar that somehow physicians are missing [7]. A modification of the technique to lower the scar at the midline has been described by Morris et al. [9].

Subjective breast and nipple sensation has been shown in the past to be relatively technique dependent, on the basis of the style of reduction used [10–12]. Other reports on decreased nipple sensation have varied from 17 to 68% [9–11]. One previous direct comparison between a bipedicled version of the modified Robertson and the McKissock technique demonstrated less loss of sensation in the former group (35 vs. 56%) [6]. The modified Robertson technique does not disrupt as much of the inferior breast tissue and skin and may thereby help to preserve sensation.

63.4 Discussion

The most significant advantage with the modified Robertson technique is the decreased amount of postoperative pseudoptosis. Estimating and correcting for anticipated bottoming-out can be very difficult and unreliable. Preservation of the skin and breast tissue below the nipple to the inframammary fold in the modified Robertson technique helps to prevent stretching of the vertical scar seen with standard inferior pedicled techniques. The inverted-T incision, inferior pedicle technique leads to a greater degree of bottoming-out type of pseudoptosis although it creates a more conical breast early post operation (a probable reason for its popularity) (Fig. 63.6). As a result, the nipple–areola complex ultimately rides higher on the breast mound than desired and leads to a poor cosmetic result. Subjectively, in our experience only a rare patient complained of the breast bottoming-out and 86% of women were happy

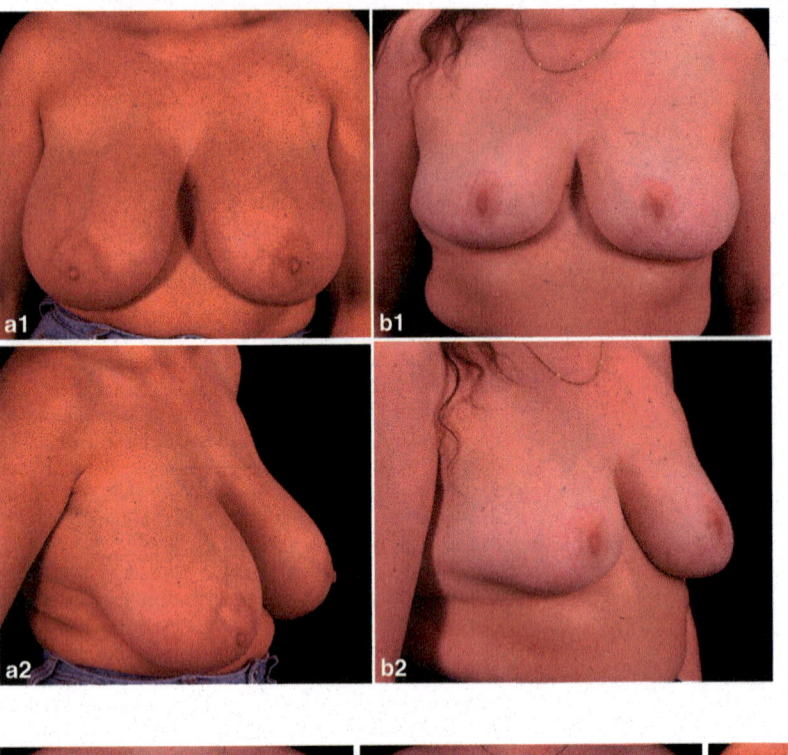

Fig. 63.7 (**a***1,2*) Preoperative. (**b***1,2*) Sixteen months postoperative after modified Robertson reduction mammaplasty with resection of 1,241 g on the left and 1,061 g on the right

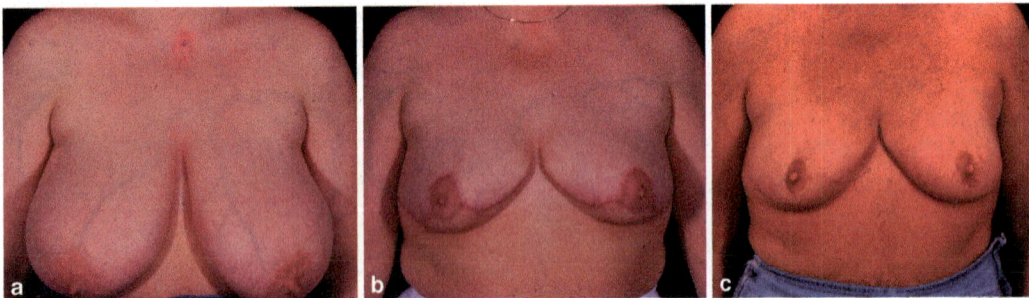

Fig. 63.8 (**a**) Preoperative reduction mammaplasty. (**b**) 3 months postoperative. (**c**) 13 years and 5 months after resection of 955 g on the left and 812 g on the right

with their nipple location with the modified Robertson technique (Fig. 63.7).

The modified Robertson technique is a reliable and consistent method of breast reduction for all sized breast reductions. It results in relief of symptoms matching or surpassing other methods of reduction and has a significant benefit in preventing pseudoptosis or bottoming-out (Fig. 63.8).

References

1. Robertson DC: Reduction mammaplasty using a large inferior flap. In Transactions of Third International Congress of Plastic Surgery. Amsterdam, Excerpta Medical Foundation 1964, p 81
2. Robertson DC: The technique of inferior flap mammaplasty. Plast Reconstr Surg 1967;40(4):372–377
3. Robertson DC: The technique of inferior flap mammaplasty. Plast Reconstr Surg 1973;52(4):438
4. Arons MS: Reduction of very large breasts: The inferior flap technique of Robertson. Br J Plast Surg 1976;29(2):137–141
5. Hurst LN, Evans HB, Murray KA: Inferior flap reduction mammaplasty with pedicled nipple. Ann Plast Surg 1983;10(6):483–485
6. Pers M, Nielsen IM, Gerner N: Results following reduction mammaplasty as evaluated by the patients. Ann Plast Surg 1986;17(6):449–455
7. Chalekson C, Neumeister M, Zook E, Russell R: Outcome analysis of reduction mammoplasty using the modified Robertson technique. J Plast Reconstr Surg 2002;110(1):71–79
8. Atterhem H, Holmner S, Janson PE: Reduction mammaplasty: symptoms, complications, and late results. Scand J Plast Reconstr Surg Hand Surg 1998;32(3):281–286
9. Morris DJ, Pribaz JJ, Abboud J: The modified Robertson breast reduction: revisited and revised. In Proceedings of the 36th Annual Meeting of the New England Society of Plastic and Reconstructive Surgeons. Boston, MA 1995
10. Davis GM, Ringler SL, Short K, Sherrick D, Bengtson BP: Reduction mammaplasty: long-term efficacy, morbidity, and patient satisfaction. Plast Reconstr Surg 1995;96(5):1106–1110
11. Hang-Fu L: Subjective comparison of six different reduction mammoplasty procedures. Aesthetic Plast Surg 1991;15(4):297–302
12. Kinell I, Beausang-Linder M, Ohlsen L: The effect on the preoperative symptoms and the late results of Skoog's reduction mammaplasty. Scand J Plast Reconstr Surg Hand Surg 1990;24(1):61–65

"Owl" Incision Technique Reduction Mammaplasty

Oscar M. Ramirez, Sung Yoon

64.1 Introduction

Reduction mammaplasty techniques continue to evolve with better understanding of the anatomy of breast which helps to incorporate improving aesthetics of breast into achieving reduction in its volume.

Reduction mammaplasty technique has two components: skin incision pattern and volume reduction pattern for which blood supply of the nipple areolar complex is based. Wise skin incision pattern with inferior pedicle technique have become standards to which all other variations are compared [1]. Reproducibility, safety, and reliability of the technique have been proved in all sizes of breast reductions, large or small [2].

Wise pattern with inferior pedicle technique does have its limitations. Resulting breasts tend to have long scars, long term boxy shape, bottoming out of breasts and lack of breast projection [3, 4].

Many variations have been proposed to try to improve upon the aesthetics of breast in both skin incision pattern and volume reduction pattern. The vertical incision pattern has been popularized to reduce length of the scar.

The "Owl" incision reduction mammaplasty combines features of a large periareolar reduction of Benelli's [5] and vertical reduction of Lassus [6], and Lejour et al [7] The name "owl" incision came from the shape of the incision pattern used. (Fig. 64.1)

The "Owl" Incision technique achieves several objectives in reduction mammaplasty. It is a shorter scar length than standard Wise skin incision pattern and it provides improved upper pole fullness and projection of breasts compared to inferior pedicle technique [8]. The "Owl" incision technique can also be used in reduction of larger breasts achieving safe, reproducible and aesthetically pleasing outcome.

64.2 Preoperative Assessment and Markings

Patients are examined and preoperative markings made with patient standing. Breast is marked with standardized reference lines (Fig. 64.1).

64.3 Taking Measurements

Measurements of breasts are taken.
1. Distance of suprasternal notch to nipple areolar complex on both sides.
2. Diameter of nipple areolar complex on both sides.
3. Distance from mid clavicle to nipple areolar complex on both sides.
4. Distance from inframammary fold to nipple on both sides.
5. Inframammary chest circumference.

64.4 Establishing the Reference Lines

The mid sternal line from the suprasternal notch to the umbilicus is marked as reference line. Then meridian of breast mound is marked from mid clavicular point and extended towards and beyond inframammary fold. This line is approximately 1 cm medial to the nipple; however if the nipple–areola complex is laterally deviating, distance from the nipple might be as wide as 2 cm (Fig. 64.1). The equator of breast mound is marked by drawing a line from medial cleavage toward the lateral breast along the curve of breast mound with surgeon's eye at the level of the patient's nipple–areola complex (Fig. 64.1).

64.5 Determining the New Nipple Position

Inframammary fold is also marked and its transposed positioned marked on the breast meridian line. This is the new nipple position.

64.6 Skin Incision Markings

For the "Owl" Skin incision pattern, a rhomboid shaped mark is outlined. Apex of the rhomboid shape is the transposed inframammary fold along the breast median

M.A. Shiffman (ed.), *Mastopexy and Breast Reduction: Principles and Practice*,
© Springer-Verlag Berlin Heidelberg 2009

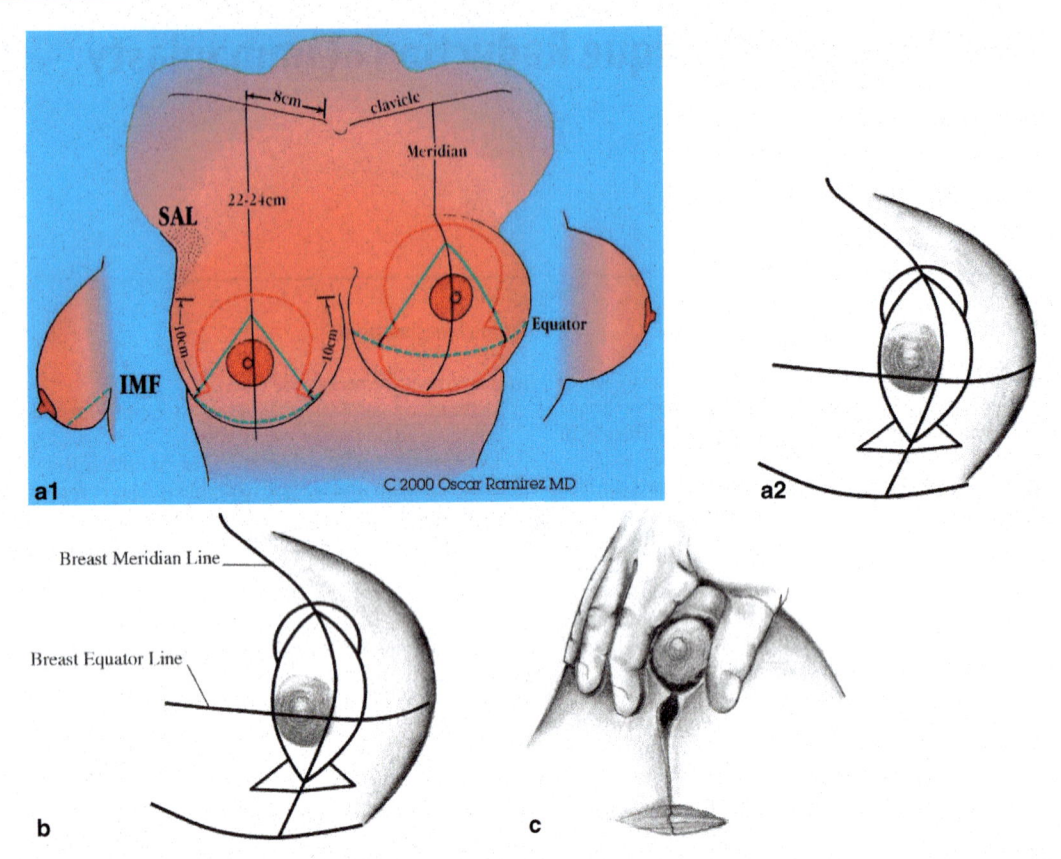

Fig. 64.1 (a) The Owl pattern has been outlined on the left breast. Observe that the nipple–areolar complex is medial to the axis of the marking (breast meridian). (b) Reference lines of breast. Breast meridian and Ecuador help to construct rhomboid pattern markings. These are reference marks over which the "Owl" outline is marked. (c) Horizontal component is short and usually stays inside hidden portion of the submammary sulcus. This is used to remove resultant dog ear that may need to have removed at a secondary stage. This does not detract from final aesthetic result

line. Along the same breast meridian line, inferior aspect of the rhomboid shape is marked by point 3 cm from inframammary fold (Fig. 64.1). Medial point of the rhomboid shape is 10 cm from the intermammary cleavage along the breast equator line. The lateral point of the rhomboid shape is 10 cm from point demarcated by the medial border of the arm as it crosses the equator of breast. Lines are drawn from the superior apex towards the medial and lateral points marked (Fig. 64.1).

Then from the superior angle of the rhomboid, mark a point of the breast meridian line located 2–3 cm above this angle. This will be the upper border of the periareolar keyhole. From this point, draw a gentle semicircle towards medial and lateral points of the already marked rhomboid. Similarly, using gentle curvilinear lines, lines are drawn from the inferior apex of the breast meridian line toward medial and lateral points along the breast equator line (Fig. 64.1).

Horizontal component of incision is made at the level of inferior aspect of the rhomboid shape 3 cm above inframammary fold (Fig. 64.1).

Areolar is marked with a diameter of 4–5 cm depending on patient's aesthetics goals and size of breast.

Using the Lassus method, markings are confirmed with the pinch method. Medial and lateral points of the breast equator line can also be checked using the Lejour mound displacement technique.

64.7 Pedicle Design

Owl incision reduction mammaplasty uses a supero-central pedicle design for volume reduction. The area of deepithelialization is marked by the semicircular line and completing it to a full circle extending approximately 2 cm below the limits of the new inferior areolar border.

64.8 Operative Technique

64.8.1 Tumescent Infiltration

To minimize blood loss, tumescent infiltration is performed on planned areas of incision on skin around the breast parenchyma. Maximum of 250 ml of volume per breast is infiltrated.

64.8.2 Deepithelialization of the Supero-Central Pedicle

Deepithelialization of the periareolar keyhole is performed with breast skin under tension. This can be done using a mammastat or similar device intended to make the breast and breast parenchyma stretched and placed under tension.

64.8.3 Supero-Central Dermoglandular Pedicle

After the supero-central dermoglandular pedicle has been deepithelialized, inferior parenchymal resection is performed starting with full thickness skin incision along the vertical component of own incision pattern. Full thickness incision continues for 2–3 cm on medial and lateral aspects of the periareolar dermoglandular flap for better skin draping. Parenchymal resection is continued perpendicular toward the chest wall and extended superiorly on medial and lateral aspect of the deepithelialized peripheral portions of the inferior portion of the supero-central dermoglandular pedicle. Care is taken now to undermine beneath the nipple areolar complex (Fig. 64.2).

To facilitate redraping of parenchyma along the areolar keyhole incision, parenchyma can be resected in a zigzag fashion especially in patients with high parenchyma to fat tissue ratio.

64.8.4 Additional Liposuction

For additional shaping and reduction of breast, liposuction of breasts along inframammary fold is performed (Fig. 64.2).

64.8.5 Insetting of the Breast

Suture closure of the periareolar and vertical components of the reduced breast is done by placing a suture in the corners of the areolar keyhole inferiorly and through the dermis of the areolar at the level of the meridian line of breast. This is done using a 4-0 polydioxanone inverted suture. The rest of the vertical limb of incision is closed with inverted suture of the dermis and the immediate adjacent parenchyma. Because the dermis will carry the parenchyma since there was no undermining medially and laterally into the parenchyma. 4-0 Prolene sutures are used if there is moderate tension for dermal layer approximation. The areolar is inset with inverted 5-0 polydioxanone sutures.

The skin is approximated with a 4-0 subcuticular Prolene sutures. Breasts are splinted with supportive sterile tape and supportive dressing. Drains can be used, but is not routine.

64.8.6 Optional Horizontal Component of the "Owl" Incision Pattern

For those cases with residual dog-ears in the vertical limb of the incision, a small horizontal component is resected at the end in an elliptical resection of skin and subcutaneous layer. Horizontal component resection is used for larger breasts reductions.

64.9 Clinical Application

The "Owl" incision technique reduction mammaplasty has been used for small to large breast reductions. The largest amount of resection was 1,900 g from one breast. This technique is so versatile that it can be used for large pendulous, wide flat, and young pubertal breasts (Figs. 64.3–64.5).

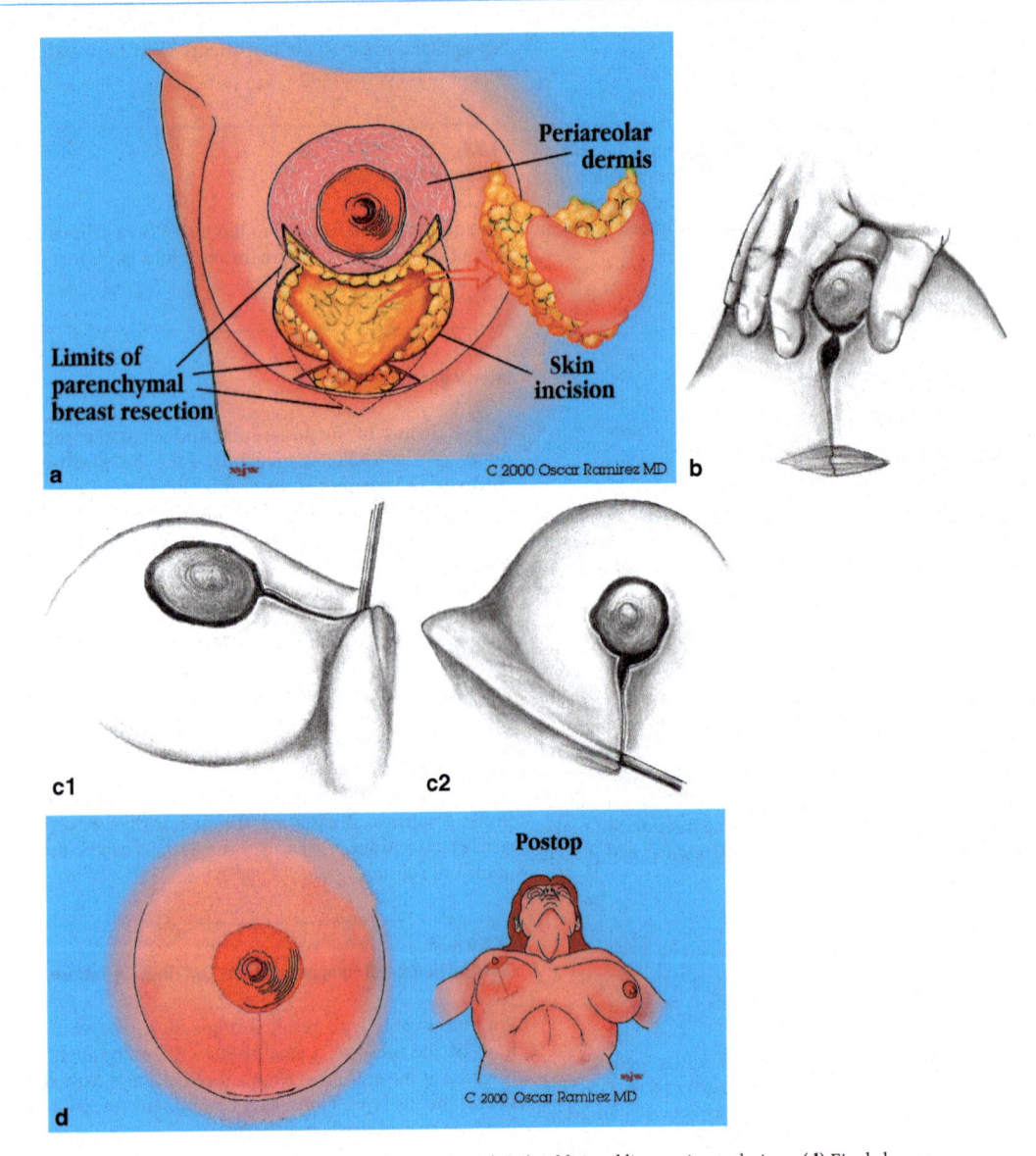

Fig. 64.2 (a) Resection of breast. (b) Horizontal component. (c1,2) Additional liposuction technique. (d) Final closure

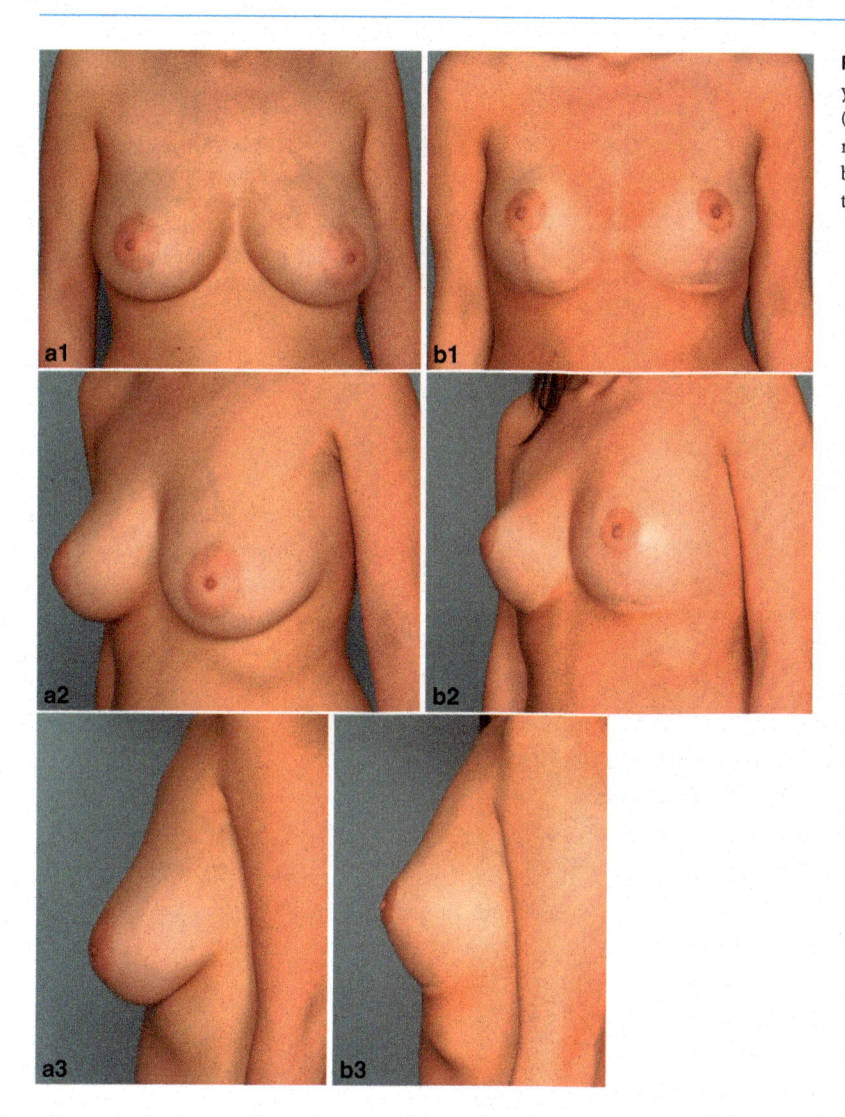

Fig. 64.3 (*a1-3*) Preoperative young female. (*b1-3*) Post-operative after resection of 460 g from each breast. Observe fullness of the upper pole

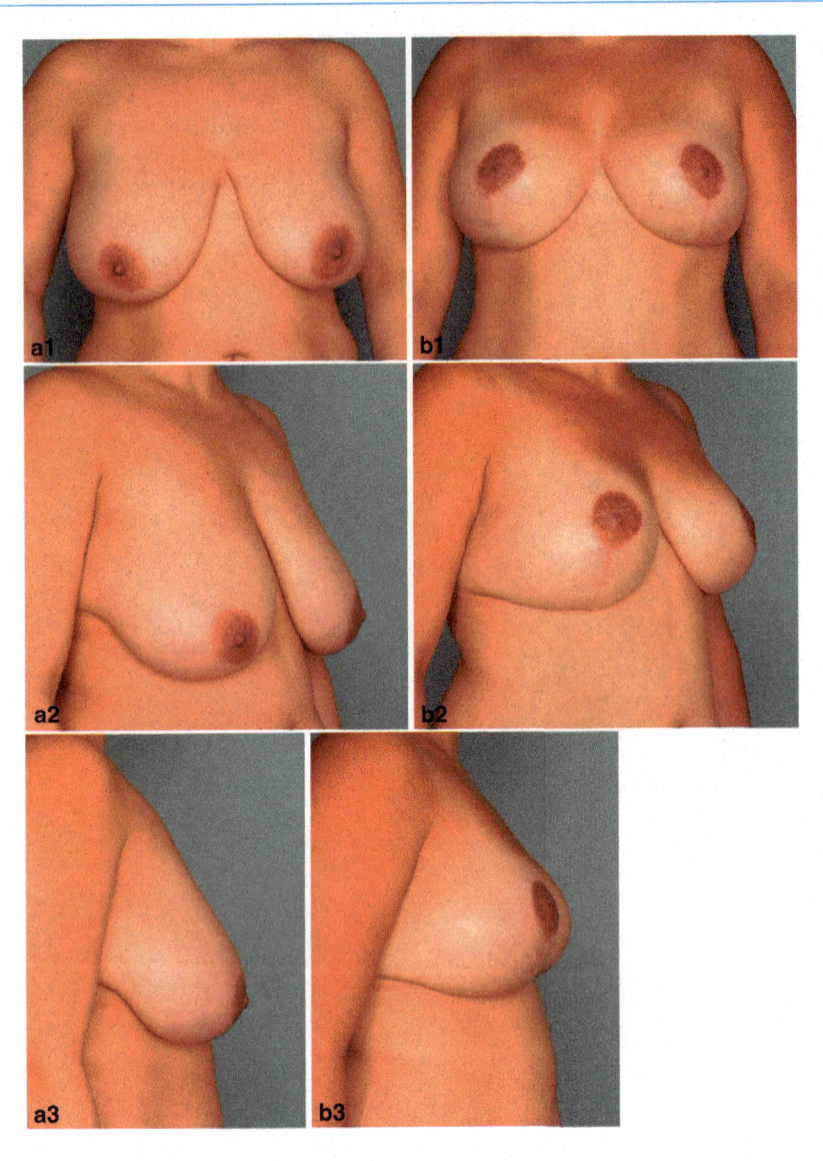

Fig. 64.4 (**a***1-3*) Preoperative patient with large pendulous breasts. (**b***1-3*) Postoperative after "Owl" reduction of 720 g of breast tissue removed from each side. Observe conical shape of breast, lifting of breast, and fullness of the upper pole

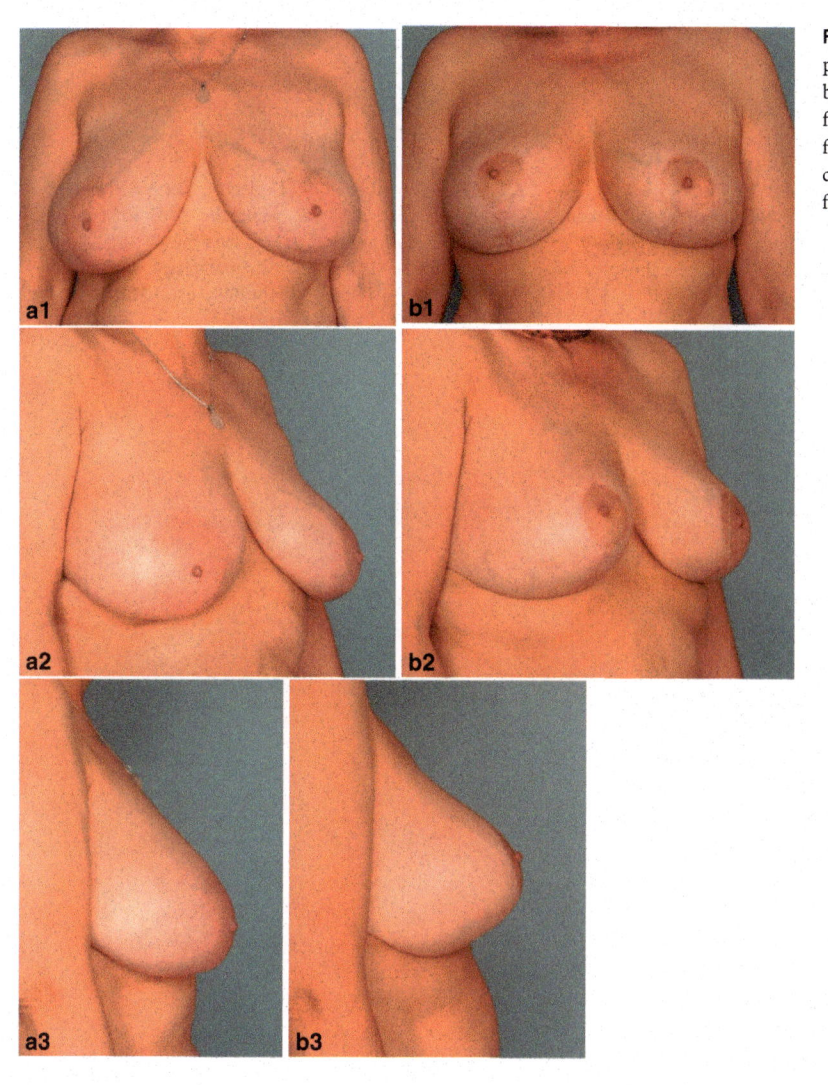

Fig. 64.5 (**a***1-3*) Preoperative patient with wide chest and breasts. (**b***1-3*) Postoperative following removal of 760 g from each breast. Note conical breast shape and fullness of the upper pole

64.10 Complications

Rate of complications has been minimal. From 100 consecutive cases analyzed retrospectively, there was only one case of partial thickness necrosis and one case of unilateral loss of nipple sensation. In about 7% there was suture extrusion that did not cause any localized infection or suture granuloma. These were excised under topical anesthesia. One obese patient requested secondary surgery to define better the submammary sulcus.

64.11 Conclusions

The "Owl" pattern of skin excision is an excellent alternative for reduction mammaplasty. It not only combines best features of the periareolar and vertical reductions but uses the superocentral pedicle removing the lower hemisphere parenchyma which is the part of breast to produce bottoming out. Resultant shape is the ideal cone. Vascularity is excellent reducing then risks of skin necrosis.

References

1. Wise RJ: Preliminary report on a method of planning the mammaplasty. Plast Reconstr Surg 1956;17:367–375
2. Hall-Findlay E: Reduction mammaplasty. In The Art of Aesthetic Surgery: Principles and Techniques. Spear S. (ed), Philadelphia, Lippincott Williams 2006
3. Mathes SJ, Nahai F, Hester TR: Avoiding the flat breast in reduction mammaplasty. Plast. Reconstr. Surg. 1980;66(1):63–70
4. Daane SP, Rockwell WB: Breast reduction techniques and outcomes: A meta-analysis. Aesthetic Surg J 1999;19:293
5. Benelli L: Technique de plastie mammaire: le "round block." Rev Fr Chir Esthet 1988;50:7
6. Lassus C: A technique for breast reduction. Int Surg 1970;53(1):69–72
7. Lejour, M., Abboud, M., Declety, A., Kertesz, P.: Reduction des cicatrices de plastie mammaire: De l'ancre courte a la verticale. Ann Chir Plast Esth 1989;35:369
8. Ramirez OM: Reduction mammaplasty with the "Owl" incision. Plast Reconstr Surg 2002;109(2):512–522

Regnault B Technique

Robert F. Garza, Patricio Andrades, Jorge I. de la Torre, Luis O. Vasconez

65.1 Introduction

Many different techniques of breast reduction have been introduced over the past 50 years. Many of the most recent techniques have attempted to improve long term outcomes of breast reduction with regard to consistency of shape, minimizing scars, and decreasing incidence of complications such as nipple sensitivity and wound dehiscence. Several of these techniques have based viability of the nipple–areolar complex on differing vascular pedicles, each one claiming to have better outcomes than the other in matters such as shape, nipple–areolar complex viability, and nipple sensitivity.

Many of the techniques can be difficult to learn while others may have shorter learning curves. Some techniques require longer operating times while others may require more secondary revisions. It is imperative for the surgeon, both experienced and inexperienced, to be familiar with several techniques so as to have an appropriate armamentarium from which to formulate an operative plan. Many patient factors must be considered, such as preoperative size of breasts, planned amount of reduction, previous breast procedures, desires of patient, and overall health of patient. All these points must be taken into consideration in the creation of an operative plan.

65.2 History

In 1974, Regnault [1] first published her technique for breast reduction, known as the "B" technique. This was a somewhat unique procedure at the time of initial publication because of following characteristics of the procedure [2]:
1. There was no skin undermining indicated.
2. Preoperative marking accurately delineated amount of skin to be resected.
3. Resection of gland was limited to inferior and deep portions of gland.
4. Scar was limited to a short curved one that did not have a medial component, which is characteristic of the classic inverted-T pattern.
5. Design of procedure took advantage of elasticity of skin by permitting approximation and suturing of two unequal lengths of incisions on the medial and lateral flaps.

Regnault's article in 1974 [1] concerned a series of 108 patients. It included detailed description of technique, resultant complications, and discussion of long-term outcomes of the technique. She continued to provide long term follow-up in literature in 1980 [3] and again in 1989 [4]. An update to the technique was provided in 1990, which included a new one for preoperative marking and excision, and a new plication procedure for mastopexy [5]. Of note, Regnault described the system of classification for breast ptosis in 1976, which is still widely in use today [6].

65.3 Technique

The original technique as outlined by Regnault [1] can be used for both mastopexy and reduction. It can also be done with simultaneous augmentation. The technique involves two stages of marking. Regnault estimated that removal of 100 cm^3 of breast tissue produced a 1-in. reduction in combined thoracic and breast girth at nipple level [2]. This allowed the surgeon to have appropriate preoperative conversation with patient regarding desired amount of breast reduction and also to compensate for asymmetric breasts.

65.4 Marking

Three basic markings are made preoperatively as patient is sitting on the edge of the bed with shoulders in upright and level position (Fig. 65.1).

M.A. Shiffman (ed.), *Mastopexy and Breast Reduction: Principles and Practice*,
© Springer-Verlag Berlin Heidelberg 2009

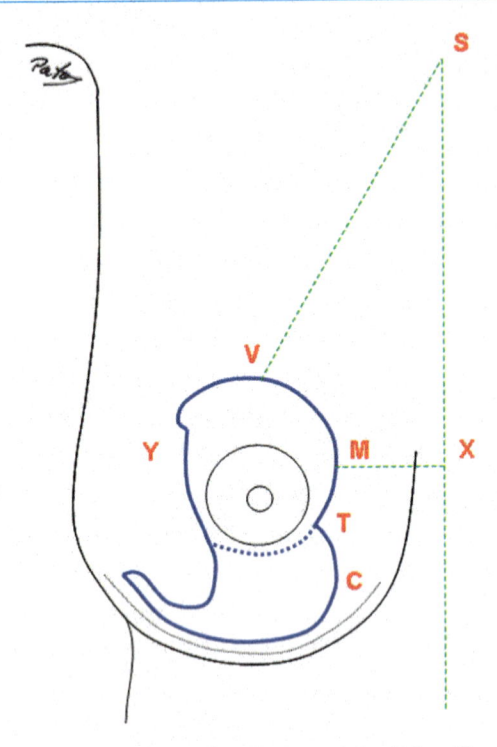

Fig. 65.1 Preoperative markings for Regnault B technique. These markings apply to both reduction and mastopexy. Note that *line XM* delineates medial border of excision, and curve C does not extend past this medial border

1. Upper limit of skin excision is marked from the sternal notch to the new upper limit of the areola. This is line marked SV.
2. Vertical and horizontal axes of the areola are marked in the sitting position to ensure proper orientation and tension of the areola at time of closure.
3. Vertical midline of chest from sternal notch to xyphoid process is also marked.

Remaining markings are then done in supine position:
1. New medial limit of the areola is marked from midline (X) to a point M, which lies on the horizontal axis perpendicular to vertical midline. This distance XM is about half of distance SV.
2. New areola is marked circumferentially, 4.5–5.5 cm in diameter.
3. A new periareolar oval is drawn, using points V and M as landmarks for a gentle curve. This oval extends to about 1 cm below current areola.
4. New inframammary fold is marked, which should lie about 1–4 cm above current inframammary fold, depending on amount of reduction to be done.
5. A curve is drawn to create lower portion of the "B," connecting the periareolar oval and the submammary fold in a gentle curve. Upper and lower curves should intersect at a 90° angle, leaving a triangular flap that is about 1 cm in length. This triangular flap is labeled T. These curves should not extend medially beyond the vertical line that includes medial limit M.
6. Originally, Regnault's description indicated a lateral gently sloping S-shaped curve to complete the marking connecting the periareolar oval with the new inframammary fold marking. However, updated technique includes a small angular flap Y, which is created in the lateral portion of the periareolar oval. It is at the level of the line horizontal to the upper limit of the current areola. It is also created at an angle of 90° with its two adjoining curves, and should also be about 1 cm in length. This angular flap will join the lower medial curve C to form the upper part of the infra-areolar vertical scar.

65.5
Surgery

Once markings are completed, patient is taken to the operating room. Procedure is carried out under general anesthesia, although smaller reduction and mastopexies can be done under local with conscious sedation. Xylocaine 0.25% with epinephrine (1:400,000) is used for infiltration of incisions and breast tissue. The technique dictates that skin incision follows all lines of preoperative marking. The periareolar area is deepithelialized, and, inferior to the areola, gland and adipose tissue are removed en bloc with skin in the case of reduction. In the mastopexy technique, only inferior and lateral portion of breast and adipose tissue is removed to lessen dog ear. Two small incisions are allowed in the dermis in the inferior aspects of the deepithelialized periareolar region, but only for a small distance (no higher than level of nipple), so as to facilitate resection of glandular tissue and later closure of breast (Fig. 65.2).

At this point, the curved lateral flap is brought medially and slightly inferior to meet with medial flap C. The medial angular flap T is brought laterally, and the lateral angular flap Y is brought medially to closely approximate the new inferior areolar curve. The areola will rotate slightly counterclockwise on the right breast and slightly clockwise on the left breast when the lateral flap is brought to the medial pillar. More tissue should be resected from medial flap than lateral flap for improved aesthetic results. All breast tissue should be removed between native inframammary fold and new marked inframammary fold. In addition, all breast tissue should

incision, provided that excision follows the natural lateral and upward curve of the given incision. The areola may need to be adjusted well to create a circular, aesthetically acceptable areola. After closure, breast will seem flat laterally and inferiorly, but will have more fullness after 3–4 weeks given effects of gravity [3].

Of note, the technique was revised in 1990 with regard to mastopexy. The upper part of the periareolar area, which has already been deepithelialized, can be undermined in the subcutaneous plane. This allows for plication sutures to be placed, usually four horizontal mattress sutures, in this upper part of the areola, providing fullness to the upper part of the finished breast. In addition, vertical plication can be done, which consists of four horizontal mattress sutures placed in the lower pole of breast in the glandular tissue. After this is completed, small resection of breast tissue is carried out according to usual technique, with the lateral skin flap brought medially and slightly downward, and subsequently sutured to the medial flap (Fig. 65.3) [5].

Sterile adhesive wound strips are applied to all incisions, and vaseline gauze and dry dressing sponges are placed on wounds. The drain is removed within 24–48 h. A bra is worn night and day for 3 weeks.

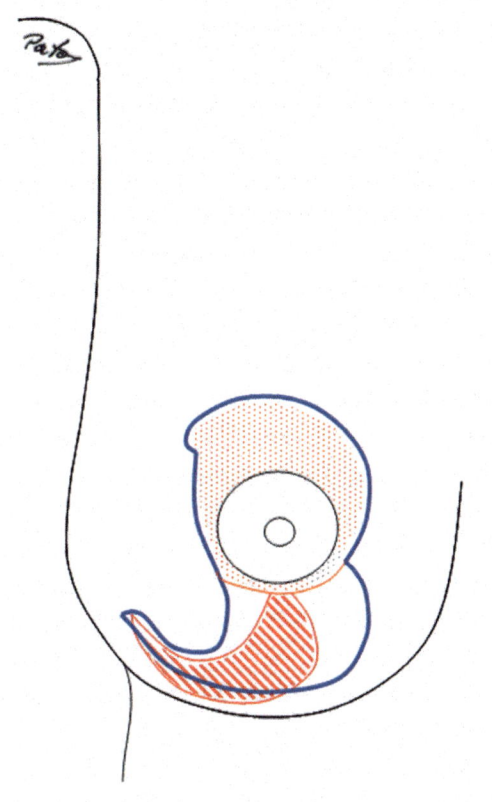

Fig. 65.2 Operative procedure. *Blue line* indicates overlying skin incision according to preoperative markings. *Dotted area* represents the periareolar area designated for deepithelialization. *Shaded area* with diagonal lines indicates area of glandular and fatty tissue resection in the reduction technique

be lifted up from the pectoral fascia up to level of the second or third rib to facilitate reshaping of new breast. Prior to suturing, the lateral flap can be brought medially, allowing the surgeon to determine line of resection of the lateral flap with respect to the medial flap in order to create an aesthetically pleasing shape without creating undue tension [4]. Medial and lateral aspects of new breast are now sutured together with absorbable suture, but are not sutured to the pectoralis fascia.

Drains are placed on individual basis when deemed necessary. Skin closure is completed in two layers with absorbable suture, first with interrupted stitches, and then with running subcuticular absorbable suture. Medial side of closure will be longer than the lateral side, and skin folds which are created by closing skin are left in place, and will flatten later. If there is a dog-ear at the end of closure, it may be excised from the lateral portion of

65.6
Complications

Early complications of this technique are similar in nature to other techniques in breast reduction and mastopexy. A hematoma takes place in 1% of all cases. Skin flap necrosis, particularly in the upper part of the lateral flap, occurs in 1.5%. Nipple–areolar complex necrosis occurs in 0.1% of cases, and tends to happen in patients who had very large reductions. Infections occur in 1% of cases are usually associated with hematoma and skin necrosis. Minimal fat necrosis is encountered with this technique.

Late complications are primarily related to the scar. Keloids are noted to occur, although rather infrequently. Sensory changes occur in 5% of patients, ranging from complete loss of feeling to diminished sensitivity [4].

Giovanoli et al. [7] prospectively studied three different techniques of reduction mammaplasty techniques in 1999. This study included a group of patients who underwent breast reduction via the B technique, and two other groups, one which underwent reduction via the Eren technique, and the other, reduction via the Frey technique. Outcomes measured included limitation in sporting activities, reduction in back pain, improvement in mastodynia, improvement in patient satisfaction, and nipple sensitivity. B technique differed

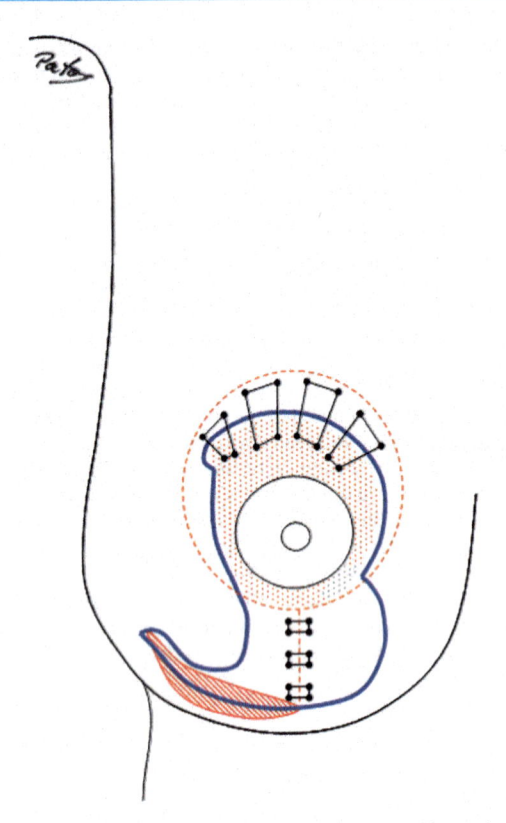

Fig. 65.3 Revised mastopexy technique. *Dotted line* indicates the nearly circumferential region of subcutaneous undermining. Note plication sutures in upper part of the periareolar area and in vertical portion of glandular tissue. Area of resection in the mastopexy is indicated by shaded area in the inferior and lateral portion of gland. Note also that *blue line* indicates skin incision and remains unchanged in this revised technique

from other two techniques in that there was no statistically significant reduction in back pain or reduction in mastodynia with this technique as opposed to other two techniques. No difference was found in patient satisfaction with regards to size, shape, and degree of ptosis. However, there was statistically significant decrease postoperatively with regard to nipple sensitivity when using B technique as measured by a subjective scale. Overall rate of minor complications, which included minimal fat necrosis, delaying wound healing, and infection, was 41.6%. Rate of major complications requiring revision was 4.7%, and 14.2% required eventual revision of scars and dog-ears. Difference in all complication rates between the three techniques was not statistically significant. Overall, B technique was favorable in small to medium size reductions because of its absence of medial scar, decreased need for secondary revisions, and retention of shape.

Peterson and Tobin retrospectively reviewed 40 patients who underwent B-technique mastopexy in 2007. Twenty-seven of these patients had simultaneous breast augmentation. Technique followed was according to Regnault's modified description published in 1990. Patients were followed for a period of 3 months. There was no incidence of hematoma, infection, or skin necrosis. Only one patient required scar revision, but none required revision of mastopexy. The authors concluded that B technique remains a viable and effective alternative for mastopexy with or without simultaneous augmentation [8].

65.7 Discussion

The Regnault technique originally met with enthusiasm on its original publication. The technique has been modified by the original author and subsequently updated in literature to accommodate experience with the technique in over 1,000 patients. The technique is versatile and can be used for both reduction and mastopexy. It can also be used with simultaneous augmentation, as indicated by the original author and by several subsequent authors [2, 8]. Although the technique is usually used for mild to moderate reductions, the author has reported its safe usage in gigantomastia (reductions larger than 800 cm^3 per breast) with minimal complications [9].

As several new techniques in breast reduction have emerged, the Regnault technique has slowly fallen out of favor. New short scar techniques, combined with new pedicle techniques, have surpassed B technique in popularity. Several newer techniques have shorter learning curve and produce consistent results. Other techniques, such as vertical scar technique, eliminate the lateral portion of the inframammary scar. However, the Regnault technique remains a very important skill in the knowledge base of the breast surgeon. Preoperative marking, once learned, easily delineates amount and location of the resection. Initial marking is reproducible, and the technique is relatively easy to learn. Resection is done en bloc, leaving a superiorly based pedicle for the nipple–areolar complex. The mastopexy technique follows same markings and excision, but with plication sutures intraoperatively to heighten aesthetic result. Use of a lateral flap initially leaves a flattened inferior pole of breast, but long-term results are very satisfactory with minimal need for revisions. Gravity provides the force needed for gradual and gentle reshaping of breast, leaving a

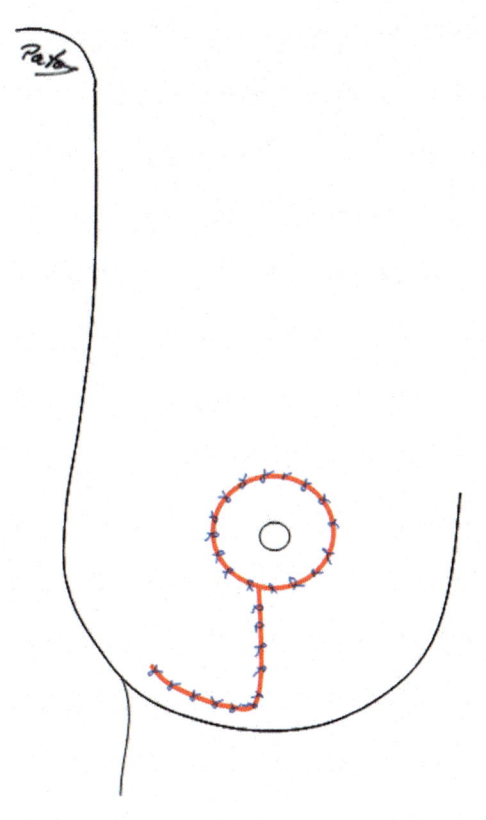

Fig. 65.4 Regnault technique final scar. Note absence of a medial scar

pleasing result. In addition, operative times for this technique are quite satisfactory, provided that time is taken outside of the operating room to perform preoperative marking [4]. The final scar pattern is quite satisfactory and does not include a medial scar in the inframammary fold (Fig. 65.4).

65.8 Conclusions

The Regnault technique remains an excellent alternative for breast reduction, mastopexy, or mastopexy/augmentation. Absence of medial scars, minimal risk of complications, and consistency of results indicate usefulness of this technique.

References

1. Regnault PC: Reduction mammaplasty by the "B" technique. Plast Reconstr Surg 1974;53(1):19–24
2. Regnault PC: Reduction mammaplasty by the "B" technique. In: Goldwyn RM (ed), Plastic and Reconstructive Surgery of the Breast. Boston, Little, Brown 1976, p 269
3. Regnault PC: Breast reduction: B technique. Plast Reconstr Surg 1980;65(6):840–845
4. Parenteau JM, Regnault PC: The Regnault "B" technique in mastopexy and breast reduction: A 12-Year Review. Aesth Plast Surg 1989;13(2):75–79
5. Regnault PC: Breast reduction and mastopexy, an old love story: B technique update. Aesthetic Plast Surg 1990;14(2):101–106
6. Regnault PC: Breast ptosis: Definition and treatment. Clin Plast Surg 1976;3(2):193–203
7. Giovanoli P, Meuli-Simmen C, Meyer VE, Frey M: Which technique for which breast? A prospective study of different techniques of reduction mammaplasty. Br J Plast Surg 1999;52(1):52–59
8. Peterson SW, Tobin HA: B mastopexy: versatility and 5-year experience. Am J Cosmetic Surg 2007; 24(2):85–90
9. Regnault PC, Hetter G: Gigantomastia: treatment by the B technique. Aesthetic Plast Surg 1977;1:115–129

Vertical (Lejour) Breast Reduction

James F. Thornton, Paul D. McCluskey

66.1
Introduction

Although a variety of skin incision patterns have been utilized with varying degrees of success, the Wise pattern inverted-T and vertical breast reduction "short scar" technique have persisted for decades. In South America and Europe, short scar or vertical methods of breast reduction have been used for many years and remain a favored method. Among these shorter scars techniques, thanks to Arie [1] and Pitanguy [2], the mosque dome pattern of skin incision has gained the greatest acceptance [3].

Understanding the technical refinements of Lejour's [4] vertical reduction mammaplasty design requires a broad understanding of the solutions that others have offered to the challenge of breast reduction and mastopexy. As multiple studies have revealed, plastic surgeons performing breast reduction typically rely on techniques learned in training or early in practice [5]. While most of these studies point to the Wise pattern inferior pedicle breast reduction as one of the preferred techniques among many plastic surgeons, vertical pattern breast reductions are increasing in popularity [5, 6].

66.2
Evolution

In 1956, Wise [7] published his experience with a refined reduction skin pattern designed in the form of a keyhole. This pattern, based on the design of commercially available brassieres at that time, has been the primary skin incision template for breast reduction for several decades. The incision leaves the classic "Inverted T" skin incision with a long horizontal or curvilinear scar at the inframammary fold (IMF), a vertical scar from the IMF to the nipple, and a periareolar scar. The technique is highly versatile and can be tailored to the needs of almost any patient desiring breast reduction or mastopexy. Despite this, a Wise pattern reduction does have limitations: Many patients do not desire the long IMF scar, the lower pole can take on a poorly rounded or flattened appearance, skin healing at the apex of the inverted "T" can be inconsistent, and over time the inferior pedicle tends to descend or "bottom-out" [8].

McKissock [9] offered a modification to Wise's technique by increasing the length of the vertical limbs to compensate for the resultant flattening of the lower pole. McKissock also employed a vertical bipedicle to enhance blood supply to the nipple–areola complex (NAC), and then imbricated the pedicle to prevent bottoming out. This technique remains popular because of the bipedicle design; however, many have noted that the longer vertical limbs actually contribute to the bottoming-out effect.

A variety of pedicle orientations can be used with either the Wise or vertical skin pattern. The initial vertical pattern mastopexies were performed by Dartigues in 1924 [10] and later by Arie in 1957 [1]. The Arie technique remains a popular alternative for mastopexy operations, but the vertical breast reduction was really popularized by Lassus in 1970 [11]. Lassus ultimately redesigned the pattern of his reduction in an effort to maintain the inferior portion of the incision at the level of the IMF.

The defining aspects of Lassus' technique include transposition of the NAC on a superiorly based dermoglandular pedicle and resection of the inferocentral portion of the gland [11–13]. The lateral composite flaps of skin and breast tissue are reapproximated centrally in a vertical scar pattern with no lateral or medial flap undermining. The initial postoperative result has a characteristic appearance of superior overcorrection that settles inferiorly over the ensuing weeks. Critics have voiced concern that the long vertical scar essentially lengthens the nipple–IMF distance, and that the superior pedicle can still bottom out. Despite its drawbacks, Lassus's contribution represented an advance in the technique of vertical breast reduction and had a strong influence on Lejour [14] and, ultimately, Elizabeth Hall-Findlay [15].

66.3
History and Physical Examination

Patients presenting with symptomatic hypermastia are often so eager to undergo breast reduction that the scarring and sensation changes associated with the operation are secondary concerns. They have suffered with back, neck, and shoulder pain, as well as shoulder notching, inframammary intertrigo, and difficulty fitting comfortably into clothes for many years, and the onus is on the surgeon to thoroughly evaluate these concerns.

A complete medical history has to be obtained. Age figures heavily into the initial workup, as it pertains to future pregnancy and breast feeding. Other critical elements of this evaluation include smoking history, family history, personal or family history of breast disease, bleeding or clotting problems in the past, history of venous thrombosis, and previous operations [16]. The physical examination should focus on vital signs, body mass index (BMI), breast masses, inframammary intertrigo, degree of breast enlargement and ptosis, skin lesions, and nipple sensation and discharge. Preoperative mammogram is recommended for patients aged 40 years and older to screen for masses and calcifications that may require further evaluation [3, 5].

Before operation, standard breast/upper torso photographs are taken, including profile, oblique, and AP views. The sternal notch-to-nipple distances and the nipple-to-IMF distances are recorded. The informed consent is then obtained, and this portion of the consultation is used as an opportunity to instruct the patient about the purpose and details of the operation. As with other plastic surgery procedures, the patient's expectations must be realistic and must be congruous with the goals of the operation with regard to the expected final shape, size, and appearance of the breasts.

Certainly, as with any operation, there are contraindications to reduction mammaplasty. Current or recent lactation and the presence of any suspicious gross or mammographic breast lesions are contraindications to surgery [17, 18]. Concern over a patient's systemic illnesses relates to anesthesia tolerance, bleeding and the ability to coagulate, recovery from surgery, and wound healing. The decision to operate on patients with multiple comorbidities is a surgeon-dependent prerogative, as is judgment of a patient's ability to understand the limitations of the procedure, or inability to accept the possible complications of the procedure [3, 8].

Key components of the informed consent should include a discussion of the risks of changes in nipples sensation, the possibility of partial or complete nipple loss, location of scars with the possibility of wound complications, as well as changes in the ability to breast-feed. The risk of deep venous thrombosis and pulmonary embolus should be discussed, especially if the breast reduction will be combined with other operations such as liposuction or abdominoplasty. In this situation, the possible need for preoperative deep vein thrombosis (DVT) prophylaxis should be addressed as well. Routine postoperative care, including presence or absence of drains, drain care, wound care, and treatment of complications should be included in the consent.

With regard to local and wound-related complications, rates of nipple necrosis and loss of nipple sensation are well documented and must be included in the preoperative discussion. The abundant blood supply to the breast is based on perforators from three major chest wall vascular routes: perforators from the internal mammary artery medially, branches from the thoracoacromial and thoracodorsal arteries superiorly, and branches from the lateral thoracic artery and intercostal perforators laterally. This rich network of perforators that arborize within the breast ultimately feeds dermal and subdermal plexuses and the periareolar plexus. Although no single vessel has been found to supply the NAC, disruption of the subdermal plexus can result in partial or total nipple loss [16].

The neurosensory supply to the breast arises from the lateral and anterior cutaneous branches of the second through sixth intercostal nerves. The nipple is supplied primarily by the fourth intercostal nerve, with contributions from the lateral third and fifth intercostal nerves and from the anterior second through fifth cutaneous nerves. It is well documented that over-dissection along the lateral border of the pectoralis major often results in an insensate nipple, and if the fourth thoracic intercostal nerve is visualized in this region it should not be skeletonized, manipulated, or divided. The multiple origins of neurosensory supply may explain how the NAC retains sensation despite the use of a variety of pedicles and degrees of undermining utilized for breast reduction [3, 19, 20].

Surgeons were initially concerned that the dissection of a superior dermoglandular pedicle transected the lateral branches of the fourth intercostal nerve posing a risk to the sensation of the NAC. The sensory branches to the NAC are now known to run deep at the level of the chest wall and perforate superficially through the breast parenchyma to reach the NAC. For this reason, keeping parenchymal resections just above the level of the chest wall preserves the nerve supply to the NAC, and therefore its sensation [20, 21].

One of the most important elements of the initial evaluation is assessing whether or not the patient is a candidate for breast reduction, and if so what skin pattern and pedicle design should be employed. Skin quality and skin elasticity are the most important factors in this determination and must be weighed with the surgeon's experience with various techniques. Although vertical breast reductions have been used successfully on all types of patients, this technique may not be ideal for every patient. Favorable candidates include younger patients with moderately enlarged or ptotic breasts. Massively overweight patients and those with poor skin elasticity may benefit from a different technique. When performing reduction mammaplasty to improve the symptoms of hypermastia, it is appropriate to suggest a trial of weight loss to the patient prior to operation. The obese patient will not only present the surgeon with much higher complication rates, but may receive little or no symptomatic benefit from breast reduction. Often in these patients, back and neck pain are associated more with the patient's BMI than with the weight of the breasts alone.

66.4 Technique

Lejour introduced her technique in 1994 with an approach highlighted by a superior dermoglandular pedicle with central breast reduction and extensive lower lateral pole undermining [14]. The mosque-pattern skin markings of the Lejour technique are adjustable, and she begins with volume-reducing liposuction. Many of her refinements borrow from the influence of Lassus, including the superior pedicle and the vertical reduction pattern which overcorrects in a superior direction allowing for settlement into the final postoperative shape (Table 66.1).

Lejour provides a detailed account of her preoperative marking process beginning with the patient in the standing position for marking. The mosque-dome skin incision and the area that represents the superior dermoglandular pedicle are marked [14]. Markings that are standard for essentially all breast reduction techniques are used, including the midline of the chest, the IMF, and the vertical axis of the breast beneath the IMF.

The position of the future NAC is marked, with care taken not to place this mark too high on the chest. Lejour positions the NAC slightly below the IMF, whereas others prefer Pitanguy's technique of transposing the new nipple position anteriorly from the level of the IMF. A hemicircle no larger than 16 cm is marked superiorly arcing downward from the new nipple position [14]. By displacing the breast medially and laterally in relation to its vertical axis, the positions of the peripheral limbs are marked. These limbs should join together no less than 5 cm above the IMF. The future areolar circumference is marked around the nipple, and a minimum of 10 cm of superior pedicle width is marked at the upper border of the future areola and continued in a conical shape down around the marked circumference (Fig. 66.1). A freehand, curvilinear marking resembling a mosque dome joins the vertical marks at a point 2 cm above the future nipple site (Fig. 66.2). This upper mark must be increased in size for larger reductions [14].

With the markings completed, the patient is taken to the operating room and placed supine on the table with

Table 66.1 Comparison of the techniques of Lassus and Lejour

Lassus	Lejour
Limited or no suction	Suction important
Round areolar deepithelialization	Mosque-dome design of de epithelialization
No undermining of skin flaps	Undermining of skin flaps from breast
No chest wall fixation	Chest wall fixation

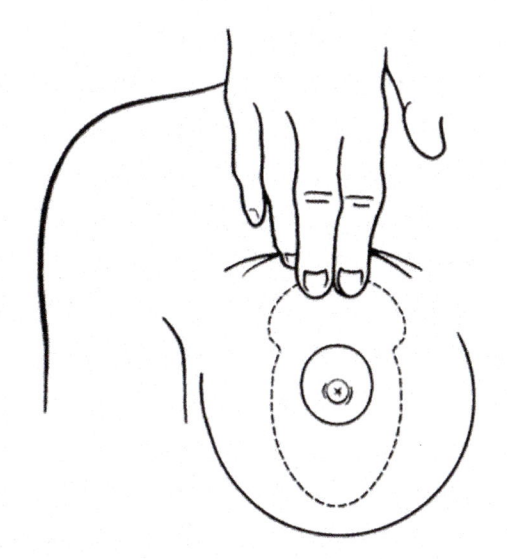

Fig. 66.1 The Lejour vertical reduction mammaplasty: Preoperative markings. Before the procedure, the breast is deviated medially and laterally and marked in line with the meridian. These lines are connected above the inframammary fold. The future position of the nipple is determined, and a free-hand mosque dome is drawn 2 cm above the nipple, connecting to the *vertical lines* (Reprinted with permission from Lejour, M. Vertical mammaplasty for breast reduction and mastopexy [22].)

arms abducted. Perioperative antibiotics are administered. The bed should be positioned (or often reversed) to allow the patient to be placed in a semisitting position intraoperatively. Lejour [14] stresses symmetry in both positioning and draping for an accurate assessment of breast symmetry with the patient on the table.

The breast parenchyma and incision lines are injected with 20–40 ml lidocaine and dilute epinephrine. The pedicle epidermis that surrounds the areola

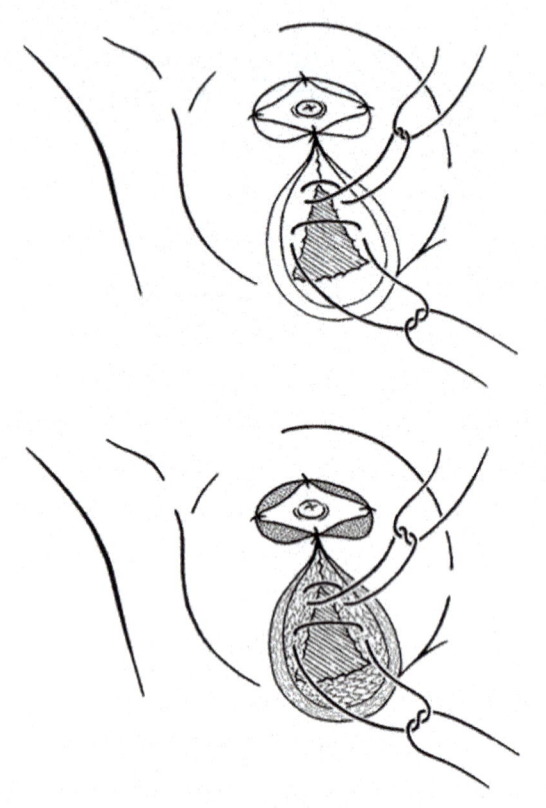

Fig. 66.2 Preoperative markings demonstrating superior periareolar pedicle and inferior skin/parenchymal resection margins of the mosque-dome pattern design

is de epithelialized to a point 2–3 cm below the areola. Suction-assisted lipectomy of the breast is then performed extending to all quadrants and levels of the breast. Only the area behind the areola is avoided. In a fatty breast, the pillars should not be oversuctioned because it will affect their ability to hold suture. Because the pillars provide the long-term support for the reduced breast, they must be left intact for suturing. Next, the medial, lower, and lateral segments of the breast are resected, with undermining of the skin below the lower curved marking [14]. Resected tissue is sent for histopathology inspection, since subclinical foci of cancer can be found in 0.1–0.9% of the specimens [17, 18].

Incisions are made along the lateral breast markings, and wide skin undermining is performed medially, laterally, and inferiorly to the level of the IMF in a plane similar to that in a subcutaneous mastectomy. This extensive undermining is one of the technical refinements, or variations, from the Lassus technique. Superficial dissection at a uniform depth allows skin redraping and contraction postoperatively. If the undermining is performed at a deeper plane, an abnormal lower breast bulge may result. No undermining is performed outside the periareolar markings. The lower central segment of the breast is elevated off the chest wall from the IMF to the upper margin of the gland, creating a 6–8-cm central tunnel. Vertical cuts are made in accordance with the degree of desired reduction, creating the new medial and lateral pillars. A 2–3-cm-thick superior dermoglandular pedicle is elevated, completing resection of the lower central segment (Fig. 66.3) [14].

A single absorbable suture elevates the nipple to its new position [14]. The suture begins at the level of the future areola on the deep surface of the pedicle and is sewn to the pectoralis fascia and muscle at the highest level of chest wall dissection. It is important to secure this suture to the deep aspect of the pedicle and not to the dermis to allow for some degree of mobility of the NAC for ease of final transposition, inset, and skin closure. The medial and lateral aspects of the pedicle are sutured to the chest wall, creating a conical underlying breast mound. Although the skin flaps may appear excessive, no further resection is performed. Rather, the skin flaps are gathered and closed in two layers. Sufficient skin gathering must be performed with this vertical suturing to reduce the closure length to 6–7 cm. A longer closure length must be avoided, as this can result in final scar extension below the IMF. The NAC is inset, and the pillars are approximated with absorbable suture. The skin is closed in two layers with dermal and subcuticular sutures. Although it is ultimately the surgeon's preference, drains can be avoided. Current evidence suggests that the incidence of seroma and wound complications in breast reduction patients is the same with and without drains [20].

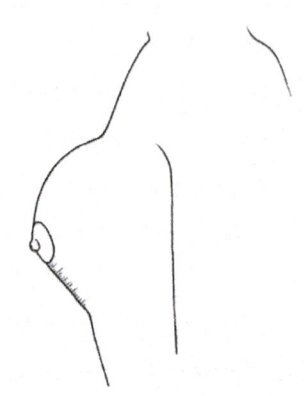

Fig. 66.3 A superior dermoglandular pedicle carries the nipple-areola complex. Volume reduction is achieved through liposuction and a central breast segment resection. (Reprinted with permission from [22])

Postoperatively, care of the Lejour breast reduction patient is surgeon dependent and does not significantly vary from the care of patients undergoing reductions by other techniques. A variety of dressings can be used, which typically include comfortable, supporting brassieres. Patients are ambulated on the day of surgery, and a light diet is resumed on the same day as well. They should avoid strenuous activity and should be advised about purchasing a comfortable sports brassiere to wear during the ensuing weeks. Regular follow-up visits are scheduled to identify and care for any possible complications. The initial follow-up visits will be used to assure the vertical breast reduction patient that the wrinkled appearance of the vertical scar will fade in 1–6 months as the breast mound settles inferiorly.

66.5
Complications

In 1999, Lejour [20] published a 10-year follow-up with a very honest and critical evaluation of her technique. This paper, which focused on complications, discussed both advantages and shortcomings of the superior pedicle vertical mammaplasty. After achieving the final postoperative shape, the reduced breast attained a stable, conical shape with minimal scarring. The internal suturing of the medial and lateral breast pillars provides postoperative breast shape and projection. According to Lejour, there is no reliance on the skin envelope to shape the postoperative breast. The use of liposuction leads to less tissue resection and, therefore, increased preservation of the nerves and vessels. Only one patient experienced permanent sensation loss in the original Lejour series. In addition, future weight loss or gain after reduction will theoretically lead to less shape change because of less fat in the postoperative breast.

Through maintenance of a wide pedicle and avoidance of any undermining of the NAC, Lejour has been able to report exceedingly low rates of nipple-related complications. In her 10 year follow-up, she noted partial areolar necrosis in 2 of 250 patients (0.8%), only one of which required surgical revision. Despite earlier concerns that creating a superior pedicle with wide subcutaneous undermining endangered NAC sensation, Lejour has reported that 7 of 170 patients experienced a reduction in sensation and only 1 of 170 had complete loss of sensation. It is possible that the sensory supply to the nipple is preserved through sources other than the lateral perforator of the fourth intercostal nerve [22].

The surgeon must provide assurance to the patient during the postoperative period in anticipation that the breast mound will settle before the final aesthetically pleasing appearance is achieved. Immediately following the operation, the breast has a characteristic shape, with exaggerated projection, and a bunched, irregular-appearing vertical scar. Patients must be counseled preoperatively about this appearance so that they may anticipate it. Fortunately, within a period of a few weeks to 6 months, the tissue settles inferiorly, giving the breast a normal, rounded form.

Secondary revision of the vertical scar is often necessary, and in many cases a horizontal component of tissue must be excised to account for inferior pole excess. The breast can be secondarily liposuctioned for volume reduction. In very large reductions or extremely ptotic breasts, a longer superior pedicle is required to transpose the nipple, which may not be reliable. Delayed healing has also been noted to occur more frequently using this method; however, wound complication rates in all breast reduction outcome studies show a strong correlation to preoperative BMI and the size or amount of reduction [3, 8].

Data regarding breast-feeding ability and nipple sensitivity are forthcoming; however, on the basis of many of Lejour's articles, the complication rate appears consistent with national averages [3, 5]. Postoperative complications in the form of seroma, wound dehiscence, hematoma, and partial nipple necrosis were seen in 10% of breasts. Liposuctioning of the breast, a technique somewhat unique to Lejour's method, was not shown to contribute to complication rates. Lejour [20] updated her experience on 324 reductions performed in 167 patients. In this study, the overall complication rate dropped to 7% of breasts. Consistent with the findings of others, she reports higher complication rates with large resections as well as in smokers and obese patients.

66.6
Conclusions

Patient satisfaction rates with breast reduction are among the highest of any procedure in plastic surgery (Fig. 66.4). In describing the relative benefits and shortcomings of the Lejour reduction mammaplasty versus other techniques and patterns, many of the aesthetic outcomes concern the surgeon's own perspective and desire for a specific postoperative appearance. In a critique of her own outcomes, Dr. Lejour cites the following potential pitfalls of the vertical design superior pedicle reduction: NAC malposition, abnormal areolar shape, hypertrophic scarring, excessive lower pole length, lower pole shape abnormalities (a flattened, boxy appearance), and lower pole redundancy (dog-ear). To be sure, Lejour is her own worst critic, and many of these characteristics are present with other techniques and can be corrected with minor secondary revisions.

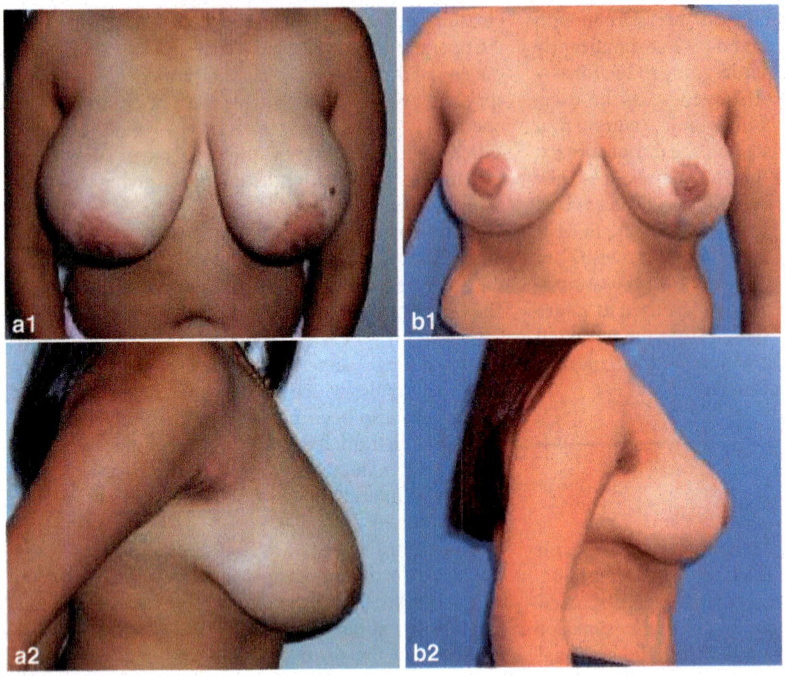

Fig. 66.4 (*a1,2*) Preoperative. (*b1,2*) Postoperative

Lejour's critique emphasizes the point that this is yet another step in the evolution of breast reduction and that innovation is required to improve aesthetic results. The effects of age and gravity are constant, and breast tissue will ultimately involute and become ptotic and the skin will lose its elastic nature. Hall-Findlay [15] and Hammond [23] offered further technical refinements to improve outcomes in vertical reduction mammaplasty. Hammond employs an inferior pedicle with his Short Scar Periareolar Inferior Pedicle Reduction, and Hall-Findlay has modified Lejour's concept by carrying the NAC on a superior–medial pedicle. Hall-Findlay cites both Lassus and Lejour as influences of her design, and because of these pioneers, residents and young plastic surgeons are learning these techniques and incorporating them into their practices. Because of this, outcome studies in vertical reduction mammaplasty will improve, leading the way for further innovation.

References

1. Arie G: Una nueva técnica de mamaplastia. Rev Lat Amer Cir Plást 1957;3:23–28
2. Pitanguy I: Mammaplstias estudio de 245 casos consecutivos e apresentacao de tecnica pessoal. Rev Bras Cir 1961;42:201–220
3. Lista F, Ahmad J: Vertical scar reduction mammaplasty: a 15-year experience including a review of 250 consecutive cases. Plast Reconstr Surg 2006;117(7):2152–2165; discussion 2166–2169
4. Lejour M: Vertical mammaplasty. Plast Reconstr Surg 1993;92(5):985–986
5. Cunningham BL, Gear AJ, Kerrigan CL, Collins ED: Analysis of breast reduction complications derived from the BRAVO study. Plast Reconstr Surg 2005;115(6):1597–1604
6. Iwuagwu OC, Stanley PW, Platt AJ, Drew PJ, Walker LG: Effects of bilateral breast reduction on anxiety and depression: results of a prospective randomized trial. Scand J Plast Reconstr Surg Hand Surg 2006;40(1):19–23
7. Wise RJ: A preliminary report on a method of planning the mammaplasty. Plast Reconstr Surg 1956;17(5):367–375
8. Miller BJ, Morris SF, Sigurdson LL, Bendor-Samuel RL, Brennan M, Davis G, Paletz JL: Prospective study of outcomes after reduction mammaplasty. Plast Reconstr Surg 2005;115(4):1025–1031; discussion 1032–1033
9. McKissock PK: Reduction mammaplasty with a vertical dermal flap. Plast Recontr Surg 1972;49(3):245–252
10. Dartigues L: Chirurgie réparatrice. In: Lépine R (ed). Plastique et Esthétique de la Poitrine et de l'Abdomen. Paris 1924, pp 44–47
11. Lassus C: A technique for breast reduction. Int Surg 1970;53(1):69–72

12. Lassus C: An "all-season" mammoplasty. Aesthetic Plast Surg 1986;10(1):9–15
13. Lassus C: Breast reduction: Evolution of a technique–a single vertical scar. Aesthetic Plast Surg 1987;11(2): 107–112
14. Lejour M: Vertical mammaplasty and liposuction of the breast. Plast Reconstr Surg 1994;94(1):100–114
15. Hall-Findlay EJ: A simplified vertical mammaplasty: shortening the learning curve. Plast Reconstr Surg 1999;104(3):748–759
16. Schumacher HH: Breast reduction and smoking. Ann Plast Surg 2005;54(2):117–119
17. Kakagia D, Fragia K, Grekou A, Tsoutsos D: Reduction mammaplasty specimens and occult breast carcinomas. Eur J Surg Oncol 2005;31(1):19–21
18. Pitanguy I, Torres E, Salgado F, Pires Viana GA: Breast pathology and reduction mammaplasty. Plast Reconstr Surg 2005;115(3):729–734; discussion 735
19. Weiner DL, Aiache AE, Silver L, Tittiranonda T: A single dermal pedicle for nipple transposition in subcutaneous mastectomy, reduction mammaplasty, or mastopexy. Plast Reconstr Surg 1973;51(2):115–120
20. Lejour M: Vertical Mammaplasty: early complications after 250 personal consecutive cases. Plast Reconstr Surg 1999;104(3):764–770
21. O'Blenes CA, Delbridge CL, Miller BJ, Pantelis A, Morris SF: Prospective study of outcomes after reduction mammaplasty: long-term follow-up. Plast Reconstr Surg 2006;117(2):351–358
22. Lejour, M: Vertical mammaplasty for breast reduction and mastopexy. In: Spear SL (ed). Surgery of the Breast: Principles and Art. Philadelphia, Lippincott-Raven 1998, p 735
23. Hammond DC: Short scar periareolar inferior pedicle reduction. Plast Reconstr Surg 1999;103(3):890–901

Liposuction and Vertical Breast Reduction

Felix Giebler

67.1 Introduction

In the search for a well-formed breast with less scaring and more symmetry, liposuction of the breast tissue is very helpful. Liposuction of the breast is an adjunctive procedure for the refinement of the form, especially the fat pads before the axilla and in the axilla that can be easily treated with liposuction, and the slight asymmetry at the end of the operation and "dog ears" may be treated as well. In specific cases it maybe an advantage to reduce the fat volume before the resection in order to make the tissue more pliable and the scars shorter.

67.2 History

The vertical resection techniques and the short scar techniques started with Dartigues [1] in 1925. This mainly conic form resection technique was generally implemented without liposuction [2].

The technique of liposuction was invented by Illouz [3], Fischer [4], and Schrudde [5]. It was only a matter of time before liposuction would be applied to the female breast. Madeleine Lejour [6] was the first surgeon who started the use of liposuction systematically. The combined operative procedures make it more possible to treat larger breast volumes with a short scar technique [7].

67.3 Technique

After defining the resection area (with a pinch test), the breasts are infiltrated. Normal blunt infiltration cannulas should be used. Infiltration is performed on each side with Klein's solution [8] with 150–500 ml depending on the size of the breasts [9]. The parenchyma of the breast should not be infiltrated or suctioned. It is wise to make sure preoperatively as to where the parenchyma is by the use of mammography and palpation and/or MRI. Ultrasound assistance can also be helpful. The injection should spread from one point with the syringe technique [10]. With the pump technique there is a greater danger of damaging the breast tissue because of the resistance of the tissue during the infiltration.

After deepithialization of the resection area (Fig. 67.1), the liposuction is started through an entry point 2 cm below the nipple–areola complex (NAC) with blunt cannulas. The placement of the cannula should be done radially and with a light touch, so as not to penetrate the gland (Fig. 67.2), which is noticeable through the resistance of the tissue and the guiding left hand. The author uses cannulas 1–3 mm in diameter with three holes. The extracted fat should be clear gold in color. At the end of the liposuction, there may be blood in the supernatant fat, which is the signal for stopping the procedure. After the liposuction and the conic formed resection of the gland, the zigzag plasty [11] on the lower pole, follows the free nipple positioning at the centre of the breast hillock (Fig. 67.3), which should be done a bit too low instead of too high. The symmetry should be checked from the foot end of the patient.

67.4 Complications

Through the liposuction manoeuvres there is traumatization of the tissue. Blunt cannulas may puncture the gland and cause bleeding or open up the gland ducts. It is a problem when an operation for aesthetics interferes with the health of the patient. Every operation on the breast leaves scars in the tissue in the subcutaneous fat or in the parenchyma. Any operation on the breast interferes with the most important screening method of mammography for breast cancer [12].

In very rare cases a severe complication may occur such as pneumothorax, when the cannula is not directed parallel to the thoracic cage by the guiding hand and penetrates the intercostal space [13].

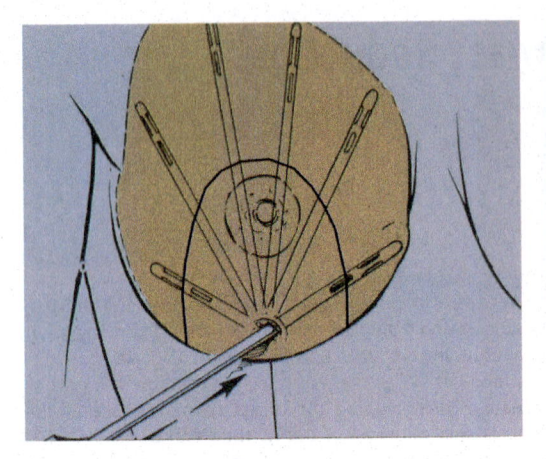

Fig. 67.1 The incision for liposuction is placed within the de-epithelialized area. Make sure not to perforate the gland

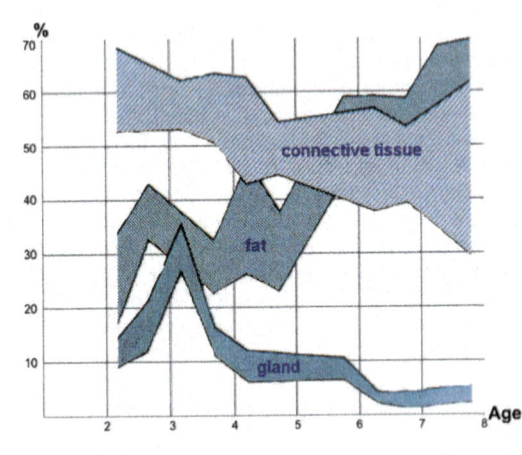

Fig. 67.2 In advanced age there is a physiological reduction of parenchyma and an increase of fat and connective tissue

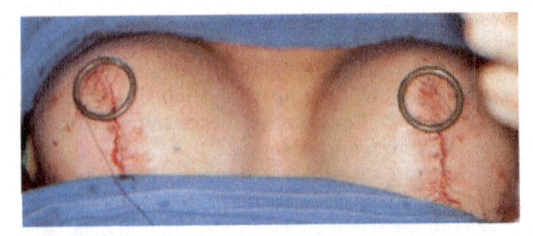

Fig. 67.3 Free nipple positioning of the nipple–areolar complex (NAC) after forming the breast hillocks. Make sure not to place the NAC to high. Check for symmetry

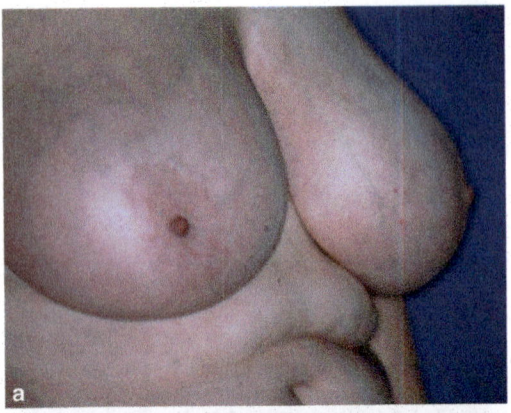

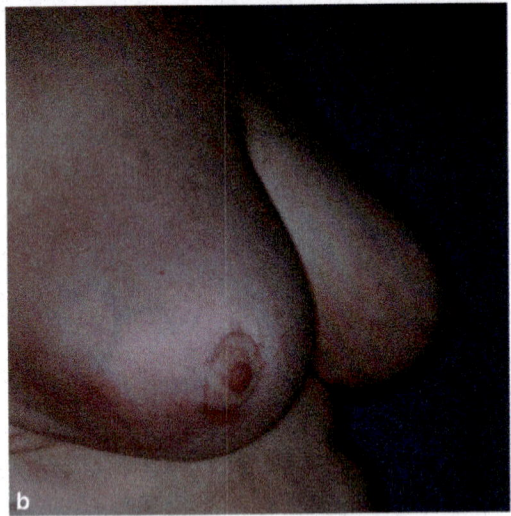

Fig. 67.4 (**a**) Preoperative 60-year-old patient. (**b**) Fourteen days after the operation. There is bruising around the NAC and the lateral pole is contoured by liposuction

67.5 Conclusions

Liposuction influences the mammogram [14] but the interpretation of a roentgenogram of an operated breast is easy for an experienced radiologist. A baseline mammography before the operation is mandatory for any cosmetic operation. In comparison to the pre- and postoperative mammogram, the changes in the mammographic pictures are obviously detectable. If there are still doubts, MRI [15], ultrasound, thermography, and stereotactic biopsy can clear the diagnosis [16]. Traumatizing of the tissue takes place in two ways, with the scalpel and with the blunt cannulas, leading to delayed healing and bruising, and the prophylactic administration of antibiotics is advisable.

Liposuction helps to refine the breast form (Fig. 67.4), especially in the area of the axilla and the sternum. Possible "dogs ears" may be flattened by liposuction. Larger breast volumes are easier to resect, and the breast is by far very pliable. Liposuction of the breast is an adjunctive procedure of the vertical resection technique and gives a better chance for the symmetry of the breast [17] (Table 67.1).

Table 67.1 Total information required by law. It is important what you tell your patients before the operation

What to tell my patients
Total information required by law
Delayed healing 10–15%
Scaring 15%
Haematoma 6–10%
Fat necrosis 2–9%
Necrosis of the NAC 0.5–7%
Loss of breast feeding 50%
Loss of sensibility of the NAC 8%
Asymmetry 10%

References

1. Dartigues L: Traitement chirurgical du prolapsus mammaire. Arch Franco-Belg Chir 1925;28:313
2. Biesenberger H: Eine neue methode der mammaplastik. Zbl Chir 1928;38:2382–2387
3. Illouz YG: Body contouring by lipolysis: a 5-year experience with over 3000 cases. Plast Reconstr Surg 1983;72(5):591–597
4. Fischer A, Fischer G: Revised techniques for cellulites fat reduction in riding breeches deformity. Bull Int Acad Cosm Surg 1977;2(4):40–43
5. Schrudde J: Lipexeresis as a means of eliminating local adiposity. Aesthetic Plast Surg 1980;4:215
6. Lejour M: Vertical Mammaplasty and Liposuction. St. Louis, Quality Medical Publishing 1994
7. Lassus C: New refinements in vertical mammaplasty. Chir Plast 1986;6:81
8. Klein, JA: The tumescent technique for liposuction surgery. Am J Cosm Surg 1987;4:263–267
9. Rygnestad T, Brevik BK, Samdal F: Plasma concentrations of lidocaine and alpha1-acid glycoprotein during and after breast augmentation. Plast Reconstr Surg 1999;103(4):1267–1272
10. Fournier P: Why the syringe and not the suction machine. J Dermatol Surg Oncol 1988;14(10):1062–1071
11. Giebler FRG: Verticale reductionplastik. Aesth Trib 7 Wiesbaden 15, 2006
12. Shwartz M: An analysis of the benefits of serial screening for breast cancer based upon a mathematical model of the disease. Cancer 1978;41(4):1550–1564
13. Coleman WP 3rd: Guidelines of care for liposuction. J Am Acad Dermatol 2001;45(3):438–447
14. Brown FE, Sargent SK, Cohen SR, Morain WD: Mammographic changes following reduction mammoplasty. Plast Reconstr Surg 1987;80(5):691–698
15. Warner E, Plewes DB, Shumak RS, Catzavelos GC, Di Prospero LS, Yafee MG, Goel V, Ramsey E, Chart PL, Cole DE, Taylor GA, Cutrara M, Samuels TH, Murphy GM, Narod SA: Comparison of breast magnetic resonance imaging, mammography, and ultrasound for surveillance of women at high risk for hereditary breast cancer. J Clin Oncol 2001;19(15):3524–3531
16. Kuhl CK, Elevelt A, Leutner CC, Gieseke J, Pakos E, Schild HH: Interventional breast MR imaging: clinical use of a stereotactic localization and biopsy device. Radiology 1997;204(3):667–675
17. Schnur PL, Hoehn JG, Ilstrup DM, Cahoy MJ, Chu CP: Reduction mammaplasty: cosmetic or reconstructive procedure? Ann Plast Surg 1991;27(3):232–237

The Circumvertical Reduction Mammaplasty

A. Aldo Mottura

68.1 Introduction

Since 20 years ago when the periareolar technique first and the vertical techniques later were introduced into plastic surgery practice, a new concept in breast reductions with fewer and smaller scars has emerged [1]. Since then, different practitioners have popularized techniques that, after the initial enthusiasm, have found their place and are now being used by many plastic surgeons. To reduce the size of a breast with small scars is not an easy task. There are many new concepts that have to be understood and experienced until good results are obtained. There is also some controversy between leaving small scars and giving a nice shape to the breast. Nowadays, periareolar [2] techniques are used mostly for small hypertrophies, whereas the vertical one can be used for moderate or big hypertrophies [3–11]. To reduce the length of the vertical scar, I began using a combination of the periareolar and the vertical techniques. For 15 years now, the evolution of the primitive circumvertical skin incisions and personal observations have allowed me to reach interesting conclusions. Circumvertical reduction mastoplasty [12–16] is a procedure that comprises concepts and principles very different from those of the vertical ones.

68.2 Surgical Technique

It is fundamental to have information on what breast size the patient wants (small or moderate) and whether she prefers a flat or a projected one. This provides an estimation of how much will be the glandular removal. The author compares the amount to be removed with the size of each breast implant. Plan to remove 300–700 g or different amounts of each according to the breast asymmetries.

With the patient in a standing position, the areola is moved to the estimated location of placement and the skin is marked at what will be the superior border of the new areola placement. Marks are made 4–6 cm medially and laterally from the nipple. Combining these three points, a semicircular inferior concave figure line is drawn, which is extended laterally downwards converging in a point 2–4 cm above the sub mammary fold (SMF). The same is done on the contralateral side.

Before beginning the surgery, each breast is thoroughly infiltrated with 250–300 ml of anesthetic solution at the submammary prepectoralis space at the subcutaneous inferior half of the breast and under the areola. The anesthetic solution is prepared with 25 ml 2% lidocaine, 25 ml 0.5% bupivacaine, and 1 ml 1:1000 adrenalin diluted in 450–550 ml of ringer lactate solution.

Once the whole periareolar skin is de-epithelialized (Fig. 68.1), the skin is undermined at the inferior half of the breast medially and laterally (Fig. 68.2). The inferior half of the breast is also detached from the pectoralis major muscle. This way, the dissected breast comes out and can be marked in a W-Wise pattern resection (Fig. 68.3) which is at the inferior quadrant and at the inferior part of the medial and lateral quadrants. After the resection, the lateral and medial glandular wedges are sutured medially in 2–3 layers (Fig. 68.4). To fix the gland to the pectoral muscle, three to four separate Vicryl 3-0 sutures are placed all along the inferior border of the pectoral muscle (Fig. 68.5). The areola is moved to the superior border of the skin and fixed with a 3-0 subdermal Vicryl suture. To finish the surgery, a suture is placed 8–10 cm from the inferior part of the skin, dividing the wound into two parts: the superior round periareolar, and the inferior vertical ellipse (Fig. 68.6). The inferior part is sutured in a vertical fashion with a 3-0 Vicryl subdermal running suture. The periareolar skin is sutured to the areolar border with another subdermal running suture. To finish the surgery, all the wounds are closed with intradermal 5-0 Vicryl suture (Fig. 68.7). Aspiration drains are placed laterally, and the wounds are fixed with paper tapes.

This technique is indicated when there is an acceptable skin quality, the amount to be removed is less than 1,000 g, and the areola elevation can be no more than 10 cm.

M.A. Shiffman (ed.), *Mastopexy and Breast Reduction: Principles and Practice*,
© Springer-Verlag Berlin Heidelberg 2009

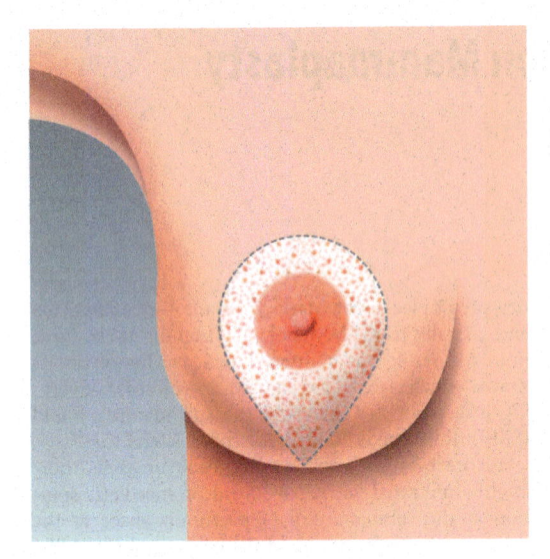

Fig. 68.1 The whole periareolar skin is de-epithelialized

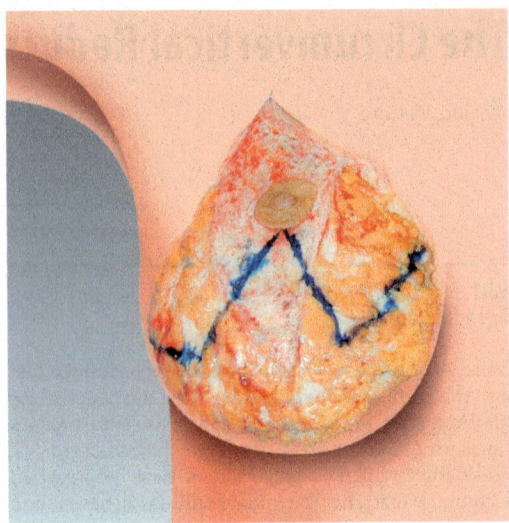

Fig. 68.3 The dissected breast can be marked in a W-Wise pattern resection

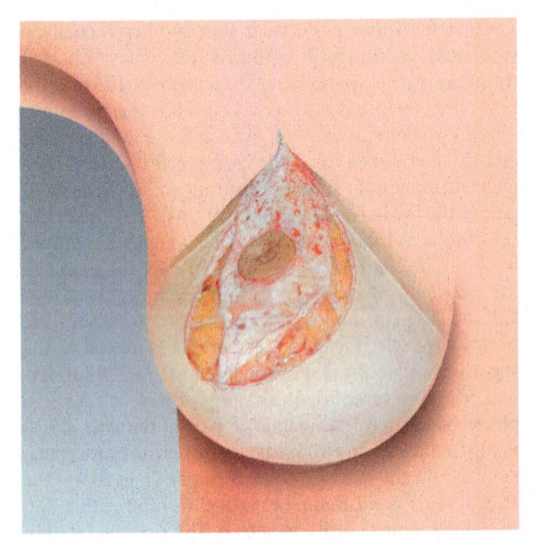

Fig. 68.2 The skin is undermined at the inferior half of the breast medially and laterally

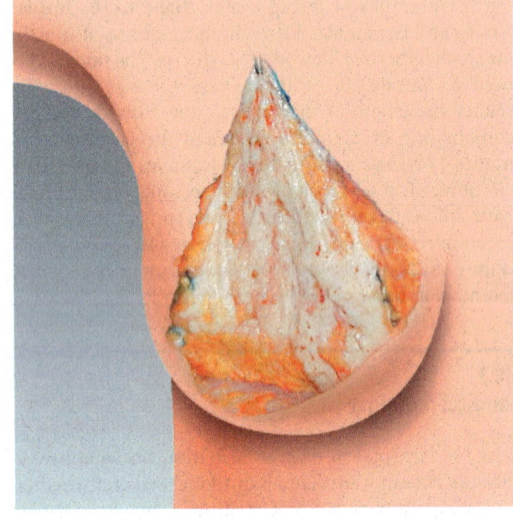

Fig. 68.4 The lateral and medial glandular wedges are sutured medially in 2–3 layers

68.3 Discussion

During surgery the marked lines are followed, and the estimation of the glandular removal is planned before surgery. This is especially important when there are asymmetries. As there is a great variety of breast hypertrophies, it is necessary to plan before surgery from which part of the breast more tissue has to be removed, and when there are difficult asymmetries, to draw a draft of the future areas to be removed as a surgical guide.

The author never uses liposuction to reduce the volume because it is better to reshape a firm breast with scalpel and sutures. Suturing the breast pillars vertically and at the base of the breast will project a flat breast (Fig. 68.8). The new conic shape of the breast is sculpted

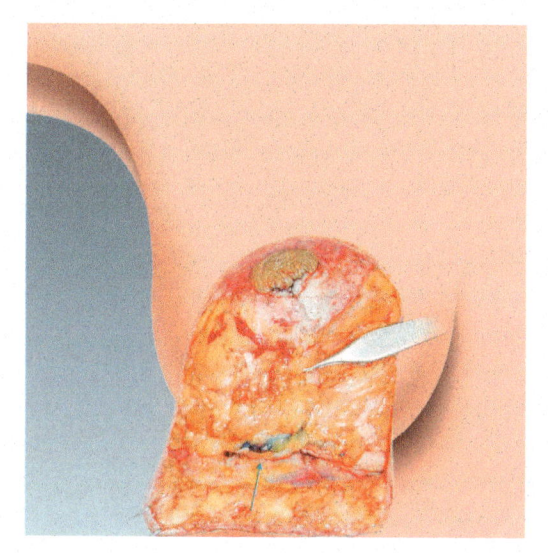

Fig. 68.5 Separate sutures are placed all along the inferior border of the pectoral muscle

in this way. By suturing the new inferior border of the breast to the pectoralis fascia, a clear SMF is defined and the gland is fixed to the muscle, thereby avoiding the possible bottoming out of the breast.

When the inferior part of the breast is removed, the skin that previously covered the breast will now attach to the thoracic wall. The suture that divides the wound can be regulated during surgery. If it is placed in a higher position, the periareolar diameter will be reduced and the vertical one enlarged, whereas if it is placed in a lower position, the periareolar diameter is wider and the vertical one is shortened (Fig. 68.9). This possibility of variations is important when a harmonic distribution of the pleats is to be achieved.

The subdermal cinching running periareolar [17] suture approximates the skin to the areola, leaving no dead spaces. As the pleats are harmonically distributed at the periareolar and vertical wounds and the undermined skin retracts during surgery, an acceptable, good result can be observed when the surgery is over.

Once the areola is moved and fixed to the superior border of the skin, all the skin moves towards the areola, and the vertical wound is also ascended this way never crossing the SMF (Fig. 68.10). The author has never had to transform a vertical into an "inverted-T" during or after surgery. As the areola is moved without any pedicle, its blood supply and the venous flow are not altered, and as the lactiferous ducts are not transected, the lactation function is not disturbed either.

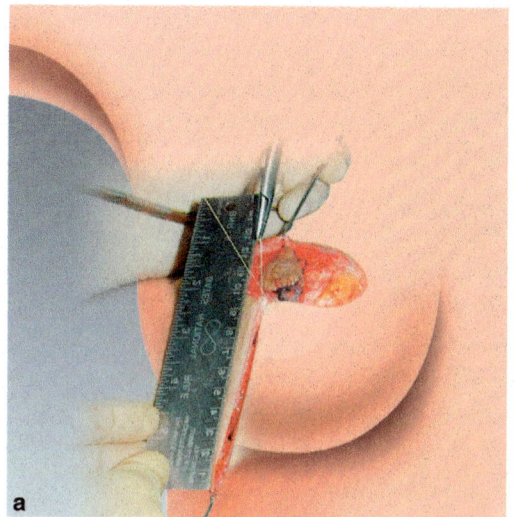

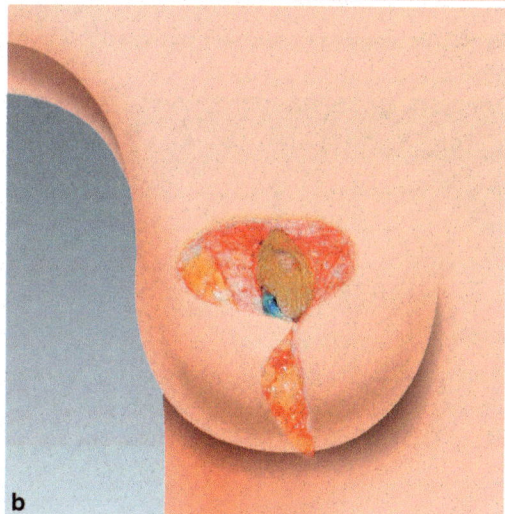

Fig. 68.6 A suture is placed 8–10 cm from the inferior part of the skin, dividing the wound into two parts. (**a**) The superior round periareolar. (**b**) The inferior vertical ellipse

This method of glandular removal at the inferior part of the breast and the areola transposition without a pedicle leaves a breast without alteration of it normal anatomy, an important factor to monitor the breast with mammograms over the years.

The use of large amounts of diluted anesthetic solution decreases the bleeding, and the hydraulic dissection facilitates the surgery and gives some hours of postoperative pain relief. All the surgeries are performed under local anesthesia and deep sedation, controlled by an anesthesiologist.

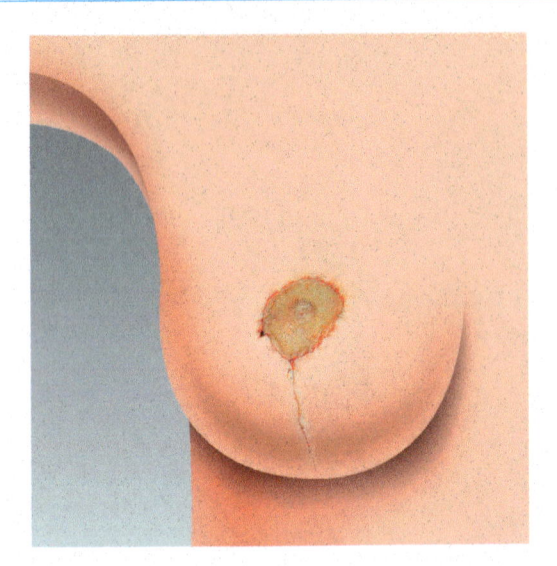

Fig. 68.7 The wounds are closed with intradermal 5–0 Vicryl suture

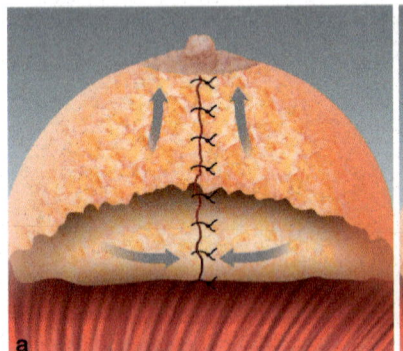

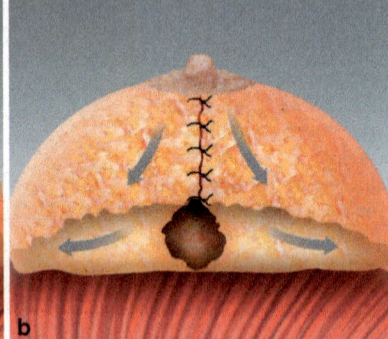

Fig. 68.8 Projecting a flat breast by (**a**) Suturing the breast pillars vertically, (**b**) Suturing at the base of the breast

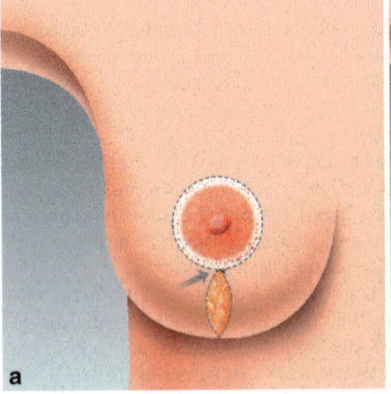

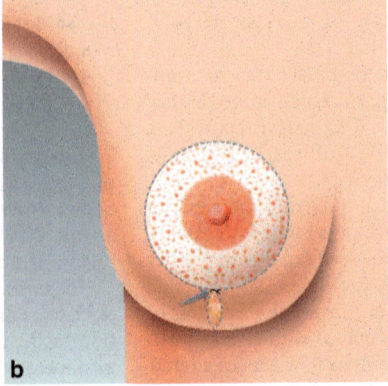

Fig. 68.9 The suture that divided the wound can be regulated during surgery. (**a**) If it is placed in a higher position, the periareolar diameter will be reduced and the vertical one enlarged. (**b**) If it is placed in a lower position, the periareolar diameter is wider and the vertical one is shortened

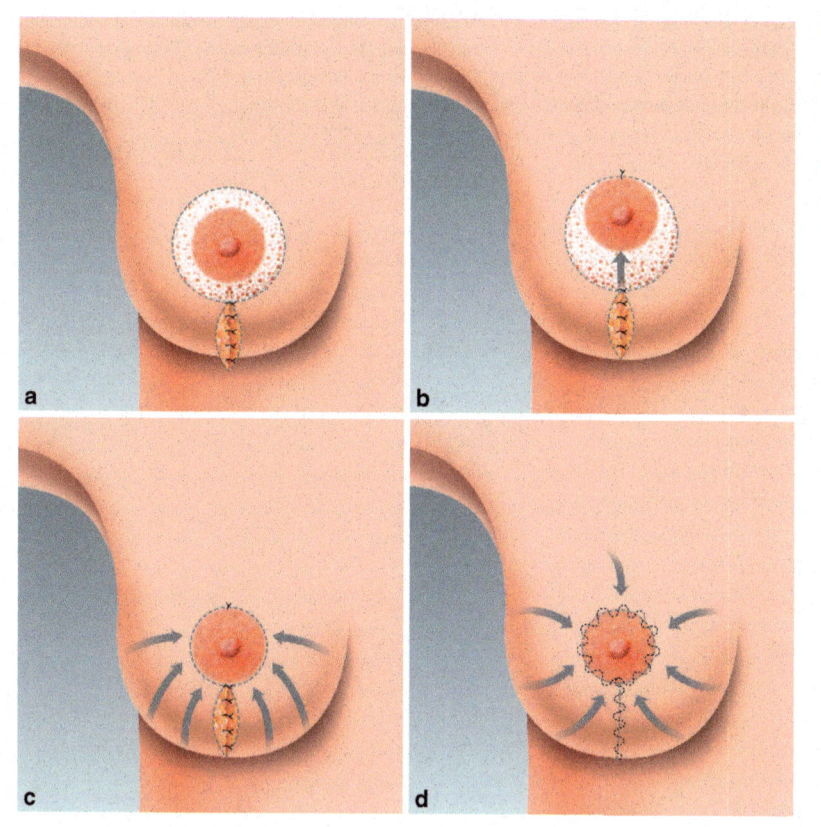

Fig. 68.10 Once the areola is moved and fixed to the superior border of the skin, all the skin moves towards the areola, thus the vertical wound is also ascended this way never crossing the submammary fold (SMF)

68.4 Conclusions

After breast removal using the circumvertical reduction mastoplasty, a conic breast is reshaped, a new SMF is defined, and the parenchyma is fixed to the pectoral fascia. Most of the skin is gathered around the areola, there is a harmonic distribution of the pleats all along the wounds, and the vertical wounds never cross the SMF. Furthermore, without any pedicle for areola transposition, its blood supply and breast-feeding function remain unaltered. An important difference from the vertical techniques is that a nice result can be observed at the end of the surgery.

References

1. Nahai F: Scar wars. Aesthet Surg 2000;24:461
2. Benelli L: A new periareolar mammaplasty: The "round block" technique. Aesth Plast Surg 1990;14(2):93–100
3. Graf R, Biggs TM: In search of better shape in mastopexy and reduction mammoplasty. Plast Reconst Surg 002;110(1):309–317
4. Graf R: Breast shape: A technique for better upper pole fullness. Aesthetic Plast Surg 2000;24(5):348–352
5. Hall-Findley EJ: A simplified vertical reduction mammaplasty: shortening the learning curve. Plast Reconst Surg 1999;104(3):748–759
6. Hammond D: The SPAIR mammaplasty. Clin Plast Surg 2002;29(3):411–421
7. Lassus C: Breast reduction: Evolution of a technique: A single vertical scar. Aesthetic Plast Surg 1987;11(2):107–112
8. Lassus C: Update on vertical mammaplasty. Plast Reconstr Surg 1999;104(7):2289–2304
9. Lejour M: Suction mammaplasty. Plast Reconstr Surg 1992;89(1):158–162
10. Lejour M: Vertical mammaplasty and liposuction of the breast. Plast Reconstr Surg 1994;94(1):100–114
11. Menke H, Restel B, Olbrisch RR: Vertical scar reduction mammaplasty as a standard procedure – Experiences in the introduction and validation of a modified reduction technique. Eur J Plast Surg1999;22:74–79

12. Mottura AA: Local anesthesia in reduction mastoplasty for out-patient surgery. Aesthetic Plast Surg 1992;16(4):309–315
13. Mottura AA: Mastoplastia reductiva con anestesia local. Rev Arg de Mastol 1990;9:56–51
14. Mottura AA, Procikieviez O: Mastoplastia reductiva periareolar. Rev Arg de Cir Plast 1996;2:195–198
15. Mottura AA: Zirkumverticale mammareduktionplastik. In: Lemperle G (ed). Aesthetische Chirurghie, 1st edn. Ecomed, Grand Werk 1998, pp 1–5
16. Mottura AA: Circumvertical Reduction mastoplasty. Aesthet Surg J 2000;20:199–204
17. Ersek RA, Ersek SL: Circular cinching stitch. Plast Reconstr Surg 1991;88(2):350–352

Eliminating the Vertical Scar in Breast Reduction

Simon G Talbot, Julian J Pribaz

69.1
Introduction

Reduction mammaplasty is one of the most commonly performed breast operations in the United States. In 2006, over 104,000 breast reductions were reported by the American Society of Plastic Surgeons, ranking it among the top five reconstructive procedures performed in the US, and representing a 162% increase from 1992 [1]. Breast reduction, in general, is associated with high patient satisfaction and significant improvements in health-related quality of life [2, 3].

Many techniques of breast reduction exist, with skin incisions including the inverted-T method, vertical-scar technique, vertical mammaplasty with short horizontal scar, periareolar technique, short-scar periareolar technique, L-short-scar mammaplasty, reduction with free nipple grafting, and liposuction alone. Each of these skin incisions has also been adapted to include a variety of pedicles such as the inferior, lateral, superomedial, central, vertical bipedicle, and horizontal. In addition, countless variations and combinations of these have been developed. The most popular technique currently is one of the various forms of inverted-T scar methods, such as the Wise-pattern reduction [4, 5].

All methods of breast reduction share several key principles: removal of excess and redundant parenchyma, removal of excess skin, preservation of the nipple–areola complex (NAC) vascularity, and reshaping of the breast [4]. Ideally, production of the "perfect" breast size and shape are achieved with minimal scarring, normal nipple vascularity and sensation, good projection, a stable inframammary fold (IMF), preservation of the ability to lactate [6], and structural stability over time. Furthermore, a method should be relatively easy to perform, reproducible by other surgeons, easy to teach, expeditious, and free from complications. However, as evidenced by the number of operations available, no one procedure has been able to reliably provide all of the above; there is no technique which is ideal "for all seasons."

While no one individual technique of breast reduction fulfills all criteria for the "perfect" operation, the key to the best result lies in correct patient selection for a particular procedure. Breast reduction without a vertical scar is no exception.

69.2
History

69.2.1
Breast Reduction

The first breast reduction likely dates to 1669, performed by William Durston [7]. Numerous techniques were developed later, many based on Schwarzmann's [8] paper from the 1930s detailing the subdermal plexus blood supply to the nipple and the concept of a de-epithelialized pedicle to maintain nipple–areolar perfusion. By 1956, Wise [9] published a detailed report on the geometry of the breast and planning of a breast reduction, from which arose the commonly known "Wise-pattern" breast reduction, commonly used today, based on an inferior de-epithelialized pedicle and inverted-T scar with excisions of "wedges of gland from one or more quadrants." Breast reduction after 1960 saw significant development in techniques using this inverted-T scar based on the Wise-pattern reduction and further modified with the use of a variety of de-epithelialized pedicles [10–12].

69.2.2
Minimizing Scarring in Breast Reduction

Minimization of scarring in breast reduction has been sought by many surgeons including Benelli (periareolar reduction) [4, 13], Lassus (vertical reduction) [10], Lejour (modification of the vertical reduction) [14, 15], Hall-Findlay (simplified vertical reduction) [16], and Ramirez [17]. However, many of these techniques have been based on periareolar scars or reduction of the horizontal/IMF scars.

While patients are generally very satisfied with breast reduction surgery, especially owing to relief from physical symptoms, cosmetic concerns from scarring remain a concern for many [3]. Notably, patients appear to be

M.A. Shiffman (ed.), *Mastopexy and Breast Reduction: Principles and Practice*,
© Springer-Verlag Berlin Heidelberg 2009

most pleased with periareolar scars. Surgeon evaluations demonstrate similar hypertrophy and color matching for periareolar, vertical, and inframammary scars, except that the vertical scar has a tendency to widen over time [3]. In addition, a well-placed inframammary scar remains in the zone 2 cosmetic unit of the breast and is typically hidden by the breast mound when viewed from the front or in a mirror [5, 18].

69.2.3
Eliminating the Vertical Scar in Breast Reduction

Several arguments can be made to eliminate the vertical scar in breast reduction surgery. First, extensive scarring due to inverted-T pattern reductions can be unaesthetic, wound complications may occur especially at the "T-intersection" of the incisions, and this region is prone to hypertrophic scarring [6, 19]. Second, loss of shape through pseudoptosis or "bottoming out" due to instability of the postoperative IMF may result in an unfavorable change in breast shape in the long term. Third, in cases of very large breast reductions, the length of a typical narrow, inverted-T-style inferior pedicle may be too long to reliably support the NAC, with some practitioners advocating free nipple grafting when a transposition of greater than 10 cm is required [20]. Breast reduction for very large breasts have been plagued by concerns over nipple vascularity and sensation, which may be compromised using techniques most suited for smaller reductions [19]. Fourth, wound-healing forces caused by contraction of the vertical scar may distort the periareolar scar, causing an ovoid shape of the areola over time [5]. For these reasons, numerous practitioners have sought to create a breast reduction operation that eliminates the vertical scar.

69.2.4
The Development of Various Methods

Passot [21] is frequently credited with developing the first breast reduction technique not requiring a vertical scar, in the 1920s. He did, however, use the technique only in cases with minimal hypertrophy and moderate ptosis, with excess tissue being removed as a wedge only from the inferior pole of the breast [22].

In 1967, Robertson [23] published a paper on a technique of breast reduction excising a wedge of breast tissue through the horizontal mid-axis of the breast. The original Robertson technique is a method of inferior flap reduction in which a central wedge of tissue comprises the reduction including the tissue underlying the nipple. This resulted in a bell-shaped, curved scar through the mid-axis and NAC, which were then re-sited with free nipple grafting. In contrast to pedicle mammaplasties, this technique removes central breast tissue, and covers the remaining breast with an inferior flap. The steep bell-shaped inferior incision and straight superior incision eliminate the discrepancy between incision lengths but leave a curved scar through the horizontal mid-axis of the breast.

Ribeiro [22] re-popularized Passot's technique in 1975. This was primarily an attempt at reducing scars visible on the breast while also maintaining NAC survival and sensation, with good breast contour produced by a conically sutured breast mound [24]. The original paper refers to a modification of the techniques used by Thorek [25], Maliniac [26], and Conway [27], all of which frequently used free nipple grafts in contrast to Ribeiro's technique. Maliniac also detailed a two-stage dissection in which NAC necrosis is prevented by "delaying" this flap rather than relying on a dermal pedicle [26]. Ribeiro placed the inferior incision 2 cm below in the IMF and, in contrast to other authors, refers to this dropping to the "proper position" after healing. He also used sutures to keep the inferior pedicle conical in shape and maintained breast shape using plaster of Paris while healing. In a later paper on this method, Ribeiro [28] detailed how the long horizontal scars and flattening of the breast led to less use of this technique, and instead continued to use an inferior glandular dermo-lipo pedicle in a modified form in inverted-T, vertical scar, and periareolar techniques.

The original Robertson technique was first modified by Hurst et al. [29], who in 1983 published a report of lowering the scar from the mid-axis of the breast to become a bell shape just inferior to the nipple, while the nipple was maintained on a broad inferior pedicle. Hurst's modification of the original Robertson technique (the modified Robertson technique) avoids free nipple grafting, which he described as "hypoesthetic" and of "poor cosmetic appearance" [29], by using an inferior dermal pedicle instead of the lower inferior breast flap described by Robertson.

Yousif et al. [18] in the early 1990s published a paper explaining their use of a no vertical scar technique for cases of very large and/or ptotic breasts, primarily to reduce unsightly scars, later termed the "apron technique" [30]. They use this method only when the edge of the NAC is greater than 7.1 cm from the center of the planned new nipple location to allow draping of a superiorly based flap over the pedicle with sufficient nonpigmented skin to form coverage over a new lower pole. Notably, they tack the superior and inferior breast tissue (which remains after a wedge excision) to one another in an axial plane. They emphasize the concept that the final shape of the breast depends on the underlying shape of the tissue and not on the skin envelope, stressing that "internal mound contouring" can help to eliminate a vertical scar by shaping the underlying breast tissue into a conical form. They also place emphasis on gathering the inferior skin excess to the center of the incision, creating several small cones, in order to maintain projection.

The no vertical scar breast reduction or Boston modification of the Robertson technique is a method designed to eliminate the visibility of the classic bell-shaped scars [6]. Both the original Robertson [23] and Hurst [29] (modified Robertson) techniques leave a scar visible from the front and through the horizontal mid-axis of the breast. On technique further lowers this scar to become a much more flattened bell shape just superior to the IMF, thereby making it far less visible while maintaining the advantage of a large and broad pyramidal NAC pedicle [6]. This broad pedicle avoids the need for free nipple grafting even in the very obese.

69.2.5
Technique (No Vertical Scar Breast Reduction or Boston Modification of the Robertson Technique)

The no vertical scar breast reduction involves a central inverted-U-shaped tissue resection and broad pyramidal pedicle (including both a central and inferior pedicle) with a low and flat bell-shaped scar just superior to the IMF. This technique is best suited to large reductions in patients with significant ptosis. The authors prefer 6–7 cm (but a minimum of 5 cm) of non-pigmented skin between the position of the inferior edge of the new areola and the superior edge of the existing pigmented areolar skin. This allows adequate coverage of the lower pole without a visible scar through the center of the breast. A lack of ptosis or a very large areola can preclude this.

Preoperative evaluation consists of examination of breast size and extent (including the size of the lateral roll), the degree of ptosis, breast consistency (fatty, fibrous, or glandular), skin quality (striae, turgor, thickness, rashes), and the size and sensibility of the NAC.

In breast hypertrophy and reduction, several important issues must be taken into consideration. First, breast hypertrophy occurs in all dimensions. Thus, a breast reduction technique must be able to manage both the vertical and transverse dimensions in order to obtain the ideal breast shape and to manage ptosis and width, respectively. Reducing a breast in the vertical dimension alone results in a "boxy" appearance. Second, as a breast hypertrophies, the NAC descends, increasing the grade of ptosis. Thus, the sternal notch (SN)-to-nipple (N) distance increases disproportionately to the IMF-to-nipple distance. This increase in SN–N to IMF–N ratio makes the nipple–areola vascularity stable when based on an inferior pedicle technique, since even with a large transposition of nipple location the inferior pedicle remains relatively short. Third, the use of a pyramidal (central and inferior) pedicle ensures maximum support of breast tissue under the NAC. This ensures good vascularity in breasts of all sizes, shapes, and degrees of ptosis. Fourth, avoiding undermining of either the pyramidal pedicle or breast tissue superior to the new nipple location (i.e., removing solely a wedge of tissue) ensures adequate vascularity of the overlying skin flaps. Fifth, excising a wedge up to, but not including, the pectoral fascia and with no undermining at this level only minimally disturbs the nerve supply to the overlying breast, helping with skin and NAC sensation. Sixth, in very large breast reductions, particularly in the obese, the roll of tissue lateral to the breast must be addressed since it appears to become part of the reduced breast when the previously larger breast is no longer able to hide this region. This is managed by using a moderate excision of tissue from the breast laterally, liposuction of this lateral roll, and quilting of the lateral skin to the chest wall to prevent fullness here or movement of the breast pedicle into this area.

The markings in the no vertical scar breast reduction are critical. They are entirely performed preoperatively, and resection adheres to these guides, making the operation predictable and expeditious (Fig. 69.1). Initial markings include the vertical and transverse mid-axial lines. The new nipple position is marked in the vertical mid-axis of the breast at the level of the IMF transposed to the anterior breast surface. The superior incision of the wedge resection (creating a 6–7 cm flap below the inferior border of the new areola) is drawn. This allows a sufficient "apron" to drape over the new inferior breast pole to hide the horizontal scar. The inferior incision of the wedge resection is drawn below this in a flattened bell-shaped curve just above the IMF. It is important to keep this above the IMF to avoid irritation from brassieres and consequent scar hypertrophy. Intraoperatively, a wide de-epithelialized pyramidal pedicle incorporating the full width of the breast is marked. Medial and lateral debulking markings are made, and the lateral roll may be marked for liposuction.

Tumescent solution is injected medially and laterally into the regions to be resected to reduce blood loss and facilitate dissection of otherwise redundant tissue. The pyramidal pedicle and new nipple–areolar site are de-epithelialized, leaving the IMF and 42 mm diameter NAC intact (Fig. 69.2). The dermis of the new areolar site is incised in a cruciate fashion to leave dermis for later suturing and to maintain a "cushion" for the new areola (Fig. 69.3). The superior incision is made (Fig. 69.4), and the flap undermined, leaving a 1.5 cm thick flap for approximately 6–7 cm up to the level of the new areolar location (Fig. 69.5). From this new nipple location, a cut is made straight down to pectoral fascia with no further superior undermining. Avoidance of undermining ensures good skin perfusion and prevents dead space which can predispose to seroma or hematoma formation. The main breast excision is done *en bloc* in a transverse inverted-U shape from the lateral, superior, and medial aspects, leaving behind a broad-based

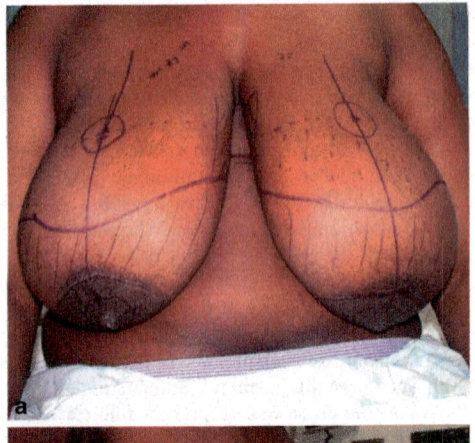

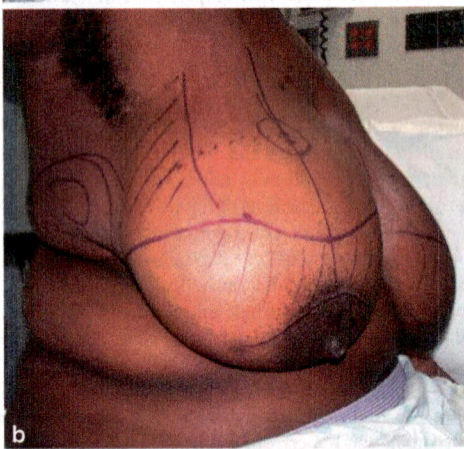

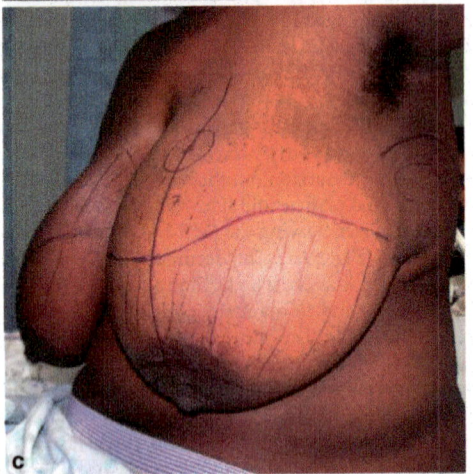

Fig. 69.1 (a) Preoperative photograph of a 34-year-old female: *left* SN–N = 43 cm, *right* SN–N = 41 cm; *left* N–IMF = 12 cm, *right* N–INF = 11 cm. SN = Sternal notch, N = Nipple, IMF = Inframammary fold. (b) Right oblique view. (c) Left oblique view

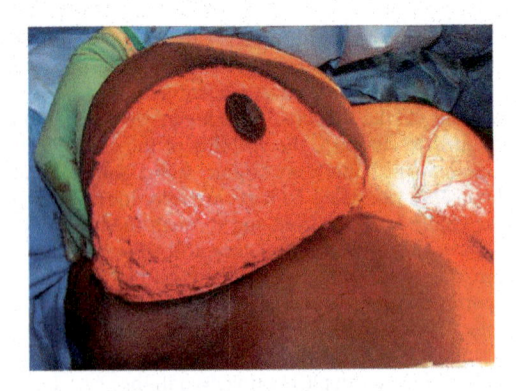

Fig. 69.2 The inferior pedicle is de-epithelialized

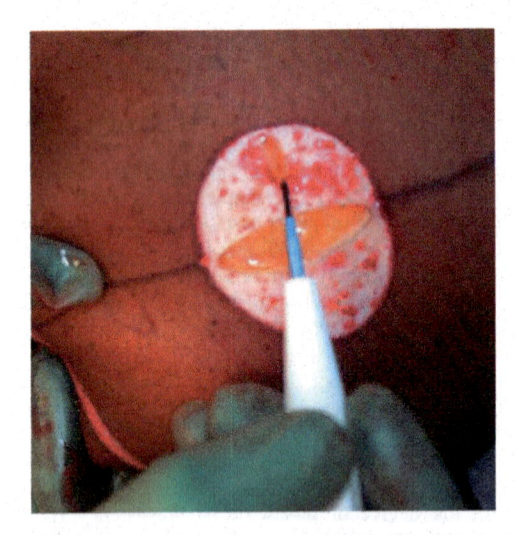

Fig. 69.3 The new nipple–areola complex site is de-epithelialized and a cruciate incision made through dermis

pyramidal de-epithelialized pedicle (Fig. 69.6). If needed, lateral fold liposuction is performed beyond the edge of the breast tissue to thin the lateral roll which otherwise becomes more pronounced with the breast reduced. This is most easily performed prior to wedge resections from this area. Following this, a larger lateral wedge (Fig. 69.7) and a smaller medial wedge (Fig. 69.8) are excised from the remaining breast and sent to pathology. Now, there remains a thinned flap with a hole for the new NAC, a superior flap narrowed in the transverse dimension, and a de-epithelialized, broad, pyramidal (central and inferior) pedicle based along the entire IMF (Fig. 69.9). After resection, lateral quilting sutures are used to obliterate the dead space and further narrow the transverse diameter of the breast

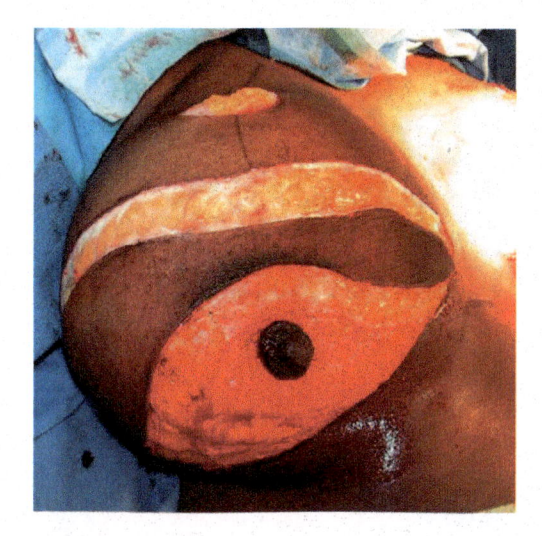

Fig. 69.4 The superior incision is made

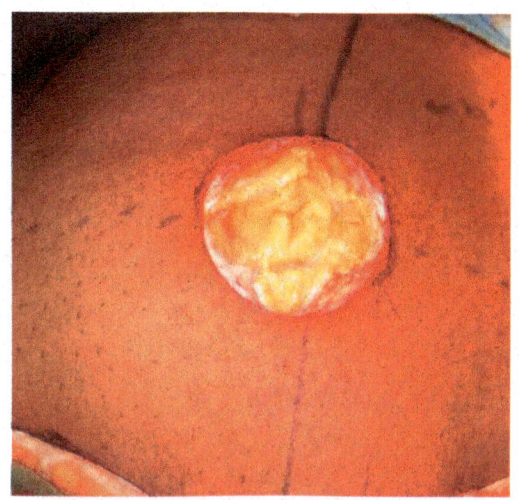

Fig. 69.5 The breast "apron" prior to resection: an inverted-U transverse breast excision and small medial with larger lateral additional wedge excisions are resected, with liposuction of the roll lateral to breast parenchyma

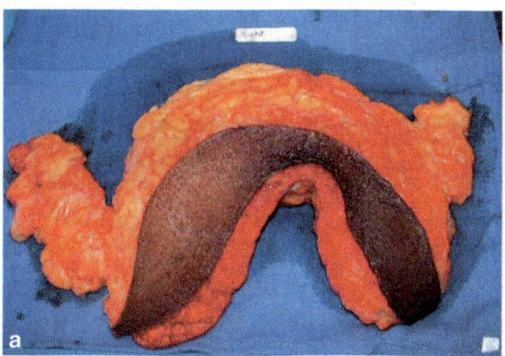

Fig. 69.6 (**a**) Excision right 1,630 g. (**b**) Excision left 2,185 g

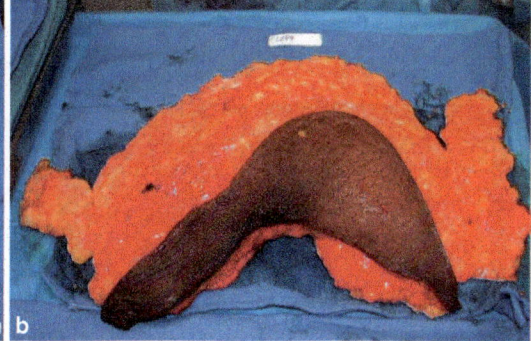

(Fig. 69.10). A suction drain is placed laterally from each breast.

The superior "apron" flap is then brought down over the inferior pedicle and preliminarily stapled, while the NAC is sutured in place with interrupted and then running absorbable sutures (Fig. 69.11). The redundancy of the longer superior flap is worked centrally to minimize "dog ears," and a running suture placed along this pleating which resolves as healing and contraction occur (Fig. 69.12).

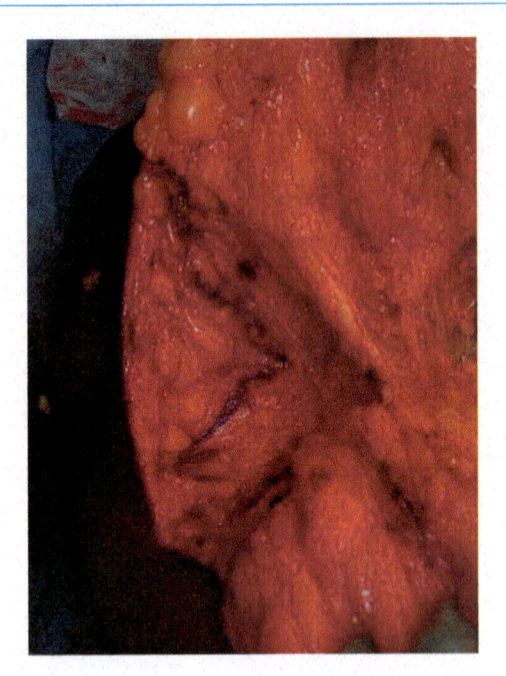

Fig. 69.7 A larger lateral wedge excision reduces the horizontal dimension of the breast, with liposuction minimizing the roll lateral to the breast

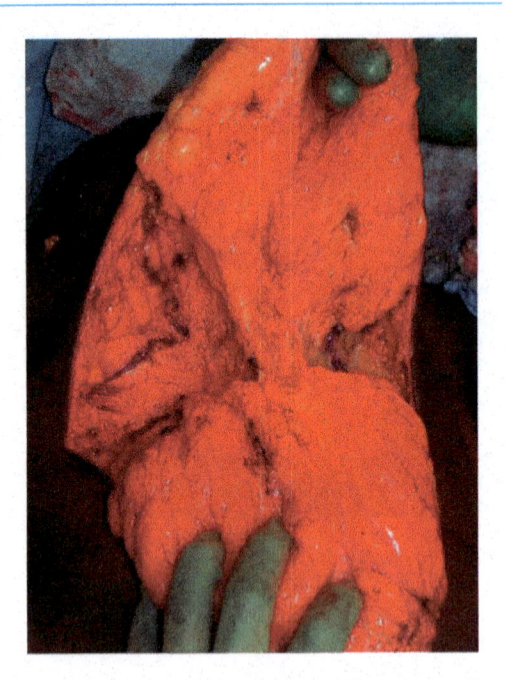

Fig. 69.9 The major wedge excision is performed in a plane straight down to the chest wall without undermining

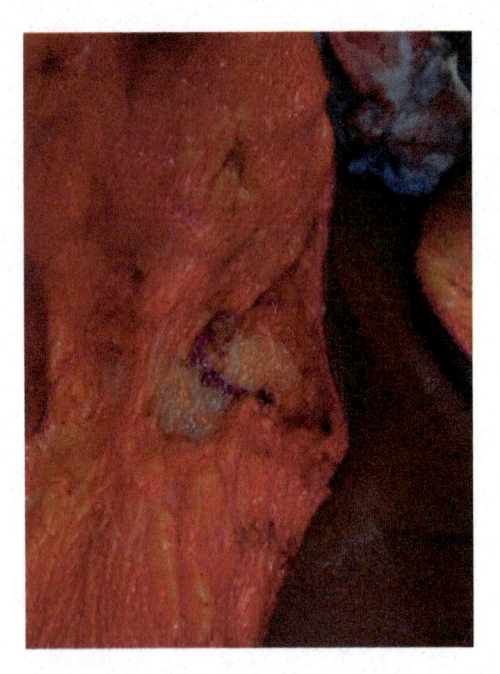

Fig. 69.8 A smaller medial wedge excision reduces the horizontal dimension of the breast without flattening the medial pole, reducing the "boxy" appearance

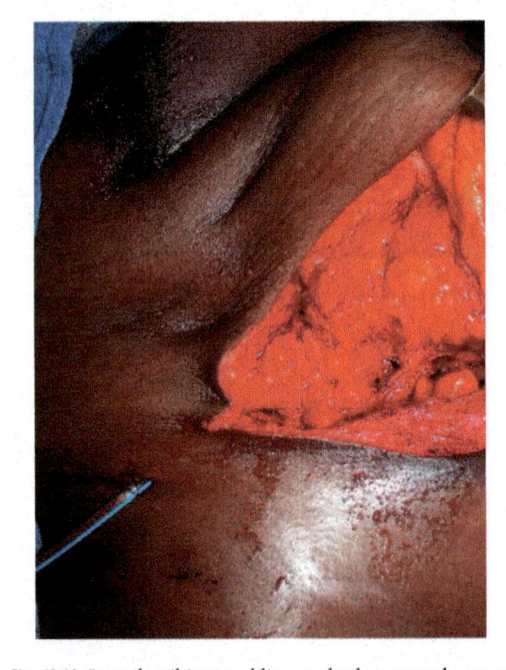

Fig. 69.10 Lateral quilting to obliterate dead space and narrow the transverse diameter of the breast

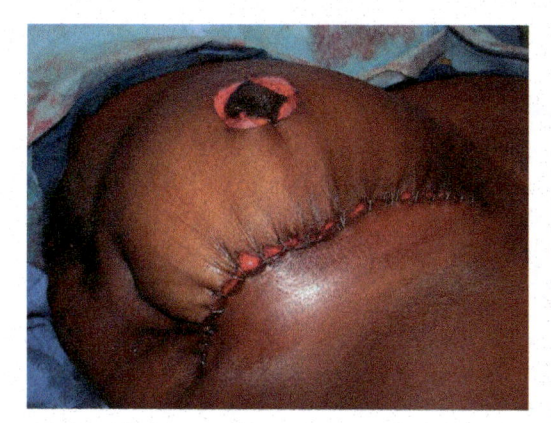

Fig. 69.11 Temporary stapling to reduce "dog ears" on final closure

69.2.6
Applications and Uses

The no vertical scar breast reduction has provided us with an effective and reliable operation for large, ptotic breasts, where a minimum of 5 cm exists below the inferior border of the new areolar site and the superior border of the old areolar skin [5, 6]. This technique eliminates a vertical scar and hides a transverse scar in inferior breast shadow. It eliminates the need for free nipple grafting owing to the wide pyramidal pedicle. By leaving the IMF intact, pseudoptosis is minimized. The superiorly based "apron" overlying the pedicle acts to support the breast tissue, like an intrinsic brassiere, thereby eliminating the stretch typically seen in inverted-T scar breast reductions and avoiding problems with dehiscence of the T-incision. This technique is reliable and easy to learn and teach, and can be safely performed in obese patients.

The technique is best applied where large excisions are required and when marked ptosis exists. It is most applicable when an inverted-T method would leave an excessively long pedicle and create concern about nipple viability or stretch on the incisions. In this technique, there must be a minimum of 5 cm, and preferably 6–7 cm, of nonpigmented skin between the inferior edge of the new nipple–areolar location and the superior edge of the existing areola to allow sufficient skin coverage for the lower pole of the breast. This technique is not effective for mastopexy alone.

This method of breast reduction is effective in operations for contralateral symmetry after autologous transverse rectal abdominus myocutaneous (TRAM) flap reconstruction. The reconstructed breast may be significantly smaller, less ptotic, and flatter, and this method allows more significant flattening of the breast, improving symmetry with the reconstructed side [19] (Fig. 69.13).

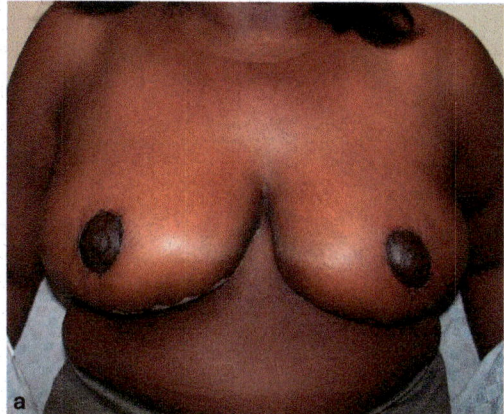

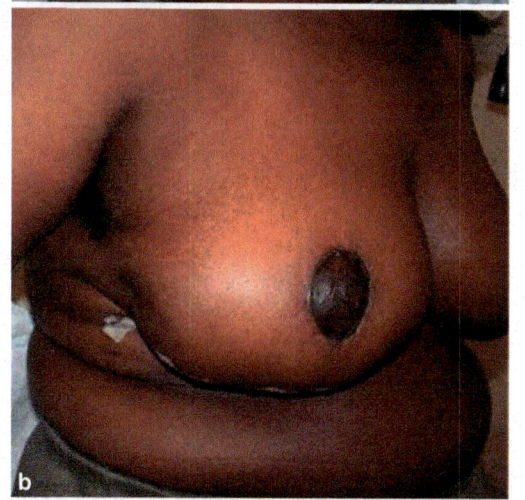

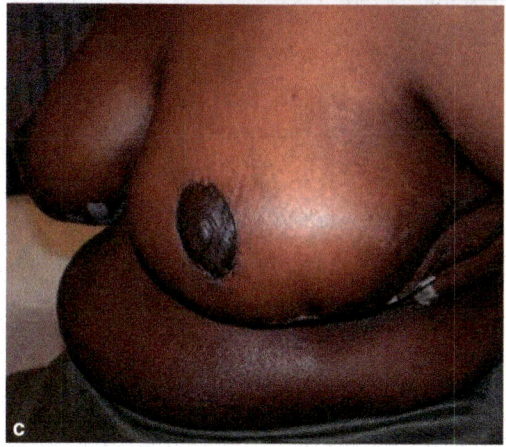

Fig. 69.12 (a) Post-operative photograph. (b) Right oblique view. (c) Left oblique view

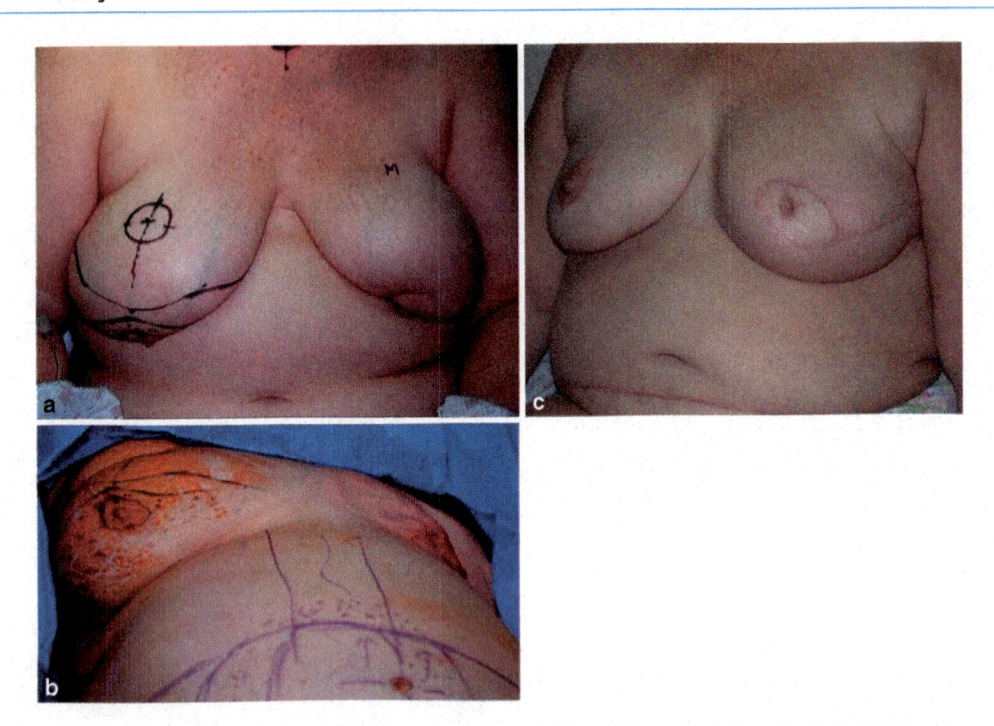

Fig. 69.13 (a) Preoperative 53-year-old female. (b) Intraoperative during left TRAM flap and right breast reduction. (c) Five years postoperative after bilateral reduction and reconstruction on left side

69.3 Outcomes and Complications

The results of various breast reductions without vertical scars have been discussed since the development of these operations. Unfavorable results include the following:

1. The transverse scar can end up too lateral on the chest wall [5]. This is especially true in obese patients with fat rolls extending onto the back [6]. Lalonde [5] minimizes this occurrence by marking the medial edge of this incision below the visible cleavage crease and keeping the incision length to 17 cm along an inferiorly curved incision similar to the wire in an underwire bra. The authors use liposuction of the lateral roll and quilting of the lateral tissues to avoid extension of this scar too far laterally.
2. The no-vertical-scar techniques can lead to a "boxy" appearance. This is especially true when medial and lateral resections are insufficient to narrow the base of the breast. Adequately resecting additional larger lateral and smaller medial wedges, performing lateral roll liposuction, and quilting the lateral skin to the chest wall minimize this problem.
3. Medial and lateral dog ears can be problems [5]. This is best dealt with by gathering the vertical pleating in the transverse incisions towards the center of the incisions [6, 19]. This problem is unique to methods in which the horizontal scar remains low on the chest wall causing a discrepancy between the superior and inferior incision lengths. The original Robertson technique avoided this by maintaining a steep bell-shaped inferior incision, similar in length to the straight superior incision; however, the location of this incision is aesthetically unfavorable [23]. We find that these pleated incisions "even out" rapidly during healing, and that dog ears and pleating rarely become a significant problem. Furthermore, dog ears can be easily revised under local anesthetic in the office, if necessary.
4. The horizontal scar can hypertrophy. We intentionally place the incision above the line of the IMF, avoiding irritation from clothing and brassieres, and consequently minimizing hypertrophy of this scar.
5. One report [5] describes two cases of skin loss on the infra-areolar skin. The authors account this to thinning the skin apron flap too much, and do not report a case after their first year of experience. They maximize perfusion to the NAC and skin by avoidance of undermining, ensuring thick skin flaps, and using a central and inferior pyramidal pedicle based on the entire IMF, as we do.

Pseudoptosis or "bottoming out," which is frequently written about in forms of inverted-T scar breast reductions, is rarely seen in the no-vertical-scar methods.

Chalekson et al. [31] support this observation after examination of 17 postoperative patients after regular modified Robertson breast reductions performed between 1987 and 1997, each of which averaged 910 g of reduction on each side and after an average of 4.7 years' follow-up. Furthermore, the bell-shaped incision just superior to the IMF allows operative versatility and good nipple projection, and reduces pseudoptosis by keeping the IMF intact. The authors' long-term results have consistently demonstrated stable long-term outcomes (Figs. 69.14, 69.15). However, in spite of breast reduction surgery, the breast will continue to "age" and the natural progression of ongoing ptosis will still occur.

Although nonrandomized, analysis of our institutional data comparing the no vertical scar breast reduction with Wise-pattern breast reductions shows several significant patient differences, reflecting contrasting patient selection. Patients were more obese and more ptotic and required larger resections. Overall, there is a lower rate of routine complications including significantly less hematoma formation and trends towards less wound dehiscence and scar hypertrophy in spite of their larger, ptotic pre-operative breasts [6].

One key paper directly compares patient satisfaction in 29 patients who underwent reduction with a no-vertical-scar technique against 24 patients with an inverted-T scar technique [11]. They state a significantly higher satisfaction with scars and a higher post-operative activity level in the no-vertical-scar group. However, the inverted-T scar patients rated nipple position as better. Groups rated their overall aesthetic satisfaction similarly.

69.4 Discussion and Other Techniques

A number of authors describe current and similar techniques of breast reduction to avoid vertical scars. Savaci [32] has described a central pedicle technique that avoids a vertical scar. The author describes a resection that "will resemble a slice of melon" being taken from between a superior incision and the inframammary sulcus. However, in this method the breast tissue is skeletonized in a conical shape, basing NAC vascularity and nerve supply on pectoral perforators. They also state that this technique is most useful in very large breasts, and necessitates a 6-cm distance between the new and old areolar sites.

Lalonde et al. [5, 33] have also written about their "no vertical scar breast reduction" using an inferior pedicle for large, ptotic breasts. They refer to the ideal candidate as having considerable ptosis and 5 cm between the lower edge of the new areola and the upper edge of the pigmented areolar skin. They also described the use of this technique in cases where less distance exists below the

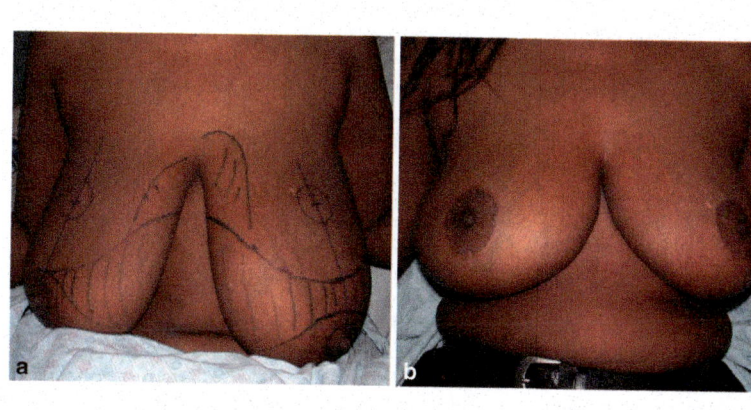

Fig. 69.14 (a) Preoperative patient. (b) Six months postoperative after reduction

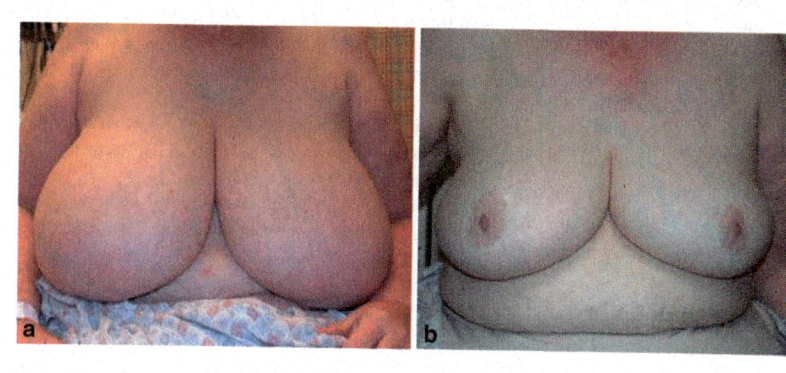

Fig. 69.15 (a) Preoperative patient. (b) Six months postoperative after reduction

new areolar site, in which case they de-epithelialize less tissue inferiorly (causing a higher scar), hide the pale areolar skin in the IMF, or wedge out the residual areolar skin in a short vertical scar. Key differences from the above-described method include a 17 cm inferiorly directed curved incision directly in the IMF to minimize its visibility. Considerable emphasis is placed on minimization of tension in the periareolar incision, principally by cutting a smaller hole in the breast flap than in the cut-out areola. In addition, "pillar sutures" may be used in the inferior pedicle to improve projection.

Thomas et al. [19] have described their experience with very large, very ptotic breasts using a "design-enhanced breast reduction" involving no vertical scar. This technique was developed because of problems with prior procedures including fat necrosis, skin and nipple necrosis, shaping difficulties, decreased nipple sensation, and bleeding. They described a technique similar to the no vertical scar breast reduction, in which they use a wide-based glandular, de-epithelialized pedicle, preservation of the fourth intercostal nerves, mesial advancement of thick skin flaps, and the use of tumescence. Similar to Lalonde's method, the design-enhanced reduction utilizes an inferior incision in the IMF.

Other authors [34, 35] have modified the long-standing amputation with free nipple–areolar grafting technique of breast reduction in order to eliminate the vertical scar. This has the merit of being a rapid operation with little blood loss. Using a back-folded dermoglandular flap de-epithelialized from the edge of the superior flap, projection is able to be maintained. However, in general, ideal cosmetic outcomes remain difficult to achieve in this operation.

69.5 Conclusions

Since the 1920s, when Passot first published his report on a reduction mammaplasty without a vertical scar, surgeons have reworked and modified various techniques of breast reduction. The quest to produce the "perfect" breast size and shape with minimal scarring, normal nipple vascularity and sensation, good projection, a stable IMF, the ability to lactate, and structural stability over time has led to many variations on a theme. The technique of the no vertical scar breast reduction or Boston modification of the Robertson method is reliable, effective, and useful in very large reductions of ptotic breasts.

Acknowledgments

The authors thank Anne Fladger and Meaghan Muir for invaluable help in obtaining the articles.

References

1. American Society of Plastic Surgery: Plastic surgery statistics: Procedural statistics trends 1992–2006. Illinois, USA, ASPS 2007
2. Thoma A, Sprague S, Veltri K, Duku E, Furlong W: A prospective study of patients undergoing breast reduction surgery: health-related quality of life and clinical outcomes. Plast Reconstr Surg 2007;120(1):13–26
3. Celebiler O, Sonmez A, Erdim M, Yaman M, Numanoglu A: Patients' and surgeons' perspectives on the scar components after inferior pedicle breast reduction surgery. Plast Reconstr Surg 2005;116(2):459–464
4. Spear S, Willey SC, Robb GL, Hammond DC, Nahabedian MY: Surgery of the Breast: Principles and Art, 2nd edn. Philadelphia, Lippincott Williams and Wilkins 2006
5. Lalonde DH, Lalonde J, French R: The no vertical scar breast reduction: a minor variation that allows to remove vertical scar portion of the inferior pedicle wise pattern T scar. Aesthetic Plast Surg 2003;27(5):335–344
6. Movassaghi K, Liao EC, Ting V, Matros E, Morris D, Orgill DP, Pribaz JJ: Eliminating the vertical scar in breast reduction – Boston modification of the Robertson technique Aesthetic Surg J 2006;26:687–696
7. Durston W: Observations about the unusual swelling of the breasts. Phil Trans Vol IV for anno 1669:1049–1050, Royal Society, London 1670
8. Schwarzmann E: Die technik der mammaplastik. Chirurgie 1930;2:932–943
9. Wise RJ: A preliminary report on a method of planning the mammaplasty. Plast. Reconstr Surg 1956;17(5): 367–375
10. Lassus C: A 30-year experience with vertical mammaplasty last. Plast Reconstr Surg 1996;97(2):373–380
11. Hosnuter M, Tosun Z, Kargi E, Babuccu O, Savaci N: No-vertical-scar technique versus inverted T-scar technique in reduction mammaplasty: a two-center comparative study. Aesthetic Plast Surg 2005;29(6):496–502
12. Greer SE: Handbook of Plastic Surgery. New York, Marcel Dekker 2004
13. Benelli L: A new periareolar mammaplasty: the "round block" technique. Aesthetic Plast Surg 1990;14(2):93–100
14. Lejour M, Abboud M, Declety A, Kertesz P: Reduction of mammaplasty scars: from a short inframammary scar to a vertical scar. Ann Chir Plast Esthet 1990;35(5):369–379
15. Lejour M: Pedicle modification of the Lejour vertical scar reduction mammaplasty. Plast Reconstr Surg 1998;101(4): 1149–1150
16. Hall-Findlay EJ: A simplified vertical reduction mammaplasty: shortening the learning curve. Plast Reconstr Surg 1999;104(3):748–759
17. Ramirez OM: Reduction mammaplasty with the "owl" incision and no undermining. Plast Reconstr Surg 2002;109(2):512–522
18. Yousif NJ, Larson DL, Sanger JR, Matloub HS: Elimination of the vertical scar in reduction mammaplasty. Plast Reconstr Surg 1992;89(3):459–467

19. Thomas WO, Moline S, Harris CN: Design-enhanced breast reduction: an approach for very large, very ptotic breasts without a vertical incision. Ann Plast Surg 1998;40(3):229–234
20. Giovanoli P, Meuli-Simmen C, Meyer VE, Frey M: Which technique for which breast? A prospective study of different techniques of reduction mammaplasty. Br J Plast Surg 1999;52(1):52–59
21. Passot R: La correction esthetique du prolapsus mammarie par le procede de la transposition du mamelon. Presse Med 1925;33:317
22. Ribeiro L: A new technique for reduction mammaplasty. Plast Reconstr Surg 1975;55(3):330–334
23. Robertson DC: The technique of inferior flap mammaplasty. Plast Reconstr Surg 1967;40(4):372–377
24. Smith GA, Schmidt GH: Experience with the Ribeiro reduction mammaplasty technique. Ann Plast Surg 1979;3(3):260–263
25. Thorek M: Possibilities in the reconstruction of the human form. N Y Med J 1922;116:572
26. Maliniac JW: Evaluation of principal mammaplastic procedures. Plast Reconstr Surg 1949;4:359
27. Conway H: Mammaplasty; analysis of 110 consecutive cases with end-results. Plast Reconstr Surg 1952;10(5): 303–315
28. Ribeiro L, Accors A Jr, Buss A, Marcal-Pessoa M: Creation and evolution of 30 years of the inferior pedicle in reduction mammaplasties. Plast Reconstr Surg 2002; 110(3): 960–970
29. Hurst LN, Evans HB, Murray KA: Inferior flap reduction mammaplasty with pedicled nipple. Ann Plast Surg 1983;10(6):483–485
30. Yousif NJ, Larson DL: The apron technique of reduction mammaplasty: elimination of the vertical scar. Perspect Plast Surg 1994;8:137–144
31. Chalekson CP, Neumeister MW, Zook EG, Russell RC: Outcome analysis of reduction mammaplasty using the modified Robertson technique. Plast Reconstr Surg 2002;110(1):71–79
32. Savaci N: Reduction mammoplasty by the central pedicle, avoiding a vertical scar. Aesthetic Plast Surg 1996;20(2): 171–175
33. Nahai F: Breast reduction with no vertical scar. Aesthetic Plast Surg 2004;28(5):354
34. Manstein ME, Manstein CH, Manstein G: Obtaining projection in the amputation free nipple/areolar graft breast reduction without a vertical scar: using breast parenchyma to create a new mound. Ann Plast Surg 1997;38(4): 421–424
35. Aydin H, Bilgin-Karabulut A, Tumerdem B: Free nipple reduction mammaplasty with a horizontal scar in high-risk patients. Aesthetic Plast Surg 2002;26(6): 457–460

The Bipolar Technique: Short Inframammary Scar Mammaplasty

Vicente De Carolis

70.1 Background

70.1.1 Rigid Versus Elastic Geometry Mammaplasty

The keyhole (Wise) [1] pattern with a superior pedicle has been until now the gold standard for breast reduction technique in terms of shape and scar quality. It corresponds to a rigid geometric design that leads directly to a pyramidal shape with high nipple projection. If properly designed and executed, the incision closure is tension-free, and therefore there is less possibility of scar dilatation and reduction of the stress stimulus for hypertrophic scarring [2].

The main drawback of this technique is that the rigid geometric design directs the horizontal scar medially towards the sternum and laterally towards the lateral thoracic wall. Despite the tension-free closure, the more the horizontal scar drifts away from the breast meridian, the more likely is the possibility of developing hypertrophic scarring.

In spite of the recognized quality of the Wise pattern mammaplasty, there is a compulsive tendency for plastic surgeons to search for alternatives to reduce the scar length in breast reduction techniques as in every other plastic surgery operation.

Two techniques, the "vertical" [3] and the "periareolar" [4, 5], have been introduced which have significantly reduced the amount of scarring. Both surgical innovations rely on the physical properties of the skin to adapt within certain limits to stress and wrinkling. The skin design of these techniques can be defined as a sort of "elastic geometry concept."

70.1.2 The Vertical Skin Excess Dilemma

Breast reduction must deal with breast parenchyma resection and the remaining skin excess which has a horizontal and a vertical component. With the classic Wise technique, the residual skin is resolved by both a vertical and horizontal wedge resection. The length of the horizontal wedge is directly proportional to the vertical skin excess (Fig. 70.1).

The main issue in the strategies for scar reduction is the way to deal with the vertical skin excess (Fig. 70.2).

The periareolar technique (Benelli's round block operation) completely absorbs the vertical and horizontal excesses.

The vertical technique absorbs all the vertical excess in the vertical scar.

Skin wrinkling, upper or lower pole compression, and further skin accommodation are the bases of these techniques.

These techniques do well in small to moderate breast reductions. However, moderate to large breast reductions establish enormous pressure to skin adjustment, and the limits for acceptable scar quality can be easily surpassed. Broadening of the scar, wrinkling permanence, and shape distortion are the main problems that can arise [6, 7].

Combining both the vertical technique and the enlarged periareolar resection is the strategy of the Lejour [8] technique, which still mainly relies on the vertical component, and the Hammond [9] technique, which relies mainly on the periareolar component.

70.1.3 The Bipolar Technique

This technique, published in 2002 [10], incorporates the essentials of the elastic geometry concept by resolving the upper pole skin excess by means of a vertically enlarged periareolar resection and the lower pole vertical skin excess by means of a small flap that replicates the same idea of concentric skin resection in the lower pole (Fig. 70.3). The inferior flap allows for the management of the vertical skin excess generated after the closure of the periareolar and vertical scar.

This technique seeks a more balanced distribution of skin tension and asserts the concept of clear geometrical

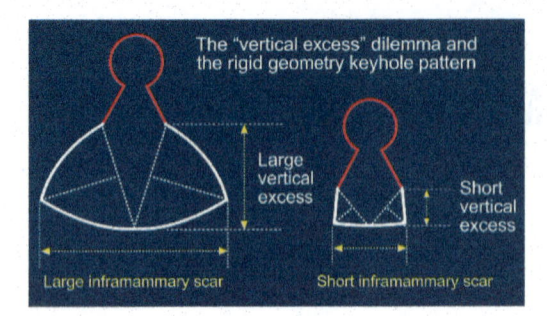

Fig. 70.1 In the rigid-geometry keyhole pattern, the length of the horizontal wedge skin resection is directly proportional to the vertical skin excess

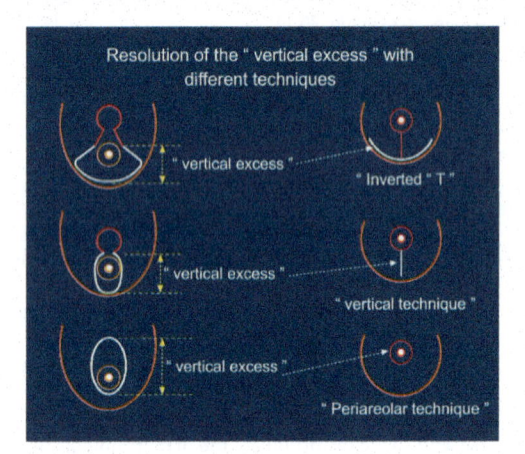

Fig. 70.2 Diagram depicting the different approaches to deal with the vertical skin excess

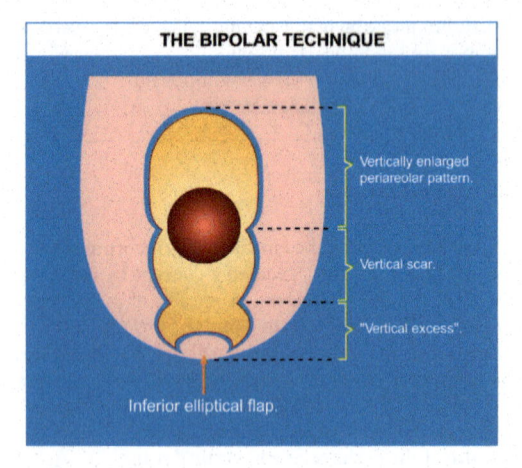

Fig. 70.3 Main technical principles involved in the bipolar technique. The vertically enlarged periareolar pattern absorbs the upper vertical skin excess. The inferior elliptical flap absorbs the lower pole vertical skin excess

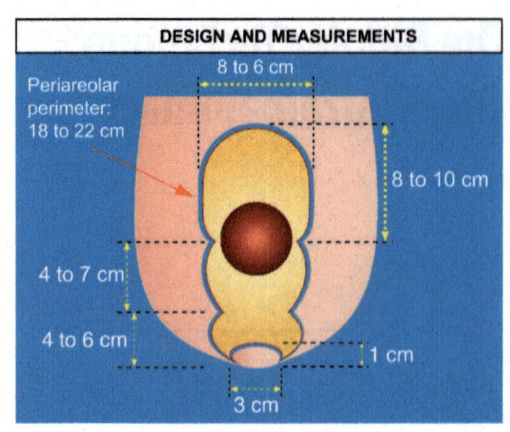

Fig. 70.4 Average measurements of the bipolar technique

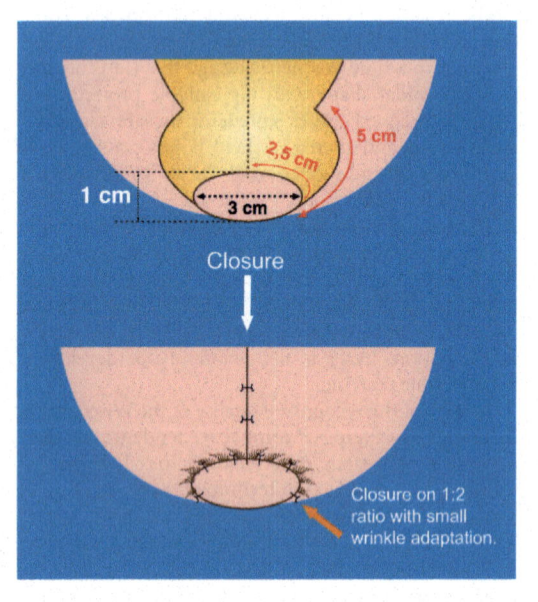

Fig. 70.5 Diagram depicting the solution for the inferior vertical excess. The elliptical flap, 1 cm high and 3 cm wide, leaves a 2.5-cm free border on each side of the flap, which can easily absorb 5–6 cm of vertical excess by means of small wrinkles. Those wrinkles disappear in a few days

limits to avoid excessive tension or wrinkling in the skin closure.

The design is related to the skin only, and it can be used with any type of parenchyma pedicle. However, when possible, the author prefers the superior pedicle technique because it results in a more aesthetic breast shape and a better nipple–areola projection.

70.1.4
Technique

The average measurements of the technique design are depicted in Figs. 70.4 and 70.5.

In the standing position, the submammary fold is outlined and the breast meridian is marked starting at the midclavicular line. The new areola position is determined according to aesthetic proportion usually leaving it about 3 cm above the submammary fold.

Operative marking is continued in the supine position with arms open (Fig. 70.6). Placement of the horizontal incision is marked 1 cm above the submammary fold. The next step is to outline the perimeter of the periareolar resection, which is a vertically enlarged design and must range from 18 to 22 cm in length. A horizontal line is marked 1 cm above the submammary fold. The elliptical flap is traced at the center of the latter line. The flap dimension is 1 cm in height and 3 cm in width leaving a 1.5 cm pedicle. The next step is to draw the medial and lateral vertical resection line connecting the end of the periareolar pattern to the extremes of the elliptical flap. The length of these vertical lines is critical in the decision regarding which horizontal scar type will remain at the completion of the procedure.

Normally, the length of the vertical scar will range from 4 to 7 cm. The distance between the ends of the planned predetermined vertical scar to the inframammary crease has been denominated as the "vertical excess." If the vertical incision is smaller than 7 cm, there is no inferior vertical excess so the final solution is a single vertical scar. If the vertical excess is less than 3 cm, the best solution is to convert it into an "inverted T," leaving a horizontal scar that is rarely longer than 3 cm. If the vertical excess is in the range of 3–6 cm, the indication is to distribute it along the elliptical flap (Fig. 70.5). This solution is the paradigm of the bipolar technique. If the vertical excess is longer than 5 or 6 cm, most of it is distributed along the inferior flap and part of it must be distributed along a small extension in the inframammary fold (Fig. 70.6).

The periareolar closure is done with a purse-string suture of 3-0 mononylon or Prolene tied around a 4-cm areola marker. The dermal plane of all the scars is closed with single 4-0 Monocryl sutures and finished with a continuous subcuticular suture.

The closure of the inferior flap is done by applying moderate tension to the horizontal extremes of the elliptical flap. The same concept of a purse-string suture is applied to the skin closure around the flap utilizing 3-0 mononylon or Prolene and completed with 4-0 Monocryl and 5-0 mononylon.

The patients are strongly encouraged to apply adhesive tape to all the scars for 6 months to help in the prevention of scar spread [11].

70.2
Clinical Series

From December 1995 to December 2007, 181 bilateral mammaplasties were performed. Of these, 21% had a vertical or inverted-T technique with a short horizontal limb. The bipolar technique was utilized in 79% of the cases. Currently, we utilize the periareolar technique only in augmentation mastopexy. Examples of clinical cases are shown in Figs. 70.9–70.11.

70.3
Evolution of the Technique

At the beginning of this series, the technique design started out with a 16-cm periareolar resection perimeter, which was progressively increased until attempting a perimeter of 26 cm. With a 23–24-cm periareolar resection perimeter, marked scar spread began to appear. Finally, a 22-cm periareolar perimeter resection was standardized as a safe measurement that guaranteed minimal scar spread. This slightly extended vertical design was preferred to a round design because it contributed more efficiently in the "absorption" of the vertical skin excess along the upper pole.

The concept involved in the inferior flap is somewhat similar to that of the periareolar technique. This elliptical flap can "absorb," with minimal wrinkling, a vertical excess of approximately twice the length of the free border of the flap. The small flap dimension was sufficient to absorb the vertical skin excess in most of the cases.

Closure of the lower flap design was performed differently from the initial description in the year 2002. After observing broadening of the scar at the inferior flap level, the closure technique was modified by incorporating a purse-string suture with 3-0 Prolene, and subsequently the scar broadening events significantly decreased.

70.4
Relevant Geometric Issues, Technical Tips and Clinical Observations

1. The length of the periareolar resection is important for good scar quality. The maximum length of the periareolar

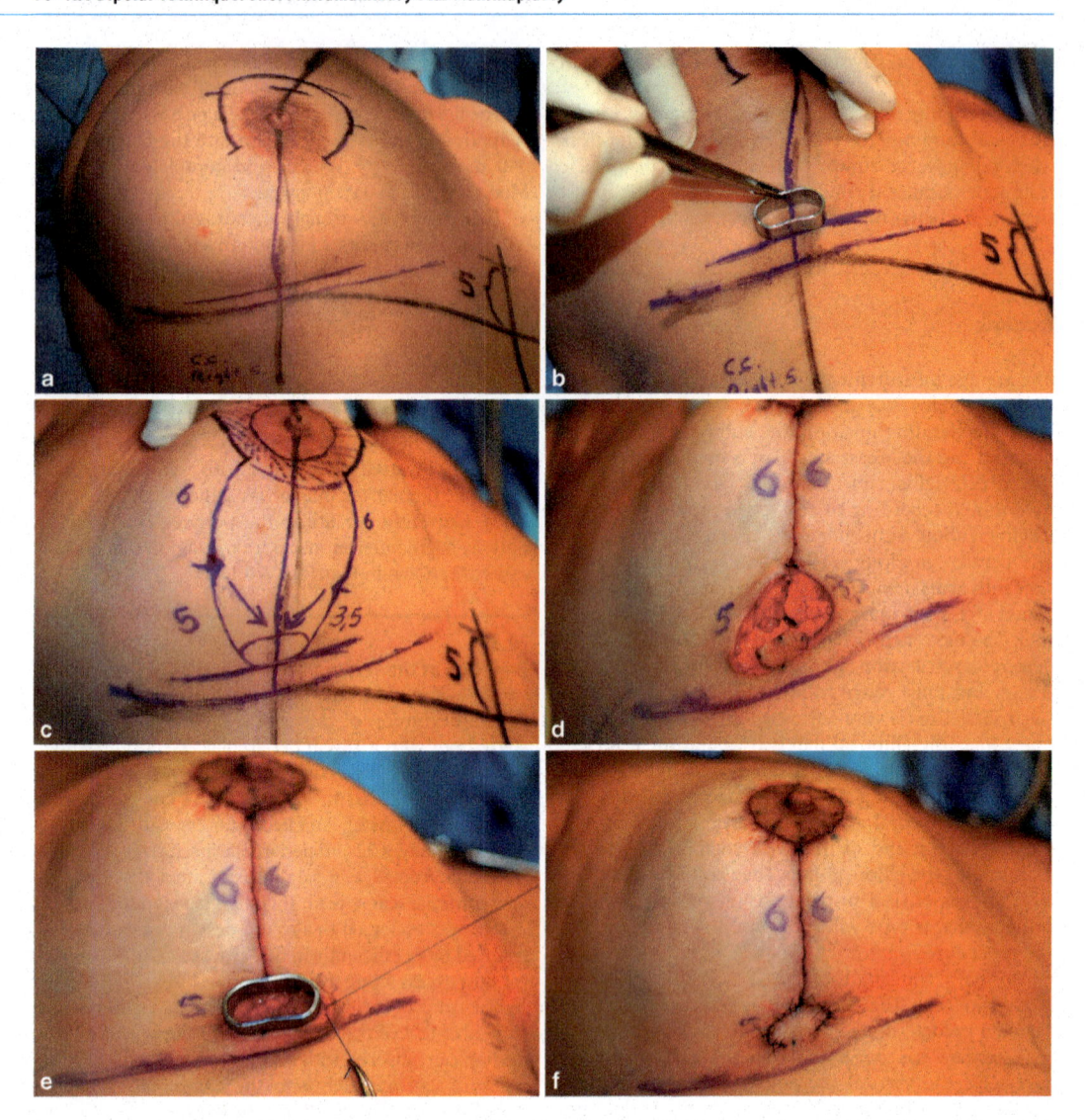

Fig. 70.6 Operative sequence: (**a**) The sub mammary incision is traced 1 cm above the submammary crease. (**b**) With the aid of a metallic pattern the elliptical inferior flap is outlined. (**c**) The *vertical incision lines* are drawn connecting the end of the periareolar pattern to the lateral endings of the inferior flap. A length of 6 cm has been assigned to the vertical scar. The remaining vertical excess is 5 cm. The *arrows* show the direction of the inferior closure. (**d**) The image shows the finished vertical scar and the vertical excess ready for closing. (**e**) A purse-string suture has been advanced along the vertical excess and the base of the flap. For precise sizing, the knot is tied on the metallic pattern of the flap. (**f**) Final view with all the incisions closed. Note the mild wrinkling at the inferior flap suture

resection that is consistent with a satisfactory scar condition is slightly less than twice the length of the areola perimeter. Spear [12] made a similar observation in an article focused on the periareolar mastopexy augmentation. Surpassing the double perimeter rule significantly leads to skin wrinkling but, more importantly, there is scar stretching that primarily affects the superior medial portion of the areola. The classic areola diameter of 4 cm has a 12.5 cm perimeter. The author has tried up to 26 cm periareolar perimeter resection, but the threshold for bad scarring clearly started just over the 22 cm periareolar perimeter resection.

2. The efficiency of the enlarged periareolar pattern to absorb the superior vertical skin excess depends on the vertical component of the periareolar pattern more than the perimeter length itself. A vertically enlarged design with an 8-cm vertical length utilizes 4 cm for the areola and recruits the other 4 cm to account for the superior vertical excess.
3. The efficiency of the inferior elliptical flap to absorb the inferior vertical skin excess requires understanding the concept that the flap must be considered as having a medial and a lateral side. A flap dimension of 1 × 3 cm leaves 2.5 cm for each side which can absorb at least twice this length. That means that each half of the flap can easily account for 5 cm of vertical excess (Fig. 70.5).
4. Understanding the amount of horizontal submammary scarring that can be avoided by the inferior flap requires an example. Considering 5 cm of vertical excess and applying the rigid geometric design of the Wise pattern, two horizontal wedge resections will be needed, one medial and one lateral, 5 cm each, which will add up to 10 cm of total scar length.

    In the same example with 5 cm vertical excess, but utilizing the bipolar technique, the inferior flap absorbs all the vertical excess. Thus, the real economy in scar length with the elliptical flap is 10 cm minus the 3 cm horizontal flap length, signifying 7 cm horizontal scar avoidance at the submammary crease.
5. The amount of breast tissue reduction compatible with a satisfactory aesthetic outcome can be determined by not trying to excise more than 40–50% of the breast volume. There are several ways to measure breast volume. The author systematically measures the breast volume with his own system, which will be described in a later publication. In general, patients requesting mastopexy have breast volumes ranging 400–800 ml. Patients with breast volume over 800 ml usually request reduction. In the author's practice, the nonobese patients of Caucasoid origin requesting breast reduction are in the range of 800–1,400 ml, and the average is close to 1,000 ml. A 40% reduction will leave the final breast volume in the range of 500–800 ml, which in fact is a very pleasing volume. Volume reduction greater than 50% usually compromises the lateral and medial pillars of the superior pedicle technique, thereby limiting the possibility to achieve high projection. Also, areola damage derived from low perfusion is dramatically increased, especially with a superior pedicle technique, when parenchyma excision is over 50%.

    Determining final breast volume must take into consideration the fact that breast tissue shrinks significantly in the following postoperative months. Perhaps this event is due to the atrophic response of the fat tissue to surgical trauma. In practical terms, when considering final breast volume the author arbitrarily assigns about 50–100 ml to account for late postoperative breast volume reduction. For example, if planning to reduce a 1,000 ml breast by 40%, which means a final volume of 600 ml, 350 ml is resected and 50–100 ml is left to account for the upcoming postoperative spontaneous breast volume reduction.

    Breasts larger than 1,400 ml usually correspond to the obese group, where a reconstructive approach is generally used that is better accomplished with a free nipple graft technique. In these cases, high aesthetic goals also become secondary, being replaced by the functional issue.
6. One has to consider planned design versus freehand adjustments. Tracing a carefully calculated geometry plan over the breast skin that directly leads to satisfactory end results is the fastest and most pleasing way to operate. However, when dealing with sagging and atrophic skin often with the presence of stretch marks, the accuracy of the geometric design can by surpassed. In the case of the bipolar technique, the planned incision at the lower pole sometimes falls into this category. To resolve this problem with a freehand approach, the vertical incision is closed with the planned length, and its end point is sutured with a single stitch to the vertex of the inferior flap. Then the vertical excess is partially trimmed out and the excess skin is sutured covering the flap with a continuous running suture and applying appropriate tension. Subsequently, a metallic pattern of the flap is applied over this area and the flap profile is outlined over the temporarily closed skin. The traced skin is excised, leaving behind the exact dimension of the flap with the appropriate tension ready for closure as described initially (Fig. 70.7).

70.5
Surgical Decision Making Based on Measurements

According to the experience attained in this clinical series, an attempt to summarize surgical decision making for scar design is presented (Fig. 70.8). The main parameter required to define which type of scar will be made is the length of the vertical resection line. This line runs from the end of the periareolar design to the center of the inframammary fold. Two basic measurements must first be considered: (a) the periareolar resection perimeter must not exceed 22 cm; and (b) the vertical scar must not exceed 7 cm. Keeping these measurements in mind, surgical decision making proceeds according to the following criteria:
1. When periareolar resection requirements exceed 22 cm, a vertical skin resection must be applied,

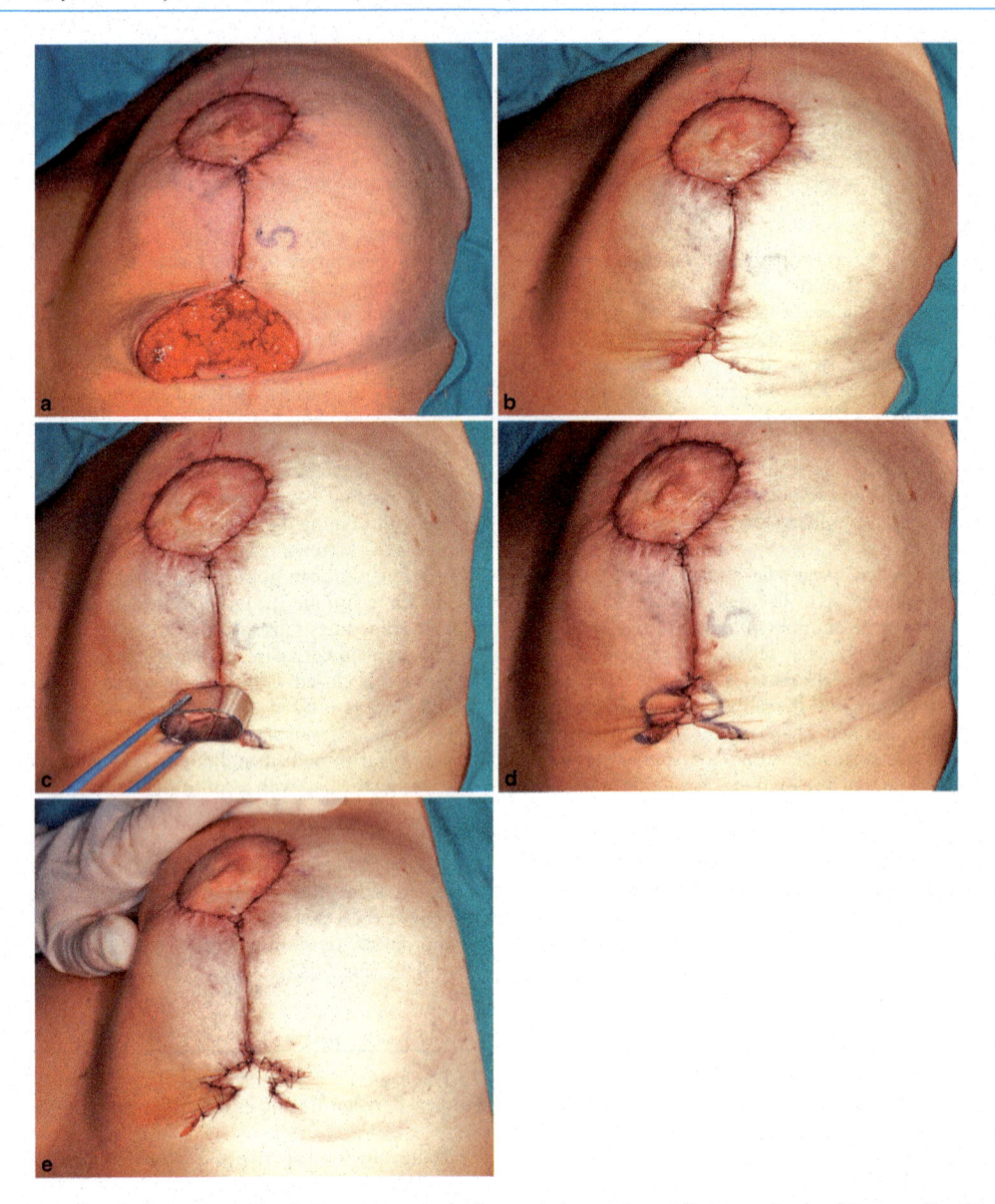

Fig. 70.7 Freehand adjustments. When dealing with sagging and atrophic skin, sometimes the accuracy of the geometric design can be surpassed. The figures show how to deal with these cases step by step. (**a**) The vertical skin excess is shown. (**b**) The vertical incision is closed with the planned length and its end point is sutured with a single stitch to the vertex of the inferior flap. The vertical excess is partially trimmed out and the exceeding skin is sutured covering the flap with a continuous running suture and applying appropriate tension. (**c, d**) The flap profile is outlined over the temporarily closed skin with the aid of a metallic pattern. (**e**) The traced skin is excised, leaving the exact dimension of the flap with the appropriate tension for skin closure

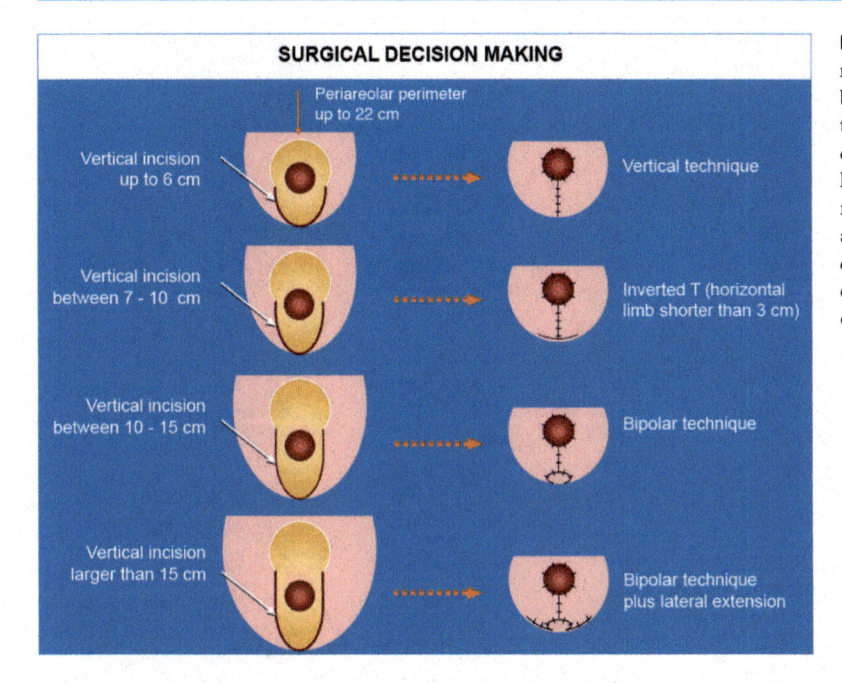

Fig. 70.8 Surgical decision making involved in the bipolar technique. There are two basic principles to be considered: (**a**) the periareolar perimeter resection must not exceed 22 cm; (**b**) the areola to inframammary crease distance must not exceed 7 cm for the average cases

making sure that the vertical scar does not exceed 7 cm in length.
2. When the vertical reduction design requirements range from 7 to 10 cm, an inverted T, with a small horizontal limb smaller than 3 cm, is indicated.
3. When the vertical reduction design requirements range from 10 to 15 cm, the inferior elliptical flap is indicated (bipolar technique).
4. When the vertical reduction design requirements exceed 15 cm, the inferior elliptical flap is indicated, but an extension toward the inframammary crease will also be necessary.

70.6 Conclusions

A mammaplasty technique focusing on the shortening of the horizontal inframammary scar is presented. This technique is based on a vertically enlarged periareolar skin resection and a small elliptical flap placed at the center of the submammary fold. The inferior flap absorbs the vertical skin excess remaining after the closure of the periareolar and vertical scar. This flap, which allows leaving the mammaplasty scars close to the breast meridian, is the fundamental contribution of this technique.

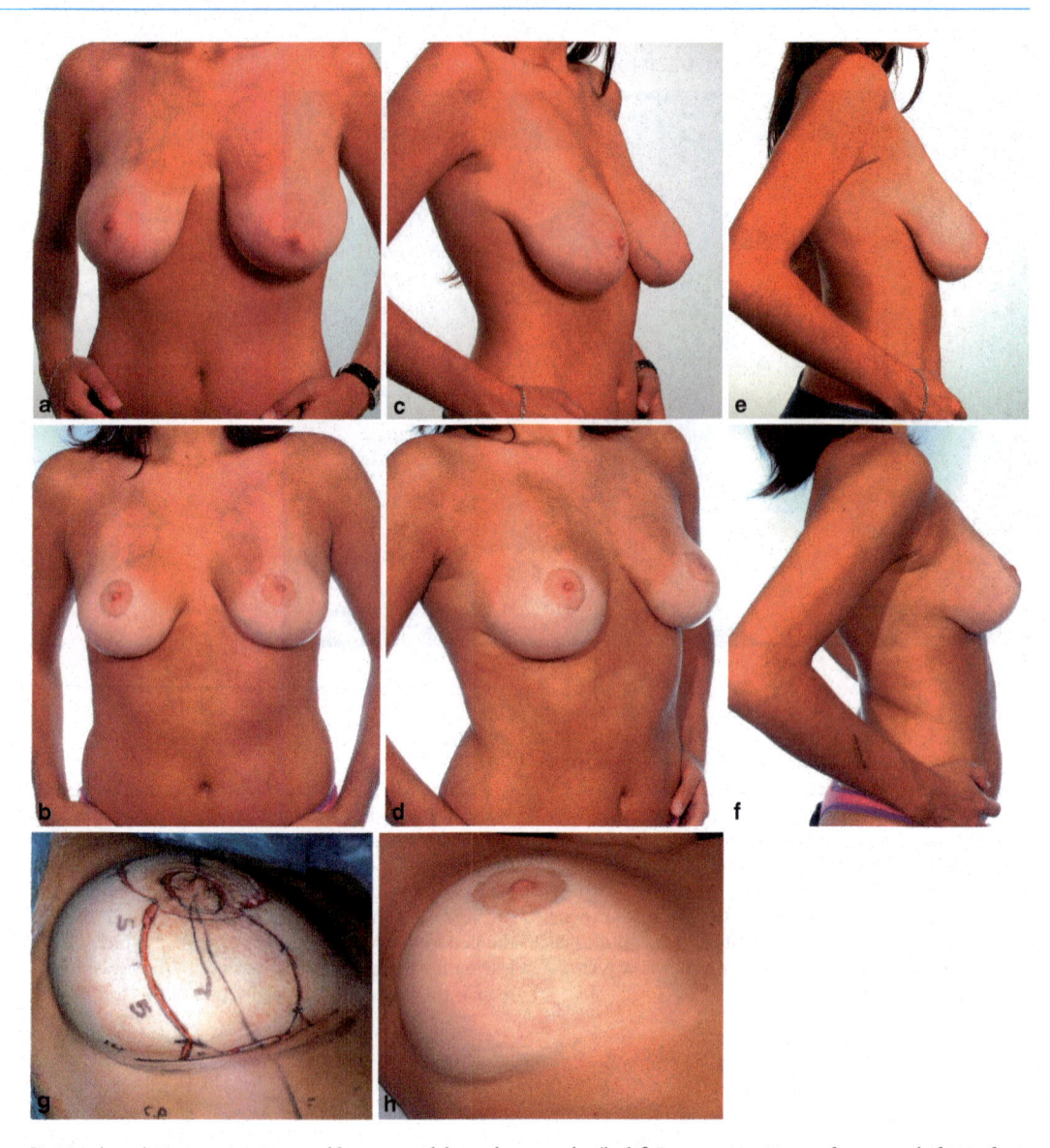

Fig. 70.9 (**a, c, e**) Preoperative 22-year-old woman with breast hypertrophy. (**b, d, f**) Postoperative 2 years after removal of 410 g from the right breast and 450 g from the left breast. (**g**) Skin markings. (**h**) Inferior elliptical scar with 1 cm lateral extension

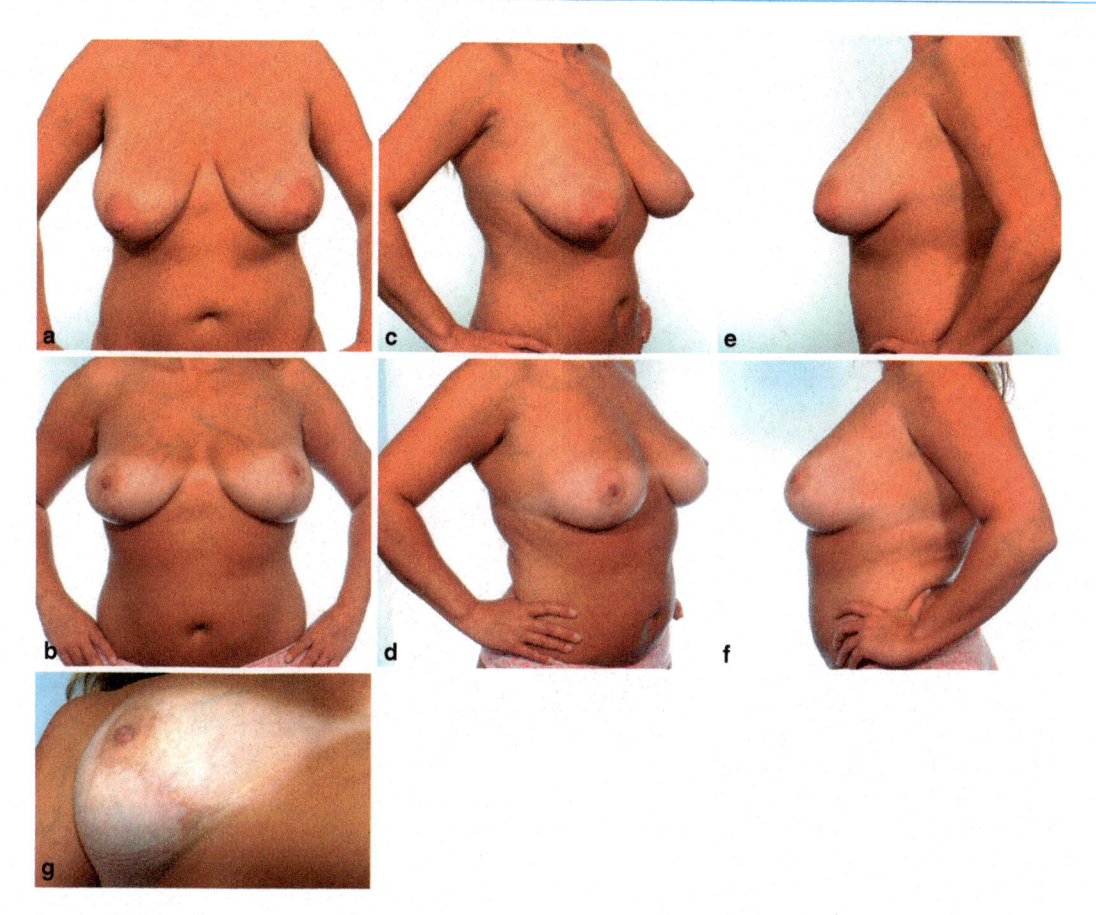

Fig. 70.10 (**a, c, e**) Preoperative 37-year-old woman with macromastia and a markedly ptotic breast. (**b, d, f**) Postoperative 10 months after removal of 390 g from the right breast and 360 g from the left. (**g**) Inferior scar. In this case, the vertical excess was easily absorbed by the inferior elliptical flap

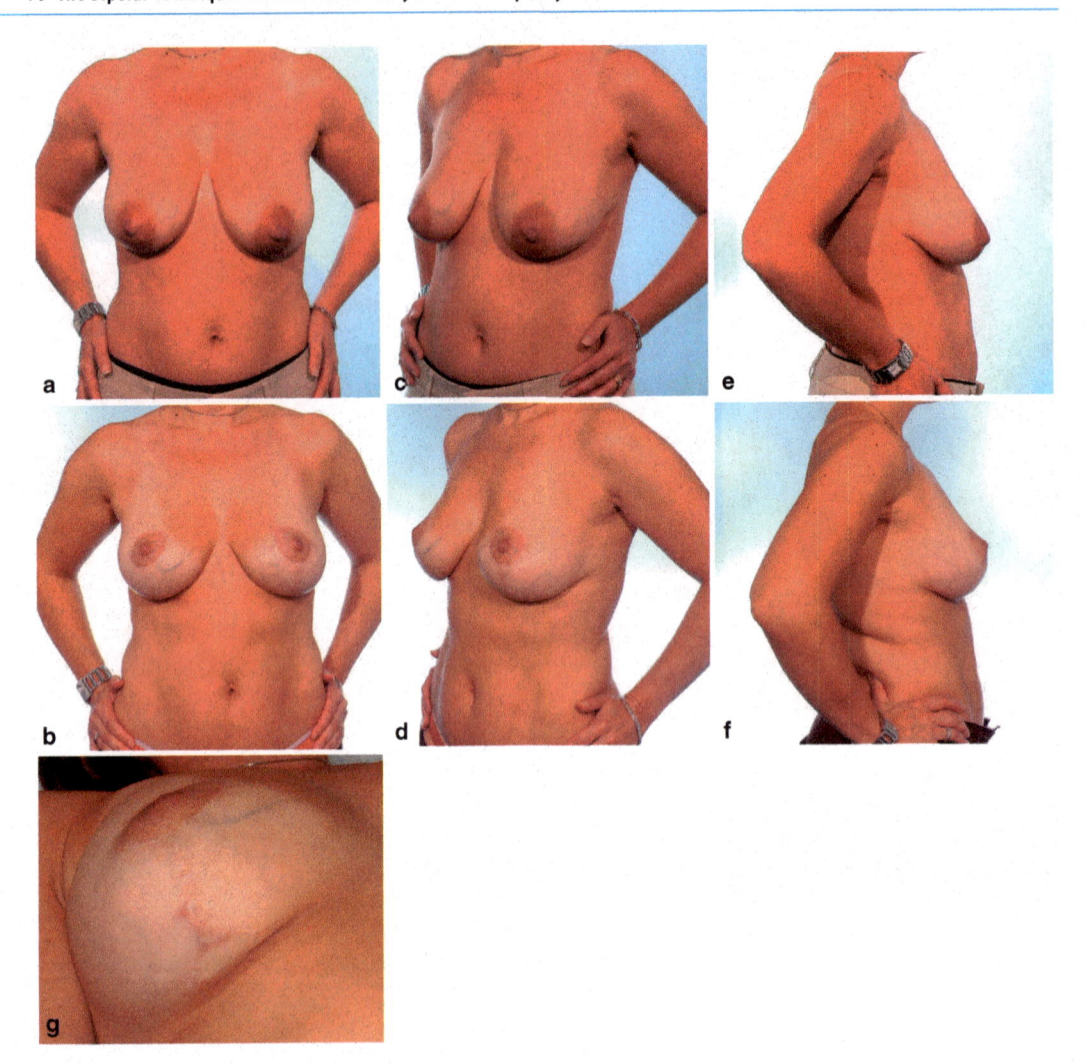

542   70 The Bipolar Technique: Short Inframammary Scar Mammaplasty

Fig. 70.11 (**a, c, e**) Preoperative 41-year-old woman with breast ptosis who requested a mastopexy. (**b, d, f**) Postoperative 20 months after mastopexy. (**g**) The vertical excess was resolved by the inferior elliptical flap without lateral extension

References

1. Wise RJ: Preliminary report on a method of planning the mammaplasty. Plast Reconstr Surg 1956;17(5):367–375
2. Hidalgo DA: Improving safety in aesthetic results in inverted T scar breast reduction. Plast Reconstr Surg 1999;103(3):874–886
3. Lassus C: A 30 year experience with vertical mammaplasty. Plast Reconstr Surg 1996;97(2):373–380
4. Benelli L: A new periareolar mammaplasty: The "round block" technique. Aesthetic Plast Surg 1990;14(2):93–100
5. Spear SL, Kassan M, Little JW: Guidelines in concentric mastopexy. Plast Reconstr Surg 1990;85(6):961–966
6. Hudson DA: Some thoughts on choosing a technique in breast reduction. (Editorial) Plast Reconstr Surg 1998;102(2): 554–557
7. Pickford MA, Boorman JG: Early experience with Lejour vertical scar reduction mammaplasty technique. Br J Plast Surg 1993;46(6):516–522
8. Lejour M: A simple device for marking the areola in Lejour's mammaplasty. (Discussion). Plast Reconstr Surg 1998;102(6):2136
9. Hammond DC: Short scar periareolar inferior pedicle reduction (SPAIR) mammaplasty. Plast Reconstr Surg 1999;103(3):890–901
10. De Carolis V: Short inframammary scar mammaplasty with an upper and lower pole encircling skin resection: "The Bipolar Technique". Plast Reconstr Surg 2002; 110(4):1092–1098
11. Reiffel RS: Prevention of hypertrophic scars by long term paper tape application. Plast Reconstr Surg 1995;96(7): 1715–1718
12. Spear S, Giese S, Ducic I: Concentric mastopexy revisited. Plast Reconstr Surg 2001;107(5):1294–1299

Breast Shaping by an Isolated Tissue Flap

Matthias Voigt, Christoph Andree

71.1 Introduction

The aim in breast reshaping surgery in tuberous breast, breast reduction, and mastopexy procedures is to keep the gained shape for a long time. One has to avoid the loss of fullness of the upper pole in breast reduction, the descent of the breast mass known as secondary dropout, and the relapse of the shape of the repaired tuberous breasts. The authors use a caudally based thoracic wall flap to avoid these problems. The blood supply of the breast comes from two main sources, the mammary internal and lateral arteries [1]. Because of invariably perforating vessels the pectoralis major muscle, it is possible to isolate a caudally based thoracic wall flap. These vessels originate from intercostal arteries as anteromedial intercostals perforators [1] and from the thoracoacromial artery like in the skin paddle of the pectoralis major muscle flap. This flap is long enough to reach every part of the breast where it is needed.

71.2 History

Breast surgery is in a constant evolution process in which scars are becoming shorter [2–8] and the shape of the breasts is better and longer lasting. Sophisticated techniques in the correction of tuberous breasts allow the patients to have a normal looking breast [9]. One of the latest modifications in breast reduction surgery is the use of a caudally based thoracic wall flap to fill up the upper quadrants and maintain the upper filling of the breast, introduced by Graf [10]. This technique follows the concept rather to resemble the breast tissue and to form a new breast than to believe in the skin belt theory. In breast reduction procedures, the breast tissue is divided actually into three parts: a lateral pillar, a medial pillar, and a caudal central part. The latter is supplied by perforating vessels emerging from the pectoralis major muscle (Fig. 71.1). The flap pedicle can be narrowed to the perforating vessels and some loose connecting tissue around the vessels, so that this tissue flap can reach nearly every part of the breast.

71.3 Technique

71.3.1 Caudally Based Thoracic Wall Flap Dimensions

The length of the caudally based thoracic wall flap changes according to the distance between the areola and the inframammary crease. Its upper limit is located 1 cm below the inferior edge of the areola, and the lateral borders extend to the medial and lateral breast contours if needed. It is advantageous to leave, laterally and medially, some breast tissue to cover the basis of the flap. The flap is 6–8 cm wide and 4 cm thick, and the vascular pedicle consists of the perforating vessels and some connecting tissue around it.

71.3.2 Breast Reduction and Mastopexy

71.3.2.1 Markings

The breast axis is found and the height of the submammary crease transferred on the outer aspect of the breast. This marking is used for the upper border of the areola. The nipple position is 2 cm lower. The medial and lateral border of the resection is found by drawing a vertical line moving the breast laterally and medially as described by Lejour et al. [6]. The skin resection ends caudally 3–4 cm above the existing submammary fold, and in larger breasts even higher. The new areola position is drawn free hand (Fig. 71.2).

71.3.2.2 Procedure

Under general anesthesia, de-epithelialization of the superior pedicle is carried out, creating the caudally based thoracic wall flap while cutting the lateral and medial line aiming away from the perforating vessels so as not to harm the blood supply. The skin stays on the tissue flap. It is possible to take some of the very caudal aspect of the flap, avoiding the supplying vessels. A bipedicled muscle sling is created out of the pectoralis major and the tissue flap is passed through the sling (Fig. 71.3). The passage should be wide so as not to constrict the blood supply. The medial and lateral breast tissue pillar is then sutured together covering the basis of the tissue flap. The areola is brought in the de-epithelialized new position. The skin is closed in two layers. In mastopexy procedures the technique is similar with or without or minimal resection of gland or fat.

71.3.2.3
Tuberous Breast Reconstruction

The marking in Type I deformities (deficient inner lower quadrant) is always for a vertical repair and in this sense similar to the planning of a vertical mastopexy. The submammary fold in Type I tuberous breasts is medially too high, and so it should be marked lower to create a round lower aspect of the breast. In Type I deformities (Fig. 71.4), a caudally based thoracic wall flap is created out of the lower, more lateral part of the breast (Fig. 71.5). The medial pillar is then freed from the muscular fascia, and the submammary fold lowered to the preoperatively marked height. The glandular flap is shifted under the mobilized skin, reaching the lowered submammary fold. Three or four Vicryl sutures hold the flap in its position. The breast tissue is sutured over the flap base so that a round breast mound is achieved. The opposite breast in four of the patients was hypoplastic, and therefore augmentation of the smaller breast through a submammary approach with anatomical gel implants that were partially submuscularly placed was performed.

In Type II deformities (deficient both lower quadrants) (Fig. 71.6), a vertical repair including the vertical scar or a periareolar repair is possible. The preoperative markings are similar to those in vertical or periareolar mastopexy. The herniated glandular tissue is separated from the upper gland and pedicled at the caudal central perforating vessels. The flap is turned over caudally and shifted under the mobilized caudal skin, reaching the lowered submammary fold. Three or four Vicryl sutures hold the flap in the desired position. If present, breast tissue is brought together over the flap basis and the skin closed in two layers. This procedure is similar to the one described by Ribeiro [9].

In all procedures, rigorous hemostasis is performed during the surgery and drains are used 24 h after the procedure. Routine follow-up controls include wound control, investigation of the nipple–areola complex (NAC) sensitivity, and sonographic check for fluids and steatonecrosis.

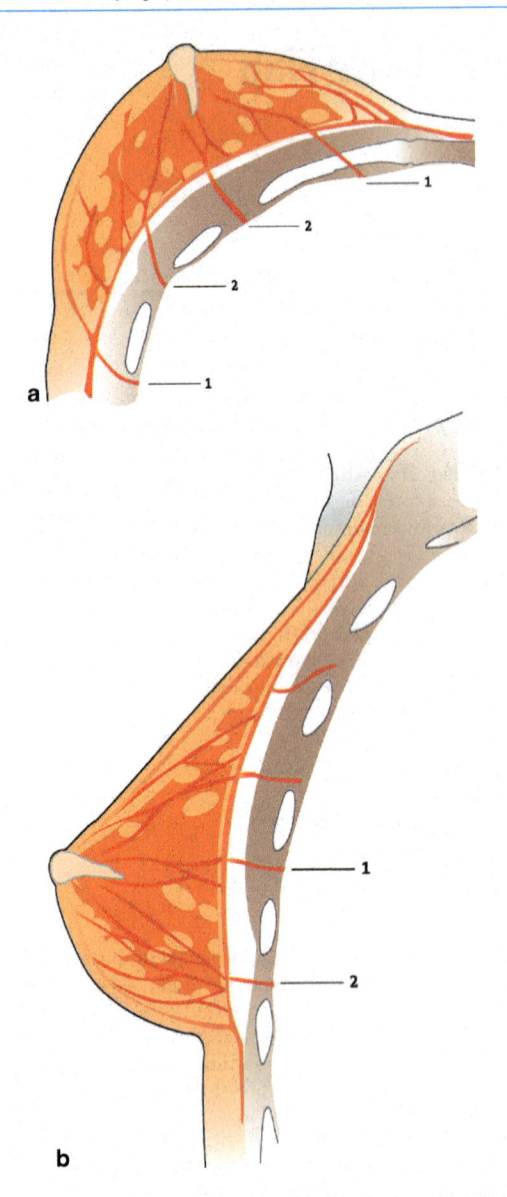

Fig. 71.1 Main sources of blood supply of the breast. (**1**) Medial and lateral perforating vessels. (**2**) Central perforating vessels through the pectoralis major muscle

flap to check the blood circulation and is removed later. The cranial breast tissue is undermined up to the second intercostal space, detaching the gland from the pectoralis major muscle fascia. Gland and fatty tissue resection can be made laterally, medially, and cranially. Care should be taken when resection takes place on the

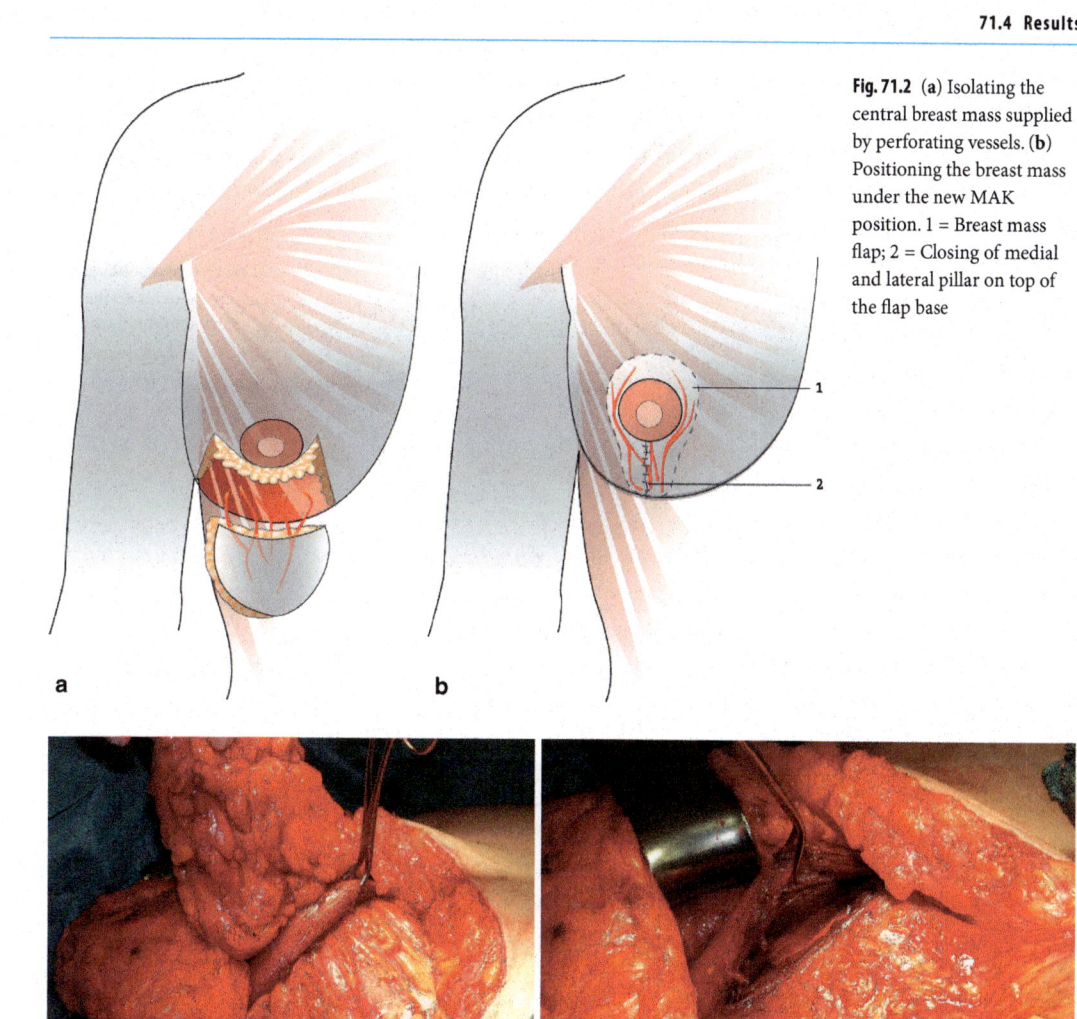

Fig. 71.2 (a) Isolating the central breast mass supplied by perforating vessels. (b) Positioning the breast mass under the new MAK position. 1 = Breast mass flap; 2 = Closing of medial and lateral pillar on top of the flap base

Fig. 71.3 Intraoperative site in breast reduction. (a) Pectoralis major muscle sling. (b) Caudally based thoracic wall flap passed under the sling

71.4 Results

The overall results are shown in Table 71.1. Between January 2002 and June 2007, 107 patients underwent procedures in which the caudally based thoracic wall flap was used. The patients' age ranged from 18 to 64 years. The follow-up period was 60 months.

The vertical scar technique was performed in patients with mild and severe breast ptosis; the best results, however, were achieved in patients with mild ptosis or hypertrophy as in every other series of breast reduction

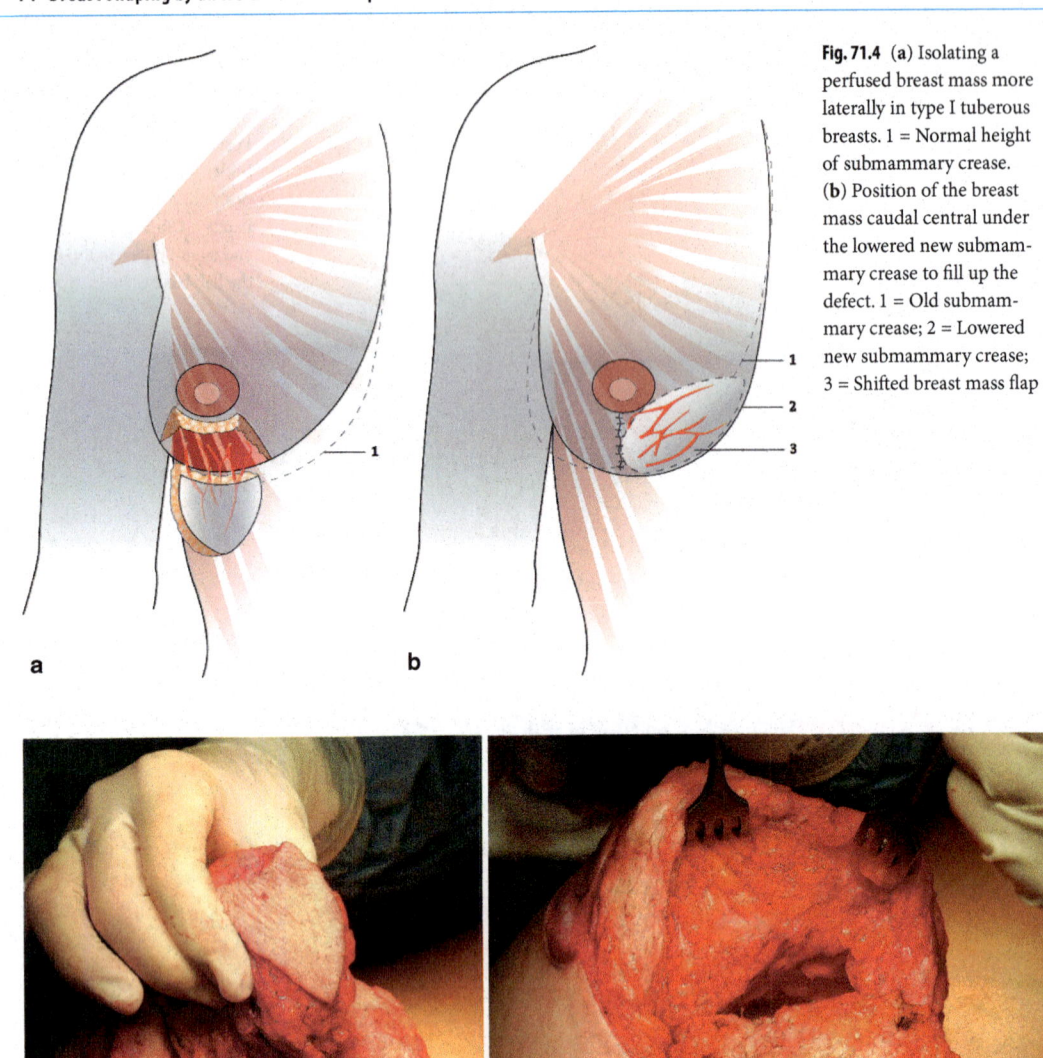

548   71 Breast Shaping by an Isolated Tissue Flap

Fig. 71.4 (**a**) Isolating a perfused breast mass more laterally in type I tuberous breasts. 1 = Normal height of submammary crease. (**b**) Position of the breast mass caudal central under the lowered new submammary crease to fill up the defect. 1 = Old submammary crease; 2 = Lowered new submammary crease; 3 = Shifted breast mass flap

Fig. 71.5 Intraoperative repair of a tuberous breast. (**a**) The caudally based thoracic wall flap is pedicled more laterally and (**b**) passed under the elevated medial pillar

techniques. Some wrinkles and excess skin were seen at the lower end of the vertical scar, which disappeared over a period of 3 months. In two patients the scar had to be revised with excision of the skin by means of a 5-cm horizontal scar. The projection of the breast in the upper quadrants, however, was lasting, especially in severe ptosis and hypertrophy (Figs. 71.7, 71.8).

With tuberous breast Type I, the missing breast tissue at the lower medial quadrant was replaced by the breast tissue flap and the regained normal breast shape did not

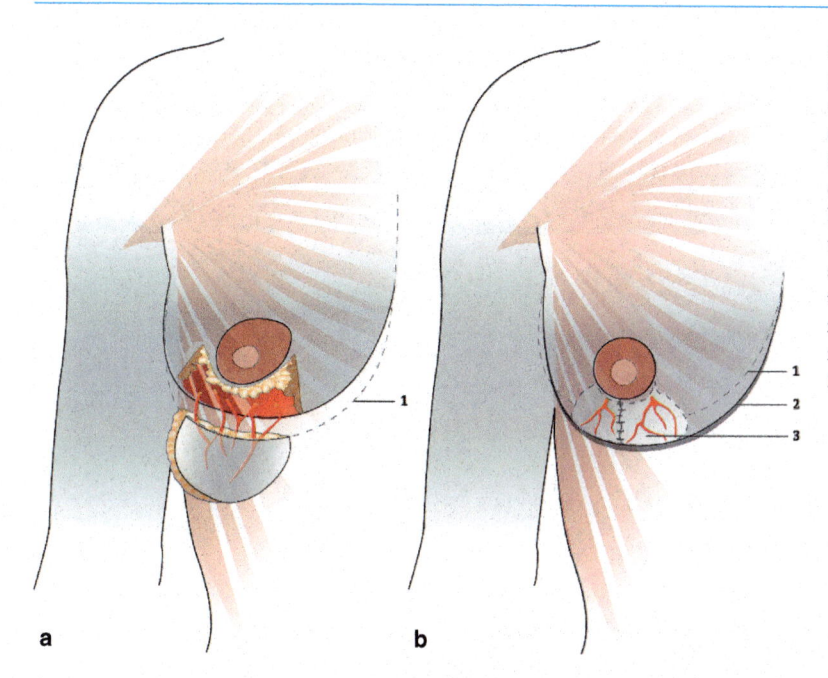

Fig. 71.6 (a) Isolating a perfused breast mass more caudal centrally in type II tuberous breasts. 1 = Normal height of submammary crease. (b) Position of the breast mass caudal central under the lowered new submammary crease to fill up the defect. 1 = Old submammary crease; 2 = Lowered new submammary crease; 3 = Shifted breast mass flap

change over the follow-up period. There were no complications (Fig. 71.9).

With tuberous breast Type II, the missing breast tissue at the lower quadrants was replaced by a turnover flap and the normal round reshaped breast contour remained over the follow-up period (Fig. 71.10).

71.5 Complications

Two hematomas had to be evacuated. There were wound-healing problems, which were solved by secondary intention in three patients, after reduction procedure in two, and after a tuberous breast repair at the lower border of the vertical scar in one. There were no instances of flap loss or steatonecrosis. There was a severe sensory change of the breast in 1 case (NAC pedicle 15 cm) and temporary decreased sensibility for 3 months in 14 patients (areola pedicle > 8 cm) (Table 71.1).

71.6 Discussion

The aim in breast reduction and mastopexy of normal-shaped or tuberous breast is to achieve a youthful, normal-shaped breast mound with moderate upper filling, short scars and a long-lasting result. Even as we try to create different, better techniques, the ideal technique has not yet been found. One of the major problems in breast shaping is the loss of upper filling, sagging of breast mass in the lower quadrants giving the NAC an upward projection, and the nipple appearing to be malpositioned too high. Short scars are now possible as we all try to use vertical techniques. Graf and Biggs [10] have improved a technique by Ribeiro [9] and later by Daniel [2], in which the breast mass is divided into three parts: a medial and a lateral pillar and a central tissue flap which is pedicled on the thoracic wall over some perforating vessels. They fixed this flap under a strip of pectoralis muscle under the new nipple position. The tissue flap acts as an autogenous implant. Obviously, the new breast mound stays divided in three parts, so the weight which hangs in the skin is less.

Another indication for this flap is in shaping tuberous breasts. In a type I tuberous breast, the lower inner quadrant is deficient. If the breast is ptotic, the central–lateral part of the breast can be isolated and put under the deficient lower–medial quadrant to gain a round breast shape.

In Type II tuberous breasts, the herniated breast mass medially and caudally can be isolated and, after the submammary fold has been lowered to a normal height, the missing caudal quadrants are filled.

Table 71.1 Overall complication rate in caudally based thoracic wall flap breast shaping procedures. There were two early cases in which both the lateral and the medial pillars were sewn over the base of the flap that was too thick resulting in overweight of the lower quadrants (bottoming out). Sensation loss was seen in one patient in whom the pedicle length of the NAC (nipple–areola complex) was 15 cm. Follow-up period ranged from 5 to 38 months with a median of 22.6 months

$N = 107$	Reduction ($N = 51$)	Mastopexy ($N = 36$)	Tub. breast Type I ($N = 12$)	Tub. breast Type II ($N = 8$)
Bottoming out	3	0	0	0
Fat necrosis	0	0	0	0
Wound healing problems	2	0	1	0
Hemorrhage	1	1	0	0
NAC blood circulation Problems	0	0	0	0
Nipple sensitivity loss	1 (NAC pedicle length 15 cm)	0	0	0

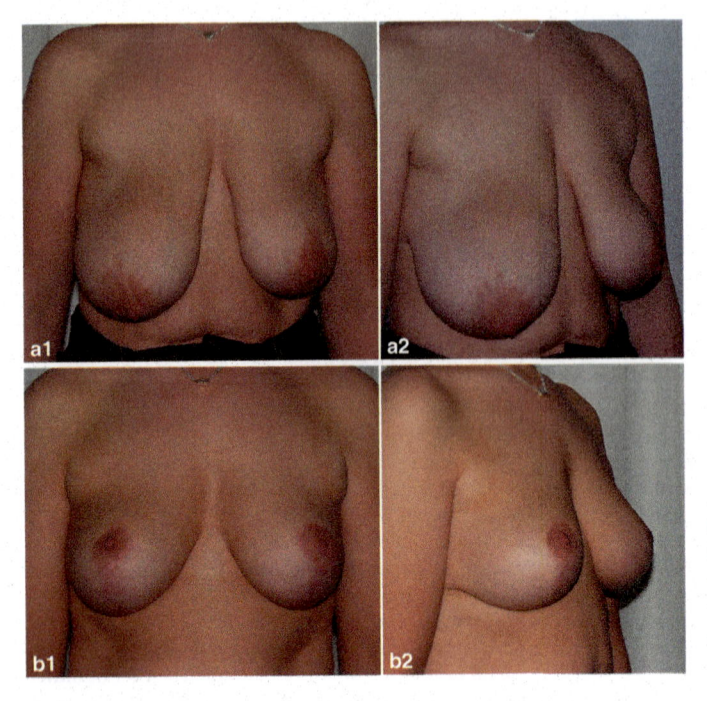

Fig. 71.7 (**a1,2**) A 38-year-old woman with marked ptosis and breast asymmetry after weight loss and breast feeding. (**b1,2**) One year after breast reduction and mastopexy with isolated caudal central breast mass to fill the upper quadrants

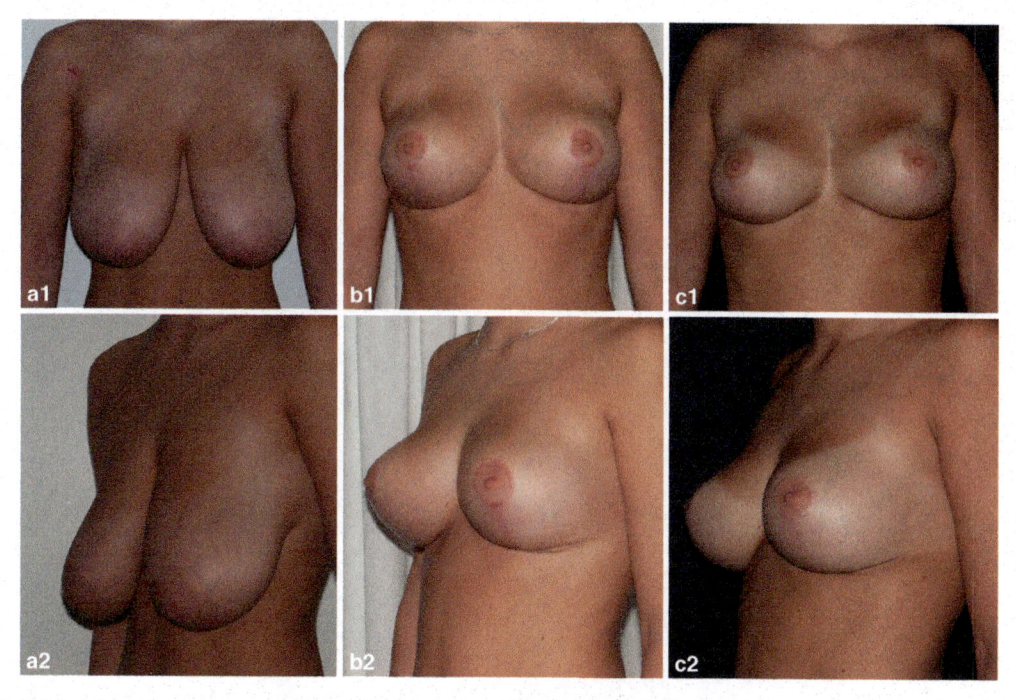

Fig. 71.8 (**a1,2**) A 22-year-old woman with juvenile hypertrophy and marked ptosis. (**b1,2**) Six months postoperative. (**c1,2**) Three years after breast reduction and mastopexy according to the described method, showing the stable projection and the upper fill of the new breast

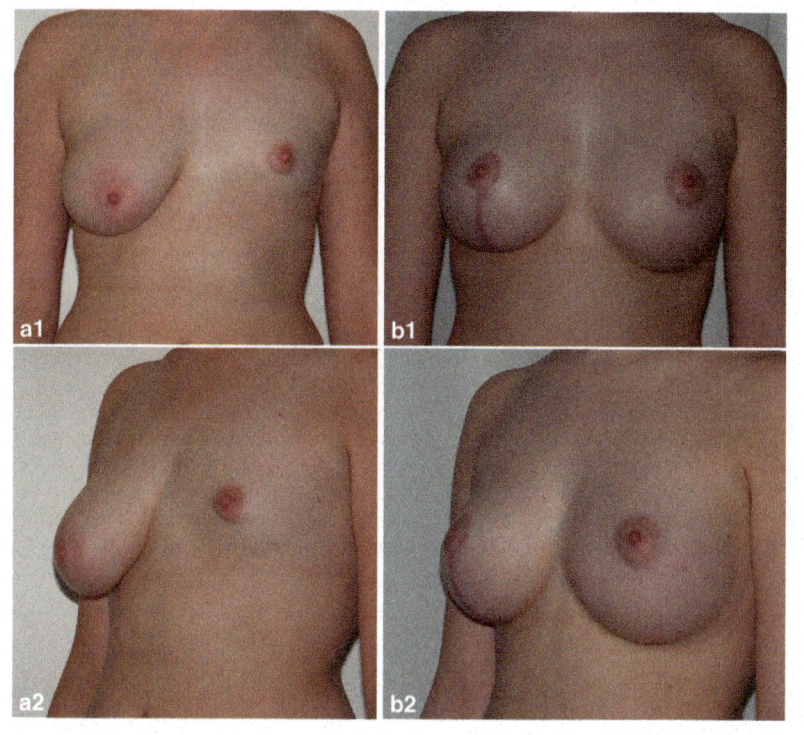

Fig. 71.9 (**a1,2**) A 20-year-old woman with tuberous breast Type I on her right and marked hypoplasia on her left. (**b1,2**) One year after breast shaping on her right with the transposed breast mass flap. Note the now round contour of the right breast. Anatomical breast implant partial subpectoral 320 ml on the left

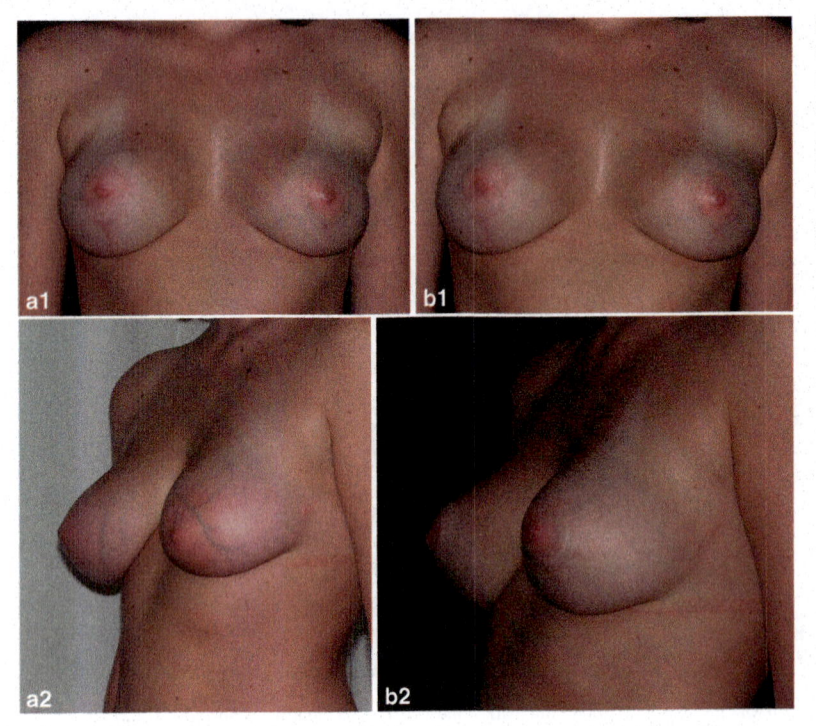

Fig. 71.10 (*a1,2*) A 21-year-old woman with tuberous breast deformity type II and marked asymmetry. (**b***1,2*) One-and-a-half years after transposing a central medial breast mass flap caudally to fill up the defect at the lower quadrants. Note the lowered submammary fold and reconstructed lower quadrants

Isolation of the tissue flap is crucial because it is the tension to other parts of the breast tissue that does not allow it to be pulled to the new position. The chance for long-lasting upper filling in breast reduction and long-lasting normal shape of a reconstructed tuberous breast is thus higher. When the isolated part of the breast is fixed under a pectoralis muscle strip, the weight on the skin is diminished and the probability of sagging is less.

Breast shaping can be performed with the caudally based thoracic wall flap in reduction procedures, mastopexy, and repair of tuberous breasts with nice and long-lasting results. The upper pole of the breast maintains a good projection, and in tuberous breast repair the normal breast mound shape is long lasting.

The length of the caudally based thoracic wall flap changes according to the distance between the areola and the inframammary crease. Its upper limit is located 1 cm below the inferior edge of the areola and the lateral borders can extend to the medial and lateral breast contours if needed. The flap is 6–8 cm wide and 4 cm thick, and the vascular pedicle consists of the perforating vessels and some connecting tissue around it. It is possible to narrow the pedicle like this to gain a greater arch of rotation without compromising the blood supply to the flap.

As in classical vertical reductions, remaining wrinkles and excess skin can be seen in the lower part of the vertical scar, which subside after 3 months without any treatment. In larger reductions, excess skin has to be removed by a short transversal resection, and compared to classic reduction procedures skin excess and dimples at the lower end of the vertical scar are less. The resection weight was lower in this technique compared to other techniques owing to the remaining flap weight left in the breast. So the resulting breast is a bit larger but with lasting projection and fullness of the upper part.

It is also possible to use these techniques in combination with a subpectoral implant, because the perforating vessels responsible for the blood supply of the flap partially originate from the thoraco-acromial vessels. These vessels can be raised like in a musculocutaneous pectoralis major flap.

There is a drawback of this technique that should be discussed preoperatively with the patient. In these techniques the breast tissue is divided, isolated, and shifted, and the lactiferous ducts are partially cut under the nipple; therefore, breast-feeding might not be possible and may be painful if it comes to mastitis due to scarified ducts.

71.7 Conclusions

The goal of every breast shaping procedure is to achieve adequate shape, nice skin coverage, NAC on the top of the created breast mound, short scars, and long-lasting results. With the caudally based thoracic wall flap technique, the breast tissue is divided into three main parts and built together afterwards. In reduction and mastopexy with this technique, the middle part of tissue is fixed under a muscle strip and so the tissue weight rests on the muscle and not on the skin or the remnant breast tissue. Therefore, the total weight of the breast tissue is diminished. This is the main cause for the minimal breast descent and long-lasting projection in the upper part of the breast.

In reshaped tuberous breasts, an isolated breast tissue flap could fill out the missing part of the breast. There is no tension on the tissue flap, so it acts as a homologous implant and stays there forever. The achieved breast shape remains.

References

1. Bostwick J III: Anatomy and physiology. In: Bostwick J III (ed), Plastic and Reconstructive Breast Surgery, 2nd edn. St. Louis, Missouri, Quality Medical 2000, pp 77–123
2. Daniel MJB: Mammaplasty with pectoral muscle flap. Presented at the 64th American Annual Scientific Meeting, Montreal 1995
3. Hall-Findlay EJ: A simplified vertical reduction mammaplasty: shortening the learning curve. Plast Reconstr Surg 1999;104(3):748–759
4. Lassus C: A technique for breast reduction. Int Surg 1970;53(1):69–72
5. Lassus C: Update on vertical mammaplasty. Plast Reconstr Surg 1999;104(7):2289–2298
6. Lejour M: Vertical mammaplasty and liposuction of the breast. Plast Reconstr Surg 1994;94(1):100–114
7. Lejour M: Vertical mammaplasty: Early complications after 250 personal consecutive cases. Plast Reconstr Surg 1999;104(3):764–770
8. Lejour M, Abboud M, Declety A, Kertesz P: Reduction of mammaplasty scars: from a short inframammary scar to a vertical scar. Ann Chir Plast Esthet 1990;35(5):369–379
9. Ribeiro L, Canzi W, Buss A Jr, Accorsi A Jr: Tuberous breast: A new approach. Plast Reconstr Surg 1998;101(1):42–50
10. Graf R, Reis de Araujo LR, Rippel R, Neto LG, Pace DT, Biggs T: Reduction mammaplasty and mastopexy using the vertical scar and thoracic wall flap technique. Aesthetic Plast Surg 2003;27(1):6–12

Free Nipple Areolar Graft Reduction Mammaplasty

Anthony Erian, Amal Dass

72.1 Introduction

Free nipple graft reduction mammaplasty describes a breast reduction technique in which the nipple–areolar complex (NAC) is transposed as a free graft to ensure its viability and to minimize complications. With advances in surgical techniques coupled with a better understanding of the vascular anatomy of the breast and the NAC, the limits at which free nipple grafting is preferred over transposition on a pedicle have been pushed further and further. However, it is still an operation that many surgeons turn to when faced with uncertainty over the viability of the NAC.

72.2 History

Breast reduction techniques had been described as early as the late nineteenth century, and Morestin's [1] report on transposing the nipple at the turn of the century. The concept of maintaining the nipple on a dermoglandular pedicle, as suggested by Strombeck in 1960 [2], revolutionized breast reduction surgery and still forms the basis of all subsequent improvements and modifications of the technique to this day. It was Thorek [3], however, who popularized free nipple grafting in 1922. Thorek combined the free nipple graft with lower pole amputation and his technique continues to this day albeit with a Wise pattern modification.

72.3 Indications

"Size and Haste" would aptly describe the most common indications for the free nipple graft reduction mammaplasty. Gigantomastia, described as a breast that requires resections in excess of 1,800 g per side, and the high risk in surgical patients [4], e.g., the elderly and those with medical comorbidities which limit the time that can be spent safely under general anesthesia, are the most common reasons for considering a free nipple graft reduction mammaplasty.

There are other indications for nipple areolar transplant in breast reduction (Table 72.1). Free nipple grafts are indicated if the NAC looks underperfused on a pedicle. This can be confirmed intraoperatively by intravenous (IV) administration of 2 g of fluorescein followed by examination under a Wood's lamp 15 min later. A yellow–green fluorescence of the NAC confirms an adequate blood supply, whereas a dark blue appearance indicates inadequate perfusion [4].

However, most surgeons would simply assess the nipple viability clinically. If there is no tension due to closure or constriction at the base of the pedicle and no hematoma or hypotension, the NAC should be removed from the pedicle and sited as a free nipple graft.

Avascular scar tissue from prior breast surgery may compromise the formation of a vascular pedicle. If this is the case, it may be prudent to consider free nipple grafting at the outset.

Male patients with severe gynecomastia may require a subtotal mastectomy which precludes keeping the NAC on an adequate dermoglandular pedicle, while the significant skin excision required in male patients following massive weight loss may mandate free nipple grafting for the best results [5]. Gender reassignment surgery to the breast involves breast amputation with free nipple grafting. The areola also has to be harvested and reduced to approximate the smaller male areola.

72.4 Vascular Anatomy of the Breast

The blood supply to the breast comes from six main sources: the internal thoracic artery, the highest thoracic artery, the anterior and posterior branches of the intercostal arteries, the thoracoacromial artery, the superficial thoracic artery, and the lateral thoracic artery. Of these, the internal thoracic vessels provide approximately 60% of the blood supply, with the lateral thoracic vessels providing approximately 30%. The tributaries of these two vessels form a rich anastomotic network around the NAC [4]. The arterial anatomy of the NAC is complex as

M.A. Shiffman (ed.), *Mastopexy and Breast Reduction: Principles and Practice,*
© Springer-Verlag Berlin Heidelberg 2009

Table 72.1 Indications for nipple areolar transplant in breast reduction

1. Gigantomastia
2. High-risk surgical candidates
3. Threatened NAC viability intraoperatively
4. Patients with previous operative scars
5. Patients with severe gynecomastia
6. Male patients after massive weight loss, resulting in severely redundant and inelastic skin
7. Female to male gender reassignment

a result of the contributions from six different sources. Various sources have identified the internal thoracic and the lateral thoracic arteries as the main blood supply routes to the NAC [6]. The reliability of the internal thoracic artery [7] as the sole blood supply route to the NAC has also been reported, as has the reliability of a lateral thoracic artery–bearing pedicle [8, 9].

The arterial supply around the NAC has recently been described as split into a superficial and deep anastomotic network [10]. The superficial system comprises tributaries of the internal thoracic, the highest thoracic and the superficial thoracic arteries, whereas the deep system is formed by the anastomoses of the lateral thoracic artery, the anterior and posterior branches of the intercostals arteries, and the thoracoacromial artery.

This may seem to suggest that the medial and lateral pedicles are the most reliable. However, the blood supply of the NAC described above fails to describe the importance of the perforators of the anterior branches of the intercostals arteries and the highest thoracic artery from the first to the fifth intercostals spaces [10]. Indeed, the perforators of the fourth and fifth intercostals vessels inferior to the NAC are remarkably consistent and of similar caliber to the internal thoracic and lateral thoracic vessels [11, 12].

Pedicle thickness and adherence to the pectoralis major muscle are also clearly important to the viability of the NAC. This may reflect on contributions from the perforators of the pectoralis major, which has been implicated in blood supply to the NAC. A thicker pedicle ensures that the vessels are enclosed safely within, thereby ensuring their viability while enhancing the reliability of the pedicle. An inferior pedicle with a base width of 8–10 cm is thought to ensure adequate perfusion for a pedicle of up to 21 cm in length [4].

While it has not been confirmed, as has been suggested, that the integrity of the NAC rests solely with the perforators rather than the subdermal plexi, there is little doubt that the perforators play an important role in NAC viability as evidenced by the success of the inferior pedicle reduction techniques as well as the fact that the most reliable pedicles are thicker and fashioned with a wider base without releasing their attachment to the pectoralis fascia.

Cadaveric anatomic studies do not take into account, however, the flow rate within these vessels in vivo and cannot be relied on solely for formulating an operative approach. However, an intimate knowledge of the vascular anatomy of the breast and its NAC can aid in ensuring nipple viability and a better aesthetic result whether it be a nipple transposition on a pedicle or a free nipple graft.

72.5
Preoperative Markings

The inferior pedicle reduction technique is most often used with free nipple grafts followed by the superior pedicle technique [13]. Other pedicles such as the superolateral and medial pedicles have also been employed. All these reductions employ standard Wise pattern markings to fashion the skin envelope over the underlying reduced breast parenchyma.

The placement of the nipple is the most vital step in preoperative planning. A superiorly displaced nipple is aesthetically unpleasant and may even peek out over the bra, causing distress to the patient. Moreover, correction of a high nipple is virtually impossible.

The breast meridian lines are drawn and the inframammary fold is transposed to the front of the breast either using calipers or the surgeon's finger within the fold. The sternal notch-to-nipple distance varies between 21 and 25 cm and should be tailored to the patient's size and reduction. This should roughly correspond to the inframammary fold. The nipple position is placed 1–2 cm below the measured nipple position along the meridian. This is to accommodate the "spring back" or McKissock effect when the weight of the breast tissue is removed and to prevent the nipple from pointing upwards secondary to lower pole fullness.

The position of the nipple can also be checked against the mid-point of the humerus ±2–3 cm as well as the internipple distance which should approximate the sternal notch-to-nipple distance.

Gradinger [14] has suggested another method of identifying the transposed nipple position (Fig. 72.1). A line is drawn from the superior point of the anterior axillary fold to the xyphoid sternum. This is to approximate the superior rim of a normal fitting brassiere. The superior rim of the areola should be 3 cm below this line along the meridian.

Gradinger also drapes a weighted tailor's tape measure around the neck and over the patient's chest, disregarding whether it falls medial or lateral to the nipple. A second tape is placed horizontally across the breast at

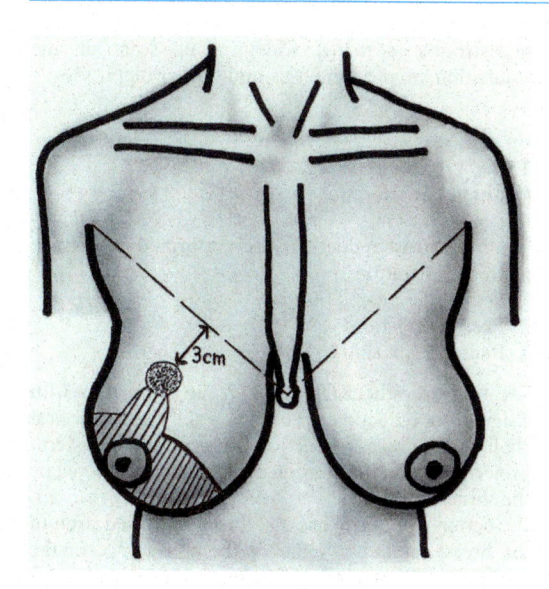

Fig. 72.1 Identifying the transposed nipple position. Adapted from [33]

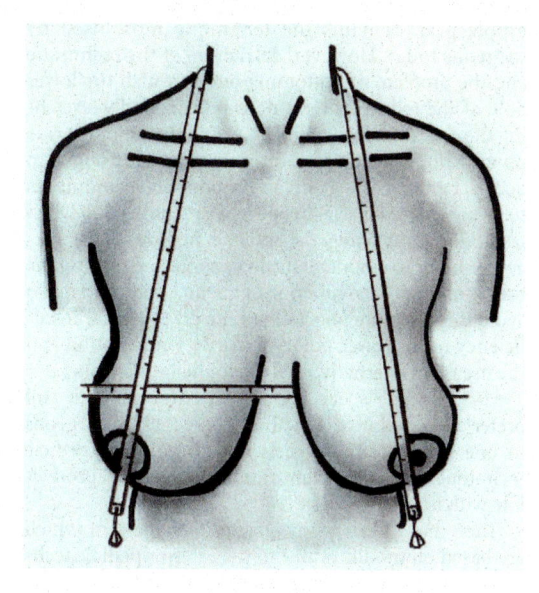

Fig. 72.2 The intersection of the two tapes is transposed onto the breast and describes the superior margin of the areola

the level of the inframammary fold. The intersection of the two tapes is transposed onto the breast and describes the superior margin of the areola (Fig. 72.2). This should correspond to a point within 1–2 cm of that described by the prior technique. The point of the weighted tape measure is to describe the true meridian to locate the nipple and to plan the operation around it rather than use the nipples of a massively hypertrophied breast to ascertain this.

The Wise pattern keyhole is then placed over the new nipple position and the template traced defining the vertical limbs. The vertical limbs vary between 5 and 9 cm with 7–7.5 cm being the most commonly used lengths. This describes the nipple-to-inframammary fold distance, which defines the lower pole of the new breast. A lazy "S" shaped incision is drawn from the lateral vertical limb to where the breast mound seems to end laterally. The process is repeated medially.

Women with gigantomastia frequently have excessively large areolas. The NAC is marked with a template prior to harvesting the free nipple graft. This usually varies from 4.2 to 4.7 cm in diameter and is chosen according to the planned reduction size.

72.6
Operative Technique: Free Nipple Grafting

The NAC is removed as a full thickness unit and thinned with a pair of scissors taking care to preserve the smooth muscle of the nipple and the dermis of the nipple and areola, as this is thought to more likely provide good postoperative projection and perhaps even erectility. It is then stored in a sponge moistened with saline.

The new nipple–areolar site is de-epithelialized. The breast reduction is then carried out according to the preoperative markings to fashion the skin envelope and the breast parenchyma reduced around the pedicle chosen.

The graft is positioned onto the recipient site with interrupted sutures and sutured into place with a running suture peripherally. A tie-over bolster dressing made up of Xerofoam gauze and mineral oil–moistened cotton is secured over the graft and left in place for 7–10 days.

72.7
Complications

Any form of breast reduction involves significant scarring which the patient must be made fully aware of. Any hesitation on the part of the patient regarding this or any of the other complication must result in postponement or cancellation of surgery until reassessment at a later date.

Criticism of the free nipple graft technique has frequently been directed at the seemingly greater postoperative loss of sensation in the NAC when compared to maintaining the NAC on a pedicle. While this may seem a reasonable conclusion, given that the NAC is severed from its vascular and nerve attachments as a free graft, recent reports contradict these earlier findings [15–17].

Studies have shown that even patients with free nipple grafts have a reasonable recovery in sensation, with erectile function persisting in most patients [18–20].

The recovery of sensation in the free nipple graft is likely multifactorial. Breast surgery by necessity divides some intercostal nerve fibers decreasing the sensation. Postoperative nipple sensibility has been shown to be inversely proportional to the amount of breast tissue resected [21]. Patients requiring free nipple graft reduction mammaplasty also tend to be older, which would also likely impair recovery in sensation [18].

Reinnervation from the intercostals and supraclavicular nerves probably explains why a large proportion of individuals regain some form of sensation after a free nipple graft [22, 23]. It has also been suggested that patients with gigantomastia have a chronic traction injury to the fourth intercostal nerve, relief of which contributes to improvement in sensation [24]. It is also noteworthy that the lack of sensation seems to bother the surgeon more than the patient.

Good recovery rates in erectile function of the nipple have also been demonstrated, which contradicts earlier conclusions by some authors that it was impossible to maintain erectile function in a free nipple graft. This could well be due to retaining a good amount of areolar smooth muscle when fashioning the graft [18, 20].

Nipple necrosis can occur with a free nipple graft, although partial loss is more common. This can be due to lack of vascularity of the parenchymal pedicle or improper harvesting and fashioning of the graft, or due to medical illnesses that limit vascularity as a whole. Partial nipple loss should be allowed to heal secondarily, with the patient warned about depigmentation. Nipple reconstruction should be planned for full nipple loss after allowing it to heal.

Hypopigmentation of the nipple is an unsightly complication which can occur even with good graft uptake. It has been well described in the literature [25] and seems more common in the darker areolas of patients of African origin. Tattooing of the hypopigmented patches is frequently unsatisfactory because of the dull-gray appearance it often takes despite the best efforts. The patient must be made aware of this and be accepting of the possibility of this complication.

Lactation is obviously compromised in a free nipple graft, as the lactiferous ducts are severed. The younger patient in whom the free nipple graft is indicated must accept this or have her surgery delayed till after childbearing.

All the other complications of breast surgery can also be encountered with a free nipple graft. These include hematomas, seromas, infections, skin necrosis, fat necrosis, and other wound complications. Complications seen in any other type of breast reduction can obviously also occur, such as breast asymmetry, over- or under-resection, a high-riding nipple or "bottoming out," hypertrophic scarring, widening of scars at the T-junction, nipple numbness, and skin or nipple loss.

72.8
Aesthetic Considerations

The best breast reductions are performed with three main considerations:
1. Pedicle design and position
2. Area of resection
3. Redraping or skin envelope design [26]

Creating an aesthetically shaped breast in a patient with a significant reduction has been one of the great surgical challenges in breast reduction surgery. Poor long-term projection is a very common complaint encountered by the surgeon [13].

Suction lipectomy has also been employed around the breast mound to enhance the appearance of the breast. Candidates for large reductions frequently tend to be overweight, and reducing the fat folds in the axilla and medial and lateral ends of the chest wall enhances the results of the surgery.

Inferior pedicle reduction mammaplasty with free nipple graft remains the technique most used by surgeons today. However, detractors of the technique cite the problem of bottoming out, in which the lower pole of the reduced breast descends gradually stretching the skin of the lower pole, causing the nipple to ride up and point upwards. Bottoming out is thought to occur at a rate of 0.44 mm a year on average and needs to be considered in the preoperative planning and when fashioning and fixing the inferior pedicle. Some surgeons prefer to amputate the lower pole and fashion the breast mound over superior or medial pedicle flaps to avoid this phenomenon. Others cite [27] vascular insufficiency of the lower pole to justify its amputation and the use of an alternative pedicle to the inferior one.

However, the sheer number of surgeons who still prefer and employ this method, some 74% of surgeons in one survey [13], suggests that the inferior pedicle technique offers consistent results which are reproducible with acceptable risks.

There have been many suggestions, most of which are based on modifications of the inferior pedicle technique, to improve the shape and projection of the breast. Most solutions to this problem have centered around retaining a dermoparenchymal flap, which can be shaped to approximate the breast mound. Traction on the lateral flap provides most of the coverage of the resultant defect. This allows flattening of the lateral pole and diminishes the need for the medial flap to be pulled excessively. Pulling the medial flap laterally in excess results in a breast that lacks the medial fullness of an unoperated breast.

Koger et al. [28] suggested preserving an inferior dermoparenchymal flap with a tapering, oblique excision of the glandular tissue to the muscle fascia to enhance the breast mound. In fashioning the flap, it is important to realize that in very large breasts frequently more than 90% of breast parenchyma is below the inframammary fold. Therefore flaps must be designed that can move cephalad and fit under skin envelope [29].

Other surgeons have suggested "staircasing" the incision and retaining glandular tissue along the excision line to help provide breast tissue for projection [30], as well as a keel-shaped excision of the keyhole to prevent excess flattening [31].

Vertical pedicle flaps are being increasingly used to shape the breast and to increase projection. A superolateral dermoparenchymal flap has been employed by Strauch et al. [25], in which the flap is rotated upwards after fashioning it to create a "periwinkle effect" by circular rotation [25] to increase projection from chest wall and create a more rounded contour (Fig. 72.3).

Hidalgo et al. [13] have suggested leaving de-epithelialized breast tissue below the 7-cm vertical limb to fold inwards to increase projection and then to bring in lateral and medial pillars to do the same.

Abramson [29] de-epithelializes the superior pedicle between the two vertical limbs of the Wise template while also maintaining an inferior dermal pedicle extending halfway between the inframammary fold and nipple. The lower flap is sutured to the pectoralis fascia and the superior flap is the folded over it while bringing in the lateral and medial flaps together (Fig. 72.4).

Ozerdem et al. [32] have also used a similar technique and suggested preserving the area between the vertical limbs of the Wise pattern even in a nonfree nipple graft reduction so that both superior and inferior dermoparenchymal flaps can be fashioned if the viability of the NAC is called into question.

Casas et al. [33] have suggested suturing the lateral and medial pillars of a superior parenchymal flap together to increase projection in a throwback to the Lejour technique of vertical mammaplasty where the medial and lateral pillars are sewn together. They also suggest intentionally creating a "dog ear" under the nipple to increase projection. However, projection and erectility are more likely a function of maintaining the areolar smooth muscle in the grafted NAC.

Breast amputation with the horizontal scar modified to include a backfolded dermoglandular superior pedicle flap with a free nipple graft after amputation of the lower pole has also been described [34]. Despite the added burden of de-epithelialization of the flap, the authors specifically cite the ease and speed of the operation (average 81 min operating time) in advocating this method.

The medial pedicle has also been used albeit less commonly, citing preservation of blood supply from the internal thoracic vessels and innervation to NAC as the advantages of this flap [35].

However, the choice of operative technique is ultimately dependent on the training and familiarity of the surgeon with it. No one technique has been shown to be markedly superior to another. As surgeons are attempting larger and larger reductions without a free nipple graft, it must always be remembered that a good number of candidates for a free nipple graft reduction mammaplasty are chosen to reduce the time spent intraoperatively. It is important not to compromise this by increasing the operative time spent by harvesting and de-epithelializing flaps. Aesthetics, while very important, should come only secondary to safety and symptom relief which are paramount.

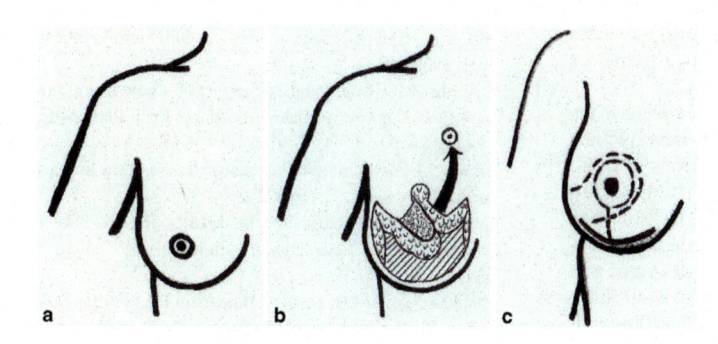

Fig. 72.3 (a–c) The flap is rotated upwards after fashioning it to create a "periwinkle effect" by circular rotation [25] to increase projection from chest wall and create a more rounded contour. Adapted from [25]

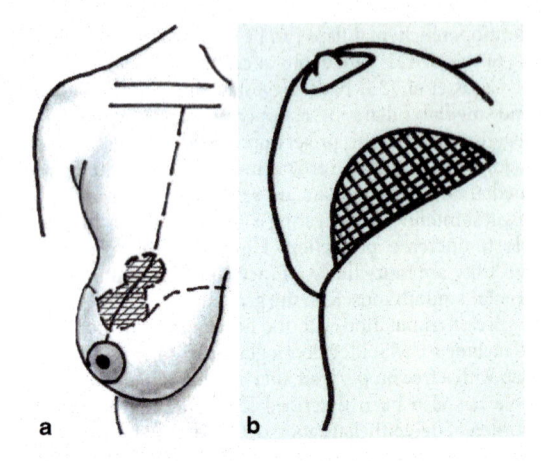

Fig. 72.4 (a,b) The superior pedicle between the two vertical limbs of the Wise template is de-epithelialized while also maintaining an inferior dermal pedicle extending halfway between the inframammary fold and nipple. The lower flap is sutured to the pectoralis fascia, and the superior flap is the folded over it while bringing in the lateral and medial flaps together. Adapted from [29]

72.9
Current Controversies with Free Nipple Graft Reduction Mammaplasty

The decision to perform a free nipple graft rests not on a set of rules but rather on arbitrary guidelines based on experience and largely anecdotal evidence. Limits for inferior pedicle reductions have been based both on reduction weights and other measurements.

The issue, of course, has been the viability of the pedicle; however, advances in the understanding of the vascular anatomy of the NAC and technical advances have challenged the limits set by the earlier experiences of surgeons.

Wise et al. [36] in a report detailing their experience with reduction mammaplasties in 1963 have recommended free nipple grafting in all reductions of more than three bra sizes. This then increased from 1,000 g (Gradinger [14]) to 1,500 g (Robbins [37], Jackson et al. [38]) to 2,500 g (Georgiade [39]). Georgiade has subsequently reported success without free nipple grafting in reductions of up to 3,300 g, while Chang et al. [40] have successfully transposed reductions of up to 5,100 g with a very low NAC necrosis rate of 1.2% over a 7-year period.

Pedicle length is a very common consideration in considering grafting over transposition of the nipple.

Common concerns are viability of the blood supply to the NAC and pedicle, folding and kinking of the pedicle, as well as excess tissue beneath and over the pedicle which can compromise it.

As with decisions based on the weight of the reduction, the recommended inferior pedicle length over which free nipple grafting should be considered has also increased over time from 15 to 25 cm [26]. This has been attributed to better handling of the pedicle, creating a pedicle with a wider base, and retaining the attachment of the base of the pedicle to the chest wall so as not to interrupt blood supply from the perforators.

Other authors cite the importance of the suprasternal notch (SSN)-to-nipple distance as most important in recommending free nipple grafting for distances exceeding 40 cm [25]. There has even been a suggestion that since the inframammary fold-to-nipple distance, which determines pedicle length, remains relatively constant when compared to the increasing SSN-to-nipple distance in progressively larger breasts, the inferior pedicle technique with transposition of the NAC on the pedicle should be applicable to all breast reductions regardless of size, rendering free nipple grafting obsolete [38].

72.10
Conclusions

There is little doubt that free nipple grafting maintains its place as a therapeutic option especially when patient fitness limits the operating time and when the NAC viability is called into question.

References

1. Morestin H: Hypertorphie mammaire. Bull Mem Soc Anat Paris 1905;80:682
2. Strombeck JO: Mammaplasty: report of a new technique based on the two pedicle procedure. Br J Plast Surg 1960;13:79–90
3. Thorek M: Possibilities in the reconstruction of the human form. N Y Med J 1922;116:572
4. Jones GE: Breast Reduction. In: Mathes SJ (ed), Plastic Surgery, 2nd edn. Philadelphia, Saunders Elsevier 2005, pp 539–584
5. Tashkandi M, Al-Qattan MM, Hassanain JM, Hawary MB, Sultan M: The surgical management of high-grade gynecomastia. Ann Plast Surg 2004;53(1):17–20; discussion 21
6. Nakajima H, Imanishi N, Aiso S: Arterial anatomy of the nipple-areola complex. Plast Reconstr Surg 1995;96(4): 843–845

7. van Deventer PV: The blood supply to the nipple-areola complex of the human mammary gland. Aesthetic Plast Surg 2004;28(6):393-390
8. Blondeel PN, Hamdi M, Van de Sijpe KA, Van Landuyt KH, Thiessen FE, Monstrey SJ: The latero-central glandular pedicle technique for breast reduction. Br J Plast Surg 2003;56(4):348-359
9. Marcus GH: Untersuchung uber die arterielle Blutversorgung der Mamilla. Arch F Klin Chir 1934;179:361
10. O'Dey D, Prescher A, Pallua N: Vascular reliability of nipple-areola complex-bearing pedicles: an anatomical microdissection study. Plast Reconstr Surg 2007;119(4):1167-1177
11. Manchot C: The Cutaneous Arteries of the Human Body. Berlin, Springer 1983
12. Corduff N, Taylor GI: Subglandular breast reduction: The evolution of a minimal scar approach to breast reduction. Plast Reconstr Surg 2004;113(1):175-184
13. Hidalgo DA, Elliot LF, Palumbo S, Casas L, Hammond D: Current trends in breast reduction. Plast Reconstr Surg 1999;104(3):806-815
14. Gradinger GP: Reduction mammoplasty utilizing nipple-areola transplantation. Clin Plast Surg 1988;15(4):641-654
15. Hoopes JE, Jabaley ME: Reduction mammaplasty: amputation and augmentation. Plast Reconstr Surg 1969;44(5):441-446
16. Craig RD, Sykes PA: Nipple sensitivity following reduction mammaplasty. Br J Plast Surg 1970;23(2):165-172
17. Courtiss EH, Goldwyn RM: Breast sensation before and after plastic surgery. Plast Reconstr Surg 1976;58(1):1-13
18. Townsend PL: Nipple sensation following breast reduction and free nipple transplantation. Br J Plast Surg 1974;27(4):308-310
19. O'Conor CM: Glandular excision with immediate mammary reconstruction. Plast Reconstr Surg 1964;33:57-60
20. Ahmed OA, Kolhe PS: Comparison of nipple and areolar sensation after breast reduction by free nipple graft and inferior pedicle techniques. Br J Plast Surg 2000;53(2):126-129
21. Gonzalez F, Brown FE, Gold ME, Walton RL, Shafer B: Preoperative and postoperative nipple-areola sensibility in patients undergoing reduction mammaplasty, Plast Reconstr Surg 1993;92(5):809-814
22. Sarhadi NS, Shaw Dunn J, Lee FD, Soutar DS: An anatomical study of the nerve supply of the breast, including the nipple and areola. Br J Plast Surg 1996;49(3):156-164
23. Farina MA, Newby BG, Alani HM: Innervation of the nipple-areola complex. Plast Reconstr Surg 1980;66(4):497-501
24. Slezak S, Lee DA: Quantitation of sensibility in gigantomastia and alteration following reduction mammaplasty. Plast Reconstr Surg 1993;91(7):1265-1269

25. Strauch B, Elkowitz M, Baum T, Herman C: Superolateral pedicle for breast surgery: an operation for all reasons. Plast Reconstr Surg 2005;115(5):1269-1277; discussion 1278-1279
26. Gerzenshtein J, Oswald T, McCluskey P, Caplan J, Angel MF: Avoiding free nipple grafting with the inferior pedicle technique. Ann Plast Surg. 2005;55(3):245-249
27. Aydin H, Bilgin-Karabulut A, Tumerdem B: Reduction mammaplasty using inferior pedicle technique combined with dermal suspension. Plast Reconstr Surg 2003;111(3):1362-1363
28. Koger KE, Sunde D, Press BH, Hovey LM: Reduction mammaplasty for gigantomastia using inferiorly based pedicle and free nipple transplantation. Ann Plast Surg 1994;33(5):561-564
29. Abramson DL: Increasing projection in patients undergoing free nipple graft reduction mammoplasty. Aesthetic Plast Surg 1999;23(4):282-284
30. McKissock P: Color Atlas of Mammaplasty. New York, Thieme 1991, pp 47-78
31. Fredricks S: Reduction mammaplasty for gigantomastia using inferiorly based pedicle and free nipple transplantation. Ann Plast Surg 1995;34(5):559
32. Ozerdem OR, Anlatici R, Maral T, Demiralay A: Modified free nipple graft reduction mammaplasty to increase breast projection with superior and inferior dermoglandular flaps. Ann Plast Surg 2002;49(5):506-510
33. Casas LA, Byun MY, Depoli PA: Maximizing breast projection after free-nipple-graft reduction mammaplasty. Plast Reconstr Surg 2001;107(4):955-960
34. Aydin H, Bilgin-Karabulut A, Tümerdem B: Free nipple reduction mammaplasty with a horizontal scar in high-risk patients. Aesthetic Plast Surg 2002;26(6):457-460
35. Nahabedian MY, McGibbon BM, Manson PN: Medial pedicle reduction mammaplasty for severe mammary hypertrophy. Plast Reconstr Surg 2000;105(3):896-904
36. Wise RJ, Gannon JP, Hill JR: Further experience with reduction mammaplasty. Plast Reconstr Surg 1963;32:12-20
37. Robbins TH: Reduction mammaplasty by the Robbins technique. Plast Reconstr Surg 1987;79(2):308-309
38. Jackson IT, Bayramicli M, Gupta M, Yavuzer R: Importance of the pedicle length measurement in reduction mammaplasty. Plast Reconstr Surg 1999;104(2):398-400
39. Georgiade GS, Riefkohl RE, Georgiade NG: The inferior dermal-pyramidal type breast reduction: Long-term evaluation. Ann Plast Surg 1989;23(3):203-211
40. Chang P, Shaaban AF, Canady JW, Ricciardelli EJ, Cram AE: Reduction mammaplasty: The results of avoiding nipple-areolar amputation in cases of extreme hypertrophy. Ann Plast Surg 1996;37(6):585-591

Liposuction Breast Reduction

Martin Jeffrey Moskovitz

73.1
Introduction

Over one hundred thousand women underwent breast reduction surgery in the United States in 2006. This represents 23% increase in the number of cases over the past 6 years [1]. Women undergoing breast reduction surgery complain of a spectrum of physical symptoms from pain in the back, neck, and shoulders, to intertrigo and hand numbness. Many social issues also come into play with women finding it difficult to buy clothing, attend social functions, and maintain a normal athletic regimen due to their large breasts. By definition, the key factors affecting breast hypertrophy sufferers are breast size and weight. It is only logical that surgical attempts at treating breast hypertrophy aim at treating breasts' size and weight issues. Traditional surgery uses a scalpel to cut skin, gland, and fat from the breast in order to achieve reduction in weight and size. Growing experience has demonstrated that liposuction alone can remove excess weight and achieve functional results similar to that of traditional breast reduction surgery.

73.2
History

Modern breast reduction surgery dates back over 50 years to the dermal pedicle techniques of Strombeck and McKissock and has moved to multiple types of parenchymal pedicle techniques popular today. Common to all these operations is the use of a scalpel to cut and remove skin, gland, and fat, of the breast and subsequently mold the breast into a smaller form. Ptosis correction and breast reduction take place concurrently since access to the breast requires incisions and those incisions may as well be used to correct skin excess.

Introduction of liposuction in the 1980s provided plastic surgeons with a powerful tool for body sculpting. Tumescent infiltration and other important advancements in liposuction technique allowed surgeons to safely and predictably address problems with localized adiposity which had been previously unsolvable or required unsightly and unacceptable scarring. Liposuction provided nearly scar-free passageway to solve issues of localized fat excess.

Use of liposuction in treatment of male breast excess (fatty gynecomastia) was rapid and multiple authors reported excellent results [2, 3]. Although efficacy in men was proved during the 1980s, liposuction was not applied to female breasts for many years and even then with severe limitations. Matarasso and Courtiss [4] advanced the concept of liposuction breast reduction but incorporated restrictions on its use that excluded the vast majority of patients. Foremost in these restrictions was exclusion of patients with any degree of breast ptosis. The concept behind the restriction was that the female breast should be corrected to a more youthful and tighter form at the same time as reduction and that liposuction alone could not achieve such a result. There are, however, errors with this concept.

The first misconception is that all women want tighter and more youthful breasts. Many women want smaller and lighter breasts. Historically, incisions needed to reduce the breast were used to concurrently lift the breast and accomplish a dual result. This result, however, comes at the cost of additional scars, longer recovery times, and higher complication rates. It is only logical that we offer an alternative to patients that reduces breast size alone without attacking the problem of ptosis in those patients unconcerned with ptosis.

The second misconception is that liposuction breast reduction will result in additional ptosis once fat has been removed. The ptosis present in macromastia patients is due to weight of the breast pulling down on breast skin. Once this weight is reduced by liposuction, skin recoils back significantly and in no case will the degree of ptosis be worse than preoperative. In many cases, skin recoil will be extreme and ptosis correction will be significant.

73.3
Patient Selection

Considering the evolution of liposuction breast reduction (LBR), the key issue in its use is patient selection. Patients whose main complaint is breast ptosis are not usually good candidates for LBR, while those who complain about breast weight symptoms such as back pain, neck pain, and difficulty buying clothing are often excellent ones.

Of course patients need to have a significant amount of breast fat to benefit from liposuction breast reduction, so assessment of breast composition needs to be considered. Patients with fat elsewhere on their bodies and normal to high body mass indices will tend to do well with LBR. Women who are thin and large breasted most likely suffer from glandular hypertrophy and will fail attempts at liposuction reduction. In general, older patients and those with children will also have higher fat content to their breasts. Key factors to examine are age, height, and weight. Ancillary testing such as mammography is minimally useful since mammograms are looking for calcifications and distortion and are poor predictors of fatty breast tissue despite the common reading of "fatty breast" or "glandular breast."

All women should have a proper preoperative workup. Mammograms are required in patients over 35 years of age and younger patients with family history of breast cancer should also have a baseline. Blood work and other tests are ordered as per usual protocols.

73.4
Technique

In general, liposuction breast reduction is treated like any other liposuction procedure. It can easily be done in the hospital or office surgery suite. Anesthesia can be general or tumescent with intravenous sedation. Tumescent solution alone is often inefficient for pain control especially when the lateral chest is being reduced at the same time.

The patient is marked in the standing position. A line is drawn one handbreadth below the clavicle bilaterally (Fig. 73.1). This marks an area with little breast tissue and a moderate amount of perforating vessels. When patients lie down the surgeon can mistakenly attempt to suction this area and will find little tissue and a higher hematoma rate. The inframammary crease is then marked and a planned insertion site is marked on each side two centimeters above the crease in the anterior axillary line (Fig. 73.2). Do not put the incision in the crease since the cannula's motion will tend to hit the ribs or abdomen and make the process much more difficult. Mark any lateral chest adiposity to be suctioned and note any breast asymmetry directly on the breast. In general, mild asymmetry will require 15–20% greater reduction on the larger side while more significant unevenness will often mandate a difference of 50–60% in the final aspirate volume.

Patients are placed prone on the operating table. Infection and deep vein thrombosis (DVT) prophylactic measures are taken as per protocol. Local anesthetic with epinephrine is injected at insertion sites and the patient is prepped and draped. Incisions are made and standard tumescent solution is placed. A "superwet" or fully tumescent technique is used and the breast is inflated until it is firm. The solution should then be allowed to take full effect for 10–15 min after which liposuction can proceed. Roughly one liter of fluid per breast is common though smaller breasts often require 500 ml and larger cases can demand 2–3 l per breast.

Liposuction is then performed with a 4 mm cannula. All planes of the breast from the pectoralis fascia to the skin are included though skin itself should not be aggressively suctioned. Superficial liposuction to skin will increase the risk of skin necrosis and minimally affect results.

If there is breast asymmetry the larger breast must be liposuctioned first since aggressive initial reduction of the smaller side could lead to a situation where the larger side can no longer be brought down in size to equal the smaller. Patients prefer two somewhat smaller, even breasts, to uneven breasts that are as small as possible. If only one breast is to be operated on, the endpoint should leave the operated breast slightly larger than the unoperated breast since swelling will mask true symmetry and the end result could be an over-resection if the breasts are made even on the table.

If liposuction of lateral chest is planned it should be done first since this area along the ribs is the most sensitive and will often require additional anesthesia. If this area is done last, additional medication can be required just before completion of surgery and the patient will need unnecessary operating room time to allow her to begin breathing and moving on her own.

Liposuction is performed until no further fat is removed or until bleeding becomes significant. Since the liposuction canister clearly measures removed amounts, even reduction is easily performed and asymmetry correction is simple. All removed material should settle for thirty minutes to assess amount of tissue removed and all tissue should be sent for pathology. The pathologist should be contacted directly so they understand the liposuction breast reduction procedure since they rarely, if ever, study liposuction aspirate specimens.

Incision sites are dressed with absorbent dressings and the patient is placed in a bra. An abdominal binder or Ace wraps are then placed for more compression.

73.5
Postoperative Care

Patients should change their dressings as needed overnight to keep dry, but must change them at least once. This is done to be sure that no areas of skin are kinked and subject to pressure necrosis.

Patients are seen in follow up the day after surgery and 1 week after surgery, and then again at 1, 6, and

12 months. Over the first 1–3 weeks ecchymosis will resolve and a mild "lumpiness" will be palpable, though not visible, in the breasts. This is due to trauma to the glandular tissue and will resolve completely in 3–6 months. Smokers can sometimes take up to 9 months to fully resolve. Breast massage may accelerate the healing process.

Patients should wear good bra support to take any tension off the skin so that skin's elasticity can maximally recoil and correct ptosis as much as possible. They should be sure that their nipples point forward or upward so that tension is taken off the skin to allow retraction.

Most patients can go back to desk work in 3–5 days and resume full exercise in 2 weeks.

Patients with significantly glandular breasts will need 3–6 months for all swelling to subside so they can see their final results. Predominantly fatty breasts will see reduction immediately and will need time only for skin retraction.

73.6
Complications

Hematoma is the most common complication with a rate of 2–4%. Bleeding will be evident in either the operating room or recovery room. The only known cases of bleeding postdischarge were in patients who drove home long distances immediately after surgery. For this reason, patients should stay in the area the night after surgery.

Most hematomas originate from perforators in the upper chest. Milking of blood followed by pressure dressing with ace wraps and gauze fluff to the bleeding area will stop progression of the hematoma. If there has already been a large amount of blood lost into the breast tissue and it does not express easily, the patient should be taken back to the operating room and blood suctioned out with the liposuction cannula. She should then be wrapped again tightly with gauze rolls to the bleeding site. There are no long term sequelae of hematoma, though the ecchymosis produced will last 1–3 months and can spread to the neck and arms.

Skin/nipple necrosis has been seen by the author only twice (<0.25% incidence) and in both cases patients were heavy smokers. In both cases patients also failed to change their dressings the night of the surgery. The cause of this limited necrosis is not certain, but it is reasonable to have smokers stop or decrease their smoking preoperatively and have patients change their dressings the night after surgery.

Infections are as rare in liposuction breast reduction as they are in other liposuction cases. I know of no cases. Antibiotic coverage should be given as per protocol, if needed.

Seromas are also very rare (<0.25%), most likely due to lymphatics of the breast area. The aggressive type of liposuction employed in LBR would have significant seroma rate if applied to other parts of the body such as the thighs, but in the breast, seromas are almost never seen. Contour deformities are equally rare. Any definite or questionable seroma should be aspirated with standard sterile technique.

Use of standard liposuction does not carry risk of carcinogenesis and mammographic breast exam is not adversely affected. Postoperative mammograms have shown benign calcifications as well as some mild scarring – both easily differentiated from a malignant processes. Ultrasonic liposuction is not advised since long term effects of ultrasound energy on breast tissue are not known and postoperative malignancy could be linked to breast reduction in litigation.

73.7
Procedural Tips

1. Choose patients with breast size/weight issues, not primarily ptosis complaints.
2. Mark the "Danger Zone" below the clavicle and avoid it during liposuction.
3. Mark incision above the inframammary fold in the anterior axillary line.
4. In asymmetry cases start liposuction on the larger side. If only one side is to be done, leave that side slightly larger than the non operated breast at the operation's conclusion to avoid over-resection. If both sides are done, look for an even endpoint.
5. Liposuction the lateral chest early in the procedure to avoid anesthesia issues.
6. Express hematomas or liposuction them – then rewrap tightly.
7. Patient should change dressings on the first postoperative night at least once.
8. Have mammograms when required and send aspirate for pathology.

73.8
Discussion

Liposuction breast reduction is a safe and efficacious procedure, yet it has been slow to move into the mainstream. The main reason for this is plastic surgeons' over appreciation for breast aesthetics and under appreciation of patient desires. During surgical training, plastic surgeons are instructed on aesthetics of the female breasts with note taken on nipple position and youthful projection. While many women do want the changes afforded by traditional surgical reduction techniques, many other women do not and strongly prefer the shorter recovery and lack of scarring of liposuction breast reduction.

Recent studies [5, 6] have demonstrated the high satisfaction rates of patients with the liposuction technique. The key factor in patient satisfaction is patient selection. Patients with standard complaints of back pain, neck pain, difficulty fitting into cloths, and general hardship with activities of daily living, will tend to do very well with liposuction breast reduction. Conversely, patients with ptosis complaints will do poorly. That is not to say that some ptosis correction does not occur with LBR. Removal of breast weight will allow skin to recoil and significant ptosis correction is possible. Sternal to nipple distance will decrease in all patients, though overall breast morphology may not change drastically. In many cases patients receive smaller version of the same breast they started with. This is opposed to traditional reduction mastopexy techniques where skin excision can lead to a dramatically different breast postoperatively. It is therefore important to discuss patient desires carefully and tailor the operation to the patient (Figs. 73.3–73.5).

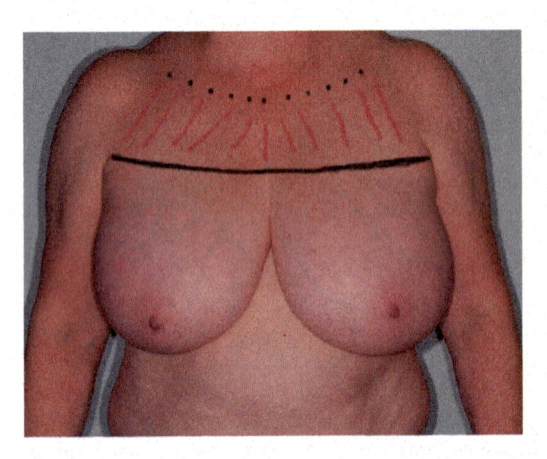

Fig. 73.1 Preoperative markings. Clavicle (*dotted lines*) and upper border of suction area (*solid line*). "Danger Zone" to be avoided hatched in *red*

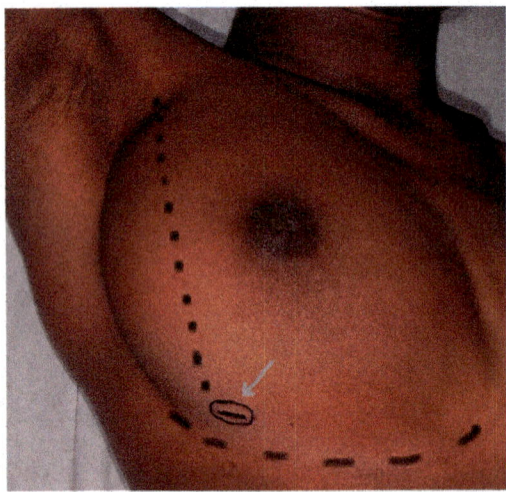

Fig. 73.2 Preoperative markings. Anterior axillary line (*dotted*) and inframammary fold (*dashed*). Incision *circled at arrow*

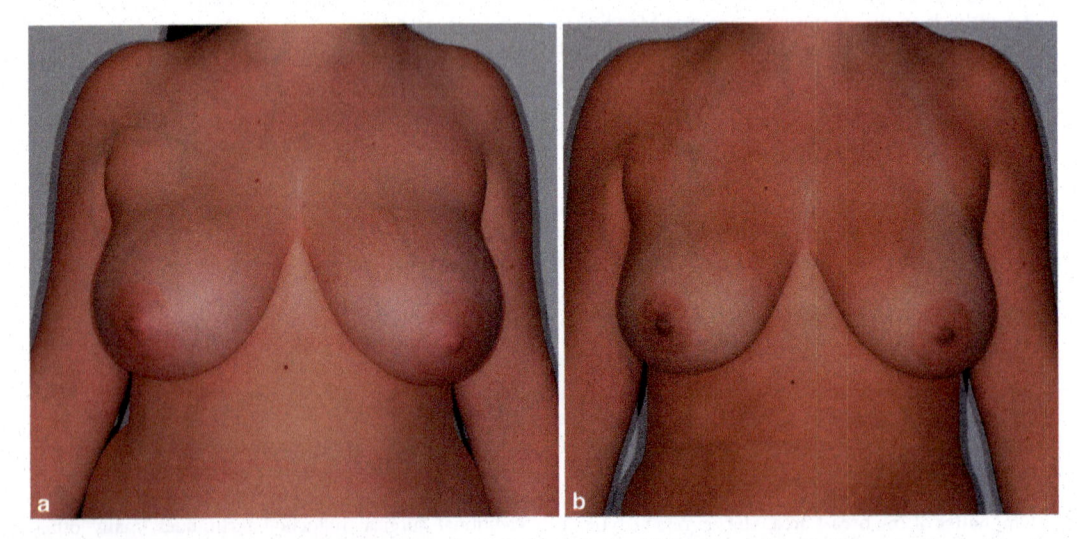

Fig. 73.3 (a) Preoperative 30-year-old female, 5′ 5″ tall, 156 lbs, 36 E cup bra. (b) Three months after liposuction breast reduction with 750 ml removed from each breast, a decrease of 2–3 cup sizes to a C cup

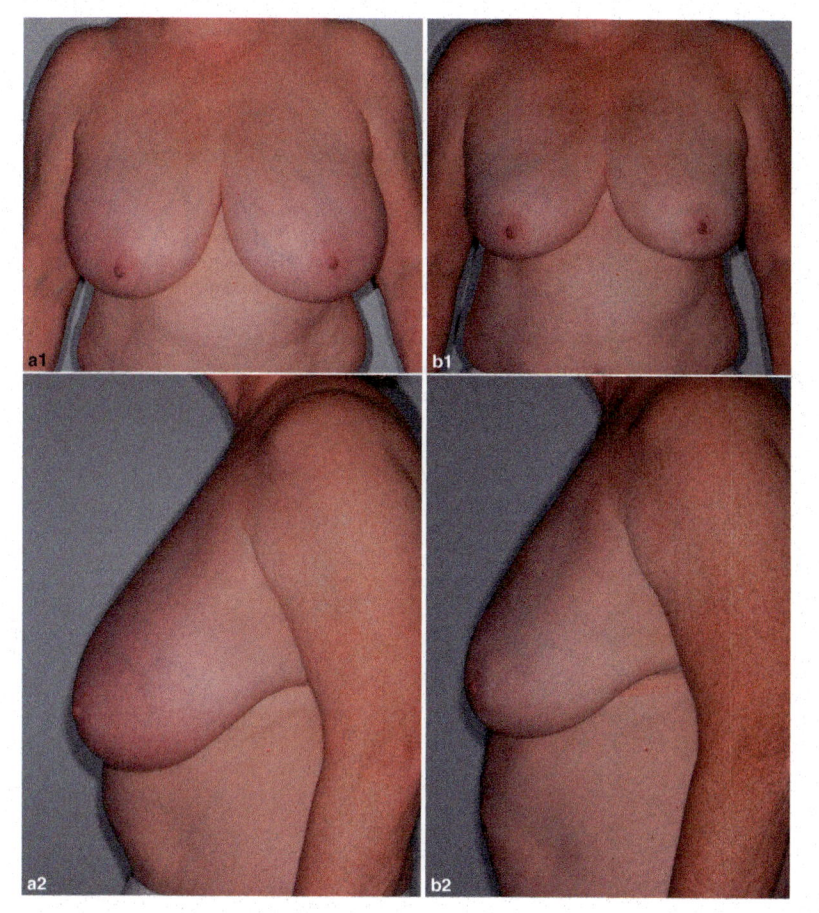

Fig. 73.4 (**a***1,2*) Preoperative 56-year-old female 5′ 2″ tall, 166 lbs. 44DDD bra. (**b***1,2*) Three months postoperative after liposuction breast reduction with 1100 ml fat removed from each breast. Now a C/D cup

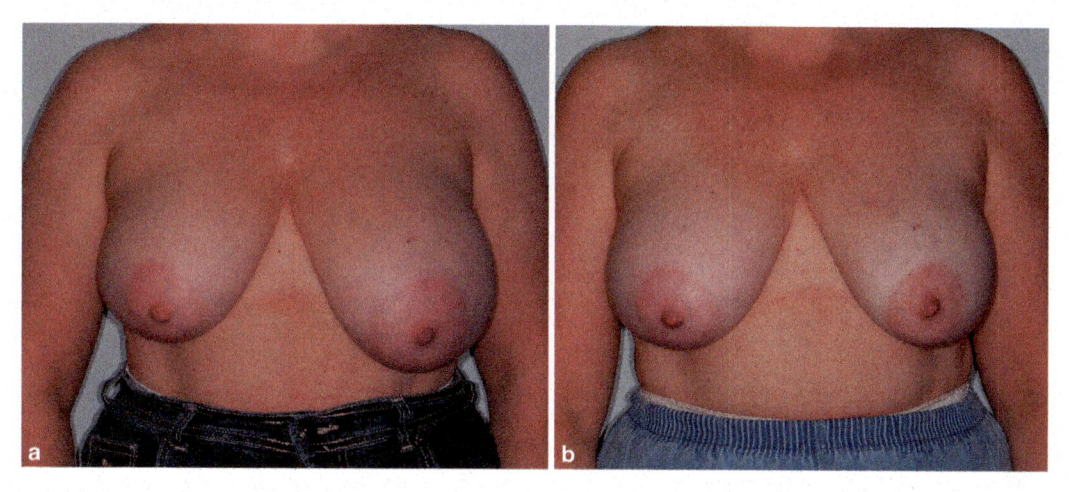

Fig. 73.5 (**a**) Preoperative 47-year-old female, 5′ 1″ tall, 140 lbs with uneven breasts since puberty. (**b**) Six months postoperatively after liposuction breast reduction on one side only with 700 ml of fat removed

73.9
Conclusions

Liposuction breast reduction is an important addition to the plastic surgeon's armamentarium. Many women with complaints of pain due to macromastia forego breast reduction surgery because they know the scars involved and will not consider the invasiveness of the procedure. These women are well served by liposuction breast reduction since it treats the cause of their discomfort while minimizing scars and recovery time. Liposuction breast reduction should not take the place of traditional techniques but should be added to the growing list of treatment options we present to our patients.

References

1. National Clearinghouse of Plastic Surgery Statistics. American Society of Plastic Surgeons. 2007
2. Courtiss EH: Gynecomastia: Analysis of 159 patients and current recommendation for treatment. Plast Reconstr Surg 1987;79(5):740–753
3. Rosenberg GJ: Gynecomastia: Suction lipectomy as a contemporary solution. Plast Reconstr Surg 1987;80(3):379–386
4. Matarasso A, Courtiss EH: Suction mammoplasty: The use of suction lipectomy to reduce large breasts. Plast Reconstr Surg 1991;87(4):709–717
5. Moskovitz MJ, Muskin E, Baxt SA: Outcome study in liposuction breast reduction. Plast Reconstr Surg 2004; 114(1):55–60
6. Moskovitz, MJ, Baxt SA, Jain AK, Housman RE: Liposuction breast reduction: a prospective trial in African American women. Plast Reconstr Surg 2007;119(2):718–726; discussion 727–728

Breast Reduction with Ultrasound-Assisted Liposuction

G. Patrick Maxwell, Allen Gabriel

74.1 Introduction

The number of breast reduction procedures performed in the United States continues to rise and the trend in plastic surgery, indeed in surgery as a whole, has been reduction in the size of skin incisions used to perform procedures. Patients with large breasts can have any of the following issues such as neck, back, and shoulder pain; intertrigo; postural imbalances; and difficulty with social situations and purchase of clothes. However, they continue to ask for minimally invasive procedures as they do not desire unwanted scars of traditional reduction mammaplasty.

An example of this paradigm shift to minimally invasive surgery is utilization of the endoscope for what were previously open procedures. The trend in surgery of the breast has been similar, as exemplified by the shorter scar techniques of Marchac [1], Lejour [2], and others, by the periareolar techniques such as those used by Goes [3] and Benelli [4], and by the use of the endoscope in breast augmentation and reconstruction.

Liposuction of the breast for purpose of breast reduction, by itself and as an adjunctive procedure, has been advocated by others [5–7], but carrying out this procedure has often been difficult and bloody, especially in younger patients whose breasts commonly contain higher proportion of breast tissue. Lejour has shown in her unique studies on composition of breast tissue that even the so called dense breast is at least 50% fatty tissue, so if this could easily and reliably be removed, small to moderate reductions could be accomplished with small incision ports alone, or perhaps with only a periareolar-type incision [8]. Larger breasts may become amenable to shorter scar techniques after reduction with ultrasound-assisted lipoplasty (UAL) as shown by Goes [9].

74.2 History

Introduction of modern liposuction techniques in the 1980s started the era of "minimally invasive" surgical procedures. Although this was widely used for body contouring procedures, its use in breast surgery was first described by Matarasso and Courtiss [10]. Liposuction mammaplasty was initially used for cases of mild hypertrophy without significant ptosis with great success [10, 11]. Increased support for advancing this procedure to more complex cases has been demonstrated successfully when used in proper patients [12–14]. This procedure gained popularity quickly in the management of gynecomastia [15, 16] and was also popularized for its ease of use through difficult fibrous tissues [17,18]. The first use of UAL in breasts was presented by Goes in 1995 [9].

Ultrasonic medical devices have been used in other fields for a number of years [19–28]. They have been used in neurosurgery, otology, ophthalmology, and urology to name a few specialties and have proved to be extremely useful and safe. UAL has been used in tens of thousand of plastic surgery cases in Europe and in other countries outside the United States for approximately 25 years [9, 17, 18, 29–31]. Plastic surgeons who have used these devices have been extremely enthusiastic about them and became more popular in the United States over the turn of the century [32–39].

74.3 Technique

74.3.1 Patient Selection

Patient selection in case of UAL mammaplasty is very important. Breast volume, soft tissue envelope, degree of ptosis, and patient expectations all need to be addressed. Ideal candidates are those with firm central glandular breasts with adipose tissue surrounding it. In addition, thick skin, good elasticity, and anatomically shaped breasts with minimal ptosis will see best results. If patients are not concerned with the preoperative degree of ptosis and are willing to except the same postoperative ptosis in exchange for scars then these patients may also be considered. Asymmetric breasts can also be successfully treated with this technique.

The following areas of the breast should be avoided with UAL for optimal results: periareolar, mammary ducts, and central breast. Define all treated areas preoperatively with intended direction of multiple parallel superficial tunnels. The tunnels should lie radial to the mammary cone, and should be placed in the lateral and upper medial quadrants.

74.3.2
Surgical Technique

This procedure is carried out under general anesthesia in the supine position. Monitored or local anesthesias are not recommended as it can very uncomfortable due to the amount of needed volume that is going to be infiltrated. In addition, the patient will be placed in 90° position several times during the case to achieve symmetry. The chest should be slightly elevated to enable assessment of the breast's anterior projection and degree of ptosis. The procedure is performed through two small incisions placed in the lateral inframammary fold (for infiltration of the hypo-osmolar solution) and within the axillary skin fold. These incisions permit easy access to the breast and allow for directional crossing of tunnels to be created by the cannula. In patients with gynecomastia, it is preferred to place incision in the periareolar margin. However, this approach should be avoided in breast reduction because the areola should always be preserved.

UAL is performed in superficial and deep planes while conventional liposuction is used only in deep planes. Deep treatment should be applied onto adipose tissue regions and should preferably be performed in the peripheral and subcutaneous layers of the breast, with conservation of the central glandular cone. In this way, the firm tissue responsible for the breast's anterior projection and the intercostal perforators which perfuse the gland are preserved. Therefore, the technique permits both volume reduction and shaping through treatment of specific areas which result in orientating the three-dimensional retraction of connective tissue and skin.

74.3.3
Postoperative Care

Suction drains are inserted through the submammary incision and placed subcutaneously along the lateral border of the breast. The drains should only be removed when output is less than 30 ml per day. A Reston occlusive compressive dressing is applied over the entire breast for seven days leaving the areola uncovered. This dressing has significantly reduced occurrence of hematoma and ecchymoses. These procedures are important to reduce edema in the early stages of healing and improve eventual retraction of connective breast tissue. Pain control is achieved with narcotics, NSAIDS, or even pulsed electromagnetic field therapy.

74.4
Complications

Most common complications are hematomas and seromas, which can be avoided by minimizing trauma during liposuction stage, utilizing effective and prolonged suction drainage, and by applying compressive dressings. Fat necrosis, which is more common in breasts with relatively less glandular tissue and in older patients, can be minimized by preventing tissue temperature from rising during application of ultrasonic energy, by performing liposuction gently, and by avoiding unnecessary tissue trauma. No cases of skin necrosis or burns have occurred that are caused by wide undermining of the sub dermal skin, local temperature rises, and persistent compression of the cannula tip onto the dermis.

74.5
Discussion

The fact that liposuction breast reduction can produce measurable and significant improvements in patients with breast hypertrophy should come as no surprise [40]. One of the principal concerns voiced by plastic surgeons regarding liposuction breast reduction is that it does not address the patient's ptosis symptoms. The key question to ask each patient considering liposuction breast reduction is whether their main complaint is weight related or ptosis related and liposuction breast reduction should be considered only in those patients where ptosis is not the main issue. No one technique is applicable to all patients and patients must be educated on the advantages and disadvantages of procedures available to them. Patients whose main complaint is breast ptosis are, by definition, poor candidates for liposuction breast reduction. Women whose complaints are weight-related are excellent candidates in many cases. Even this latter group of patients must understand, however, that the breast gland may be a significant part of their problem and will not be treated by liposuction breast reduction because liposuction can only remove fat, not gland. Thin patients with large breasts are often predominantly glandular and will fail liposuction breast reduction.

Other advantages of liposuction in breast reduction have been discussed by Matarasso and Courtiss [10], and Lejour [5]. Selective removal of fat from the breast should leave structures that are most important for breast survival, function, and sensation, and possibly make reduction more stable and less likely to be affected by fluctuations in weight during the postoperative period. Breast liposuction additionally makes achieving symmetry, even secondarily, quite easy as it has been demonstrated by several authors [9, 13, 31, 32, 40].

Ultrasound Assisted Liposuction, offers clear cut advantages over traditional liposuction in several ways: (1) UAL appears to be less trauma to surrounding tissues and structures and appears to target fat cells alone respecting vessels, nerves, and other tissue types; (2) It is physically much easier to perform liposuction with UAL, and UAL cannulas slide easily and atraumatically through even dense fibrous tissues; (3) There appears to be less blood loss, and the emulsion removed is essentially yellow–white in color; (4) There appears to be improved skin retraction over the area suctioned, but whether this is caused by thermal trauma to the underside of the dermis (an "internal peel") or by easily accomplished superficial fat removal as hypothesized by Illouz [41], is yet undetermined; (5) Results of UAL as compared with traditional liposuction appear to be much smoother, probably because of even emulsification and removal of fat as compared with irregular removal of chunks of tissue by the suction cannulas.

The authors have performed reduction mammaplasties on patients using UAL alone. Results have been quite good, with minimal bruising and actual reduction of the suprasternal notch to nipple distances of 2–3 cm. Postoperative mammograms were obtained at 12 months. Comparison with preoperative radiographs shows only increased density of the breast tissue, which might have been predicted after removal of the fatty tissues. There were no abnormal calcifications or any changes that could be misinterpreted as breast cancer. On examination, all breasts were soft without areas of skin changes or firmness. One of the primary initial concerns with liposuction was the possibility of inducing fat necrosis leading to inframammary calcification. A 2-year follow-up of Courtiss' original patients has failed to demonstrate any traumatic calcification [42]. This observation has been corroborated by Lejour [43], who performed extensive whole breast liposuction in her series of vertical reductions without evidence of traumatic calcification. Concern has been voiced about the use of UAL in the breast. Calcification has not been seen as cause for concern after either suction modality. The role of ultrasonic energy in inducing malignant change remains unclear, although this is probably more theoretical than practical. Calcification can occur with any type of breast surgery and are usually associated with fat necrosis and ischemia. Changes noted after traditional reduction mammaplasty have been seen to be predictable and usually distinguishable from breast cancer [44, 45]. Abboud et al. [44], published a study which concurs with this. Liposuction in conjunction with surgery was used to perform reduction in 250 breasts, and 13% developed calcifications that were benign in appearance. Liposuction in general and UAL in particular should be less traumatic to the vasculature of the breast, and we would expect to see fewer calcifications. Walgenbach et al. [46] compared breast tissue treated only with conventional lipectomy to breast tissue treated with UAL. Results showed stronger destruction of the cellular structure of adipocytes in the conventional treated group. Destruction was visible even in areas more distant from the aspiration channel. In contrast, breast tissue treated with UAL was mostly intact, without signs of ultrasonic-induced cellular destruction. The glandular structure was kept intact. Besides direct mechanical destruction by the probe and the cannula, no further alterations of cellular integrity of the glandular parts were visible. This study conclusively indicated that UAL is a safe technique for use in breast surgery. Besides easy handling and improved modeling, the destructive effect of ultrasound does not include the glandular breast tissue (Fig. 74.1).

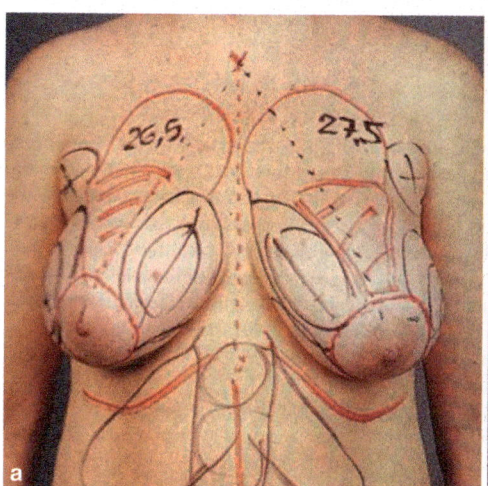

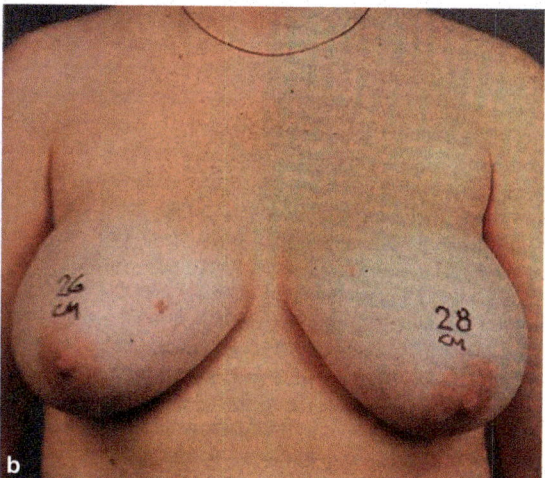

Fig. 74.1 (a) A 33-year-old woman with preoperative markings. (b) Six months after removal of 425 ml from each breast using ultrasound-assisted liposuction

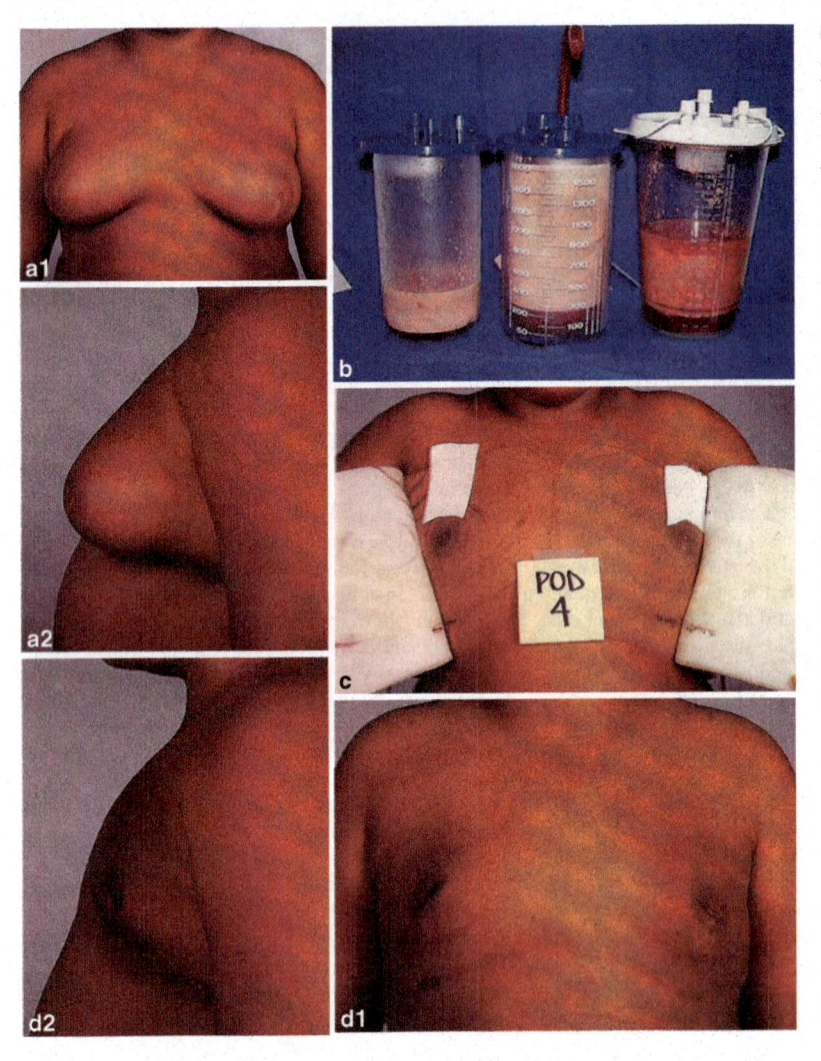

Fig. 74.2 (a) Preoperative appearance of a 10-year-old boy with severe gynecomastia. (b) One thousand six hundred ml and 1,800 ml were removed from the right and left sides, respectively, via a single port in each inframammary fold. The canisters on the *left* show typical material obtained with UAL. That on *the right* shows material that was removed at the end of the procedure using traditional liposuction to remove any fluid left behind after UAL was completed. (c) Four days after surgery at the time of the removal of his dressings. Note lack of bruising. (d) Four weeks after UAL-only procedure showing excellent resolution of the patient's gynecomastia

Concern has been expressed about the possibility of UAL interfering with detection of occult breast cancers, because the emulsion cannot be sent for pathological evaluation. In the study by Abboud et al. [43], the aspirate from traditional liposuction of the breasts was sent for histological exam, and only one of 170 specimens contained breast cells. The remainders of the cells were adipocytes and because of this insignificant yield, they have even stopped sending specimens for histology. If UAL indeed affects only the fatty tissues, then breast cancers should not be affected. The resultant denser reduced breast does not appear to be more difficult to patrol either radiologically or with physical examinations.

The authors have found UAL to be a useful adjunct in other forms of breast surgery, such as primary traditional breast reduction, secondary breast reductions, and second stage breast reconstructions. Whereas many of these results could be accomplished perhaps with traditional liposuction, UAL can be used with much less effort and trauma. The authors have tried using traditional liposuction in areas such as the axillary regions for purposes of comparison and were virtually unable to pass the cannulas. In contrast, UAL cannulas of the same diameter can be passed with only two fingers and a light touch.

Another area of breast surgery where UAL has gained popularity is the treatment of gynecomastia. Authors have reported improved management of this with suction alone or with suction and skin excision depending on the level of ptosis and need for skin excision [30].

The fact that patients are happy following liposuction breast reduction should come as no surprise, since most patients are always worried about external scarring in cases of these procedures. Women desire an operation to treat their primary problem, breast hypertrophy, and are willing to forego treatment of their secondary breast ptosis. These reports also infer that many women may avoid traditional breast reduction surgery because of inherent permanent scars, invasive nature of procedure, and recovery time required. In practice, the authors have found that many women, especially older patients, desire to relieve themselves of breast hypertrophy symptoms and are happy to continue to wear a bra for their ptosis issues. Similarly, many younger patients are content to reduce their bra size by limited amount, provided they do not encounter noticeable breast scarring (Fig. 74.2).

74.6
Conclusions

Use of UAL in surgery of the breast has provided an alternative to patients seeking minimal invasive or minimally scarring procedure. In selected cases, UAL is a valuable adjunct to procedures such as correcting symmetry, reduction mammaplasty, and breast reconstruction permitting both volume reduction and shaping through three-dimensional retraction of connective tissue and skin.

References

1. Marchac D, de Olarte G: Reduction mammaplasty and correction of ptosis with a short inframammary scar. Plast Reconstr Surg 1982;69(1):45–55
2. Lejour M: Vertical mammaplasty. Plast Reconstr Surg 1993;92(5):985–986
3. Goes JC: Periareolar mammoplasty: double skin technique with application of polyglactin or mixed mesh. Plast Reconstr Surg 1996;97(5):959–968
4. Benelli L: A new periareolar mammaplasty: The "round block" technique. Aesthetic Plast Surg 1990;14(2):93–100
5. Lejour M: Vertical mammaplasty and liposuction of the breast. Plast Reconstr Surg 1994;94(1):100–114
6. Teimourian B, Massac E Jr, Wiegering CE: Reduction suction mammoplasty and suction lipectomy as an adjunct to breast surgery. Aesthetic Plast Surg 1985;9(2):97–100
7. Toledo LS, Matsudo PK: Mammoplasty using liposuction and the periareolar incision. Aesthetic Plast Surg 1989;13(1):9–13
8. Lejour M: Evaluation of fat in breast tissue removed by vertical mammaplasty. Plast Reconstr Surg 1997;99(2):386–393
9. Goes JC: The use of UAL in breast surgery. In: Inaugural meeting of the International Society of Ultrasonic Surgery. Portugal, Algarve 1995
10. Matarasso A, Courtiss EH: Suction mammaplasty: the use of suction lipectomy to reduce large breasts. Plast Reconstr Surg 1991;87(4):709–717
11. Matarasso A: Suction mammaplasty: The use of suction lipectomy to reduce large breasts. Plast Reconstr Surg 2000;105(7):2604–2607; discussion 2608–2610
12. Gray LN: Liposuction breast reduction. Aesthetic Plast Surg 1998;22(3):159–162
13. Gray LN: Update on experience with liposuction breast reduction. Plast Reconstr Surg 2001;108(4):1006–1010; discussion 1011–1013
14. Moskovitz MJ, Muskin E, Baxt SA: Outcome study in liposuction breast reduction. Plast Reconstr Surg 2004;114(1):55–60; discussion 61
15. Courtiss EH: Gynecomastia: Analysis of 159 patients and current recommendations for treatment. Plast Reconstr Surg 1987;79(5):740–753
16. Rosenberg GJ: Gynecomastia: Suction lipectomy as a contemporary solution. Plast Reconstr Surg 1987;80(3):379–386
17. Zocchi M: Ultrasonic liposculpturing. Aesthetic Plast Surg 1992;16(4):287–298
18. Zocchi ML: Ultrasonic assisted lipoplasty. Technical refinements and clinical evaluations. Clin Plast Surg 1996;23(4):575–598
19. Young W, Cohen AR, Hunt CD, Ransohoff J: Acute physiological effects of ultrasonic vibrations on nervous tissue. Neurosurgery 1981;8(6):689–694
20. Chopp RT, Shah BB, Addonizio JC: Use of ultrasonic surgical aspirator in renal surgery. Urology 1983;22(2):157–159
21. Tranberg KG, Rigotti P, Brackett KA, Bjornson HS, Fischer JE, Joffe SN: Liver resection. A comparison using the Nd-YAG laser, an ultrasonic surgical aspirator, or blunt dissection. Am J Surg 1986;151(3):368–373
22. Derderian GP, Walshaw R, McGehee J: Ultrasonic surgical dissection in the dog spleen. Am J Surg 1982;143(2):269–273
23. Flamm ES, Ransohoff J, Wuchinich D, Broadwin A: Preliminary experience with ultrasonic aspiration in neurosurgery. Neurosurgery 1978;2(3):240–245
24. Richmond IL, Hawksley CA: Evaluation of the histopathology of brain tumor tissue obtained by ultrasonic aspiration. Neurosurgery 1983;13(4):415–419
25. Hodgson WJ, Bakare S, Harrington E, Finkelstein J, Poddar PK, Loscalzo LL, Weitz J, McElhinney AJ: General surgical evaluation of a powered device operating at ultrasonic frequencies. Mt Sinai J Med 1979;46(2):99–103
26. Weitz J, Hodgson WJ, Loscalzo LJ, McElhinney AJ: A bloodless technique for tongue surgery. Head Neck Surg 1981;3(3):244–246
27. Fasano VA, Zeme S, Frego L, Gunetti R: Ultrasonic aspiration in the surgical treatment of intracranial tumors. J Neurosurg Sci 1981;25(1):35–40

28. Eguaras MG, Saceda JL, Luque I, Concha M: Mitral and aortic valve decalcification by ultrasonic energy. Experimental report. J Thorac Cardiovasc Surg 1988;95(6):1038–1040
29. Millan Mateo J, Vaquero Perez MM: Systematic procedure for ultrasonically assisted lipoplasty. Aesthetic Plast Surg 2000;24(4):259–269
30. Zocchi ML: Basic physics for ultrasound-assisted lipoplasty. Clin Plast Surg 1999;26(2):209–220
31. Goes JC, Landecker A: Ultrasound-assisted lipoplasty (UAL) in breast surgery. Aesthetic Plast Surg 2002;26(1):1–9
32. Di Giuseppe A: Breast reduction with ultrasound-assisted lipoplasty. Plast Reconstr Surg 2003;112(1):71–82
33. Gingrass MK, Kenkel JM: Comparing ultrasound-assisted lipoplasty with suction-assisted lipoplasty. Clin Plast Surg 1999;26(2):283–288
34. Hultman CS, McPhail LE, Donaldson JH, Wohl DA: Surgical management of HIV-associated lipodystrophy: role of ultrasonic-assisted liposuction and suction-assisted lipectomy in the treatment of lipohypertrophy. Ann Plast Surg 2007;58(3):255–263
35. Nahai F: Positioning for ultrasound-assisted lipoplasty. Clin Plast Surg 1999;26(2):235–243
36. Rohrich RJ, Beran SJ, Kenkel JM, Adams WP Jr, DiSpaltro F: Extending the role of liposuction in body contouring with ultrasound-assisted liposuction. Plast Reconstr Surg 1998;101(4):1090–1102; discussion 117–119
37. Rohrich RJ, Gosman AA, Brown SA, Tonadapu P, Foster B: Current preferences for breast reduction techniques: a survey of board-certified plastic surgeons 2002. Plast Reconstr Surg 2004;114(7):1724–1733; discussion 34–36
38. Rohrich RJ, Ha RY, Kenkel JM, Adams WP Jr: Classification and management of gynecomastia: defining the role of ultrasound-assisted liposuction. Plast Reconstr Surg 2003;111(2):909–923; discussion 24–25
39. Rohrich RJ, Raniere J, Jr., Beran SJ, Kenkel JM: Patient evaluation and indications for ultrasound-assisted lipoplasty. Clin Plast Surg 1999;26(2):269–278
40. Moskovitz MJ, Baxt SA, Jain AK, Hausman RE: Liposuction breast reduction: a prospective trial in African American women. Plast Reconstr Surg 2007;119(2):718–726; discussion 27–28
41. Illouz YG: UAL panel discussion. In: Inaugural meeting of the International Society of Ultrasonic Surgery. Algarve, Portugal 1995
42. Courtiss EH: Reduction mammaplasty by suction alone. Plast Reconstr Surg 1993;92(7):1276–1284; discussion 85–89
43. Lejour M: Vertical mammaplasty. Plast Reconstr Surg 1993;92(5):985–986
44. Abboud M, Vadoud-Seyedi J, De Mey A, Cukierfajn M, Lejour M: Incidence of calcifications in the breast after surgical reduction and liposuction. Plast Reconstr Surg 1995;96(3):620–626
45. Brown FE, Sargent SK, Cohen SR, Morain WD: Mammographic changes following reduction mammaplasty. Plast Reconstr Surg 1987;80(5):691–698
46. Walgenbach KJ, Riabikhin AW, Galla TJ, Bannasch H, Voigt M, Andree C, Horch RE, Stark GB: Effect of ultrasonic assisted lipectomy (UAL) on breast tissue: histological findings. Aesthetic Plast Surg 2001;25(2):85–88

Vaser-Assisted Breast Reduction

Alberto Di Giuseppe

75.1 Introduction

Ultrasound energy has been applied to the adipose component of the breast parenchyma in case of breast hypertrophy to reduce the volume of the breast mold.

As is known, ultrasound energy was initially used by Zocchi [1–6] to emulsify fat.

A special instrument composed of an ultrasound generator, a crystal piezoelectric transducer, and a titanium probe transmitter, it is utilized to target adipocyte cells.

This new technology was first applied to body fat to emulsify only fat cells while sparing the other supporting vascular and connective components of the cutaneous vascular network. More recently, Goes [7], Zocchi [1–6], Benelli [8] and the author [9–12], have started to apply this technology to the breast tissue to achieve breast reduction and correction of mild to medium-degree breast ptosis.

75.2 Patient Selection

The ideal candidate for a breast reduction with ultrasound-assisted lipoplasty (UAL) is a patient with juvenile breasts, which are usually characterized by fatty parenchyma, or a patient with postmenopausal involution parenchyma, with good skin tone and elasticity present. Between 60 and 70% of women with large breasts are candidates for reduction with UAL. Preoperative assessment includes a mammographic study, breast clinical history, evaluation of breast ptosis, and evaluation of the consistency of breast parenchyma.

75.3 Preoperative Mammography

Preoperative mammograms (anteroposterior and lateral views), the so-called Eklund view, are taken to evaluate the nature and consistency of the breast tissue (fibrotic, mixed or fatty parenchyma), the distribution of the fat, the presence of calcifications, and areas of dysplasia or nodularity that might necessitate further study or biopsy (Fig. 75.1). The presence of fibroadenomas, calcifications, and other suspected or doubtful radiologic findings should be double-checked with ultrasound and a radiologist experienced in breast-tissue resonance.

75.4 Contraindications

Patients with a history of breast cancer or mastodynia and fearful of potential sequelae from this new technique were not considered for the author's study. Furthermore, because the amount of fat in the breast is variable as is its distribution, not all women are candidates for breast volume reduction with UAL. If fat tissue and glandular tissue are mixed, penetration of the tissue may be impossible, as noted by Lejour [13] and Lejour and Abboud [14]. If the breast tissue is primarily glandular, the technique is not indicated.

75.5 Infiltration

Infiltration should be divided into the three different layers of the breast: deep, intermediate, and superficial (Fig. 75.2). In the deeper and intermediate layers there should be a 1.5:1 ratio between infiltration and aspirate. In the superficial layer the author normally infiltrates twice of what is expected to be extracted (2:1 ratio). A blunt infiltration cannulas, 15–20 cm long, is used, as described by Klein. It is essential to make a meticulous infiltration of the superficial layers, then wait for 15 min minimum to allow adrenaline make its effect, before starting the ultrasound. A total of 500 ml of infiltration fluid is infused; normally 400 ml is for the deeper and intermediate layers and 100 ml for the superficial.

M.A. Shiffman (ed.), *Mastopexy and Breast Reduction: Principles and Practice*,
© Springer-Verlag Berlin Heidelberg 2009

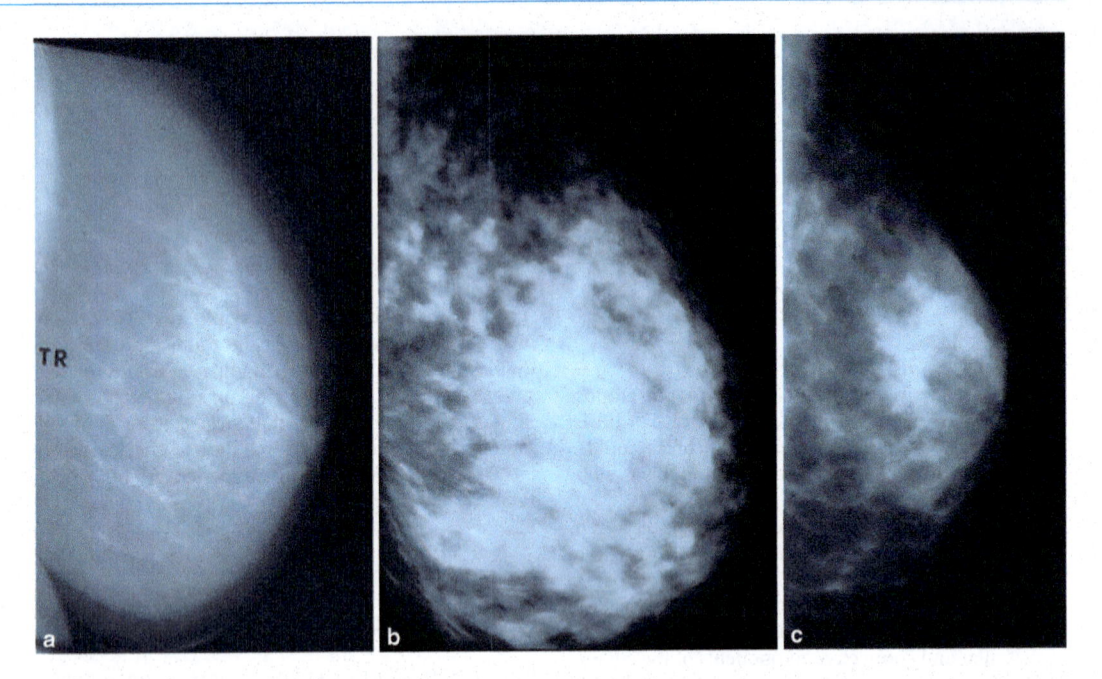

Fig. 75.1 Mammographic evaluation of candidates for breast reduction with the use of ultrasound-assisted lipoplasty (UAL). (**a**) A typical fatty breast. This patient is an ideal candidate for UAL. (**b**) Fibrotic glandular tissue is a contraindication for UAL. (**c**) Fibrotic mixed tissue. This patient is a candidate for UAL of the posterior upper and lower cone

75.6
Technique

The operation begins with the introduction of the skin protector placed at the incision site, normally 1 cm below the inframammary crease (Fig. 75.3). This skin port is designed to protect against friction injuries of the solid titanium probe during its continuous movement.

The fatty breast is emulsified in the lateral and medial compartments, the upper quadrants and the inferior aspect of the periareolar area. All the periareolar area, where most of the glandular tissue is localized (5 cm circumference around the nipple areola complex) is preserved.

The deep portion, mostly fat, is also emulsified, allowing the breast mold to regain a natural shape through upward rotation thus increasing the elevation from initial position, taken from the midclavicular notch. Up to 4 cm of breast elevation is obtained after proper reduction and stimulation to allow skin retraction and correction of the ptosis.

75.7
Incisions

Two 1.5–2.0 cm stab incisions, one at the axillary line and the other 2 cm below the inframammary crease, are made to allow for the entrance of the titanium probe. A periareolar incision can be made in patients with very lax skin for further subcutaneous stimulation.

Through these incisions the surgeon can reach all the breast tissues, working in a crisscross manner. The skin is protected from friction injuries with a specially made skin protector. Recently, the ultrasound device software has been upgraded to provide the same degree of cavitation with less power, which reduces the risk of friction injury and burn at the entrance site, which even allows discontinuing the use of the skin protector.

75.8
Probes

With the existing technology, a solid probe has been found to be more efficacious than a hollow probe for cavitation, which is the physics phenomenon that allows fat fragmentation and destruction. Moreover, the level of ultrasound energy, conveyed by a hollow probe is limited, and consequently the level of the cavitations obtained in the tissue is diminished.

The Vaser system (Sound Surgical Technologies, Denver, CO, US) provides for solid titanium probes of different sizes and length, expressively designed to fulfill all purposes in body contouring, as well in the capability

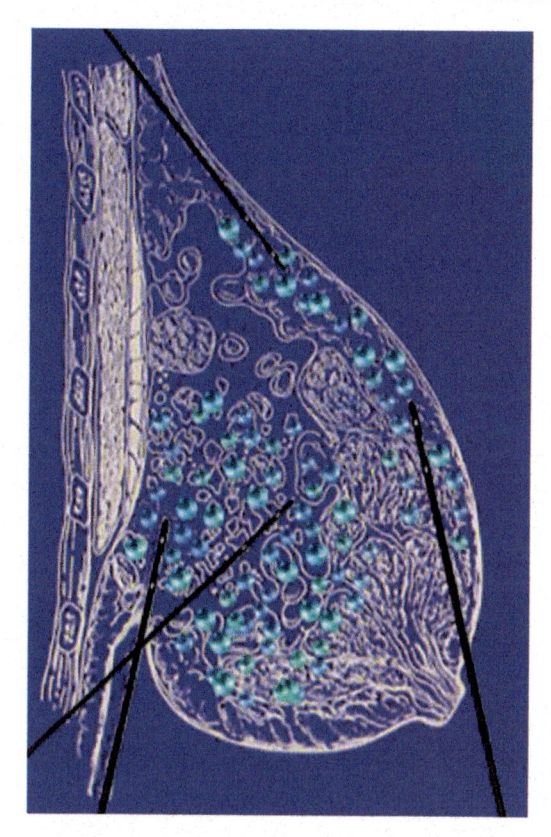

Fig. 75.2 Infiltration divided into three different layers: deep, intermediate, superficial (1.5:1/2:1 ratio)

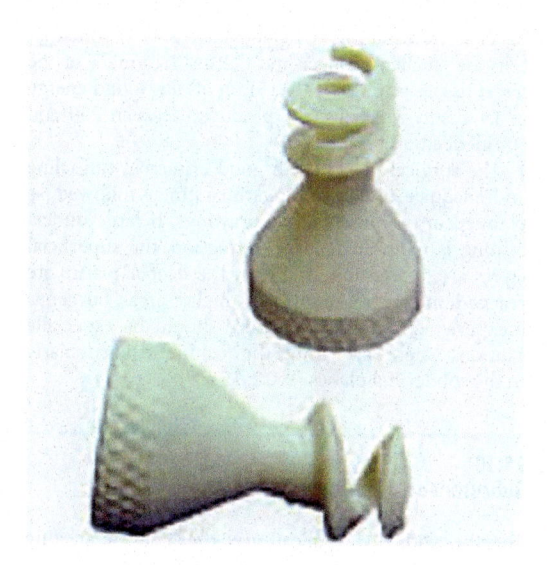

Fig. 75.3 Skin Ports

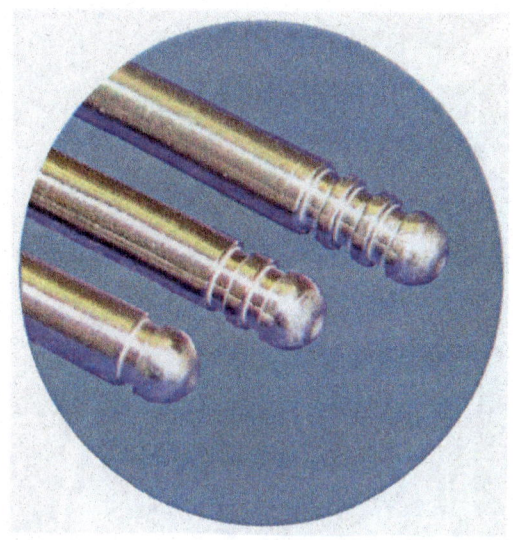

Fig. 75.4 Probes

of emulsification through the cavitation effect produced by the ultrasound energy (Fig. 75.4). The piezoelectric transducer transforms electric energy into "vibration energy," thus allowing the solid titanium probe to emulsify the target fat cells. Four different probe diameters are actually provided by the manufacturers:

1. 2.2 mm diameter, for face.
2. 2.9–3.7 mm diameter, for body contouring, including breasts.
3. 4.1 mm diameter, for larger areas and big volumes of fat. 3.7 mm diameter probe with a special "cone tip" designed to emulsify male breasts, but very aggressive also in fibrous tissue.

The efficacy of these probes, which are narrower than the previous technologies available on the market, is connected with their design, as they are provided with rings (one-two-three) at the tip of each probe.

Rings have two special scopes:

1. To enhance the efficiency of the emulsification that is not limited to the tip, but extended to the last 1.5 cm of the shaft.
2. To allow for a larger selection of options, for targeting the various types of tissues (purely fat, mixed, fibrotic), by utilizing different probes.

The number of rings to be chosen depends on the types of tissue encountered: the most fibrotic is treated with one ring, the less dense tissue (pure fat) with the three rings.

These options are not purely an academic difference: the energy and the wave length of each probe is selected for the target tissue, avoiding unnecessary extra power, thus energy which is useless and a potential cause of secondary unwanted complications (already seen with previous

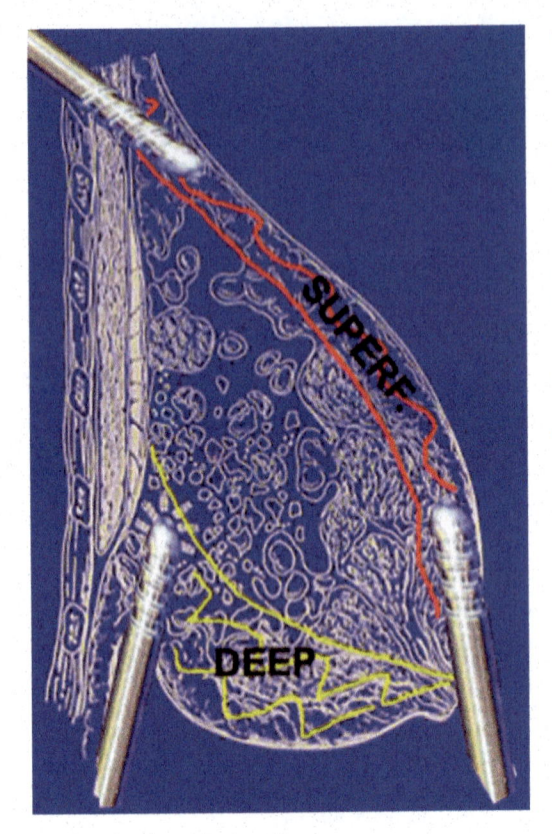

Fig. 75.5 Technique: 2.9 mm probe, one ring for deep layers and 3.7 mm probe, three rings for superficial layers

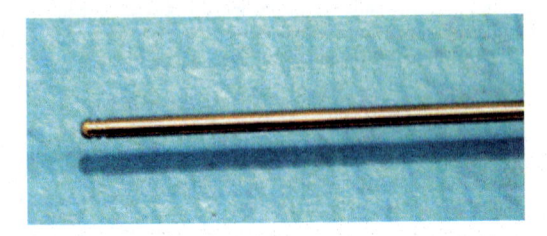

Fig. 75.6 New probe

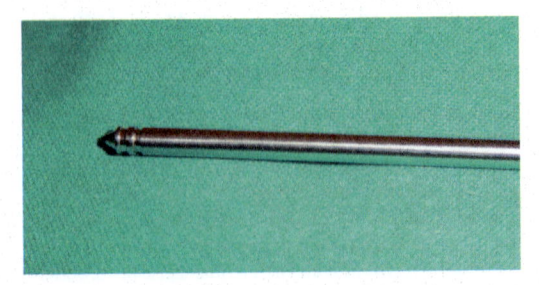

Fig. 75.7 One ring: 4.1 mm

technologies). In breast reduction with pure Vaser, the author prefers the 2.9 mm probe, one ring, for deep layers, and the 3.7 mm, three rings for superficial layers (Fig. 75.5).

Recently, the Vaser surgeon may utilize two further options: (1) The 4.1 mm large probe, for larger volumes, which has a higher percentage of fat emulsification for a minute of time depending on the diameter of the probe (Fig. 75.6) and (2) the "cone" tip probe, which is very aggressive in fibrous tissue, and has been designed for the male breast (gynecomastia) for breast tissue destruction (Fig. 75.7).

The author recommends the larger probe in all massive volume cases, including big breasts, and the cone tip in really fibrotic breast.

75.9
Fat Emulsification

In breast reduction with UAL, the duration of the procedure varies depending on the volume of reduction, the type of breast tissue encountered, and the amount of skin retraction required. A breast with purely fatty tissue is easier to treat than one with mixed glandular tissue, in which fat cells are smaller, stronger and denser.

The author started utilizing the Vaser ultrasound device with solid probes (2.9–3.7 mm wide). It delivers 50% of the ultrasound energy in comparison with the older Sculpture unit (by SMEI, Casale Monferrato, Italy), which was used from 1990 to 2001, while emulsifying fatty tissue much more efficiently. The duration of the procedure and the amount of energy required to liquefy the excess fat may vary depending on the characteristics of the tissues encountered, the volume of the planned reduction, and the type of the breast tissue. Purely fatty breast tissue is easier to treat than mixed glandular tissue, in which fat cells are smaller, stronger and denser. Treatment of the target tissues starts with 10–15 min of ultrasound energy in fat tissue, which usually produces between 250 and 300 ml of emulsion (Fig. 75.8).

The surgical planes, with good crisscross tunneling and adequate undermining, are routinely followed, as planned in the preoperative drawings. If large undermining is required for skin retraction, the superficial layers are treated initially. Then the deeper planes are reached, more time is spent in thicker areas. Surgeons inexperienced in the procedure should be especially cautious when performing the technique, particularly in the subdermal planes [9–12, 15–19].

75.10
Subcutaneous UAL Undermining

Together with UAL application to the fat layers, starting from the deeper layers and progressing to the more superficial ones, it is advisable to thin the superficial layer of the subcutaneous tissue of the upper and lower quadrants by using a different angles pattern, as in a standard lipoplasty [20, 21]. This superficial undermining with low-frequency ultrasound energy helps to enhance the retraction of the breast skin and to redrape the breast skin to the newly shaped and reduced mammary cone (Fig. 75.8).

To facilitate these maneuvers, I often place a second tiny incisions at the axilla, and (sometimes) at the areola border. This helps the superficial work of the probe. The undermining has to be complete, with full liberation of all adherences with the deeper layers. The purpose is to thin the dermal flap all over the breast tissue, thus maintaining its vascularity, sensibility, etc.

Vaser is selective, does not interfere with the vascular network of the dermal tissue, if properly made. It spares the connective and supporting structures of the skin. Gibson and Kenedi [22] showed the great potential of the dermal layer in wound contracture. The resulting contraction is as much as the thinning of the dermis, providing the tissue vascularization to be preserved. This is what happens in all tissue when superficial dermal thinning is accomplished. Tissues contract more easily, and combined with the forces of gravity which help the upward rotation of the gland (when decreased in weight), the final result is a greater contraction of the breast, with a superior antigravity effect.

75.11
Postoperative Care

Suction drainage is routinely applied in the breast for at least 24–48 h. A custom-made elastic compression support (silicone-backed adhesive foam pads) is applied for 7–10 days and a brasserie completes the dressing. These items together with skin redraping help support the breast in the immediate postoperative period.

75.12
Clinical Results

Results are visible immediately after surgery; the skin envelope the redrapes nicely and contours the new breast shape and mold. The skin and treated breast tissue appear soft and pliable. The elevation of the nipple–areola-complex resulting from skin contraction and the rotation of the breast mold was immediately visible. The major postoperative nipple–areola complex elevation was 5 cm.

Emulsification of fatty breast tissue ranged from a minimum of 300 ml per breast in mild reductions and breast lifts to a maximum of 1,200 ml of aspirate for each breast in large breasts. The author was able to easily obtain a mean of 500 ml of fat emulsion from each breast, after infiltration of 700 ml of Klein's modified solution for tumescence, followed by wide thinning of the subcutaneous breast envelope, to allow skin redraping. Elevation of the nipple–areola complex up to 5 cm was obtained in large-volume reductions in combination with thinning of the subcutaneous layer.

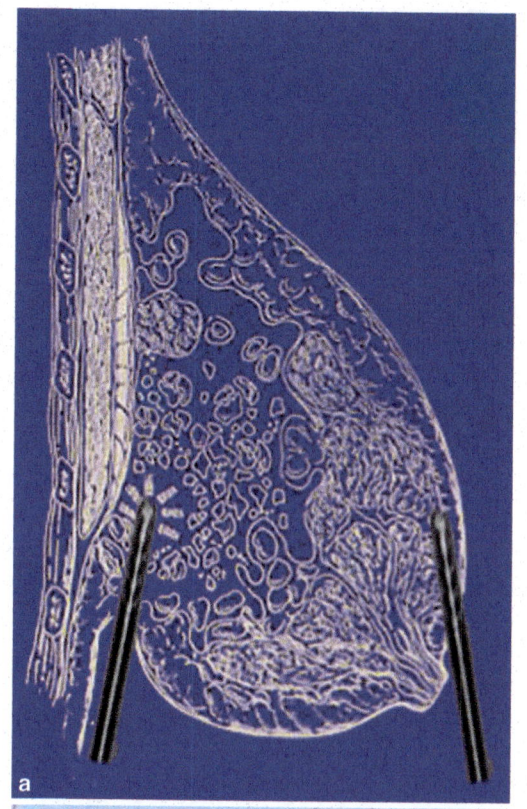

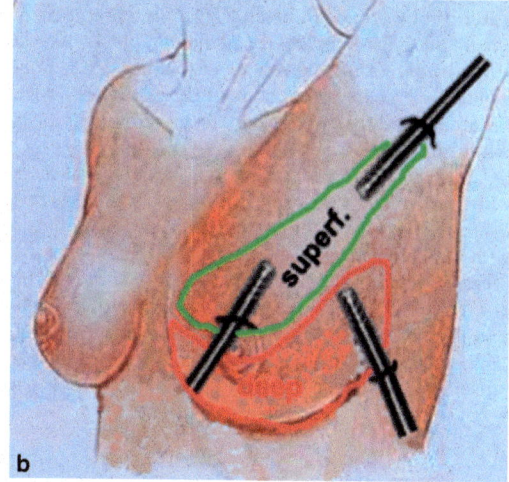

Fig. 75.8 Time of procedure. *Upper quadrants*, superficial layer, 2–3 min. *Lower quadrants*, deep layer, 7–20 min

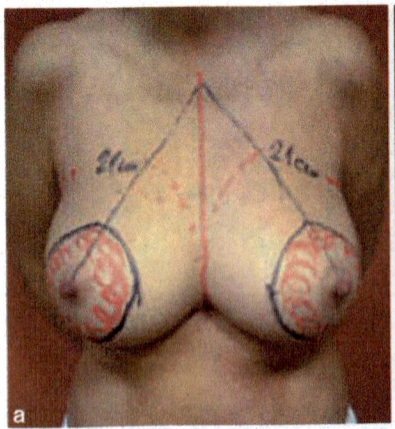

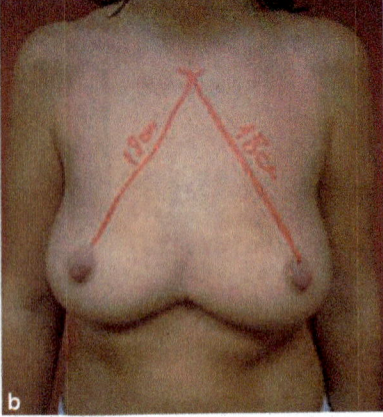

Fig. 75.9 (a) Preoperative breast hypertrophy and planning. *Red dotted area* indicates fibrotic breast tissue not to be addressed. (b) One year postoperative. Breast nipple raised from 21 to 18 cm from suprasternal notch

There was no evidence of suspicious calcifications resulting from surgery at the 5-years postoperative follow-up. Essentially, an increase in breast-tissue fibrosis was noticeable in the postoperative mammograms, which was responsible for the new consistency, texture and tone of the breasts. The increase was also responsible for the lifting of the breasts (Fig. 75.9).

75.13
Mastopexy

Vaser can be applied in breast surgery in clinical cases which present minor degree glandular ptosis. As we know, by decreasing the volume of the breast, it is normal to have an upward rotation of the gland itself. Also the areola tends to shrink when the underlying tissue is diminished in size and volume.

The author has applied the technique in clinical cases with the patient who expressly refused visible breast cutaneous scars and the potential correction of ptosis with an anatomical implant. The upward rotation of the breast and the retraction can finally elevate the breast by 2–4 cm from initial position. The result is readily visible a week after surgery, with minimal bruising and edema.

A supporting bra has to be applied for the first 4 weeks after surgery, although I strongly believe that a similar bra should be advised for ever in patients with large breast or a tendency to ptosis, which is common with age to a majority of females.

75.14
Histological Changes

The breast tissue that underwent emulsification with ultrasound assisted lipoplasty with the Genesis Contour device (Mentor HS, Santa Barbara, CA) has been analyzed histologically. No gross pathological changes were noted at the time of surgery and microscopic diagnosis included fibrocystic change of stromal fibrosis [23]. No atypia or malignancy was found. With long term follow-up, it was shown that the emulsified fat, when not aspirated, will eventually dissolve in few days or weeks.

Areas of relative fibrosis may appear at 1 or 2 months interval; palpable nodes or lumps were a rare event in a survey of 200 patients with breast reduction and/or mastopexy that were performed alone or in combination with other body contouring procedures.

Nagy and McCraw [24] presented the combination of breast fat emulsification by Vaser with open surgery breast reduction. They reintroduced the technique of

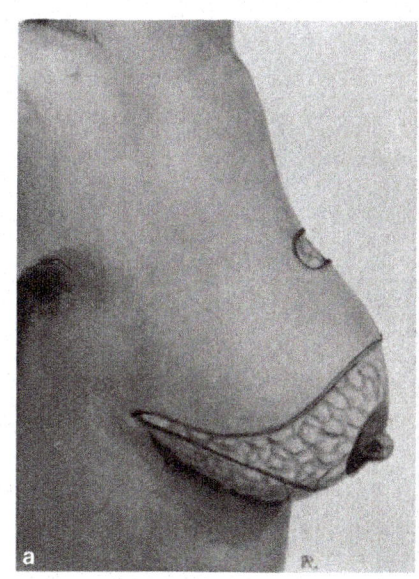

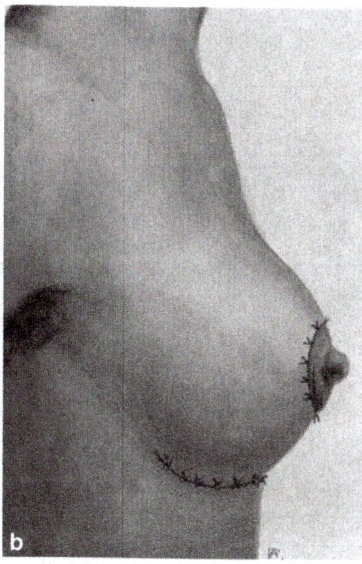

Fig. 75.10 Passot's Button mammaplasty

Passot [25] who in 1925 published the so-called "Button" mammoplasty or the "no vertical scar" reduction that became the most common method of breast shaping in Europe before World War II (Fig. 75.10).

75.15 Marking

The new nipple-position is marked that is between 19 and 21 cm from the midclavicular point (as in all classic measurement – it is the Pitanguy referral point).

The existing inframammary and new inframammary folds (ranging from 15 to 23 cm), the flap margin 8–9 cm below the new nipple site, and the medial and lateral points are marked (Fig. 75.11).

The upper quadrants of the breast are infiltrated with tumescent solution, then Vaser is applied to emulsify the fat of this area (Fig. 75.12). In this case, no skin protector is applied, as the skin in this area is due to be deepithelialized for breast reduction.

After completing aspiration of emulsified fat, the lower flap is detached from the chest wall, with a central large inferior pedicle based on perforators from the pectoralis muscle (Fig. 75.13).

The upper quadrants, already treated with Vaser, show the network of the subcutaneous breast tissue, as it appears after emulsification of fat and aspiration (Fig. 75.14). All the supporting structures of the skin, as elastic bundles, vessels, nerves, connective supports, are conserved. This pattern is similar to what happens in closed breast reduction. As the flap is reduced, it is advanced to fill the empty space (Fig. 75.15). The new nipple is positioned and centered on its pedicle (Fig. 75.16).

The Passot technique combined with Vaser has been applied to several types of breast ptosis. With this technique, the author has performed, large reductions (up to 2,900 g from each side) (Fig. 75.17), and operated on the so-called "long breasts" (Fig. 75.18) with 1,500 g removal from each side.

The typical case where the author actually combines the Passot technique with Vaser is a moderate degree ptosis, 26–28 cm from middle-clavicular point, with mild to moderate hypertrophy. Results are satisfactory and tend to improve over time.

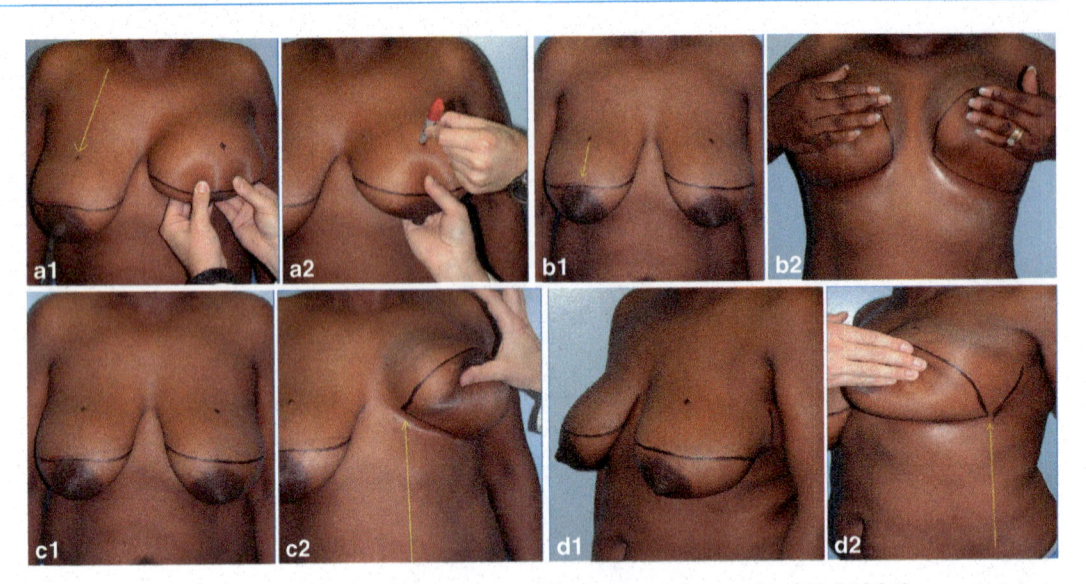

Fig. 75.11 (a) [1] Inframammary fold ranges from 15 to 23 cm. [2] Pointing to inframammary fold. (b) [1] Flap margin 8–9 cm. [2] Inframammary fold. (c1,2) Medial point. (d1,2) Lateral point. From Dr. Nagy and Dr. McCraw, Mississipi University Medical Centre–MS. USA

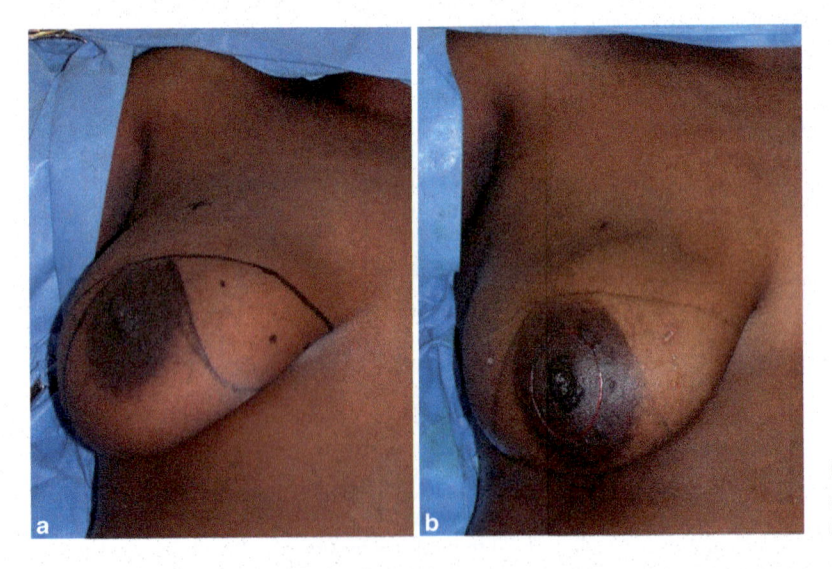

Fig. 75.12 (a) Prior to infiltration. (b) After Vaser and 500 ml aspiration

The secrets of the success of the Passot technique combined with the breast reduction are:
1. Shaping the upper and lower quadrants of breast under control.
2. Maintaining the vascularization of the upper quadrants by using Vaser, as it is a selective technique of emulsification.
3. Repositioning of nipple–areola complex without tension, which ensures good scar (no distortion, no widening).
4. Surgeons must possibly reconsider the priority in scar selection for breast reduction. For most women, the inframammary scar is preferable to the vertical scar, as less visible, despite longer. This could be a

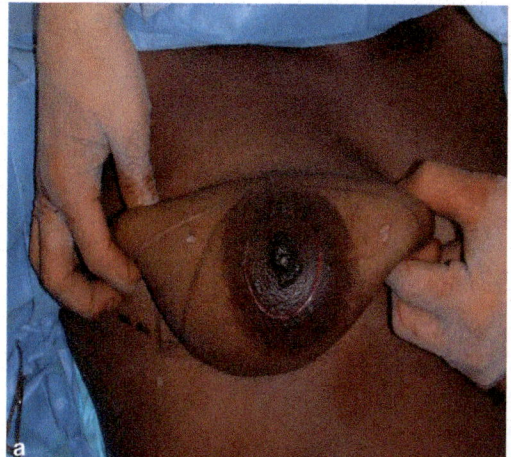

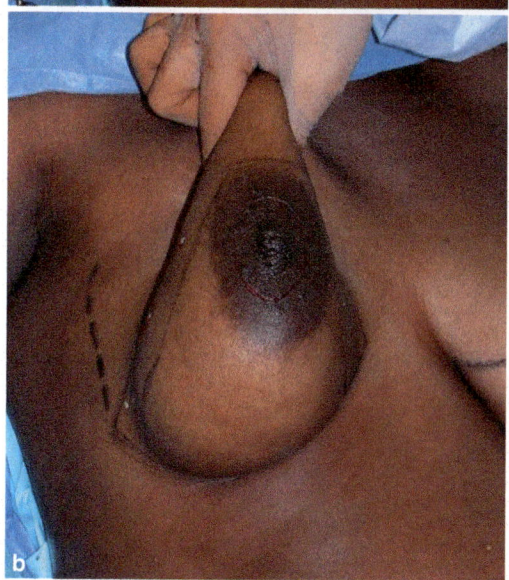

Fig. 75.13 Following 500 ml aspiration

subject of debate among modern plastic surgeon who advocated the short vertical scar techniques for all types of breast reduction.

75.16 Complications

No major complications occurred in the author's series of patients. It should be emphasized that such good results require extensive experience with UAL. As stated by a task force on UAL established by the American Society for Aesthetic Plastic Surgery (ASAPS), the Plastic Surgery Educational Foundation (PSEF), the Lipoplasty Society of North America (LSNA), the Aesthetic Society Education and Research Foundation (ASERF), the learning curve for UAL is longer than that for standard lipoplasty.

Specifically, practitioners must learn how to work close to the subdermal layer with a solid titanium probe to defat this layer and obtain good skin retraction while avoiding complications, such as skin burns and skin necrosis. To safely work close to the skin, two conditions are mandatory. The surgeon must be experienced in ultrasound-assisted body contouring and the correct ultrasound device (one that is able to maximize the cavitations effects while minimizing the thermal effects) must be selected.

75.16.1 Skin Necrosis

Fat necrosis with secondary tissue induration is a typical sequela of ultrasound surgery. When it is localized in small areas, such necrosis can be treated with massage or local infiltration of corticosteroids to soften the area. Skin necrosis can occur (Fig. 75.19).

75.16.2 Loss of Sensation

Loss of sensation is generally limited to the first 3 weeks after surgery. Recovery is rapid because the central cone of the breast is composed mainly of pure parenchyma and is not touched during surgery. Skin sensation is recovered in a few weeks time.

75.16.3 Hematoma

Hematoma formation is another potential complication, though no such cases occurred in this series. In a case of hematoma in a patient treated by another surgeon (Fig. 75.20), the hematoma was localized in the subaxillary region, where the tumescent infiltration was initially administered. The surgeon who performed the operation revealed that the anesthesiologist, who regularly performed the tumescent anesthesia infiltration, incorrectly used standard sharp needles rather than blunt infiltration cannulas. The formation of the hematoma, which appeared immediately after the infiltration, was thus related to an incorrect tumescent infiltration technique and not to the breast reduction with UAL.

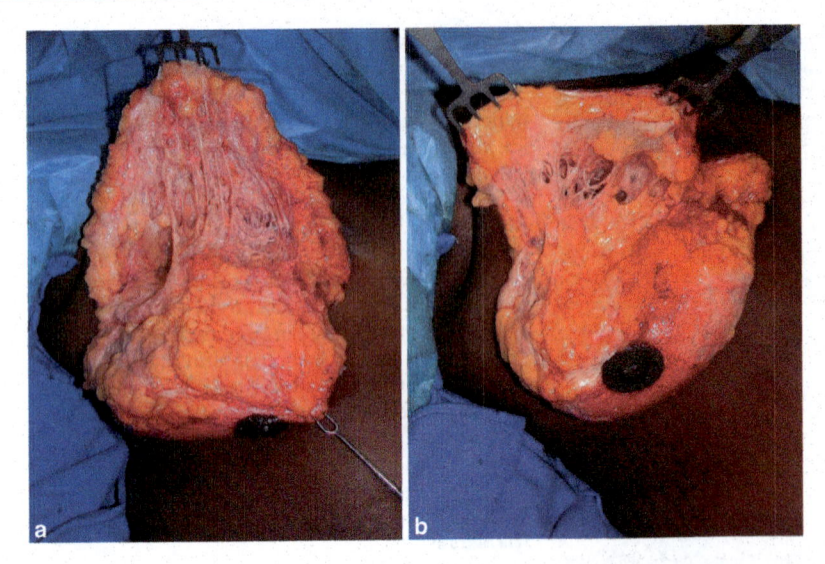

Fig. 75.14 Vaser effect with fat loss

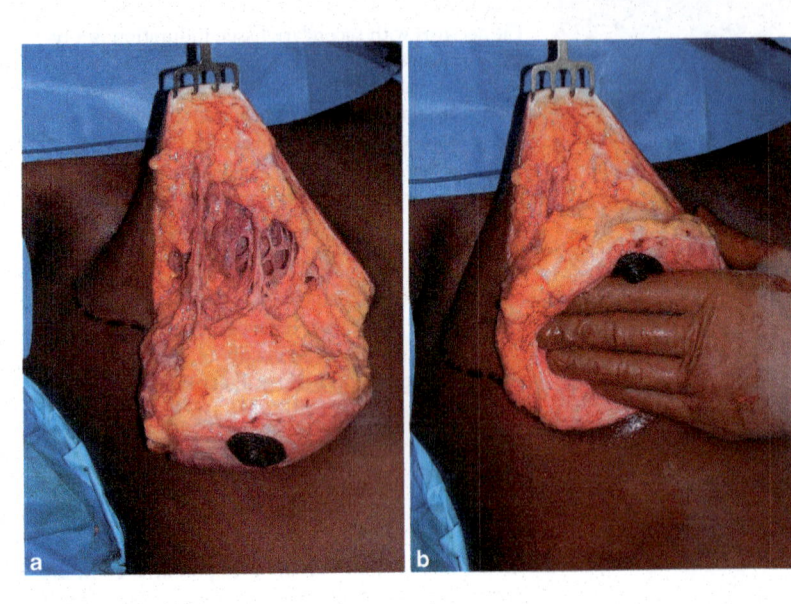

Fig. 75.15 After 500 ml aspiration

75.16.4
Mastitis

Mastitis, an inflammatory response of the breast parenchyma to surgery, occurred in a few patients early in the series. Once surgery was avoided for patients at or near heir menstrual period, only a minor inflammatory response was noted. When encountered, mastitis rapidly subsided with immediate treatment consisting of oral antiinflammatory drugs and wide-spectrum antibiotics for 3 days.

75.16.5
Seroma

Seroma formation is a potential complication of any breast surgery. Regular application of suction drainages

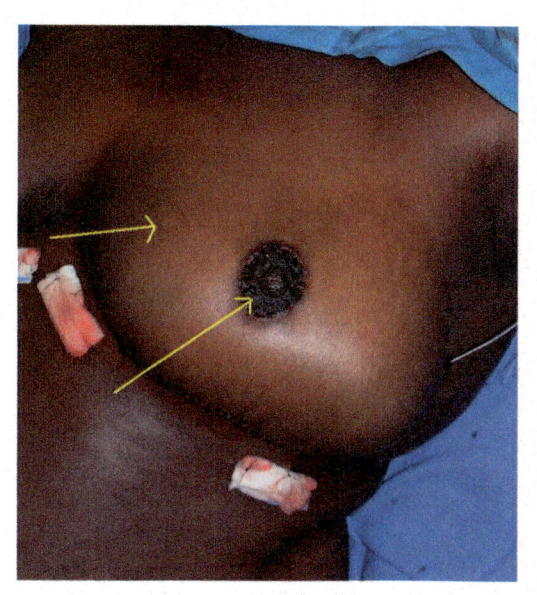

Fig. 75.16 Accentuated medial fullness and center nipple on pedicle

and breast compression for several days with a foam pad and a bra prevent this event.

75.16.6
Selectivity and Specificity of Ultrasound

Large amounts of fat are often found in patients with breast hypertrophy, even among thin adolescents. Lejour and Abboud [14] emphasized that once the fat is removed by lipoplasty before breast reduction, the proportion of glandular tissue, connective tissue vessels, and nerves is increased. These structures are important for maintaining vascularity, sensitivity, and lactation potential. Unlike fat, they are not likely to be affected by patient weight fluctuations. Lejour [13] affirmed that if the breasts contain substantial fat, weight loss may result in breast ptosis. The degree of recurrent ptosis can be minimized if lipoplasty is performed preoperatively to reduce the fatty component of the breasts. This observation anticipated the great potential of UAL for breast surgery.

The clear limits of standard lipoplasty with mechanical indiscriminate destruction of fat and surrounding elements followed by power aspiration of the destroyed tissue are particularly enhanced in breast surgery, where specialized structures (e.g., lactation ducts, vessels, sensitive nerves, elastic bounding structures of the subcutaneous tissue) have to be carefully preserved.

Because it is a selective technique, Vaser UAL may be applied in breast surgery to destroy and emulsify only the fatty component of the breast tissue without affecting the breast parenchyma for which the ultrasound energy has no specificity. The specificity of the technique is connected with the cavitation phenomenon and the efficiency of the system hinges on the type of the titanium probe used and the energy level selected. Lejour [13] argued that the suctioning of breast fat also made the breast suppler and more pliable, which facilitates shaping, especially when the areola pedicle was long. This consideration is particularly important with fatty breasts, which have a less reliable blood supply. These benefits are significantly increased by the use of UAL because the specificity of this technique spares the vessel network.

The selectivity of UAL was demonstrated by Fisher [26, 27], and Palmieri [28] in their studies on the action

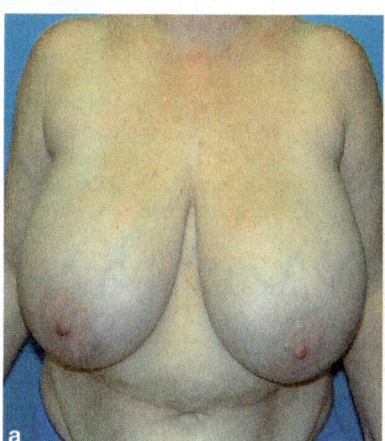

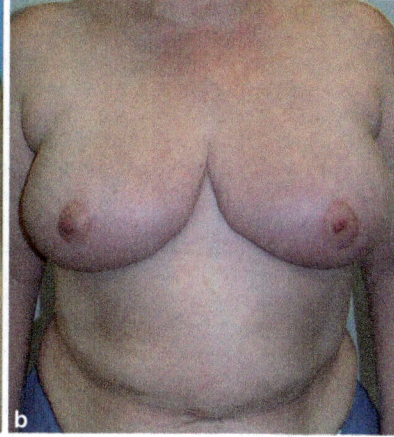

Fig. 75.17 (a) Preoperative large breasts. (b) Following reduction by removing 2,900 g from each side. From Nagy and McCraw

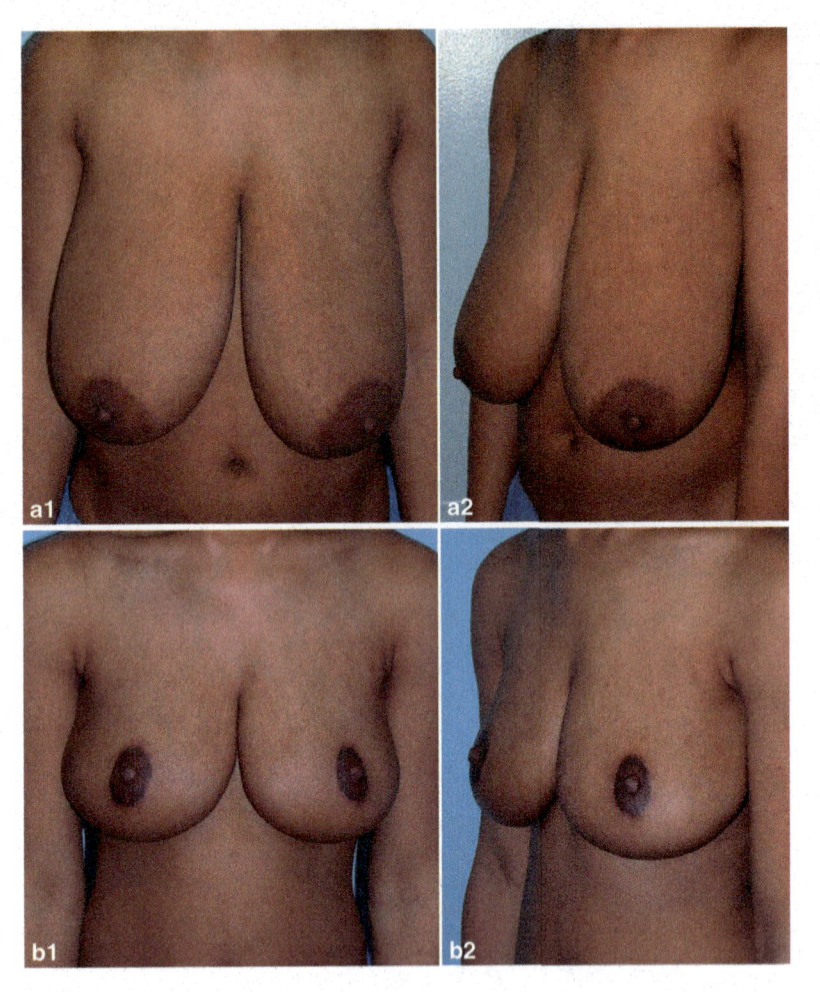

Fig. 75.18 (a) Preoperative long breast. (b) Five months postoperatively after removal of 1,500 g from each side. From Nagy and McCraw

of the ultrasound probe in rat mesenteric vessels. Later Maillard et al. [29] introduced endoscopic evaluation of UAL. They used a Stortz endoscopic system and camera (Stortz, Tuttlingen, Germany) to videotape the action of the titanium probe within the ultrasound device in the superficial layers of the subcutaneous fat, verified by needle depth, after standard infiltration with the tumescent technique. UAL was performed with crisscross tunnels, and the procedure was recorded on videotape. An adjacent area was treated with standard lipoplasty. The technique was compared with standard lipoplasty, which was also endoscopically assisted and monitored. The authors found that standard lipoplasty appears to be the more aggressive technique, characterized by the mechanical destruction of the subcutaneous tissue, including vessels, nerves and supporting structures, despite the use of 2–3 mm wide blunt cannulas.

By contrast, UAL spared vessels, nerves, and elastic supporting fibers. Alteration in breast tissue resulting from the use of UAL were a thickened dermal undersurface, markedly thickened vertical collagenous fibers, intact lymphatic vessels, and intact blood vessels. The horizontal and vertical thickening and shortening of the collagen in the dermis and ligamentous fibers are responsible for the remarkable skin tightening that follows subcutaneous stimulation with the ultrasound probe. The closer to the skin and the more complete the removal of fat from the intermediate subdermal space, the greater the skin-tightening effect. This is of great value in breast surgery, where volume reduction has to be accomplished by skin redraping and recontouring of the breast shape.

As noted by Lejour [13], retraction of the skin after standard lipoplasty cannot be expected to be sufficient to

75.16 Complications

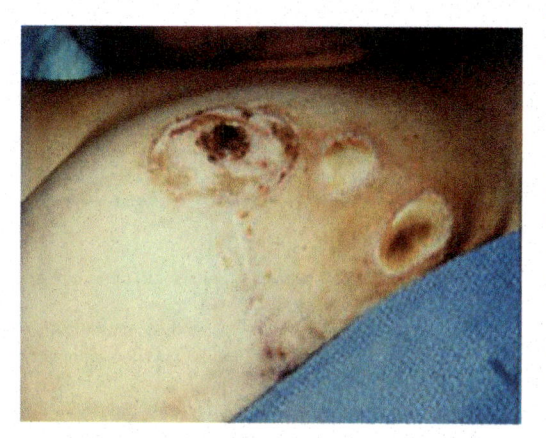

Fig. 75.19 Skin necrosis of the breast medial flap. The surgeon performed a standard breast reduction and then attempted to debulk the medial flap without infiltration of tumescent solution. Skin necrosis resulted, with spontaneous healing after 3 weeks

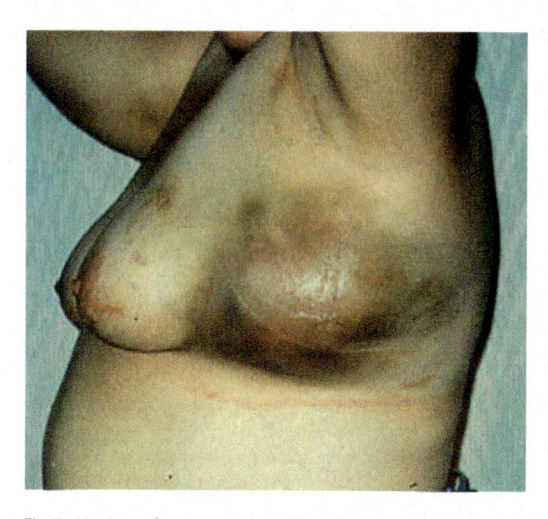

Fig. 75.20 Breast hematoma caused by infiltration of Klein's solution with sharp needle instead of the classic atraumatic blunt needle. The hematoma required evacuation after which regular healing followed

produce a satisfactory breast shape. Subcutaneous aspiration must be extensive to obtain the necessary skin retraction, and the risk of localized skin necrosis resulting from excessive superficial liposuction cannot be ignored [30].

75.16.7
Calcifications

Lejour [13] and Lejour and Abboud [14] argued that the risk of postoperative fat necrosis or calcifications was the reason many surgeons avoided the use of lipoplasty in the breast. The main cause of fat necrosis is breast ischemia brought about by extensive dissection or mechanical direct damage, with resultant venous drainage. This phenomenon is typical in open breast surgery. Calcification in breast-reduction surgery may derive from area of fat necrosis or breast necrosis and subsequent scarring. Such calcifications are most often located at the incision lines (periareolar, or vertical scar in the inverted-T approach), where more tension is placed in approximating the lateral and medial flaps. However, when the tension is too high, areas of necrosis could arise from the approximating suture and later cause calcifications that are visible on mammography. However the risk of such complications in UAL procedures is quite low.

Calcifications in breast parenchyma are to be expected after any mammoplasty procedure. In reduction mammoplasty, it is preferable that they be localized along the breast scars [31]. When lipoplasty is performed in addition to the mammoplasty procedure, benign macro-calcifications are slightly more numerous in the parenchyma than they are in breasts reduced without lipoplasty. This may occur because of the trauma caused by lipoplasty or because lipoplasty suction is applied to the most fatty breasts, which are more prone in liponecrosis [32]. However 1 year after fatty-breast reduction with UAL, follow-up mammography revealed only a slight increase of small microcalcifications, similar to those found after other mammary procedures.

75.16.8
Potential Risks

Topaz [33] speculated that the thermal effect of UAL and the free radicals generated during UAL might result in neoplastic transformation and other long-term complications as a consequence of the physical effect known as sonoluminescence. Since then, it has been generally agreed that some individuals do not understand the mechanism of UAL action, though multiple mechanisms are probably involved, such as mechanical forces, cavitation, and thermal effects.

Additional research has revealed that long-term complications or negative bioeffects (including DNA damage and oxidation- free radical attack) are probably not serious safety concerns for UAL.

With reference to the application of UAL to breast surgery, Young and Schorr [34] investigated the histology of the breast fat tissue before and after UAL breast surgery (with serial biopsies at 6 months and 1 year after surgery) and the mammographic appearance of the breast before and 1, 2, and 3 years after surgery, particularly with respect to calcification. The results were evaluated by a senologist not directly involved with the clinical research. Histological studies revealed an increased fibrotic response to thermal insult, with a prevalence of fatty scar tissue, in all specimens evaluated.

Mammography showed a significant increase in breast parenchymal fibrosis, with a denser consistency and thicker breast trabeculae that were constant over time. The calcifications that appeared were benign and were typically small, round, less numerous, and more regular than those characteristic of malignancy. Comparison of the mammographic results typical of a standard breast reduction and those typical of breast reduction with UAL showed that microcalcifications are less likely to develop with UAL. It is likely that the scared tissue caused by breast reduction with electrocautery or by necrosis resulting from the tension of internal sutures may more frequently cause calcifications or irregular mammographic aspects of the operated parenchyma. Particularly, in standard breast-reduction surgery, they can appear at the areola line and at the site of the vertical scar.

From a mammographic viewpoint, the typical appearance of a breast reduction with UAL demonstrates predictably less scarring and fewer calcifications than occur in the standard open technique. Courtiss [35] reported similar mammographic evidence in a denser breast after breast reduction by lipoplasty alone. No malignancies were reported.

The question of whether potential lactation is affected by UAL remains unanswered. The technique has been used for breast reduction and mastopexy in young and older patients and there has been no problem in lactation reported.

75.17
Conclusions

The use of UAL for reduction of fatty breasts and mastopexy is effective and safe when applied in selected patients and performed by a surgeon with expertise in ultrasound assisted body contouring. The selectivity of UAL enables emulsification of the fatty component of the breast parenchyma while sparing the glandular tissue and vascular network. Furthermore, long-term mammographic studies have revealed no alteration of the morphology of the breast parenchyma resulting from this technique. The typical mammographic appearance of breast tissue after UAL is a denser breast.

Acknowledgment

Portions of this work are reprinted from [32] with permission from the International Journal of Cosmetic Surgery and Aesthetic Dermatology, Mary Ann Liebert, Inc.

References

1. Zocchi M: Clinical aspects of ultrasonic liposculpture. Perspect Plast Surg 1993;7:153–174
2. Zocchi M: The ultrasonic assisted lipectomy (U.A.L): Physiological principles and clinical application. Lipoplasty 1994;11:14–20
3. Zocchi M: Ultrasonic assisted lipectomy advances. In: Plastic and Reconstructive Surgery. St Louis, MO, Mosby Year Book 1995
4. Zocchi M: The ultrasonic assisted lipectomy, instructional course. Am Soc Aesthetic Plast Surg (ASAPS) Annual Meeting, San Francisco, March 1995
5. Zocchi M: The treatment of axillary hyperadenosis and hyperhidrosis using ultrasonically assisted lipoplasty. Meeting of the International Society of Ultrasonic Surgery, Faro, Portugal, November 1995
6. Zocchi ML: Basic physics for ultrasound assisted lipoplasty. Clin Plast Surg 1999:26(2):209–220
7. Goes JC: Periareolar mammoplasty: Double skin technique with application of polyglactine or mixed mesh. Plast Reconstr Surg 1996;97(5):959–968
8. Benelli L: A new periareolar mammaplasty: round block technique. Aesthetic Plast Surg 1990;14(2):93–100
9. Di Giuseppe A: Mammoplasty reduction and mastopexy utilizing ultrasound liposuction. Mammographic study preoperative. Abstract from 46th National Congress of Italian Society of Plastic Reconstructive and Aesthetic Surgery. Venice, Italy, June 1997
10. Di Giuseppe A: Ultrasonically assisted liposculpturing. Am J Cosm Surg 1997;14(3):317–327
11. Di Giuseppe A: Reducion mamaria y pexia con la asistencia de la lipoplastia ultrasonida. Lipoplastia 1998;1(1):16–26
12. Di Giuseppe A: UAL for Face-Lift and Breast Reduction. Abstract for World Congress on Liposuction Surgery. Pasadena, California, October 1998
13. Lejour M: Reduction of large breasts by a combination of liposuction and vertical mammoplasty. In: Cohen M (ed). Master of Surgery: Plastic and Reconstructive Surgery. Boston, Little, Brown 1994
14. Lejour M, Abboud M: Vertical mammoplasty without inframammary scar and with liposuction. Perspect Plast Surg 1990;4:67
15. Di Giuseppe A: Ultrasound assisted for body contouring, breast reduction and face lift. How to do it? Abstract at the 3rd European Congress of Cosmetic Surgery. Themes: Berlin, 23–25 April 1999

16. Di Giuseppe A: Ultrasonic assisted lipoplasty of the breast (Poster). Abstract at the XV Congress of the International Society of Aesthetic Plastic Surgery (ISAPS). Tokyo, April 2000
17. Di Giuseppe A: Ultrasonically assisted breast reduction and mastopexy. Int J Cosm Surg Aesthet Derm 2001;3(1):23–29
18. Di Giuseppe A: Ultrasound assisted breast reduction and mastopexy. Aesthet Surg J 2001;21(6):493–506
19. Di Giuseppe A: Breast reduction with ultrasound assisted lipoplasty. Reconstr Surg J 2003;112(1):71–82
20. Teimourian B: Suction Lipectomy and Body Sculpturing. St. Louis, MO, CV Mosby 1987, pp 219–251
21. Teimourian B, Massac E Jr, Wiegering CE: Reduction suction mammoplasty and suction lipectomy as an adjunct to breast surgery. Aesthetic Plast Surg 1985;9(2):97–100
22. Gibson T, Kenedi RM: Factors affecting the mechanical characteristics of human skin. In: Proceedings of the Centennial Symposium on Repair and Regeneration, New York, Mc Graw-Hill 1968, p 87
23. Gibson T, Stark H, Kenedi RM: The significance of Langer's lines. In Hueston JT (ed). Transactions of the Fifth International Congress of Plastic and Reconstructive Surgery. Australia, Butterworths 1971, p 1213
24. Nagy M, McCraw J: Presented at the Amer Soc Aesthet Plast Surg (ASAPS) meeting in Orlando, FL, May 2006
25. Passot R: La correction esthetique du prolapsus mammaire par le procede de la transposition du mamelon. Presse Med 1925;33:317
26. Fischer PD, Narayanan K, Liang MD: The use of high frequency ultrasound for the dissection of small diameter blood vessels and nerves. Ann Plast Surg 1992;28(4):326–330
27. Fischer PD: Revised technique for cellulitis reduction in riding breeches deformity. Bull Int Acad Cosm Surg 1977;2:26–38
28. Palmieri B: Studio sull' azione degli ultrasuoni sul tessuto vasculare del ratio. Riv Ital Chir Plast 1994:9:635- 639
29. Maillard GF, Schleflan M, Bussein R: Ultrasonically assisted lipectomy in aesthetic breast surgery. Plast Reconstr Surg 1997;100(1):238–241
30. Becker H: Liposuction of the breast. Presented at the Lipoplasty Society of North America meeting, September 1992
31. Mitnick JS, Roses DF, Harris MN, Colen SR: Calcifications of the breast after reduction mammoplasty. Surg Gynecol Obstet 1990;171(5):409–412
32. Di Giuseppe A, Santoli M: Ultrasonically assisted breast reduction and mastopexy. Int J Cosm Surg Aesth Derm 2001;3(1):23–29
33. Topaz M: Possible long-term complications in U.A.L. induced by sonoluminescence, sonochemistry, and thermal effects. Aesthetic Surg J 1998;18:19–24
34. Young VL, Schorr MV: Report from the conference on ultrasound assisted liposuction safety and effects. Clin Plast Surg 1999:26(3):481–524
35. Courtiss EH: Breast reduction by section alone. In: Spear S (ed). Surgery of the Breast: Principles and Art. Philadelphia, Lippincott-Raven 1998

Part VI
Complications of Breast Reduction and Mastopexy

Complications of Breast Reduction

Melvin A. Shiffman

76.1 Introduction

Complications following breast reduction can be difficult to prevent and should be timely diagnosed so that proper treatment can be instituted. The surgeon should be aware of the means to avoid complications and as to how to treat those complications that occur, in a timely fashion.

76.2 Complications

76.2.1 Calcifications

Yalin et al. [1] reported on mammographic and ultrasonographic findings of calcifications following breast reduction. Masses were seen with coarse and thick spiculations, irregular margins, central radiolucencies, and amorphous and pleomorphic, dystrophic, coarse and branching microcalcifications. There were eggshell-like oil cyst calcifications. Fat necrosis and oil cysts are associated with all types of surgical procedures in the breast (Fig. 76.1).

Parenchymal redistribution, asymmetry, scarring, parenchymal or retroareolar linear bands and calcifications, high position of the nipple, and discontinuity of the ducts were reported by Brown [2] and Miller [3].

Mendelson [4] noted skin thickening of the lower pole of the breast around the incision sites in the periareolar area and inframammary fold. Spicules were thicker and more curvilinear than the fine and straight speculations of breast cancer. There were needle-like calcifications.

Mitnick et al. [5] reported that calcifications following breast reduction were found within the skin of the breast, mainly at a periareolar location.

Mitnick et al. [6] noted suspicious mammographic findings including 31 stellate lesions, 20 regions of grouped calcifications, 2 nodules, and 1 area of trabecular markings. Adenocarcinoma was diagnosed by fine needle biopsy in 5 patients. There was a higher incidence of contralateral breast cancer in patients who had cancer on one side and breast reduction on the other side.

Heywang-Kobrunner [7] reported calcifications of fat necrosis and oil cysts that are round and have ring or eggshell-like wall calcifications with radiolucent centers.

76.2.2 Cancer

Breast cancer has been diagnosed intraoperatively [8–10] and in the postoperative specimen following reduction [11]. This is the reason that all patients for breast reduction should have a preoperative mammogram.

Lund et al stated that breast reduction may reduce the incidence of future breast cancer [12]. Of 1,245 cases having breast reduction followed for over 10 years after surgery there were 18 cases of breast cancer. The expected number for the incidence of breast cancer in the normal population would be 30.28 cases.

76.2.3 Cyanotic Nipple–Areolar Complex

The patient should be seen on the first postoperative day in order to evaluate the nipple–areolar complex for cyanosis. If there is any question of the blood supply to the nipple areolar complex, test for capillary refill that should be less than 6 s. Six seconds or more requires that the wound sutures be removed to relieve the tension and check the pedicle for rotation. With an "anchor" incision, the sutures can be removed along the lower half of the areola and along the vertical portion of the wound. If necessary remove all sutures and allow secondary healing. Nitropaste has not been effective in preventing necrosis. Continued cyanosis with refill of six seconds or more may be best treated with nipple areola transplant.

76.2.4 Excessive Breast Reduction

Some surgeons use techniques that consistently reduce the breast excessively. A patient with a DD should not be changed into an A cup but a cup size that is adequate for the height and weight should be made. Agarwal [13]

M.A. Shiffman (ed.), *Mastopexy and Breast Reduction: Principles and Practice*,
© Springer-Verlag Berlin Heidelberg 2009

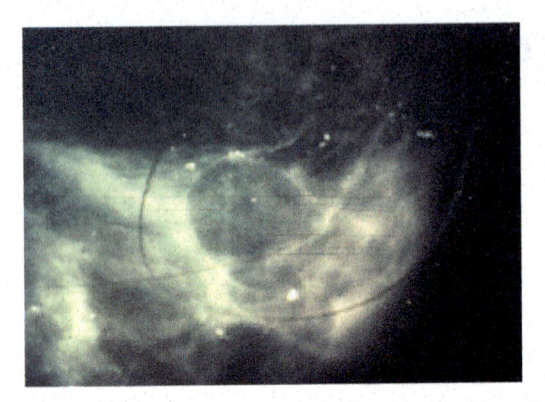

Fig. 76.1 Calcifications following breast reduction

has described a flap augmentation for excessive breast reduction. Most of the time implants can be used to augment the breast to a proper size.

76.2.5
Fat Necrosis

As with any necrosis problem there can be loss of vascular supply to parts of the fat along the incision sites. This can result in postoperative drainage of an oily substance or a mass that may have to be treated with excision or drainage. An untreated area of fat necrosis may result in a fat cyst followed by calcification.

76.2.6
Hematoma

Excessive bleeding with hematoma should be treated with exploration, evacuation of the hematoma, and coagulation of any bleeders. It is probably prudent to place a suction catheter or penrose in the space for at least 24 h.

76.2.7
High Nipple–Areolar Complex

The cause of a postoperative high nipple–areolar complex is either "bottoming out" of the breast where the breast falls behind the nipple–areolar complex to a more inferior position or because the surgeon has not adjusted to a lower position for the large breast weight stretching the skin. The new nipple point, instead of being at the inframammary fold, should be adjusted 1–2 cm lower for the heavy breast (Fig. 76.2).

76.2.8
Infection

Infection should be treated with proper antibiotics, if possible, following culture and sensitivity. Cellulitis is most often a Strep infection. An abscess needs an open drainage with culture and sensitivity.

76.2.9
Methcillin-Resistant *Staphylococcus aureus*

Methcillin-resistant *Staphylococcus aureus* is now the most common contaminant of surgical infections. Previously it was *Staphylococcus aureus* and the Pseudomonas.

76.2.9.1
Community-Acquired Methicillin-Resistant *Staphylococcus aureus* (CA-MRSA)

CA-MRSA is becoming an increasingly important, major pathogen[24–26]. Particular strains of MRSA have

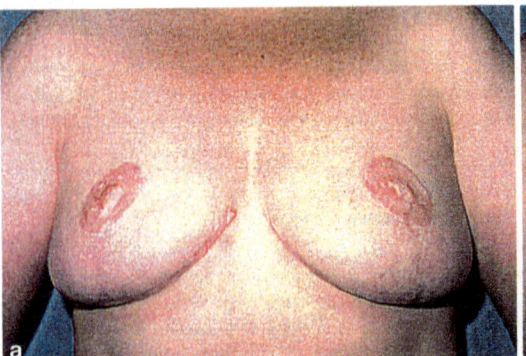

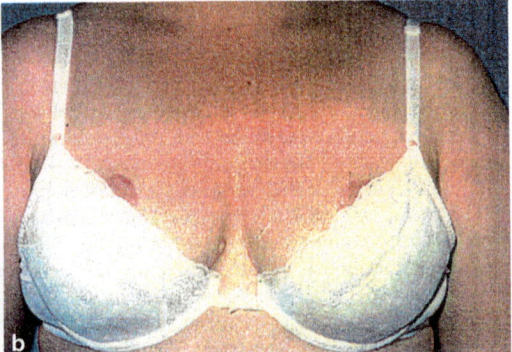

Fig. 76.2 High nipple areolar complexes secondary to "bottoming out"

recently arisen in CA-MRSA that have been identified by pulsed field gel electrophoresis typing as USA300 that have genetic differences from the typical strain that has been circulating.[27]

The USA300 and USA400 strains are quite different from the typical Hospital-acquired Methicillin resistant *Staphylococcus aureus* (HA-MRSA).[28, 29] The USA300 strain occurs in diverse regions of the United States,[30] while the USA400 strain has been found in several outbreaks and "endemic" CA-MRSA infections in the US Midwest.[31]

CA-MRSA accounts for 59% of skin infections (ranges from 15 to 74% in different cities). The drug-resistant strain can cause painful skin lesions that resemble infected spider bites, necrotizing pneumonia, and toxic shock syndrome. CA-MRSA is resistant to erythromycin, cephalexin (Keflex), and dicloxacillin (Diclocil) and more or less susceptible to clindamycin, fluoroquinolones, tetracycline, rifampin, and trimethoprim-sulfamethoxazole (TMP–SMX)[28, 29, 32]

Moran et al.[32] studied skin and soft tissue infections seen in the emergency room in Los Angeles, California, with cultures and clinical information. *Staphylococcus aureus* isolates were characterized by antimicrobial-susceptibility testing, pulsed-field gel electrophoresis, and detection of toxin genes. On MRSA isolates, typing of the staphylococcal cassette chromosome mec (SCCmec), the genetic element that carries the mecA gene encoding methicillin resistance, was performed The presence of MRSA was overall 57% (ranging from 15 to 74%). Pulsed-field type USA300 isolates accounted for 97% of MRSA isolates; 74% of these were a single strain (USA300–0114). SCCmec type IV and the Panton-Valentine leukocidin (PVL) toxin gene were detected in 98% of MRSA. Among the MRSA isolates, 100% were susceptible to rifampin and trimethoprim–sulfamethoxazole, 95% to clindamycin, 92% to tetracycline, and 60% to fluoroquinolones. When antimicrobial therapy is indicated for the treatment of skin and soft-tissue infections, clinicians should consider obtaining culture and modifying empirical therapy to provide MRSA coverage.

76.2.9.2
Virulence

Virulence factors may allow pathogens to adhere to surfaces and invade or avoid the immune system, while causing toxic effects to the host.[33] There may be the production of exotoxins related to the infection.[34] Superantigens that have been identified include TSST-1 (toxic shock syndrome toxin-1), staphylococcal enterotoxin serotype B (SEB), or staphylococcal enterotoxin serotype C (SEC). Along with PVL these toxins are associated with toxic shock syndrome, pupura fulminans, and hemorrhagic, necrotizing MRSA pneumonia.[34–36] The superantigens induce massive cytokine release from the T cells and macrophages. The ensuing hypotension and shock are believed to be the result of tumor necrosis factor α and β (TNF-α and TNF-β)-mediated activity.[34] There is a 70% mortality rate from community-acquired pneumonia caused by PVL-positive CA-MRSA.[36]

PVL has a possible role in virulence either directly or as a marker for closely associated pathogenic factors. PVL is a 2-component staphylococcal pore-forming membrane cytotoxin that operates by targeting mononuclear and polymorphonuclear cells producing severe inflammatory lesions, capillary dilation, chemotaxis, polymorphonuclear karyorrhexis, and tissue necrosis.[28, 33]

76.2.9.3
Reservoirs and Transmission

Humans serve as a reservoir for *Staphylococcus aureus* through asymptomatic colonization.[28] Higher carriage rates of *Staphylococcus aureus*, compared to the general population, are associated with intravenous drug users, insulin-dependent diabetes, patients with dermatologic conditions, patients with indwelling catheters, and healthcare workers.[28, 37]

76.2.9.4
Prevention and Management

To prevent spread of MRSA in hospitals it is recommended that those at higher risk for MRSA carriage be screened at admission and isolated if found to be colonized.[38] Surfaces in examination rooms should be cleaned with commercial disinfectants or diluted bleach (1 tablespoon to 1 quart of water) and wound dressings and other materials that cone into contact with pus, nasal discharge, blood, and urine should be disposed of carefully.[25] Healthcare providers need to wash their hands between contacts with patients[25] and should use barrier precautions and don fresh gowns and gloves for contact with each patient.[39, 40]

Guidelines have been developed by the Centers for Disease Control (CDC) for prevention of infection among members of competitive sports teams and others in close contact. These include avoid sharing equipment and towels, common surfaces should be cleaned on a regular basis, wounds should be covered, individuals with potentially infectious skin lesions should be excluded from practice and competition until the lesions have healed or are covered, and frequent showering and use of soap and hot water should be encouraged.[26]

A rapid, easy to use identification of MRSA in nasal carriers has been developed that consists of real-time polymerase chain reaction (PCR) assay.

76.2.9.5
Clinical Management

The CDC has recommended guidelines for CA-MRSA (Table 76.1).[41]

Once an infection has been established, wound cultures should be obtained, ideally from pus or grossly infected tissue. Cultures form ulcers are of dubious value since bacteria isolated may be due to colonizing strains and not pathogens.[42] Antibiotics may not be needed in SSTIs when adequate surgical drainage can be achieved.[42–44] When antibiotics are not prescribed, patients should have follow-up care and be instructed to seek medical care if symptoms worsen or do not resolve. When antibiotics are used, local patterns of antibiotic susceptibility among CA-MRSA should be used to help direct empiric therapy against this pathogen.

76.2.9.6
Antibiotics

Antimicrobial therapy is critical.[45] Vancomycin has been a mainstay of treatment for serious infections that are resistant to β-lactams.[46] However, in the treatment of methicillin sensitive *Staphylococcus aureus* (MSSA), Vancomycin has been associated with a slower clinical response and longer duration of bacteremia compared to β-lactams.[29] There has been a recent emergence of Vancomycin-resistant *Staphylococcus aureus* (VRSA) and Vancomycin-intermediate susceptible *Staphylococcus aureus* (VISA).[29]

Fluoroquinolones have variable activity against CA-MRSA strains and in some locales there has been over 40–50% fluoroquinolones resistance among MRSA strains.[47–49] Susceptibility to ciprofloxacin indicates that low-level or partial fluoroquinolones resistance is probably not present. There is little clinical data on the use of moxifloxacin and gemifloxacin for the treatment of CA-MRSA.

Clindamycin has been useful to treat CA-MRSA disease,[41,50,51] but greater than 10%–15%.[28,47,48] resistance has been encountered In a Taiwan study the resistance was 93%.[52] Some strains that are Clindamycin susceptible and erythromycin resistant can develop resistance when exposed to Clindamycin (lincosamide), erythromycin (macrolide), and quinupristin/dalfopristin (streptogramin B). This inducible resistance can be detected by the D-test that, if positive, is considered diagnostic for inducible resistance.[53] It is believed that Clindamycin should not be used to treat D-test-positive strains, especially in a serious syndrome.[53]

For multidrug-resistant infections caused by MRSA that require parenteral therapy, Vancomycin, linezolid, Daptomycin, and quinupristin/dalfopristin are the only agents that are reliably active against many HA-MRSA infections.[51] TMP-SMX, tetracyclines, Clindamycin, and fluoroquinolones may be alternatives if susceptibility to these agents is documented.

76.2.9.7
Guidelines

The CDC[54] developed, with internationally recognized experts, guidelines to control MRSA through hospitals and healthcare facilities. These include:
1. Ensure prevention programs are funded and adequately staffed.
2. Carefully track infection rates and related data to monitor the impact of prevention efforts.
3. Ensure that staff use standard infection control practices and follow guidelines regarding the correct use of antibiotics.
4. Promote the best practices with health education campaigns to increase adherence to established recommendations.
5. Designing robust prevention programs customized to specific settings and local need.

76.2.9.8
Definitions

CA-MRSA: Community-Acquired MRSA
HA-MRSA: Hospital-Acquired MRSA
PCR: Polymerase Chain Reaction
PVL: Panton-Valentine Leukocidin
MRSA: Methicillin Resistant *Staphylococcus aureus*
MSSA: Methicillin-Susceptible *Staphylococcus aureus*
SCC: Staphylococcus Cassette-Chromosome
SSTI: Skin and Soft-Tissue Infection
TMP-SMX: Trimethoprim-Sulfamethoxazole
TNF: Tumor Necrosis Factor
TSST: Toxic Shock Syndrome Toxin
VISA: Vancomycin-Intermediate Susceptible *Staphylo-coccus aureus*
VRSA: Vancomycin-Resistant *Staphylococcus aureus*

76.2.10
Necrosis

Necrosis of skin flaps can occur from inadequate blood supply, torsion of the pedicle, excessive tension on the skin or compression of the pedicle, thin flaps, hematoma causing excessive tension, smoking, and uncontrolled diabetes especially with infection (Fig. 76.3). Necrotizing ulceration was reported by Berry et al. [14].

Treatment consists of debriding the necrotic areas, keeping the open wounds clean with saline soaks, and secondary closure when the granulations have properly formed. If secondary closure fails, then the wound should be left open to close on its own.

76.2.11
Neurological

Pressure sensation (using the Pressure-Specified Sensory Device) of the breast was measured at nine points of the breast by Ferreira et al. [15]. All 25 patients had decreased sensation in all points measured when the upper medial pedicle technique was used.

Hamdi et al. [16] noted loss of sensitivity of nipple areolar complex (NAC) with superior and inferior pedicle techniques that resolved with the change to the laterocentral pedicle technique.

76.2.12
Pain

Gonzalez et al. [17] reported that headache, neck pain, back pain, shoulder pain, and bra strap groove pain was present in 60–92% of patients and 97% of patients had at least three of these pain symptoms preoperatively. All patients had reduction of their pain and 25% had complete elimination of pain symptoms after reduction mammaplasty.

Chronic breast pain can occur following breast reduction [18].

76.2.13
Phantom Breast Pain

Phantom breast pain at the site of the original nipple locations has been reported following breast reduction [19]. This was resolved with explanation to the patient of the origin of the pain and with nonsteroidal antiinflammatory analgesics.

76.2.14
Retained Excess Areola

In patients for breast reduction with very large areolas, the Wise pattern has to be modified to allow removal of all of the excess areola. Otherwise the pigmented area of the residual areola will mar the cosmetic result (Fig. 76.4).

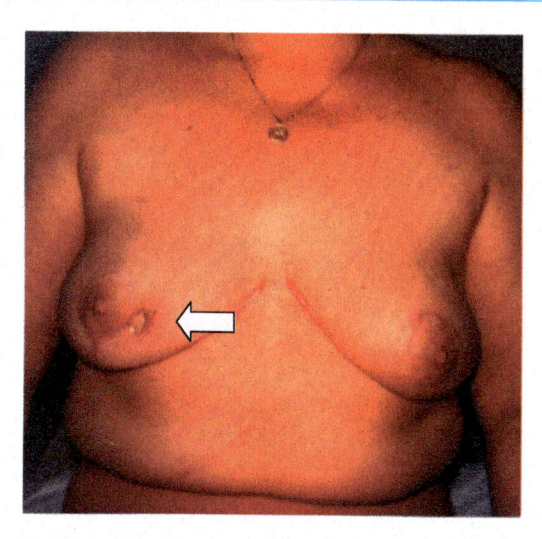

Fig. 76.3 Postoperative necrosis following breast reduction in a diabetic with infection

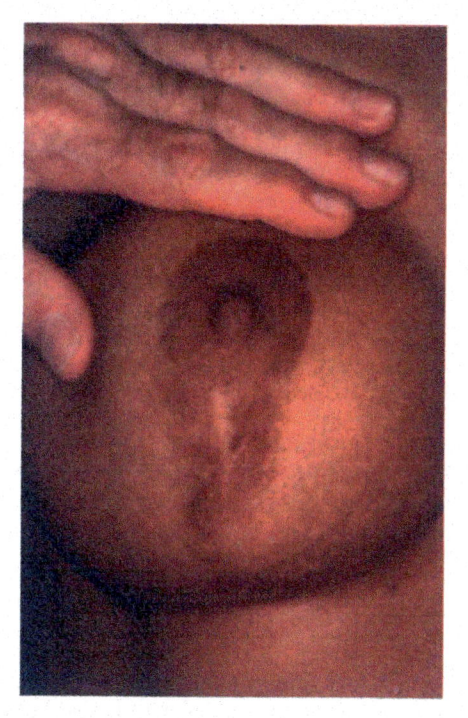

Fig. 76.4 Residual pigmented areola tissue along the vertical scar following breast reduction

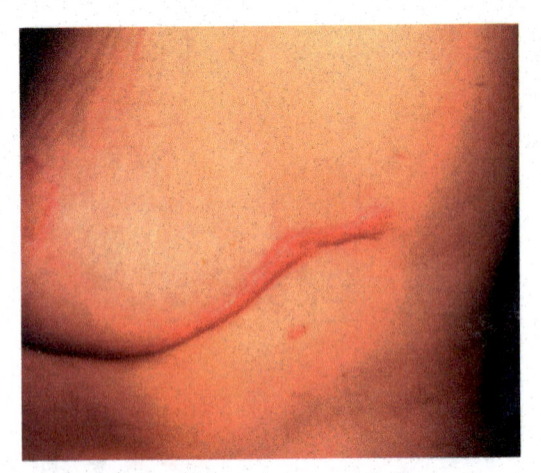

Fig. 76.5 Hypertrophic scar

76.2.15
Scar

Hypertrophic (Fig. 76.5) and keloid scars can occur with any surgical wound.

76.2.16
Pathology

Hypertrophic scars can be distinguished from keloid scars microscopically. Both are characterized by excessive deposits of collagen in the dermis and subcutaneous tissues following trauma or surgical injuries with collagen bundles that appear stretched and aligned in the same plane. Collagen bundles in keloids are thicker and more abundant and form acellular node-like structures in the deep dermis.

76.2.17
Clinical Manifestations

Keloids may have a genetic predisposition and occur in 15–20% of blacks, Hispanics, and Asians. Hypertrophic scars are confined to the area of injury while keloids grow beyond the confines of the original wound and can appear nodular. Hypertrophic scars may regress without treatment while keloids rarely regress. The scars can cause disfigurement, contractures, pain, and itching.

76.2.18
Treatment

Keloids and hypertrophic scars can be treated with intralesional corticosteroids alone or in combination with surgical excision, superficial radiation, laser, cryotherapy, or pressure therapy. Silicone sheeting used 8 h daily for 3–6 months is helpful in reducing the height of a thickened scar. Keloids tend to recur in about 80% of patients with most types of treatment.

Other therapeutic agents [20] include 5-fluorouracil, verapamil (calcium blocker), Bleomycin, interferon-α-2β, histamine antagonist, or colchicine (with or without penicillamine and β-aminopropionitrile).

Surgical excision of keloids followed by superficial radiotherapy for 2 treatments, one per day, is very helpful. The best way to remove the keloid surgically is to excise the scar leaving about 1 mm of scar circumferentially and closing the wound with sutures in the scar edges. The use of steroids in the edges of the wound closure may be helpful in reducing the amount of scarring.

In using corticosteroids care should be taken to inject the drug into the middle of the lesion. If injected too superficially, there may be visible spots of chalky material. There may be pain with injecting steroids into the scar because there is very little give to the tissues and local anesthesia may be necessary. The author uses a combination of Triamcinolone (40 mg cc^{-1}), 0.2–0.4 cc, 5-fluorouracil, 1 cc (50 mg), and 1 cc 0.5% lidocaine with epinephrine for the injection. Hypopigmentation in the scar may occur. Inadvertent injection of steroids deep to the scar may result in steroid fat atrophy.

76.2.19
Steroid Fat Atrophy

The treatment for fat atrophy secondary to steroid injection has usually been with the use of fillers, including autologous fat.

The author has a patient who was a post reduction mammoplasty with implant augmentation with postoperative hypertrophic scars that had been treated in the inferior medial aspect of both breasts with steroids resulting in complete loss of the fat of the inferior medial portions of the breast fat one year before being seen (Fig. 76.6). While performing a capsulotomy for capsule contracture of the right breast, 300 ml of saline was injected as tumescent fluid into the inferior medial quadrants of both breasts for a total of 600 ml. Thirty days after the procedure the inferior medial quadrants

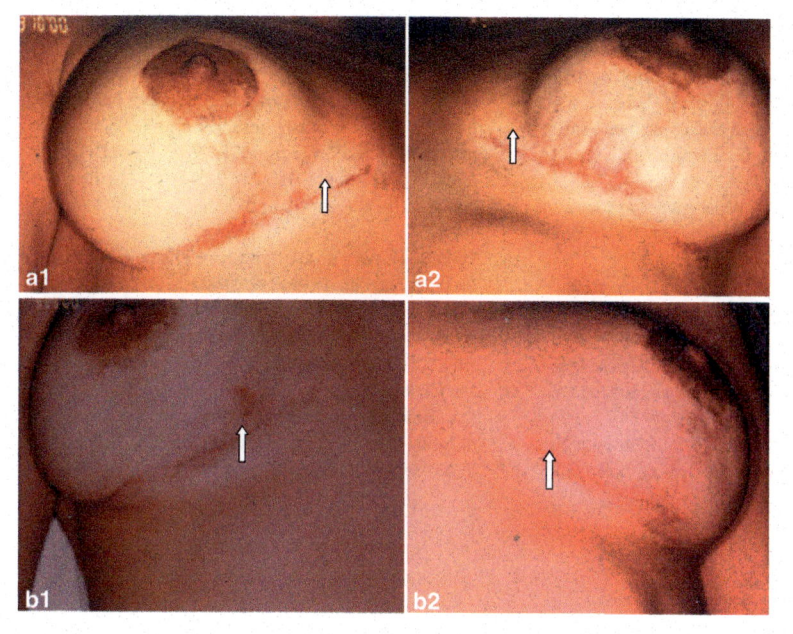

Fig. 76.6 (*a1,2*) Fat atrophy of the inferior medial quadrants of both breasts following steroid injections of the scars. (*b1,2*) Thirty days after tumescence with 300 ml saline on each side showing the fat content of the inferior medial quadrants to be normal

of the breast were found to be filled out to normal proportions with fat.

Apparently, the steroids cause loss of the fat in the cell but do not destroy the fat cells. Placing the steroid crystals back in the emulsion form allows the body to remove these as foreign substances.

76.3 Discussion

Some form of complication occurs in about 10% of patients. Mandrekas [21] reported the incidence percentage of some complications as given below.
Hematoma 0.3%
Nipple and/or pedicle necrosis 0.8%
Wound dehiscence 4.6%
Hypertrophic scars 3.3%
Loss of sensitivity of the nipple 1.3%

References

1. Yalin CT, Bayrak IK, Katranci S, Belet U: Breast changes after breast reduction mammaplasty: A case report with mammographic and ultrasonographic findings and a literature review. Breast J 2003;9(2):133–137
2. Brown FE, Sargent SK, Cohen SR, Morain WD: Mammographic changes following reduction mammoplasty. Plast Reconstr Surg 1987;80:691–698
3. Miller CL, Freog SA, Fox JW: Mammographic changes after reduction mammoplasty. Am J Roentgenol 1987;149:35–38
4. Mendelson EB: Evaluation of the postoperative breast. Radiol Clin N Am 1992;30:107–138
5. Mitnick JS, Roses DF, Harris MN, Colen SR: Calcifications of the breast after reduction mammoplasty. Surg Gynecol Obstet 1990;171(5):409–412
6. Mitnick JS, Vazquez MF, Plesser KP, Pressman PI, Harris MN, Colen SR, Roses DF: Distinction between Postsurgical changes and carcinoma by means of stereotactic fine-needle biopsy after reduction mammaplasty. Radiology 1993;188(2):457–462
7. Heywang-Kobrunner SH, Scheer I, Dershaw DD: Diagnostic Breast Imaging. Stuttgart, Thieme 1997, pp 280–315
8. Butler CE, Hunt KK, Singletary SE: Management of breast carcinoma identified intraoperatively during reduction mammaplasty. Ann Plast Surg 2003;50(2):193–197
9. Snyderman RK: Breast carcinoma found in association with reduction mammaplasty. Plast Reconstr Surg 1990;83(1):153–154
10. Dinner MI, Sheldon J: Carcinoma of the breast occurring in routine reduction mammaplasty. Plast Reconstr Surg 1989;83(6):1042–1044

11. Keleher AJ, Langstein HN, Ames FC, Ross M I, Chang DW, Reece GP, Singletary SE: Breast cancer in reduction mammaplasty specimens: Case reports and guidelines. Breast J 2003;9(2):120–125
12. Lund K, Ewertz M, Schou G: Breast cancer incidence subsequent to surgical reducing of the female breast. Scand J Plast Reconstr Surg 1987;21;209–212
13. Agarwal AK, Ali SN, Erdmann MW: Free DIEP flap breast augmentation following excessive reduction. Br J Plast Surg 2003;56(2):191–193
14. Berry M.G, Tavakkolizadeh A, Sommerlad C: Necrotizing ulceration after breast reduction. J R Soc Med 2003;96(4): 186–187
15. Ferreira MC, Costa MP, Cunha MS, Sakae E, Fels KW: Sensibiltiy of the breast after reduction mammaplasty. Ann Plast Surg 2003;51(1):1–5
16. Hamdi M, Blondeel P, Van de Sijpe K, Van Landuyt K, Monstrey S: Evaluation of nipple-areola complex sensitivity after the latero-central glandular pedicle technique in breast reduction. Br J Plast Surg 2003;56(4):360–364
17. Gonzalez F, Walton RL, Shafer B, Matory WE Jr, Borah GL: Reduction mammaplasty improves symptoms of macromastia. Plast Reconstr Surg 1993;91(7):1270–1276
18. Wallace MS, Wallace AM, Lee J, Dobke MK: Pain after breast surgery: A survey of 282 women. Pain 1996;66(2): 195–205
19. Tytherleigh MG, Koshy C, Evans J: Phantom breast pain. Plast Reconstr Surg 1998;102(3):921
20. Al-Attar A, Mess S, Thomassen JM, Kauffman CL, Davison SP: Keloid pathogenesis and treatment. Plast Reconstr Surg 2006;117(1):286–300
21. Mandrekas AD, Zambacos GJ, Anastasopoulos A, Hapsas DA: Reduction mammaplasty with the inferior pedicle technique: early and late complications in 371 patients. Br J Plast Surg 1996;49(7):442–446

Late Sequelae of Breast Reduction

Nicholas G. Economides

77.1 Introduction

Reduction mammoplasty has evolved as a procedure of necessity for the treatment of mammary hypertrophy or mammary gigantism. Either condition is the cause of physical discomfort in the "over 30" population of women and additional severe psychological distress in females of teenage and prepregnancy years.

Several techniques are available; however the long-term surgical goals are common to all: (a) reduce the volume and hence the symptoms, (b) preserve the functionality; i.e., breast-feeding, (c) create a desirable appearance, (d) produce acceptable scars, (e) minimize long-term sequelae. Although the variety of surgical alternatives mostly achieves the first three goals, it behooves the plastic surgeon to be aware of the latter as he or she communicates the procedure to the candidate patient.

77.2 History

The author used the McKissock technique until 1984 and then changed to the inferior-lateral pedicles as described by Robbins [1] and Georgiade [2] to preserve sensation in the areola and to provide better blood supply to the pedicle and support the nipple with breast parenchyma for future breast-feeding.

77.3 Technique

The breast is marked by first identifying the axis of the gland and the anterior projection of the inframmary fold. The new areola site is marked at equal distance from the midline. A Greek capitol Lambda (Γ) is designed originating from the mark and extending 7 cm down. The width of the limbs is adjusted upwards from 7 cm according to the amount of skin that needs to be removed from the medial and lateral meridians. The pedicle is drawn 2.5 cm above the new areolar border and is 5–6 cm wide. If the length exceeds 15 cm a free nipple graft will be contemplated. For patients who are postmenopausal, have gigantomastia (over 1,000 g per side), or want to have small breasts after the procedure, the author uses a superior pedicle as described by Spear and Little [3], with the exception of making the pedicle narrower and longer for improved postoperative appearance.

There are a few cases where liposuction accomplished at least four out of the five goals of breast reduction. The patients selected were younger or did not develop hypertrophy until after they had gained weight later in life. The lateral projection of the nipple areolar complex has to be at, above, or 2 cm below the inframammary fold. The author utilizes a small infraareolar incision, and a "pancake" resection of the breast tissue lying directly over the pectoralis major muscle and tumescent liposuction of the breasts to include the axillary tail and the infraclavicular space. The expectation is to stimulate shrinkage of the skin of the upper pole, a condition desired for correction of mild ptosis (Fig. 77.1).

77.4 Complications

There have been a total of 1,055 reduction procedures all performed by the author (Table 77.1). The vast majority was bilateral. One hundred and fifty three reductions were performed for a matching procedure associated with breast reconstruction or unilateral for a congenital asymmetry (Table 77.2). The free nipple areolar graft technique was used in 131 cases (Fig. 77.2). Liposuction with pancake resection was reserved for 52 cases. The rest were performed using the inferior pedicle option (Table 77.3). Complications occurring in the early postoperative period are listed in Table 77.4.

77.5 Late Sequelae

Following the initial postoperative period of 6 months, the plastic surgeon should anticipate and expect various conditions related to reduction mammoplasty.

M.A. Shiffman (ed.), *Mastopexy and Breast Reduction: Principles and Practice*,
© Springer-Verlag Berlin Heidelberg 2009

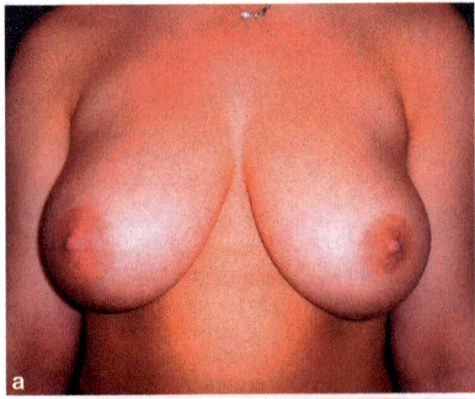

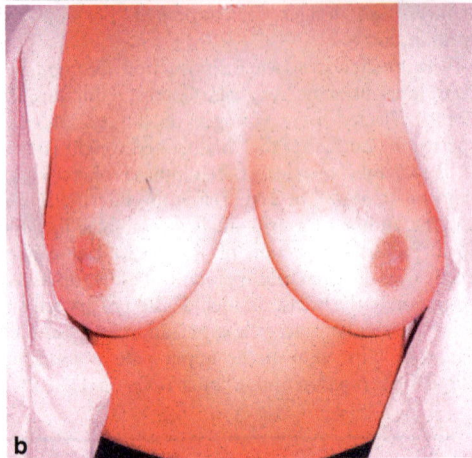

Table 77.1 Breast reduction: Number of cases

Years	Number of cases (Bilateral)	Number of cases (Unilateral)
1981–1985	73	24
1986–1995	180	50
1995–2002	129	16
2002–2007	520	63
Total	902	153

Table 77.2 Bilateral breast reduction: Condition

Condition	Number of cases
Matching reconstructed breast	106
Breast asymmetry	47

Table 77.3 Various techniques utilized

	Bilateral	Unilateral	Total
Inferior Pedicle	770	103	883
Free Areolar Graft	130	1	131
Liposuction/ Pancake	49	2	51
Total	949	106	1055

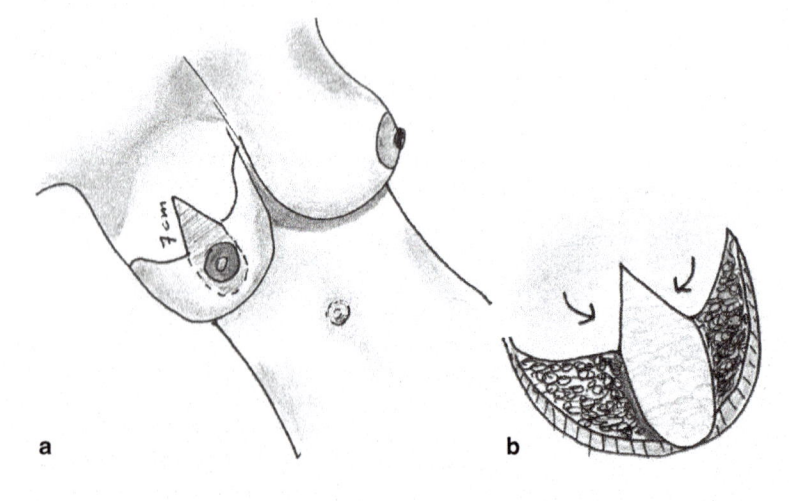

Fig. 77.1 (a) Preoperative patient. (b) Postoperative after liposuction

Fig. 77.2 Superior pedicle reduction when nipple/areolar graft is required

Table 77.4 Complications

1. Nipple-areolar partial loss
2. Nipple-areolar full loss
3. Wound infection (localized)
4. Minor dehiscence (5 cm or less)
5. Hematoma
6. Numbness of fingers
7. Hypertrophic scars

Table 77.5 Late sequelae

1. Asymmetry, inferior displacement
2. Unsightly scars
3. Fat necrosis
4. Hypomastia
5. Keloids
6. Recurrence
7. Lateral fullness
8. Areolar depigmentation
9. Breast cancer
10. Lack of lactation
11. Litigation (malpractice)

Table 77.6 Treatment of sequelae

1. Revision scars, asymmetry inferior displacement	71
2. Revision lateral breast	34
3. Nipple areolar tattooing	17
4. Augmentation	6
5. Subcutaneous mastectomy	8
6. Open excisional biopsy	36
7. Second reduction	4
8. Irradiation	3
Total	179

Tables 77.5 and 77.6 reflect the outcomes and additional surgeries that were performed.

77.5.1
Scars, Asymmetry, Inferior Displacement

The usual patient who does not like the scars or complains of asymmetry will also likely have displacement of the majority of the remaining volume to the inferior pole. This is associated mainly to either an early wound dehiscence or widening of the horizontal scar. The condition can be minimized preventively by assuring a short vertical incision (less than 4.5 cm) and by placing nonabsorbable sutures between the pedicle and the pectoralis fascia. Indiscriminate use of intralesional steroid injections for hypertrophic scarring in the early postoperative period may also contribute to the condition.

Surgical correction is relatively easy. Retightening by removal of the excess skin and the scars will result in significant improvement if there is adequate breast volume; if not, insertion of implants will definitely improve the situation.

77.5.2
Lateral Breast Fullness

This condition is usually the result of obesity in patients either at the time of the surgery or who gain weight later. Patients with massive weight loss prior to the surgery also end up with excess skin laterally due to the intraoperative positioning and the entrapment of the skin posteriorly. Some prevention may be obtained by performing lateral liposuction at the time of the reduction. The author prefers syringe liposuction that minimizes alteration of the blood supply to the areola. Secondary lateral excisions are always highly successful.

77.5.3
Areolar Depigmentation

Medical tattooing of both areolas with a seven prong needle tip alleviates the problem of depigmentation that occurs commonly on dark skinned patients and mostly with free nipple graft (Fig. 77.3).

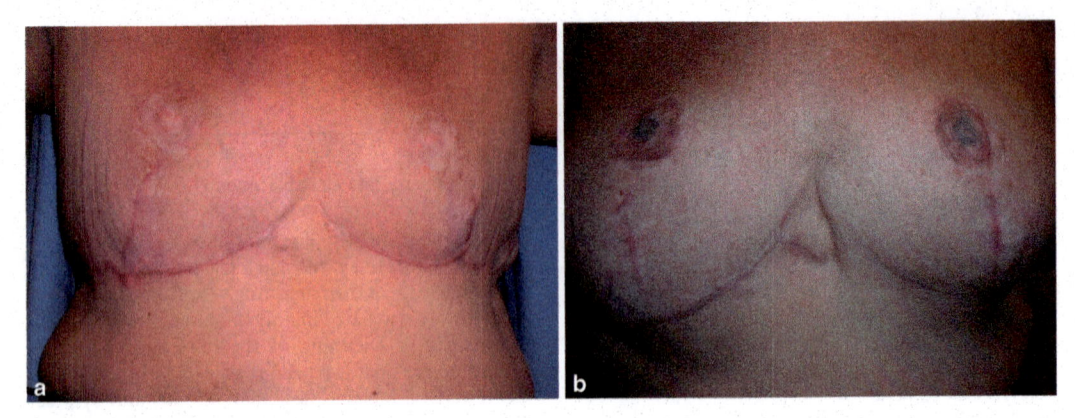

Fig. 77.3 (a) Depigmentation of grafted areolar complex. (b) Improvement with tattooing

77.5.4
Fat Necrosis

It is most likely to occur with large reductions. Although always characteristic to the surgeons, it needs excisional biopsy to eliminate any anxiety from the patient's standpoint. A preoperative mammogram and ultrasound is recommended. For extensive segments of necrosis a biopsy of a smaller area will suffice. This particular late complication tends to improve with time and massaging.

77.5.5
Keloids

This complication may be identified prior to the surgery if there have been other incidents of keloid formation on the patient's skin. The only treatment available is irradiation [4] soon after the primary procedure or a re-excision is performed. Intrakeloid injection 4–6 weeks prior to re-excision is recommended (Fig. 77.4).

77.5.6
Recurrence

Patients who have virginal hypertrophy and are less than 25 years of age are more likely to have a recurrence. "Superimposed" reduction reusing the inferior pedicle is feasible. Areolar compromise has not been observed. It is important however to investigate the technique used with the primary procedure. Liposuction can be considered if the areola remains above the inframammary fold.

77.5.7
Breast Cancer

Reduction mammoplasty will neither increase nor decrease the risk of breast cancer. The volume reduction however allows the gland to be more accessible radiologically and for examination. Detection is heightened. Some cases with insitu cancers are amenable to subcutaneous mastectomy as a primary treatment or as a matching procedure for the opposite breast. There is a high risk however for partial skin loss due to the previous scarring. Therefore, a tissue expander is recommended in lieu of permanent prosthesis in the case where reconstruction is desired.

77.5.8
Lack of Lactation

The patients who receive free nipple areolar grafts will be unable to breast feed. It is important however to tell patients who undergo the procedure using the inferior pedicle that lactation following pregnancy may be impaired or inadequate.

77.5.9
Hypomastia

There are women who will lose or gain weight in the subsequent years, causing changes to the breasts. Similar situations occur with pregnancies. When the volume involutes, the patients will need augmentation either with implants or autogenous tissue (Fig. 77.5).

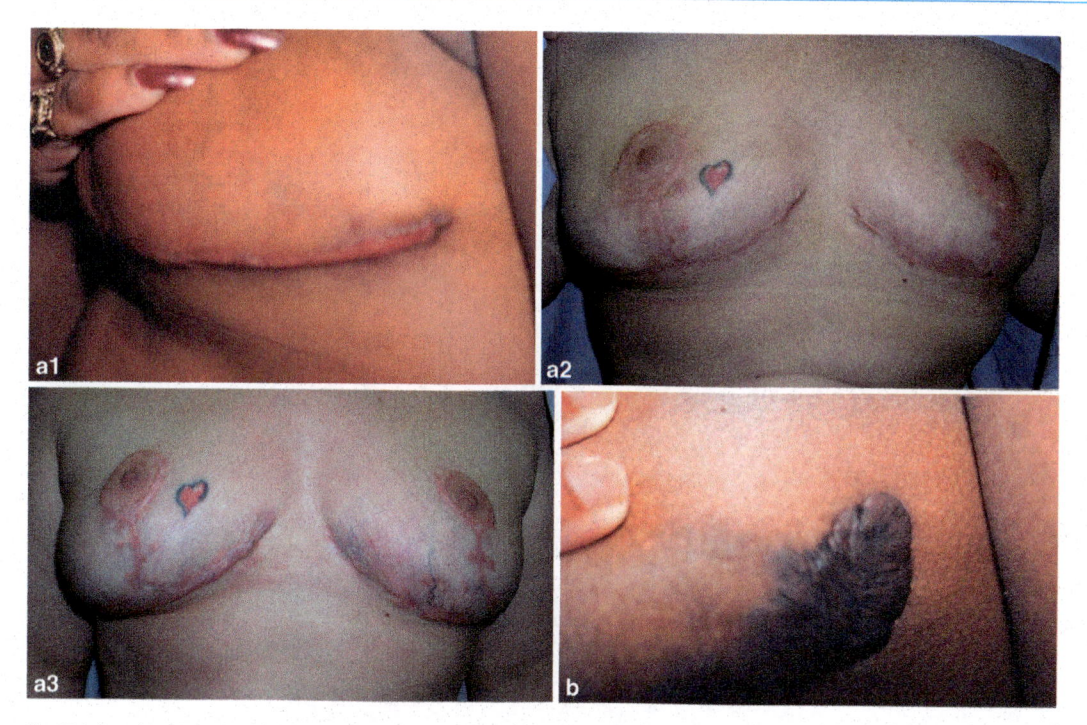

Fig. 77.4 (*a1-3*) Beginning of keloid 2 months following surgery [5]. Keloid scar after steroid injection [6]. After re-excision and irradiation [1]. (**b**) Fully developed keloid 2 years following reduction

77.5.10 Litigation

Most malpractice suits in cases of breast reduction are generated because of late sequelae although the issues could be resolved very early with proper communication with the patient. The complaints almost never address "failure to cure" the symptoms that drive the patients to the plastic surgeon. The dissatisfaction is because of scars, asymmetry, nipple areolar malposition, inadequate remaining volume, need for more surgery and additional cost to the patients (Fig. 77.6). The cases are easily defended if the surgeon adheres to the indications, planning, execution and follow-up while openly communicating with the patient. Documentation and consent are of great importance. There have been proportionally very few awards of small amounts (ProAssurance letter).

77.6 Discussion

It has been well established that the medical reasons and necessity for reduction mammoplasty are neck and shoulder pain, shoulder furrows from the support bras and anterior chest wall syndrome. These symptoms coupled with hypertrophy and ptosis lead the patients to surgery. The reversal of symptoms occurs in over 95% of the patients who would also recommend it to others [7].

The early complication rate has been found to be at around 12% [8]. Patients with over 2,000 g total volume reduction or who are overweight have a higher rate and are two times more prone to postoperative risks. The most significant risk in the author's opinion is partial or full nipple–areolar necrosis, wound dehiscence, infections, and scarring.

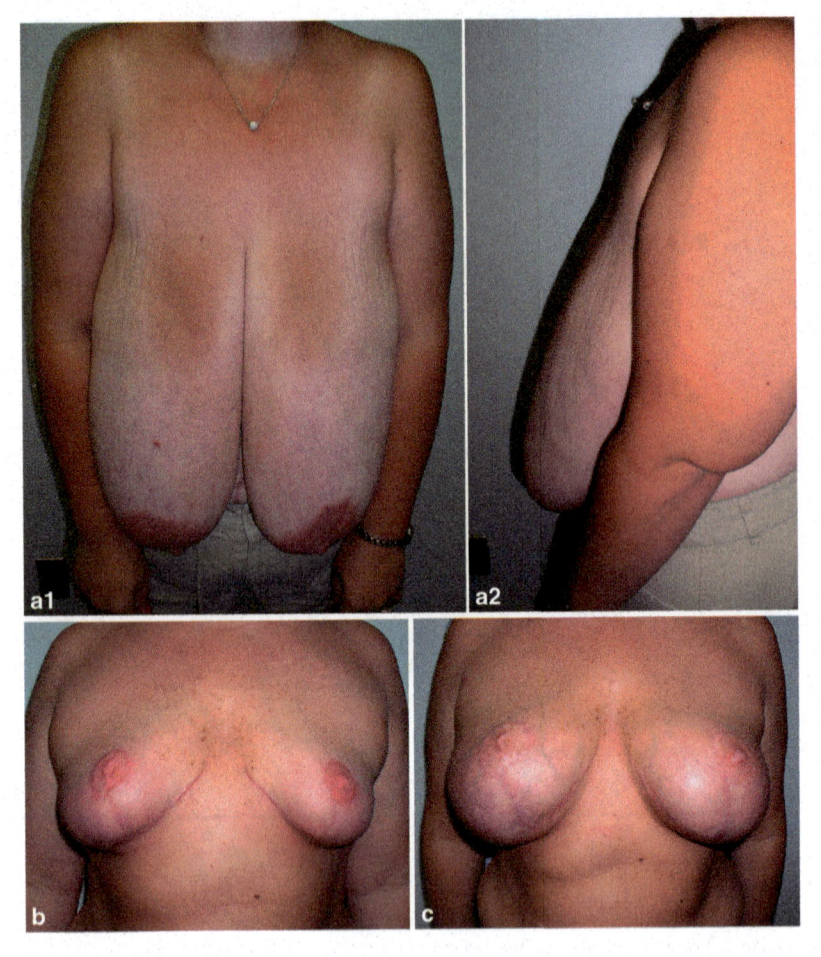

Fig. 77.5 (**a1-2**) Preoperative patient. (**b**) One year postoperative with complaints that breasts need shape. (**c**) Augmentation with 350 ml high profile saline implants

There is a discrepancy between expectation and reality concerning the understanding of the procedure as is perceived by the potential patient. There should be clarity in terms of what the procedure will do as it relates to symptoms and what the ultimate relief will be, vis á vi the appearance of the breast in the future as affected by inevitable chronological changes. The relief is permanent, but the cosmetic result is not and hence the importance of recognizing the long-term effects (sequelae) of the procedure. In the authors experience there were an additional 179 procedures or 18.1% in the years following reduction mammoplasties (Table 77.6). There were none when liposuction with "pancake" excision was performed.

Scarring, asymmetry and residual tissue along with weight changes comprised the majority of the additional operations. Fortunately, the secondary procedures are of low risk with the exception of a "new" reduction where the nipple–areolar complex needed to be repositioned. The author has not experienced any significant tissue loss. Reversible epidermolysis has been observed in three cases.

Areolar sensation was addressed in a prior report [9]. Patients should be instructed about experiencing temporary or even permanent loss of sensibility. Preservation is likely with short pedicles. Grafted areolar complexes eventually recover the sense of temperature and pain. Lack of erectile ability is perceived as loss of nipple by a significant number of patients.

The likelihood of litigation following reduction mammoplasty falls within the usual risks for plastic surgery. Informed consent, adherence to the indications and operative management according to the standard of care is of utmost importance. Preoperative and postoperative photos and factual medical records will offer additional protection to the defendant physician.

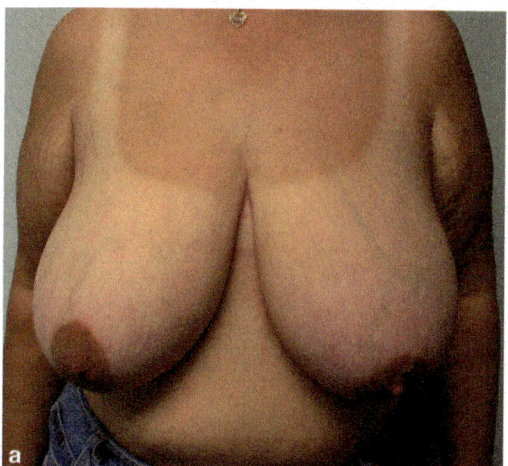

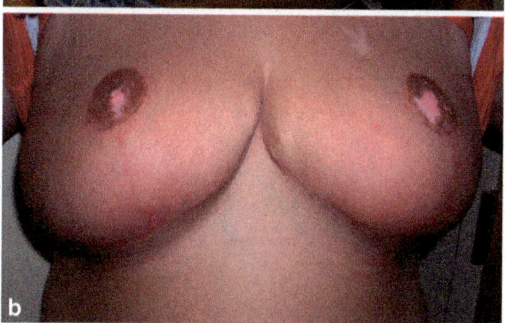

Fig. 77.6 (a) Preoperative patient. (b) Postoperative patient unhappy with scars and depigmentation. Malpractice case verdict in favor of defendant

77.7 Conclusions

Reduction mammoplasty remains a procedure designed to relieve skeletal symptoms to patients with very large breasts. The success rate is over 95%. Following the procedure and past the initial period of 6 months that carries a 12% complication rate, there is an 18.1% incidence for further surgery. Late sequelae include scars, residual tissue, recurrence, atrophy, breast cancer (not related) and litigation. It is important that both the surgeon and the patient are aware of the long term potential outcomes, both favorable and unfavorable [10–12].

References

1. Rubin LR: Surgical treatment of the massive hypertrophic breast. In: Georgiade NG (ed). Reconstructive Breast Surgery. St. Louis, Mosby 1976
2. Georgiade NG, Serafin D, Morris R, Georgiade G: Reduction mammoplasty utilizing an inferior pedicle nipple-areola flap. Ann Plast Surg 1979;3(3):211–218
3. Spear SL, Little JW III: Reduction mammoplasty and mastopexy. In: Aston SJ, Beasley RW, Thorne CHM (eds). Grabb and Smith's Plastic Surgery, 5th edn. Philadelphia, Lippincott-Raven 1997, pp 725–752
4. Norris JE: Superficial x-ray therapy in keloid management: A retrospective study of 24 cases and literature review. Plast Reconstr Surg 1995;95(6):1051–1055
5. McKissock PK: Reduction mammoplasty with a vertical dermal flap. Plast Reconstr Surg 1972;49(3):245–252
6. Strömbeck JO: Mammoplasty: Report of a new technique based on the two pedicle procedure. Br J Plast Surg 1960;13:79–90
7. Queens County, NY Newson v Defendant: Defendant's verdict; alleged ischemia resulting in loss of nipple. Zarin's Med Liability Alert 2006;15(3):32
8. Bergen County, NJ. Paker vs. Dr. M,.Docket No. L-008710-04: Surgeon fails to disclose alleged known risk of necrosis in area of nipple prior to breast reduction and liposuction. Zarin's Med Liability Alert 2007;15(9):31
9. Economides NG: Reduction mammoplasty; a study of sequelae. Breast J 1997;3(2):69–73
10. Miller BJ, Morris SF, Sigurdson LL, Bendor-Samuel RL, Brennan M, Davis G, Paletz JL: Prospective study of outcomes after reduction mammoplasty. Plast Reconstr Surg 2005;115(4):1025–1031
11. Wagner DS, Alfonso DR: The influence of obesity and volume of resection on success in reduction mammoplasty: an outcomes study. Plast Reconstr Surg 2005;115(4):1034–1038
12. Hawtof DB, Levine M. Kapetansky DI, Pieper D: Complications of reduction Mammoplasty: comparison of nipple-areolar graft and pedicle. Ann Plast Surg 1989;23(1):3–10

Breast Feeding After Breast Reduction

Arnis Freiberg

78.1 Introduction

"Will I be able to breast feed after my reduction mammaplasty?" is a commonly asked question by patients in the child bearing age group. This question has been asked ever since the introduction of the now very popular reduction mammaplasty operation. Unfortunately, and in view of the present day principles of stressing the importance of evidence based medicine, there are no definitive answers, and because of the nature of the problem, which is multifactorial, there may never be one!

In 1990 the author presented the results of studying this question and reviewing the literature [1]. The purpose of this article is to look at this problem once more and to review and update the current literature.

78.2 History

Some of the well known authors, like Pitanguy (1962) [2], McKissock (1972) [3], Pontes (1973) [4], who described their procedures and others reporting on large series, make no mention of breast feeding. Some series mention lactation but no numbers on breast feeding. Strombeck [5] in a 1980 publication reported that out of 726 patients, 118 had become pregnant postoperatively, and 33 breast fed.

In the author's study [1] 73 patients between ages of 18–40 who had previously undergone an inferiorly based pedicle reduction mammaplasty between 1977 and 1989 were reviewed by a telephone interview. 29% (20 out of the 68 patients who responded) who had become pregnant indicated that all lactated. Seven women (35%) successfully breast fed for at least 2 months. Nine others (45%) breast fed for up to 2 weeks but failed to continue for a variety of reasons. The remaining four women (20%) did not breast feed for a variety of reasons and since all lactated, it is presumed that they, at least theoretically, could have breast fed.

In 1992 Caouette-Laberge and Duranceau, [6] reviewed 243 women who had undergone a pedicle technique breast reduction between 1967 and 1987 at the ages between 15 and 35 years. Out of the 234 they were able to reach 98. Eighteen out of the 98 had become pregnant after their surgery. Eight out of the 18 (45%) nursed their children for up to 32 weeks (mean 11 weeks). Only one mother had to supplement nursing with a formula. Ten of 18 mothers (55%) did not breast feed for the following reasons: six by personal choice, two due to premature delivery, one was advised that nursing was not feasible, and one had no lactation. The authors concluded that nursing capacity of the breast is preserved after a breast reduction and that women should be encouraged to nurse their children.

A study by Marshall et al. [7] in 1994 studied 30 women who had undergone breast reduction and subsequently wished to breast feed. Since 18 patients out of 19 were able to breast feed, they concluded that breast feeding is possible following a physiological type of operation. They strongly suggested that all functioning breast tissue that remains after reduction should be left attached to the nipple in a physiological manner.

In 1996 Mandrekas et al. [8] reviewed 371 patients who had undergone an inferior pedicle technique over 10 years before to look at late complications. They stated that 72% of the patients who had become pregnant were able to lactate.

In 2000 Tairych et al. [9] reported on a long term outcome of six techniques of breast reduction in 192 patients between 1973 and 1993. They concluded that breast feeding was possible after all the techniques except for free nipple grafting.

The most comprehensive review on breast feeding following reduction mammaplasty is by Brzozowski, et al. [10] in 2000. Like most of these studies, it is a retrospective study. The study involved 554 patients between the ages of 15–35 who were operated upon by the inferior pedicle technique between 1984 and 1994. They were able to contact 334 patients. They defined breast feeding success if the patient was able to breast feed for up to or more than 2 weeks. Seventy-eight of these patients had children. Fifteen out of 78 mothers (19.2%) breast fed exclusively. Eight out of 78 (10.3%) patients breast fed with formula supplement. Fourteen out of 78 (17.9%) were unsuccessful in breast feeding attempts. Forty one out of 78 (52.5%) did not attempt breast feeding. Nine of the 41 were discouraged about breast feeding by a health care professional! Of the 78 women who had children postoperatively, a total of 27 were discouraged from breast feeding by a health care professional. In comparison, 26 patients were encouraged to breast feed; nineteen (73.1%) subsequently attempted breast feeding. Thirty one of the 41 patients not attempting to breast feed, experienced breast engorgement and lactation. The authors concluded that by the use of the inferior flap technique and professional encouragement, the breast feeding rate falls near the breast feeding rate found in the population not having undergone breast reduction surgery, according to an article published in the Canadian Journal of Public Health [11].

An article by Zambacos et al. in 2001 [12] commented on the study by Brzozowski and presented the results of their own study using the inferior pedicle technique. Although the numbers were comparatively small, they stated that 72% of their patients were able to breast feed. They argued that the inferior pedicle procedure by design, leaves the nipple in continuity with the glandular tissue and spares the important nerves required to supply the nipple for successful breast feeding, and therefore should allow for breast feeding.

In 2002 Aillet et al. [13] studied breast feeding after reduction mammaplasty performed during adolescence. The purpose of the study was to determine surgical factors influencing the outcome and patient perception of information concerning breast feeding. A questionnaire was sent to 109 women between the ages of 15 and 17 who had undergone reduction mammaplasty between 1981 and 1997. Sixty five questionnaires (60%) could be analyzed. Seventeen women (26%) had delivered 25 infants over this period of time. Five women (29%) nursed their first infant for a mean of 11.3 days. None of the women interrupted breast feeding for a reason related to nipple anomaly or difficulty in suckling. Although information on breast feeding was systematically delivered, 41 women (63%) stated that they had not been informed. The authors concluded that adolescents who undergo reduction mammaplasty can nurse their future infants with a complication rate similar to that in the general population. Special attention must be given to the delivery of information on breast feeding.

In 2003 Hefter et al. [14] studied lactation and breast feeding following lateral pedicle mammaplasty. They considered breast feeding successful if it was performed exclusively without supplementation for 2 months. Thirteen of the women who replied had given birth after surgery. To preserve lactation, a technique leaving structures untouched within the pedicle with increased dimensions was used. Seven women (54%) breast fed successfully for between 2 and 14 months. Two women (16%) were classified as unsuccessful and four women (30%) did not breast feed at all. The authors concluded that breast feeding was limited by nonsurgical factors, including the influence of medical personnel.

In 2004 Cruz-Korchin et al. [15] studied breast feeding after vertical mammaplasty with medial pedicle. They compared breast feeding success between two groups of women in child bearing age (15–40 years) with macromastia. The control group of 149 had been evaluated for possible breast reduction surgery and who had children before the consultation. The study group of 58 women had had children after their vertical mammaplasty. A period of 2 weeks or more was chosen as the duration for successful breast feeding attempt. The results demonstrated that 61% in the control group and 65% in the study group were successful, with no statistical difference between the two groups. They concluded that there was no significant difference in the rate of breast feeding success between women who had a medial pedicle vertical reduction mammaplasty and women who had no prior breast surgery.

A 2005 study by Kakagia et al. [16] studied breast feeding after reduction mammaplasty, comparing three different techniques. A questionnaire was sent to 178 patients, 106 patients of the patients who replied had given birth after the reduction mammaplasty. Breast feeding was considered successful if it was performed for at least 3 weeks without supplementation. The success rates were as follows: 71% for superior pedicle, 77% for inferior pedicle and 63% following horizontal bipedicled reduction mammaplasty. The postoperative ability to breast feed was not found to relate to the amount of resected breast tissue or the time elapsing between operation and delivery. They concluded that as long as the nipple–areola complex transposition preserved adequate subareolar breast tissue, the ability to breast feed depends on the encouragement and support offered to women rather than the choice of operation.

78.3
Discussion

There has been an increasing interest in breast feeding after reduction mammaplasty during the past decade. Most authors agree that a pedicled flap reduction, leaving sufficient or extra breast tissue behind the nipple–areola complex, is essential for patients in the child bearing age group who are interested in breast feeding following their reduction mammaplasty. Although there are only a few studies comparing the ability to breast feed following different procedures, it appears that the origin of the pedicle is not important. It appears that the inferior pedicle and the Wise pattern techniques have become very popular in the United States. Rohrich et al. [17] in 2002 surveyed 1,500 members of the American Society for Aesthetic Surgery. Five hundred and fifty four members returned the survey. Fifty six percent of the respondents use only the inferior pedicle and the Wise pattern procedure, as compared to 6.9% who use only the limited incision techniques. Although the majority of surgeons reported that they did not anticipate changing their practices to accommodate advances in limited excision techniques, 89% reported that the new limited incision techniques and liposuction are trends that are here to stay. It is only hoped that those surgeons will keep in mind the importance of breast feeding while changing their techniques!

A survey of Canadian plastic surgeons in 1993 by Carr et al. [18] found that 65% of surgeons used the inferior pedicle technique. Most surgeons also altered their procedures in special clinical situations. The author's personal choice of alteration was to leave excess breast tissue behind the nipple in young patients, regardless of whether they indicated a desire to breast feed postoperatively or not, allowing them to make that choice postoperatively. Although the majority of studies reviewed indicate that breast feeding is possible following reduction mammaplasty, a paper by Souto et al. [19], after comparing a group of 49 women who had undergone breast reduction surgery using the transposition technique with 96 controls concluded that breast reduction may have a negative impact on breast feeding performance.

In this day and age of evidence based medicine, the question of breast feeding after reduction mammaplasty may be difficult, if not impossible, to answer. There are two main problems: because of the multitude of variables, socio-economic and technical, a large number of patients would be required to satisfy statistical requirements. The other problem deals with the multitude of reasons for not breast feeding, especially in the control group. There are other problems, such as the definition of successful breast feeding: the time, the use of supplements, and the reasons for discontinuance.

78.4
Conclusions

Breast feeding after reduction mammaplasty by pedicled techniques is possible in the majority of patients. Health care professionals, and more specifically surgeons, should discuss this aspect with patients preoperatively and encourage breast feeding. Although there is at least anecdotal evidence from studies around the world about successful breast feeding after reduction mammaplasty, a large, well controlled study, perhaps involving multiple centers, would lead to more convincing evidence.

References

1. Harris L, Morris SF, Freiberg A: Is breast feeding possible after reduction mammaplasty? Plast Reconstr Surg 1992; 89(5):836–939
2. Pitanguy I: Une nouvelle technique de plastie mammaire. Etude de 245 cas consecutifs et presentation d'une technique personelle. Ann Chir Plast 1962;7:199
3. McKissock PK: Reduction mammaplasty with a vertical dermal flap. Plast Recontr Surg 1972;49(3):245–252
4. Pontes R: A technique of reduction mammaplasty. Br J Plast Surg 1973;26(4):365–370
5. Strombeck JO: Late results after reduction mammaplasty. In: Goldwyn RM (ed). Long-Term Results in Plastic and Reconstructive Surgery. Boston, Little Brown 1980, p 723
6. Caouette-Laberge L, Duranceau LA: Breast feeding after reduction. Ann Chir 1992;46(9):826–829
7. Marshall DR, Callan PP, Nicholson W: Breast feeding after reduction mammaplasty. Br J Plast Surg 1994;47(3): 167–169
8. Mandrekas AD, Zambacos GJ, Anastasopoulos A, Hapsas DA: Reduction mammaplasty with the inferior pedicle technique: early and late complications in 371 patients. Br J Plast Surg 1996;49(7):442–446
9. Tairych G, Worseg A, Kuzbari R, Deutinger M, Holle J: A comparison of long–term outcome of 6 techniques of breast reduction. Handchir Mikrochir Plast Chir 2000; 32(3):159–165
10. Brzozowski D, Niessen M, Evans HB, Hurst LN: Breastfeeding after inferior pedicle reduction mammaplasty. Plast Reconstr Surg 2000;105(2):530–534
11. Matthews MK, Webber K, Mc Kim E, Banoub-Baddour S, Laryea M: Infant feeding practices in Newfoundland and Labrador. Can J Public Health 1995;86:296
12. Zambacos GJ, Mandrekas AD: Breast feeding after inferior pedicle reduction mammaplasty. Plast Reconstr Surg 2001;107(1):294–295
13. Ailett S, Watier E, Chevrier S, Pailheret JP, Grall JY: Breast feeding after reduction mammaplasty performed during adolescence. Eur J Obstet Gynecol Reprod Biol 2002;101:79–82
14. Hefter W, Lindholm P, Elvenes OP: Lactation and breast feeding ability following lateral pedicle mammaplasty. Br J Plast Surg 2003;56(8):746–751

15. Cruz-Korchin N, Korchin L: Breast feeding after vertical mammaplasty with medial Pedicle. Plast Reconstr Surg 2004;114(4):890–894
16. Kakagia D, Tripsiannis, G, Tsoutsos, D: Breast-feeding after reduction mammaplasty: a comparison of 3 techniques. Ann Plast Surg 2005;55(4):343–345
17. Rohrich RJ, Gosman AA, Brown SA, Tonadapu P, Foster B: Current preferences for breast reduction techniques: a survey of board-certified plastic surgeons. Plast Reconstr Surg 2004;114(7):1724–1733
18. Carr MM, Freiberg A: Canadian survey of reduction mammaplasty techniques. Canad J Plast Surg 1996;3: 199–201
19. Souto GC, Giugliani ERJ, Giugliani C, Schneider MA: The impact of breast reduction surgery on breast feeding performance. J Hum Lact 2003;19(1):43–49

Alteration of Nipple and Areola Sensitivity by Reduction Mammaplasty

Schlenz Ingrid, Rigel Sandra, Schemper Michael, and Kuzbari Rafic

Breast hypertrophy can cause physical, psychological, and cosmetic discomfort. More than 100 different operative techniques have been described to reduce the size and to relieve the symptoms. For many years, shape, length of scars, and low complication rates were the major goals in breast reduction surgery. However, during the last years, attention has been directed towards the nerves supplying the breast, and hence the preservation of the sensibility of the nipple–areola complex has become a criterion in evaluating the different reduction techniques [1–9].

The sensitivity of the nipple and the areola of the nonoperated breast was investigated by several authors, and from these studies it became clear that there is an inverse relationship between the size of the breast and the sensitivity of the nipple–areola complex [2,3,5,8,10–20]. There is also an inverse relationship between breast ptosis and the sensitivity of the nipple–areola complex [14,18]. Thus patients with hypertrophic and ptotic breasts have a significantly diminished sensibility of the nipple–areola complex. However, 79% of these patient rated nipple–areola sensitivity as very important or important for their sexual life [8] and therefore it should be preserved during the operation.

In the past, several reports have attributed loss of sensitivity to the weight of resection rather than to the surgical technique [2,3,11,20]. In the recent literature, however, there have been claims that the postoperative sensory outcome is dependent on the reduction technique. Some authors have associated the inferior pedicle techniques with a better preservation of nipple and areola sensitivity than the superior pedicle techniques [1,5,16, 21,22], while others found no differences between the techniques [4,15]. In a prospective study, we assessed the influence of the surgical technique and resection weight on the postoperative sensitivity of the nipple–areola complex by comparing five different reduction techniques [8].

In 80 patients, the sensitivity of the nipple and the cardinal points of the areola was tested with Semmes Weinstein monofilaments before surgery and 3 weeks, 3, 6, and 12 months after surgery. Patients were operated according to the original techniques of Lassus (10 patients), Lejour (13 patients), McKissock (18 patients), Würinger (20 patients), and Georgiade (19 patients).

The value of the lightest monofilament recognized by the patient was recorded. If the largest monofilament (6.65) was applied without its pressure being sensed by the patient, the area was touched with the fingertip. If the touch of the fingertip was not felt by the patient, then the area was considered insensate.

Patient characteristics and preoperative sensitivity were similar in all groups. When questioned preoperatively, all patients stated that the nipple was the most sensitive part of their breast and this was confirmed by the sensory testing. Every postoperative change of the sensitivity of the nipple, the cardinal points of the areola, or the breast skin that amounted to two or more monofilaments was noticed and mentioned by the patients before the testing was done. All patients who had an insensate nipple also reported a loss of the erectile function of the nipple. Until the sixth postoperative month, patients did not mind any alteration of the sensitivity of the nipple or the areola. At 12 months postoperatively, 50% of the patients suffering from a decreased nipple sensitivity and 75% of the patients with complete loss of nipple sensitivity were bothered by the changes.

The mean resection weight was statistically less in the Lassus (540 ± 123 g) and the Lejour (390 ± 112 g) groups compared with the Georgiade (935 ± 460 g) group ($p < 0.05$); it was also significantly less in the Lejour group compared with the McKissock (730 ± 315 g) and the Würinger (740 ± 315 g) groups ($p < 0.05$) (values given are means ± SD).

The sensitivity of the nipple (Fig. 79.1) was found to be significantly lower after a superior pedicle technique (Lassus, Lejour) than after any other technique at 3 weeks, and 3, 6, and 12 months postoperatively ($p < 0.001$). Three weeks postoperatively, 47.8% of the patients operated by a superior pedicle technique were found to have insensate nipples. Most insensate nipples were bilateral (72.7%). In 27.3%, the insensate nipple was unilateral, but the sensitivity of the contralateral side was also severely compromised as the patients could only feel

M.A. Shiffman (ed.), *Mastopexy and Breast Reduction: Principles and Practice,*
© Springer-Verlag Berlin Heidelberg 2009

the largest monofilament. The sensitivity of the nipple was unchanged or sometimes even slightly improved in patients operated with an inferior (Georgiade, McKissock) or inferocentral (Würinger) pedicle technique. Between 3 and 6 months after surgery, sensitivity of the nipple started improving in most patients. However, even at 12 months, preoperative values of nipple and areola sensitivity were not reached in 69.5% of the patients operated with a superior pedicle technique and insensate nipples were found in 13% of the patients.

The sensitivity of the areola (Fig. 79.2) was decreased in all patients 3 weeks after surgery. Patients operated with an inferior pedicle technique reached preoperative values between 6 and 12 months postoperatively. Patients of the Georgiade group with resections higher than 700 g even showed a slight improvement of the sensitivity of the inferior and lateral rim of the areola at 12 months. Patients operated with a superior pedicle technique had a significantly reduced sensitivity of the inferior and lateral part of the areola at 3 weeks, 3, 6, and 12 months postoperatively ($p < 0.05$). A complete loss of sensitivity of the areola was also found only in the Lassus and Lejour groups. These were all temporary and resolved between 3 and 6 months postoperatively.

The sensitivity of the breast skin (Fig. 79.3) was unchanged or slightly improved after breast reduction by the Georgiade, Würinger, McKissock, and Lassus techniques. At 3 weeks postoperatively, the sensitivity of the inferiolateral and inferiomedial quadrants was significantly reduced after a reduction mammaplasty by the Lejour technique ($p < 0.05$). However, this resolved between 6 and 12 months postoperatively. At 12 months postoperatively, the sensitivity of the upper medial and upper lateral quadrant of the breast of the patients of the Lejour group was slightly improved compared with the preoperative values, but the changes were not statistically significant.

The superimposition of the most common nerve pathways on the plane of tissue resection helps to explain the differences in postoperative sensitivity. The superior pedicle reduction techniques (Lassus, Lejour)

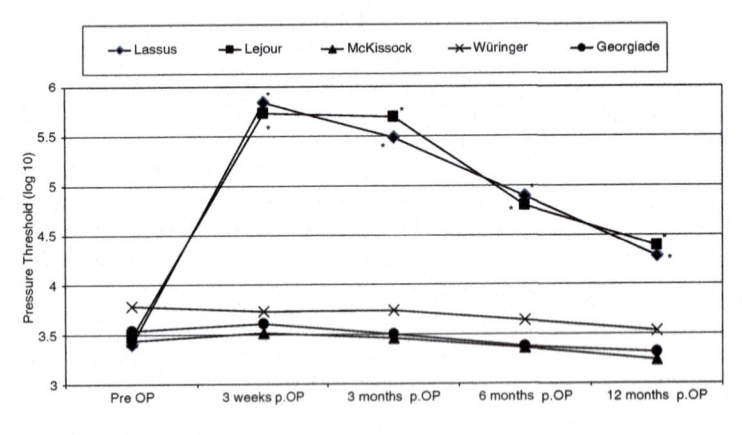

Fig. 79.1 Alteration of nipple sensitivity. $^*p < 0.001$

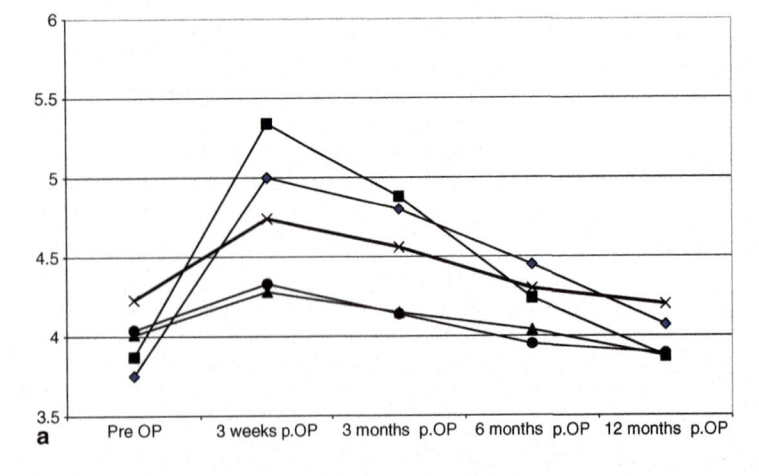

Fig. 79.2 Alteration of the sensitivity of the areola. $^*p < 0.05$

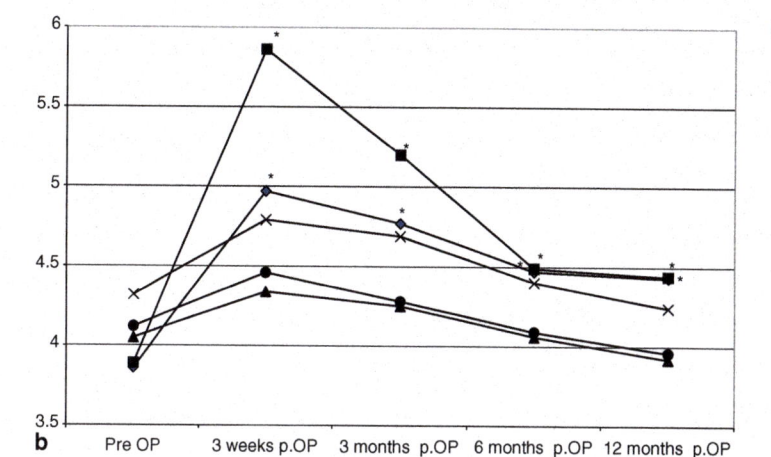

Fig. 79.2 (continued)

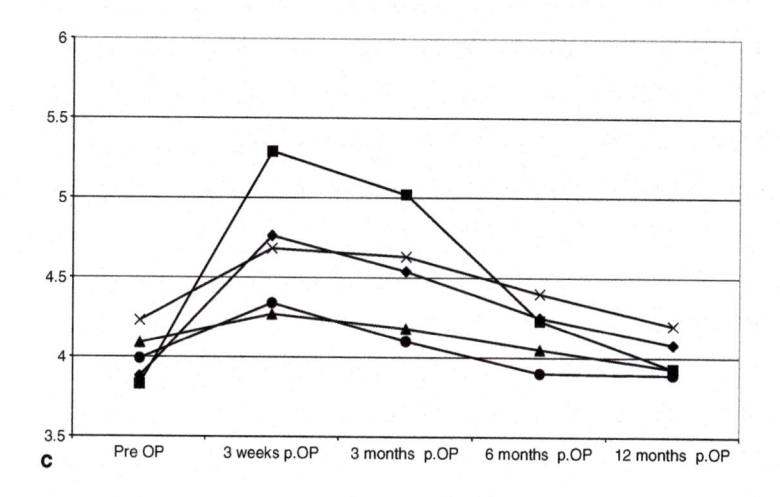

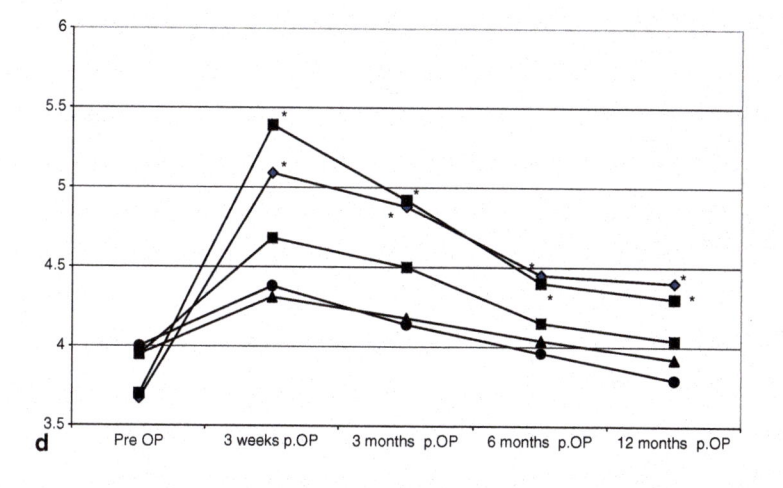

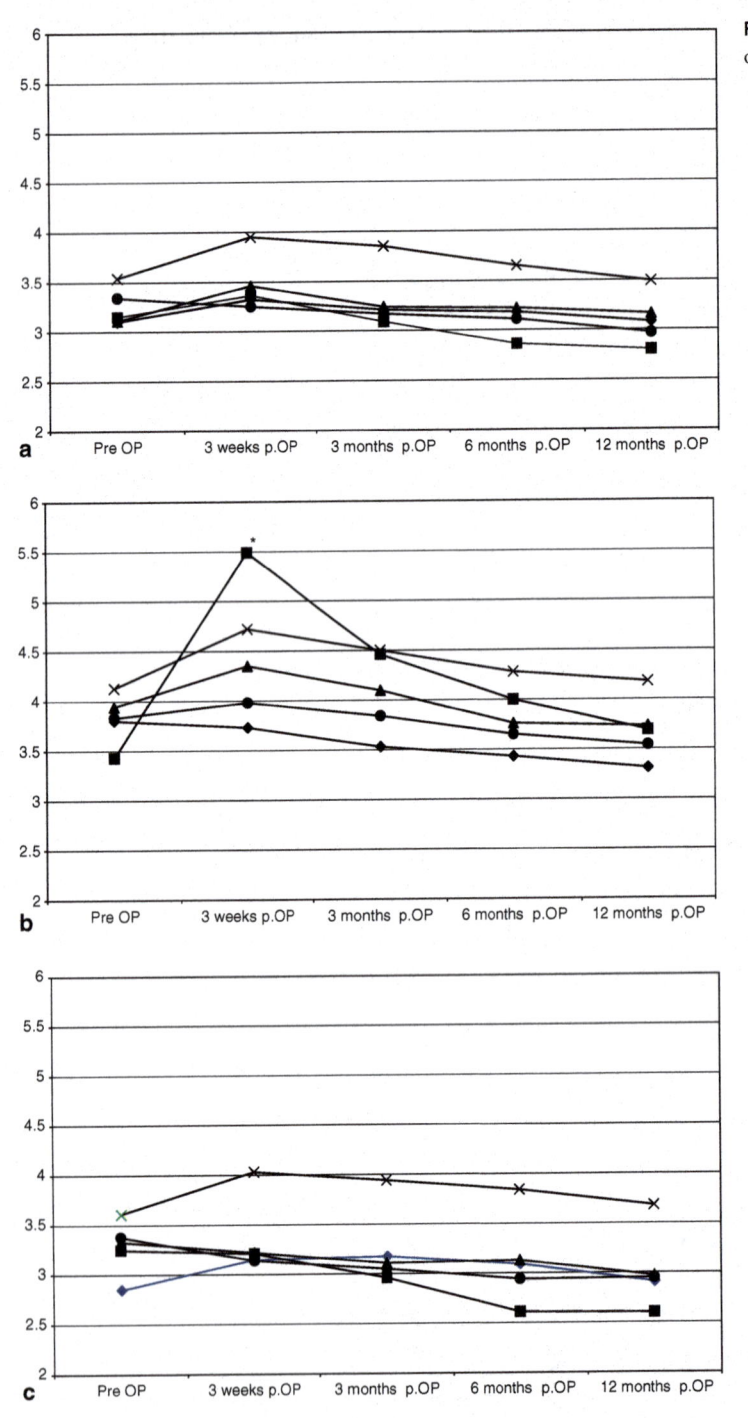

Fig. 79.3 Alteration of the sensitivity of the breast skin. $^*p < 0.05$

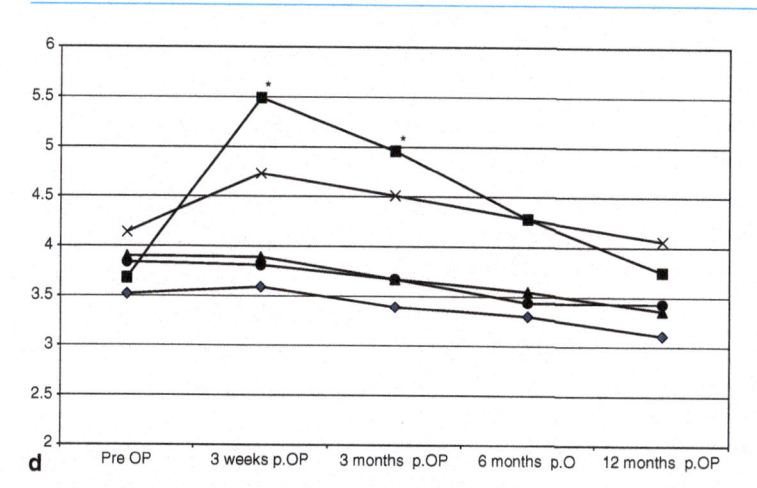

Fig. 79.3 (continued)

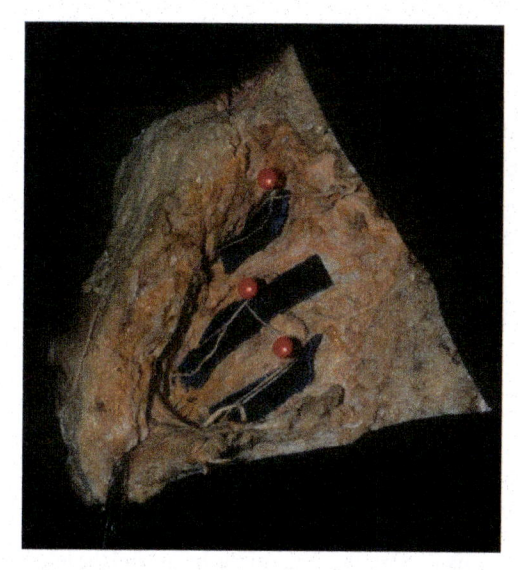

Fig. 79.4 Anterior view of a left breast (*Arrows*: third and fourth anterior cutaneous branch terminating at the medial border of the areola)

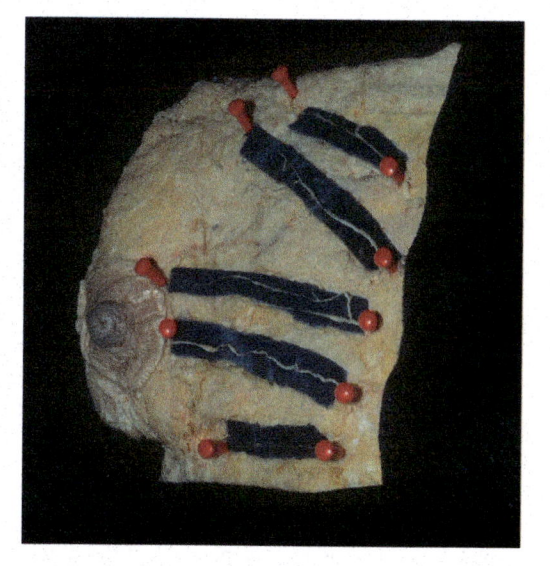

Fig. 79.5 Lateral view of a left breast (*Double Arrow*: Lateral cutaneous branch of the fourth intercostal nerve reaching the posterior surface of the nipple; *Arrow*: Cutaneous branch of the lateral cutaneous branch terminating in the skin of the lower lateral quadrant)

that require tissue resections at the base of the breast are associated with a significantly higher risk of injury to the nerves supplying the nipple–areola complex than the inferior (McKissock, Georgiade) or inferocentral (Würinger) pedicle techniques. Even 1 year after surgery, 69.5% of the patients operated with a superior pedicle technique did not regain the preoperative sensitivity of their nipple and areola and 13% had insensate nipples.

The nipple–areola complex is innervated by the lateral and anterior cutaneous branches of the third, fourth, and fifth intercostal nerves as shown in an earlier study [23]. The anterior cutaneous branches take a superficial course within the subcutaneous tissue and terminate at the medial areola border (Fig. 79.4) – some of their terminal branches are injured when the size of the areola is reduced and probably account for the postoperatively diminished sensitivity of the medial and superior part of the areola (Fig. 79.2). The lateral cutaneous branches take a deep course within the pectoral fascia and reach the nipple from its posterior surface in 93% of the patients (Fig. 79.5). These nerves are easily injured when the tissue is resected in this area as done by the superior

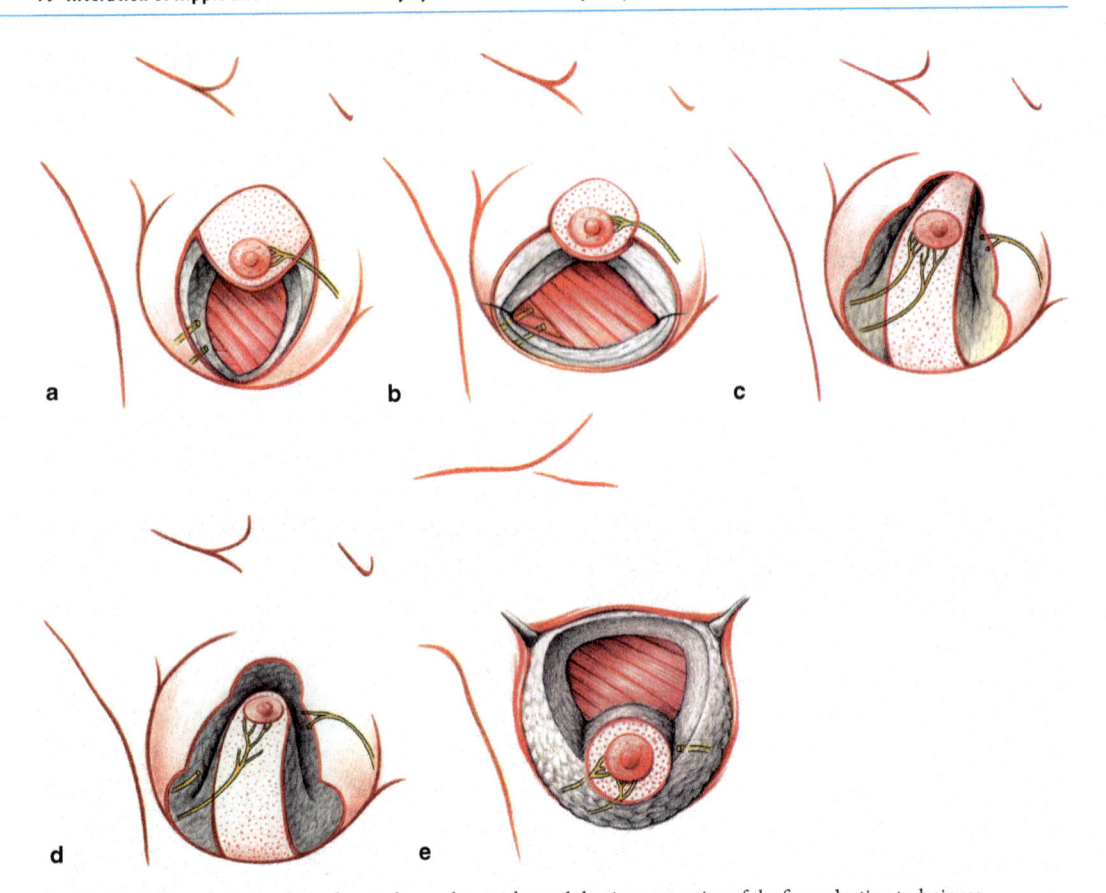

Fig. 79.6 (a–e) The nerves supplying the nipple–areola complex and the tissue resection of the five reduction techniques

pedicle techniques (Fig. 79.6a, b). Injury of the lateral nerves, which are the dominant nerves for the innervation of the nipple and the lateral and inferior part of the areola, results in an insensate nipple and loss of sensitivity of the inferior and lateral part of the areola (Figs. 79.1 and 79.2). Improvement of the sensitivity of the nipple and areola after 6 months is either due to the recovery of the medial nerves from neuropraxia or due to the nerve regeneration of the lateral nerves [11,20,24].

Breast reduction by an inferior pedicle technique such as the McKissock or Georgiade techniques results in an injury to the medial nerves, while the dominant lateral nerves are well protected along their course within the pectoral fascia. They leave the thoracic wall at the height of the pedicle and are not endangered by the resection (Fig. 79.6c, d). Thus, the sensitivity of the nipple and the lateral and the inferior part of the areola of the patients operated by an inferior pedicle technique remains unchanged.

The resection of the cranial part of the breast as done by the Würinger technique also does not endanger the lateral nerves (Fig. 79.6e). Thus, sensitivity of the nipple is unchanged after this operation (Fig. 79.1).

79.1 Discussion

For many years, the shape of the breast and the length of the scars were the major topics of papers on breast reduction. Now that several reduction techniques that offer a long lasting aesthetic result with few complications have evolved, the preservation of nipple sensitivity has shifted into the center of interest. Several papers with contradictory results have been published on postoperative nipple and breast skin sensitivity to pressure, static, and moving two point discrimination, temperature, and vibration [1–5,11,15,16,20–22]. However, it is still unclear whether changes in the sensitivity of the nipple–areola complex are related to the resection weight or the surgical technique. Furthermore, none of the studies has ever evaluated how the sensory changes of the nipple and areola complex affect the patients and which type of changes the patients really mind.

In the present study, we analyzed the influence of reduction weight and surgical technique on the postoperative sensory outcome of the nipple and areola complex, and for the first time documented how patients were affected by these changes [8].

The nipple is subjectively and objectively the most sensitive part of the breast and important for women's sexual life [2,3,12,13,21]. Loss of sensitivity and erectile function can be dramatic for some women, while others do not complain about it. We found that in the first 6 months after the reduction mammaplasty, none of the patients minded a decrease or loss of sensitivity of the nipple. Satisfaction with the new size and shape of the breast and relief from preoperative symptoms such as neck and shoulder pain are overwhelming in this period [16]. Between the 6th and the 12th postoperative month, women tend to forget their preoperative symptoms and start focusing on sensitivity changes of the nipple. Fifty percent of the patients with reduced sensitivity of the nipple and 75% of the patients with complete loss of sensitivity and erectile function of the nipple started being bothered after 6 months [8]. Any decrease or loss of sensitivity to light touch was accompanied by a decrease or loss of erectile function in our patients [8]. These are the sensory changes that matter to a woman. Changes in the sensitivity of the nipple to vibration, temperature, and one or two point moving pressure perception may also occur, but are of minor importance for a woman.

Greuse et al. [15] and Hamdi et al. [4] also found a reduced nipple sensitivity in 52% of their patients 6 months after breast reduction using the Lejour technique. Hamdi et al. [4] also reported that 40% of the patients operated with an inferior pedicle technique showed reduced nipple sensitivity. We compared two different inferior pedicle and one inferocentral pedicle technique and found no insensate nipple or diminished sensitivity of the nipple in any of our patients. In contrast, half of our patients operated with an inferior pedicle technique showed slight improvement of their nipple sensitivity as early as 3 weeks after surgery. This is in keeping with the results of Slezak and Dellon [2] (Mc Kissock), Mofid et al. [5] (Robbin), Harbo et al. [16] (Robbin), and Wechselberger et al. [22] (Robbin), who found unchanged or even improved sensitivity of the nipple after an inferior pedicle reduction mammaplasty.

In the past, high resection weights have been associated with a diminished nipple sensitivity. Thus Gonzales et al. [3], Slezak and Dellon [2], Craig and Sykes [20], and Mitrofanoff et al. [25] have reported a higher risk of nerve injury in patients with gigantomastia, but did not either differentiate between the used techniques [3] or examine very few patients [2,20]. Greuse et al. [15] and Wechselberger et al. [22] assessed their patients in two groups depending on the amount of tissue resection and found no difference in nipple sensitivity after reductions of less or more than 500 g per breast. We compared five different reduction techniques and found that a loss or diminished nipple sensitivity was not associated with reduction weight. On the contrary, the superior pedicle techniques, which were used for smaller resections, were the only ones that resulted in a loss or diminished postoperative sensitivity of the nipple [8]. Therefore, the surgical technique is more important for the postoperative sensory outcome than the resection weight.

79.2
Conclusion

Changes of nipple and areola sensitivity after reduction mammaplasty do not depend on the weight of resection but on the surgical technique [8]. The superior glandular pedicle techniques with tissue resections at the base of the breast are associated with a higher risk of injury to the nerves supplying the nipple–areola complex. Although sensitivity starts improving between 3 and 6 months after surgery, it does not recover fully in 69.5% of the patients even 12 months after the operation [8]. Although relief from physical symptoms is the major goal of patients undergoing reduction mammaplasty, sensitivity of the nipple–areola complex is very important for the majority of the patients. They are very much aware of any sensory changes and complain of loss of sensitivity to light touch and erectile function. Therefore, the importance of nipple sensitivity to the individual patient should be taken into account when choosing a reduction technique.

References

1. Serletti JM, Reading G, Caldwell E, Wray RC: Long-term patient satisfaction following reduction mammoplasty. Ann Plast Surg 1992;28:363
2. Slezak S, Dellon AL: Quantitation of sensibility in gigantomastia and alteration following reduction mammaplasty. Plast Reconstr Surg 1993;92:809
3. Gonzalez F, Brown FE, Gold WE, et al.: Preoperative and postoperative nipple-areola sensibility in patients undergoing reduction mammaplasty. Plast Reconstr Surg 1993;91:1265
4. Hamdi M, Greuse M, DeMey A, Webster MHC: A prospective quantitative comparison of breast sensation after superior and inferior pedicle mammaplasty. Br J Plast Surg 2001;54:39
5. Mofid MM, Dellon AL, Elias JJ, et al.: Quantitation of breast sensibility following reduction mammaplasty: A comparison of inferior and medial pedicle techniques. Plast Reconstr Surg 2002;109:2283
6. Nahabedian MY, Mofid MM: Viability and sensation of the nipple-areola complex after reduction mammaplasty. Ann Plast Surg 2000;49:24

7. Ahmed OA, Kohle PS: Comparison of nipple and areola sensation after breast reduction by free nipple graft and inferior pedicle techniques. Br J Plast Surg 2001;53:126
8. Schlenz I, Rigel S, Schemper M, Kuzbari R: Alteration of nipple and areola sensitivity by reduction mammaplasty: a prospective comparison of five different techniques. Plast Reconstr Surg 2005;115:743
9. Sandsmark M, Amland PF, Abyholm F, et al.: Reduction mammaplasty: a comparative study of the Orlando and Robbins methods in 292 patients. Scand J Reconstr Hand Surg 1993;91:1265
10. Kuzbari R, Schlenz I: Reduction mammaplasty and sensitivity of the nipple–areola complex: sensuality versus sexuality? Ann Plast Surg 2007;58(1):3
11. Courtiss EH, Goldwyn RM: Breast sensation before and after plastic surgery. Plast Reconstr Surg 1976;58:1
12. Jäger K, Schneider B: Die Innervation und Durchblutung der Mamille im Hinblick auf die Perimamilläre Incision. Chirurg 1982;53:525
13. Terzis JK, Vincent MP, Wilikins LM, et al.: Brest sensibility: a neurophysiological appraisal in the normal breast. Ann Plast Surg 1987;19:318
14. Tairych GV, Kuzbari R, Rigel S, et al.: Normal cutaneous sensibility of the breast. Plast Reconstr Surg 1998;102:701
15. Greuse M, Hamdi M, DeMey A: Breast sensitivity after vertical mammaplasty. Plast Reconstr Surg 2001;107:970
16. Harbo SO, Jorum E, Roald HE: Reduction mammaplasty: a prospective study of symptom relieve and alteration of skin sensibility. Plast Reconstr Surg 2003;111:103
17. Ferreira MC, Cost MP, Cunha MS, et al.: Sensibility of the breast after reduction mammaplasty. Ann Plast Surg 2003;51:1
18. Godwin Y, Valassiadou K, Lweis S, et al.: Investigation into the possible cause of subjective decreased sensory perception the nipple–areola complex of women with macromastia. Plast Reconstr Surg 2004;113:1598
19. DelVecchyo C, Caloca J Jr, Calca J, et al.: Evaluation of breast sensibilità using dermatomal somatosensory evoked potentials. Reconstr Surg 2004;113:1975
20. Craig RD, Sykes PA: Nipple sensitivity following reduction mammaplasty. Br J Plast Surg 1970;23:165
21. Temple CL, Hurst LN: Reduction mammaplasty improves breast sensibility. Plast Reconstr Surg 1999;104:72
22. Wechselberger G, Stoß S, Schoeller T, et al.: An analysis of breast sensation following inferior pedicle mammaplasty and the effect of the volume of the resected tissue. Aesth Plast Surg 2001;25:443
23. Schlenz I, Kuzbari R, Gruber H, Holle J: The sensitivity of the nipple-areola complex: an anatomical study. Plast Reconstr Surg 2000;105:905
24. Slezak S, McGibbon B, Dellon AL: The sensational transverse rectus abdominis musculocutaneous (TRAM) flap: return of sensibility after TRAM breast reconstruction. Ann Plast Surg 1992;28:210
25. Mitrofanoff M, Dallassera M, Bourkis T, Baruch J: Clinical study of breast sensitivity before and after reduction mammaplasty. An Chir Plast Esthet 1997;42:314

Prevention of the Inverted Teardrop Areola Following Mammaplasty

Geoffrey G. Hallock, John A. Altobelli

80.1 Introduction

Although the major objective of mammaplasty is to produce a breast mound of the desired size, position, and projection, oftentimes minor nuances can make the difference between just a good clinical result and a superior aesthetic outcome acceptable to the patient. Since the nipple–areola complex usually becomes the focal point when evaluating the operated breast, its location, size, sustained viability, scar visibility, and geometry become extremely important secondary characteristics when seeking the excellent result. In this regard, we have been asked to update our modification of just one such simple technique to minimize the risk of creating an iatrogenic inverted teardrop areolar deformity [1].

The inverted teardrop or comma-shaped areola is a documented sequela of breast reduction following horizontal or vertical bipedicled nipple-bearing flaps [2] or a single inferior pedicle technique, as we still most commonly utilize (Fig. 80.1) [3]. This can also occur after a vertical mastopexy, without reduction (Fig. 80.2) [4]. This deformity occurs at the junction of the vertical line of the breast closure with the areola. Many theories have been advanced to explain its pathogenesis. Some believe that it is inevitable with a circular areolar design to have such distortion, and so an oval shape with a larger horizontal axis is intentionally made from the outset [5]. Scalloping the edges of the areola and the corresponding recipient keyhole intentionally by distorting the entire perimeter of the areola so as to make it more subtly blend-in with the surrounding paler breast skin will hide any such malformation, yet the entire result can be so distorted [6]. A tight closure of the breast envelope below the nipple, whether due to excessive medial or lateral skin or breast tissue excision, will pull in the direction of that excessive resection, also pulling the areola with it [2]. A most plausible explanation is that the tightness of the vertical scar alone due to contraction pulls the areola down with it, which is simply prevented by minimizing tension by the usual subcuticular running closure at least in the superior portion of the vertical limb closure [4]. Whatever the actual cause of the inverted teardrop shape of the areola, we have found that our technique of insetting the nipple–areolar complex has permitted us to avoid this deformity in all the cases which we have performed over the past 20 years since our introduction of this idea [1].

80.2 Technique

The preoperative design and operative steps, whether for inferior pedicled breast reduction [7] or mastopexy [8] as we commonly use, do not differ from that described better by others. Location of the nipple usually will be at the point of greatest projection of the newly transformed breast mound, on a vertical line coinciding with that of the vertical closure of the breast flaps beneath it. Rather than creating a circular areola as we and others used to do, we can't design on the recipient platform that will be deepithelialized, centered at the nipple, on an axis slightly oblique, so that the superior pole points closer to the chest midline. We agree that this will provide a more natural appearance [6].

The areola is then retrieved as usual, and inset with single simple sutures at all quadrants except at the inferior or 6 o'clock margin. If this was done as we did previously, obvious vertically oriented deforming forces will occur, which we believe predisposes to the inverted teardrop deformity (Fig. 80.3). Instead, the dermis is split here under the areola for about a centimeter (Fig. 80.4), which should not by itself compromise vascularity, while immediately demonstrating the desired oval shape of the areola (Fig. 80.5). In our original description [1], the deeper dermis left behind at the 6 o'clock area was sutured to the dermis of the lower breast flaps at their superior juncture, which is still done by the senior author. An alternative is to altogether avoid any connection with the vertical line of the flap closure,

M.A. Shiffman (ed.), *Mastopexy and Breast Reduction: Principles and Practice,*
© Springer-Verlag Berlin Heidelberg 2009

622 80 Prevention of the Inverted Teardrop Areola Following Mammaplasty

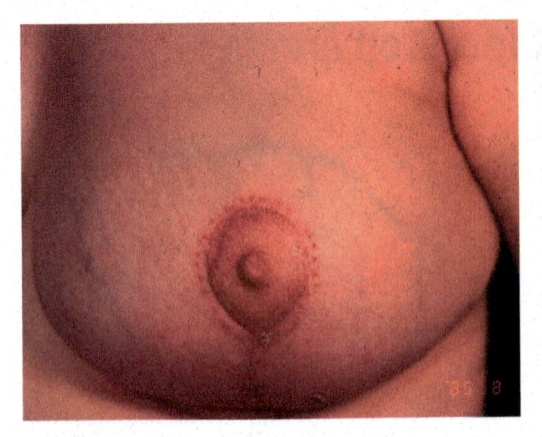

Fig. 80.1 Inverted teardrop deformity where the inferior half of the areola has been stretched downward, following inferior pedicled breast reduction

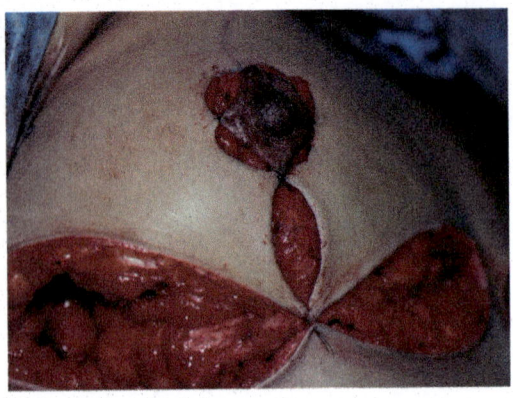

Fig. 80.3 Preliminary tacking of the areola at all quadrants of the keyhole window following inferior pedicled breast reduction results in obvious vertical deforming forces

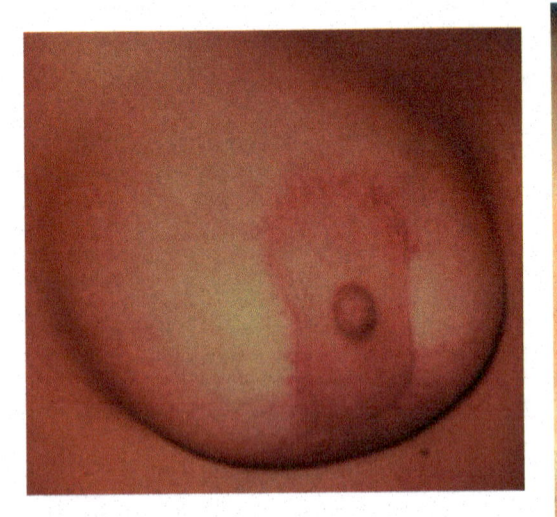

Fig. 80.2 Exaggerated stretching of the areola following mastopexy (Figure donated by Shiffman MA)

placing instead a skin suture at the 5 o'clock and 7 o'clock points on the areola followed by subcuticular closure of the rest of its perimeter (Fig. 80.6). An inferior gap is intentionally left open to close by itself, with minimal risk that the areola itself will be pulled down by the vertical scar of the breast when they both heal, as they are not directly connected (Fig. 80.6).

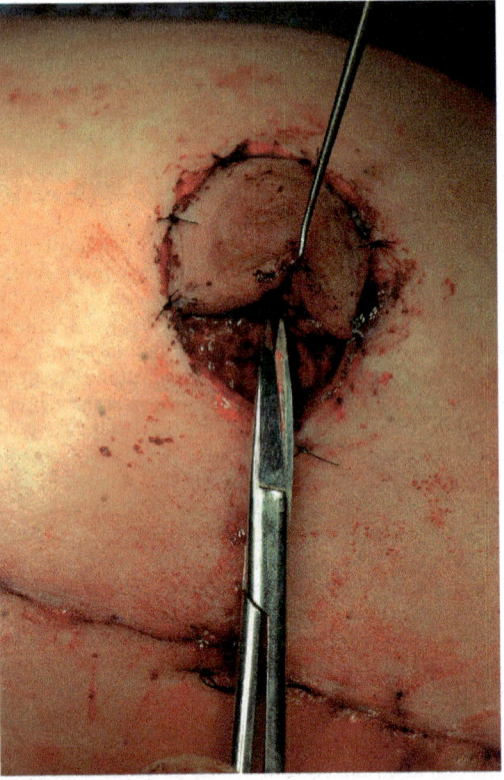

Fig. 80.4 The inferior centimeter of the areola is released by splitting the underlying dermis

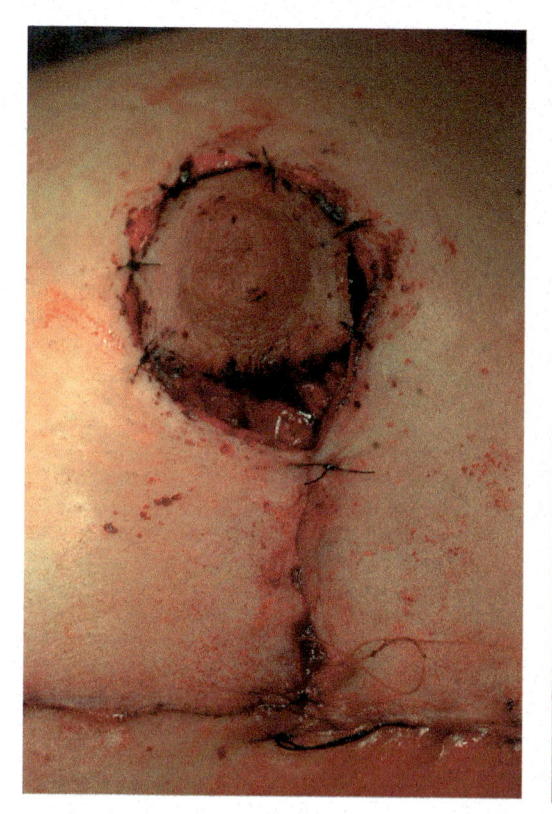

Fig. 80.5 The desired oval appearance of the areola is immediately assumed

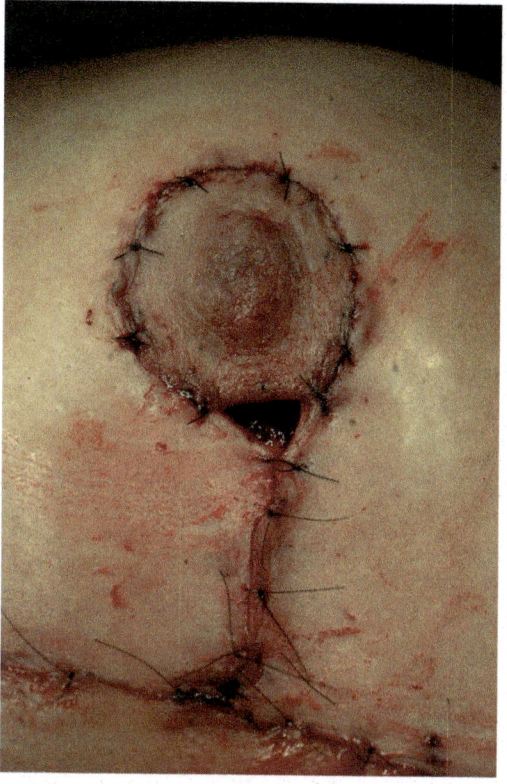

Fig. 80.6 Sentinel sutures are placed at the 5 o'clock and 7 o'clock margins, and the rest of the perimeter of the areola is closed with a subcuticular non-cinching suture, leaving a gap open below

80.3 Discussion

A youthful breast lift or sheer reduction of volume following breast reduction is often enough to satisfy most women. Sometimes the demand for greater perfection is more of a burden for the surgeons themselves. Even a minimal geometrical defect of the areola such as the inverted teardrop deformity can be a distraction (Figs. 80.1 and 80.2). Our technique [1] that has evolved over the past two decades is one solution. We have postulated that it is the downward distracting forces of the vertical scar under the areola that is the culprit. Redistributing this vector so that there is no direct connection to the areola itself by splitting the dermis has consistently prevented this problem (Figs. 80.7 and 80.8). It is a simple maneuver that adds almost nothing to the overall operative time, and should not jeopardize vascularity to the robust nipple–areola complex. If there are such concerns, our adjunct should be avoided, and perhaps other risk factors corrected.

80.4 Conclusions

Maximizing the result of any mammaplasty can require mastering even the most minor of minutia. Prevention of areolar deformity, and particularly the inverted teardrop areola, can be systematically avoided following the simple areolar dermal splitting maneuver that we have consistently found useful over the past few decades. There really are no complications associated with the judicious application of this useful adjunct, as long as the vascularity of the nipple–areolar complex is satisfactory.

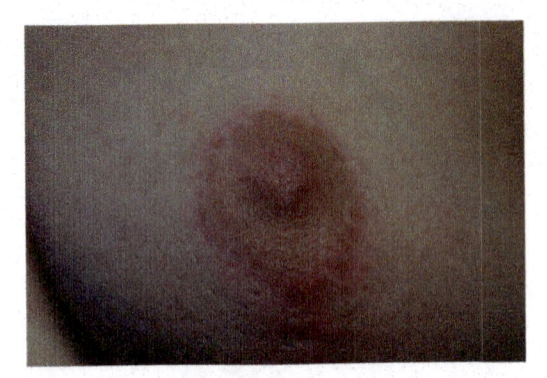

Fig. 80.7 The final result without inverted teardrop deformity 4 months later

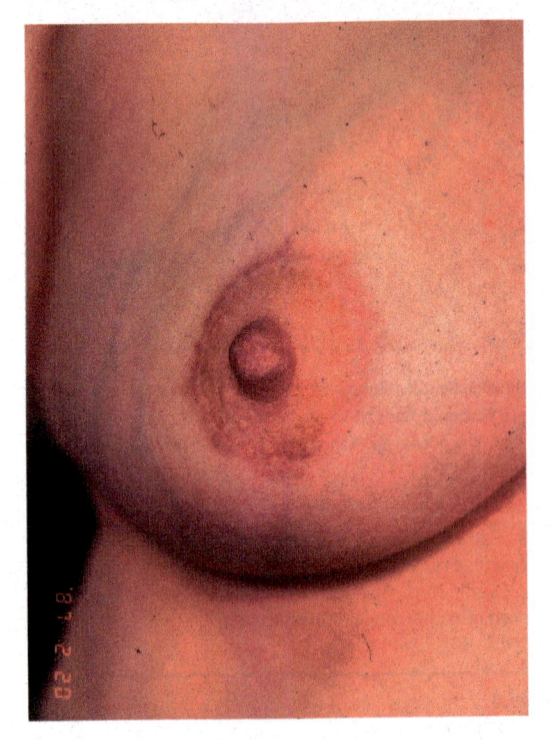

Fig. 80.8 Circular areolar maintained, after inferior pedicled breast reduction performed 20 years ago with our adjunctive technique

References

1. Courtiss EH, Goldwyn RM: Reduction mammaplasty by the inferior pedicle technique. Plast Reconstr Surg 1977;59:500–507
2. Labandter HP, Dowden RV, Dinner MI: The inferior segment technique for breast reduction. Ann Plast Surg 1982;8:493–503
3. Crepeau R, Klein HW: Reduction mammaplasty with inferiorly based glandular pedicle flap. Ann Plast Surg 1982;8:463–470
4. McKissock PK: Complications and undesirable results with reduction mammaplasty. In: Goldwyn RM (ed). The Unfavorable Result in Plastic Surgery, 2nd edn. Little, Brown, Boston 1984, pp 751–752
5. Hallock GG, Altobelli JA: Prevention of the teardrop areola following the inferior pedicle technique of breast reduction. Plast Reconstr Surg 1988;82:531–534
6. Pandya AN, Arnstein PM: Refinement of nipple areolar placement in breast surgery. Plast Reconstr Surg 1998;101:806–807
7. Lejour M: Vertical mammaplasty: update and appraisal of late results. Plast Reconstr Surg 1999;104:771–781
8. Wallach SG: Avoiding the teardrop-shaped nipple–areola complex in vertical mammaplasty. Plast Reconstr Surg 2000;106:1217–1218

Prevention of Teardrop Areola and Increasing Areola Projection in Inferior Pedicle Reduction Mammoplasty

Meltem Ayhan, Metin Görgü, Bulent Erdoğan, Zeynep Sevým

81.1 Introduction

When the inferior pedicle technique is used, a deformity sometimes occurs at the junction of the areola with the vertical line of breast closure with medial and lateral flaps. There have been multiple hypotheses to explain the pathogenesis of the distortion [1–3]. If the areola window is not circular on being closed, the deformity is bound to occur. To prevent this, Labandter et al. (1982) [1] designed a keyhole pattern with an oval window, with the major axis lying horizontal. If the vertical midline closure is skewed away from the midpoint to the right or left side beneath the areola, comma deformity will occur (Fig. 81.1) [2]. A too tight vertical closure, usually caused by excessive lateral flap excision, will result in areola tethering [3]. If the breast tissue is over resected, the central inferior-based pedicle may move to the lateral side (Fig. 81.2) owing to excessive skin envelope. These deformities are aesthetically undesirable.

81.2 Technique

With the patient standing upright, the midsternal and midclavicular lines are marked passing over the nipple. The base of the inferior dermal pedicle is marked 0.5 cm over the actual inframammary sulcus. The new nipple position is marked 18–21 cm from the midsternal line and the areola is marked with a diameter of 4.5–5.0 cm. The inferior pedicle is marked with a width of 6–9 cm and 1 cm above the new areola. After deepithelialization, breast tissue is excised at the lateral and medial parts. One centimeter from the circular margin of the keyhole pattern is left denuded and the rest of the keyhole is excised (Fig. 81.3). The margin of the keyhole that is left denuded is incised to the subcutaneous tissue at the 9, 12, and 3 o'clock positions (Fig. 81.4). The medial and lateral components are sutured and the superior part of the areola is sutured subcutaneously to the incised part of the margin at the 12 o'clock position. Subcutaneous sutures are placed at the 3 o'clock and 9 o'clock positions. The dermis of the inferior pedicle is incised 0.5 cm horizontally to move the inferior areola slightly away from the pedicle (Fig. 81.5). Sutures are placed under the split at the 6 o'clock level and the areola skin is closed.

Twelve patients had this procedure to implement the inferior pedicle technique and all had projected, circular, and properly positioned nipple–areola complexes (Fig. 81.6).

81.3 Discussion

Those patients who had teardrop-shaped areola after inferior pedicle reduction mammaplasty were evaluated by the authors for the causes. These patients had large breasts and lateral and medial components were 6 cm long. Following suturing the lateral and medial elements without tension to prevent necrosis at the junction of the inverted T, there was retraction at the junction of the inferior pedicle with the areola. This deformity also occurred when the vertical closure line was skewed to the right or left side. Even when all measures were taken to prevent it, the deformity occurred. Using the incision to move the inferior part of the areola away from the pedicle [4] did not prevent the deformity in all cases. In the cases where a circular areola was obtained, it was not projected enough. The authors proceeded to denude the inner 1 cm of the keyhole, creating an area where the areola could expand taking into account the following factors:

1. In large breasts, the lateral and medial flap length was not very short, 4.5–5.0 cm. When the flaps were shortened to prevent high-riding deformity, excessive excision at the lateral side was necessary for easy closure and prevention of necrosis at the inverse T junction, which in turn caused the midline to skew to the medial

M.A. Shiffman (ed.), *Mastopexy and Breast Reduction: Principles and Practice*,
© Springer-Verlag Berlin Heidelberg 2009

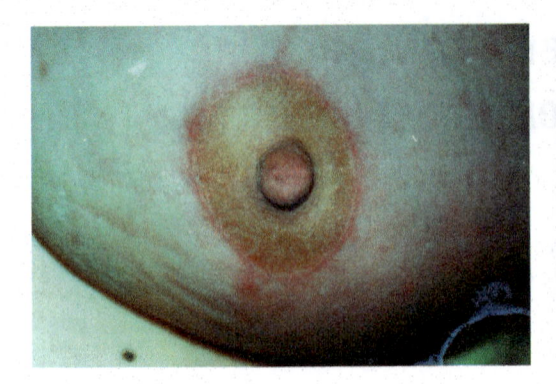

626 81 Prevention of Teardrop Areola and Increasing Areola Projection in Inferior Pedicle Reduction Mammoplasty

Fig. 81.1 Comma deformity of the nipple areola complex

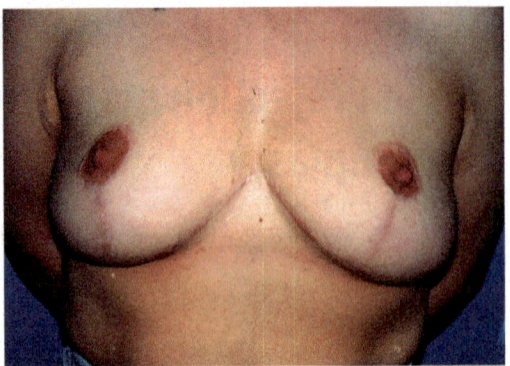

Fig. 81.2 The areola is displaced and oval

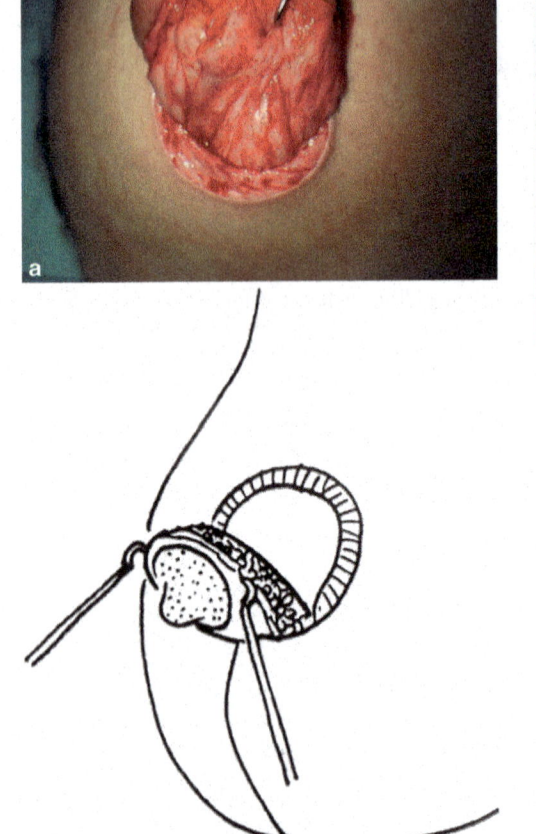

Fig. 81.3 1 cm inner edge of the keyhole is left denuded

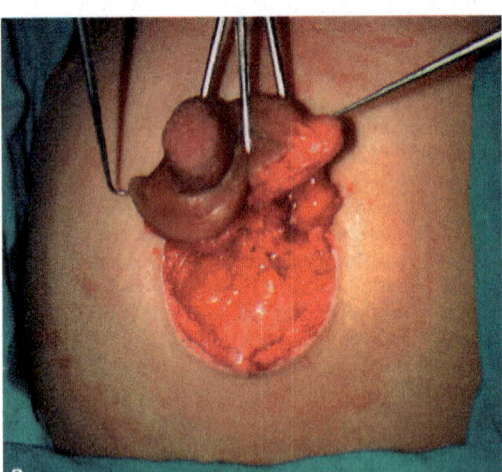

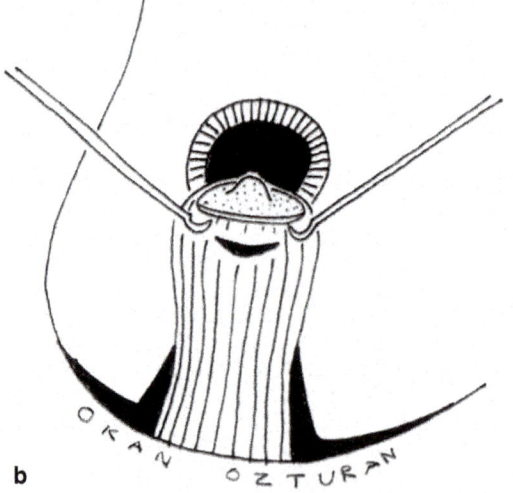

Fig. 81.4 (a) Inferior pedicle. (b) Inferior pedicle incised

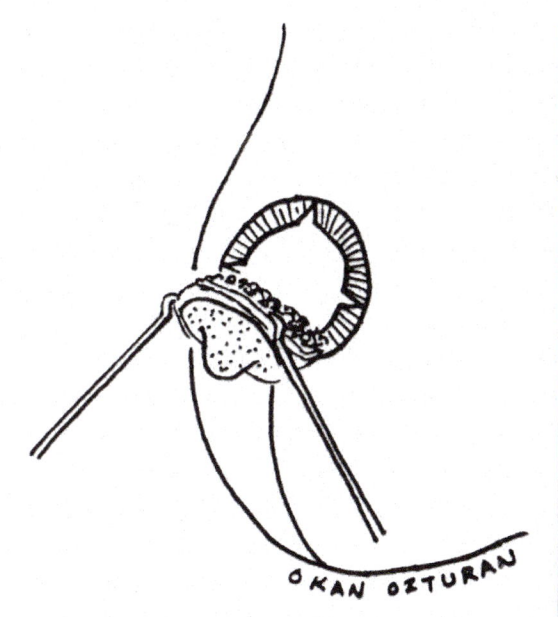

Fig. 81.5 The denuded 1 cm inner edge is incised into the subcutaneous tissues at the 9, 12, and 3 o'clock positions

side with contracture at the leg of the T and caused the areola to be misshapen following healing.
2. A circular areola was obtained in all cases by denuding 1 cm of the keyhole, producing an area where the areola could expand, and by incising dermis inferior to the areola to prevent the pedicle from retracting the areola.

81.4 Conclusions

The technique described results in uniform circular areolas and better projection of the nipple–areola complex over the long term.

Acknowledgment

We thank Okan Özturan for his original drawings.

References

1. Labandter HP, Dowden RV, Dinner MI: The inferior segment technique for breast reduction. Ann Plast Surg 1982;8(6):493–503
2. McKissock PK: Reduction mammaplasty. In: Courtiss EH (ed). Aesthetic Surgery, St. Louis, Mosby 1978, pp 197–198
3. McKissock PK: Complications and undesirable results with reduction mammaplasty. In: Goldwyn RM (ed). The Unfavorable Result in Plastic Surgery, 2nd edn. Boston, Little, Brown and Co. 1984, pp 751–752
4. Hallock G, Altobelli JA: Prevention of the teardrop areola following the inferior pedicle technique of breast reduction. Plast Reconstr Surg 1988;82(3):531–534

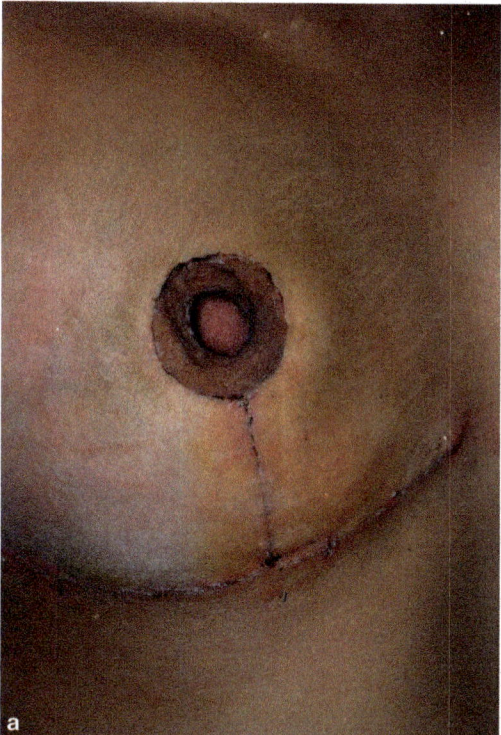

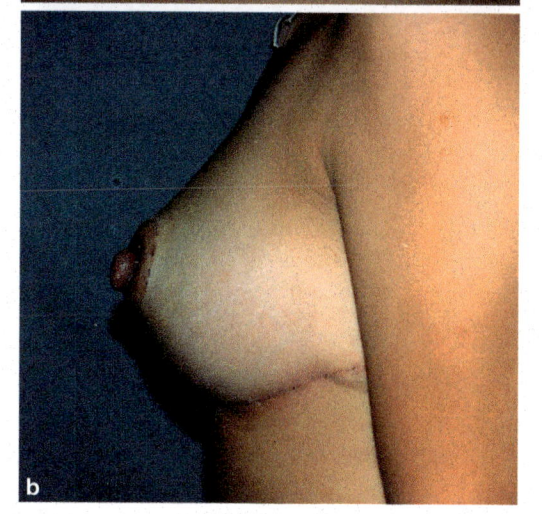

Fig. 81.6 (a) Postoperative anterior view with author's technique (b) Postoperative lateral view with author's technique

Correction of the High-Riding Nipple After Breast Reduction

Greg Chernoff

82.1 Introduction

Reduction mammaplasty and mastopexy are common procedures that typify the congruity between reconstruction and aesthetic concepts. When properly planned and executed, these procedures provide patients with viable options for changing the size or the shape of the breast. Lifting the breast and raising the nipple–areola complex also provide for a more youthful appearance. Improper planning or execution can result in several problems. One of the most devastating problems is placement of the nipples in an unnaturally high position. For the patient, this is difficult, and in some cases, impossible to camouflage. This leads to unhappiness and a loss of confidence in the doctor. Few reports in the literature offer the physician options for reconstruction of this challenging problem [1–6].

82.2 History

As problematic as this can be for the patient, it is surprising how little has been written on the subject. Strombeck [5] warned that a high nipple is almost impossible to correct at a later time. The defect may be unilateral or bilateral. It can be evident immediately postoperatively, or several months afterwards, due to the gravitational effects on the breast tissue, leaving the relatively fixed nipples at a higher location. Most of the publications concerning breast reduction deal with flap and pedicle types.

82.3 Discussion

High-riding nipples following breast reduction or mastopexy remain a problem with few surgical solutions. The cause of nipple elevation and the degree of severity affect the management. To add clarity to the therapeutic decision, Colwell and May [6] categorized the problem. Grade 1 elevation or "pseudo elevation" is defined as inferior pole decent or "bottoming out," although the nipple remains in a relatively fixed position. Treatment of Grade 1 nipple elevation involves lower pole remodeling. Grade 2 nipple elevation is defined as mild superior displacement, with or without inferior pole descent. Treatment of Grade 2 elevation involves a variety of techniques, including skin excision, scar revision, and inferior pole remodeling. Grade 3 elevation is classified as severe elevation, not improved by skin excision and inferior pole remodeling. Severity of nipple elevation can be assessed by skin manipulation in the lower pole of the breast or tacking skin along the inframammary fold to determine if this yields the desired shift in nipple position.

A recent report [6] utilizes infraclavicular tissue expansion to increase skin at the superior pole and lower the nipple position. This inclusion of skin to the upper pole of the breast results in an increase in the absolute notch-to-nipple distance. This technique results in lowering the nipple position by 2–6 cm. Expanders are placed in the infraclavicular region through periareolar incisions or old scars, avoiding any new scars being placed on the breast. Crescent-shaped or round expanders are used. This position optimally recruits superior skin without thinning breast tissue or creating irregularities occurring due to submammary expansion. Expander dimension is matched with the base breast diameter in width. Superior placement has not met with significant skin recoil subsequent to expander removal.

Elsahy [1] described an inferior pole triangular resection for types 1 and 2, which can lower the nipple between 90 and 110°. This technique involves creating a triangular resection around the old vertical scar, with the apex at the lower end of the areola. If more skin needs resecting, the triangle is made wider. An ellipse is then made around the horizontal scar. The width of this excision will determine the degree to which the nipple is lowered. If the nipple requires additional lowering, the horizontal lines of the ellipse are drawn further apart, bearing in mind that the upper line of the ellipse is approximately 5 cm from the lower end of the areola. Excising the skin inside the aforementioned triangle and ellipse will lower the nipple, get rid of the scar, and tighten the skin around the breast.

82.4
Conclusions

The high-riding nipple post breast reduction or mastopexy is a difficult problem. The stress to the patient is significant. The stress to the surgeon who takes pride in his work is no less. The surgical solutions while viable cause the patient with significant healing time. This problem underscores the necessity and benefit of proper planning, execution, and as always, doing it "right" the first time.

References

1. Elsahy NI: Correction of abnormally high nipples after reduction mammaplasty. Aesthetic Plast Surg 1990;14(1): 21–26
2. Millard DR Jr, Mullin WR, Lesavoy MA: Secondary correction of the too high areola and nipple after a mammaplasty. Plast Reconstr Surg 1976;58(5):568–572
3. Radovan C: Tissue expansion in soft-tissue reconstruction. Plast Reconstr Surg 1984;74(4):482–492
4. Raffel B: Technique for correction of areola misplacement with no new scars. Plast Reconstr Surg 1991;88(5): 895–897
5. Strombeck JO: Reduction mammaplasty: some observations and reflections. Aesthetic Plast Surg 1983;7(4): 249–251
6. Colwell AS, May JW, Slavin SA: Lowering the postoperative high-riding nipple. Plast Reconstr Surg 2007;120(3): 596–599

Zigzag Glanduloplasty to Reduce Flatness of Lower Pole of Breast Following Breast Reduction

Felix Giebler

83.1 Introduction

Most of the reduction mammoplasties comprised of a cone-form resection of the lower pole of the breasts [1–3]. On looking critically through the literature you may find certain flatness, here and there, on the lower pole of the breast. This flatness is often corrected by itself but may stay as a telltale sign of the mammoplasty for years after. The additional zigzag resection of the lower pole tissue by inner plasty may help to avoid this problem.

83.2 History

There are many resection techniques available, most of them with a superior pedicle [4], because the main vascularization of the breasts comes from the cranial direction [5]. The overwhelming problem of breast surgery is how to attain symmetry and how to divide the breast into four equal quarters, which only the radiologist can do. Drawing an exact pattern on the breast makes good drawing, but not automatically a good postoperative result. The most common resection of the gland is still by the procedure of Strömbeck [6]. In the last years, there has been a wide development of the vertical resection techniques of the breast. The vertical reduction mammoplasty leaves fewer scars, especially at the critical location over the sternum [7] (high incidence hypertrophic scars). The vertical reduction (Lejour [8] and Lassus [9]) is still combined with a keyhole pattern, which may hamper the centralization of the nipple–areola complex (NAC) after breast formation. A good reduction plasty shows good symmetry and a symmetric central positioning of the NAC. This is made more possible by using free nipple positioning after glanduloplasty.

Prevalence of the symmetric and aesthetic formation of the breast led the author to the inner zigzag plasty. The conic form resection of the gland compromises the roundness of the lower pole that leads to flatness in the lower breast after suturing the gland. This flatness may settle down of its own accord but it is not always the case. The zigzag plasty technique solves this problem (Fig. 83.1–83.3).

83.3 Technique

For an inexperienced surgeon, the zigzag plasty is a difficult procedure to plan and execute [10]. The following guidelines will be helpful. First mark a vertical line from the NAC to the inframammary fold down the middle of the deepithelialized area. Mark the zigzags, two to three limbs, in ink. Cut through the pattern forming flaps of 2 cm of superficial tissue. The flaps should never be undermined beyond their base. Then carry out the deep resection of the gland. After connecting the medial and lateral pillars with inverted sutures, one can feel the inverted "T" flatness of the parenchyma.

Before suturing the flaps in the transposed position, check the transfer of the limbs. If the caudal flaps are raised first, this may easily influence the lateral or the medial pole of the breast by traction, using a 4-0 resorbable suture. Although usually no skin undermining is advised, detachment of the skin for 0.5–1.0 cm may be helpful for running the intradermal suture.

At the end of the mammoplasty, put the NAC complex on top of the breast, after defining the location, with an appropriate sizer [11].

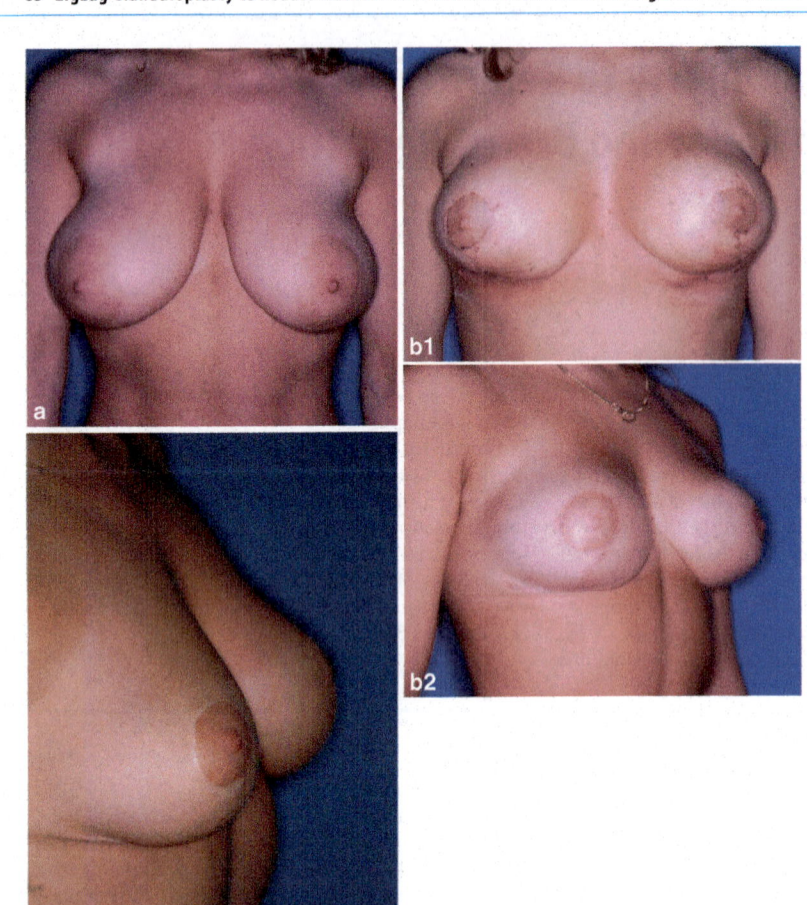

Fig. 83.1 (a) Preoperative 20-year-old female. (b) Immediately postoperative showing flattening of the lower pole following vertical reduction of 280 g on each side. (c) Ten years postoperative with persistent flattening of the lower pole on the right

83.4 Discussion

Result of the cone-shaped resection of the gland is often an inverted "T" flatness of the lower pole. The superficial zigzag glandoplasty covers this defect using a double layer of the tissue, reshaping the natural roundness of the lower breast. The zigzag subcutaneous mammoplasty can influence the lateral and medial lower pole of the breasts, depending on the traction and the positioning of the tips of the triangular flaps. This additional superficial plasty is an inner bra maneuver and improves the projection of the breast, underlying the effect of the vertical resection technique.

83.5 Complications

There may be buckling of the skin in the lower pole area that settles down of its own accord after removing the skin sutures.

83.6 Conclusions

The aim of the reduction mammoplasty is to achieve an aesthetic smaller breast with a good projection and with a nonoperated appearance [12]. Another goal is to decelerate the signs of age, the ptosis of the breast. With improvement in the support of tissue in the lower pole, you act against the gravitational pull. The vertical scarring and the zigzag plasty are solid supports against the settling down of the tissue. The inner bra technique seems [13], through this second layer of tissue as crossed arms, to give a longer lasting stable result.

Breast reduction is a compromised procedure. It is not really cosmetic, but we try to make it so. Vertical breast resection along with superficial zigzag-plasty is a way to eliminate much of the scarring and to refine the form defects due to resection.

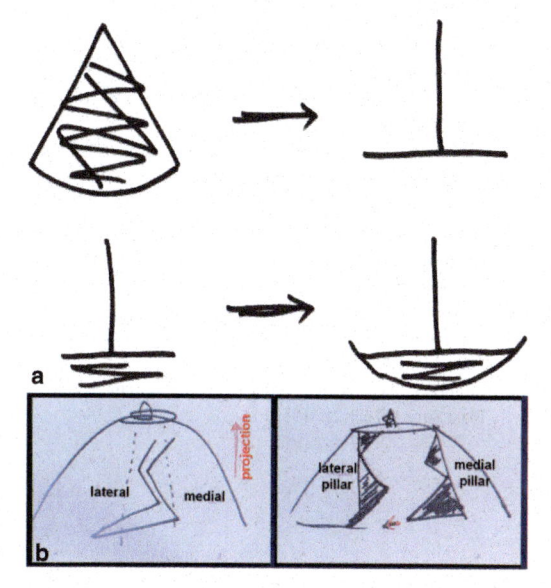

Fig. 83.2 (**a**) Resection of cone form segment of the breast leading to flatness of the breast because of the lack of roundness. (**b**) The superficial zigzag plasty adds roundness to the lower pole

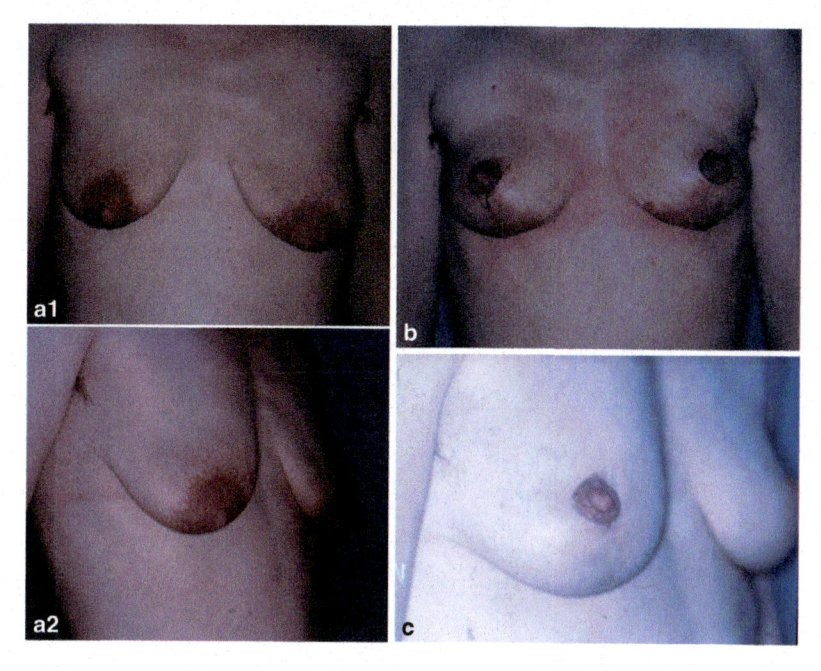

Fig. 83.3 (**a1,2**) Preoperative 38-year-old female. (**b**) Immediately postoperative after resection of 110 g each side using vertical resection zigzag glanduloplasty and good roundness. (**c**) One year postoperative showing unchanged roundness of the lower pole

References

1. Schorcher F: Brustplastik in Kosmetische Operationen. Munich, F. Lehman 1955, pp 108–113
2. Strombeck JO: Mammaplasty: report of a new technique based on the two pedicle procedure. Br J Plast Surg 1960;13:79–90
3. Pitanguy I: Surgical treatment of breast hypertrophy. Br J Plast Surg 1967;20(1):78–85
4. McKissock PK: Reduction mammaplasty with a vertical dermal pedicle flap. Plast Reconstr Surg 1972;49(3):245–252
5. Maliniac JW: Arterial blood supply of the breast. Arch Surg 1943;47:329
6. Menke H, Olbrisch RR, Bahr C: Standard technique of breast reduction surgery with vertical scar. Handchir Mikrochir Plast Surg 1999;31(2):134–136
7. Morris AM: Complications of Breast Surgery, London, Bailliere Tindall 1989
8. Lejour M: Vertical mammaplasty. Plast Reconstr Surg 1993;92(5):985–986
9. Lassus C: Personal method of reduction mammaplasty. In: Goldwyn M (ed). Reduction Mammaplasty, Boston, Little Brown and Co. 1990:441–467
10. Zolton J: Atlas der Chirurgischen Schnitt und Nahttechnik, Basel, S. Karger 1980
11. Giebler FRG: Vertikale reduktionplastik. Aesthetic Tribune 2006;7:15
12. Giebler FRG: Creating invisible scars. Aesthet Derm 2002;4(2):105–107
13. Hinderer UT: The dermal brassiere mammaplasty. Clin Plast Surg 1976;3(2):349–370

Recurrent Deformities after Breast Reduction and Mastopexy

Saul Hoffman

84.1
Introduction

Breast reduction and mastopexy are two of the most common operations performed by plastic surgeons. The results are satisfactory in the majority of cases, but problems do occur even with the most careful planning.

84.2
History

In 1976, Goldwyn [1] covered the history of breast surgery dating back to Hippocrates. In 1990 [2], he included chapters on history and various techniques as well as complications and problems that can occur.

In 1990, Georgiade [3] described the techniques used in reduction mammaplasty and mastopexy. Many of these techniques are of historical interest only, but he points out the fact that an ideal method is not yet available. However, many of the operations are similar and have a similar revision rate. In 1991, Noone [4] edited a book with sections on developmental deformities, augmentation and reduction mammaplasty, and breast reconstruction.

In 1991, Strombeck [5] described his horizontal pedicle technique consisting of 375 cases. Eleven percent of patients were not satisfied with the operation, and breast size was satisfactory in 83%, too large in 13%, and too small in 4%.

In 1987, a questionnaire was sent to the members of the American Society of Plastic and Reconstructive Surgery in an effort to determine the degree of patient satisfaction and the complication rate [6, 7]. Thirty-eight percent of the membership responded. The most frequent complaint was the appearance of the scars. In 11% of the responding surgeons, a malpractice suit had been precipitated by a dissatisfied reduction mammaplasty patient.

In 1999, a report by Hudson and Skoll [8] discussed repeat reduction mammaplasty. Sixteen patients out of a total of 467 underwent repeat reduction in an 11-year period. The interval between operations varied from 13 months to 10 years. Several different pedicles were used. The nipple to inframammary fold distance was 7 cm initially, but had increased to an average of 11.4 cm. In 2002, Graf et al. [9] described a technique designed to minimize bottoming-out and reduce visible scarring. The technique involved a shortened lateral incision in the inframammary fold. A loop of pectoral muscle is used to support the inferior pedicle and maintain superior fullness. A good result is shown with a 2 year follow-up.

In 1975, Herman et al. [10] described the problems that can occur after a reduction mammaplasty. Correction of these complications was also discussed.

84.3
Problems that May Occur and Require Revision

1. Residual asymmetry
2. Insufficient reduction
3. Over reduction
4. Loss of nipple
5. Loss of sensation
6. Hypertrophic scarring
7. Lengthening of the vertical scar – bottoming out

A result that appears satisfactory initially may change in time and require revision (Figs. 84.1–84.6). The final result may not be apparent for several months or even longer. Aging, pregnancy, weight gain or loss, and nursing will affect the outcome. The patient must be informed of the postoperative changes and the possible need for revision.

In reviewing cases in which the patient was not happy, it was common to hear, "the surgeon didn't tell me that this could happen." Photographs may be helpful to show average results and especially the location and type of scarring that can occur.

In revising a reduction it is important to maintain the same pedicle that was used in the initial procedure,

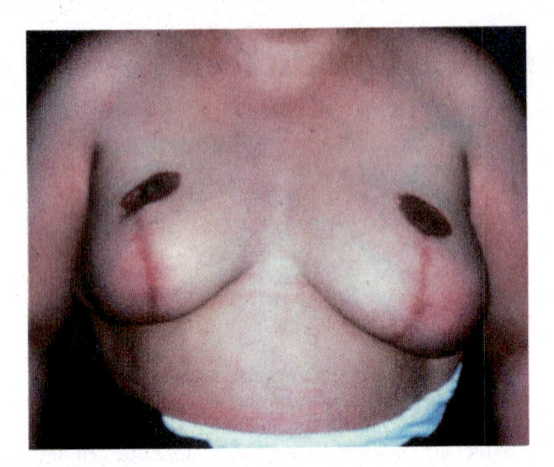

Fig. 84.1 Bottoming out after breast reduction

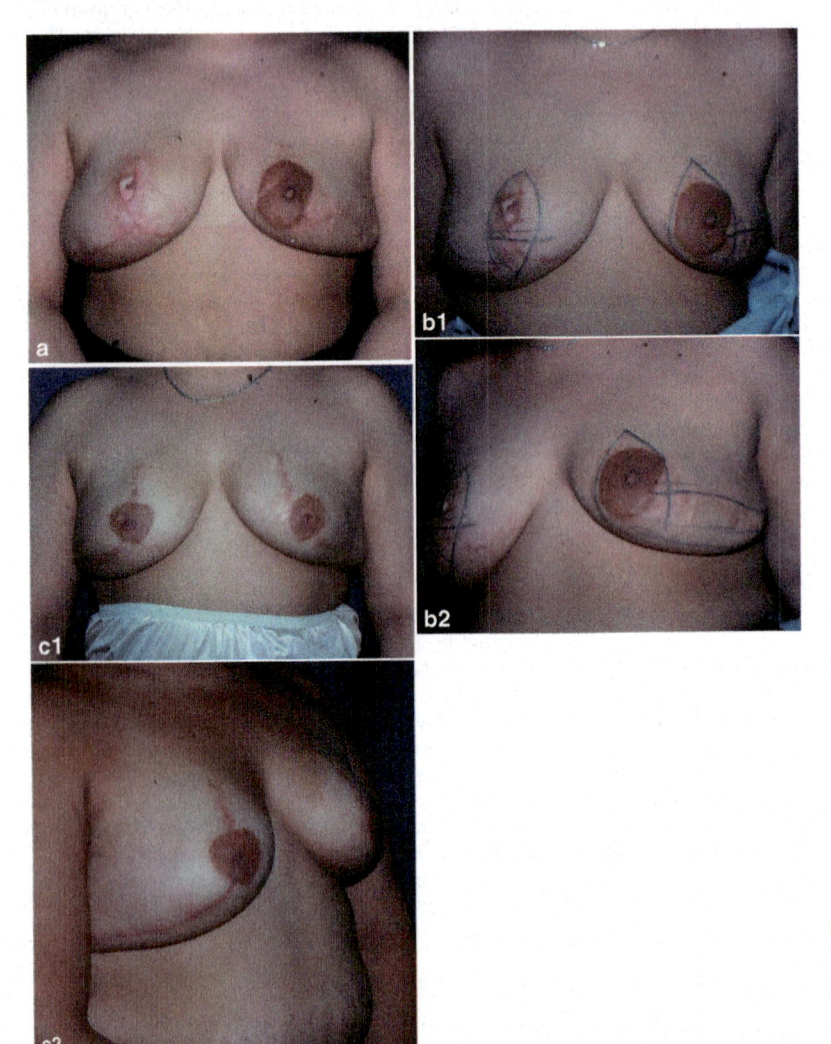

Fig. 84.2 (a) Poor result after breast reduction. (b1,2) Preoperative marking. (c1,2) Result after revision surgery

84.3 Problems that May Occur and Require Revision 637

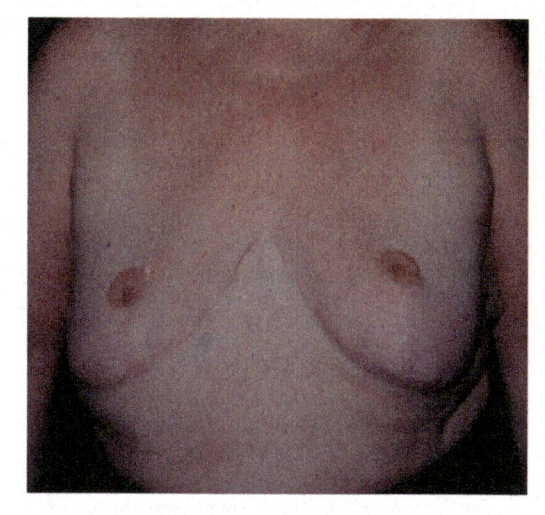

Fig. 84.3 Excessive breast reduction

Fig. 84.5 Wound breakdown after breast reduction

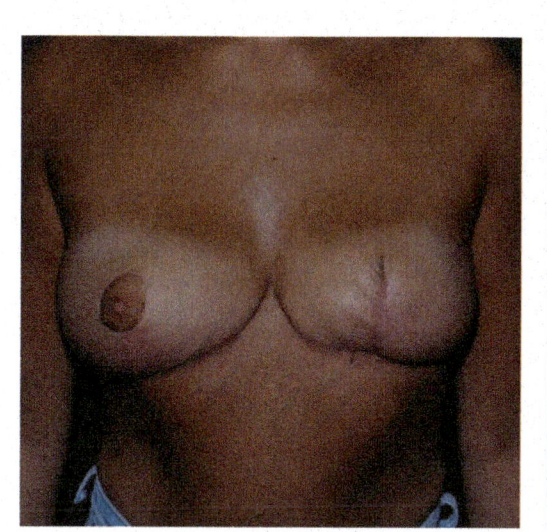

Fig. 84.4 Loss of nipple–areolar complex after breast reduction

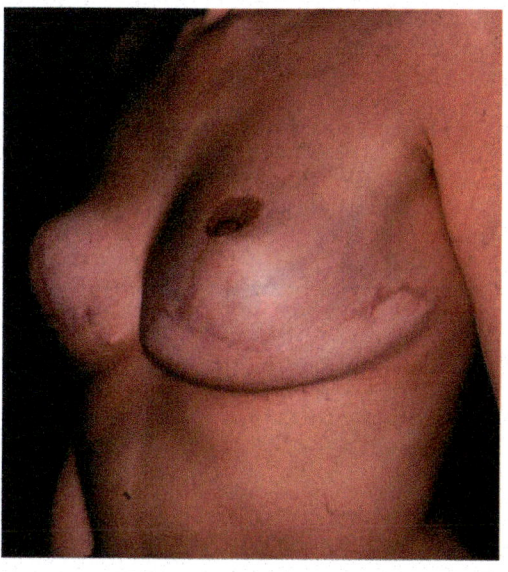

Fig. 84.6 Poor preoperative marking for breast reduction

as there is a possibility of interfering with the blood supply to the nipple. If the type of pedicle is not known, a free nipple graft may be the best option. It is also important to get an idea of the size that the patient has in mind. An elderly woman with very large and uncomfortable breasts complained that the surgeon made her breast too small even though the result was excellent.

While a reduction mammaplasty is often performed to make the patient more comfortable, a mastopexy is a more cosmetic procedure. The patient must decide if the scarring and possible loss of nipple sensation is worth the trade off. The procedure has become increasingly popular; the number of mastopexies has increased over 500% in the past 10 years. Stevens et al. [11] reviewed a series of 100 cases to determine the complication rate. Their revision rate was 8.6%. They concluded that mastopexy is a safe and effective procedure.

In 1968, Kahn [12] stated that the Strombeck technique was the safest method, as it involved very little undermining and preserved the pedicles. He showed satisfactory results after 3 weeks but bottoming out in 1 year.

Another method involved wide undermining of the skin, but this technique resulted in more complications.

Lassus, in 1977 [13], was the first person to describe the vertical mammaplasty. He reported that complications were few and far between, but he pointed out that scar revisions may be necessary. In very large breasts, a short transverse incision might be necessary in the inframammary fold. Lejour [14] followed up with the vertical mammaplasty. The operation is now referred to as the Lejour technique. Keck et al. [15] discussed the postoperative changes, complications, and patient evaluation of the vertical mammaplasty. Between 2002 and 2005, 72 patients underwent the procedure. They were followed up to 1 year. The main changes took place during the first 3 months after surgery. The nipple diameter increased by 28% and the nipple to inframammary fold distance increased by 17% in 3 months and by 22% after a year. The complication rate was low and the patient satisfaction was high.

Asymmetry was the next most common concern. In spite of these complaints, most of the respondents to the questionnaire stated that reduction mammaplasty is one of the most satisfying procedures they performed.

If optimum results are to be achieved, careful preoperative evaluation, accurate measurements, and correct markings are important. A detailed informed consent is essential. The patient must accept the negative aspects of the operation, which include scarring, possible loss of nipple sensation, and the possibility of a revision.

References

1. Goldwyn RM (ed): Plastic and Reconstructive Surgery of the Breast. Little Brown and Co., Boston 1976
2. Goldwyn RM (ed): Reduction Mammaplasty, Boston, Little Brown and Co. 1990
3. Georgiade NG, Georgiade GS, Riefkohl R: Aesthetic Surgery of the Breast. W.B. Saunders London 1990
4. Noone RB (ed): Plastic and Reconstructive Surgery of the Breast, B.C. Decker, Philadelphia 1991
5. Strombeck JO: Reduction mammaplasty with horizontal pedicle technique. In: Noone RB (ed). Plastic and Reconstructive Surgery of the Breast. B.C. Decker, Philadelphia 1991, p 195
6. Hoffman S: Reduction mammaplasty: a medicolegal hazard? Aesthetic Plast Surg 1987;11(2):113–116
7. Hoffman S: Medicolegal aspects of reduction mammaplasty. In: Goldwyn RM (ed). Reduction Mammaplasty. Boston, Little Brown and Co. 1989, p 59
8. Hudson DA, Skoll PJ: Repeat reduction mammaplasty. Plast Reconstr Surg 1999;104(2):401–408
9. Graf RM, Auersvald A, Bernardes A, Biggs TM: Reduction mammaplasty and mastopexy with shorter scar and better shape. Aesthetic Surgery 2002;20:99
10. Herman S, Hoffman S, Kahn S: Revisional surgery after reduction mammaplasty. Plast Reconstr Surg 1975;55(4):422–427
11. Stevens WG, Stoker DA, Freeman ME, Quardt SM, Hirsch EM: Mastopexy revisited: a review of 150 consecutive cases for complication and revision rates. Aesthetic Surg 2007;27(2):150
12. Kahn S, Hoffman S, Simon B: Correction of non-hypertrophic ptosis of the breasts. Plast Reconstr Surg 1968;4(3):244–147
13. Lassus, C. New refinements in vertical mammaplasty. Presented at the 2nd Congress of the Asian Section of International Plastic Reconstructive Surgery, Tokyo 1977
14. LeJour M: Vertical mammaplasty: early complications after 250 personal consecutive cases. Plast Reconstr Surg 1999;104(3):764–770
15. Keck M, Kaye K, Thieme I, Ueberreiter K: Vertical mammaplasty: postoperative changes, complications and patient evaluation. Canadian J Plast Surg 2007;15:41–43

Recurrent Mammary Hyperplasia

James F. Thornton, Paul D. McCluskey

85.1 Introduction

Reduction mammaplasty is now one of the most commonly performed operations in plastic surgery. Patient satisfaction with breast reduction is high regardless of pedicle choice or incision pattern, a fact that has now been well elucidated by multiple outcome studies [1, 2]. In addition, the operation carries a relatively low incidence of complications. Prevention and treatment of some of the most devastating complications such as nipple loss has also been well described [2–4]. One of the least frequent complications of breast reduction surgery is recurrent hyperplasia of the breast. This diagnosis presents many unique challenges to both the patient and the surgeon and heavy emphasis must therefore be placed on preoperative counseling [5, 6].

Symptomatic hypermastia, the condition of breast enlargement which most frequently leads the patient to reduction surgery, is characterized by a group of symptoms stemming from the excess weight and muscle strain of enlarged breasts. Common symptoms presented include neck, back, and shoulder pain, as well as shoulder notching and intertriginous rashes. Many of these patients are obese and may not experience resolution of symptoms such as back and neck pain following breast reduction. Despite this, patient satisfaction remains well over 80% among reduction mammaplasty patients [1, 2, 7].

Occasionally, patients present with postoperative concerns that are aesthetic in nature and are caused by asymmetry, scarring, and/or shape of the breast mound. Inadequate excision and recurrent hypermastia are more complex concerns, which require careful evaluation and treatment. Analysis of both the presented deformity and the original surgical approach is critical in determining an operative plan [8].

A woman may be disappointed with her postoperative result because of scarring, asymmetry, and odd-shaped or boxy breasts; rarely is the disappointment due to inadequate excision [7]. Loss of nipple sensation and inability to breast-feed are infrequent complaints because patients often expect this postoperatively if properly counseled. Informed consent with proper communication preoperatively usually prevents unrealistic expectations. Recurrence should be mentioned in preoperative discussions, but is primarily a risk in patients with juvenile hypertrophy [9].

Long-term scars are one of the tradeoffs of reduction mammaplasty [10]. Although various techniques have been designed to minimize scarring, complete elimination of scars is clearly impossible. On follow-up, physical examination is important to ensure that incisions are healing appropriately and patients are counseled on realistic expectations for ultimate scar maturation. Postoperative massage and silicone pressure sheeting can be encouraged, and time is allowed for scar maturation. Occasionally, scar revision is undertaken after the patient is counseled that the scar may not improve even with surgical intervention. The psychological impact of poor scarring should not be underestimated.

Breast asymmetry is a norm and should be pointed out preoperatively to the patient. If only a slight undesirable asymmetry exists, liposuction can be performed with good results [10]. If a larger discrepancy exists, surgical revision can be considered. An appropriate interval usually a minimum of 6 months for swelling to resolve and wound maturation to occur should be allowed before revision is considered.

Preoperative expectations clearly influence a patient's satisfaction with shape. Patients need to be counseled preoperatively that the initial result is designed to both allow for and minimize the inevitable "bottoming out" that occurs over time [11]. The goal of breast reduction should not be to create a virginal-appearing breast but rather a mature, slightly pendulous breast that will persist proportional to the patient's build [12, 13].

Inadequate excision is a rare complaint and must be distinguished from recurrent hypertrophy as an indication for repeat breast reduction [2]. Preoperative expectations should be openly discussed. This is imperative to avoid misunderstandings and disappointments between surgeon and patient. Regnault and Daniel [14] described the amount of excised tissue needed to decrease breast size in various chest circumferences (Table 85.1). Acutely, hematomas or seromas may be the culprit for size discrepancies and likely need drainage. In addition, infection and swelling need to be considered. Operative

M.A. Shiffman (ed.), *Mastopexy and Breast Reduction: Principles and Practice*,
DOI 10.1007/978-3-540-89873-3_85, © Springer-Verlag Berlin Heidelberg 2009

Table 85.1 Amount of tissue removed for each change in cup size*

Chest circumference (in.)	For each cup size of desired reduction, remove (g)
32–34	100
36–38	200
42–44	300
44–46	400

*Adapted from [14]

re-excision should be performed if there is a gross discrepancy in size immediately postoperatively. In this case, reopening of incisions should allow dissection along previous planes without compromising the known pedicles.

85.2 Pathophysiology

Breast growth is an end-organ response to circulating estrogens. This explains the rapid periods of breast growth during puberty and pregnancy; however, many patients with normal levels of circulating estrogens experience abnormal breast hypertrophy. Jabs et al. [15] studied breast hypertrophy and found that breast enlargement typically consists of fibrous tissue and fat. Contrary to what was previously believed, the glandular elements of the breast remain essentially normal in size and distribution. This study also revealed normal levels of estrogen and the usual number of estrogen receptors in women with mammary hypertrophy, and concluded that this is instead evidence of a condition of hypersensitivity to the hormone.

Juvenile virginal hypertrophy of the breast was first described by Durston in 1670 [16], and was initially termed gigantomastia. This condition is marked by massive enlargement of the breasts, and is often asymmetric. When the condition manifests, typically in early puberty, it can present as an extreme and debilitating level of hypertrophy. It does not regress, and in some, breast growth continues from the age of 11 into the teen years. Kupfer and Dingman [17] studied juvenile hypertrophy of the breast and found a mother–daughter pair with the condition, suggesting a familial inheritance.

Breast enlargement in juvenile hypertrophy is often asymmetric and can sometimes be completely unilateral [18]. In these cases, it is critical to distinguish this condition from other causes of unilateral breast enlargement. Tumors such as fibroadenoma, cystosarcoma phyllodes, and breast hamartoma readily present as asymmetric breast enlargement [19, 20].

All studies pertaining to virginal hypertrophy and recurrent hypermastia deal with relatively small patient populations. For this reason, it is difficult to assess the risk of recurrence of hypermastia or gigantomastia after breast reduction. Recurrence is a recognized risk, particularly among pregnant women. Many of these patients have experienced extreme recurrent mammary hypertrophy, returning to or exceeding their pre-reduction size [21]. There is no known medical therapy to this condition and surgery is essentially the only option. One exception is a case described by Taylor et al. [22], in which D-penicillamine-induced hypermastia was treated with danazol. The most extreme option for treating this condition is bilateral mastectomy with reconstruction [9]. Because of the young age of the typical patient and the potential psychological impact of this operation, most patients choose to undergo bilateral reduction mammaplasty, despite the risk of recurrence [8, 16].

Many surgeons fear the untoward sequelae of repeat or secondary breast reduction. Repeat operation puts the pedicle and the nipple areolar complex (NAC) at risk, and although it is best to use the previous pedicle for dissection, details of the initial operation are not always available. Hudson and Skoll [8] reviewed an 11 year experience with repeat reduction mammaplasty that consisted of 16 patients (28 breasts). The Nipple to IMF (inframammary fold) mean was 11.4 cm, considered to be elongated from the 7 cm average during the first operation. In the second surgery, two patients had their initial pedicles transected and vascular compromise of the NAC developed in both. Of the five patients in whom the same pedicle was used, one had unilateral nipple necrosis. The authors recommend reusing the initial pedicle when possible. If the original pedicle is unknown, a free nipple graft is the next best option. The complication rate in secondary reduction is higher than during the first surgery. The same pedicle should be used if at all possible [4, 13].

Postoperatively the breast will often undergo morphological changes that impact final appearance [11, 12]. Patients often request smaller revisions, including correction of size discrepancies, correction of nipple asymmetry, scar revisions, or excision of necrotic fat. These procedures do not qualify as secondary breast reduction, which, as defined by Hudson and Skoll [8], requires re-elevation of the NAC on a vascular pedicle.

These authors [8] identified an additional indication for repeat breast reduction: pseudoptosis. They state that performing a mastopexy for pseudoptosis not requiring transposition of the nipple can be completed via an inferior pole wedge excision. Patients requested secondary reduction mammaplasty for the following reasons: (1) progressive ptosis or pseudoptosis, (2) recurrent breast hypertrophy, and (3) asymmetric breast size.

Recurrent hypermastia is a complex problem and an algorithm is described for its management (Fig. 85.1) [23]. A careful history must be obtained from the patient. Important factors include details of the breast before initial operation, along with the immediate, initials, postoperative result. If photographs are available, they are invaluable in this regard. Medical record photographs along with a chart review provide useful information and details that the patient may not recall, especially if the first procedure was performed by a different surgeon. Preoperative measurements along with the gross mass excised can be compared with current findings. Have the breasts continued to enlarge postoperatively, or were they inadequately reduced? The patient should be asked her preoperative, postoperative, and current bra size. The patient should also be questioned about a history of overall weight gain, pregnancies, and medication or drug use [16, 22]. A mammogram should also be obtained.

Most important is whether the growth has been symmetric or is limited to one breast. A careful physical examination to detect palpable masses must be performed. It is imperative to rule out malignancy with any complaints of recurrent hypermastia. A good history, a careful physical examination, and a mammogram must be obtained. Baseline-screening mammograms are recommended for all postoperative reduction mammaplasty patients. Consideration should be given to the areas of

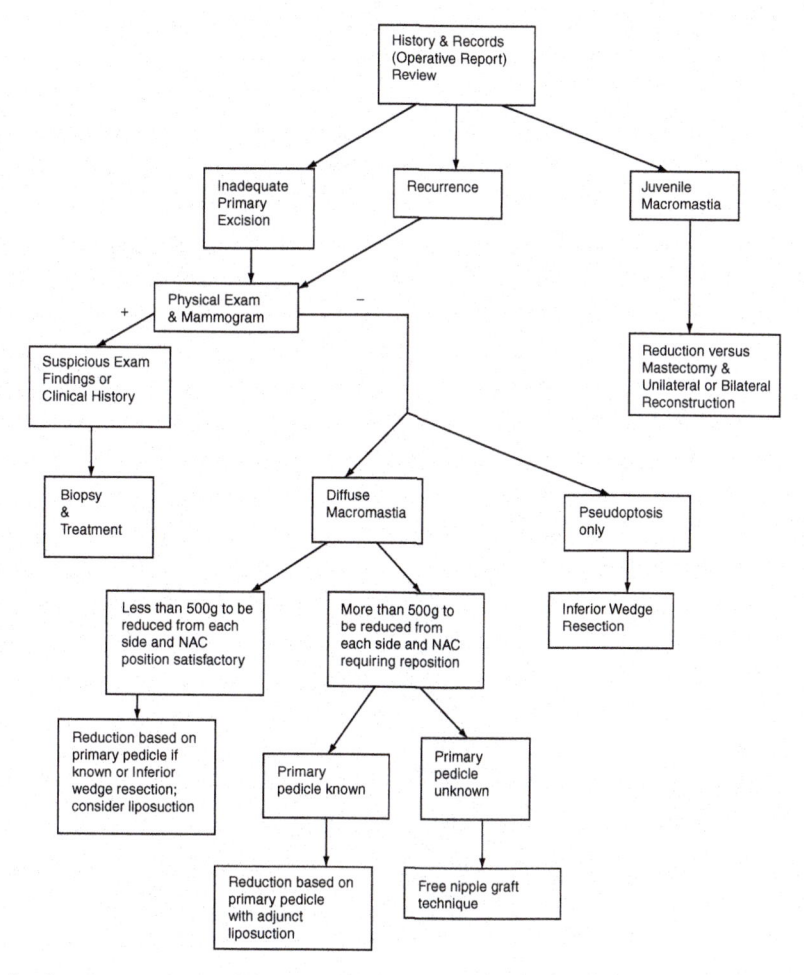

Fig. 85.1 Algorithm for recurrent mammary hypermastia (NAC, nipple-areola complex)

excess breast tissue. Does the breast have diffuse tissue hypertrophy or localized areas of excess? Is the excess located laterally or inferiorly? Is the breast ptotic or pseudoptotic? After reduction mammaplasty, bottoming out often leads to pseudoptosis where the nipple is at or above the inframammary fold.

85.3 Case Reports

85.3.1 Case 1

A 44-year-old woman presented with complaining of recurrent symptomatic hypermastia, including back and shoulder pain. She had a reduction mammaplasty and noted that she never obtained relief of the symptoms. She believed that the primary operation had not removed adequate breast tissue. Breast examination was notable for well-healed but slightly widened scars in an inverted T pattern (Fig. 85.2). She had bilateral ptosis, and the right breast was larger than the left. The breasts were soft, and no palpable masses or lymphadenopathy was appreciated. Nipple sensation was grossly intact. Screening mammography was within normal limits.

Because no operative report was available and the breasts demonstrated marked pseudoptosis, inferior wedge resection was performed, incorporating the original transverse incisions (Fig. 85.3) [24]. Liposuction was used laterally, with the removal of 425 g from the right breast and 375 g from the left breast. As shown in the algorithm presented, this patient was in the pathway of inadequate excision → small planned reduction → unknown primary pedicle. Therefore, inferior wedge resection was performed with adjunctive contouring liposuction. She tolerated the procedure well and postoperatively was satisfied with the resolution of long-term back and shoulder pain at 9 months.

85.3.2 Case 2

A 40-year-old Caucasian woman with a history of reduction mammaplasty 16 years before presentation noted a history of fluctuating weight loss and presented complaining of both recurrent macromastia and nipple asymmetry (Fig. 85.4). At examination, she was noted to

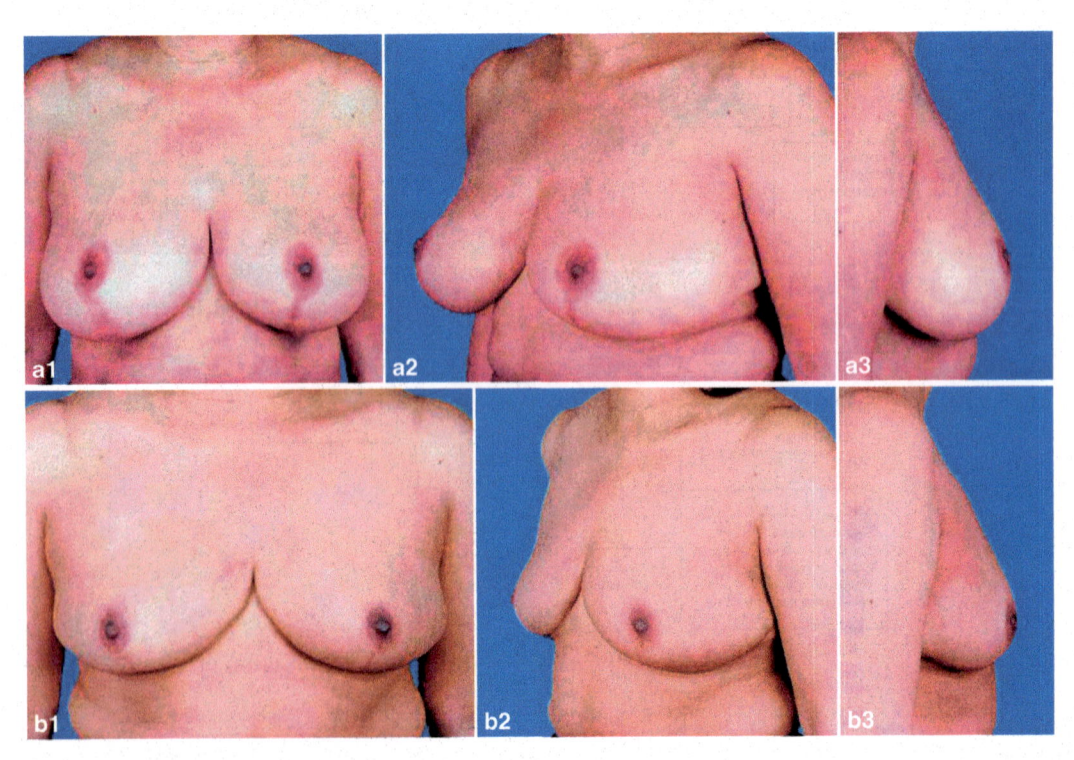

Fig. 85.2 (a*1-3*) Preoperative. (b*1-3*) Nine months postoperative

have well-healed scars and grade III ptosis with pseudoptosis. In addition, she had nipple asymmetry, with a larger left areola. Her physical examination was unremarkable for masses or nipple discharge. A mammogram was obtained and was normal.

In the operating room, secondary reduction mastopexy was performed using the previous T incisions in an inferior wedge design. Liposuction was performed, with the removal of 525 and 600 g from the right and left breasts, respectively, followed by wedge resection of 142 and 128 g. Circumareolar and periareolar mastopexy was performed to address asymmetry. Based on the algorithm, this patient followed the pathway recurrent hypermastia → negative mammogram → pseudoptosis → inferior wedge resection with mastopexy for areolar asymmetry. The patient got healed without complication and was well satisfied with her result at 6 months.

The algorithm presented divides recurrent hypermastia into three basic categories [23]. In both the recurrent and the inadequate primary excision groups, operative planning should be based on the amount of the planned excision. In small reductions and in cases of pseudoptosis, inferior wedge resection or a fleur-de-lys type of excision (if volume reduction in both vertical and horizontal vectors is required) can be safely performed. Alternatively, if the original pedicle is known, re-excision can be performed using the original pedicle. Larger excisions (greater than 500 g) are more complex. In these cases, if the primary pedicle is known, this is the safest technique. When the pedicle is unknown and the planned resection is large, free nipple grafting must be considered [23].

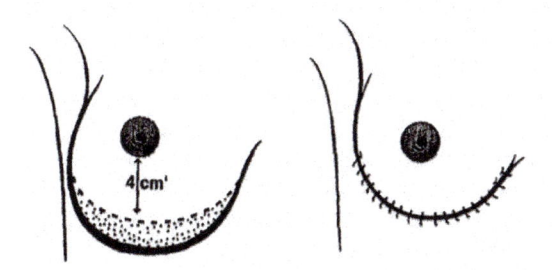

Fig. 85.3 Technique of inferior wedge resection. From [8]

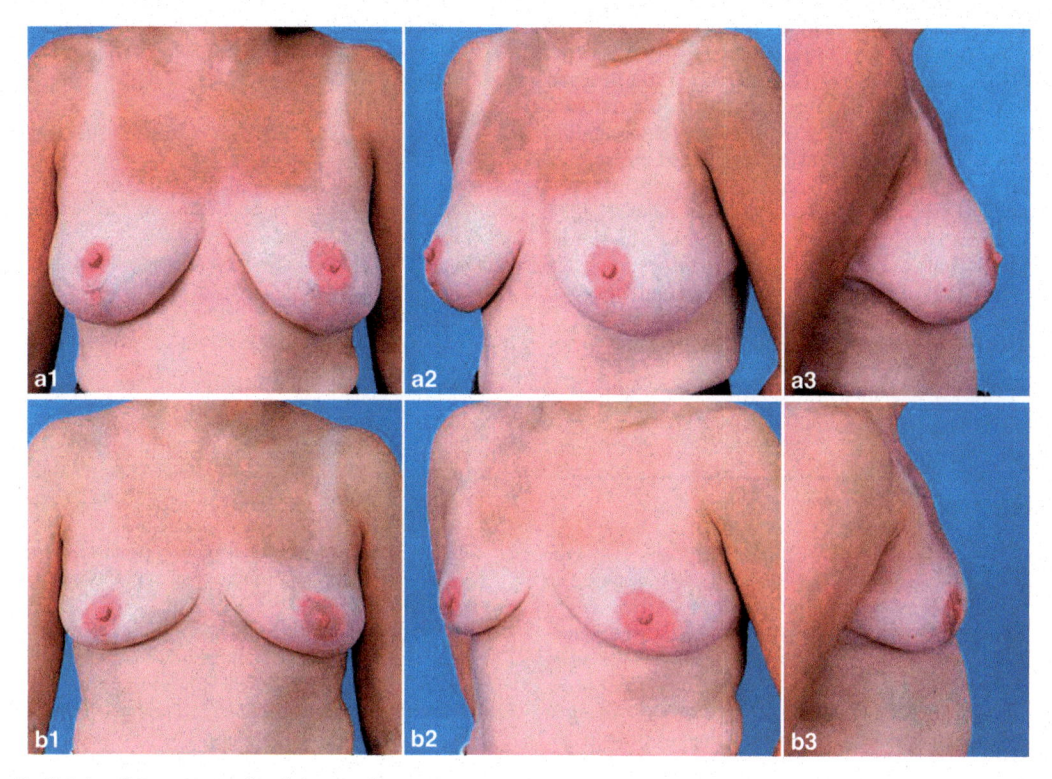

Fig. 85.4 (*a1-3*) Preoperative. (*b1-3*) Six months postoperative

Important considerations in designing a surgical plan include the location of the previous incisional scars, the location of the NAC, assessment of the degree of pseudoptosis, and the altered blood supply to the breast. Reviewing the surgical technique used is important in formulating a new surgical plan. Blood supply to the NAC will consist of the original pedicle along with neovascularization from the surrounding breast tissue. If the nipple needs to be transposed and the pedicle is known, then reconstruction based on this pedicle can be performed. Knowledge of the original pedicle is important because transection has resulted in nipple–areola ischemia.

Cases of true juvenile macromastia are rare and should be aggressively treated with early reduction and planned revision as the macromastia recurs. This should be discussed with the young patient and her parents during early consultations. The psychological impact of multiple procedures and the resulting deformity must be addressed, and psychological referral may be necessary. Mastectomy and reconstruction is occasionally necessary in aggressive cases.

Reduction mammaplasty is a highly successful operation that results in a high level of patient satisfaction. Most complaints are because of small aesthetic problems that can easily be addressed. Recurrent hypermastia is a more complex problem and the authors present an algorithm (Fig. 85.1) that is useful when patients desire revision reduction. Consideration must be given to the reasons for the recurrent breast hypertrophy. Different operative strategies will be useful, depending on the structure of the previously operated breast.

Important principles in recurrent mammary hyperplasia and repeat breast reduction include the following [23]:
1. Review of history of breasts since the initial operation
2. Careful examination for asymmetries and masses
3. Mammographic radiological evaluation
4. Review of operative technique used from the operative report, if available
5. Choice of operative technique based of examination findings and amount of reduction to be performed.

References

1. Dabbah A, Lehman JA Jr, Parker MG, Tantri D, Wagner DS: Reduction mammaplasty: An outcome analysis. Ann Plast Surg 1995;35(4):337–341
2. Boschert MT, Barone CM, Puckett CL: Outcome analysis of reduction mammaplasty. Plast Reconstr Surg 1996;98(3):451–454
3. Gonzalez F, Walton RL, Shafer B, Matory WE Jr, Borah GL: Reduction mammaplasty improves symptoms of macromastia. Plast Reconstr Surg 1993;91(7):1270–1276
4. Klassen A, Jenkinson C, Fitzpatrick R, Goodacre T: Patient's health related quality of life before and after aesthetic surgery. Br J Plast Surg 1996;49(7):433–438
5. Raispis T, Zehring RD, Downey DL: Long-term functional results after reduction mammaplasty. Ann Plast Surg 1995;34(2):113–116
6. Kinnell I, Beausang-Linder M, Ohlsen L: The effect on the preoperative symptoms and late results of Skoog's reduction mammaplasty. Scand J Plast Reconstr Surg Hand Surg 1990;24:61
7. Davis GM, Ringler SL, Short K, Sherrick D, Bengtson BP: Reduction mammaplasty: Long-term efficacy, morbidity, and patient satisfaction. Plast Reconstr Surg 1995;96(5):1106–1110
8. Hudson DA, Skoll PJ: Repeat reduction mammaplasty. Plast Reconstr Surg 1999;104(2):401–408
9. Samuelov R, Siplovich L: Juvenile gigantomastia. J Pediatr Surg 1988;23(11):1014–1015
10. Hidalgo DA: Improving safety and aesthetic results in inverted T scar breast reduction. Plast Reconstr Surg 1999;103(3):874–886
11. Schwartz M, Rohrich RJ, Singer D: The UT Southwestern approach to reduction mammaplasty. Presented at the Annual Meeting of the Texas Society of Plastic Surgeons, San Antonio, Texas, November 7–9, 1997
12. Penn J: Breast reduction. Br J Plast Surg 1955;7:357–371
13. Berry EP: Geometric planning in reduction mammaplasty. Plast Reconstr Surg 1968;42(3):232–2236
14. Regnault P, Daniel RK: Breast reduction. In: Regnault P, Daniel RK (eds). Aesthetic Plastic Surgery, Principles and Techniques. Little, Brown and Co., Boston 1984, pp 499–538
15. Jabs AD, Frantz AG, Smith-Vaniz A, Hugo NE: Mammary hypertrophy is not associated with increased estrogen receptors. Plast Reconstr Surg 1990;86(1):64–66
16. Ryan RF, Pernoll ML: Virginal hypertrophy. Plast Reconstr Surg 1985;75(5):737–742
17. Kupfer D, Dingman D, Broadbent R: Juvenile breast hypertrophy: report of a familial pattern and review of the literature. Plast Reconstr Surg 1992;90(2):303–309
18. Griffith JR: Virginal breast hypertrophy. J Adolesc Health Care 1989;10(5):423–432
19. Beer GM, Kompatscher P, Hergan K: Diagnosis of breast tumors after breast reduction. Aesthetic Plast Surg 1996;20(5):391–397
20. Durston, W. Concerning a very sudden and excessive swelling of a woman's breasts. Phil Trans Vol IV for anno 1669:1047–1049, Royal Society, London 1670
21. Ship AG: Virginal and gravid mammary gigantism: recurrence after reduction mammaplasty. Br J Plast Surg 1971;24(4):396–401
22. Taylor PJ, Cumming DC, Corenblum B: Successful treatment of D-penicillamine-induced breast gigantism with danazol. Br Med J 1981;282(6261):362–363
23. Rohrich RJ, Thornton JF, Sorokin ES: Recurrent mammary hyperplasia: current concepts. Plast Reconstr Surg 2003;111(1):387–394
24. Rohrich RJ, Beran SJ, Restifo RJ, Copit SE: Aesthetic management of the breast following explantation: evaluation and mastopexy options. Plast Reconstr Surg 1998;101(3):827–837

Repeat Reduction Mammaplasty

Donald A Hudson

86.1
Introduction

The author is not addressing minor aesthetic deformities such as dog ears, unsightly scars, or breast asymmetry, but rather addresses the uncommon problem of a patient presenting and requesting further reduction of an enlarged breast after a previous reduction mammaplasty.

Repeat breast reduction appears to have been an uncommonly performed procedure before the 1990s as there was almost no literature on the subject. Probably the changes in techniques of breast reduction, particularly the popularising of short scar techniques, combined with advances in breast reconstruction are partly responsible for these changes [1].

The reasons for patients seeking repeat breast reduction remains poorly defined, although logically it is either recurrence of the hypertrophy or inadequate primary excision [2]. Obviously, a reduction performed as an adolescent for virginal hypertrophy may require repeating when the person reaches adulthood. One of the problems of the short scar techniques is to under resect breast tissue at reduction, whereas other patients put on weight leading to a repetition of mammary hypertrophy. The role of pregnancy, drugs and changes in weight are unknown factors in this entity.

Pseudoptosis is not an uncommon consequence of a previous breast reduction. The problem may be aggravated where the nipple is placed too high, above the inframammary fold (IMF) in the original reduction. With the passage of time and the effect of gravity, breast tissue descend inferiorly. This lengthens the distance from the inframammary fold to the nipple, often originally set at 5 cm. This excess tissue now situated in the inferior pole of the breast may result in the nipple pointing towards the ceiling and also impairs the aesthetics of the reduced breast.

The key issue to consider relates to the blood supply of the nipple–areola complex (NAC). Almost all modern techniques of breast reduction employ a pedicle. Necrosis of the NAC is a feared complication in the first procedure. The risk is even greater in the second procedure. The NAC blood supply, previously rich and derived from a number of different sources, is now axial via the pedicle, although some neovascularization from the surrounding tissue also contributes. This axial supply must be retained to prevent nipple necrosis, especially if the position of the NAC is to be moved.

86.2
Clinical Assessment

86.2.1
History

This is aimed at finding the reason for seeking secondary surgery and also trying to assess whether the present problem arises from recurrence or inadequate primary excision. As in the initial procedure, risk factors also need to be obtained.

86.2.2
Examination

The breast needs to be assessed similarly to a patient presenting with macromastia for the first time. The body mass index (BMI) is measured. The degree of asymmetry is assessed.

The breast is palpated for lumps and the standard measurements of distance from the suprasternal notch to nipple and nipple to inframammary fold are measured. A mammogram may be considered prudent in the older patient.

A key point in the clinical assessment is to evaluate the position of the nipple. If there is a "true" secondary macromastia, the breast is globally enlarged and the NAC needs to be transposed superiorly to a new position. Alternatively, is the nipple position adequate and the problem really one of pseudoptosis? If it is the former and the nipple needs to be transposed again, the pedicle used in the initial procedure needs to be determined if possible. This approach allows for a safe and reliable surgical plan to be formulated. An algorithm (Fig. 86.1) helps in this regard.

Preoperative photographs are taken.

M.A. Shiffman (ed.), *Mastopexy and Breast Reduction: Principles and Practice*,
© Springer-Verlag Berlin Heidelberg 2009

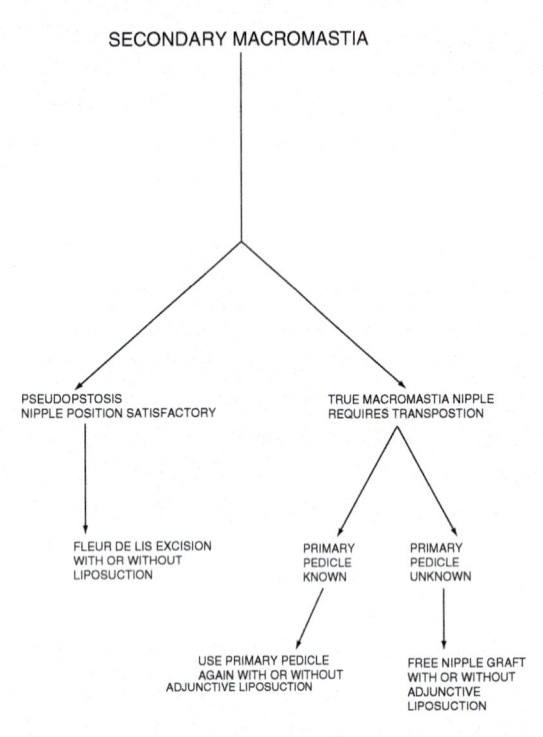

Fig. 86.1 Secondary macromastia algorithm

Clearly the patient also needs careful counselling not only regarding the risk of nipple necrosis (which, with careful planning should be unlikely) but also warned about nipple sensation and the potential for breast feeding. The issue of scar maturation and realistic expectations are important in every consultation.

86.3 Management

A period of at least 6–9 months after the initial surgery should elapse before contemplating further surgery. If the problem is that of pseudoptosis and the nipple position is adequate, the excess tissue in the inferior pole of the breast can be excised, either using a fleur-de-lis pattern, or by just removing a large horizontal ellipse- with the inferior limb of the ellipse extending along the inframammary fold. The previous pedicle used is irrelevant in this procedure.

However, if the nipple needs to be transposed, the previous pedicle used is important. If the previous pedicle used is known, it must be reused to avoid the risk of NAC necrosis. It must be remembered that the initial pedicle would have been covered by skin flaps in the previous procedure; hence the pedicle should not be too thin or too narrow.

If the initial pedicle is not known, then the safe option is a breast reduction using a free nipple graft. Transection and transposition of a previously used pedicle leads to risks in nipple necrosis in over 50% of the cases.

Liposuction can be used as an adjunctive procedure in all cases. Where the nipple is transposed on a known pedicle, it is prudent to avoid liposuction of the pedicle.

References

1. Hudson DA, Skoll PJ: Repeat reduction mammaplasty. Plast Reconstr Surg 1999;104:401–408
2. Rohrich RJ, Thornton JF, Sorokin ES: Recurrent mammary hyperplasia: Current Concepts. Plast Reconstr Surg 2003;111:387–394

Breast Reduction and Cancer in the Gland Remnant

Beniamino Palmieri, Giorgia Benuzzi, Alberto Costa

87.1
Introduction

Breast reduction (BR) operation is a plastic procedure based on different surgical techniques, aiming at reducing the breast volume when it has reached an excessive size, thus worsening the quality of life of the affected women. The problem of cancer either as an incidental finding during operation or in the long term after surgery has been widely investigated in the last 20 years; specifically, the management of unexpected tumours, and the relationship between the amount of tissue removed and the cancerogenesis of the remnant gland, with or without a case-control comparison, have been the focus.

The up-to-date literature concerning extra-cosmetic outcome of breast reduction surgery emphasizes improvement of both physical and psychological postoperative symptoms. The problem of occult synchronous cancer and cancer occurring in the scarred mammary gland in the long-term follow up is a very intriguing issue. In the last 20 years, some studies both on animals and humans have been addressed to the relationship between the amount of tissue removed and cancerogenesis of the remnant gland, with or without case-control investigation. Our review evaluates the incidence and relationship between breast reduction and cancer, either in terms of intra-postoperative cancer observation or of the curative potential of breast reduction techniques when cancer arises in hypertrophied glands. There is some significant evidence that breast reduction surgery does decrease the risk for breast (up to 48%) and other types of cancers in many cases, the actual risk being lower for patients older than 40-years-old, and depending on the amount of tissue removed.

Breast reduction surgery is, partially, a tumour preventive operation in those patients presenting various degrees of breast hypertrophy and some evidence of breast cancer in parents or relatives, and also allows contralateral symmetry after mastectomy and reconstruction. Its tumour-preventing potential would hopefully be increased, if a subcutaneous nipple sparing mastectomy might be enclosed in the reduction protocol, with a suitable technique.

The authors reviewed the available clinical studies (Tables 87.1–87.3) trying to outline an adequate pre-intraoperative diagnostic protocol, and to design the future trends of the procedure from the oncologic point of view.

87.2
Clinical Studies

The first report from Lund et al. (1987) [1] (Table 87.1) describes 1,245 women aged between 20 and 70 years, who underwent breast reduction in Denmark between 1943 and 1971 with different surgical procedures. They observed 18 cases of breast cancer and expected 30.28, for a relative risk (R.R.) (defined as the ratio between observed and expected cancers) of 0.39. In the first 10 years of follow up, 5 cases were detected, and 7.11 expected; after 10 years 13 cases were observed versus the 23.17 expected. The greatest advantage in reducing cancer risk was experienced in those women with 600 g or more tissue removed (R.R = 0.31, 95% confidence interval 0.06–0.91).

Nine years later Baasch et al. (1996), [2] following up the original group of Lund et al. up to 1990, fixed the relative risk at 0.61, and supported Lund's observation that 600 g weight or more was the critical resected specimen mass needed to achieve a significant cancer risk reduction. This long run follow up (19 years) on 1,240 patients gave 32 observed cancers versus the 52.55 expected; the women operated on at age 20 or less had a substantial but nonstatistically significant risk of malignancy compared to the general populations or other age groups. In his Copenhagen series there was a 30% reduction in risk seen among women aged between 21 and 40 in the long term follow-up with 20.7% of the group of patients 40-years-old or more being nulliparous, compared with the 20% in the general population, and with the number of children being 1.7 and mean age 24.0 at the first birth, similar to the general population. The long-term follow up did not show any specific trend toward cancer occurrence. The population compliance to X-rays screening for preoperatively detecting small cancers in women over 50-years-old should

M.A. Shiffman (ed.), *Mastopexy and Breast Reduction: Principles and Practice*,
Springer-Verlag Berlin Heidelberg 2009

Table 87.1 Previous studies concerning clinical data[a]

First author (year)	T_N (age)	C_r	C_E[b]	Relative risk (C.I.)	Follow-up (year) and R.R.	Risk factors (R.R.)
Lund [1] (1987)	1,245 (20–70)	18	30.28	0.59 (0.35–0.94)	10 years: R.R. = 0.70	N.R.
Baasch [2] (1996)	1,240 Lund's patients	32 [1]	52.55	0.61 (0.42–0.86)	10 or more years later: R.R. = 0.56 As the previous study, up to 1990 (19 further years)	N.R.
Brinton [3] (1996)	2,174 cases 2,009 controls (<55) 10 cases with MR vs. 13 controls	N.R.	N.R.	0.5% of N had MR got R.R. = 0.7 (0.3–1.6)	< 5 years: R.R. = 0 5–9 years: R.R. = 1.44 10 + years: R.R. = 0.69	race: RR = 1.2 late age at first birth: RR = 1.6 for 30 + vs. < 20 years old. biopsy or benign breast disease: RR = 1.4 mother or sister's breast cancer: RR = 2.3 long-term use of oral contraceptives: RR = 1.3 for 10 + years vs. < 6 months
Boice [4] (1997)	7,720 (13–79)	182	209	0.9 (0.7–1.0)	0–17 (Average 7.5)	Significantly reduced risk only among 40 + years old women (RR = 0.5) especially > 50 (RR = 0.3)
Brown [5] (1999)	27,500 (15–60+)	Breast 101	165.8[d]	Breast cancer 0.61 (0.50–0.74)	Average 6.5 years At 10 years: 86 observed vs. 147.0 expected (R.R. = 0.59); the remaining 15 cases occurred 10 to 14 years post op. (R.R. = 0.80)	Decrease in risk not highly correlated with age: 15–29 years old. R.R. = 0.47 (0.01–2.37) 30–49 years old. R.R. = 0.53 (0.36–0.75) 50 + years old. R.R. = 0.66 (0.51–0.83)

(continued)

Boice [6] (2000)	31910 (11–87)	662 different types: breast 161	729 223.9	0.91 (0.84–0.98) 0.72 (0.61–0.84)	0–30 (Average 7.5)	Risk reduced especially for 50 + years old. (R.R. = 0.57) and for those followed for 5 + years (R.R. = 0.68)
Brinton [7] (2001)	31910 (11–87) 161 developed subsequently breast cancer	137 compared with 422 controls	223.9	0.72 (0.61–0.84)	Up to 28 years (1965–1993)[e]	Height weight, Body Mass Index, Parity, N. of children, Oral contraceptive use, Hormone replacement therapy

[a]Abbreviations:
- T_N: total number of analysed cases
- C_F: number of breast cancers found among T_N
- C_E: number of breast cancers expected among T_N
- N.R.: not explicitly reported

[b]*Note*: the expected number of breast cancers was estimated, if anything is explicitly said, by multiplying age and calendar-time specific breast cancer incidence rates from a specific Registry by the appropriate person-years follow-up

[c]R.R.: ratio of observed and expected numbers of breast cancers *(useful as a measure of correlation between mammaplasty and risk of B.C.)* C.I. = confidence interval, calculated at 95%

[d]Calculated by using the PERSON YEARS program [8]

[e]This study was accomplished by calculating the person-years of observation, begun at 3 months after the date of BR and ended either at the date of death, migration or December 31,1993

Table 87.2 Comparison between the studies performed by Jansen et al. (1998) [9] and Snyderman and Lizardo (1960) [10]

	Jansen et al. [9]	Snyderman and Lizardo [10]
Total number of cases	2,576	5,008
Breast carcinoma diagnosed during the preoperative work-up	0	5
Breast carcinoma diagnosed from surgical specimen	4	14
Total breast carcinomas detected	5	19
Incidence of malignancy in operative findings	0.16%	0.38%

explain the substantial tumour incidence reduction in the 5 years follow-up: two cancers observed versus the 12 expected, but under 50-years-old this effect has not been seen, the overall observed tumours being 12 against the 12.2 expected. No significant variations were observed with any type of technique, date of operation, place of surgery and quadrant.

As to the relationship between the incidence of cancer and age, it has to be stressed that younger females are usually slimmer compared to the older ones with large breasts; older women are often overweight or frankly obese: this might increase the risk of tumourigenesis, and also the protection offered by breast reduction surgery. In fact, not only is the glandular mass that is potentially expected to become malignant reduced, but so also are a large number of adipocytes in the fat tissue, that are responsible for enhancing hormone co-carcinogenic potential transforming androstenedione into estrogens through aromatase.

A small population-based case-control report on BR ad cancer, by Brinton et al. (1996) [3] was part of an investigation on surgical breast enlargement which included 2,174 patients and 2,009 controls with previous breast implants but only 10 reductive mastoplasties and 13 controls. In the prosthesis group the observed percentage of cancers was 36 cases (1.1%) versus 44 (2.%) of the controls who showed a risk reduction, R.R., of 0.2 and an R.R. of 0.8 for both localized and distant tumours: the risk reduction in reductive mastoplasties was 0.7% (95% CI 0.4–1.0).

Boice et al. (1997) [4] examined 7,720 women from the Danish hospital discharge registry, who had undergone breast reduction between 1977 and 1992, with specific focus on risk by age and time since surgery. The median age at the time of surgery was 46 years and the mean follow-up was 7.5 years. One hundred eighty two various types of cancer were observed in the follow-up, compared with the 209 expected (standardized incidence ratio SIR = 0.9, 95% CI 0.7–1.0). Specifically, breast cancers were reduced roughly to 50% (29 observed vs. the 53.9 expected with R.R. = 0.54). Patients' age at surgery was meaningful in that the risk reduced at the age of 40, and subsequently at 50 to an overall of 70%.

Jansen et al. (1998) [9], from a retrospective study of 2,576 breast reductions, reported 4 cases (0.16%) of intra operative cancer detection, that had escaped routine mammography, self examination and physical examination by the surgeons. This different rate of incidental tumour finding at the time of reduction surgery might be explained on the basis of different accuracy in preoperative breast examination. Nearly 660 patients with preexisting breast cancer with the risk for the contralateral operated breast, exposed to high risk of cancer before the operation was subsequently found not at risk.

Brown et al. (1999) [5] using the Canadian Institute for Health databank identified 30,137 women submitted to bilateral (94.7%) or unilateral (5.3%) breast reduction between 1979 and 1992. The final eligible cases were 26,567 bilateral and 933 unilateral reductions; of this latter group 412 patients had prior breast cancer, 314 had prior or synchronous cancer, and 87 of these (27.7%) had specific breast cancer, with 18 cases detected during the operation.

Among the 26,567 operated women, 101 cancers were observed compared with the expected 165.8, yielding a R.R. of 0.61 (95% CI 0.50–0.74). As to all the other primary cancers, there were 285 cases observed and 372.5 expected with R.R. = 0.77 (95% CI 0.68 –0.86). Lung cancer, cervical carcinoma and non colorectal gastrointestinal tract tumours were most frequently observed, but they also presented a well defined reduced risk to 0.59, 0.51 and 0.58 respectively; probably this benefit was due to postoperative lifestyle changes, such as stopping smoking, increasing physical activity and weight reduction. Evaluating the breast cancer incidence, in the first 10 postoperative years, 86 were observed versus the 147 expected; the remaining 15 cases occurred 10–14 years after the initial surgery; thus the relative risk in the first 10 years was 0.59 (95% CI 0.47–0.72): for the remaining 4 years it rose up to 0.80 (95% CI 0.45–1.32). No difference in risk between groups evaluated on decades of age was observed.

Tang et al. (1999) [16] reported a cohort study of breast cancer risk in breast reduction patients (27,500 cases and cancers found 101) following a contemporary Tang et al. [17] report that had shown a 40% reduction in the risk of developing breast cancer after breast reduction. In his retrospective survey, the author describes the diagnosis of cancer between 3 months and

Table 87.3 Combination of reduction mastoplasty with mastectomy and other oncologic procedures

First author (year)	T_N (age)	Surgical procedure	Follow-up	Breast tissue removed (g)	Complication rates	Cosmetic result	Oncologic result
Shestak [11] (1993)	4 with macromastia-hypertrophy and breast carcinoma	Wise pattern: 2 inferior pedicle 2 resection and transplantation of the nipple	7–43 months	825 on average	N.R.	N.R	All patients are alive and without disease
Clough [12] (1995)	20 with lower quadrant breast cancer (41–70)	Wide lumpectomy combined with superior pedicle mastoplasty and pre-op (9) and post-op (11) irradiation	1–7.5 years (mean 4.5) At a mean 4 years follow up: 17 out of 20 are in complete remission, 1 is treated for metastases and 2 died from metastases	248 on average	1 case: local recurrence 4 cases: metastases (same oncologic results as lumpectomy and irradiation)	At 1 year: Very Good: 75% Moderate: 20% Poor: 5% (nipple areola necrosis)	3 years after surgery: Only one distant recurrence
Cothier-Savey [13] (1996)	70	RM contralateral mastopexy	9–43 months (mean 21)	120–440 (mean 350)	N.R.	N.R	N.R
Smith [14] (1998)	10 RM for breast cancer followed by irradiation (59 years old., on average)	Bilateral RM Radiotherapy: 4 weeks after surgery	8–37 months (no recurrence)	945 on average	No complications arising from the surgery or radiation therapy	From good to excellent	N.R
Spear [15] (1998)	3 cases of RM with previous radiation and mastectomy (average age: 46.3 years old)	RM performed 3–16 months after surgery Lumpectomy and axillary dissection	3 to 18 months (reported only for 1 case)	711.7 on average	fibrous mastopathy fibrocystic changes and apocrine metaplasia edematous breast for several months; stromal fibrosis	N.R	N.R

13 years after mammaplasty with a median of 5 years. The median age of the patients when submitted to reduction was 50 years, and their average age at cancer detection was 55, a significantly younger age if compared with 61 of the average cancer detection in the general population. This difference might be explained in terms of more attention and awareness that the breast-reduced women focused on their gland health, with an easier physical and instrumental exploration of the reduced parenchyma. Histology and distribution were similar to control cases, as well as surgical and oncologic protocols: the survival rate at 5 years was 70% in the reduced breast and 77 in the control group, a not significant difference confirmed also by the overlapping of the lower and upper confidence level.

Boice et al. (2000) [6] investigated the oncologic impact of breast reduction on 31,910 women, excluding cancers occurring before and within 3 months of surgery. The mean age at surgery was 33 years and the mean length of follow-up was 7.5 years. Six hundred and sixty-two cancers were observed and 729 were expected (SIR = 0.91, 95% CI 0.84–0.98) with a 28% breast cancer reduction (161 detected vs. 223 expected, SIR=0.72, 95% CI 0.61–0.84). Lung cancer was also reduced (SIR = 0.73) as well as melanoma (SIR = 0.72). Corpus uteri cancer (SIR = 1.37), thyroid (SIR = 1.39), other endocrine tumours (SIR = 1.55), parathyroid adenomas (SIR = 1.51) were found increased post operatively. The inverse association between age at surgery with cancer risk is also confirmed in this study: in fact it was reduced 24 and 43% between the group 40–49, and the group over 50 respectively.

Brinton et al. (2001) [7] focused their investigation on the amount of tissue removed during reduction mastoplasty toward breast cancer risk: they examined 137 breast reduction specimens and 422 control patients: subjects with more than 800 g removed had a 76% decreased risk relative to those who had more than 400 g of tissue removed from either breast, irrespective of the age at surgery. Probably the weak protection from cancer in patients operated before 40 years should be related to the lower volume of tissue removed due to the minor weight of young women compared with older ones, but also to the genetic impact of cancer early in life; thus a longer follow-up would allow to correctly evaluate the life span.

87.3
Breast Reduction and Cancer: Incidental Findings and Intentional Treatment

The incidental finding of breast cancer during cosmetic or symmetrical reconstructive breast reduction (Table 87.3), has been reported by some authors, [9, 16, 18–20] but it has to be stressed adequately in order to achieve a preoperative diagnosis and correct planning of tumour surgery. Rees et al. (1972) [20] some years ago outlined the opportunity of careful macroscopic intra operative fat and gland examination, with further microscopic inspection to detect unrecognized tumours. Petit et al. (1997) [18] who operated on 440 contralateral breasts for symmetric correction observed 22 (4.4%) occult undetected cancers in the surgical specimen, which were located in the lower quadrant-central area in 70% of the cases. Their size ranged between 3 and 16 mm, 12 of the tumours were in situ and 10 ductal infiltrating neoplasms. The author stresses the opportunity of performing this reconstructive procedure, from the oncologic point of view, to achieve symmetry of the breast area, thus preventing further tumour incidence on the other side.

Jansen et al. (1998) [9] starting from occult breast carcinoma occurring during surgical practice collected a questionnaire from the 43% of the plastic surgeons in New Orleans area. In 2,576 BR patients, no carcinomas were detected in the preoperative evaluation (self breast exam, physician exam and preoperative mammography). There were four malignancies in the surgical specimens with a rate of 0.16% of breast carcinoma. This incidental finding is significantly lower than the 0.38% of Syndeman and Lizardo [10] (Table 87.4). This difference might be due to a better mammographic screening that has 85% sensitivity in detecting carcinomas in all the age groups. Keleher et al. (2003) [19] reported from M.D Anderson Cancer Centre that incidental breast cancer was found in 4 patients who underwent BR, three of whom had no preoperative mammogram. All the patients underwent modified radical mastectomy. In order to improve cancer detection at the time of BR surgery, the authors suggested the following guidelines for different protocols on the basis of the women's age; accordingly the American Cancer Society [21] recommends (1) breast examination with ultrasound every 1–3 years by a doctor for patients between 20 and 39, with repeated self breast exam regularly in between and (2) early physical breast examination, screening mammography and breast self-examination for patients at 40 years or above regularly. The women who have high risk of developing cancer are further subdivided into four groups:

(a) Group with previous thoracic irradiation: annual mammography and breast examination every 6 months by a doctor, to begin 10 years after radiotherapy and not before 35 years.
(b) Women with a prospective 5-year risk of invasive breast carcinoma ≥ 1.7%: according to Gail model: medical examination every 1–3 years and regular breast self-exam.
(c) Women ≥ 35 years of age with risk > 1.7%: mammography and physical examination plus breast self-examination are prescribed.
(d) Women at genetic risk for breast cancer (at least 2 breast cancers and 1 or more ovarian cancer in

Table 87.4 Breast cancer found at the time of reduction mammaplasty

First author (year)	T_N (age range)	C_L and cancer location	Surgical procedure	Follow-up
Petit [18] (1997)	440	In RM 20 occulte 4.6%	813 (total Contralateral BR)	N.R.
		In lower and central quadrants (70%)	440 RM 373 Mastopexies	
Jansen [9] (1998)	2576	2 cases not found preoperatively by mammography and self exam	Case 1: unilateral modified radical mastectomy and immediate reconstruction	2 years free of cancer 1.5 years
			Case 2: right: bilateral modified radical mastectomy; left: total mastectomy and immediate reconstruction with TRAM flap	
Tang [17] (1999)	27500 105 controls 17 (incidence 0.06%) had breast cancer at the time of RM (49 years old, average)	Breast cancer found at 49 years old for women undergoing RM, while the average age at diagnosis is 61 years old	Bilateral BR: All 17 with breast cancer found at the time of RM	8 years
Brown [5] (1999)	27500 18 cases of incidental finding out of 314 bilateral RM	Breast cancer	Bilateral (96.7% of eligible cases)	Average 6.5 years
			Unilateral (3.4% of eligible cases)	
Keleher [19] (2003)	Incidental findings	4 cases not found preoperatively by mammography and self exam at M.D. Anderson Cancer	Case 1: secondary skin sparing modified lateral mastectomy	Two months
			Case 2: skin sparing modified mastectomy and expander reconstruction	One month
			Case 3: classic bilateral breast reduction	Six months
			Case 4: modified radical mastectomy without reconstruction	N.R. follow-up

parents and relatives; incidence of breast cancer in sisters before 50-years-old, and various penetrance of ovarian mixed with breast cancer in the family). In these cases annual mammography and medical breast examination every 6 months have to be started 5–10 years before the age of the youngest relative affected. BRCA-1 BRCA-2 mutations can involve multiple genes and thus show different expressions of tumours and their follow-up has to be individualized.

The surgical technique in case of incidental finding of cancer has to have extensive dissection performed in order to leave at least 1 cm of tumour-free breast tissue. The suspected specimen margins have to be marked with ink for correct pathological orientation.

Different containers for the specimen from each breast quadrant have to be sent to the pathologist, and if the diagnosis of suspected tissues is confirmed, a radical modified mastectomy with node dissection and potential reconstruction should be considered. In this case Keleher suggests approaching mastectomy through the keyhole incision of breast reduction technique, removing a block of the nipple–areola complex with a final vertical and horizontal scar. If the tumour is multicentric and cannot be safely and completely removed with the previously planned incision, the operation can be converted to a standard mastectomy with a different final scar. Tang et al. (1999) [16] identified 17 women with breast cancer at the time of BR out of 27,500 (incidence 0.06%), patients enrolled with over 13 years and 6 months of follow-up. The average age of this intra-operative cancer group was 49 years and all the patients underwent bilateral operation. The follow-up of this specific cohort was 8 years. 35% of the cancers were suspected at the operating table and 65% were identified by the pathologist. 65% were ductal and 35% lobular carcinomas. 29% were lymph node positive. In the control group (105 women) selected from Ontario Canada Cancer Registry Database between 1979 and 1993 the mean age of the patients was 61 years and 86% had ductal carcinoma, 10% lobular and 4% ductal and lobular mixed; they had 42% lymph node metastases.

Thirty-three percent of the breast reduction group had partial mastectomy at the time of breast reduction without any further operation; 67% had modified radical mastectomy. In the control groups there were 48 partial mastectomies and 32 radical modified mastectomies. Radiotherapy was performed in 50% of the BR group and 71% of the comparison group. 25% were treated with chemotherapy and hormonal therapy compared with 60% of the comparison group. The 5-year survival rate for breast cancer was 88% in the breast reduction and 67% in the comparison group. The explanation for the high incidence of lobular carcinoma (35%) compared with 11% of the control, should be due to the fact that this multicentric tumour is more difficult to detect either clinically or mammographically. Tang [16] suggests that the gold standard treatment of intra operative detected breast cancer should be mastectomy, because typical breast reduction rotates the quadrants and modifies the anatomy of the area to be treated with radiation, with further risk of tumour seeding. The cancer found during reductive surgery in this report affects younger women with earlier diagnosis and a minor number with involved lymph nodes and a better than 5-year survival.

87.4
Breast Reduction as First Choice Oncologic Procedure

Other authors [12–15] have emphasized the role of reduction mammaplasty (RM) in cancer operated breast remodelling, either contralaterally, or on the same side of a previous quadrantectomy, which is usually cosmetically quite unpleasant (Table 87.2).

Shestak et al. (1993) [11] were the first to suggest RM in four patients with macromastia or mammary hypertrophy and simultaneous carcinoma of the breast. The operation consisted of keyhole markings and wide mammary gland resection with two inferior pedicle reconstruction, and two resections and transplantation of the nipple with an average specimen weight of 825 g. The follow-up between 7 and 43 months was disease-free, and in the author's opinion, this strategy is very well accepted for cosmetic reasons, and it is also quite effective in terms of radiation target and easier postoperative self-examination.

Cothier-Savey et al. (1996) [13] suggested RM as a safe procedure for breast cancer instead of quadrantectomy, followed by chemo and radiotherapy. She evaluated 70 patients operated upon between 1983 and 1991 with breast reduction and contralateral mastopexy. The cases were matched as to age, history, stage, pathology of the tumours, etc. The 5 year overall survival was 85% with 5% local relapses (detected in an interval of 9–43 months, 21 months on average) and 81% patient satisfaction. The morbidity–mortality rate was not superior to the quadrantectomy, and postoperative treatment was the same. The difference of survival and relapse, based on histology and tumour size led to the observation that of the 36 patients with a tumour of diameter more than 3 cm, local relapses were 3% and actuarial survival 79%. Among all the patients an actuarial rate of 8.5% of local relapses was globally found at 5 years, next to an average delay of illness appearance of 21 months. In situ cancers were found in 24.2% of the cases, while the remaining were infiltrating cancers; this last group showed local relapse in 8% of the cases with an actuarial survival of 84% at 5 years. The cosmetic outcome was judged to be very good in 39% of the cases, fair in 36%, acceptable in

24% and poor in 1%. The reduction specimens weighed between 120 and 440 g with an average of 350 g, and nipple areola complex was always evaluated with frozen sections, in order to exclude any cancer infiltration.

Clough et al. (1995) [12] described 20 patients with lower quadrant cancers between 1983 and 1993, treated with remodelling mammaplasty with nipple bearing superior pedicle, preceded (9 cases) or followed (11 cases) by radiation. Contralateral breast was rendered symmetrical at the same time. The mean resection weight was 248 g (40–540 g).

Pathologic examination showed free margins and contralaterally fibrocystic disease in 13 patients and a single case of epithelial proliferation. The only one serious postoperative complication was nipple areola necrosis that required debridement and full thickness skin graft. With a mean follow up of 4.5 years there were 1 local recurrence and 4 distant metastasis with no difference from the oncologic point of view in comparison to similar stage-size cancers.

Between 1996 and 1998 Smith et al. (1998) [14], performed 10 bilateral breast reductions for breast malignancy followed by radiation therapy. The average amount of tissue removed was 945 g per breast; radiotherapy started 4 weeks after surgery with 50 Gy in 25 sessions. Follow up was for 37 months, without recurrence. The cosmetic outcome was excellent, and in the authors' opinion, in suitable women with large ptotic breast and cancer the reductive choice should be primarily considered.

Spear et al. (1998) [15] describe the RM procedure in three cases conservatively operated and radiated for breast cancer. The reductive procedure was performed 3–16 months after surgery; the technical note in this very selected cohort of patients was to prepare wide and short flaps, with very little undermining of the skin to avoid dehiscence and ulceration due to post radiation fibrosis.

The overall number of patients treated for cancer is not large enough to give evidence that this treatment can have a specific role in breast surgery oncologic protocols.

These anecdotic reports cautiously emphasize the cosmetic role of the reducing technique in supporting the psychological distress of women toward amputation perspective introducing a single bilateral procedure.

87.5
Discussion

The problem of breast reduction is really not only actually cosmetic, but also oncologic in perspective; thus we do have evidence, based on the literature reports, that a critical reduction of the amount of gland and fat tissue significantly lowers, in the long run, the breast cancer incidence in the operated cohort of patients (Table 87.3).

Symmetric reduction after contralateral modified mastectomy and breast reconstruction is an advisable procedure: in fact the increased risk of the patient due to impending exposure to carcinogenic factors is counteracted by gland tissue subtraction.

The breast reduction technique as a specific oncologic procedure in some types of cancer developed in the lower quadrants in hypertrophic glands should be cautiously considered, on the basis of wider and accurate case-control investigations: these preliminary literature reports might be the pilot background for a multicenter surgical trial: the psychological comfort of the patients submitted to such a procedure, and followed by radiotherapy and chemotherapy without cosmetically devastating effects, is an adequate stimulus to follow this method.

As to the incidental findings of cancer during breast reduction procedure, the authors think that with a more accurate screening policy, and with the plastic surgeon's sensitization toward careful preoperative planning of physical and instrumental investigation, they should virtually disappear; in fact the unexpected cancer identification is a source of distress to the patient, and creates sudden management problems to the surgeon: the gland specimens, individually for each quadrant, must be anyway submitted to detailed pathological examination.

If an occult breast carcinoma is microscopically identified the reductive mastoplasty will anyway mean an early and effective oncologic strategy. The breast reduction, when its enlargement has reached a symptomatic clinical level, should therefore be emphasized not only as a restorative procedure for the patient's fitness and wellness, as was demonstrated by the authors in a previous extensive literature review, but also as an effective subtraction of the aging gland tissue inhibiting potential cancerization.

Women should be made aware of undergoing a total subcutaneous mastectomy, targeted to specific physical improvement, and also to cancer prevention, with some scars on the breast, but with a marked substantial cosmetic outcome. Many women probably might take the challenge to submit themselves to this procedure, if oncologic prevention has to be achieved; in the RM operated women, cancer risk reduction has otherwise also been observed, for other types of tumours, such as lung or G.I. We do not take note of a genetic relationship that might exist between breast gland plus fat tissue reduction and cancer growth in general: the role of the changes in lifestyle, probably related to improved self-esteem and image, as well as to the improvement or disappearance of arthro-muscular pain and discomfort, might actually be the up-to-date reasonable explanation of this phenomenon.

We should encourage breast reduction in order to improve the well-being status of the patients and also in an oncologic preventive perspective. Our suggestion is to remove as much of the gland tissue as possible during breast reduction converting the classic pedicle, and partial gland resection technique, in a formal nipple sparing "radical" modified subcutaneous mastectomy; the preliminary nipple–areola complex vascular autonomization is obtained with a further mini-invasive "office" procedure that has to be done 2–4 weeks before the main operation.

This strategy of a more appealing middle-aged woman on the background of completely preventing the breast cancer should be very well accepted, especially by patients with various degrees of breast hypertrophy, and some evidence of breast cancer in parents or relatives.

References

1. Lund K, Ewertz M, Schou G: Breast cancer incidence subsequent to surgical reduction of the female breast. Scand J Plast Reconstr Surg Hand Surg 1987;21(2):209–212
2. Baasch M, Nielsen SF, Engholm G, Lund K: Breast cancer incidence subsequent to surgical reduction of the female breast. Br J Cancer 1996;73(7):961–963
3. Brinton LA, Malone KE, Coates RJ, Schoenberg JB, Swanson CA, Daling JR, Stanford JL: Breast enlargement and reduction: results from a breast cancer case-control study. Plast Reconstr Surg 1996;97(2):269–275
4. Boice JD Jr, Friis S, McLaughlin JK, Mellemkjaer L, Blot WJ, Fraumeni JR, Olsen JH: Cancer following breast reduction surgery in Denmark. Cancer Causes Control 1997;8(2):253–258
5. Brown MH, Weinberg M, Chong N, Levine R, Holowaty E: A cohort study of breast cancer risk in breast reduction patients. Plast Reconstr Surg 1999;103(6):1674–1681
6. Boice JD Jr, Persson I, Brinton LA, Hober M, McLaughlin JK, Blot WJ, Fraumeni JF Jr, Nyren O: Breast cancer following breast reduction surgery in Sweden. Plast Reconstr Surg 2000;106(4):755–762
7. Brinton LA, Persson I, Boice JD Jr, McLaughlin JK, Fraumeni JF Jr: Breast cancer risk in relation to amount of tissue removed during breast reduction operations in Sweden. Cancer 2001;91(3):478–483
8. Coleman M, Douglas A, Hermon C, Peto J: Cohort study analysis with a FORTRAN computer program. Int J Epidemiol 1986;15(1):134–137
9. Jansen DA, Murphy M, Kind GM, Sands K: Breast cancer in reduction mammoplasty: Case reports and a survey of plastic surgeons. Plast Reconstr Surg 1998;101(2): 361–364
10. Snyderman RK, Lizardo JG: Statistical study of malignancies found before, during, or after routine breast plastic operations. Plast Reconstr Surg 1960;25:253–256
11. Shestak KC, Johnson RR, Greco RJ, Williams SL: Partial mastectomy and breast reduction as a valuable treatment option for patients with macromastia and carcinoma of the breast. Surg Gynecol Obstet 1993;177(1):54–56
12. Clough KB, Nos C, Salmon RJ, Soussaline M, Durand JC: Conservative treatment of breast cancers by mammaplasty and irradiation: a new approach to lower quadrant tumors. Plast Reconstr Surg 1995;96(2):363–370
13. Cothier-Savey I, Otmezguine Y, Calitchi E, Sabourin JC, Le Bourgeois JP, Baruch J. Value of reduction mammoplasty in the conservative treatment of breast neoplasms. Apropos of 70 cases. Ann Chir Plast Esthet 1996;41(4):346–533
14. Smith ML, Evans GR, Gurlek A, Bouvet M, Singletary SE, Ames FC, Janjan N, McNeese MD: Reduction mammaplasty: its role in breast conservation surgery for early-stage breast cancer. Ann Plast Surg 1998;41(3):234–239
15. Spear SL, Burke JB, Forman D, Zuurbier RA, Berg CD: Experience with reduction mammaplasty following breast conservation surgery and radiation therapy. Plast Reconstr Surg 1998;102(6):1913–1916
16. Tang CL, Brown MH, Levine R, Sloan M, Chong N, Holowaty E: A follow-up study of 105 women with breast cancer following reduction mammaplasty. Plast Reconstr Surg 1999;103(6):1687–1690
17. Tang CL, Brown MH, Levine R, Sloan M, Chong N, Holowaty E: Breast cancer found at the time of breast reduction. Plast Reconstr Surg 1999;103(6):1682–1686
18. Petit JY, Rietjens M, Contesso G, Bertin F, Gilles R: Contralateral mastoplasty for breast reconstruction: a good opportunity for glandular exploration and occult carcinomas diagnosis. Ann Surg Oncol 1997;4(6): 511–515
19. Keleher AJ, Langstein HN, Ames FC, Ross, MI, Chang DW, Reece GP, Singletary SE: Breast cancer in reduction mammaplasty specimens: Case reports and guidelines. Breast J 2003;9(2):120–125
20. Rees TD, Coburn R: Breast reduction: is it an aid to cancer detection? Br J Plast Surg 1972;25(2):144–146
21. Smith RA, Mettlin CJ, Davis KJ, Eyre H: American Cancer Society guidelines for the early detection of cancer. CA Cancer J Clin 2000;50(1):34–49

Breast Cancer and Reduction Mammoplasty

David A. Jansen, Mary Catherine Ghere, Mark Lee, Madeline O. Jansen

88.1 Introduction

An age specific algorithm for preoperative work up, intraoperative considerations, and necessary histopathology for surgical specimens:

> The diagnosis of invasive carcinoma presents a surgical dilemma when discovered incidentally at breast reduction mammoplasty. Subsequent surgical and therapeutic management for such cases have not been established. Although management and treatment may very according to patient preference, a review of the literature of the past four decades yielded scant discussion of the topic.
> Rudolph and Niedbala [1].

Breast reduction is an extremely common procedure with around 100,000 cases performed annually in the United States. A growing number of women are having the surgery for a variety of reasons. Classically breast reduction is indicated for women with macromastia, who often complain of associated neck, back, or other musculoskeletal pain. These women may also progress to more debilitating ailments such as kyphosis, deep furrows with possible excoriations from bra straps, chronic intertrigo in the folds beneath the breasts, and ulnar nerve paresthesias from traction on the ulnar nerve. Large breasts become pendulous and can hinder physical exercise and daily function as well. Other reasons women desire the procedure are purely cosmetic for symmetry or what they perceive as more appropriately sized breasts. Breast reduction is also often employed for symmetry of the contralateral breast following mastectomy and breast reconstruction.

Despite the frequency of this procedure, guidelines for preoperative work-up, intraoperative tissue removal, marking, and consistent histopathological analysis have not been established. This chapter will provide a review of the literature and establish what is the best preoperative workup for women of different age groups undergoing reduction mammoplasty, will discuss techniques for marking removed tissue in different risk groups for the purpose of maintaining orientation during histopathology and possibly for future treatment decisions and will detail the ideal histopathology that surgical specimens should receive following excision as this is a unique opportunity to thoroughly examine the breast tissue.

Any surgeon who operates on the breast must be prepared to deal with potential breast pathology, especially cancer of the breast. Breast cancer is the leading cancer of women excluding cancers of the skin. It represents one in three cancer diagnoses in US women, with a lifetime incidence of 13.2% or roughly one in eight women [2]. Over 200,000 cases are diagnosed annually. Of these roughly 40,000 die each year [2]. Though the incidence increases with age, breast cancer affects women of all ages. The median age of onset is 61 years [2]. With half of the breast cancers occurring in women under 61, this poses unique considerations for surgeons performing elective breast reductions as most women opting for this surgery are in the age group of 20–50.

A limited number of case reports and statistical analyses have brought to light the need for the surgeon to have breast cancer in mind before, during and after breast reduction surgery. Snyderman and Lizardo (1959) [3] were the first to give a statistical study of malignancies found before, during, or after routine breast plastic operations. They found the breast cancer incidence to be 0.3% overall and 0.4% when narrowed to breast reduction alone. In 1963 Pitanguy [4] revisited the concept of discovering breast pathology from elective breast surgery. In his series he looked at 181 consecutive elective breast operations performed by plastic surgeons where breast tissue was removed for, "functional, aesthetic, and psychological reasons." He determined the cancer incidence to be 1.5%. In the author's survey in 1998 [5] based on a questionnaire given to plastic surgeons in the New Orleans area, the cancer incidence was found to be 0.16%. In the author's review of the literature, the incidence of breast cancer discovered via reduction mammoplasty is somewhere between 0.16 and 1.6%.

In 2004 a report by Hage and Karim [6] provided a summary of the breast cancer incidence found in the literature, and their results are similar to the author's findings. They determined the incidence to be somewhere between 0.05 and 1.66%.

When reviewing several of these studies, Colwell et al. [7] commented on the wide ranges of the incidence

M.A. Shiffman (ed.), *Mastopexy and Breast Reduction: Principles and Practice*,
© Springer-Verlag Berlin Heidelberg 2009

determined from different researchers, pointing out that not all used the same criteria for patient inclusion. In particular Synderman and Lizardo [3] included those with cancer detected in the preoperative workup, perhaps falsely elevating their incidence, while Tang et al. [8] only included invasive cancers leaving out ductal carcinoma in situ. Colwell et al. [7] also point out that there were probable differences in pathological assessment given that it was performed at different facilities. Furthermore, there is also a possible difference in incidence due to an inherent bias with different patient populations.

Colwell et al. [7] found the incidence to be 0.8% in their own study based on a review of 800 reduction mammoplasties over a 14-year period from the same institution. One pathology department performed all histopathological assessments. In addition to their hypotheses as to why studies reveal such a wide range of incidence, they also propose that the incidence may vary depending on the indication for surgery and stratified their patient population accordingly. They included those diagnosed during surgery and from the histopathology of the removed tissue.

It is clear from the above studies, as well as others not mentioned, that breast cancer being discovered from elective breast reduction is a rare and a distinct possibility for surgeons performing these operations. So why hasn't there been a consensus regarding what to do prior to, during, and after reaching breast reduction? In the author's opinion it is related to the fact that it is rare that the surgeon encounters this problem. Other possible reasons are that screening for breast cancer is a constantly evolving target, with the guidelines frequently changing. Complicating matters more is the age group of women that undergo breast reduction. Though the age is rising, they still tend to be younger women under the age of 40 where breast cancer screening is even more controversial and a relatively gray area.

What to do when cancer is discovered during breast reduction is extremely difficult to standardize as these surgeries are performed in many different settings such as outpatient surgery centers and university hospitals. There is a big difference in what these institutions can offer the patient. Additionally if women have not been counseled before the surgery as to the possibility of carcinoma, a surgeon's hands are tied should mastectomy or more extensive dissection or tissue removal be indicated.

For those cancers found from the histopathological review of removed tissue, determining the next step for the patient can be difficult for several reasons. Most surgeons separate right from left breast when sending tissue to pathology, but there may be no other tissue orientation. A pathologist will not know what quadrant the pathology is in or what the margins are. These are two things that can have a major role in determining treatment options. With all these things in mind, it is easy to see why no solid rules have been standardized regarding pre, intra, and postoperative considerations in breast reduction.

88.2
Preoperative Considerations

…the chance of finding breast cancer in a reduction specimen is affected by the level of scrutiny of preoperative workup to detect breast cancer. [6]

In general it has been advocated that for women undergoing breast reduction, the surgeon should focus on predisposing factors as well as a personal or family history of breast cancer. Along with the above, most encourage a thorough physical examination as well. Recognizing the limitation of the physical examination when it comes to small tumors, some surgeons recommend mammography. Mammography can be controversial and its indications and utility are unclear in women under 40. Ultrasonography is utilized by some for women under 30, but is by no means employed universally. Even for those physicians using both modalities there is a gap for those women aged between 30 and 39. What is best for this age group is open for debate. In recent years magnetic resonance imaging (MRI) has emerged as another possible tool for detecting breast cancer. Cost and ease of use with MRI must be considered, and its use as a screening tool in asymptomatic women is still being evaluated.

88.2.1
Family/Past Medical History

The use of the patients past medical history and her family history cannot be underestimated. A previous personal breast cancer diagnosis obviously should raise a red flag for the surgeon. According to the American Cancer Society, a woman with a previous breast cancer has a 3–4 times increased risk for developing cancer in the opposite breast or in a different location of the same breast. This refers to an increase in the occurrence of new cancers not recurrence of past disease [2]. Those surgeons performing reduction mammoplasty for symmetry of the contralateral breast after mastectomy and breast reconstruction must be acutely aware of this increased risk. The next question to ask is as to how this changes what the surgeon will do from their standpoint.

A link between a positive family history and a patient's own breast cancer risk has long been appreciated. Approximately 20–30% of women who are diagnosed with breast cancer have a family member with the disease [2]. The extent of how much family history contributes to an individual's risk is known for certain hereditary breast cancers. However there is also a strong association of cancer risk in those with a family history of other breast cancer types for which the heredity is unknown.

Specifically 5–10% of breast cancers are related to mutated BRCA1 or BRCA2 genes. Research indicates that women with either of these mutations have an 80% lifetime breast cancer risk. Cancer also tends to occur at younger ages in these women making this group even more pertinent to our discussion. The BRCA mutations tend to occur in women of Ashkenazi Jewish descent, but are also seen in African–American, and Hispanic women [2].

There are other women who fall into a different category. These women are negative for BRCA1 and BRCA2 mutations but still have immediate family members with a history of breast cancer. Several other genes have been indicated in the development of breast cancer and may explain this other group of women. However at this time it appears that these other gene mutations are extremely rare causes of familial breast cancer and more research is needed to further elucidate their relationship to breast cancer [2].

What we do know for sure is that the family history of a female undergoing breast surgery is very important, whether it be positive or negative. The surgeon should get a thorough history that covers the known risk factors for breast cancer. Any first degree relative with a history of breast cancer should be elucidated. This includes mothers, sisters, and daughters. Having a first-degree relative with breast cancer roughly doubles a woman's risk of developing breast cancer. A history in two first-degree relatives increases her risk five fold. Though rare, breast cancer can occur in men. There is an increased risk for women who have a first-degree male relative with breast cancer, though the exact risk is unknown. In addition to the above, surgeons should inquire as to the following according to the American Cancer Society;

1. Do you have two or more relatives with breast or ovarian cancer?
2. Has breast cancer occurred on either side of the family before the age of 50?
3. Do you have a relative with both breast and ovarian cancer?
4. Do you have a relative with two cancers, in both breasts or breast and ovarian?
5. Do you have a male relative with breast cancer?
6. Do you have a Ashkenazi Jewish heritage?
7. Do you have a family history of Li-Fraumeni or Cowden syndrome?

In today's modern age of DNA technology and genetic screening the question can be posed as to whether women with a strong family history undergo genetic screening for BRCA1 and BRCA2 mutations prior to elective breast surgery. Should all women undergo genetic screening? Would this knowledge affect how the surgeon proceeds or how the pathology specimens are scrutinized? It is hard to know what the repercussions of this knowledge are. Knowing ones genetic risk can have a major impact on a person's life. Not to minimize the emotional significance, already in some states patients have to worry about getting and maintaining health insurance if they have a positive genetic screen. As you can imagine this is a controversial area. It is not the intent of this chapter to embark on an ethical debate. What seems a more realistic approach is to consider women who know their BRCA status already, and to use that knowledge to help further striate them in to different risk groups. The author considers women who know they have a positive mutation and are seeking reduction mammoplasty to be at high risk.

Like others in the high risk group BRCA positive women should have their breast tissue removed in a fashion that maintains orientation of breast, quadrant, and margin. In addition they should have a thorough histopathological analysis as if the tissue were a biopsy for a cancer workup.

88.2.2
The Clinical Exam

One would imagine that any surgeon performing an operation on a patient would have examined the patient clinically before operating on her/him. Results from a survey of plastic surgeons and trainees in the Netherlands found that this was not always the case. In fact 10% of those responding to the questionnaire said they never examined the breast [6]. It seems that not much argument need be made for the necessity of the clinical breast examination prior to elective breast surgery. In the very least the surgeon should be familiar with the patient's anatomy. Research has shown that a significant number of breast cancers are in fact palpable masses at the time of diagnosis. The clinical breast examination is an easy tool that should always be employed. It is also an opportunity for the physician to educate the patient about the operation and possible outcomes as it pertains to her particular breast.

Different guidelines exist about when women should begin to have a breast examination, but we recommend that all preoperative patients be examined for the reasons mentioned above. In young women undergoing reduction mammoplasty this may be all that is needed as the incidence of carcinoma in these women is extremely low. Though recent literature indicates that self-breast examination may not affect morbidity or mortality and probably increases the number of clinical assessments and biopsies, we still suggest that patients be familiar with their breast so that they recognize changes when they occur [9].

88.2.3
Mammography

Perras [10] reviewed 1,149 cosmetic surgery cases performed on the breast between 1973and 1989. Early diagnosis of breast cancer was discovered in 34 patients. Specifically 7 cancers out of 204 breast reduction cases were found preoperatively. From this research they stated that, "We strongly recommend that our policy of preoperative mammography be implemented so that patients can be protected from a lethal disease that has a far better prognosis when detected early." Most would not argue with this logic. However in this series all the mammograms were done on women over the age of 35 years. Multiple studies over the past 50 years have proven mammography to be an effective tool in screening women aged 40 and over. The American Cancer Society officially recommends that a baseline mammogram be done at 40 and then annually thereafter. Additionally they recommend screening mammography for high-risk women from the age of 30.

Due to these general guidelines, mammography in women aged 40 and over is done prior to breast reduction by most surgeons. The aforementioned gray area arises in low-risk women under 40 where mammography is controversial for several reasons.

One of the biggest problems with screening for breast cancer in women under 40 years of age is a lack of studies in this age group. Large screening trials do not invite these women to participate due to the low carcinoma incidence in this age group. Most research in the literature compares and contrasts screening modalities in symptomatic women under 40. In other words they already have a breast complaint, which is defined slightly differently depending on the study you read. Most include a breast mass, and skin changes.

Snodgrass and Yu [11] detailed the argument against mammography in women under 35 based on a retrospective study of 208 patients having elective breast surgery. Of these women 51 had mammography with no malignancies found. They stated, "It remains unclear whether preoperative mammograms are necessary in young patients having nononcologic breast surgery. Various authors have recommended mammography in such cases. We believe mammograms are not routinely needed before elective breast surgery in patients under 35 years of age." Problematic considerations regarding mammography in women under 40 years of age according to Yu and Snodgrass is that young breast tissue is dense and can obscure small lesions, breast cancer is rare in this age group, and the risk–benefit ratio is low. In this series only 59 women underwent reduction mammoplasty. Of these, only 21 had a preoperative mammogram.

In a retrospective study performed by Foxcraft and Porter [12] 239 patients under the age of 40 with a history of breast cancer were reviewed and compared to 2,101 women over 40 with a history of breast cancer. Of the younger age group 222 were referred with symptoms, 9 had symptoms that were unrelated, and 7 were asymptomatic but referred due to a strong family history. In 24 cases mammography was not done, but of the 215 remaining, 207 mammograms were available for review. Abnormalities were present in 149 of the reviewed films, 72% of the abnormalities included calcifications, stellate lesions, irregular mass, rounded or lobulated mass, and asymmetric density. Twelve lesions showed a multicentric pattern on mammography. The authors classified breast parenchymal patterns based on the Breast Imaging Reporting and Data System, BI-RADS. In summary they found that mammography in younger women was less likely to detect lesions and that a lesion was more likely to be determined as benign in this age group. They propose that a patient's age may greatly influence the radiologist's interpretation. This was especially true in women with very dense breast. There were however 10 women under 40 with impalpable cancers diagnosed solely via microcalcifications manifest on mammography.

In addition [12] ultrasound was performed on 230 of the 239 young cancer patients, and an abnormality was detected in 92.2%. Ultrasound was found to be useful for determining ultimate tumor size and multifocality. Like mammography ultrasound fell short in some patients in this age group. Specifically 18 cancers would have been missed if ultrasound alone was the only diagnostic modality employed. Based on their data ultrasound and mammography should be used in conjunction to evaluate the symptomatic women under 40. The authors define 'symptomatic' as a breast mass or thickening. Only seven women in this series were asymptomatic and the authors make no conclusion on what to do for screening in this situation even though these women were reviewed in their study. Though mammography was less sensitive and less specific in this age group the smallest of lesions were detected as microcalcifications. In addition mammography can help the sonographer target suspicious areas.

It is widely accepted that ultrasound is useful in young women. Ultrasound and mammography were compared in women between 30 and 39. [13] This retrospective study showed that ultrasound was more sensitive than mammography for detecting breast cancer in this age group, 95% vs. 85%. In particular ultrasonography was more sensitive in detecting invasive carcinomas, 99% vs. 85%, in mammography. However mammography was much more sensitive in detecting DCIS, 89% compared to the 68% with ultrasound. This information echoes the Wesley Breast Clinic study [12] in the sense that they feel there is utility to using both modalities. Twenty four tumors evaluated by ultrasound alone would have been misdiagnosed as fibroadenomas, had mammography not been done in conjunction. Both studies conclude that the combination of the modalities is best with follow up of suspicious lesions with FNA, the standard triple therapy.

88.2.4
MRI

MRI is increasingly being used as a screening tool for breast cancer. Recently the American Cancer Society (ACS) has recommended MRI for high-risk women generally beginning at the age of 30. MRI does not replace the need for mammography and should be done in conjunction with traditional screening modalities on an annual basis. In particular an MRI is better at evaluating denser breasts. The ACS also suggests that the physician discuss the pros and cons of MRI with moderate-risk women as well. With this imaging modality there are more false positives and subsequent unnecessary invasive tests. A prudent point, also made by the ACS, is that ideally a woman who requires MRI for screening should have it done at a facility where MRI guided biopsy is available to avoid the need of a second MRI at a different location [2].

The CDC reports [14] that 1/250 women who are 30 will develop breast cancer in the next 10 years. There are case reports of carcinoma discovered from reduction mammoplasty in adolescent females. Dinner and Sheldon [15] reported diffuse bilateral cribiform carcinoma in an 18-year-old girl discovered during postoperative pathology from a reduction specimen. There is one report that discusses a cancer diagnosis in a 16-year-old female who underwent reduction mammoplasty [16].

Given the above, it is the author's opinion that a mammogram be done on all preoperative women thirty and above. The author did not consider digital verses traditional mammography. Many feel that digital mammography is more sensitive and may have a role in younger women. Recent studies have shown that digital mammography has a higher cancer detection rate and is particularly effective in women under 50, women with dense breasts, and in pre and peri-menopausal women [17]. There is also some evidence that there are fewer patient recalls when this modality is employed [18]. At this time it seems that digital mammography would be preferable especially in the above subcategories of women. What to do regarding screening asymptomatic women under 40 is controversial. It is the author's position at this time that there is enough variability in the literature to erron the side of an over aggressive assessment. All women thirty and over should have a mammogram prior to surgery, digital mammography is ideal. Ultrasound should be used in conjunction with mammography in women aged thirty to forty. Low risk women under thirty can be evaluated by clinical examination alone, though we do not feel it would be unreasonable to use ultrasound in this group especially with the adolescent case reports in the literature. The indication for the surgery can help the surgeon determine the need for ultrasound screening in low risk women of this age group. For example if the surgeon is concerned about recent changes in breast symmetry or some pattern of breast development in the young low risk patient, whole breast ultrasound prior to elective surgery would be an effective tool to help rule out pathology. Women under thirty who are at moderate to high risk should have an ultrasound, and in accordance with the ACS guidelines [2] the author also advocates a screening MRI for all high-risk women regardless of age before they undergo elective breast surgery.

88.2.5
What to Do with the Preoperative Work-Up

If in your preoperative workup a cancer is discovered, these women should be referred to a surgical oncologist for management of their disease. For women whose family history raises concern of possible BRCA mutations it is suggested they be counseled regarding the possibility of cancer and given the opportunity to consider genetic screening. Positive mutations may affect their surgery choices. For other women with a negative workup we suggest that they be considered low risk, moderate risk, or high risk based on a combination of their age and the details of their preoperative analysis. By doing so, the surgeon can then tailor his approach to the patient's risk category. So, what constitutes low risk, moderate risk, and high risk?

88.2.6
Risk Groups

In general the author's risk groups echo those of the American Cancer Society with some exception (Table 88.1). They are based primarily on family history and

Table 88.1 Summary of risk groups

High risk	Personal history of breast cancer in either breast
	BRCA mutations
	Fraumeni or Cowden syndrome
Moderate risk	Family history of breast cancer
	Personal breast disease
Low risk	No family history of breast cancer
	Age under 30

personal history of breast cancer. The ACS established a lifetime risk of 20% as high risk, women with a 15–20% lifetime risk are considered as moderate risk, and those under 15% considered as low risk. There are several risk assessment tools available to help physicians estimate a patient's risk, the Claus model or BRCAPRO. A thorough past medical and family history should reveal the necessary information. These tools only provide estimates, and there is no way to precisely determine an individual's risk, with this in mind we recognize the value of clinical experience and the physician's judgment where the risk category is not obvious.

1. High Risk

Personal history of breast cancer either in the same breast or in the contralateral breast (note ACS considers these women moderate risk)
   A. Known BRCA1 or BRCA2 mutations
   B. First degree relative with a known BRCA1 or BRCA2 mutation, but the patient has not been tested themselves
   C. History of radiation to the chest between the ages of 20 and 30
   D. Personal history of a cancer syndrome, or a first degree relative with a cancer syndrome (Li-Fraumeni, Cowden, Bannayan–Riley–Ruvalcaba syndromes)
2. Moderate Risk

Family history other than BRCA1 or BRCA2.
   A. Personal history of breast biopsy
   B. Extremely dense breasts or unevenly dense breasts when viewed via mammography
3. Low Risk

No family history
   A. No personal history
   B. Patient under the age of 30

88.2.7
Intraoperative Considerations

88.2.7.1
Intraoperative Discovery of Carcinoma with a Previous Negative Workup

During breast reduction, the surgeon should palpate the breast parenchyma for any suspicious lesions. The elevation of skin flaps and resection of breast tissue allows the surgeon a better tactile examination than the normal screening breast examination. This is a direct examination and allows the surgeon to send lesions with a wide gross margin for a frozen section to the pathologist. In the event a malignancy is discovered early in the course of the reduction mammaplasty, the procedure should be aborted and the patient referred to a surgical oncologist. If the cancer is discovered later in the procedure with the flap elevated and most of the reduction completed, a surgical oncologist should also be consulted intraoperatively if available. If an adequate oncologic resection with clear marked margins and correct orientation can be achieved, then the reduction mammaplasty should be completed. Some studies advocate specimen radiography to direct histopathologic examination by the pathologist.

In the past decade, sentinel node mapping and biopsy of the axillary node became an established practice in staging breast cancer; thereby sparing some patients the morbidity of an axillary node dissection. However, with the extensive resection and flap elevation that occurs in breast reduction, the sentinel node mapping and biopsy become unreliable. When one discovers the malignancy after the completion of the reduction by a pathology report, the opportunity of the sentinel node biopsy may be compromised due to the disruption of lymphatics, as well as the scarring that occurs as a direct result of surgery. A history of breast reduction has traditionally been considered a contraindication to sentinel node biopsy. However, Golshan et al. [19] recently reported a series of six sentinel node biopsies performed successfully after breast reduction and suggest that a history of breast reduction should not be a contraindication to sentinel node biopsy.

In the event that sentinel node biopsy cannot be achieved, an axillary node dissection may be necessary to adequately stage the cancer. However the decision to undertake an axillary dissection will also depend on tumor biology, grade, and invasiveness.

To the author's knowledge there is no literature regarding a sentinel node biopsy at the time of breast reduction. The author would like the opportunity to prevent patients from having to have a second surgery in the event that carcinoma is discovered during breast reduction. Sentinel node biopsy at this time will most likely be dependent on how far along the reduction is and whether or not the patient was counseled before surgery as to this possibility.

88.2.8
Techniques for Tissue Marking

Most plastic surgeons resect the breast reduction specimen and place them into two containers, one for the right breast and one for the left breast. The author advocates that the specimens be further divided into more segments and sent in individual containers. For example, one should have a total of six containers for a breast reduction based on an inferior pedicle. Segments should be divided into lateral segments, superior segments and the medial segments of each side.

88.2 Preoperative Considerations

Furthermore, each segment should be marked for orientation and the margins should be inked. By convention, the area is marked on the specimen facing the nipple with dye. (Figs. 88.1–88.4) If in an area near a previous cavity, tumor or new suspicious area, then mark and clearly document this to the pathologist.

Since the author's method of marking and separating each segment of the resected breast tissue is time consuming, most plastic surgeons would be reluctant to invest this time into marking and orientating each specimen. This is especially true when combined with the low incidence of finding occult malignancy. Therefore, the following recommendations are made based on the risk factors:

1. In high-risk patients, the surgeons should operate in an institution where surgical oncology, and pathology is readily available, and each specimen should be appropriately marked, oriented, and divided into individual containers per segment resected (lateral, medial, and superior for each breast, 6 total).
2. In moderate risk patients, the surgery should be performed as above, but the inking of the margins may

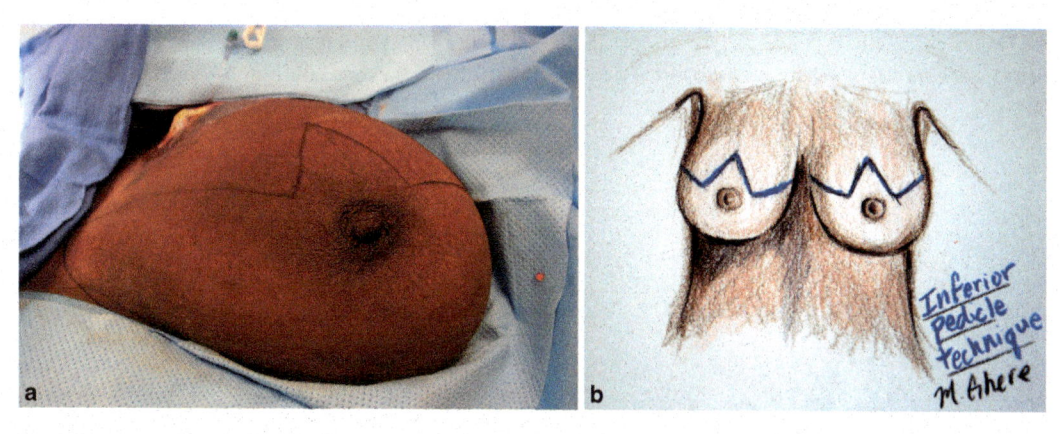

Fig. 88.1 Wise pattern marked on the left breast

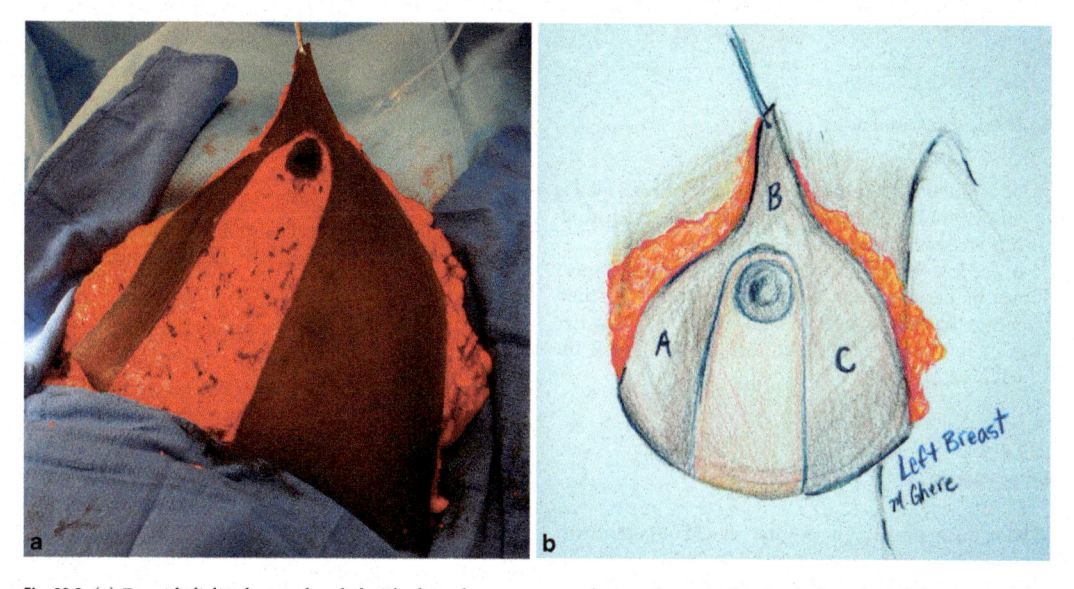

Fig. 88.2 (a) Deepithelialized central pedicle. The lateral segments are about to be excised and inked on the border closest to the nipple. (b) The segments inked correctly

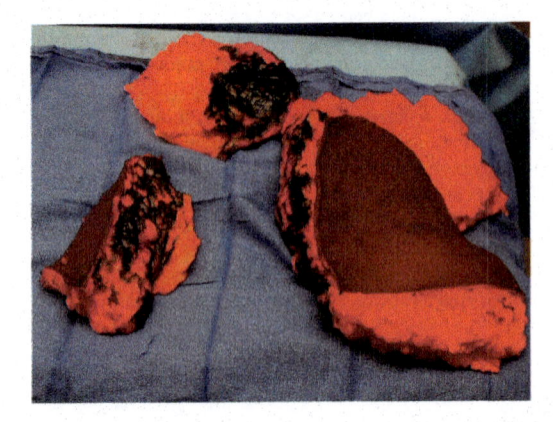

Fig. 88.3 Segments excised with the margins closest to the nipple inked

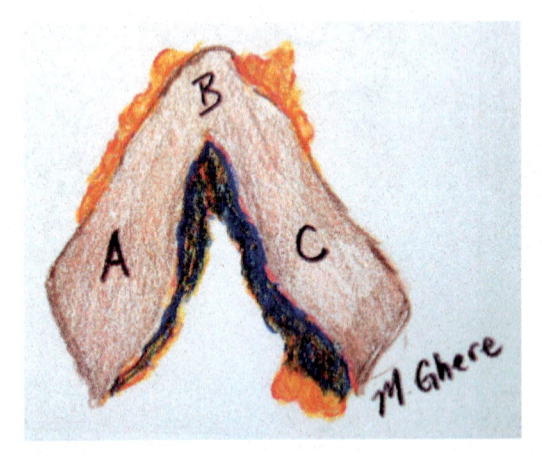

Fig. 88.4 Reduction segments

be omitted. Also, the surgery should be performed at an institution where surgical oncology and pathology are readily available.
3. In the low risk patients, the breast reduction surgery can be performed at an out patient center. Furthermore, the breast specimen can be sent in just two containers, one for the right breast and one for the left breast.

88.2.9 Histopathology

What is the minimal pathology that should be performed?

Although reduction specimens are recommended to undergo pathological examination, the ideal extent of specimen dissection and histopathologic sampling remains undefined, and cost factors may limit the extent of analysis of a large volume of grossly normal-appearing tissue from a seemingly healthy patient. [20]

Pitanguy et al. [21] advocate careful histopathologic examination of the breast specimen obtained from breast reduction. In a retrospective study of 2,488 patients who underwent breast reduction from 1957 to 2002, researchers found the frequency of occult breast cancer to be 0.5%. The most common malignancy in this series was invasive ductal carcinoma (seven cases, 0.3%). All breast tissues were sent to the pathologist. The specimens were placed in 10% buffered formalin for fixation. Each breast tissue specimen were serially sectioned at 0.5 mm intervals and grossly examined. Any suspicious area identified by appearance or tactile sensation was excised for histological examination. All suspected areas were fixed in paraffin and formaldehyde for 24 h before being sectioned and stained for routine hematoxylin and eosin. Once the malignancy is identified further pathologic studies can be obtained per the pathologist, including immunohistochemical staining, ER and PR receptor status, and her-2-neu status.

Should aggressiveness of the histopathological examination differ with age group or other risk modifiers?

In Pitanguy et al. [21], all specimens were treated equally regardless of age or risk modifiers. Only 91 of the 2,488 women had completely normal breast parenchyma leaving 2,497 abnormalities in the remaining 2,397 women to be discovered. Of course most abnormalities were benign lesions with fibrocystic disease accounting for 80.8% of breast pathology.

In a follow up study, Viana et al. [22] divided a total of 274 consecutive asymptomatic patients who had undergone breast reduction from January 1987 to December 2002. These women were stratified into three groups as per age. Group I (13– 35 years), Group II (36– 49) and Group III (50 and older) and they examined the incidence of malignancy for each age group (Table 88.2). All malignancies occurred in women 50 years or older in a population of women with no family history and no personal history, physical or radiographic examination suggestive of any breast disease. The incidence of breast cancer in this population was 1.1%.

However, not all patients fall into such a low risk category. In patients needing reconstruction after a breast malignancy, it is not uncommon for these women to undergo reduction of the contralateral or nondiseased breast to attain better symmetry. These women form a higher risk group (therapeutic breast reduction). Ramakrishnan et al. [23] looked at 81 patients undergoing therapeutic breast reduction and found the incidence of occult breast malignancy to be higher than Viana's [22] "cosmetic reductions." The median age of the patients was 49. They found one grade II invasive ductal carcinoma and five cases of DCIS in their 81 women. The incidence of occult malignancy was 6% in

Table 88.2 Histopathologic findings in surgical specimens obtained from reduction mammaplasties (Pires et al.) [20]

	Group 1 Ages 13–35	Group 2 Ages 36–49	Group 3 Ages 50 and over	Total
Ductal Carcinoma	–	–	1	1
Lobular carcinoma in situ	–	–	1	1
Ductal carcinoma in situ	–	–	1	1
Total	10	4	4	18

Table 88.3 Occult breast carcinoma in reduction mammaplasty specimens: 14-year experience, Colwell et al. (2004) [7]

Indication	Invasive cancer	DCIS	Total cancer Detection
Macromastia	0.3% (2/611)	0.3% (2/611)	0.7% (4/611)
Asymmetry	0% (0/19)	0% (0/19)	0% (0/19)
Reconstruction	0.6% (1/170)	0.6% (1/170)	1.2% (2/170)
Total indication	0.4% (3/800)	0.4% (3/800)	0.8% (6/800)

women undergoing therapeutic breast reduction. In a larger study, Petit et al. [24] looked at 813 therapeutic breast reduction and found 20 (4.6%) occult contralateral cancer in the reduction specimen. Colwell et al. [7] (Table 88.3) stratified their 14-year experience into three groups: Breast reconstruction, macromastia, and congenital asymmetry and made a comparison. The therapeutic occult malignancy incidence is higher in comparison to the cosmetic reductions.

Although these various studies indicate different risk modifiers of occult malignancy in breast reduction depending on age and indications for reduction mammaplasty, there is always an exception. A case report [25] presented an 18-year-old adopted women with unknown family history. She underwent a reduction mammaplasty for macromastia with removal of 750 g from each side. Pathology revealed a diffuse bilateral cribiform DCIS.

Ishag et al. [26] urges all breast reduction specimens undergo pathological examination for breast carcinoma. Although the pathology may yield benign disease, it will help identify lesions associated with mildly increased carcinoma risk such as moderate/ florid ductal hyperplasia, sclerosing adenosis, and nonsolitary papillomas. Marsh looked at their institution's experience from July 1989 to December 2000 with a total of 560 patients who had undergone breast reduction, 503 bilateral and 57 unilateral. He identified 4 cases of occult malignancy (0.7%), 8 cases of atypical hyperplasia (1.4%), and 52 cases of lesions with mildly increased risk of cancer (9.3%). Of the 4 cases of occult malignancy only one patient had a family history of breast cancer.

In terms of pathology cost, Ishag et al. [26] based all costs on actual expenses reported in the fiscal year of 2000. The total technical cost of performing a pathological examination on a unilateral breast reduction was $41. This includes costs associated with wages, benefits, supplies, services and overhead costs. Marsh estimates, based on his experience, that in order for a large academic center to perform the same pathological screening of 560 specimens over an 11.5 year period, the technical would be $44,000. This is significant when contrasted to the technical cost of treating a woman with stage 1 breast cancer over one a 1 year period. Ishag et al. determined this cost at Ohio State to be from $15,000 to $33,000.

In a contrasting article by Olack et al. [27], he found that a significant savings could be had by restricting pathological screening of reduction specimens to those from women over 40. However in their retrospective chart review of 300 women who underwent breast reduction from 1991 to 1999, if they had limited sending specimens to those that came from women over 40, they would have missed 20% of moderate to high risk pathology. They concluded this to be an unacceptable risk.

Cook and Fuller [28] in response to the Royale College of Pathologists document, "Histopathology of limited or no clinical value" published in 2002, looked retrospectively at the histology reports of every breast reduction performed at Salisbury District Hospital from January 1992 to December 2001. They reviewed a total of 1,289 patients ranging from 14 to 78 years of age. The average age was 36.8 years. The overwhelming majority of patients. 97.6%, had histologically normal appearing breast tissue, Twenty six cases showed lesions of uncertain malignant potential, 4 cases showed DCIS, and there was one case of invasive malignancy (.1%) All specimens received by the pathologist were sliced and examined macroscopically. If no lesions were identified two random blocks were taken from each breast and submitted for microscopy. Otherwise microscopy was directed at macroscopic lesions as necessary.

In their discussion Cook and Fuller [28] commented on the development of breast cancer. "It is thought that there is a stepwise progression from normal epithelium via nonatypical hyperplasia and atypical hyperplasia, to in situ carcinoma. Studies have shown an increased relative risk of developing invasive carcinoma of four to five times that of the normal population in patients with a biopsy diagnosis of ADH or ALH. This risk is doubled if there is also a positive family history of breast carcinoma. The presence of an intraductal papilloma has also been reported to be associated with an increased relative risk of cancer of three times that of the normal population. Both LCIS and DCIS are estimated to incur a relative risk of double that of atypical hyperplasia—that is, a relative risk of eight to 10 times. Molecular pathology studies have shown that shared genetic alterations may be found within cases of ADH, DCIS, and invasive carcinoma. Similarly, shared genetic alterations may be found within cases of ALH, LCIS, and invasive carcinoma."

With the above in mind combined with the findings in their analysis, Cook and Fuller [28] concluded that histopathological analysis of reduction specimens may reveal pathological diagnoses that have prognostic relevance. They discovered important pathology in 2.4% of their patients. Important diagnoses were made in 2.1% of patients who had no macroscopic abnormalities. This discrepancy is not a problem that could be overcome unless the whole specimen was processed for microscopy, which would create problems with time and cost. From their research they suggest that the Royal College of Pathologists provide guidelines regarding the histopathological analysis of breast reduction specimens, and that guidelines also be put in place for plastic surgeons managing this pathology.

Although the risk of finding occult malignancy varies between different patient populations, we think that it is prudent that all specimens be carefully examined by the pathologist for potential suspicious lesions. The same histopathological standard should be used regardless of age or risk modifiers. From the author's review of the literature it is not totally clear whether this is cost effective or not, but as Olack et al. [27] discovered in their research, if all specimens are not sent, a significant amount of pathology would be missed. In the very least, breast reduction specimens should be examined macroscopically for any lesions. There is no current standard for how large the slices should be. Viana et al. [22] cut their specimens into 0.5 cm slices; Snyderman and Lizardo [3] used 1 cm, and Cook and Fuller [28] suggest it might be necessary to send the entire specimen for microscopy. The author suggests that sampling of any solid part be routine.

What should be done with carcinoma discovered from pathology specimen?

Malignancy detected by pathology should follow the same oncologic guidelines established for breast cancer. In the modern era, the trend toward breast conservation therapy has been established by numerous controlled studies. The excision of the primary tumor with a surrounding rim of grossly clear margins has been termed as lumpectomy, partial mastectomy, or segmentectomy. When a rim of 1–2 cm clear margin plus overlying skin is obtained, this more aggressive local excision is termed quadrantectomy.

NSABP B-06 trial [29] compared mastectomy, lumpectomy and lumpectomy with radiation in 1,851 patients with tumor size up to 4 cm and clinically negative nodes. All positive patients with positive nodes received chemotherapy and a boost of radiation, but did not undergo complete axillary dissection. After a 25 year follow up, the overall survival rates were the same in all three arms of the study; about 46%. The disease free survival rate (survival without reoccurrence of breast cancer) was about 35% in all three groups. The emphasis of the trial focused on lumpectomy versus lumpectomy combined with radiation. Lumpectomy alone had a reoccurrence rate of 39.2% versus the 14.3% for lumpectomy combined with radiation.

The Milan Cancer Institute Trial of Breast Conserving Surgery was begun in 1973 and finished in 1982 [30]. The trial only permitted cancers less than 2 cm and all local excision was a quadrantectomy, which removed a large amount of tissue and overlying skin to achieve a widely clear margin. A total of 701 women were randomly divided into two arms, a radical mastectomy versus post operative radiation. All BCT underwent an axillary node dissection. Positive nodes received chemotherapy. At 20 years the deaths due to breast cancer occurred in 24.3% in the radical mastectomy and in 26.1% in the BCT group. Local failure rate for mastectomy was 2.3% while local failure rate was 8.8% in the BCT group over 20 years.

The Institut Gustave-Roussy trial [31] of breast conservation versus mastectomy was a small trail with only 179 patients accrued between 1972 and 1979. The study looked at lumpectomy with a 2 cm margin combined with radiation versus modified radical mastectomy in tumor less than 2 cm. All pathologically positive nodes in each group were randomized to receive radiation. No differences were observed between two surgical groups for risk of death, or for local–regional recurrence a at 15 year follow up. The survival was about 75% in both groups.

In terms of whether these studies apply to occult breast cancer found in breast reduction is up to debate. Colwell et al. [7] advocated a total mastectomy, axillary lymph node dissection, chemotherapy and radiation for patients with invasive carcinomas. For patients with small DCIS that is completely excised, she recommends observation. For LCIS, Coldwell advocates close observation.

Careful labeling of breast reduction specimens with proper ink markings, orientation, and separation of different segments into individual containers is more time consuming for the surgeons than the traditional separation of specimen by right breast or left breast. However, it allows more data and possible location of the tumor, and allows the oncologist to treat the resection as a quadrantectomy.

If the margins are positive, one may not be able to treat the breast reduction as a quadrantectomy. The idea of resection of new margins and postoperative radiation for positive margins in a lumpectomy does not apply because the rotation of the breast parenchyma places the tumor bed in a different location. Furthermore, there is the added concern of seeding the incisions and surgical bed with malignancy.

Tang et al. [8] identified 27,500 women who underwent breast reduction surgery in Ontario using the Canadian Institute of Health Information database and the Ontario Cancer registry database between April 1979 and December 1992. They found 17 patients, making the incidence of occult breast cancer in reduction mammaplasty 0.06%. The incidence is lower in this study because she excluded carcinoma in situ from

Table 88.4 Algorithm for treatment of breast cancer

```
                    Preoperative Assessment
                              ⇓
                    Risk Group Assignment
                 ⇓            ⇓             ⇓
             High Risk   Moderate Risk   Low Risk
                 ⇓            ⇓             ⇓
```

High Risk	Moderate Risk	Low Risk
Make sure all appropriate screening is complete. MRI is most likely indicated before surgery. Perform surgery in a center where a surgical oncologist and pathology are available. Margins and resected sections should be marked and sent to pathology individually.	Operate where surgical oncology and pathology are readily available. No need to mark margins.	Okay to operate at any capable center including outpatient surgery centers. Tissue should be sent to pathology asight and left breast.

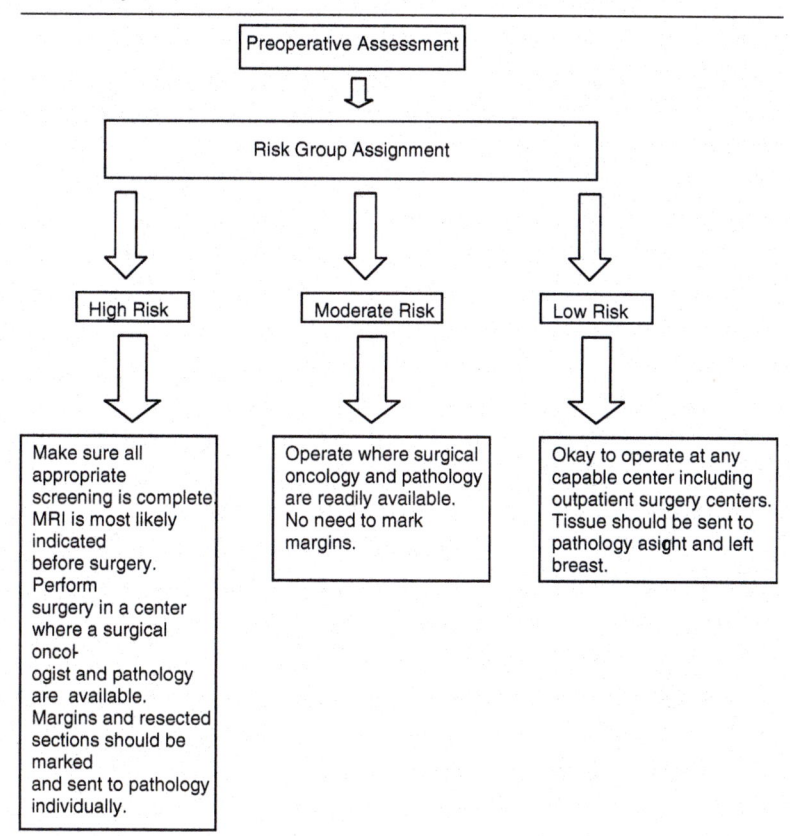

Note: Moderate and high-risk patients should be counseled in detail about the possibility of the discovery of carcinoma prior to surgery. All of their surgical options should be discussed based on the current standard of care

her data. Of these patients 67% underwent mastectomy while 33% underwent lumpectomies. 50% of the breast reduction group received post operative radiation and 25% received chemotherapy. The 5 year survival rate of patients treated for breast cancer discovered at the time of breast reduction is better than the 5 year survival rate of breast cancer in the general population; 88% versus 77%.

The decision of modified radical mastectomy versus lumpectomy combined with axillary node dissection, post operative radiation and chemotherapy should not be made by the plastic surgeon alone. It should be made through a multidisciplinary approach with a surgical oncologist, oncologist, pathologist, radiation oncologist and the desires of the patient. Once an occult malignancy is discovered, the treatment for breast cancer for patient survival with local and regional control becomes the foremost priority (Table 88.4).

Any suspicious areas noticed during surgery should be aggressively assessed by a pathologist regardless of the patient's preoperative risk group assignment.

88.3
Conclusions

With careful preoperative assessment women undergoing breast reduction can be stratified into different risk profiles. By doing so the surgeon can maximize the outcome for patients, especially those at high risk for carcinoma. The surgeon will also minimize the chance of encountering the complicating picture of carcinoma discovered from pathology after breast reduction or during the operation as well. Though the incidence is rare a thorough review of the literature suggests that discovery of breast cancer via breast reduction is a real possibility for surgeons performing this operation on a regular basis. It is imperative that surgeons be prepared to deal with breast cancer in the elective breast surgery setting. With the emphasis put on the preoperative assessment, we feel the surgeon can striate their patients and tailor to their particular risk profile. The possible discovery of carcinoma should be discussed when counseling patients in the preoperative setting, especially those in the moderate to high-risk categories. Covering this information will allow the surgeon and the patient to know their options and have a game plan that possibly can avoid additional surgeries or loss of orientation should cancer be discovered.

Areas of future study are given below.

88.3.1
Sentinel Node Biopsy (SNB) Following Reduction Mammoplasty

Thoughts on sentinel node biopsy following reduction mammoplasty are evolving. Historically sentinel node biopsy following reduction mammoplasty has been contraindicated. Recent reports in the literature suggest that this may no longer be the case. These are very limited however and report a very small number of patients. More powerful research is needed in this area before a reasonable conclusion can be drawn.

88.3.2
SNB at the Time of Reduction Mammoplasty

To our knowledge this has never been reported. It would rarely be needed, but would be a nice option for women who were candidates because it would spare them a second operation as well as provide earlier staging of their disease.

References

1. Rudolph R, Niedbala AR: Surgical management of the patient with invasive carcinoma discovered at reduction mammoplasty. Am Surg 2003;69(11):1003–1005
2. www.cancer.org, American Cancer Society
3. Snyderman R, Lizardo J: Statistical study of malignancies found before, during, and after routine breast plastic operations. Plast Reconstr Surg Transplant Bull 1960;25: 253–256
4. Pitanguy I, Torres E: Histopathological aspects of mammary gland tissue in cases of plastic surgery of breast. Br J Plast Surg 1964;17:297–302
5. Jansen D, Murphy M, Kind G, Sands K: Breast cancer in reduction mammoplasty: case reports and a survey of plastic surgeons. Plast Reconstr Surg 1998;101(2): 361–364
6. Hage JJ, Karim RB: Risk of breast cancer among reduction mammaplasty patients and the strategies used by plastic surgeons to detect such cancer. Plast Reconstr Surg 2006;117(3):727–735
7. Colwell AS, Kukreja J, Breuing KH, Lester S, Orgill DP: Occult breast carcinoma in reduction mammaplasty specimens: 14-year experience. Plast Reconstr Surg 2004;113(7): 1984–1988
8. Tang C, Brown M, Levine R, Sloan M, Chong N, Holowaty E: Breast cancer found at the time of breast reduction. Plast Reconstr Surg 1999;103(6):1682–1686
9. Screening for Breast Cancer, Recommendations and Rationale, U.S. Preventive Task Force, 2002

10. Perras C: Fifteen years of mammography in cosmetic surgery of the breast. Aesthetic Plast Surg 1990;14(2):81-84
11. Snodgrass K, Yu J, Doster E, Camp M, Moody D, Given K: The value of preoperative mammograms in nononcologic breast surgery. South Med J 1997;90(4):402-404
12. Foxcroft LM, Evans EB, Porter AJ: The diagnosis of breast cancer in women younger than 40. Breast 2004;13(4):297-306
13. Osako T, Takahashi K, Iwase T, Lijima K, Miyagi Y, Nishimura S, Tada K, Makita M, Akiyama F, Sakamoto G, Kasumi F: Diagnostic Ultrasonography and Mammography for Invasive and Noninvasive Breast Cancer in Women Aged 30 to 39 Years. Breast Cancer 2007;14(2):229-233
14. www.cdc.gov/cancer/breast
15. Dinner MI, Artz JS: Carcinoma of the breast occurring in routine reduction mammaplasty. Plast Reconstr Surg 1989;83(6):1042-1044
16. Sergent B, Aldana Ubillus C: Discovery of breast cancer in adolescent during the plastic surgery: a case report. Ann Chir Plast Esthet 2007 in publication
17. Pisano ED, Gatsonis C, Hedrick E, Yaffe M, Baum JK, Acharyya S, et al.: Diagnostic performance of digital versus film mammography for breast-cancer screening. N Engl J Med 2005;353(17):1773-1783
18. Vigeland E, Klassen H, Klingen TA, Hofvind S, Skaane P: Population-based screening using full field digital mammography with soft copy reading; First year experience from Vestfold County Norway. [abstr] Radiological Society of N Am, scientific assembly and annual meeting program, Oak Brook Ill. Radiological Society of North America 2005:287
19. Golshan M, Lesnikoski BA, Lester S: Sentinel lymph node biopsy for occult breast cancer detected during breast reduction surgery. Am Surg 2006;72(5):397-400
20. Blansfield JA, Kukora JS, Goldhahn RT Jr, Buinewicz BR: Suspicious findings in reduction mammaplasty specimens: Review of 182 consecutive patients. Ann Plast Surg 2004;52(2):126-130
21. Pitanguy I, Torres E, Salgado F, Pires Viana GA: Breast pathology and reduction mammoplasty. Plast Reconstr Surg. 2005;115(3):729-734
22. Viana G, Pitanguy I, Torres E: Histopathological findings in surgical specimens obtained from reduction mammaplasties. Breast 2005;14(3):242-248
23. Ramakrishnan R, Bhandare D, Fine N, Khan SL, Lal A, Nayar R: Pathologic findings in contralateral reduction mammaplasty specimens Breast J 2005;11(5):372-373
24. Petit JY, Rietjens M, Contesso G, Bertin F, Gilles R: Contralateral mastoplasty for breast reconstruction: a good opportunity for glandular exploration and occult carcinoma diagnosis. Ann Surg Oncol 1997;4(6):511-515
25. Snyderman R: Breast carcinoma found in association with reduction mammaplasty. Plast Reconstr Surg 1990;85(1):153-154
26. Ishag MT, Baschinsky DY, Beliaeva IV, Niemann TH, Marsh WL Jr: Pathologic findings in reduction mammaplasty specimens. Am J Clin Path 2003;120(3):377-380
27. Olack J, Martin T, Tirabassi M, Stueber K: Cost-benefit analysis for pathologic examination of reduction mammoplasty specimens. Plastic Surgery Abstract supplement 2005:136-138
28. Cook IS, Fuller CE: Does histopathological examination of breast reduction specimens affect patient management and clinical follow up? J Clin Path 2004;57(3):286-289
29. Fisher B, Anderson S, Bryant J, Margolese RG, Deutsch M, Fisher ER, Jeong JH, Wolmarck N: Twenty Year follow up of a randomized trial comparing total mastectomy, lumpectomy and lumpectomy plus radiation for treatment of invasive breast cancer. N Engl J Med 2002;347(16):1237-1241
30. Veronesi U, Cascinelli N, Mariani L, Greco M, Saccozzi R, Luini A, Aguilar M, Marubini E: Twenty-year follow up of a randomized study comparing breast cancer surgery with radical mastectomy for early breast cancer. N Eng J Med 2006;347(16):1227-1232
31. Arriagada R, Le MG, Rochard F, Contesso G: Conservative treatment versus mastectomy in early breast cancer: patterns of failure with 15 year follow-up data. Institut Gustave-Roussy Breast Cancer Group. J Clin Oncol 1996;14(5):1558-1564

Skin Circulation in the Nipple After Bipedicle Dermal Flap Reduction

Leif Perbeck

89.1 Introduction

Avascular necrosis of the nipple is a serious complication of reduction mammaplasty with nipple transposition. A frequency of fat necrosis of 2.1% and a total or partial necrosis of 0.3% has been reported in the literature [1]. In performing reduction mammaplasty different kinds of pedicles can be used such as the horizontal bipedicle, medial or lateral or vertical bipedicle, or inferior based pedicles. The perfusion of the nipple–areola complex is especially important while performing operations for cosmetic purposes. Its blood supply arises medially and cranially from the internal thoracic artery, and laterally and inferiorly from the lateral thoracic artery and the intercostal arteries. By a combination of two techniques, laser Doppler flowmetry (LDF) and fluorescein flowmetry (FF), it is possible to measure the changes in blood flow at the different operative steps and also to determine whether the blood flow in the nipple is homogeneous. LDF measures the product of the number of erythrocytes and their velocity in arbitrary units within a sphere of a radius of 1–2 mm [2]. FF is so far based on a photographic procedure and measures the transca-pillary exchange of sodium fluorescein, expressed as a fluorescence index, within a circular area of a diameter of 2 mm on the film negative, corresponding to 1 cm in natural size. The fluorescence is emitted from a tissue depth of 0.6 mm [3]. Nowadays, adrenaline is used to reduce blood loss which also temporarily influences the blood flow.

The blood flow during the different steps in the operative procedure in performing a reduction mammaplasty was studied.

89.2 Techniques

The blood flow was measured by LDF (Periflux® PF 1c. Järfälla, Stockholm Sweden) which measures the circulation down to 1–2 mm in the tissue (Figs. 89.1, 89.2) and FF (Fig. 89.3). Results for three bipedicle operations – horizontal pedicle (A), bipedicle vertical dermal flap without adrenaline (B) and with adrenaline (C) – are given below.

89.2.1 Horizontal Flap [4]

As measured by LDF, the blood flow in the nipple increased after the deepithelialization to 204% of the preoperative blood flow (100%). After the upper and lower glandular reduction, the blood flow in the nipple of the dermal bridge was reduced by 115–90% of the preoperative blood flow. There was no measurable change in the blood flow in the nipple after the division of the lateral pedicle, the value being 85%. When the skin had been sutured postoperatively, the blood flow in the nipple was 72% of the preoperative blood flow. The blood flow one to four days postoperatively again normalized to 100% of the preoperative value.

At FF, the postoperative fluorescence index was 0.0034 ± 0.0008 density unit/s, with a range of 0.0012–0.010 density unit/s (n =18). Homogeneous fluorescence was observed in the nipple in all the patients except two. In one of the patients, there was no fluorescence at all in one of the nipples and this nipple was not viable. The preoperative LDF value in this nipple was 40 V and the postoperative value 12 V, thus a reduction to 30% of the preoperative value. In another patient, there was no fluorescence in the medial area of the nipple and this area was not viable. The preoperative LDF value in this area was 10 V and the postoperative value 8 V correspondoing to 80% of the preoperative value.

89.2.2 Bipedicle Vertical Flap without Adrenaline [5]

As measured by LDF, the blood flow in the nipple increased after the deepithelialization to 245% of the preoperative blood flow (100%). After the medial and lateral glandular resection, the blood flow in the nipple

M.A. Shiffman (ed.), *Mastopexy and Breast Reduction: Principles and Practice*,
© Springer-Verlag Berlin Heidelberg 2009

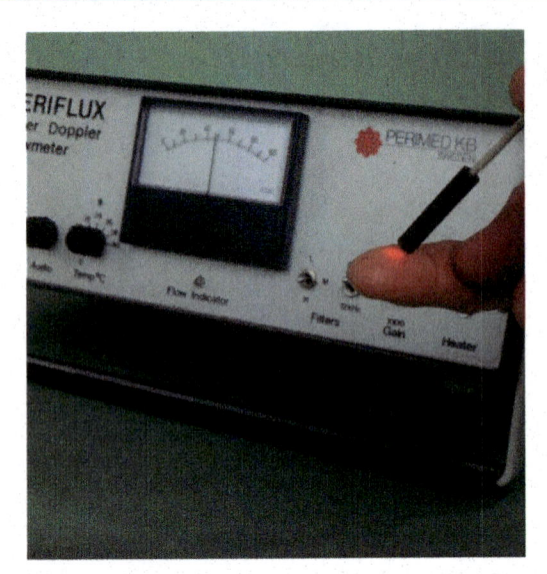

Fig. 89.1 The blood flow was measured by laser Doppler flowmetry (Periflux® PF 1c. Järfälla, Stockholm Sweden) which measures the circulation down to 1–2 mm in the tissue

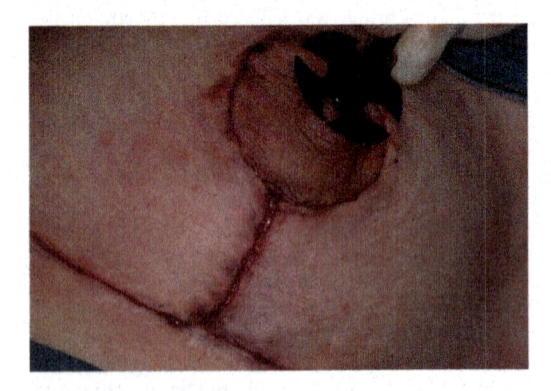

Fig. 89.2 Laser Doppler flowmetry measured on the nipple by a handheld concave adapter

of the vertical dermal bridge reduced by 128% of the blood flow after deepithelialization to 125% of the preoperative blood flow. One to four days postoperatively, the blood flow was 123% of the preoperative blood flow.

At FF, the postoperative fluorescence index was 0.007 ± 0.003 density unit/s, with a range of 0.001–0.032 density unit/s (n=12).

89.2.3
Bipedicle Vertical Flap with Adrenaline [5]

In the group that received adrenaline, the blood flow in the nipple increased after deepithelialization to 156% of the preoperative blood flow (100%). After the medial and lateral glandular resection, the blood flow in the nipple of the vertical dermal bridge reduced by 74% of the blood flow obtained after the deepithelialization to 79% of the preoperative blood flow measured after the adrenaline injection in the incision lines. Postoperative blood flow was 177% of the preoperative blood flow after the administration of adrenaline. One to four days postoperatively, the blood flow was 130% of the preoperative blood flow measured before adrenaline was given.

At FF, the postoperative fluorescence index of the breast that received adrenaline was 0.007 ± 0.004 density unit/s, with a range of 0.000–0.055 (n=13). Homogeneous fluorescence was observed in the nipple in all patients except in one. In this patient, a glandular resection of 2,197 g was performed and the patient also received adrenaline. There was no visible fluorescence, but the LDF signal was 6 corresponding to 75% of the preoperative value after adrenaline was given. On the fourth day, it was obvious that the nipple was not viable and became necrotic, most likely as a result of a strangulation of the approximately 20-cm-long distal vertical pedicle.

89.3
Discussion

The increase in blood flow by more than 150%, after the deepithelialization of the area around the nipple, was most probably because of hyperaemia caused by the operative trauma. In the breast that received adrenaline at the beginning of the operation, this increase was less pronounced, about 50%. The blood flow reduced by 100% in the dermal bridges after the medial and lateral glandular resections. However, the blood flow in the vertical bridge was of the same magnitude as the preoperative value. These findings strongly indicate that there is a great reserve capacity in the tissue regarding the blood flow to the nipple. The flow in the vertical pedicle was of the same magnitude or even higher as in the lateral and medial pedicles when the horizontal pedicle was preserved. After the skin has been sutured, 125% compared with 90% of the preoperative value and 130% compared with 70% by the

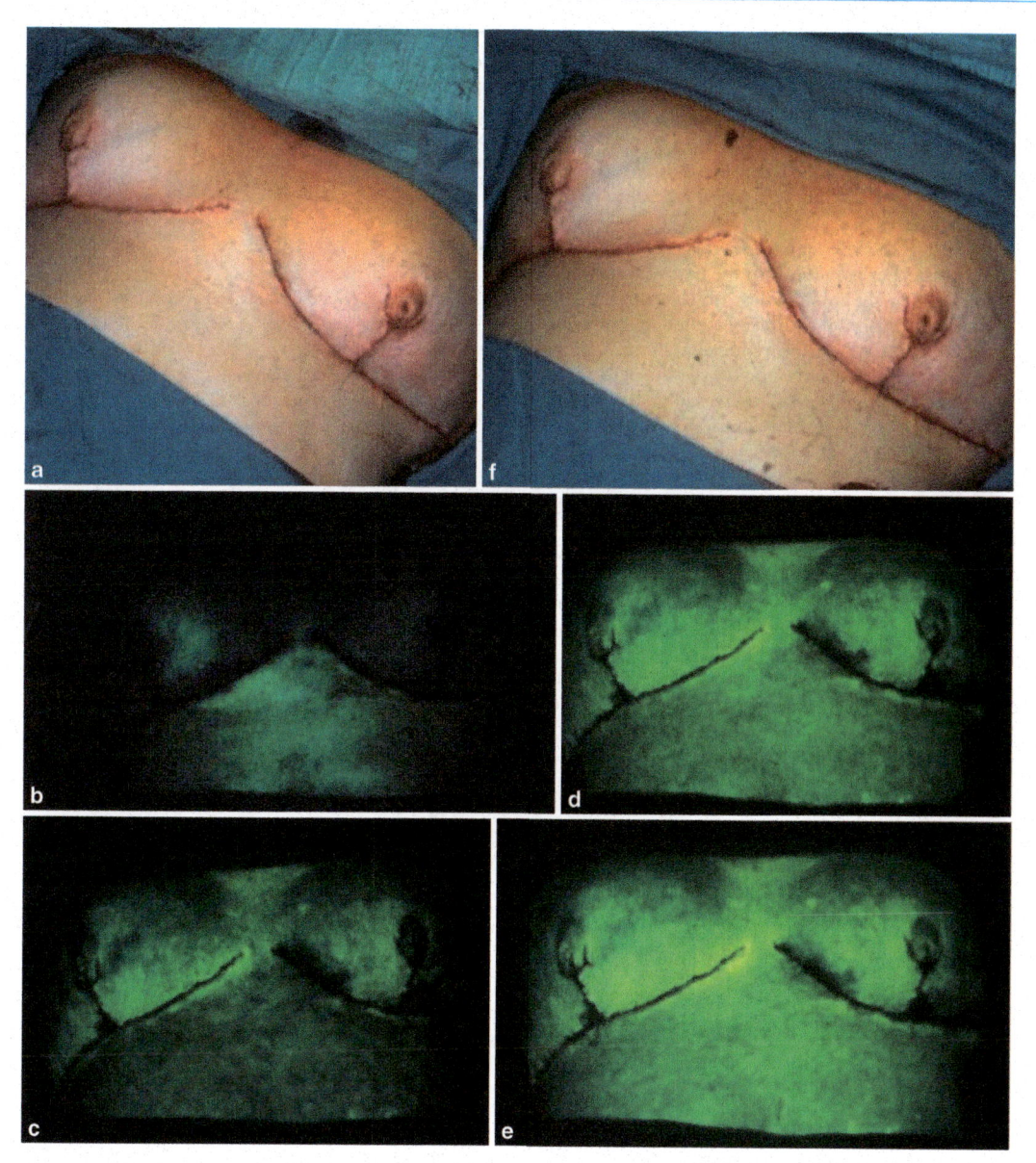

Fig. 89.3 Seven mg kg^{-1} sodium fluorescein was given intravenously as a bolus after completion of reduction mammaplasty. (**a**) Before injection of sodium fluorescein in daylight. (**b**) With light switched off. (**c**) Sixty seconds after injection. (**d**) Three minutes after injection. (**e**) Five minutes after injection. (**f**) Five minutes after injection in daylight

horizontal method. In our material concerning the bipedicle vertical flap, one case of total necrosis of the nipple occurred. In this patient, fluorescence was not at all seen in the nipple with FF, whereas LDF showed low voltage values. This discre-pancy is most likely explained by the difficulties in measuring low blood flow by the LDF method because of a certain amount of background tissue activity, which influences the zero value of the LDF signal. Moreover, LDF measures a slightly deeper blood flow in the tissue compared to FF, including a shunt blood flow which is not nutritive. A number of factors may probably influence the blood flow in the nipple after reduction mammaplasty, such as crinkling and compression of the pedicle. The blood flow in the nipple still increased within the first four days of postoperation, most likely because of hyperemia. Tracy et al. [6] have also studied the circulation in the nipple 2 weeks postoperatively and found a 12% below baseline (Skoog technique) in eight patients, 2% above baseline (central pedicle) in six patients and 44% below baseline (inferior pyramidal) in two patients. However, the use of adrenaline to diminish blood loss during the operation results in a temporary decrease in the blood flow, sometimes to such an extent that the tissue would seem not to be viable. After 3–4 h, the influence of adrenaline of the microcirculation has ceased and the blood flow increased. This makes an evaluation of the microcirculation more difficult in low-flow states when adrenaline has been given and must be postponed during this time period.

89.4
Conclusions

Vascular necrosis of nipple is a serious, but a rare complication, after bipedicle dermal flap reduction.

References

1. Strömbeck JO: Mammaplasty. Report of a new technique based on the two pedicle procedure. Br J Plast Surg 1960;13:79–90
2. Nilsson GE, Tenland T, Öberg PÅ: A new instrument for continuous measurement of tissue blood flow by light beating spectroscopy. IEEE Trans Biomed Eng 1980;27(1):12–19
3. Perbeck L, Lund F, Svensson L, Thulin L: Fluorescein flowmetry: a method for measuring relative capillary blood flow in the intestine. Clin Physiol 1985;5(3):281–292
4. Perbeck L, Alveryd A, Määttänen H, Wallberg H: Skin circulation in the nipple after reduction mammaplasty by upper and lower glandular resections. Scand J Plast Reconstr Surg 1988;22(3):237–240
5. Perbeck L, Proano E, Määttänen H: Skin circulation in the nipple after reductaction mammaplasty with a bipedicle vertical dermal flap. Scand J Plast Reconstr Hand Surg 1991;25(1):41–45
6. Tracy CA, Pool R, Gellis M, Vasileff W: Blood flow of the areola and breast skin flaps during reduction mammaplasty as measured by laser Doppler flowmetry. Ann Plast Surg 1992;28(2):160–166

Complications in Augmentation Mastopexy

Mervin Low, MD

90.1 Introduction

Breast augmentation with concurrent or secondary mastopexy is a common, yet complex, operation [1, 2]. It is discussed frequently at national and international meetings and in the plastic-surgery literature. Despite its success in improving the overall aesthetic appearance of the breast, caution is advised in the use of the procedure [3, 4]. Augmentation with mastopexy remains one of the most frequently litigated operations in plastic surgery, primarily because of the litany of complications that can arise following this procedure [5]. This chapter will review such complications and provide clinical some pearls for their avoidance.

Full uplifted breasts with the nipple–areolar complex situated above the inframammary fold are the aesthetic destination of virtually all plastic surgery of the breast. On the one hand, fullness achieved by breast augmentation stretches the breast and areolar skin. In contradistinction, mastopexy is designed to reduce skin envelope excess while repositioning the nipple–areolar complex. These two operations have competing yet necessary goals, as volume deficiency and skin excess with ptosis are common clinical findings. A multitude of variables, associated with augmentation and mastopexy in addition to late changes following such operations, challenge the surgeon and can make it difficult, if not impossible, to predict the outcomes in certain cases. These factors lead to the numerous complications seen with augmentation mastopexy. Some of these concerns occur in the immediate perioperative period while others occur in the long term. A complication rate of 17% and revision rate of 8% by an experienced academic surgeon has been quoted for primary simultaneous augmentation mastopexy [5]. Another retrospective review of simultaneous breast augmentation with mastopexy demonstrated a 14.6% revision rate with the majority of complications being implant-related rather than tissue-related [6].

90.2 Preoperative Disclosure

Preoperative disclosure and education is of the utmost importance in providing complete informed consent to patients. Patients must be aware that although breast augmentation alone or mastopexy alone are relatively simple operations, combining the two can exponentially increase the number and magnitude of potential complications as well as the attendant risk of revision. Breast augmentation makes mastopexy more difficult. Mastopexy makes breast augmentation more difficult.

90.3 Complications

The following complications can occur in augmentation mastopexy including: increased risks of infection, implant and nipple malposition, implant exposure and extrusion, loss of nipple sensation, and misshapen breasts; insufficient soft-tissue coverage; devascularization of the breast with partial or total skin flap or nipple loss; and poor scarring [7].

The increased risk of infection and implant exposure with subsequent extrusion are due to the increased soft-tissue rearrangement and resulting tension and incisions overlying the implant (Figs. 90.1, 90.2). Nipple sensation can be impaired and/or lost because of the soft-tissue surgery around the nipple–areolar complex. Malposition of the nipple can occur because of the simultaneous placement of the implant and repositioning of the nipple. Planning errors in placement of nipple position relative to the implant and implant descent, can result in the nipple being too high or too low. Interestingly, in guarding against placing a nipple too high, the nipple is much more commonly placed too low [8]. Implant malposition can occur following the repositioning of the breast by the mastopexy performed on top of the previously placed implant. The implant can settle in a position below the inframammary fold or unnaturally well above it.

M.A. Shiffman (ed.), *Mastopexy and Breast Reduction: Principles and Practice,*
© Springer-Verlag Berlin Heidelberg 2009

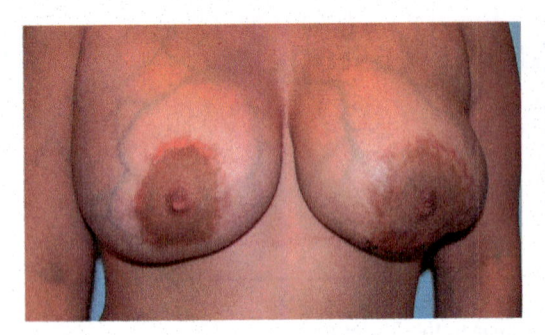

Fig. 90.1 Misshapen breasts following breast augmentation with simultaneous circumareolar mastopexy

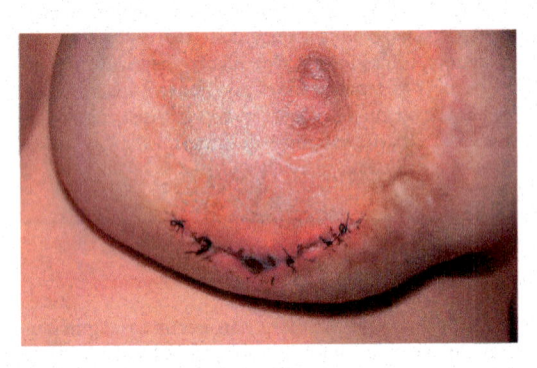

Fig. 90.2 Impending implant extrusion following breast augmentation with simultaneous circumareolar mastopexy

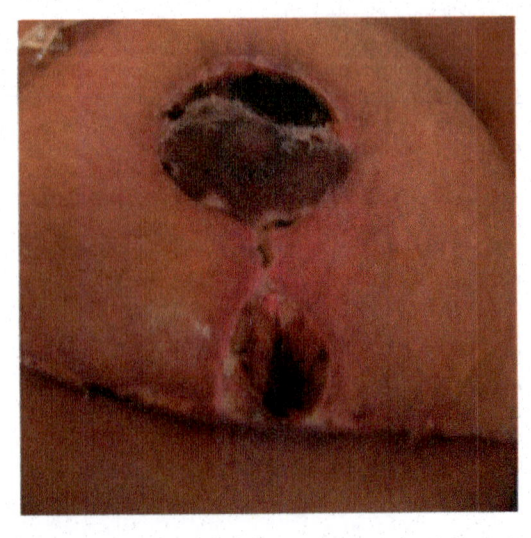

Fig. 90.3 Nipple and skin flap necrosis following breast augmentation with simultaneous Wise pattern mastopexy

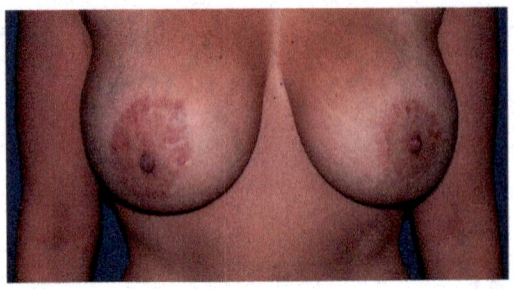

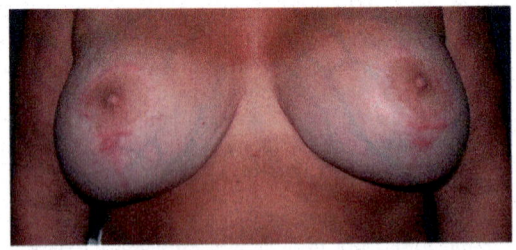

Fig. 90.4 Poor scarring following breast augmentation with simultaneous circumareolar mastopexy

Fig. 90.5 Poor scarring following breast augmentation with simultaneous circumvertical mastopexy

The combination of skin envelope expansion due to breast augmentation and mastopexy related skin envelope reduction can lead to a situation where insufficient soft-tissue coverage exists for the placed implant. This unfortunate situation is further worsened by the tension that exists on the skin envelope and breast parenchyma. Pocket dissection can further devascularize the breast (subglandular positioning being worse than subpectoral and wider dissections being worse than lesser dissections). The use of large implants can and will impair blood supply. The risk of skin flap and nipple necrosis, and poor scarring are consequently increased (Fig. 90.3). Poor scarring related to tension upon closure can further distort the nipple–areolar complex (Figs. 90.4, 90.5).

90.4 Discussion

Clinical pearls to reduce the above mentioned complications include first and foremost an understanding and appreciation of the magnitude of the potential complications. While the technical details of augmentation mastopexy are beyond the scope of this chapter, care in the design and execution of the operation, conservative skin excision and meticulous multilayer closure are crucial. Measure twice and cut once planning is particularly applicable in simultaneous augmentation mastopexy. Staging the operation, with mastopexy performed first or deferred until after the augmentation may be prudent in certain patients. While these options may be financially prohibitive to some patients, the ultimate emotional and financial savings of an uneventful complication free operation will be attractive to the patient and surgeon alike.

The complications seen with augmentation mastopexy predictably will lead to the need for revisions. A retrospective review performed by myself and others highlights the frequency of such complications and adverse outcomes following augmentation mastopexy [8]. At that time, the frequency, indications, techniques and outcomes of revision augmentation mastopexy were never formally addressed in the plastic surgery literature. This review demonstrated that revision following augmentation mastopexy is not only likely but common. Multiple indications for revision existed. These indications included: nipple malposition, implant malposition, poor scars, and recurrent ptosis. Each of the patients reviewed had multiple indications for revision.

While difficulties with augmentation with simultaneous mastopexy have been addressed, mastopexy following augmentation can also be problematic. Only recently has this topic been addressed [9]. However, the problems posed will become increasingly frequent as generations of augmented women age and present with unsatisfactory appearance of their breasts. These patients, will have usually undergone breast augmentation in their early twenties and thirties. While initially content with the outcome of their original operation, they will frequently develop ptosis and desire a mastopexy. Pregnancy, breastfeeding, weight fluctuations, tissue thinning and atrophy related to the implant and the undeniable gravitational effects will lead to the clinical changes. The triad of ptosis, tissue atrophy and capsular contracture pose additional challenges to the plastic surgeon. The additional operative hazards can be attributed to the inevitable changes to the breast following placement of implants. In addition to the initial operation, further impairments in blood supply to the breast can occur with subsequent capsule-related operations prior to the definitive mastopexy procedure.

Five surgical options are available for the ptotic augmented breast [9]: explantation alone, capsular surgery alone (capsulotomy or capsulectomy), mastopexy alone, explantation with mastopexy and explantation with mastopexy, and reaugmentation.

Mastopexy alone may be the optimal solution if the implant is located in a satisfactory position and no capsular contracture exists. In this particular situation, superficial and judicious dissection of the mastopexy skin flaps and care to maintain an intact vascular pedicle are critical. In those patients who undergo explantation with mastopexy, there also exists an increased risk of complications, particularly if an aggressive capsulectomy with breast parenchymal trauma is simultaneously performed. Initial pocket dissection, tissue atrophy, capsulectomy and mastopexy flap dissection can compromise blood supply to the skin and nipple. As such, the least aggressive mastopexy that will achieve the necessary nipple elevation and breast reshaping is preferred. The combination of explantation with mastopexy and reaugmentation poses the greatest risk of complications. Capsulectomy can impair an already tenuous blood supply. Superficial flap undermining, a conservative mastopexy with the nipple and areolar complex based on a superior pedicle and the use of an appropriate (preferably smaller) implant are clinical pearls that will minimize, or eliminate adverse outcomes.

The major issue in the secondary augmentation mastopexy patient is the relative uncertainty in the vascularity of the breast and nipple. In general, it is safe to assume that these patients will have altered vascular flow within the breast from the original augmentation surgery and the subsequent thinning of the breast parenchyma, especially inferiorly. Details regarding the original procedure will be helpful to obtain and will facilitate surgical planning. The priority is identifying the vascular pedicle for the nipple and areola. Transecting the only available blood supply will lead to inevitable ischemia. An appreciation and understanding of these factors can reduce the risk of devastating complications.

90.5 Conclusions

While it has been established that mastopexy performed with augmentation, whether simultaneously or at a secondary operation, can be generally successful, it can also be complication and revision prone. One stage augmentation mastopexy is a difficult operation and delaying the mastopexy may lead to a more stable result. However, the latter sequence of operations can also be a treacherous endeavor. The desire of patients for fuller lifted breasts after one or two operations will continue to vex and challenge surgeons for years to come. The goal of acknowledging and identifying the possible factors leading to adverse outcomes will undoubtedly reduce the need for revisions.

References

1. American Society of Aesthetic Plastic Surgery 2006. Cosmetic Surgery National Data Bank 2006
2. Hammond DC: Augmentation mastopexy: general considerations. In Spear SL (ed). Surgery of the Breast: Principles and Art, Vol. 2, 2nd Edn. Philadelphia, Lippincott Williams and Wilkins 2006, pp 1403–1416
3. Spear SL et al.: Simultaneous breast augmentation and mastopexy. Aesthet Surg J 2000;20:155
4. Spear SL et al.: One-stage augmentation combined with mastopexy: aesthetic results and patient satisfaction. Aesthetic Plast Surg 2004 ;28(5):259–67
5. Spear SL et al.: Augmentation/mastopexy: A 3-year review of a single surgeon's practice. Plast Reconstr Surg 2006;118 (7 Suppl):136S–147S
6. Stevens WG et al.: One-stage mastopexy with breast augmentation: A review of 321 patients. Plast Reconstr Surg 2007;120(6):1674–1679
7. Spear SL: Augmentation/mastopexy: Surgeon, Beware. Plast Reconstr Surg 2006;118(7 Suppl):133S–134S
8. Spear SL et al.: Revision augmentation mastopexy: Indications, operations, and outcomes. Ann Plast Surg 2003;51(6):540–546
9. Handel N: Secondary mastopexy in the augmented patient: A recipe for disaster. Plast Reconstr Surg 2006;118(7 Suppl):152S–163S

Part VII
Miscellaneous

Medical Legal Aspects

Melvin A. Shiffman

91.1 Introduction

Medical malpractice suits are upsetting, depressing, and frustrating for surgeons in cosmetic breast surgery who have done the "best they can" and still get complications or a dissatisfied patient. Surgeons must understand the medical legal consequences of their practice, especially when, in cosmetic surgery, an elective surgery is performed and there follows litigation. Patients expect near perfection without complications and surgeons should try to make them understand the realistic expectations.

91.2 Requirements for Medical Negligence

The plaintiff's attorney must establish all the four aspects of negligence in order to pursue a case of medical negligence.

91.2.1 Duty

When the physician establishes a relationship with a patient, the physician has a duty of due care in the care and treatment of that patient.

91.2.2 Breach of Duty

The physician may breach that duty by not using adequate skill and knowledge in treating a patient. This breach may be established by an expert witness testifying to the opinion that the defendant failed to follow the standard of care. The types of breaches may also include lack of informed consent. A lay jury may establish the standard if the facts are within the knowledge and experience of lay persons. This can best be seen in the case where a foreign body (sponge, instrument) is left in the surgical wound.

91.2.3 Injury

An injury, physical or mental, to the plaintiff must be shown by the facts of the case, usually through medical records.

91.2.4 Causation

Causation requires that the injury be caused by the breach of duty.

91.2.5 Standard of Care

The standard of care is what a reasonably prudent (careful) physician would do under the same or similar circumstances. The court considers expert testimony to establish the standard of care in most instances except if the circumstances are in the purview of a lay person. Also, the court may consider what a responsible minority of physicians would do under the same or similar circumstances. Medical literature may help to establish standard of care.

91.3 Informed Consent

91.3.1 Definition

The patient has the absolute right to receive enough information about his diagnosis, proposed treatment, prognosis, alternatives, and possible risks and complications of proposed therapy and alternatives to enable the patient to make a knowledgeable decision. The patient is the one who makes all the decisions in opposition to the old paternalistic theory that gave the physician

M.A. Shiffman (ed.), *Mastopexy and Breast Reduction: Principles and Practice*,
© Springer-Verlag Berlin Heidelberg 2009

complete control over all decisions. A physician would now have to prove that the decision he made was because of the patient's inability to make the decision or because there was an extreme emergency.

Other requirements of the "Informed Consent" doctrine in law require that a complication which was not explained to the patient did in fact occur and that the patient would not have agreed to have the surgery if informed of that particular risk or complication.

91.3.2
Legal Definition

In terms of surgical procedures, the surgeon must have explained to the patient the nature and purpose of any proposed operation or treatment, any viable alternatives, and the material risks and benefits of both. All questions must be answered.

In order for the plaintiff to succeed in a complaint for lack of informed consent, he must show
1. That the risk or complication, which was not explained to him, indeed did occur
2. That if he had been informed of that particular risk, he would not have consented to the surgical procedure

There are different means of proof at trial depending upon the jurisdiction (state). The opinion as to what risks is "material" to the patient in order to make his decision, under the same or similar circumstances, can be that of:
1. A reasonably prudent physician: This allows a physician to testify as to what is material.
2. A reasonably prudent patient: This allows the jury to decide what a reasonably prudent patient would consider material risks.
3. The plaintiff patient: This places the onus on the plaintiff to decide what would be the material risks. The cosmetic surgery patient may be unique because cosmetic surgeries are elective procedures and not medically required except, perhaps, for the patient's mental well being.

91.4
Patient Rapport

There is nothing as important as a good doctor–patient relationship before performing cosmetic breast surgery. This requires careful discussion with the patient concerning the surgical procedure proposed, viable alternatives, and the potential risks and complications of each by a caring empathetic staff person or the doctor. The surgeon must, at the very least, give the patient the opportunity to ask questions of him/her to allow the patient to feel more comfortable with the person carrying out the surgery. Surgeon must be careful when the patient is first seen by him on the day of surgery. This is not a good idea if ultimate litigation is to be avoided. If a patient is coming in from a long distance or from another state, a consultation can usually be performed at least the day or night before surgery.

There should be strict control of all staff persons involved in the patient's care so that incorrect information is not given to the patient and that the patient is not told "do not worry." This requires detailed training of each of the office staff from receptionist to scrub tech and registered nurse on what to say and what not to say to patients and how to respond to patient's problems.

No one should get angry with a patient or appear rushed. The patient should be treated with respect and dignity. Questions must be answered and phone calls returned in a timely fashion.

91.5
Complications

If a complication occurs, the surgeon should be available to talk to the patient, examine the wound, and explain how long it will take for the complication to subside. Every complication seen by the office personnel should be reported to the surgeon and the surgeon should decide what to do.

Any complication can lead to a lawsuit; even though it appears minor because the patient may think it is major. Surgeon should remember that the cosmetic surgery patient, despite all the warnings about possible complications, feels that there will be no complications and that the/she will look much better than they did before surgery.

91.6
The Angry Patient

If a patient shows anger, whatever the cause, the surgeon should try to handle the problem in an expeditious manner. That means speaking with the patient to find out the cause of the anger and figure out ways to satisfy the patient. Avoiding this type of patient after surgery will frequently lead to litigation. This means answering all phone calls in a timely fashion, showing a truthful caring attitude, and seeing the patient frequently enough to satisfy the patient's needs.

91.7
Medical Record

Handwriting that cannot be deciphered should be avoided. Not only is this irritating to the attorneys and expert witnesses, but the State Medical Board may find this to be inadequate records and thus unprofessional conduct, and loss of medical license may ensue. Handwritten notes are a continuous problem, especially when years later the doctor who wrote the note cannot read it.

Typewritten notes are easy to read and usually contain much more information than written notes. This author dictates all of the medical record notes. The cost to get a microcassette for dictation and hire someone to take down the dictation will save the surgeon time with minimal cost including maintaining the medical license.

91.8
Legal Aspects

The first thing an attorney thinks is that a bad result is the fault of the surgeon because of a negligent act. This may include claims of poor training, lack of skill, or inattention during surgery. The attorney will seek out an "expert witness" to show a breach in the standard of care. The standard of care is essentially a legal term meaning what a reasonable prudent (careful) physician would do under the same or similar circumstances. The defendant surgeon's attorney will try to find an expert witness to show that there was no breach in the standard of care. The surgeon should be realistic because everyone makes mistakes and the expert witness should not be biased and should give an honest opinion as to whether or not the standard of care has been breached.

91.9
The Misinformed Expert Witness

There are times when the expert witness in medical malpractice litigation is not aware of advances made in mastopexy and/or breast reduction or what standard of care really means. When this happens, misinformation may be provided to the court and may be difficult to refute. There are also instances where different training and experience comes into play.

For instance, there are different classifications for ptosis and, therefore, the Benelli or "Round Block" mastopexy may or may not be indicated, which would depend on the ptosis classification used by the surgeon. There are so many types of breast reduction with different pedicles that the expert should be familiar with before giving an expert opinion.

The expert opinion should not be biased no matter which side he/she is testifying for, plaintiff or expert. The expert who testifies only for the defense or only for the plaintiff would be suspect for possible bias.

91.10
Legal Cases

Mitchell v. Forshell, Cook County (IL) Circuit Court, Case No. 03L-13594. In Med Malpr Verdicts Settlements Experts 2007;23(6):41.

The 32-year-old plaintiff had bilateral breast reduction in 1996. The plaintiff alleged that the defendant removed an excessive amount of tissue from the breasts causing an uneven and asymmetrical result with the nipples to high and not level and hypertrophic scarring of the wounds. The defendant claimed that the procedure was performed properly, the results were known complications of the procedure, and the plaintiff had two pregnancies since the procedure. There was a verdict for $800,000.

Comment: The complaint of removal of excessive amount of tissue is a result of the patient not being forewarned about this possibility and for the physician's failure to ask the patient what cup size she would desire after surgery. There have been many cases where the surgeon reduces the breast to an A cup without regard to the patient's wishes. The surgeon should understand that the procedure should result in breasts that are adequate for the patient's size and shape and choose a technique that would produce this result since this is a cosmetic procedure as well as a procedure to resolve pain. Asymmetry and hypertrophic scarring are know risks of breast reduction but the surgeon should mark the patient preoperatively to obtain the best symmetry possible.

Hawkins v. Guinn, Jackson County (MO) Circuit Court, Case No. 04CV221063. In Med Malpr Verdicts Settlements Experts 2007;23(6):41.

The 25-year-old plaintiff had breast reduction in 2002 to alleviate back pain. The plaintiff alleged that the nipple–areolar complexes were placed too high on the breast resulting in incorrect appearance. The plaintiff underwent two corrective procedures preformed by another doctor. The defendant claimed that the surgery had been successful because the plaintiff's back pain was reduced. There was a verdict for $253,000.

Comment: Breast reduction surgery for relief of pain is also a cosmetic procedure that should result in the nipple–areolar complexes being in a normal position. The most common error resulting in high nipples is the failure to take into consideration the stretching of skin while marking the patient with large breast in a standing position. The point marked at the inframammary fold will then be too high when the patient is reclining. This point should be moved inferiorly 1–2 cm for the final nipple position. However, it is also possible to have high-riding nipples if pseudoptosis occurs after surgery and the breast parenchyma falls behind and below the nipple areola complexes. This can be resolved by securing the breast in a higher position with permanent sutures.

Allis v. Boemi, Collier County (FL) Circuit Court Case, Case No. 04-0031-35. In Med Malpr Verdicts Settlements Experts 2007;23(5):41.

The 28-year-old plaintiff had breast lift with augmentation by the defendant in 2003. The day after surgery the plaintiff had intense pain in the breasts and was seen by the defendant. Hard tissue in the breasts developed that turned black and necrotic resulting in the bilateral loss of the nipple areola complexes. Thirteen surgeries were necessary to repair wounds and reshape the breasts. The plaintiff alleged that a lift and an implant should not have been performed in the same surgery and that implants were used without her consent. The defendant claimed that the procedure was proper and that the outcome was an unfortunate result that had nothing to do with how the surgery was performed. There was a judgment for $8,250,000.

Comment: The performance of breast lift and augmentation at the same time is within the standard of care. However, the use of implants without the consent of the patient is a "battery" with possible punitive damages. The nipple areolar necrosis was a known risk of breast lift with augmentation.

Wrede v. Marfuggi, Morris County (NJ) Superior Court, Case No. MRS-L-120605. In Med Malpr Verdicts Settlements Experts 2007;23(2):42-43.

The 49-year-old plaintiff had breast reduction surgery to decrease back pain. Nine pounds of breast tissue were removed. The plaintiff alleged that the breasts are disfigured and that she looks like she has had a double mastectomy. The defendant claimed that the plaintiff was morbidly obese and had a history of smoking and circulatory problems which led him remove less skin underneath her breasts to avoid further compromise of her vascular system. There was a defense verdict.

Comment: Excessive removal of breast tissue without regard to the patient's desires is a recurring problem with surgeons. Certain reduction techniques are prone to allow excessive removal. Chronic smoking can be a cause of postoperative necrosis following breast reduction and surgeons should forewarn the patient of the risks and consider avoiding the patient who will not quit smoking for 2 weeks before and 2 weeks after surgery. Asymmetry and breast deformity are known risks of breast reduction.

Smith v. Vu, Orange County (CA) Superior Court, Case No. 02CC10689. In Med Malpr Verdicts Settlements Experts 2005;21(1):41.

The plaintiff had breast reduction surgery performed by the defendant. The central pedicle technique was used with placement of implants. The plaintiff began to show signs of necrosis, infection, loss of nipple-areolar complex, and disfigurement of the left breast. The plaintiff alleged that the procedure was unorthodox, performed without informed consent, failure to schedule an appointment within 24h of surgery, and failure to provide timely treatment that resulted in left nipple-areolar loss and extensive scarring. There was a $250,000 settlement.

Comment: Although necrosis and infection are known risks of breast reduction, the failure to follow up the patient in a timely manner can be considered negligence. At an early stage of cyanotic changes, nipple-areolar (NA) transplant is possible and may have saved the NA complex. The patient should be seen early in the postoperative period to observe for any changes in nipple-areolar color.

McMillan v. Dow Corning, New York (NY) Supreme Court, Index No. 26858/92. In Med Malpr Verdicts Settlements Experts 2005;21(5):36-37.

The 30-year-old plaintiff had breast lift and augmentation in 1990. The plaintiff alleged that there was too much pressure applied on the tissues and this created excessive scars, too much tissue was removed, and the nipples were not raised. The defendant claimed that the plaintiff had good results, her nipples placed in a proper position, and the plaintiff had a tattoo placed on her chest which countered the argument that the plaintiff was embarrassed by her appearance. There was a defense verdict.

Comment: There was evidence that the patient lied by the fact that she had a tattoo placed on the chest after surgery and was not ashamed and distressed about her breasts. Scarring and asymmetry are known risks of mastopexy and augmentation.

Karachun v. Wasserstrum, Bergen County (NJ) Superior court. In Med Malpr Verdicts Settlements Experts 2005;21(6):38.

The 40-year-old plaintiff had breast reduction to improve her appearance and reduce discomfort from 48H cup size breasts. The plaintiff alleged that the defendant promised she would be a C or D cup following surgery and that she had asymmetric nipples and scarring. The defendant claimed that asymmetric nipples and scarring are known surgical risks. There was a verdict for $1,500,000.

Comment: Reducing the breasts to an A cup after estimating a C or D cup result is a breach of the standard of care. The estimate acts almost like a warranty of the results. Failure to make the breasts the proper size is negligence on the part of the surgeon. It would be rare that a large breasted female undergoing breast reduction would be happy with an A cup. The patient wishes to be normal in appearance postoperatively which includes the breast size to be consistent with her body size.

Terminelle v. Tornambe, Bronx County (NY) Supreme Court, Index No. 8221/99. In Med Malpr Verdicts Settlements Experts 2006;22(11):42.

The 23-year-old plaintiff had breast reduction for chronic pain. Keloid scar developed after the procedure.

The plaintiff alleged lack of informed consent and should have been informed of the risk of keloids due to her dark skin pigmentation as a Puerto Rican. The defendant claimed that nationality had no bearing on the type of information she needed and the scarring was a known complication of the procedure. There was a defense verdict.

Comment: It is not true that nationality has no bearing on the type of information that the patient needed. The risk of keloid scarring is 15% in Hispanics, Asians, and blacks. The patient should have been forewarned that she ran a higher risk of keloid scars (15%) than Caucasian patients.

Shorter v. Reichel, Roanoke City (VA) Circuit Court, Case No. CL03000133-00. In Med Malpr Verdicts Settlements Experts 2006;22(5):44.

The 60-year-old plaintiff went to the defendant plastic surgeon for the removal of a benign lipoma under the arm. The defendant indicated to the plaintiff that breast reduction (weight was 250 lb and breast size 46DD) would alleviate her ongoing shoulder and back pain. Breast reduction was performed followed by multiple complications including wound dehiscence around the nipple–areola complexes and inframammary areas of both breasts. The wounds were resutured, but the sutures tore through the skin. Skin grafts were ultimately applied but there was further separation of the grafts. The plaintiff developed masses from the scar tissue under the nipple–areolar areas. The defendant recommended the masses be surgically removed. The plaintiff underwent multiple corrective surgeries by another surgeon that included breast reconstruction with implants. The plaintiff alleged that the defendant incorrectly marked her breast in preparation for surgery which led to the removal of too much skin and tissue resulting in wound separation, and there was too much tension at the surgical site which caused wound separation and reduction of blood supply to the nipple–areola area and caused the formation of scar tissue. The defendant claimed that there was no negligence, the plaintiff had an old scar on the right breast which complicated the procedure and had a history of poor recovery following surgeries, and wound dehiscence and fat necrosis are recognized complications of the procedure. There was a verdict for $1,500,000.

Comment: Wound dehiscence and fat necrosis are known complications of breast reduction. It is not clear whether the defendant talked to the plaintiff on the breast reduction procedure; she initially was seen for a lipoma and was not seeing the defendant for breast reduction. Complications in this situation almost always end up with litigation. Juries end to be swayed by the severity of the injuries and the need for multiple corrective surgeries rather than seriously considering whether there was a breach of the standard of care. The reasoning by the plaintiff's "expert" was that dehiscence occurred; therefore, the wound must have been closed too tightly because too much skin and tissue were removed. There was Opinion only without proof.

Evans v. Leighton, Maricopa County (AZ) Superior Court, Case No. CV 2003-092169. In Med Malpr Verdicts Settlements Experts 2005;21(12):43.

The 43-year-old plaintiff had a breast lift by the defendant. A postoperative hematoma developed and there was asymmetry. The plaintiff alleged that the defendant either negligently measured the breast position prior to surgery or negligently deviated from the plan during surgery to cause the asymmetry and that the deformity was so severe that the plaintiff suffered pot-traumatic stress disorder and depression. The defendant claimed that there was no deviation in the standard of care and postoperative hematoma resulted in "bottoming out" of the right breast which resulted in the right nipple rising significantly higher than the left nipple. There was a defense verdict.

Comment: The plaintiff's expert was manufacturing, as opinion without proof, the possible cause of the asymmetry without taking into consideration "bottoming out."

91.11
Discussion

Prevention of malpractice litigation should be kept in mind by keeping more than adequate medical records especially with all informed consent discussions and their contents. Physicians may have difficulty recalling discussions with patients unless it is in writing. Patients have to understand that complications occur even in elective cases such as mastopexy and breast reduction and more than one procedure may be necessary. It is possible that the patient may not remember all the risks and complications discussed previously by the surgeon months or years back and may think that some of the complications were not discussed [1]. It is also necessary for the patient to state that if the complication had been discussed, she would not have had the surgery.

Timely diagnosis and treatment of complications are essential to limit any damage. The surgeon must be prepared to discuss with the patient the cause of the complication, the treatment, how long it will take for healing to occur, and what further surgery might be necessary.

For mastopexy or breast reduction, chronic smokers should be either avoided or the record must show reasonable efforts to have the patient stop smoking and that the patient complied. It should be explained to the patient that smoking, even in decreased amounts, will likely result in poor and delayed healing, possible tissue necrosis, and significantly increased scarring.

The surgeon should be aware that trials are unpredictable as to the results and depend quite a bit on the skilled attorney and the persuasive expert witness.

Arbitration, as an alternative to trial, is less emotionally charged and shorter in time but associated with more likelihood of payment to the plaintiff but usually less an amount than at trial.

Mediation is a method for the court to reduce the number of cases going to trial. In this instance, the judge will have the attorneys argue both sides of the case in the absence of witnesses. The attorneys will try to wear each other down for a final settlement. In the meantime, the defendant and plaintiff sit outside the courtroom and their attorneys bring them the offers for them to decide. This may go on for days.

Reference

1. Shiffman MA: Cognitive dysfunction in the postoperative patient. Plast Reconstr Surg 2001;107(4):1079–1080

CHAPTER 92

Editor's Commentary

Melvin A. Shiffman

92.1 Introduction

The Editor's Commentary allows me to express some of my opinions in an informal manner. After over 44 years of practice in the field of oncologic surgery, reconstructive surgery, and cosmetic surgery and over 32 years in the medical legal arena, there is some experience and knowledge gained in the field of cosmetic surgery that I would like to share with those who may be interested.

92.2 Mastopexy

1. Any surgeon performing mastopexy should be aware of and experienced in some of its more important aspects such as the standard mastopexy with anchor scar, vertical mastopexy, Benelli "round block" mastopexy, and the crescent mastopexy. There are some variations of these mastopexies that are of interest but not quite as important as those mentioned.
2. Periareolar or "round block" mastopexy
   a. The subcuticular pursestring should always be with a nonabsorbable suture and not with absorbable suture because when the suture is absorbed the scar will spread.
      i. Interrupted permanent suture in the subcuticular layer may be used but takes somewhat longer to perform.
   b. When augmentation mammoplasty is added, the amount of skin to be removed would best be decided upon after the implant is in place.
      i. This may prevent skin necrosis from too tight a closure.
   c. The amount of ptosis that will be corrected by this procedure is limited; mild to moderate ptosis.
   d. A lift of over 4 cm (inframammary fold to lowest part of breast) will almost always result in permanent pleating that will have to be corrected surgically.
3. Crescent mastopexy
   a. A crescent excision of 3 cm will lift the breast approximately 1 cm.
4. Severe ptosis (Grade III) usually needs a definitive procedure such as the standard mastopexy with a T scar or vertical mastopexy.
   a. Consideration should also be given to the techniques of mastopexy without a vertical scar.

92.3 Breast Reduction

1. When the nipple–areola complex (NAC) is too high after reduction mammoplasty, the surgeon should distinguish between "bottoming out," where the breast falls inferiorly behind the NAC and surgical misplacement.
   a. A surgically misplaced NAC is usually the result of marking the patient in a sitting position and not taking into account the weight of the large breast that should be countered by lowering the premarked position 1–2 cm below the inframammary fold (to account for skin stretch).
2. Postoperative cyanotic changes in the NAC should be examined carefully for venous refill that should be under six seconds.
   a. For refill of over six seconds, immediate treatment would consist of removing sutures around the areola and the vertical incision to relieve tension, and perhaps to allow a twisted pedicle to loosen and straighten.
   b. If venous refill persists over 6 s, consideration should be given to transplant of the NAC to the lower abdomen or upper thigh and then transfer to the nipple–areola area after granulations have formed or after healing.
3. The surgeon should be careful that the type of breast reduction to be performed does not reduce the breast to an A cup. Patients expect to appear normal after surgery and going from a DD to A cup can be devastating to the patient.
   a. A breast reduction with breast augmentation sounds like an oxymoron. Most of the time, with breast reduction breast fullness can be maintained with a C or B cup without the need for excessive resection. However, there may still be

M.A. Shiffman (ed.), *Mastopexy and Breast Reduction: Principles and Practice*,
© Springer-Verlag Berlin Heidelberg 2009

lack of fullness in the superior portion of the breast that can be treated with fat transfer or breast implant.

It is better to remove too little than too much. A prosthesis is not a substitute for normal breast tissue.

4. Nipple Level
   a. The normal nipple level is considered to range from 19 to 23 cm from the midclavicular point or the sternal notch to the nipple. This is difficult to be used for deciding on the nipple level when performing a mastopexy or breast reduction. Which centimeter level to use is a guesswork according to the experience of the surgeon. If the patient's height is 5 ft or less, this measurement may be shorter than 19 cm in the normal individual; if 5 ft 9 in. or more, this measurement may be longer (over 23 cm) in the normal individual. Some believe that the nipple level is approximately at the mid humerus, measured from below the acromion process to the olecranon process. The best measurement is still the level of the inframammary fold with lowering up to 2 cm for the excess weight of the breast (again some guesswork).

5. Vertical Mastopexy
   a. The vertical mastopexy eliminates the scar in the inframammary fold. Most patients who are concerned about the mastopexy scar and refuse the procedure are concerned about the vertical scar. The proper procedure, for aesthetic purposes in patients concerned about the scar, is avoiding the vertical scar in mastopexy procedures.

6. Combined Mastopexy and Breast Augmentation
   a. The higher risk of complications in combined mastopexy and breast augmentation may be prevented by avoiding tension on the wound closure by not using an excessively large implant (sometimes it may be prudent for the surgeon to determine the final implant size according the skin tension at closure), and by planning skin resection (deepithelialization) less wide than usual.
   b. It is necessary, because of the medical literature showing excessive complications, that patients be forewarned about the possibility of complication in overperformance of either procedure alone. However, carrying out the procedures separately at different times will not change the risk of increased complications.
   c. This author has performed over 200 combined mastopexy and breast augmentations without any complications.

92.4 Discussion

There is nothing more important that a complete and accurate medical record since the medical record is the physician's best defense. If something is omitted, then it may be presumed that the discussion, observation, or event did not occur. Unreadable records may require translation by the physician who wrote the record and there are times when even the physician who wrote the record cannot understand what is written.

Medical record should never be changed except to run a line through the erroneous entry, and then date and initial the new entry. Deleting portions of the record or adding portions to the record after the litigation is started may be considered legally as spoliation. In the event of spoliation, the court may deem that the party who did the spoliation is wrong and everything that the opposing party states is correct.

Subject Index

A
Abboud, M. 38, 251, 568, 571, 583
Abramo, A.C. 348
Abramson, D.L. 455, 555
Aillet, S. 606
Ancef 431
Andrews, J.M. 73, 323
Andrews, J.U. 189
Arie, G. 103, 121, 249, 267, 323, 337, 348, 473, 499
Aspirin 12
Asymmetry 73, 85, 93, 106, 112, 125, 135, 136, 142, 159, 164, 176, 195, 271, 273, 291, 307, 310, 315, 323, 343, 360, 386, 441, 457, 476, 509, 511, 546, 560, 599, 601, 602, 634, 635, 637, 638, 641, 661, 679–681
Atrophy 603
Aubert, V. 55, 249
Aufricht, G.L. 249

B
Baasch, M. 643, 644
Balch, C. 383
Bames, H. 249
Bannayan–Riley–Ruvalcaba syndromes 658
Bartels, R.J. 149, 151
Becker, H. 19
Benelli, L. 44, 51, 58, 66, 67, 70, 73, 149, 151, 168, 179, 189, 201, 202, 251, 517, 529, 565, 571
Berry, M.G. 592
Biesenberger, H. 55, 103, 207, 249, 323, 337, 411, 437, 461, 466, 473
Biggs, T.M. 136, 545
Bilgen, I.G. 38
Bleeding 190, 195, 315, 387, 413, 437, 500, 526
Bleomycin 594
Body mass index (BMI) 24, 27, 280, 387, 500, 501, 503, 641
Boice, J.D. 644–646, 648
Botti, G. 217, 218, 227
Bottoming out 68, 73, 74, 101, 125, 195, 233, 238, 271, 395, 412, 482, 485, 546, 554, 625, 633, 681, 683
Boustos technique 201, 202
Brachial plexus 23, 43
Brantner, J.N. 257

BRCA 39, 650, 655, 658
Breast
– hypertrophy 109, 258, 262, 285, 313, 323, 337, 344, 347, 349, 354, 367
– tuberous 166, 177
Bretteville-Jensen, G. 257
Brink, R. 51, 73
Brinton, L.A. 644–646, 648
Brown, F.E. 38
Brown, M.H. 644, 646, 649
Bruhlmann, Y. 31
Brzozowski, D. 605, 606
Bustos, R.A. 67

C
Calcifications 38, 39, 315, 500, 560, 561, 567, 576, 583, 584, 589
Camper's fascia 56
Caouette-Laberge, L. 605
Capsular contracture 158
Cardoso, A.D. 251
Cardoso de Oliveira, M 103
Carpal tunnel syndrome 11, 23, 24, 25, 26, 27, 33
Carreras 70
Carr, M.M. 607
Caruso, M.K. 19
Casas, L.A. 555
Cefazolin 391
Celebiler, O. 267
Cellulitis 393
Ceydeli, A. 427
Chalekson, C.P. 525
Chassaignac 204
Chiari, A. Jr 73
Chong, J. 251
Cimino, W.W. 179
Cinelli, P.B. 189
Cipro 431, 433
Circumareolar incision 57
Clindamycin 592
Clough, K.B. 647, 651
Collins, E.D. 29
Colwell, A.S. 653, 654, 663
Conway, H. 249, 518

Cook, I.S.   661, 662
Cooper, A.P.   369
Cooper's ligaments   3, 43, 61, 104, 118, 136, 215, 216
Cothier-Savey, I.   647, 650
Courtiss, E.H.   97, 239, 251, 261, 265, 266, 348, 411, 559, 565, 566, 567
Cowden syndrome   655, 658
Craig, R.D.   615
Cramer, L.   251
Cruz-Korchin, N.   606
Cunningham, B.L.   376
Cyanosis   433
Cystosarcoma phyllodes   636
Cysts   177, 589

D
Dacron   202, 206
Daniel, M.J.B.   97, 545
Daniel, R.K.   635
Daptomycin   592
Dartigues, L.   121, 267, 323, 472, 499
Davidson, B.A.   189
De Araujo Cerqeira, A.   97
de Castro, C.C.   251
Deep vein thrombosis   117, 393, 494, 500, 560
Dehiscence   60, 158, 271, 315, 457, 493, 503, 525, 595, 601, 681
De la plaza, R.   427
Dellon, A.L.   615
de Olarte, G.   97, 121, 207, 251, 426
Dexon   444
Diabetes   26, 121, 592
Dieffenbach, J.F.   65, 97, 249, 447
Di Giuseppe, A.   179, 265
Dingman, D.   636
Dog ears   73, 392, 486, 487, 496, 503, 509, 521, 524, 555, 641
Doppler   667, 668
Dufourmental, L.   189
Dufourmentel, C.   250, 323, 466, 473
Duranceau, L.A.   605
Durston, W.   249, 323, 517, 636

E
Eed, M.D.   97
Eklund view   571
Elsahy, N.I.   625
Endoscope   231, 565
Endoscopy   307, 310, 312
Epifoam   243
Eren technique   495
Erythema   177

Estrogens   12
Ethibond   145
Exner, K.   426

F
Faivre, J.   201
Fat necrosis   38
Fayman, M.S.   73
Ferreira, M.C.   593
Fibroadenoma   636
Finger, R.   361
Fischer, A.   507
Fischer, G.   179
Flowers, R.S.   97
Fluorescein   354, 551, 667, 669
Fluoroquinolones   592
5-Fluorouracil   594
Fournier, P.   324
Foxcraft, L.M.   656
Free nipple areolar graft   456, 459, 551–556, 597
Free nipple graft   519, 552, 554, 556, 599, 633
Frey, M.   233
Frey technique   495
Fuller, C.E.   661, 662

G
Galvao, M.S.L.   251
Georgiade, G.S.   556
Georgiade, N.G.   251, 411, 455, 597, 609, 610, 613, 631
Gibson, T.   575
Gigantomastia   124, 262, 370, 448, 449, 454, 456, 457, 459, 476, 496, 551, 552, 554, 597, 615
Gillies, H.   106, 249, 411, 438, 454, 455, 461
Giovanoli, P.   233, 495
Glatt, B.S.   31
Goes, J.C.S.   73, 97, 251, 262, 265, 426, 565, 571
Goldwyn, R.H.   266
Goldwyn, R.M.   19, 97, 103, 251, 261, 348, 411, 631
Golshan, M.   658
Gonzalez, F.   593, 615
Gore-Tex   270, 420, 421
Gossman–Rowdner device   19, 20
Gradinger, G.P.   552, 556
Graf, R.M.   46, 136, 139, 141, 541, 545, 631
Gray, L.   265
Greuse, M.   615
Gsell, F.   251
Guinard, A.   249
Gulyas, G.   73
Guthrie, R.H.   251, 447
Gynecomastia   189, 190, 191, 239, 243, 244, 245, 365, 552, 559, 568, 574

H

Hage, J.J. 653
Hall–Findlay, E.J. 45, 73, 97, 133, 261, 262, 266, 269, 383, 385, 499, 504, 517
Hamartoma 636
Hamdi, M. 593, 615
Hammond, D.C. 73, 417, 426, 504
Hammond technique 529
Harbo, S.O. 615
Hauben, D.J. 447
Hefter, W. 455, 606
Hematoma 55, 61, 85, 99, 117, 125, 135, 184, 195, 244, 265, 271, 315, 360, 393, 394, 437, 457, 496, 503, 525, 545, 551, 554, 561, 579, 583, 590, 592, 595, 599, 635, 681
Hemorrhage 546
Herman, S. 631
Hester, T.R. 251, 391, 448
Heywang-Kobrunner, S.H. 589
Hidalgo, D.A. 555
Hinderer, U.T. 65, 68, 70, 97, 250, 426
Hoffman, L.A. 449
Höhler, H. 303
Hollander, E. 249
Hoopes, J.E. 250
Hudson, D.A. 631, 636
Hurst, L.N. 519
Hypermastia 635, 636, 637, 639, 640
Hyperpigmenation 60
Hyperplasia 635
Hypertrophy 439, 448, 454, 455, 457, 458, 459, 471, 475, 476, 518, 544, 547, 559, 560, 576, 581, 597, 601, 609, 635, 636, 637
Hypesthesia 341
Hypomastia 600
Hypopigmentation 60, 347, 554, 594
Hypoplasia 66
Hypotension 551
Hypothyroidism 26

I

Illouz, Y.G. 507, 567
Infection 55, 61, 135, 190, 195, 265, 315, 387, 393, 447, 457, 491, 496, 554, 560, 561, 590, 599, 601, 671, 680
Informed consent 677–678
Inframammary crease ligament 216
Inframammary fold (IMF) 15, 16, 49, 65, 66, 70, 85, 93, 101, 106, 111, 115, 122, 133, 134, 147, 153–155, 160, 164–167, 170–174, 181, 184, 203, 207, 208, 209, 210, 211, 217, 218, 219, 220, 229, 230, 232, 235, 236, 239, 255, 261, 262, 265, 266, 268, 269, 277, 278, 280, 286, 291, 303, 304, 308, 309, 315, 316, 330, 331, 334, 340, 348, 349, 371, 372, 383, 384, 386, 391, 392, 393, 398, 399, 400, 412, 417–419, 421, 425, 426, 431, 433, 442, 447, 449, 450, 452, 453, 468, 470, 471, 476, 485, 487, 491, 494, 497, 499, 501, 502, 511, 513, 518, 519, 520, 524, 525, 526, 531, 535, 541, 542, 544, 545, 548, 553, 561, 562, 566, 572, 578, 600, 621, 627, 631, 634, 636, 638, 641, 642, 671, 683
Intertrigo 266, 447, 449, 500
Ischemia 341, 413
Ishag, M.T. 661

J

Jabaley, M.E. 250
Jabs, A.D. 636
Jackson, I.T. 556
Jansen, D.A. 646, 648, 649
Jones, G. 449
Joseph, J. 189

K

Kahn, S. 633
Kakagia, D. 606
Karim, R.B. 653
Karp, N. 19
Keck, M. 634
Keflex 238
Keleher, A.J. 648. 649
Kenedi, R.M. 575
Kesselring, U. 251
Keyhole pattern 13, 97, 256, 262, 291, 292, 295, 296, 349, 453, 530, 621, 627
Khan, U.D. 45
Kinoshita, T. 38
Klein, H.W. 571, 575
Klein, J.A. 257, 357
Klein's solution 507
Koger, K.E. 555
Kornstein, A.N. 189
Kraske, H. 44, 103, 109, 112, 357
Kraske, I.I. 249, 261
Kupfer, D. 636
Kurono, Y. 319

L

Labandter, H.P. 621
Lactation 554, 584
Lalardrie, J.P. 250, 251
Lalonde, D.H. 524, 525, 526
Lassus, C. 45, 56, 73, 97, 121, 129, 149, 151, 261, 267, 357, 368, 369, 473, 486, 499, 501, 504, 517, 609, 610, 613, 627, 634
LaTrenta, G.S. 449
Lejour, M. 45, 62, 73, 97, 104, 149, 151, 180, 235, 251, 262, 269, 271, 357, 413, 418, 448, 473, 486, 499, 501–504, 507, 517, 565, 566, 567, 571, 581, 582, 583, 609, 610, 613, 627, 634

Subject Index

Lejour technique 529, 555, 634
Lexer, E. 97, 103, 109, 112, 261, 337, 357, 411
Li-Fraumeni syndrome 655, 658
Linezolid 592
Lizardo, J. 653, 662
Lockhart, R.D. 348
Lockwood, T. 137
Longacre reverse flap 467
Loustau, H.D. 45
Luce, E.A. 354
Lund, K. 643, 644

M
Macromastia 262, 358, 640, 641, 653
Magnetic resonance imaging 19, 37, 509, 654, 657
Maiman 315
Maliniac, J.W. 249, 518
Mammaplasty
- bipedicle 431
- inferior pedicle 417, 554
- vertical 135, 269, 421, 423, 555, 617
- vertical scar 121

Mammary
- hypertrophy 23, 27
- hypoplasia 163

Mammary innervation 5
Mammograms 37, 39, 49, 360, 560, 637, 656
Mammography 19, 70, 507, 509, 584, 638, 640, 657
Mammoplasty 44
Mammostat 385, 487
Mandrekas, A.D. 595, 605
Maneuver of Claoué 442
Marc, H. 437
Marchac, D. 73, 97, 121, 207, 251, 426, 565
Marcos 32
Marcus, G.H. 369
Marfan's syndrome 4
Marino, H. 249
Marlex mesh 129
Marshall, D.R. 605
Martins, P.A. 189, 190
Mastitis 184, 447, 548, 580
Mastopexy
- circumareolar 65, 157, 159
- crescent 51, 52, 53, 54, 56, 57, 59–62, 67, 68, 70, 71, 683
- eccentric 67
- hyperplasia 215w
- inferior pedicle 45
- vertical 45, 52, 55, 73, 74, 80, 81, 93, 94, 180, 183

Matarasso, A. 265, 559, 565, 566
Mathes, S. 449, 454
McCraw, J. 576
McIndoe, A.H. 411, 461

McKissock, P.K. 13, 44, 97, 115, 215, 235, 250, 348, 368, 383, 426, 431, 434, 441, 448, 455, 499, 552, 559, 605, 609, 610, 613
McKissock technique 481, 597, 615
McMahan, J.D. 33
Medical negligence 677
Mendelson, E.B. 589
Menderes, A. 426
Menesi, L. 251
Methcillin-resistant *Staphylococcus aureus* 590
Methylene blue 399
Meyer, R. 251
Micropore 310, 311, 333
Miller, A.P. 29, 32
Miller, C.L. 38
Mitnick, J.S. 589
Mitrofanoff, M. 615
Mofid, M.M. 615
Monocryl 58, 166, 168, 170, 172, 173, 175, 232, 236, 237, 269, 317, 323, 375, 377, 393, 400, 413, 531
Morestin, H. 97, 249, 447, 551
Morris, D.J. 481
Moskovitz R. 265
Mouly, R. 250, 466
Mouly, R.Y. 323, 473

N
Nagy, M. 576
Nahabedian, M.Y. 455
Nahai, F. 121
Nakajima, H. 369
Necrosis 55, 109, 124–125, 136, 158, 176, 184, 196, 214, 237, 267, 347, 352, 360, 393, 397, 435, 437, 457, 491, 495, 496, 500, 503, 509, 526, 546, 554, 561, 579, 583, 589, 590, 592, 593, 599–601, 621, 636, 641, 642, 668, 670, 680, 681, 683
Nedhoff 261
Neurovascular bundle 399
Neuro-vascular structures 454
Neurovascular supply 397
Niedbala, A.R. 653
Nipple–areola graft 347, 365, 438
Nipple–areolar complex (NAC) 13, 14, 16, 45, 51, 54–58, 61, 65, 68–71, 73, 74, 76, 80, 82, 84, 86, 87, 93, 94, 97–99, 101, 116, 122, 123, 126, 129, 130, 133, 136, 137, 163–171, 173, 181, 182, 189, 203, 214–216, 218, 219, 223, 225–227, 255, 261, 270, 316, 334, 338–340, 342, 344, 357–362, 368–371, 373, 377, 380, 384–386, 389, 391, 394, 395, 397, 398, 400, 412, 413, 419, 425, 431, 433, 435, 447, 448, 451–456, 459, 461, 464, 465, 479, 485, 493, 495, 499–502, 504, 507, 508, 517–521, 524, 542, 545, 546, 549, 551–553, 556, 572, 575, 578, 589, 593, 602, 606, 609, 613, 614, 616, 617, 619, 621, 622, 625, 627, 633, 636, 641, 642, 652, 667, 679–681, 683

Nitropaste 589
Nonsteroidal anti-inflammatory drugs (NSAIDs) 12
Nydick, M. 239

O

Obesity 26, 31, 239, 449, 457
O'Dey, D. 348, 369
Olack, J. 661, 662
Orlando, J.C. 251, 447
Owl-technique 45
Ozerdem, O.R. 555

P

Palmer, J.H. 262
Passot, R. 44, 180, 181, 183, 518, 526, 577
Passot technique 577, 578
Paulus of Aegina 189
Pectoral fascia 215, 350, 363, 412
Pectoralis fascia 115, 137, 155, 216, 392, 393, 426, 427, 431, 456, 502
Pectus excavatum 4
Peixoto, G. 73, 97, 104, 323, 329, 332
Peled, I.J. 66, 68, 149, 151
Penn, J. 43
Perras, C. 39, 656
Peterson, H.D. 257
Peterson, S.W. 496
Petit, J.Y. 648, 649, 661
Phalen test 24
Pinch test 153, 170, 172, 177, 280–283, 315
Pitanguy, I. 55, 97, 101, 103, 164, 189, 207, 250, 303, 305, 323, 330, 333, 337, 342, 343, 344, 357, 441, 447, 449, 461, 466, 473, 499, 605, 660
Pleating 196, 197, 236, 422, 513, 524
Pneumothorax 507
Poland's syndrome 4
Pontes, R. 250, 605
Porter, A.J. 656
Pousson, M. 44, 249
Prepectoral fascia 131, 134
Prolene 106, 177, 487, 531
Pseudoptosis 45, 51, 52, 73, 171, 217, 482, 637, 639, 641, 679
Ptosis 16, 45, 49, 51–54, 60, 61, 65, 70, 73, 93, 94, 97, 101, 109, 135, 149, 152–157, 163–165, 176, 197, 211, 213, 215, 217, 218, 221, 223, 226, 227, 235, 239, 250, 255, 258, 262, 273, 278, 279, 285, 311–313, 323, 333, 334, 338, 347, 349, 354, 365, 368, 384, 388, 426, 429, 439, 442, 449, 455, 464, 476, 503, 519, 523, 537, 544, 547, 559, 565, 568, 597, 601, 609, 637, 638, 673, 679, 683
Pulmonary embolus 117, 387
Pulsed electromagnetic field therapy 566

Q

Qiao, Q. 73, 97
Quardt, M.D. 31

R

Ramakrishnan, R. 660
Ramirez, O.M. 517
Reduction
– vertical bipedicle 44
Rees, T.D. 648
Regnault B technique 45, 426, 494
Regnault, P.C. 43, 51, 153, 229, 232, 251, 384, 493, 494, 496, 635
Regnault technique 496, 497
Renault, P. 65, 66
Renó, W.T. 251
Reston 566
Reverse-Phalen test 24
Reverse Trendelenburg position 384
Rhomboid technique 341, 342
Ribeiro, L. 97, 189, 201, 202, 250, 251, 266, 383, 448, 518, 542, 545
Ribeiro's technique 518
Robbins, T.H. 251, 261, 266, 303, 305, 556, 597
Robbin technique 615
Robertson, D.C. 250, 480–482, 518, 519, 525
Robertson technique 479, 481, 482, 518, 519, 523, 525, 526
Rohrich, R.J. 91, 607
Rosenberg, G.J. 239, 241
Rudolph, R. 243, 653

S

Sampaio-Goes, J.C. 67, 251
Savaci, N. 525
Scarpa's fascia 56, 270
Scars 73, 124, 125, 136, 149, 150, 160, 168, 176, 177, 189, 197, 202, 212, 215, 225, 231, 233, 238, 266, 267, 270, 271, 304, 307, 310, 311, 315, 323, 324, 329, 334, 337, 340, 344, 360, 368, 372, 386, 394, 450, 472, 475, 481, 485, 493, 496, 499, 507, 509, 517, 518, 524, 525, 531, 533, 537, 544, 545, 552, 554, 555, 564, 565, 569, 578, 583, 584, 597, 600–603, 614, 629, 633, 634, 635, 636, 641, 651, 671–673, 684
– hypertrophic 59, 85, 92, 100, 106, 123, 158, 159, 503, 518, 524, 525, 594, 595, 599, 631
– hypertrophy 65–67, 69, 71
– keloid 158, 327, 495, 594, 680, 681
Scheufler, O. 426
Schlenz, I. 348, 369
Schnur, E. 19
Schnur, P. 19
Schrudde, J. 507
Schwartzmann's maneuver 338, 339

Schwarzmann, E. 51, 129, 249, 250, 261, 348, 383, 411, 517
Seitchik, M.W. 19
Semmes–Weinstein monofilaments 347
Sentinel node biopsy 664
Serafin, D. 348
Seroma 55, 61, 85, 99, 106, 184, 190, 265, 315, 387, 394, 457, 503, 554, 561, 580, 635
Shestak, K.C. 647, 650
Sigurdson, L. 32
Simon, B.E. 189
Skoll, P.J. 631, 636
Skoog, T. 44, 97, 250, 289, 348, 369, 370, 373, 383, 441, 447
Slezak, S. 615
Smith, E.M. Jr 97
Smith, J. 249
Smith, M.L. 647, 651
Smokers 85, 449, 457, 561
Smoking 12, 49, 121, 363, 500, 592, 680, 681
Snodgrass, K. 656
Snyderman, R. 653, 662
Sommer, N.Z. 20
Spear, S.L. 149, 163, 454, 532, 647, 651
Spector, J. 19
Spoliation 684
Standard of care 677
Steatonecrosis 99, 542, 545
Steroid fat atrophy 594
Stevens, W.G. 633
Stortz endoscopic system 582
Streptogramin B 592
Striae 519
Strömbeck, J.O. 44, 97, 215, 250, 289, 323, 348, 357, 376, 383, 437, 438, 439, 441, 443, 445, 447, 551, 559, 605, 625, 627, 631
Strömbeck technique 438, 439, 444, 633
Subcutaneous musculoaponeurotic system (SMAS. 217
Submammary fold 205
Supernumerary nipples 3
Suture granuloma 491
Sykes, P.A. 615

T
Tail of Spence 3
Tairych, G. 605
Tang, C.L. 646, 649, 650, 663
Taylor, G.I. 262
Tebbetts, J.B. 149, 151, 176
Thomas, W.O. 526
Thoracic outlet syndrome 26

Thorek, M. 249, 383, 437, 438, 447, 518, 551
Thorek technique 439
Thromboembolism 12, 449
Tinel test 24
Tobin, H.A. 496
Topaz, M. 583
Triamcinolone 594
Tuberous breast 541, 542, 544, 545, 547, 548, 549

U
Ulnar nerve paresthesia 447
Ultrasound 37, 168, 657

V
Vancomycin 592
Vechere, F. 44
Velpeau, A.A.L.M. 43
Viana, G. 660, 662
Vicryl 58, 98, 99, 106, 116, 202, 206, 224, 323, 326, 511, 542
Villarde, I. 97
Visual analogue scale (VAS) pain testing 258

W
Walgenbach, K.J. 567
Webster, J.P. 189
Webster, M.H.C. 335
Wechselberger, G. 615
Weiner, D.L. 44, 250, 251, 348, 383, 447
Wise keyhole pattern 289, 290, 291
Wise pattern 29, 88, 130, 138, 139, 160, 185, 250, 269, 362, 363, 368, 411, 412, 431, 432, 454, 485, 499, 511, 525, 529, 553, 593, 607, 672
Wise, R.J. 73, 130, 249, 250, 289, 383, 411, 485, 499, 517, 529, 556
Wise technique 529
Wise template 556
Wood's lamp 551
Wray, R.C. 354
Würinger, E. 216, 609, 610, 613

Y
Yalin, C.T. 589
Yousif, N.J. 181, 518
Yu, J. 656

Z
Zambacos, G.J. 606
Zocchi, M.L. 179, 265, 571

Printed by Printforce, United Kingdom